Second Edition

HARRISON'S Endocrinology

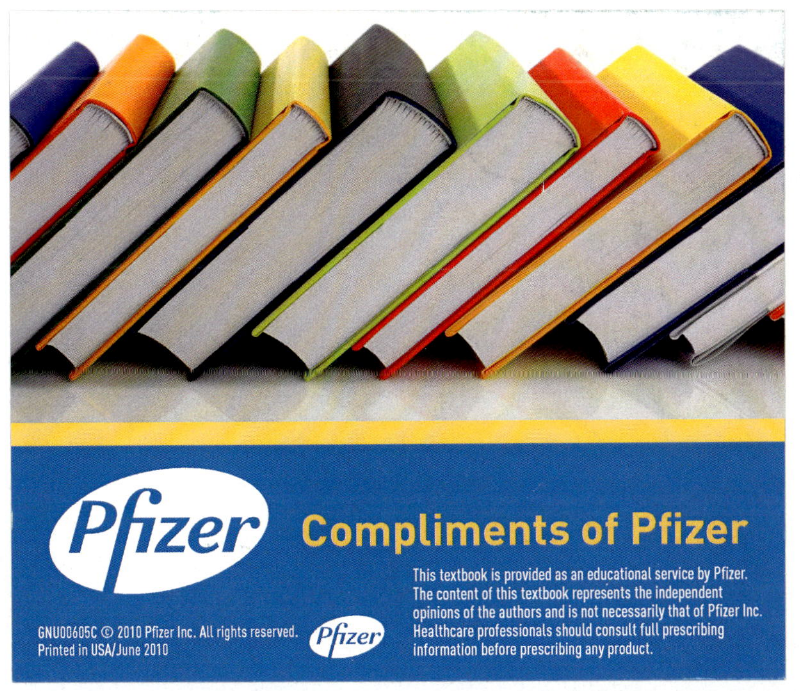

Derived from Harrison's Principles of Internal Medicine, 17th Edition

Editors

ANTHONY S. FAUCI, MD
Chief, Laboratory of Immunoregulation;
Director, National Institute of Allergy and Infectious Diseases,
National Institutes of Health, Bethesda

DENNIS L. KASPER, MD
William Ellery Channing Professor of Medicine, Professor of
Microbiology and Molecular Genetics, Harvard Medical School;
Director, Channing Laboratory, Department of Medicine,
Brigham and Women's Hospital, Boston

DAN L. LONGO, MD
Scientific Director, National Institute on Aging,
National Institutes of Health,
Bethesda and Baltimore

EUGENE BRAUNWALD, MD
Distinguished Hersey Professor of Medicine,
Harvard Medical School; Chairman, TIMI Study Group,
Brigham and Women's Hospital, Boston

STEPHEN L. HAUSER, MD
Robert A. Fishman Distinguished Professor and Chairman,
Department of Neurology, University of California, San Francisco

J. LARRY JAMESON, MD, PhD
Professor of Medicine;
Vice President for Medical Affairs
and Lewis Landsberg Dean,
Northwestern University Feinberg
School of Medicine, Chicago

JOSEPH LOSCALZO, MD, PhD
Hersey Professor of Theory and Practice of Medicine,
Harvard Medical School; Chairman, Department of Medicine;
Physician-in-Chief, Brigham and Women's Hospital, Boston

Second Edition

HARRISON'S Endocrinology

Editor

J. Larry Jameson, MD, PhD
Professor of Medicine;
Vice President for Medical Affairs and Lewis Landsberg Dean,
Northwestern University Feinberg School of Medicine, Chicago

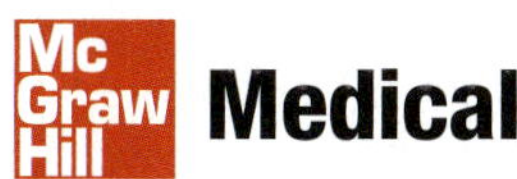

New York Chicago San Francisco Lisbon London Madrid Mexico City
Milan New Delhi San Juan Seoul Singapore Sydney Toronto

The McGraw-Hill Companies

Harrison's Endocrinology, Second Edition

Dr. Fauci's and Dr. Longo's works were performed outside the scope of their employment as U.S. government employees. These works represent their personal and professional views and not necessarily those of the U.S. government.

1 2 3 4 5 6 7 8 9 0 CTP/CTP 14 13 12 11 10

ISBN 978-0-07-174144-6
MHID 0-07-174144-5

This book was set in Bembo by Glyph International. The editors were James F. Shanahan and Kim J. Davis. The production supervisor was Catherine H. Saggese. Project management was provided by Arushi Chawla of Glyph International. The cover design was by Thomas DePierro.

China Translation & Printing Services, Ltd. was the printer and binder.

Library of Congress Cataloging-in-Publication Data

Harrison's endocrinology / editor, J. Larry Jameson. —2nd ed.
p. ; cm.
Expansion of the endocrinology section of Harrison's principles of internal medicine.
Includes bibliographical references and index.
ISBN-13: 978-0-07-174144-6 (pbk. : alk. paper)
ISBN-10: 0-07-174144-5 (pbk. : alk. paper)
1. Endocrinology. 2. Endocrine glands—Diseases. 3. Metabolism—Disorders.
I. Jameson, J. Larry, II. Harrison's principles of internal medicine. III. Title: Endocrinology.
[DNLM: 1. Endocrine System Diseases. 2. Metabolic Diseases.
WK 140 H323 2010]
RC648.H27 2010
616.4—dc22

2009045956

CONTENTS

CONTRIBUTORS

Numbers in brackets refer to the chapter(s) written or co-written by the contributor.

JOHN C. ACHERMANN, MD
Lecturer in Endocrinology, UCL Institute of Child Health, University College, London, United Kingdom [7]

SHARI S. BASSUK, ScD
Epidemiologist, Division of Preventive Medicine, Brigham and Women's Hospital, Boston [12]

SHALENDER BHASIN, MD
Chief and Professor, Department of Endocrinology, Diabetes, & Nutrition, Boston University, Boston [8]

GERALD BLOOMFIELD, MD, MPH
Department of Internal Medicine, The Johns Hopkins University School of Medicine, Baltimore [Review and Self-Assessment]

GEORGE J. BOSL, MD
Chairman, Department of Medicine, Memorial Sloan-Kettering Cancer Center; Professor of Medicine, Joan and Sanford I. Weill Medical College of Cornell University, New York [9]

F. RICHARD BRINGHURST, MD
Senior Vice President for Medicine and Research Management, Massachusetts General Hospital; Associate Professor of Medicine, Harvard Medical School, Boston [25]

CYNTHIA D. BROWN, MD
Department of Internal Medicine, The Johns Hopkins University School of Medicine, Baltimore [Review and Self-Assessment]

FELICIA COSMAN, MD
Associate Professor of Clinical Medicine, Columbia University College of Physicians and Surgeons; Medical Director, Clinical Research Center, Helen Hayes Hospital, West Haverstraw, New York [28]

PHILIP E. CRYER, MD
Irene E. and Michael M. Karl Professor of Endocrinology and Metabolism in Medicine, Washington University, St. Louis [20]

MARIE B. DEMAY, MD
Associate Professor of Medicine, Harvard Medical School; Associate Physician, Massachusetts General Hospital, Boston [25]

ROBERT G. DLUHY, MD
Program Director, Fellowship in Endocrinology; Professor of Medicine, Brigham and Women's Hospital, Harvard Medical School; Associate Editor, *New England Journal of Medicine,* Boston [5]

ROBERT H. ECKEL, MD
Professor of Medicine, Division of Endocrinology, Metabolism and Diabetes, Division of Cardiology; Professor of Physiology and Biophysics; Charles A. Boettcher II Chair in Atherosclerosis; Program Director, Adult General Clinical Research Center, University of Colorado at Denver and Health Sciences Center; Director, Lipid Clinic, University Hospital, Aurora [18]

DAVID A. EHRMANN, MD
Professor of Medicine; Associate Director, University of Chicago General Clinical Research Center, Chicago [13]

MURRAY J. FAVUS, MD
Professor of Medicine, Interim Head, Endocrine Section; Director, Bone Section, University of Chicago Pritzker School of Medicine, Chicago [29]

DANIEL J. FINK,† MD, MPH
Associate Professor of Clinical Pathology, College of Physicians and Surgeons, Columbia University, New York [Appendix]

JEFFREY S. FLIER, MD
Caroline Shields Walker Professor of Medicine, Harvard Medical School; Dean of the Faculty of Medicine, Harvard School of Medicine, Boston [16]

ROBERT F. GAGEL, MD
Professor of Medicine and Head, Division of Internal Medicine, University of Texas MD Anderson Cancer Center, Houston [23]

JANET E. HALL, MD
Associate Professor of Medicine, Harvard Medical School; Associate Physician, Massachusetts General Hospital, Boston [10, 11]

HELEN H. HOBBS, MD
Investigator, Howard Hughes Medical Institute; Professor of Internal Medicine and Molecular Genetics, University of Texas Southwestern Medical Center, Dallas [21]

J. LARRY JAMESON, MD, PhD
Professor of Medicine; Vice President for Medical Affairs and Lewis Landsberg Dean, Northwestern University Feinberg School of Medicine, Chicago [1, 2, 4, 7, 8, 24]

ROBERT T. JENSEN, MD
Chief, Digestive Diseases Branch, National Institute of Diabetes, Digestive and Kidney Diseases, National Institutes of Health, Bethesda [22]

CAMILO JIMENEZ, MD
Assistant Professor, Department of Endocrine Neoplasia & Hormonal Disorders, The University of Texas MD Cancer Center, Houston [23]

SUNDEEP KHOSLA, MD
Professor of Medicine and Physiology, Mayo Clinic College of Medicine, Rochester [26]

STEPHEN M. KRANE, MD
Persis, Cyrus and Marlow B. Harrison Distinguished Professor of Medicine, Harvard Medical School, Massachusetts General Hospital, Boston [25]

ALEXANDER KRATZ, MD, PhD, MPH
Assistant Professor of Clinical Pathology, Columbia University College of Physicians and Surgeons; Associate Director, Core Laboratory, Columbia University Medical Center, New York-Presbyterian Hospital; Director, Allen Pavilion Laboratory, New York [Appendix]

HENRY M. KRONENBERG, MD
Chief, Endocrine Unit, Massachusetts General Hospital; Professor of Medicine, Harvard Medical School, Boston [25]

†Deceased.

ROBERT F. KUSHNER, MD
Professor of Medicine, Northwestern University Feinberg School of Medicine, Chicago [17]

ROBERT LINDSAY, MD, PhD
Professor of Clinical Medicine, Columbia University College of Physicians and Surgeons; Chief, Internal Medicine, Helen Hayes Hospital, West Havershaw, New York [28]

JOANN E. MANSON, MD, DrPH
Professor of Medicine and the Elizabeth Fay Brigham Professor of Women's Health, Harvard Medical School; Chief, Division of Preventive Medicine, Brigham and Women's Hospital, Boston [12]

ELEFTHERIA MARATOS-FLIER, MD
Associate Professor of Medicine, Harvard Medical School; Chief, Obesity Section, Joslin Diabetes Center, Boston [16]

KEVIN T. MCVARY, MD
Associate Professor of Urology, Northwestern University Feinberg School of Medicine, Chicago [15]

SHLOMO MELMED, MD
Senior Vice President, Academic Affairs; Associate Dean, Cedars Sinai Medical Center, David Geffen School of Medicine at UCLA, Los Angeles [2]

ROBERT J. MOTZER, MD
Attending Physician, Department of Medicine, Memorial Sloan-Kettering Cancer Center; Professor of Medicine, Weill Medical College of Cornell University, New York [9]

HARTMUT P. H. NEUMANN, MD
Head, Section Preventative Medicine, Department of Nephrology and General Medicine, Albert-Ludwigs-University of Freiburg, Germany [6]

MICHAEL A. PESCE, PhD
Clinical Professor of Pathology, Columbia University College of Physicians and Surgeons; Director of Specialty Laboratory, New York Presbyterian Hospital, Columbia University Medical Center, New York [Appendix]

JOHN T. POTTS, JR., MD
Jackson Distinguished Professor of Clinical Medicine, Harvard Medical School; Director of Research and Physician-in-Chief Emeritus, Massachusetts General Hospital, Charlestown [27]

ALVIN C. POWERS, MD
Joe C. Davis Chair in Biomedical Science; Professor of Medicine, Molecular Physiology and Biophysics; Director, Vanderbilt Diabetes Research and Training Center; Director, Vanderbilt Diabetes Center, Nashville [19]

DANIEL J. RADER, MD
Cooper-McClure Professor of Medicine, University of Pennsylvania School of Medicine, Philadelphia [21]

GARY L. ROBERTSON, MD
Emeritus Professor of Medicine, Northwestern University Feinberg School of Medicine, Chicago [3]

JOSHUA SCHIFFER, MD
Department of Internal Medicine, The Johns Hopkins University School of Medicine, Baltimore [Review and Self-Assessment]

ADAM SPIVAK, MD
Department of Internal Medicine, The Johns Hopkins University School of Medicine, Baltimore [Review and Self-Assessment]

TAMARA J. VOKES, MD
Associate Professor, Section of Endocrinology, University of Chicago, Chicago [29]

ANTHONY P. WEETMAN, MD, DSc
Professor of Medicine and Dean of the School of Medicine and Biomedical Sciences, University of Sheffield, Sheffield, United Kingdom [4]

CHARLES WIENER, MD
Professor of Medicine and Physiology; Vice Chair, Department of Medicine; Director, Osler Medical Training Program, The Johns Hopkins University School of Medicine, Baltimore [Review and Self-Assessment]

GORDON H. WILLIAMS, MD
Professor of Medicine, Harvard Medical School; Chief, Cardiovascular Endocrinology Section, Brigham and Women's Hospital, Boston [5]

ROBERT C. YOUNG, MD
Chancellor, Fox Chase Cancer Center, Philadelphia [14]

PREFACE

The editors of *Harrison's Principles of Internal Medicine* refer to it as the "mother book," a description that confers respect but also acknowledges its size and its ancestral status among the growing list of Harrison's products, which now include *Harrison's Manual of Medicine*, *Harrison's Online*, and *Harrison's Practice,* an online highly structured reference for point-of-care use and continuing education. This book, *Harrison's Endocrinology,* second edition, is a compilation of chapters related to the specialty of endocrinology.

Our readers consistently note the sophistication of the material in the specialty sections of *Harrison's*. Our goal was to bring this information to readers in a more compact and usable form. Because the topic is more focused, it was possible to increase the presentation of the material by enlarging the text and the tables. We have also included a Review and Self-Assessment section that includes questions and answers to provoke reflection and to provide additional teaching points.

The clinical manifestations of endocrine disorders can usually be explained by considering the physiologic role of hormones, which are either deficient or excessive. Thus, a thorough understanding of hormone action and principles of hormone feedback arms the clinician with a logical diagnostic approach and a conceptual framework for treatment approaches. The first chapter of the book, Principles of Endocrinology, provides this type of "systems" overview. Using numerous examples of translational research, this introduction links genetics, cell biology, and physiology with pathophysiology and treatment. The integration of pathophysiology with clinical management is a hallmark of *Harrison's*, and can be found throughout each of the subsequent disease-oriented chapters. The book is divided into five main sections that reflect the physiologic roots of endocrinology: (I) Pituitary, Thyroid, and Adrenal Disorders; (II) Reproductive Endocrinology; (III) Diabetes Mellitus, Obesity, Lipoprotein Metabolism; (IV) Disorders Affecting Multiple Endocrine Systems; and (V) Disorders of Bone and Calcium Metabolism.

While *Harrison's Endocrinology* is classic in its organization, readers will sense the impact of the scientific renaissance as they explore the individual chapters in each section. In addition to the dramatic advances emanating from genetics and molecular biology, the introduction of an unprecedented number of new drugs, particularly for the management of diabetes and osteoporosis, is transforming the field of endocrinology. Numerous recent clinical studies involving common diseases like diabetes, obesity, hypothyroidism, osteoporosis, and polycystic ovarian syndrome provide powerful evidence for medical decision-making and treatment. These rapid changes in endocrinology are exciting for new students of medicine and underscore the need for practicing physicians to continuously update their knowledge base and clinical skills.

Our access to information through web-based journals and databases is remarkably efficient. While these sources of information are invaluable, the daunting body of data creates an even greater need for synthesis and for highlighting important facts. Thus, the preparation of these chapters is a special craft that requires the ability to distill core information from the ever-expanding knowledge base. The editors are therefore indebted to our authors, a group of internationally recognized authorities who are masters at providing a comprehensive overview while being able to distill a topic into a concise and interesting chapter. We are grateful to Emily Cowan for assisting with research and preparation of this book. Our colleagues at McGraw-Hill continue to innovate in health care publishing. This new product was championed by Jim Shanahan and impeccably produced by Kim Davis.

We hope you find this book useful in your effort to achieve continuous learning on behalf of your patients.

J. Larry Jameson, MD, PhD

Review and self-assessment questions and answers were taken from Wiener C, Fauci AS, Braunwald E, Kasper DL, Hauser SL, Longo DL, Jameson JL, Loscalzo J (editors) Bloomfield G, Brown CD, Schiffer J, Spivak A (contributing editors). *Harrison's Principles of Internal Medicine Self-Assessment and Board Review*, 17th ed. New York, McGraw-Hill, 2008, ISBN 978-0-07-149619-3.

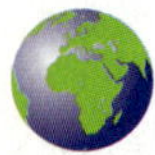
The global icons call greater attention to key epidemiologic and clinical differences in the practice of medicine throughout the world.

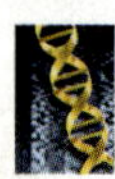
The genetic icons identify a clinical issue with an explicit genetic relationship.

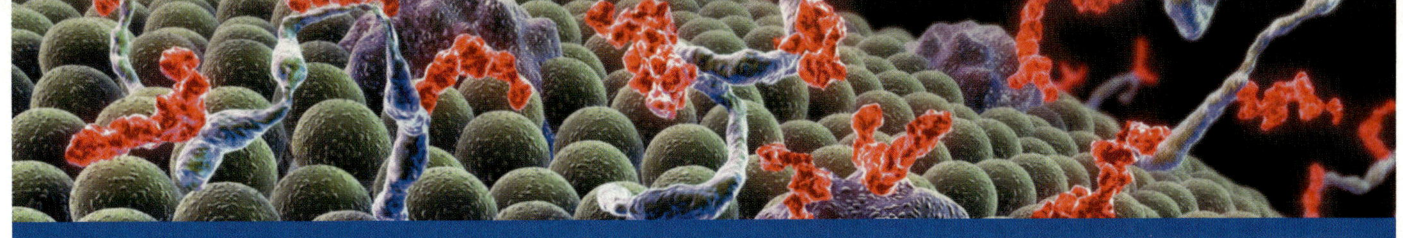

CHAPTER 1

PRINCIPLES OF ENDOCRINOLOGY

J. Larry Jameson

The management of endocrine disorders requires a broad understanding of intermediary metabolism, reproductive physiology, bone metabolism, and growth. Accordingly, the practice of endocrinology is intimately linked to a conceptual framework for understanding hormone secretion, hormone action, and principles of feedback control. The endocrine system is evaluated primarily by measuring hormone concentrations, thereby arming the clinician with valuable diagnostic information. Most disorders of the endocrine system are amenable to effective treatment, once the correct diagnosis is determined. Endocrine deficiency disorders are treated with physiologic hormone replacement; hormone excess conditions, usually due to benign glandular adenomas, are managed by removing tumors surgically or by reducing hormone levels medically.

SCOPE OF ENDOCRINOLOGY

The specialty of endocrinology encompasses the study of glands and the hormones they produce. The term *endocrine* was coined by Starling to contrast the actions of hormones secreted internally (endocrine) with those secreted externally (*exocrine*) or into a lumen, such as the gastrointestinal tract. The term *hormone*, derived from a Greek phrase meaning "to set in motion," aptly describes the dynamic actions of hormones as they elicit cellular responses and regulate physiologic processes through feedback mechanisms.

Unlike many other specialties in medicine, it is not possible to define endocrinology strictly along anatomic lines. The classic endocrine glands—pituitary, thyroid, parathyroid, pancreatic islets, adrenal, and gonads—communicate broadly with other organs through the nervous system, hormones, cytokines, and growth factors. In addition to its traditional synaptic functions, the brain produces a vast array of peptide hormones, spawning the discipline of neuroendocrinology. Through the production of hypothalamic releasing factors, the central nervous system (CNS) exerts a major regulatory influence over pituitary hormone secretion (Chap. 2). The peripheral nervous system stimulates the adrenal medulla. The immune and endocrine systems are also intimately intertwined. The adrenal glucocorticoid, cortisol, is a powerful immunosuppressant. Cytokines and interleukins (ILs) have profound effects on the functions of the pituitary, adrenal, thyroid, and gonads. Common endocrine diseases, such as autoimmune thyroid disease and type 1 diabetes mellitus, are caused by dysregulation of immune surveillance and tolerance. Less common diseases such as polyglandular failure, Addison's disease, and lymphocytic hypophysitis also have an immunologic basis.

The interdigitation of endocrinology with physiologic processes in other specialties sometimes blurs the role of hormones. For example, hormones play an important role in maintenance of blood pressure, intravascular volume, and peripheral resistance in the cardiovascular system. Vasoactive substances such as catecholamines, angiotensin II, endothelin, and nitric oxide are involved in dynamic changes of vascular tone, in addition to their multiple roles in other tissues. The heart is the principal source of atrial natriuretic peptide, which acts in classic endocrine fashion to induce natriuresis at a distant target organ (the kidney). Erythropoietin, a traditional circulating hormone, is made in the kidney and stimulates erythropoiesis in the bone marrow. The kidney is also integrally involved in the renin-angiotensin axis (Chap. 5) and is a primary target of several hormones, including parathyroid hormone (PTH), mineralocorticoids, and vasopressin. The gastrointestinal tract produces a surprising number of peptide hormones such as cholecystokinin, ghrelin, gastrin, secretin, and vasoactive intestinal peptide, among many others. Carcinoid and islet tumors can secrete excessive amounts of these hormones, leading to specific clinical syndromes (Chap. 22). Many of these gastrointestinal hormones are also produced in the CNS, where their functions remain poorly understood. As new hormones such as inhibin, ghrelin, and leptin are discovered, they become integrated into the science and practice of medicine on the basis of their functional roles rather than their tissues of origin.

Characterization of hormone receptors frequently reveals unexpected relationships to factors in nonendocrine disciplines. The growth hormone (GH) and leptin receptors, for example, are members of the cytokine receptor family. The G protein–coupled receptors (GPCRs), which mediate the actions of many peptide hormones, are used in numerous physiologic processes, including vision, smell, and neurotransmission.

NATURE OF HORMONES

Hormones can be divided into five major classes: (1) *amino acid derivatives* such as dopamine, catecholamine, and thyroid hormone (TH); (2) *small neuropeptides* such as gonadotropin-releasing hormone (GnRH), thyrotropin-releasing hormone (TRH), somatostatin, and vasopressin; (3) *large proteins* such as insulin, luteinizing hormone (LH), and PTH produced by classic endocrine glands; (4) *steroid hormones* such as cortisol and estrogen that are synthesized from cholesterol-based precursors; and (5) *vitamin derivatives* such as retinoids (vitamin A) and vitamin D. A variety of *peptide growth factors*, most of which act locally, share actions with hormones. As a rule, amino acid derivatives and peptide hormones interact with cell-surface membrane receptors. Steroids, thyroid hormones, vitamin D, and retinoids are lipid-soluble and interact with intracellular nuclear receptors.

HORMONE AND RECEPTOR FAMILIES

Many hormones and receptors can be grouped into families, reflecting their structural similarities (Table 1-1). The evolution of these families generates diverse but highly selective pathways of hormone action. Recognizing these relationships allows extrapolation of information gleaned from one hormone or receptor to other family members.

The glycoprotein hormone family, consisting of thyroid-stimulating hormone (TSH), follicle-stimulating hormone (FSH), LH, and human chorionic gonadotropin (hCG), illustrates many features of related hormones. The glycoprotein hormones are heterodimers that have the α subunit in common; the β subunits are distinct and confer specific biologic actions. The overall three-dimensional architecture of the β subunits is similar, reflecting the locations of conserved disulfide bonds that restrain protein conformation. The cloning of the β-subunit genes from multiple species suggests that this family arose from a common ancestral gene, probably by gene duplication and subsequent divergence to evolve new biologic functions.

As the hormone families enlarge and diverge, their receptors must co-evolve if new biologic functions are to be derived. Related GPCRs, for example, have evolved for each of the glycoprotein hormones. These receptors are structurally similar, and each is coupled to the $G_s\alpha$ signaling pathway. However, there is minimal overlap of hormone binding. For example, TSH binds with high specificity to the TSH receptor but interacts minimally with the LH or the FSH receptor. Nonetheless, there can be subtle physiologic consequences of hormone cross-reactivity with other receptors. Very high levels of hCG during pregnancy stimulate the TSH receptor and increase TH levels, resulting in a compensatory decrease in TSH.

Insulin, insulin-like growth factor (IGF) type I, and IGF-II share structural similarities that are most apparent when precursor forms of the proteins are compared. In contrast to the high degree of specificity seen with the glycoprotein hormones, there is moderate cross-talk among the members of the insulin/IGF family. High concentrations of an IGF-II precursor produced by certain tumors (e.g., sarcomas) can cause hypoglycemia, partly because of binding to insulin and IGF-I receptors (Chap. 24). High concentrations of insulin also bind to the IGF-I receptor, perhaps accounting for some of the clinical manifestations seen in severe insulin resistance.

Another important example of receptor cross-talk is seen with PTH and parathyroid hormone–related peptide (PTHrP) (Chap. 27). PTH is produced by the parathyroid glands, whereas PTHrP is expressed at high levels during development and by a variety of tumors (Chap. 24). These hormones share amino acid sequence similarity, particularly in their amino-terminal regions. Both hormones bind to a single PTH receptor that is expressed in bone and kidney. Hypercalcemia and hypophosphatemia may therefore result from excessive production of either hormone, making it

TABLE 1-1

MEMBRANE RECEPTOR FAMILIES AND SIGNALING PATHWAYS

RECEPTORS	EFFECTORS	SIGNALING PATHWAYS
G Protein–Coupled Seven-Transmembrane (GPCR)		
β-Adrenergic	$G_s\alpha$, adenylate cyclase	Stimulation of cyclic AMP production, protein kinase A
LH, FSH, TSH		
Glucagon		
PTH, PTHrP	Ca^{2+} channels	Calmodulin, Ca^{2+}-dependent kinases
ACTH, MSH		
GHRH, CRH		
α-Adrenergic	$G_i\alpha$	Inhibition of cyclic AMP production
Somatostatin		Activation of K^+, Ca^{2+} channels
TRH, GnRH	G_q, G_{11}	Phospholipase C, diacylglycerol, IP_3, protein kinase C, voltage-dependent Ca^{2+} channels
Receptor Tyrosine Kinase		
Insulin, IGF-I	Tyrosine kinases, IRS	MAP kinases, PI 3-kinase; AKT, also known as protein kinase B, PKB
EGF, NGF	Tyrosine kinases, ras	Raf, MAP kinases, RSK
Cytokine Receptor–Linked Kinase		
GH, PRL	JAK, tyrosine kinases	STAT, MAP kinase, PI 3-kinase, IRS-1
Serine Kinase		
Activin, TGF-β, MIS	Serine kinase	Smads

Note: IP_3, inositol triphosphate; IRS, insulin receptor substrates; MAP, mitogen-activated protein; MSH, melanocyte-stimulating hormone; NGF, nerve growth factor; PI, phosphatylinositol; RSK, ribosomal S6 kinase; TGF-β, transforming growth factor β. For all other abbreviations, see text.

difficult to distinguish hyperparathyroidism from hypercalcemia of malignancy solely on the basis of serum chemistries. However, sensitive and specific assays for PTH and PTHrP now allow these disorders to be separated more readily.

Based on their specificities for DNA binding sites, the nuclear receptor family can be subdivided into type 1 receptors (GR, MR, AR, ER, PR) that bind steroids and type 2 receptors (TR, VDR, RAR, PPAR) that bind TH, vitamin D, retinoic acid, or lipid derivatives. Certain functional domains in nuclear receptors, such as the zinc finger DNA-binding domains, are highly conserved. However, selective amino acid differences within this domain confer DNA sequence specificity. The hormone-binding domains are more variable, providing great diversity in the array of small molecules that bind to different nuclear receptors. With few exceptions, hormone binding is highly specific for a single type of nuclear receptor. One exception involves the glucocorticoid and mineralocorticoid receptors. Because the mineralocorticoid receptor also binds glucocorticoids with high affinity, an enzyme (11β-hydroxysteroid dehydrogenase) located in renal tubular cells inactivates glucocorticoids, allowing selective responses to mineralocorticoids such as aldosterone. However, when very high glucocorticoid concentrations occur, as in Cushing's syndrome, the glucocorticoid degradation pathway becomes saturated, allowing excessive cortisol levels to exert mineralocorticoid effects (sodium retention, potassium wasting). This phenomenon is particularly pronounced in ectopic adrenocorticotropic hormone (ACTH) syndromes (Chap. 5). Another example of relaxed nuclear receptor specificity involves the estrogen receptor, which can bind an array of compounds, some of which share little structural similarity to the high-affinity ligand estradiol. This feature of the estrogen receptor makes it susceptible to activation by "environmental estrogens" such as resveratrol, octylphenol, and many other aromatic hydrocarbons. On the other hand, this lack of specificity provides an opportunity to synthesize a remarkable series of clinically useful antagonists (e.g., tamoxifen) and selective estrogen response modulators (SERMs) such as raloxifene. These compounds generate distinct conformations that alter receptor interactions with components of the transcription machinery, thereby conferring their unique actions.

HORMONE SYNTHESIS AND PROCESSING

The synthesis of peptide hormones and their receptors occurs through a classic pathway of gene expression: transcription → mRNA → protein → posttranslational protein processing → intracellular sorting, membrane integration, or secretion.

Many hormones are embedded within larger precursor polypeptides that are proteolytically processed to yield the biologically active hormone. Examples include proopiomelanocortin (POMC) → ACTH; proglucagon → glucagon; proinsulin → insulin; and pro-PTH → PTH, among others. In many cases, such as POMC and proglucagon, these precursors generate multiple biologically active peptides. It is provocative that hormone precursors are typically inactive, presumably adding an additional level of regulatory control. This is true not only for peptide hormones but also for certain steroids (testosterone → dihydrotestosterone) and thyroid hormone [L-thyroxine (T_4) → triiodothyronine (T_3)].

Hormone precursor processing is intimately linked to intracellular sorting pathways that transport proteins to appropriate vesicles and enzymes, resulting in specific cleavage steps, followed by protein folding and translocation to secretory vesicles. Hormones destined for secretion are translocated across the endoplasmic reticulum under the guidance of an amino-terminal signal sequence that is subsequently cleaved. Cell-surface receptors are inserted into the membrane via short segments of hydrophobic amino acids that remain embedded within the lipid bilayer. During translocation through the Golgi and endoplasmic reticulum, hormones and receptors are also subject to a variety of posttranslational modifications, such as glycosylation and phosphorylation, which can alter protein conformation, modify circulating half-life, and alter biologic activity.

Synthesis of most steroid hormones is based on modifications of the precursor, cholesterol. Multiple regulated enzymatic steps are required for the synthesis of testosterone (Chap. 8), estradiol (Chap. 10), cortisol (Chap. 5), and vitamin D (Chap. 25). This large number of synthetic steps predisposes to multiple genetic and acquired disorders of steroidogenesis.

Although endocrine genes contain regulatory DNA elements similar to those found in many other genes, their exquisite control by other hormones also necessitates the presence of specific hormone response elements. For example, the TSH genes are repressed directly by thyroid hormones acting through the thyroid hormone receptor (TR), a member of the nuclear receptor family. Steroidogenic enzyme gene expression requires specific transcription factors, such as steroidogenic factor-1 (SF-1), acting in conjunction with signals transmitted by trophic hormones (e.g., ACTH or LH). For some hormones, substantial regulation occurs at the level of translational efficiency. Insulin biosynthesis, while requiring ongoing gene transcription, is regulated primarily at the translational level in response to elevated levels of glucose or amino acids.

HORMONE SECRETION, TRANSPORT, AND DEGRADATION

The circulating level of a hormone is determined by its rate of secretion and its circulating half-life. After protein processing, peptide hormones (GnRH, insulin, GH) are stored in secretory granules. As these granules mature, they are poised beneath the plasma membrane for imminent release into the circulation. In most instances, the stimulus for hormone secretion is a releasing factor or neural signal that induces rapid changes in intracellular calcium concentrations, leading to secretory granule fusion with the plasma membrane and release of its contents into the extracellular environment and bloodstream. Steroid hormones, in contrast, diffuse into the circulation as they are synthesized. Thus, their secretory rates are closely aligned with rates of synthesis. For example, ACTH and LH induce steroidogenesis by stimulating the activity of *st*eroidogenic *a*cute *r*egulatory (StAR) protein (transports cholesterol into the mitochondrion) along with other rate-limiting steps (e.g., cholesterol side-chain cleavage enzyme, CYP11A1) in the steroidogenic pathway.

Hormone transport and degradation dictate the rapidity with which a hormonal signal decays. Some hormonal signals are evanescent (e.g., somatostatin), whereas others are longer-lived (e.g., TSH). Because somatostatin exerts effects in virtually every tissue, a short half-life allows its concentrations and actions to be controlled locally. Structural modifications that impair somatostatin degradation have been useful for generating long-acting therapeutic analogues, such as octreotide (Chap. 2). On the other hand, the actions of TSH are highly specific for the thyroid gland. Its prolonged half-life accounts for relatively constant serum levels, even though TSH is secreted in discrete pulses.

An understanding of circulating hormone half-life is important for achieving physiologic hormone replacement, as the frequency of dosing and the time required to reach steady state are intimately linked to rates of hormone decay. T_4, for example, has a circulating half-life of 7 days. Consequently, >1 month is required to reach a new steady state, but single daily doses are sufficient to achieve constant hormone levels. T_3, in contrast, has a half-life of 1 day. Its administration is associated with more dynamic serum levels and it must be administered two to three times per day. Similarly, synthetic glucocorticoids vary widely in their half-lives; those with longer half-lives (e.g., dexamethasone) are associated with greater suppression of the hypothalamic-pituitary-adrenal (HPA) axis. Most protein hormones [e.g., ACTH, GH, prolactin (PRL), PTH, LH] have relatively short half-lives (<20 min), leading to sharp peaks of secretion and decay. The only accurate way to profile the pulse frequency and amplitude of these hormones is to measure levels in frequently sampled blood (every 10 min or less) over long durations (8–24 h). Because this is not practical in a clinical setting, an alternative strategy is to pool three to four samples drawn at about 30-min intervals, recognizing that pulsatile secretion makes it difficult to establish a narrow normal range. Rapid hormone decay is useful in certain clinical settings. For example, the short half-life of PTH allows the use of intraoperative PTH determinations to confirm successful removal of an adenoma. This is particularly valuable diagnostically when there is a possibility of multicentric disease or parathyroid hyperplasia, as occurs with multiple endocrine neoplasia (MEN) or renal insufficiency.

Many hormones circulate in association with serum-binding proteins. Examples include (1) T_4 and T_3 binding to thyroxine-binding globulin (TBG), albumin, and thyroxine-binding prealbumin (TBPA); (2) cortisol binding to cortisol-binding globulin (CBG); (3) androgen and estrogen binding to sex hormone–binding globulin (SHBG) (also called testosterone-binding globulin, TeBG); (4) IGF-I and -II binding to multiple IGF-binding proteins (IGFBPs); (5) GH interactions with GH-binding protein (GHBP), a circulating fragment of the GH receptor extracellular domain; and (6) activin binding to follistatin. These interactions provide a hormonal reservoir, prevent otherwise rapid degradation of unbound hormones, restrict hormone access to certain sites (e.g., IGFBPs), and modulate the unbound, or "free," hormone concentrations. Although a variety of binding protein abnormalities have been identified, most have little clinical consequence, aside from creating diagnostic problems. For example, TBG deficiency can greatly reduce total TH levels, but the free concentrations of T_4 and T_3 remain normal. Liver disease and certain medications can also influence binding protein levels (e.g., estrogen increases TBG) or cause displacement of hormones from binding proteins (e.g., salsalate displaces T_4 from TBG). In general, only unbound hormone is available to interact with receptors and thereby elicit a biologic response. Short-term perturbations in binding proteins change the free hormone concentration, which in turn induces compensatory adaptations through feedback loops. SHBG changes in women are an exception to this self-correcting mechanism. When SHBG decreases because of insulin resistance or androgen excess, the unbound testosterone concentration is increased, potentially leading to hirsutism (Chap. 13). The increased unbound testosterone level does not result in an adequate compensatory feedback correction because estrogen, and not testosterone, is the primary regulator of the reproductive axis.

An additional exception to the unbound hormone hypothesis involves megalin, a member of the low-density lipoprotein (LDL) receptor family that serves as an endocytotic receptor for carrier-bound vitamins A and D, and SHBG-bound androgens and estrogens. Following internalization, the carrier proteins are degraded in lysosomes and release their bound ligands within the cells. Megalin deficiency in mice impairs androgen-dependent testis descent and estrogen-mediated vaginal opening, confirming a functional role in these steroid-dependent events.

HORMONE ACTION THROUGH RECEPTORS

Receptors for hormones are divided into two major classes—membrane and nuclear. *Membrane receptors* primarily bind peptide hormones and catecholamines. *Nuclear receptors* bind small molecules that can diffuse across the cell membrane, such as TH, steroids, and vitamin D. Certain general principles apply to hormone-receptor interactions, regardless of the class of receptor. Hormones bind to receptors with specificity and an affinity that generally coincides with the dynamic range of circulating hormone concentrations. Low concentrations of free hormone (usually 10^{-12} to 10^{-9} *M*) rapidly associate and dissociate from receptors in a bimolecular reaction, such that the occupancy of the receptor at any given moment is a function of hormone concentration and the receptor's affinity for the hormone. Receptor numbers vary greatly in different target tissues, providing one of the major determinants of specific cellular responses to circulating hormones. For example, ACTH receptors are located almost exclusively in the adrenal cortex, and FSH receptors are found only in the gonads. In contrast, insulin and TRs are widely distributed, reflecting the need for metabolic responses in all tissues.

MEMBRANE RECEPTORS

Membrane receptors for hormones can be divided into several major groups: (1) seven transmembrane GPCRs, (2) tyrosine kinase receptors, (3) cytokine receptors, and (4) serine kinase receptors (**Fig. 1-1**). The *seven transmembrane GPCR family* binds a remarkable array of hormones, including large proteins (e.g., LH, PTH), small peptides (e.g., TRH, somatostatin), catecholamines (epinephrine, dopamine), and even minerals (e.g., calcium). The extracellular domains of GPCRs vary widely in size and are the major binding site for large hormones. The transmembrane-spanning regions are composed of hydrophobic α-helical domains that traverse the lipid bilayer. Like some channels, these domains are thought to circularize and form a hydrophobic pocket into which certain small ligands fit. Hormone binding induces conformational changes in these domains, transducing structural changes to the intracellular domain, which is a docking site for G proteins.

The large family of *G proteins*, so named because they bind guanine nucleotides (GTP, GDP), provides great diversity for coupling receptors to different signaling pathways. G proteins form a heterotrimeric complex that is composed of various α and βγ subunits. The α subunit contains the guanine nucleotide–binding site and hydrolyzes GTP → GDP. The βγ subunits are tightly associated and modulate the activity of the α subunit, as

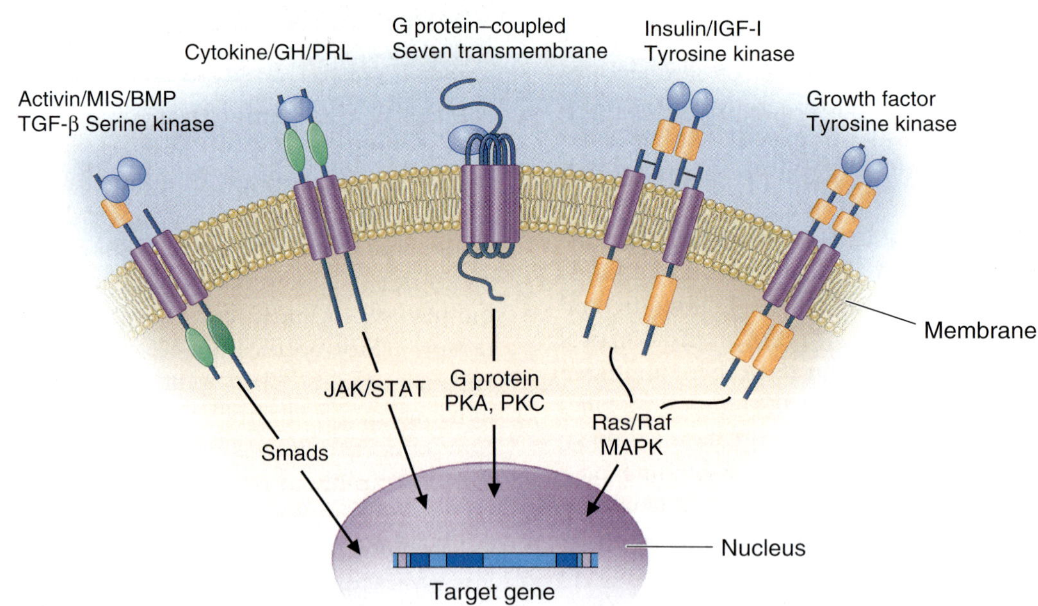

FIGURE 1-1

Membrane receptor signaling. MAPK, mitogen-activated protein kinase; PKA, -C, protein kinase A, C; TGF, transforming growth factor. For other abbreviations, see text.

well as mediating their own effector signaling pathways. G protein activity is regulated by a cycle that involves GTP hydrolysis and dynamic interactions between the α and βγ subunits. Hormone binding to the receptor induces GDP dissociation, allowing Gα to bind GTP and dissociate from the βγ complex. Under these conditions, the Gα subunit is activated and mediates signal transduction through various enzymes such as adenylate cyclase or phospholipase C. GTP hydrolysis to GDP allows reassociation with the βγ subunits and restores the inactive state. As described below, a variety of endocrinopathies result from G protein mutations or from mutations in receptors that modify their interactions with G proteins.

There are more than a dozen isoforms of the Gα subunit. $G_s\alpha$ stimulates, whereas $G_i\alpha$ inhibits, adenylate cyclase, an enzyme that generates the second messenger, cyclic AMP, leading to activation of protein kinase A (Table 1-1). G_q subunits couple to phospholipase C, generating diacylglycerol and inositol triphosphate, leading to activation of protein kinase C and the release of intracellular calcium.

The *tyrosine kinase receptors* transduce signals for insulin and a variety of growth factors, such as IGF-I, epidermal growth factor (EGF), nerve growth factor, platelet-derived growth factor, and fibroblast growth factor. The cysteine-rich extracellular ligand-binding domains contain growth factor–binding sites. After ligand binding, this class of receptors undergoes autophosphorylation, inducing interactions with intracellular adaptor proteins such as Shc and insulin receptor substrates. In the case of the insulin receptor, multiple kinases are activated, including the Raf-Ras-MAPK and the Akt/protein kinase B pathways. The tyrosine kinase receptors play a prominent role in cell growth and differentiation as well as in intermediary metabolism.

The GH and PRL receptors belong to the *cytokine receptor* family. Analogous to the tyrosine kinase receptors, ligand binding induces receptor interaction with intracellular kinases—the Janus kinases (JAKs), which phosphorylate members of the signal transduction and activators of transcription (STAT) family—as well as with other signaling pathways (Ras, PI3-K, MAPK). The activated STAT proteins translocate to the nucleus and stimulate expression of target genes.

The *serine kinase receptors* mediate the actions of activins, transforming growth factor β, müllerian-inhibiting substance (MIS, also known as anti-müllerian hormone, AMH), and bone morphogenic proteins (BMPs). This family of receptors (consisting of type I and II subunits) signals through proteins termed *smads* (fusion of terms for *Caenorhabditis elegans* sma + mammalian mad). Like the STAT proteins, the smads serve a dual role of transducing the receptor signal and acting as transcription factors. The pleomorphic actions of these growth factors dictate that they act primarily in a local (paracrine or autocrine) manner. Binding proteins, such as follistatin (which binds activin and other members of this family), function to inactivate the growth factors and restrict their distribution.

NUCLEAR RECEPTORS

The family of nuclear receptors has grown to nearly 100 members, many of which are still classified as orphan receptors because their ligands, if they exist, remain to be identified (Fig. 1-2). Otherwise, most nuclear receptors are classified based on the nature of their ligands. Though all nuclear receptors ultimately act to increase or decrease gene transcription, some (e.g., glucocorticoid receptor) reside primarily in the cytoplasm, whereas others (e.g., thyroid hormone receptor) are always located in the nucleus. After ligand binding, the cytoplasmically localized receptors translocate to the nucleus. There is growing evidence that certain nuclear receptors (e.g., glucocorticoid, estrogen) can also act at the membrane or in the cytoplasm to activate or repress signal transduction pathways, providing a mechanism for cross-talk between membrane and nuclear receptors.

The structures of nuclear receptors have been extensively studied, including by x-ray crystallography. The DNA-binding domain, consisting of two zinc fingers, contacts specific DNA recognition sequences in target genes. Most nuclear receptors bind to DNA as dimers. Consequently, each monomer recognizes an individual DNA motif, referred to as a "half-site." The steroid receptors, including the glucocorticoid, estrogen, progesterone, and androgen receptors, bind to DNA as homodimers. Consistent with this twofold symmetry, their DNA recognition half-sites are palindromic. The thyroid, retinoid, peroxisome proliferator–activated, and vitamin D receptors bind to DNA preferentially as heterodimers in combination with retinoid X receptors (RXRs). Their DNA half-sites are arranged as direct repeats. Receptor specificity for DNA sequences is determined by (1) the sequence of the half-site, (2) the orientation of the half-sites (palindromic, direct repeat), and (3) the spacing between the half-sites. For example, vitamin D, thyroid, and retinoid receptors recognize similar tandemly repeated half-sites (TAAGTCA), but these DNA repeats are spaced by three, four, and five nucleotides, respectively.

The carboxy-terminal hormone-binding domain mediates transcriptional control. For type 2 receptors, such as TR and retinoic acid receptor (RAR), co-repressor proteins bind to the receptor in the absence of ligand and silence gene transcription. Hormone binding induces conformational changes, triggering the release of co-repressors and inducing the recruitment of coactivators that stimulate transcription. Thus, these receptors are capable of mediating dramatic changes in the level of gene activity. Certain disease states are associated with defective regulation of these events. For example, mutations in the TR prevent co-repressor dissociation, resulting in a dominant form of hormone resistance (Chap. 4). In promyelocytic leukemia, fusion of RARα to other nuclear proteins causes aberrant gene silencing and prevents normal cellular differentiation. Treatment with retinoic acid reverses this repression and allows cellular differentiation and apoptosis to occur. Most type 1 steroid receptors interact weakly with co-repressors, but ligand binding still induces interactions with an array of coactivators. X-ray crystallography shows that various SERMs induce distinct estrogen receptor conformations. The tissue-specific responses caused by these agents in breast, bone, and uterus appear to reflect distinct interactions

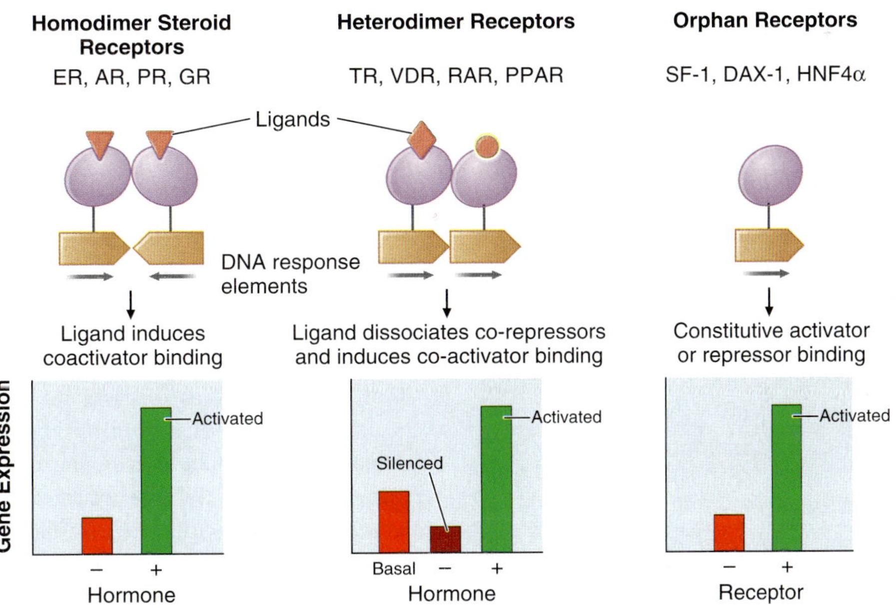

FIGURE 1-2

Nuclear receptor signaling. ER, estrogen receptor; AR, androgen receptor; PR, progesterone receptor; GR, glucocorticoid receptor; TR, thyroid hormone receptor; VDR, vitamin D receptor; RAR, retinoic acid receptor; PPAR, peroxisome proliferator activated receptor; SF-1, steroidogenic factor-1; DAX, *d*osage-sensitive sex reversal, *a*drenal hypoplasia congenita, *X* chromosome; HNF4α, hepatic nuclear factor 4α.

with coactivators. The receptor-coactivator complex stimulates gene transcription by several pathways, including (1) recruitment of enzymes (histone acetyl transferases) that modify chromatin structure, (2) interactions with additional transcription factors on the target gene, and (3) direct interactions with components of the general transcription apparatus to enhance the rate of RNA polymerase II–mediated transcription. Studies of nuclear receptor–mediated transcription show that these are dynamic events involving relatively rapid (e.g., 30–60 min) cycling of transcription complexes on any given target gene.

FUNCTIONS OF HORMONES

The functions of individual hormones are described in detail in subsequent chapters. Nevertheless, it is useful to illustrate how most biologic responses require integration of several different hormone pathways. The physiologic functions of hormones can be divided into three general areas: (1) growth and differentiation, (2) maintenance of homeostasis, and (3) reproduction.

GROWTH

Multiple hormones and nutritional factors mediate the complex phenomenon of growth (Chap. 2). Short stature may be caused by GH deficiency, hypothyroidism, Cushing's syndrome, precocious puberty, malnutrition, chronic illness, or genetic abnormalities that affect the epiphyseal growth plates (e.g., *FGFR3* or *SHOX* mutations). Many factors (GH, IGF-I, TH) stimulate growth, whereas others (sex steroids) lead to epiphyseal closure. Understanding these hormonal interactions is important in the diagnosis and management of growth disorders. For example, delaying exposure to high levels of sex steroids may enhance the efficacy of GH treatment.

MAINTENANCE OF HOMEOSTASIS

Though virtually all hormones affect homeostasis, the most important among these are the following:

1. TH—controls about 25% of basal metabolism in most tissues
2. Cortisol—exerts a permissive action for many hormones in addition to its own direct effects
3. PTH—regulates calcium and phosphorus levels
4. Vasopressin—regulates serum osmolality by controlling renal free-water clearance
5. Mineralocorticoids—control vascular volume and serum electrolyte (Na^+, K^+) concentrations
6. Insulin—maintains euglycemia in the fed and fasted states

The defense against hypoglycemia is an impressive example of integrated hormone action (Chap. 20). In response to the fasted state and falling blood glucose, insulin secretion is suppressed, resulting in decreased glucose uptake and enhanced glycogenolysis, lipolysis, proteolysis, and gluconeogenesis to mobilize fuel sources. If hypoglycemia develops (usually from insulin administration or sulfonylureas), an orchestrated counterregulatory response occurs—glucagon and epinephrine rapidly stimulate glycogenolysis and gluconeogenesis, whereas GH and cortisol act over several hours to raise glucose levels and antagonize insulin action.

Although free-water clearance is primarily controlled by vasopressin, cortisol and TH are also important for facilitating renal tubular responses to vasopressin (Chap. 3). PTH and vitamin D function in an interdependent manner to control calcium metabolism (Chap. 25). PTH stimulates renal synthesis of 1,25-dihydroxyvitamin D, which increases calcium absorption in the gastrointestinal tract and enhances PTH action in bone. Increased calcium, along with vitamin D, feeds back to suppress PTH, thereby maintaining calcium balance.

Depending on the severity of a given stress and whether it is acute or chronic, multiple endocrine and cytokine pathways are activated to mount an appropriate physiologic response. In severe acute stress such as trauma or shock, the sympathetic nervous system is activated and catecholamines are released, leading to increased cardiac output and a primed musculoskeletal system. Catecholamines also increase mean blood pressure and stimulate glucose production. Multiple stress-induced pathways converge on the hypothalamus, stimulating several hormones including vasopressin and corticotropin-releasing hormone (CRH). These hormones, in addition to cytokines (tumor necrosis factor α, IL-2, IL-6), increase ACTH and GH production. ACTH stimulates the adrenal gland, increasing cortisol, which in turn helps to sustain blood pressure and dampen the inflammatory response. Increased vasopressin acts to conserve free water.

REPRODUCTION

The stages of reproduction include (1) sex determination during fetal development (Chap. 7); (2) sexual maturation during puberty (Chaps. 8 and 10); (3) conception, pregnancy, lactation, and child-rearing (Chap. 10); and (4) cessation of reproductive capability at menopause (Chap. 12). Each of these stages involves an orchestrated interplay of multiple hormones, a phenomenon well illustrated by the dynamic hormonal changes that occur during each 28-day menstrual cycle. In the early follicular phase, pulsatile secretion of LH and FSH stimulates the progressive maturation of the ovarian follicle. This results in gradually increasing estrogen and progesterone levels, leading to enhanced pituitary sensitivity to GnRH, which, when combined with accelerated GnRH secretion, triggers the LH surge and rupture of the mature follicle. Inhibin, a protein produced by the granulosa cells, enhances follicular growth and feeds back to the pituitary to selectively suppress FSH, without affecting LH. Growth factors such as EGF and IGF-I modulate follicular responsiveness to gonadotropins. Vascular endothelial growth factor and prostaglandins play a role in follicle vascularization and rupture.

During pregnancy, the increased production of prolactin, in combination with placentally derived steroids (e.g., estrogen and progesterone), prepares the breast for lactation. Estrogens induce the production of progesterone receptors, allowing for increased responsiveness to progesterone. In addition to these and other hormones involved in lactation, the nervous system and oxytocin mediate the suckling response and milk release.

HORMONAL FEEDBACK REGULATORY SYSTEMS

Feedback control, both negative and positive, is a fundamental feature of endocrine systems. Each of the major hypothalamic-pituitary-hormone axes is governed by negative feedback, a process that maintains hormone levels within a relatively narrow range (Chap. 2). Examples of hypothalamic-pituitary negative feedback include (1) thyroid hormones on the TRH-TSH axis, (2) cortisol on the CRH-ACTH axis, (3) gonadal steroids on the GnRH-LH/FSH axis, and (4) IGF-I on the growth hormone–releasing hormone (GHRH)-GH axis (**Fig. 1-3**).

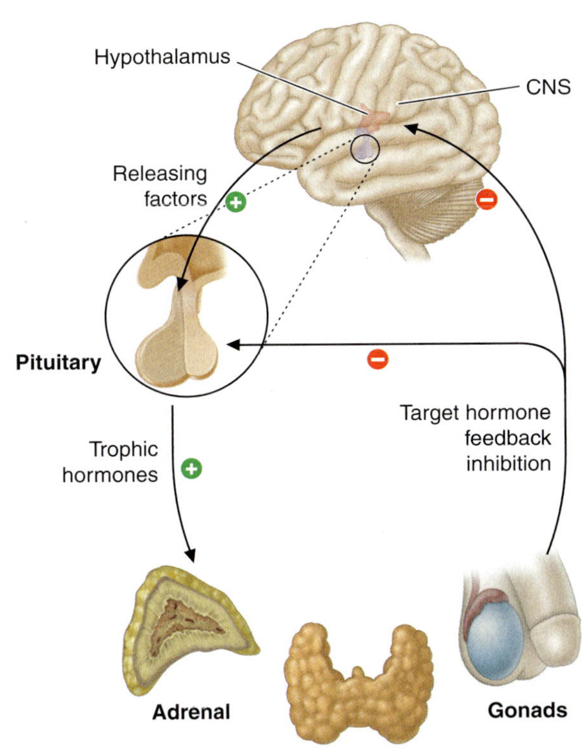

FIGURE 1-3
Feedback regulation of endocrine axes. CNS, central nervous system.

These regulatory loops include both positive (e.g., TRH, TSH) and negative components (e.g., T_4, T_3), allowing for exquisite control of hormone levels. As an example, a small reduction of TH triggers a rapid increase of TRH and TSH secretion, resulting in thyroid gland stimulation and increased TH production. When the TH reaches a normal level, it feeds back to suppress TRH and TSH, and a new steady state is attained. Feedback regulation also occurs for endocrine systems that do not involve the pituitary gland, such as calcium feedback on PTH, glucose inhibition of insulin secretion, and leptin feedback on the hypothalamus. An understanding of feedback regulation provides important insights into endocrine testing paradigms (see below).

Positive feedback control also occurs but is not well understood. The primary example is estrogen-mediated stimulation of the midcycle LH surge. Though chronic low levels of estrogen are inhibitory, gradually rising estrogen levels stimulate LH secretion. This effect, which is illustrative of an endocrine rhythm, involves activation of the hypothalamic GnRH pulse generator. In addition, estrogen-primed gonadotropes are extraordinarily sensitive to GnRH, leading to a ten- to twentyfold amplification of LH release.

PARACRINE AND AUTOCRINE CONTROL

The aforementioned examples of feedback control involve classic endocrine pathways in which hormones are released by one gland and act on a distant target gland. However, local regulatory systems, often involving growth factors, are increasingly recognized. *Paracrine regulation* refers to factors released by one cell that act on an adjacent cell in the same tissue. For example, somatostatin secretion by pancreatic islet δ cells inhibits insulin secretion from nearby β cells. *Autocrine regulation* describes the action of a factor on the same cell from which it is produced. IGF-I acts on many cells that produce it, including chondrocytes, breast epithelium, and gonadal cells. Unlike endocrine actions, paracrine and autocrine control are difficult to document because local growth factor concentrations cannot be readily measured.

Anatomic relationships of glandular systems also greatly influence hormonal exposure—the physical organization of islet cells enhances their intercellular communication; the portal vasculature of the hypothalamic-pituitary system exposes the pituitary to high concentrations of hypothalamic releasing factors; testicular seminiferous tubules gain exposure to high testosterone levels produced by the interdigitated Leydig cells; the pancreas receives nutrient information from the gastrointestinal tract; and the liver is the proximal target of insulin action because of portal drainage from the pancreas.

HORMONAL RHYTHMS

The feedback regulatory systems described above are superimposed on hormonal rhythms that are used for adaptation to the environment. Seasonal changes, the daily occurrence of the light-dark cycle, sleep, meals, and stress are examples of the many environmental events that affect hormonal rhythms. The *menstrual cycle* is repeated on average every 28 days, reflecting the time required for follicular maturation and ovulation (Chap. 10). Essentially all pituitary hormone rhythms are entrained to sleep and to the *circadian cycle*, generating reproducible patterns that are repeated approximately every 24 h. The HPA axis, for example, exhibits characteristic peaks of ACTH and cortisol production in the early morning, with a nadir during the night. Recognition of these rhythms is important for endocrine testing and treatment. Patients with Cushing's syndrome characteristically exhibit increased midnight cortisol levels when compared to normal individuals (Chap. 5). In contrast, morning cortisol levels are similar in these groups, as cortisol is normally high at this time of day in normal individuals. The HPA axis is more susceptible to suppression by glucocorticoids administered at night as they blunt the early morning rise of ACTH. Understanding these rhythms allows glucocorticoid replacement that mimics diurnal production by administering larger doses in the morning than in the afternoon. Disrupted sleep rhythms can alter hormonal regulation. For example, sleep deprivation causes mild insulin resistance and hypertension, which are reversible at least in the short term.

Other endocrine rhythms occur on a more rapid time scale. Many peptide hormones are secreted in discrete bursts every few hours. LH and FSH secretion are exquisitely sensitive to GnRH pulse frequency. Intermittent pulses of GnRH are required to maintain pituitary sensitivity, whereas continuous exposure to GnRH causes pituitary gonadotrope desensitization. This feature of the hypothalamic-pituitary-gonadotrope axis forms the basis for using long-acting GnRH agonists to treat central precocious puberty or to decrease testosterone levels in the management of prostate cancer.

It is important to be aware of the pulsatile nature of hormone secretion and the rhythmic patterns of hormone production when relating serum hormone measurements to normal values. For some hormones, integrated markers have been developed to circumvent hormonal fluctuations. Examples include 24-h urine collections for cortisol, IGF-I as a biologic marker of GH action, and HbA1c as an index of long-term (weeks to months) blood glucose control.

Often, one must interpret endocrine data only in the context of other hormones. For example, PTH levels are typically assessed in combination with serum calcium concentrations. A high serum calcium level in association with elevated PTH is suggestive of hyperparathyroidism, whereas a suppressed PTH in this situation is more likely to be caused by hypercalcemia of malignancy or other causes of hypercalcemia. Similarly, TSH should be elevated when T_4 and T_3 concentrations are low, reflecting reduced feedback inhibition. When this is not the case, it is important to consider secondary hypothyroidism, which is caused by a defect at the level of the pituitary.

PATHOLOGIC MECHANISMS OF ENDOCRINE DISEASE

Endocrine diseases can be divided into three major types of conditions: (1) hormone excess, (2) hormone deficiency, and (3) hormone resistance (**Table 1-2**).

CAUSES OF HORMONE EXCESS

Syndromes of hormone excess can be caused by neoplastic growth of endocrine cells, autoimmune disorders, and excess hormone administration. Benign endocrine tumors, including parathyroid, pituitary, and adrenal adenomas, often retain the capacity to produce hormones, perhaps reflecting the fact that they are relatively well differentiated. Many endocrine tumors exhibit subtle defects in their "set points" for feedback regulation. For example, in Cushing's disease, impaired feedback inhibition of ACTH secretion is associated with autonomous function. However, the tumor cells are not completely resistant to feedback, as evidenced by ACTH suppression by higher doses of dexamethasone (e.g., high-dose dexamethasone test) (Chap. 5). Similar set point defects are also typical of parathyroid adenomas and autonomously functioning thyroid nodules.

The molecular basis of some endocrine tumors, such as the MEN syndromes (MEN 1, 2A, 2B), have provided important insights into tumorigenesis (Chap. 23). MEN 1 is characterized primarily by the triad of parathyroid, pancreatic islet, and pituitary tumors. MEN 2 predisposes to medullary thyroid carcinoma, pheochromocytoma, and hyperparathyroidism. The *MEN1* gene, located on chromosome 11q13, encodes a putative tumor-suppressor gene, menin. Analogous to the paradigm first described for retinoblastoma, the affected individual inherits a mutant copy of the *MEN1* gene, and tumorigenesis ensues after a somatic "second hit" leads to loss of function of the normal *MEN1* gene (through deletion or point mutations).

In contrast to inactivation of a tumor-suppressor gene, as occurs in MEN 1 and most other inherited cancer syndromes, MEN 2 is caused by activating mutations in a single allele. In this case, activating mutations of the *RET* protooncogene, which encodes a receptor tyrosine kinase, leads to thyroid C cell hyperplasia in childhood before the development of medullary thyroid carcinoma. Elucidation of this pathogenic mechanism has allowed early genetic screening for *RET* mutations in individuals at risk for MEN 2, permitting identification of those who may benefit from prophylactic thyroidectomy and biochemical screening for pheochromocytoma and hyperparathyroidism.

TABLE 1-2

CAUSES OF ENDOCRINE DYSFUNCTION

TYPE OF ENDOCRINE DISORDER	EXAMPLES
Hyperfunction	
Neoplastic	
Benign	Pituitary adenomas, hyperparathyroidism, autonomous thyroid or adrenal nodules, pheochromocytoma
Malignant	Adrenal cancer, medullary thyroid cancer, carcinoid
Ectopic	Ectopic ACTH, SIADH secretion
Multiple endocrine neoplasia	MEN 1, MEN 2
Autoimmune	Graves' disease
Iatrogenic	Cushing's syndrome, hypoglycemia
Infectious/inflammatory	Subacute thyroiditis
Activating receptor mutations	LH, TSH, Ca^{2+} and PTH receptors, $G_s\alpha$
Hypofunction	
Autoimmune	Hashimoto's thyroiditis, type 1 diabetes mellitus, Addison's disease, polyglandular failure
Iatrogenic	Radiation-induced hypopituitarism, hypothyroidism, surgical
Infectious/inflammatory	Adrenal insufficiency, hypothalamic sarcoidosis
Hormone mutations	GH, LH β, FSH β, vasopressin
Enzyme defects	21-Hydroxylase deficiency
Developmental defects	Kallmann syndrome, Turner syndrome, transcription factors
Nutritional/vitamin deficiency	Vitamin D deficiency, iodine deficiency
Hemorrhage/infarction	Sheehan's syndrome, adrenal insufficiency
Hormone Resistance	
Receptor mutations	
Membrane	GH, vasopressin, LH, FSH, ACTH, GnRH, GHRH, PTH, leptin, Ca^{2+}
Nuclear	AR, TR, VDR, ER, GR, $PPAR_\gamma$
Signaling pathway mutations	Albright's hereditary osteodystrophy
Postreceptor	Type 2 diabetes mellitus, leptin resistance

Note: AR, androgen receptor; ER, estrogen receptor; GR, glucocorticoid receptor; PPAR, peroxisome proliferator activated receptor; SIADH, syndrome of inappropriate antidiuretic hormone; TR, thyroid hormone receptor; VDR, vitamin D receptor. For all other abbreviations, see text.

Mutations that activate hormone receptor signaling have been identified in several GPCRs. For example, activating mutations of the LH receptor cause a dominantly transmitted form of male-limited precocious puberty, reflecting premature stimulation of testosterone synthesis in Leydig cells (Chap. 8). Activating mutations in these GPCRs are predominantly located in the transmembrane domains and induce receptor coupling to $G_s\alpha$, even in the absence of hormone. Consequently, adenylate cyclase is activated, and cyclic AMP levels increase in a manner that mimics hormone action. A similar phenomenon results from activating mutations in $G_s\alpha$. When these occur early in development, they cause McCune-Albright syndrome. When they occur only in somatotropes, the activating $G_s\alpha$ mutations cause GH-secreting tumors and acromegaly (Chap. 2).

In autoimmune Graves' disease, antibody interactions with the TSH receptor mimic TSH action, leading to hormone overproduction (Chap. 4). Analogous to the effects of activating mutations of the TSH receptor, these stimulating autoantibodies induce conformational changes that release the receptor from a constrained state, thereby triggering receptor coupling to G proteins.

CAUSES OF HORMONE DEFICIENCY

Most examples of hormone deficiency states can be attributed to glandular destruction caused by autoimmunity, surgery, infection, inflammation, infarction, hemorrhage, or tumor infiltration (Table 1-2). Autoimmune damage to the thyroid gland (Hashimoto's thyroiditis) and pancreatic islet β cells (type 1 diabetes mellitus) is a prevalent cause of endocrine disease. Mutations in a number of hormones, hormone receptors, transcription factors, enzymes, and channels can also lead to hormone deficiencies.

HORMONE RESISTANCE

Most severe hormone resistance syndromes are due to inherited defects in membrane receptors, nuclear receptors, or the pathways that transduce receptor signals. These disorders are characterized by defective hormone action, despite the presence of increased hormone levels. In complete androgen resistance, for example, mutations in the androgen receptor lead to a female phenotypic appearance in genetic (XY) males, even though LH and testosterone levels are increased (Chap. 7). In addition to these relatively rare genetic disorders, more common acquired forms of functional hormone resistance include insulin resistance in type 2 diabetes mellitus, leptin resistance in obesity, and GH resistance in catabolic states. The pathogenesis of functional resistance involves receptor downregulation and postreceptor desensitization of signaling pathways; functional forms of resistance are generally reversible.

Approach to the Patient: ENDOCRINE DISEASE

Because endocrinology interfaces with numerous physiologic systems, there is no standard endocrine history and examination. Moreover, because most glands are relatively inaccessible, the examination usually focuses on the manifestations of hormone excess or deficiency, as well as direct examination of palpable glands, such as the thyroid and gonads. For these reasons, it is important to evaluate patients in the context of their presenting symptoms, review of systems, family and social history, and exposure to medications that may affect the endocrine system. Astute clinical skills are required to detect subtle symptoms and signs suggestive of underlying endocrine disease. For example, a patient with Cushing's syndrome may manifest specific findings, such as central fat redistribution, striae, and proximal muscle weakness, in addition to features seen commonly in the general population, such as obesity, plethora, hypertension, and glucose intolerance. Similarly, the insidious onset of hypothyroidism—with mental slowing, fatigue, dry skin, and other features—can be difficult to distinguish from similar, nonspecific findings in the general population. Clinical judgment, based on knowledge of disease prevalence and pathophysiology, is required to decide when to embark on more extensive evaluation of these disorders. Laboratory testing plays an essential role in endocrinology by allowing quantitative assessment of hormone levels and dynamics. Radiologic imaging tests, such as CT scan, MRI, thyroid scan, and ultrasound, are also used for the diagnosis of endocrine disorders. However, these tests are generally employed only after a hormonal abnormality has been established by biochemical testing.

HORMONE MEASUREMENTS AND ENDOCRINE TESTING

Radioimmunoassays are the most important diagnostic tool in endocrinology, as they allow sensitive, specific, and quantitative determination of steady-state and dynamic changes in hormone concentrations. Radioimmunoassays use antibodies to detect specific hormones. For many peptide hormones, these measurements are now configured to use two different antibodies to increase binding affinity and specificity. There are many variations of these assays; a common format involves using one antibody to capture the antigen (hormone) onto an immobilized surface and a second antibody, coupled to a chemiluminescent (ICMA) or radioactive (IRMA) signal, to detect the antigen. These assays are sensitive enough to detect plasma hormone concentrations in the picomolar to nanomolar range, and they can readily distinguish structurally related proteins, such as PTH from PTHrP. A variety of other techniques are used to measure specific hormones, including mass spectroscopy, various forms of chromatography, and enzymatic methods; bioassays are now rarely used.

Most hormone measurements are based on plasma or serum samples. However, urinary hormone determinations remain useful for the evaluation of some conditions. Urinary collections over 24 h provide an integrated assessment of the production of a hormone or metabolite, many of which vary during the day. It is important to ensure complete collections of 24-h urine samples; simultaneous measurement of creatinine provides an internal control for the adequacy of collection and can be used to normalize some hormone measurements. A 24-h urine free cortisol measurement largely reflects the amount of unbound cortisol, thus providing a reasonable index of biologically available hormone. Other commonly used urine determinations include 17-hydroxycorticosteroids, 17-ketosteroids, vanillylmandelic acid, metanephrine, catecholamines, 5-hydroxyindoleacetic acid, and calcium.

The value of quantitative hormone measurements lies in their correct interpretation in a clinical context. The normal range for most hormones is relatively broad, often varying by a factor of two- to tenfold. The normal ranges for many hormones are gender- and age-specific. Thus, using the correct normative database is an essential part of interpreting hormone tests. The pulsatile nature of hormones and factors that can affect their secretion, such as sleep, meals, and medications, must also be considered. Cortisol values increase fivefold between midnight and dawn; reproductive hormone levels vary dramatically during the female menstrual cycle.

For many endocrine systems, much information can be gained from basal hormone testing, particularly when different components of an endocrine axis are assessed simultaneously. For example, low testosterone and elevated LH levels suggest a primary gonadal problem, whereas a hypothalamic-pituitary disorder is likely if both LH and testosterone are low. Because TSH is a sensitive indicator of thyroid function, it is generally recommended as a first-line test for thyroid disorders. An elevated TSH level is almost always the result of primary hypothyroidism, whereas a low TSH is most often caused by thyrotoxicosis. These predictions can be confirmed by determining the free thyroxine level. Elevated calcium and PTH levels suggest hyperparathyroidism, whereas PTH is suppressed in hypercalcemia caused by malignancy or granulomatous diseases. A suppressed ACTH in the setting of hypercortisolemia, or increased urine free cortisol, is seen with hyperfunctioning adrenal adenomas.

It is not uncommon, however, for baseline hormone levels associated with pathologic endocrine conditions to overlap with the normal range. In this circumstance, dynamic testing is useful to further separate the two groups. There are a multitude of dynamic endocrine tests, but all are based on principles of feedback regulation, and most responses can be remembered based on the pathways that govern endocrine axes. *Suppression tests* are used in the setting of suspected endocrine hyperfunction. An example is the dexamethasone suppression test used to evaluate Cushing's syndrome (Chaps. 2 and 5). *Stimulation tests* are generally used to assess endocrine hypofunction. The ACTH stimulation test, for example, is used to assess the adrenal gland response in patients with suspected adrenal insufficiency. Other stimulation tests use hypothalamic-releasing factors such as TRH, GnRH, CRH, and GHRH to evaluate pituitary hormone reserve

(Chap. 2). Insulin-induced hypoglycemia evokes pituitary ACTH and GH responses. Stimulation tests based on reduction or inhibition of endogenous hormones are now used infrequently. Examples include metyrapone inhibition of cortisol synthesis and clomiphene inhibition of estrogen feedback.

SCREENING AND ASSESSMENT OF COMMON ENDOCRINE DISORDERS Many endocrine disorders are prevalent in the adult population (Table 1-3) and can be diagnosed and managed by general internists, family practitioners, or other primary health care providers. The high prevalence and clinical impact of certain endocrine

TABLE 1-3

EXAMPLES OF PREVALENT ENDOCRINE AND METABOLIC DISORDERS IN THE ADULT

DISORDER	APPROX. PREVALENCE IN ADULTS[a]	SCREENING/TESTING RECOMMENDATIONS[b]	CHAPTER
Obesity	31% BMI ≥30 65% BMI ≥25	Calculate BMI Measure waist circumference Exclude secondary causes Consider comorbid complications	17
Type 2 diabetes mellitus	>7%	Beginning at age 45, screen every 3 years, or earlier in high-risk groups: Fasting plasma glucose (FPG) >126 mg/dL Random plasma glucose >200 mg/dL An elevated HbA1c Consider comorbid complications	19
Hyperlipidemia	20–25%	Cholesterol screening at least every 5 years; more often in high-risk groups Lipoprotein analysis (LDL, HDL) for increased cholesterol, CAD, diabetes Consider secondary causes	21
Hypothyroidism	5–10%, women 0.5–2%, men	TSH; confirm with free T_4 Screen women after age 35 and every 5 years thereafter	4
Graves' disease	1–3%, women 0.1%, men	TSH, free T_4	4
Thyroid nodules and neoplasia	5% palpable >25% by ultrasound	Physical examination of thyroid Fine-needle aspiration biopsy	4
Osteoporosis	5–10%, women 2–4%, men	Bone mineral density measurements in women >65 years or in postmenopausal women or men at risk Exclude secondary causes	28
Hyperparathyroidism	0.1–0.5%, women > men	Serum calcium PTH, if calcium is elevated Assess comorbid conditions	27
Infertility	10%, couples	Investigate both members of couple Semen analysis in male Assess ovulatory cycles in female Specific tests as indicated	8, 10
Polycystic ovarian syndrome	5–10%, women	Free testosterone, DHEAS Consider comorbid conditions	10
Hirsutism	5–10%	Free testosterone, DHEAS Exclude secondary causes Additional tests as indicated	13
Menopause	Median age, 51	FSH	12
Hyperprolactinemia	15% in women with amenorrhea or galactorrhea	PRL level MRI, if not medication-related	2
Erectile dysfunction	20–30%	Careful history, PRL, testosterone Consider secondary causes (e.g., diabetes)	15
Gynecomastia	15%	Often, no tests are indicated Consider Klinefelter syndrome Consider medications, hypogonadism, liver disease	8
Klinefelter syndrome	0.2%, men	Karyotype Testosterone	7
Turner syndrome	0.03%, women	Karyotype Consider comorbid conditions	7

[a]The prevalence of most disorders varies among ethnic groups and with aging. Data based primarily on U.S. population.

[b]See individual chapters for additional information on evaluation and treatment. Early testing is indicated in patients with signs and symptoms of disease or in those at increased risk.

Note: BMI, body mass index; CAD, coronary artery disease; DHEAS, dehydroepiandrosterone; HDL, high-density lipoprotein; LDL, low-density lipoprotein. For other abbreviations, see text.

diseases justify vigilance for features of these disorders during routine physical examinations; laboratory screening is indicated in selected high-risk populations.

FURTHER READINGS

DeGroot LJ, Jameson JL (eds): *Endocrinology*, 5th ed. Philadelphia, Elsevier, 2006

Gereben B et al: Cellular and molecular basis of deiodinase-regulated thyroid hormone signaling. Endocr Rev 29:898, 2008

Golden SH et al: Clinical review: Prevalence and incidence of endocrine and metabolic disorders in the United States: A comprehensive review. J Clin Endocrinol Metab 94:1853, 2009

Hammes A et al: Role of endocytosis in cellular uptake of sex steroids. Cell 122:751, 2005

Inagaki T et al: Inhibition of growth hormone signaling by the fasting-induced hormone FGF21. Cell Metab 8:77, 2008

Kleinau G et al: Thyrotropin and homologous glycoprotein hormone receptors: Structural and functional aspects of extracellular signaling mechanisms. Endocr Rev 30:133, 2009

Marx SJ, Simonds WF: Hereditary hormone excess: Genes, molecular pathways, and syndromes. Endocr Rev 26:615, 2005

Smith CL et al: Coregulator function: A key to understanding tissue specificity of selective receptor modulators. Endocr Rev 25:45, 2004

Veldhuis JD et al: Motivations and methods for analyzing pulsatile hormone secretion. Endocr Rev 29:823, 2008

SECTION I

PITUITARY, THYROID, AND ADRENAL DISORDERS

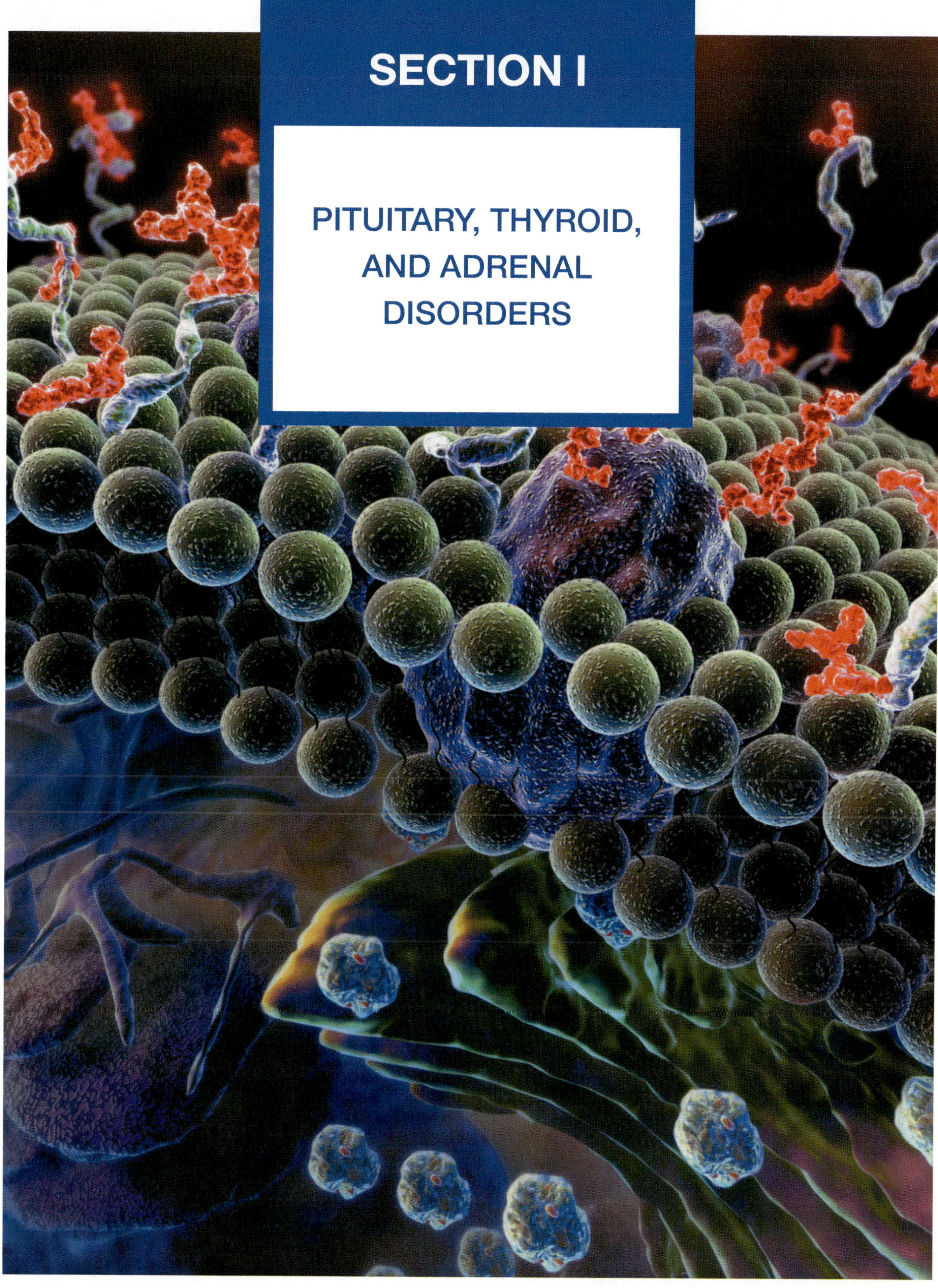

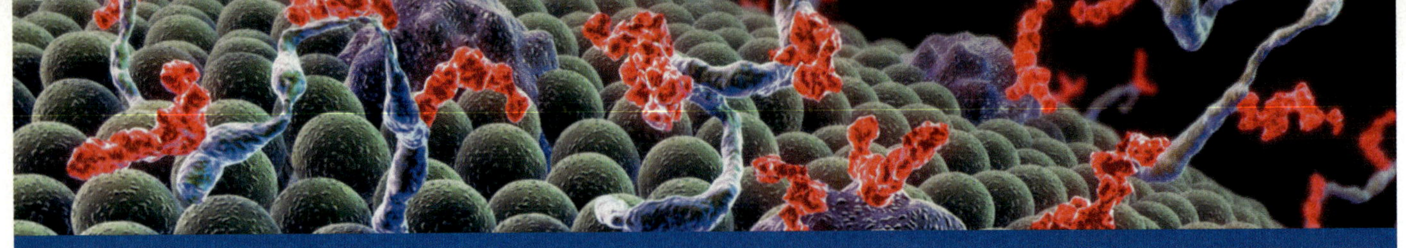

CHAPTER 2

DISORDERS OF THE ANTERIOR PITUITARY AND HYPOTHALAMUS

Shlomo Melmed ■ J. Larry Jameson

The anterior pituitary is often referred to as the "master gland" because, together with the hypothalamus, it orchestrates the complex regulatory functions of multiple other endocrine glands. The anterior pituitary gland produces six major hormones: (1) prolactin (PRL), (2) growth hormone (GH), (3) adrenocorticotropin hormone (ACTH), (4) luteinizing hormone (LH), (5) follicle-stimulating hormone (FSH), and (6) thyroid-stimulating hormone (TSH) (**Table 2-1**). Pituitary hormones are secreted in a pulsatile manner, reflecting stimulation by an array of specific hypothalamic releasing factors. Each of these pituitary hormones elicits specific responses in peripheral target tissues. The hormonal products of these peripheral glands, in turn, exert feedback control at the level of the hypothalamus and pituitary to modulate pituitary function (**Fig. 2-1**). Pituitary tumors cause characteristic hormone excess syndromes. Hormone deficiency may be inherited or acquired. Fortunately, efficacious treatments exist for the various pituitary hormone excess and deficiency syndromes. Nonetheless, these diagnoses are often elusive, emphasizing the importance of recognizing subtle clinical manifestations and performing the correct laboratory diagnostic tests.

For discussion of disorders of the posterior pituitary, or neurohypophysis, see Chap. 3.

TABLE 2-1

ANTERIOR PITUITARY HORMONE EXPRESSION AND REGULATION

CELL	CORTICOTROPE	SOMATOTROPE	LACTOTROPE	THYROTROPE	GONADOTROPE
Tissue-specific transcription factor	T-Pit	Prop-1, Pit-1	Prop-1, Pit-1	Prop-1, Pit-1, TEF	SF-1, DAX-1
Fetal appearance	6 weeks	8 weeks	12 weeks	12 weeks	12 weeks
Hormone	POMC	GH	PRL	TSH	FSH LH
Chromosomal locus	2p	17q	6	α-6q; β-1p	β-11p; β-19q
Protein	Polypeptide	Polypeptide	Polypeptide	Glycoprotein α, β subunits	Glycoprotein α, β subunits
Amino acids	266 (ACTH 1–39)	191	199	211	210 204
Stimulators	CRH, AVP, gp-130 cytokines	GHRH, Ghrelin	Estrogen, TRH, VIP	TRH	GnRH, activins, estrogen
Inhibitors	Glucocorticoids	Somatostatin, IGF-I	Dopamine	T_3, T_4, dopamine, somatostatin, glucocorticoids	Sex steroids, inhibin
Target gland	Adrenal	Liver, other tissues	Breast, other tissues	Thyroid	Ovary, testis
Trophic effect	Steroid production	IGF-I production, growth induction, insulin antagonism	Milk production	T_4 synthesis and secretion	Sex steroid production, follicle growth, germ cell maturation
Normal range	ACTH, 4–22 pg/L	<0.5 μg/L[a]	M <15; F < 20 μg/L	0.1–5 mU/L	M, 5–20 IU/L, F (basal), 5–20 IU/L

[a]Hormone secretion integrated over 24 h.

Note: M, male; F, female. For other abbreviations, see text.

Source: Adapted from I Shimon, S Melmed, in S Melmed, P Conn (eds): *Endocrinology: Basic and Clinical Principles*. Totowa, NJ, Humana, 2005.

ANATOMY AND DEVELOPMENT

ANATOMY

The pituitary gland weighs ~600 mg and is located within the sella turcica ventral to the diaphragma sella; it comprises anatomically and functionally distinct anterior and posterior lobes. The sella is contiguous to vascular and neurologic structures, including the cavernous sinuses, cranial nerves, and optic chiasm. Thus, expanding intrasellar pathologic processes may have significant central mass effects in addition to their endocrinologic impact.

Hypothalamic neural cells synthesize specific releasing and inhibiting hormones that are secreted directly into the portal vessels of the pituitary stalk. Blood supply of the pituitary gland is derived from the superior and inferior hypophyseal arteries (Fig. 2-2). The hypothalamic-pituitary portal plexus provides the major blood source for the anterior pituitary, allowing reliable transmission of hypothalamic peptide pulses without significant systemic dilution; consequently, pituitary cells are exposed to releasing or inhibiting factors and in turn release their hormones as discrete pulses (Fig. 2-3).

The posterior pituitary is supplied by the inferior hypophyseal arteries. In contrast to the anterior pituitary, the posterior lobe is directly innervated by hypothalamic neurons (supraopticohypophyseal and tuberohypophyseal nerve tracts) via the pituitary stalk (Chap. 3). Thus, posterior pituitary production of vasopressin [antidiuretic hormone (ADH)] and oxytocin is particularly sensitive to neuronal damage by lesions that affect the pituitary stalk or hypothalamus.

PITUITARY DEVELOPMENT

The embryonic differentiation and maturation of anterior pituitary cells have been elucidated in considerable detail. Pituitary development from Rathke's pouch involves a complex interplay of lineage-specific transcription factors expressed in pluripotent stem cells and gradients of locally produced growth factors (Table 2-1). The transcription factor Pit-1 determines cell-specific expression of GH, PRL, and TSH in somatotropes, lactotropes, and thyrotropes. Expression of high levels of estrogen receptors in cells that contain Pit-1 favors PRL expression, whereas thyrotrope embryonic factor (TEF) induces TSH expression. Pit-1 binds to GH, PRL, and TSH gene regulatory elements, as well as to recognition sites on its own

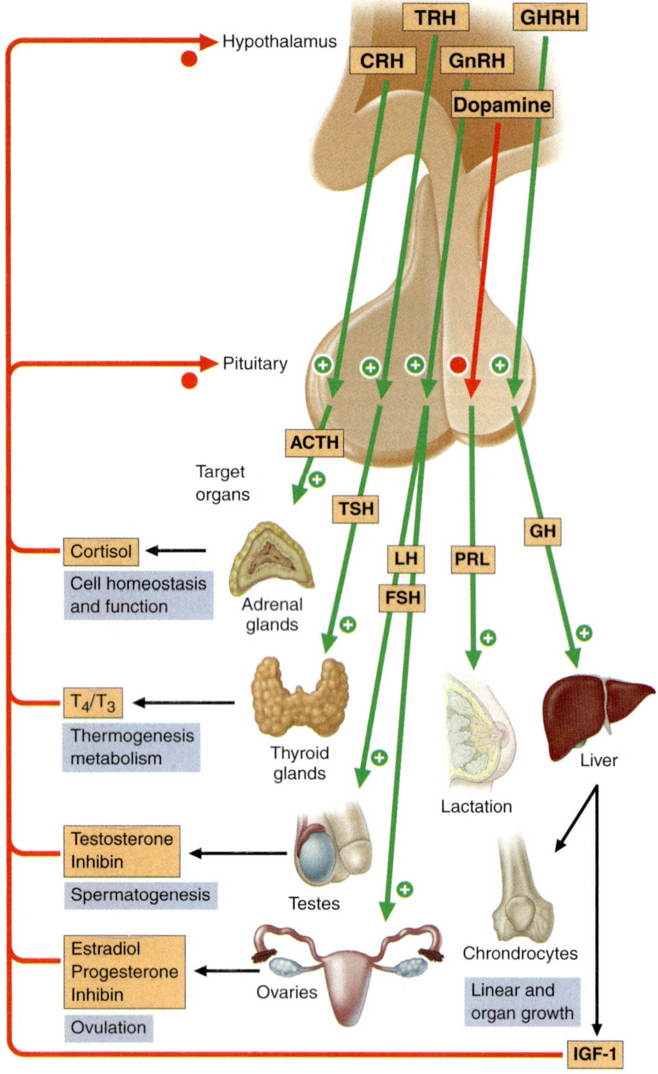

FIGURE 2-1

Diagram of pituitary axes. Hypothalamic hormones regulate anterior pituitary trophic hormones that, in turn, determine target gland secretion. Peripheral hormones feed back to regulate hypothalamic and pituitary hormones. For abbreviations, see text.

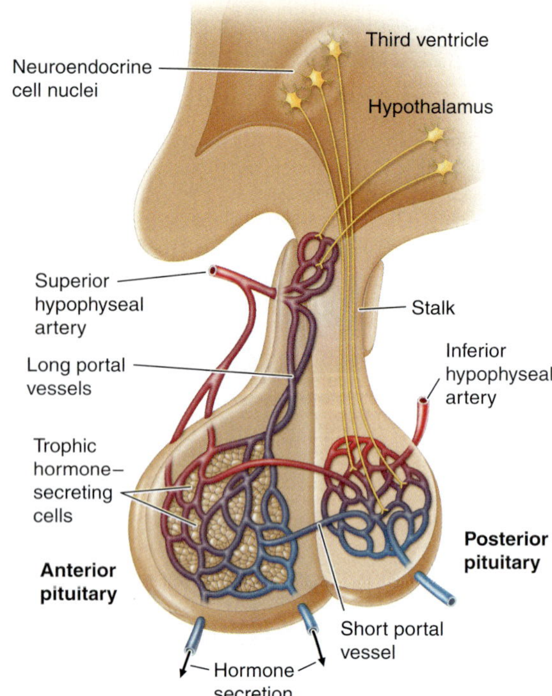

FIGURE 2-2

Diagram of hypothalamic-pituitary vasculature. The hypothalamic nuclei produce hormones that traverse the portal system and impinge on anterior pituitary cells to regulate pituitary hormone secretion. Posterior pituitary hormones are derived from direct neural extensions.

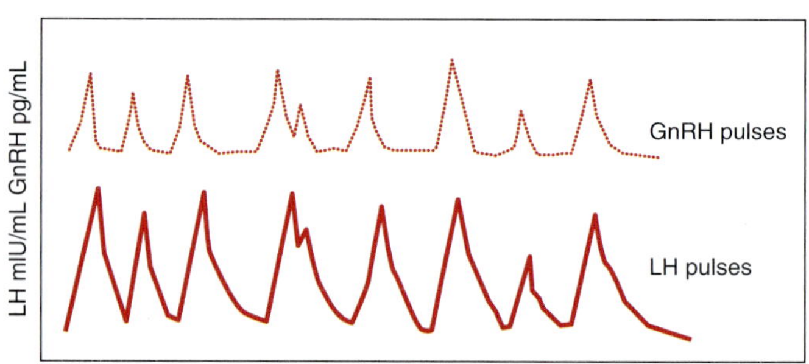

FIGURE 2-3

Hypothalamic gonadotropin-releasing hormone (GnRH) pulses induce secretory pulses of luteinizing hormone (LH)

promoter, providing a mechanism for perpetuating selective pituitary phenotypic stability. The transcription factor Prop-1 induces the pituitary development of Pit-1-specific lineages, as well as gonadotropes. Gonadotrope cell development is further defined by the cell-specific expression of the nuclear receptors, steroidogenic factor (SF-1) and DAX-1. Development of corticotrope cells, which express the proopiomelanocortin (POMC) gene, requires the T-Pit transcription factor. Abnormalities of pituitary development caused by mutations of Pit-1, Prop-1, SF-1, DAX-1, and T-Pit result in a series of rare, selective or combined, pituitary hormone deficits.

HYPOTHALAMIC AND ANTERIOR PITUITARY INSUFFICIENCY

Hypopituitarism results from impaired production of one or more of the anterior pituitary trophic hormones. Reduced pituitary function can result from inherited disorders; more commonly, it is acquired and reflects the mass effects of tumors or the consequences of inflammation or vascular damage. These processes may also impair synthesis or secretion of hypothalamic hormones, with resultant pituitary failure (Table 2-2).

TABLE 2-2

ETIOLOGY OF HYPOPITUITARISM[a]
Development/structural
Transcription factor defect
Pituitary dysplasia/aplasia
Congenital CNS mass, encephalocele
Primary empty sella
Congenital hypothalamic disorders (septo-optic dysplasia, Prader-Willi syndrome, Laurence-Moon-Biedl syndrome, Kallmann syndrome)
Traumatic
Surgical resection
Radiation damage
Head injuries
Neoplastic
Pituitary adenoma
Parasellar mass (meningioma, germinoma, ependymoma, glioma)
Rathke's cyst
Craniopharyngioma
Hypothalamic hamartoma, gangliocytoma
Pituitary metastases (breast, lung, colon carcinoma)
Lymphoma and leukemia
Meningioma
Infiltrative/inflammatory
Lymphocytic hypophysitis
Hemochromatosis
Sarcoidosis
Histiocytosis X
Granulomatous hypophysitis
Vascular
Pituitary apoplexy
Pregnancy-related (infarction with diabetes; postpartum necrosis)
Sickle cell disease
Arteritis
Infections
Fungal (histoplasmosis)
Parasitic (toxoplasmosis)
Tuberculosis
Pneumocystis carinii

[a]Trophic hormone failure associated with pituitary compression or destruction usually occurs sequentially GH > FSH > LH > TSH > ACTH. During childhood, growth retardation is often the presenting feature, and in adults hypogonadism is the earliest symptom.

DEVELOPMENTAL AND GENETIC CAUSES OF HYPOPITUITARISM

Pituitary Dysplasia

Pituitary dysplasia may result in aplastic, hypoplastic, or ectopic pituitary gland development. Because pituitary development requires midline cell migration from the nasopharyngeal Rathke's pouch, midline craniofacial disorders may be associated with pituitary dysplasia. Acquired pituitary failure in the newborn can also be caused by birth trauma, including cranial hemorrhage, asphyxia, and breech delivery.

Septo-Optic Dysplasia

Hypothalamic dysfunction and hypopituitarism may result from dysgenesis of the septum pellucidum or corpus callosum. Affected children have mutations in the *HESX1* gene, which is involved in early development of the ventral prosencephalon. These children exhibit variable combinations of cleft palate, syndactyly, ear deformities, hypertelorism, optic atrophy, micropenis, and anosmia. Pituitary dysfunction leads to diabetes insipidus, GH deficiency and short stature, and, occasionally, TSH deficiency.

Tissue-Specific Factor Mutations

Several pituitary cell–specific transcription factors, such as Pit-1 and Prop-1, are critical for determining the development and function of specific anterior pituitary cell lineages. Autosomal dominant or recessive Pit-1 mutations cause combined GH, PRL, and TSH deficiencies. These patients present with growth failure and varying degrees of hypothyroidism. The pituitary may appear hypoplastic on magnetic resonance imaging (MRI).

Prop-1 is expressed early in pituitary development and appears to be required for Pit-1 function. Familial and sporadic *PROP1* mutations result in combined GH, PRL, TSH, and gonadotropin deficiency. Over 80% of these patients have growth retardation; by adulthood, all are deficient in TSH and gonadotropins, and a small minority later develop ACTH deficiency. Because of gonadotropin deficiency, they do not enter puberty spontaneously. In some cases, the pituitary gland is enlarged. *TPIT* mutations result in ACTH deficiency associated with hypocortisolism.

Developmental Hypothalamic Dysfunction

Kallmann Syndrome

This syndrome results from defective hypothalamic gonadotropin-releasing hormone (GnRH) synthesis and is associated with anosmia or hyposmia due to olfactory bulb agenesis or hypoplasia (Chap. 8). The syndrome may also be associated with color blindness, optic atrophy, nerve deafness, cleft palate, renal abnormalities, cryptorchidism, and neurologic abnormalities such as mirror movements. Defects in the *KAL* gene, which maps to chromosome Xp22.3, prevent embryonic migration of GnRH neurons from the hypothalamic olfactory placode to the hypothalamus. Genetic abnormalities, in addition to *KAL* mutations, can also cause isolated GnRH deficiency, as autosomal recessive (i.e., *GPR54*) and dominant (i.e., *FGFR1*) modes of transmission have been described. GnRH deficiency prevents progression through puberty. Males present with delayed puberty and pronounced hypogonadal features, including micropenis, probably the result of low testosterone levels during infancy. Female patients present with primary amenorrhea and failure of secondary sexual development.

Kallmann syndrome and other causes of congenital GnRH deficiency are characterized by low LH and FSH levels and low concentrations of sex steroids (testosterone or estradiol). In sporadic cases of isolated gonadotropin deficiency, the diagnosis is often one of exclusion after eliminating other causes of hypothalamic-pituitary dysfunction. Repetitive GnRH administration restores normal pituitary gonadotropin responses, pointing to a hypothalamic defect.

Long-term treatment of men with human chorionic gonadotropin (hCG) or testosterone restores pubertal development and secondary sex characteristics; women can be treated with cyclic estrogen and progestin. Fertility may also be restored by the administration of gonadotropins or by using a portable infusion pump to deliver subcutaneous, pulsatile GnRH.

Bardet-Biedl Syndrome

This is a rare, genetically heterogeneous disorder characterized by mental retardation, renal abnormalities, obesity, and hexadactyly, brachydactyly, or syndactyly. Central diabetes insipidus may or may not be associated. GnRH deficiency occurs in 75% of males and half of affected females. Retinal degeneration begins in early childhood, and most patients are blind by age 30. Ten subtypes of Bardet-Biedl syndrome (BBS) have been identified with genetic linkage to nine different loci. Several of the loci encode genes involved in basal body cilia function, which may account for the diverse clinical manifestations.

Leptin and Leptin Receptor Mutations

Deficiencies of leptin, or its receptor, cause a broad spectrum of hypothalamic abnormalities including hyperphagia, obesity, and central hypogonadism (Chap. 16). Decreased GnRH production in these patients results in attenuated pituitary FSH and LH synthesis and release.

Prader-Willi Syndrome

This is a contiguous gene syndrome resulting from deletion of the paternal copies of the imprinted *SNRPN* gene, the *NECDIN* gene, and possibly other genes on chromosome 15q. Prader-Willi syndrome is associated with hypogonadotropic hypogonadism, hyperphagia-obesity, chronic muscle hypotonia, mental retardation, and adult-onset diabetes mellitus. Multiple somatic defects also involve the skull, eyes, ears, hands, and feet. Diminished hypothalamic oxytocin- and vasopressin-producing nuclei have been reported. Deficient GnRH synthesis is suggested by the observation that chronic GnRH treatment restores pituitary LH and FSH release.

ACQUIRED HYPOPITUITARISM

Hypopituitarism may be caused by accidental or neurosurgical trauma; vascular events such as apoplexy; pituitary or hypothalamic neoplasms such as pituitary adenomas, craniopharyngiomas, lymphoma, or metastatic tumors; inflammatory diseases such as lymphocytic hypophysitis; infiltrative disorders such as sarcoidosis, hemochromatosis, and tuberculosis; or irradiation.

Increasing evidence suggests that patients with brain injury including trauma, subarachnoid hemorrhage, and irradiation have transient hypopituitarism and require intermittent long-term endocrine follow-up, as permanent hypothalamic or pituitary dysfunction will develop in 25–40% of these patients.

Hypothalamic Infiltration Disorders

These disorders—including sarcoidosis, histiocytosis X, amyloidosis, and hemochromatosis—frequently involve both hypothalamic and pituitary neuronal and neurochemical tracts. Consequently, diabetes insipidus occurs in half of patients with these disorders. Growth retardation is seen if attenuated GH secretion occurs before pubertal epiphyseal closure. Hypogonadotropic hypogonadism and hyperprolactinemia are also common.

Inflammatory Lesions

Pituitary damage and subsequent dysfunction can be seen with chronic infections such as tuberculosis, with opportunistic fungal infections associated with AIDS, and in tertiary syphilis. Other inflammatory processes, such as granulomas or sarcoidosis, may mimic the features of a pituitary adenoma. These lesions may cause extensive hypothalamic and pituitary damage, leading to trophic hormone deficiencies.

Cranial Irradiation

Cranial irradiation may result in long-term hypothalamic and pituitary dysfunction, especially in children and adolescents, as they are more susceptible to damage following whole-brain or head and neck therapeutic irradiation. The development of hormonal abnormalities correlates strongly with irradiation dosage and the time interval after completion of radiotherapy. Up to two-thirds of patients ultimately develop hormone insufficiency after a median dose of 50 Gy (5000 rad) directed at the skull base. The development of hypopituitarism occurs over 5–15 years and usually reflects hypothalamic damage rather than primary destruction of pituitary cells. Although the pattern of hormone loss is variable, GH deficiency is most common, followed by gonadotropin and ACTH deficiency. When deficiency of one or more hormones is documented, the possibility of diminished reserve of other hormones is likely. Accordingly, anterior pituitary function should be evaluated over the long term in previously irradiated patients, and replacement therapy instituted when appropriate.

Lymphocytic Hypophysitis

This often occurs in postpartum women; it usually presents with hyperprolactinemia and MRI evidence of a prominent pituitary mass often resembling an adenoma, with mildly elevated PRL levels. Pituitary failure caused by diffuse lymphocytic infiltration may be transient or permanent but requires immediate evaluation and treatment. Rarely, isolated pituitary hormone deficiencies have been described, suggesting a selective autoimmune process targeted to specific cell types. Most patients manifest symptoms of progressive mass effects with headache and visual disturbance. The erythrocyte sedimentation rate is often elevated. As the MRI image may be indistinguishable from that of a pituitary adenoma, hypophysitis should be considered in a postpartum woman with a newly diagnosed pituitary mass before embarking on unnecessary surgical intervention. The inflammatory process often resolves after several months of glucocorticoid treatment, and pituitary function may be restored, depending on the extent of damage.

Pituitary Apoplexy

Acute intrapituitary hemorrhagic vascular events can cause substantial damage to the pituitary and surrounding sellar structures. Pituitary apoplexy may occur spontaneously in a preexisting adenoma; post-partum (Sheehan's syndrome); or in association with diabetes, hypertension, sickle cell anemia, or acute shock. The hyperplastic enlargement of the pituitary during pregnancy increases the risk for hemorrhage and infarction. Apoplexy is an endocrine emergency that may result in severe hypoglycemia, hypotension, central nervous system (CNS) hemorrhage, and death. Acute symptoms may include severe headache with signs of meningeal irritation, bilateral visual changes, ophthalmoplegia, and, in severe cases, cardiovascular collapse and loss of consciousness. Pituitary computed tomography (CT) or MRI may reveal signs of intratumoral or sellar hemorrhage, with deviation of the pituitary stalk and compression of pituitary tissue.

Patients with no evident visual loss or impaired consciousness can be observed and managed conservatively with high-dose glucocorticoids. Those with significant or progressive visual loss or loss of consciousness require urgent surgical decompression. Visual recovery after surgery is inversely correlated with the length of time after the acute event. Therefore, severe ophthalmoplegia or visual deficits are indications for early surgery. Hypopituitarism is very common after apoplexy.

Empty Sella

A partial or apparently totally empty sella is often an incidental MRI finding. These patients usually have normal pituitary function, implying that the surrounding rim of pituitary tissue is fully functional. Hypopituitarism, however, may develop insidiously. Pituitary masses may undergo clinically silent infarction with development of a partial or totally empty sella by cerebrospinal fluid (CSF) filling the dural herniation. Rarely, small but functional pituitary adenomas may arise within the rim of pituitary tissue, and these are not always visible on MRI.

PRESENTATION AND DIAGNOSIS

The clinical manifestations of hypopituitarism depend on which hormones are lost and the extent of the hormone deficiency. GH deficiency causes growth disorders in children and leads to abnormal body composition in adults. Gonadotropin deficiency causes menstrual disorders and infertility in women and decreased sexual function, infertility, and loss of secondary sexual characteristics in men. TSH and ACTH deficiency usually develop later in the course of pituitary failure. TSH deficiency causes growth retardation in children and features of hypothyroidism in children and in adults. The secondary form of adrenal insufficiency caused by ACTH deficiency leads to hypocortisolism with relative preservation of mineralocorticoid production. PRL deficiency causes failure of lactation. When lesions involve the posterior pituitary, polyuria and polydipsia reflect loss of vasopressin secretion. Epidemiologic studies have documented an increased mortality rate in patients with longstanding pituitary damage, primarily from increased cardiovascular and cerebrovascular disease.

LABORATORY INVESTIGATION

Biochemical diagnosis of pituitary insufficiency is made by demonstrating low levels of trophic hormones in the setting of low target hormone levels. For example, low free thyroxine in the setting of a low or inappropriately normal TSH level suggests secondary hypothyroidism. Similarly, a low testosterone level without elevation of gonadotropins suggests hypogonadotropic hypogonadism. Provocative tests may be required to assess pituitary reserve (Table 2-3). GH responses to insulin-induced hypoglycemia, arginine, l-dopa, growth hormone–releasing hormone (GHRH), or growth hormone–releasing peptides (GHRPs) can be used to assess GH reserve. Corticotropin-releasing hormone (CRH) administration induces ACTH release, and administration of synthetic ACTH [cosyntropin (Cortrosyn)] evokes adrenal cortisol release as an indirect indicator of pituitary ACTH reserve (Chap. 5). ACTH reserve is most reliably assessed during insulin-induced hypoglycemia. However, this test should be performed cautiously in patients with suspected adrenal insufficiency because of enhanced susceptibility to hypoglycemia and hypotension. Insulin-induced hypoglycemia is contraindicated in patients with active coronary artery disease or seizure disorders.

℞ Treatment: HYPOPITUITARISM

Hormone replacement therapy, including glucocorticoids, thyroid hormone, sex steroids, growth hormone, and vasopressin, is usually safe and free of complications. Treatment regimens that mimic physiologic hormone production allow for maintenance of satisfactory clinical homeostasis. Effective dosage schedules are outlined in Table 2-4. Patients in need of glucocorticoid replacement require careful dose adjustments during stressful events such as acute illness, dental procedures, trauma, and acute hospitalization (Chap. 5).

TABLE 2-3

TESTS OF PITUITARY SUFFICIENCY

HORMONE	TEST	BLOOD SAMPLES	INTERPRETATION
Growth hormone	Insulin tolerance test: Regular insulin (0.05–0.15 U/kg IV)	–30, 0, 30, 60, 120 min for glucose and GH	Glucose <40 mg/dL; GH should be >3 μg/L
	GHRH test: 1 μg/kg IV	0, 15, 30, 45, 60, 120 min for GH	Normal response is GH >3 μg/L
	L-Arginine test: 30 g IV over 30 min	0, 30, 60, 120 min for GH	Normal response is GH >3 μg/L
	L-dopa test: 500 mg PO	0, 30, 60, 120 min for GH	Normal response is GH >3 μg/L
Prolactin	TRH test: 200–500 μg IV	0, 20, and 60 min for TSH and PRL	Normal prolactin is >2 μg/L and increase >200% of baseline
ACTH	Insulin tolerance test: Regular insulin (0.05–0.15 U/kg IV)	–30, 0, 30, 60, 90 min for glucose and cortisol	Glucose <40 mg/dL Cortisol should increase by >7 μg/dL or to >20 μg/dL
	CRH test: 1 μg/kg ovine CRH IV at 0800 h[D3]	0, 15, 30, 60, 90, 120 min for ACTH and cortisol	Basal ACTH increases two- to fourfold and peaks at 20–100 pg/mL Cortisol levels >20–25 μg/dL
	Metyrapone test: Metyrapone (30 mg/kg) at midnight	Plasma 11-deoxycortisol and cortisol at 8 A.M.; ACTH can also be measured	Plasma cortisol should be <4 μg/dL to ensure an adequate response Normal response is 11-deoxycortisol >7.5 μg/dL or ACTH >75 pg/mL
	Standard ACTH stimulation test: ACTH 1-24 (Cosyntropin), 0.25 mg IM or IV	0, 30, 60 min for cortisol and aldosterone	Normal response is cortisol >21 μg/dL and aldosterone response of >4 ng/dL above baseline
	Low-dose ACTH test: ACTH 1-24 (Cosyntropin), 1 μg IV	0, 30, 60 min for cortisol	Cortisol should be >21 μg/dL
	3-day ACTH stimulation test consists of 0.25 mg ACTH 1-24 given IV over 8 h each day		Cortisol >21 μg/dL
TSH	Basal thyroid function tests: T_4, T_3, TSH	Basal tests	Low free thyroid hormone levels in the setting of TSH levels that are not appropriately increased
	TRH test: 200–500 μg IV	0, 20, 60 min for TSH and PRL[a]	TSH should increase by >5 mU/L unless thyroid hormone levels are increased
LH, FSH	LH, FSH, testosterone, estrogen	Basal tests	Basal LH and FSH should be increased in postmenopausal women Low testosterone levels in the setting of low LH and FSH
	GnRH test: GnRH (100 μg) IV	0, 30, 60 min for LH and FSH	In most adults, LH should increase by 10 IU/L and FSH by 2 IU/L Normal responses are variable
Multiple hormones	Combined anterior pituitary test: GHRH (1 μg/kg), CRH (1 μg/kg), GnRH (100 μg), TRH (200 μg) are given IV	–30, 0, 15, 30, 60, 90, 120 min for GH, ACTH, cortisol, LH, FSH, and TSH	Combined or individual releasing hormone responses must be elevated in the context of basal target gland hormone values and may not be uniformly diagnostic (see text)

[a]Evoked PRL response indicates lactotrope integrity.
Note: For abbreviations, see text.

TABLE 2-4

HORMONE REPLACEMENT THERAPY FOR ADULT HYPOPITUITARISM[a]

TROPHIC HORMONE DEFICIT	HORMONE REPLACEMENT
ACTH	Hydrocortisone (10–20 mg A.M.; 5–10 mg P.M.) Cortisone acetate (25 mg A.M.; 12.5 mg P.M.) Prednisone (5 mg A.M.; 2.5 mg P.M.)
TSH	L-Thyroxine (0.075–0.15 mg daily)
FSH/LH	Males Testosterone enanthate (200 mg IM every 2 weeks) Testosterone skin patch (5 mg/d) Females Conjugated estrogen (0.65–1.25 mg qd for 25 days) Progesterone (5–10 mg qd) on days 16–25 Estradiol skin patch (0.5 mg, every other day) For fertility: Menopausal gonadotropins, human chorionic gonadotropins
GH	Adults: Somatotropin (0.1–1.25 mg SC qd) Children: Somatotropin (0.02–0.05 mg/kg per d)
Vasopressin	Intranasal desmopressin (5–20 μg twice daily) Oral 300–600 μg qd

[a]All doses shown should be individualized for specific patients and should be reassessed during stress, surgery, or pregnancy. Male and female fertility requirements should be managed as discussed in Chaps. 8 and 10.

Note: For abbreviations, see text.

HYPOTHALAMIC, PITUITARY, AND OTHER SELLAR MASSES

PITUITARY TUMORS

Pituitary adenomas are the most common cause of pituitary hormone hypersecretion and hyposecretion syndromes in adults. They account for ~15% of all intracranial neoplasms. At autopsy, up to one-quarter of all pituitary glands harbor an unsuspected microadenoma (<10 mm diameter). Similarly, pituitary imaging detects small, clinically inapparent pituitary lesions in at least 10% of individuals.

Pathogenesis

Pituitary adenomas are benign neoplasms that arise from one of the five anterior pituitary cell types. The clinical and biochemical phenotype of pituitary adenomas depend on the cell type from which they are derived. Thus, tumors arising from lactotrope (PRL), somatotrope (GH), corticotrope (ACTH), thyrotrope (TSH), or gonadotrope (LH, FSH) cells hypersecrete their respective hormones (Table 2-5). Plurihormonal tumors that express combinations of GH, PRL, TSH, ACTH, and the glycoprotein hormone α subunit may be diagnosed by careful immunocytochemistry or may manifest as clinical syndromes that combine features of these hormonal hypersecretory syndromes. Morphologically, these tumors may arise from a single polysecreting cell type or comprise cells with mixed function within the same tumor.

Hormonally active tumors are characterized by autonomous hormone secretion with diminished responsiveness to physiologic inhibitory pathways. Hormone production does not always correlate with tumor size. Small hormone-secreting adenomas may cause significant

TABLE 2-5

CLASSIFICATION OF PITUITARY ADENOMAS[a]

ADENOMA CELL ORIGIN	HORMONE PRODUCT	CLINICAL SYNDROME
Lactotrope	PRL	Hypogonadism, galactorrhea
Gonadotrope	FSH, LH, subunits	Silent or hypogonadism
Somatotrope	GH	Acromegaly/gigantism
Corticotrope	ACTH	Cushing's disease
Mixed growth hormone and prolactin cell	GH, PRL	Acromegaly, hypogonadism, galactorrhea
Other plurihormonal cell	Any	Mixed
Acidophil stem cell	PRL, GH	Hypogonadism, galactorrhea, acromegaly
Mammosomatotrope	PRL, GH	Hypogonadism, galactorrhea, acromegaly
Thyrotrope	TSH	Thyrotoxicosis
Null cell	None	Pituitary failure
Oncocytoma	None	Pituitary failure

[a]Hormone-secreting tumors are listed in decreasing order of frequency. All tumors may cause local pressure effects, including visual disturbances, cranial nerve palsy, and headache.

Note: For abbreviations, see text.

Source: Adapted from S Melmed, in JL Jameson (ed): *Principles of Molecular Medicine*, Totowa, NJ, Humana Press, 1998.

clinical perturbations, whereas larger adenomas that produce less hormone may be clinically silent and remain undiagnosed (if no central compressive effects occur). About one-third of all adenomas are clinically nonfunctioning and produce no distinct clinical hypersecretory syndrome. Most of these arise from gonadotrope cells and may secrete small amounts of α- and β-glycoprotein hormone subunits or, very rarely, intact circulating gonadotropins. True pituitary carcinomas with documented extracranial metastases are exceedingly rare.

Almost all pituitary adenomas are monoclonal in origin, implying the acquisition of one or more somatic mutations that confer a selective growth advantage. In addition to direct studies of oncogene mutations, this model is supported by X-chromosomal inactivation analyses of tumors in female patients heterozygous for X-linked genes. Consistent with their clonal origin, complete surgical resection of small pituitary adenomas usually cures hormone hypersecretion. Nevertheless, hypothalamic hormones, such as GHRH or CRH, also enhance mitotic activity of their respective pituitary target cells, in addition to their role in pituitary hormone regulation. Thus, patients harboring rare abdominal or chest tumors elaborating ectopic GHRH or CRH may present with somatotrope or corticotrope hyperplasia.

Several etiologic genetic events have been implicated in the development of pituitary tumors. The pathogenesis of sporadic forms of acromegaly has been particularly informative as a model of tumorigenesis. GHRH, after binding to its G protein–coupled somatotrope receptor, utilizes cyclic AMP as a second messenger to stimulate GH secretion and somatotrope proliferation. A subset (~35%) of GH-secreting pituitary tumors contain sporadic mutations in $G_s\alpha$ (Arg 201 → Cys or His; Gln 227 → Arg). These mutations inhibit intrinsic GTPase activity, resulting in constitutive elevation of cyclic AMP, Pit-1 induction, and activation of cyclic AMP response element binding protein (CREB), thereby promoting somatotrope cell proliferation and GH secretion.

Characteristic loss of heterozygosity (LOH) in various chromosomes has been documented in large or invasive macroadenomas, suggesting the presence of putative tumor suppressor genes at these loci. LOH of chromosome regions on 11q13, 13, and 9 is present in up to 20% of sporadic pituitary tumors including GH-, PRL-, and ACTH-producing adenomas and in some nonfunctioning tumors.

Compelling evidence also favors growth factor promotion of pituitary tumor proliferation. Basic fibroblast growth factor (bFGF) is abundant in the pituitary and has been shown to stimulate pituitary cell mitogenesis. Other factors involved in initiation and promotion of pituitary tumors include loss of negative-feedback inhibition (as seen with primary hypothyroidism or hypogonadism) and estrogen-mediated or paracrine angiogenesis. Growth characteristics and neoplastic behavior may also be influenced by several activated oncogenes, including *RAS* and pituitary tumor transforming gene (*PTTG*).

Genetic Syndromes Associated with Pituitary Tumors

Several familial syndromes are associated with pituitary tumors, and the genetic mechanisms for some of these have been unraveled.

Multiple endocrine neoplasia (MEN) 1 is an autosomal dominant syndrome characterized primarily by a genetic predisposition to parathyroid, pancreatic islet, and pituitary adenomas (Chap. 23). MEN 1 is caused by inactivating germline mutations in *MENIN*, a constitutively expressed tumor-suppressor gene located on chromosome 11q13. Loss of heterozygosity, or a somatic mutation of the remaining normal *MENIN* allele, leads to tumorigenesis. About half of affected patients develop prolactinomas; acromegaly and Cushing's syndrome are less commonly encountered.

Carney syndrome is characterized by spotty skin pigmentation, myxomas, and endocrine tumors including testicular, adrenal, and pituitary adenomas. Acromegaly occurs in about 20% of patients. A subset of patients have mutations in the R1α regulatory subunit of protein kinase A (*PRKAR1A*).

McCune-Albright syndrome consists of polyostotic fibrous dysplasia, pigmented skin patches, and a variety of endocrine disorders, including GH-secreting pituitary tumors, adrenal adenomas, and autonomous ovarian function (Chap. 10). Hormonal hypersecretion is the result of constitutive cyclic AMP production caused by inactivation of the GTPase activity of $G_s\alpha$. The $G_s\alpha$ mutations occur postzygotically, leading to a mosaic pattern of mutant expression.

Familial acromegaly is a rare disorder in which family members may manifest either acromegaly or gigantism. The disorder is associated with LOH at a chromosome 11q13 locus distinct from that of *MENIN*.

OTHER SELLAR MASSES

Craniopharyngiomas are benign, suprasellar cystic masses that present with headaches, visual field deficits, and variable degrees of hypopituitarism. They are derived from Rathke's pouch and arise near the pituitary stalk, commonly extending into the suprasellar cistern. Craniopharyngiomas are often large, cystic, and locally invasive. Many are partially calcified, providing a characteristic appearance on skull x-ray and CT images. More than half of all patients present before age 20, usually with signs of increased intracranial pressure, including headache, vomiting, papilledema, and hydrocephalus. Associated symptoms include visual field abnormalities, personality changes and cognitive deterioration, cranial nerve damage, sleep difficulties, and weight gain. Hypopituitarism can be documented in about 90% and diabetes insipidus occurs in about 10% of patients. About half of affected children present with growth retardation. MRI is generally superior to CT to evaluate cystic structure and tissue components of craniopharyngiomas. CT is useful to define calcifications and to evaluate invasion into surrounding bony structures and sinuses.

Treatment usually involves transcranial or transsphenoidal surgical resection followed by postoperative radiation of residual tumor. Surgery alone is curative in less than half of patients because of adherence to vital structures or because of small tumor deposits in the hypothalamus or brain parenchyma. The goal of surgery is to remove as much tumor as possible without risking complications associated with efforts to remove firmly adherent or inaccessible tissue. In the absence of radiotherapy, about 75% of tumors recur, and 10-year survival is less than 50%. In patients with incomplete resection, radiotherapy improves 10-year survival to 70–90% but is associated with increased risk of secondary malignancies. Most patients require lifelong pituitary hormone replacement.

Developmental failure of Rathke's pouch obliteration may lead to *Rathke's cysts*, which are small (<5 mm) cysts entrapped by squamous epithelium, and are found in about 20% of individuals at autopsy. Although Rathke's cleft cysts do not usually grow and are often diagnosed incidentally, about a third present in adulthood with compressive symptoms, diabetes insipidus, and hyperprolactinemia due to stalk compression. Rarely, internal hydrocephalus develops. The diagnosis is suggested preoperatively by visualizing the cyst wall on MRI, which distinguishes these lesions from craniopharyngiomas. Cyst contents range from CSF-like fluid to mucoid material. *Arachnoid cysts* are rare and generate an MRI image isointense with cerebrospinal fluid.

Sella chordomas usually present with bony clival erosion, local invasiveness, and, on occasion, calcification. Normal pituitary tissue may be visible on MRI, distinguishing chordomas from aggressive pituitary adenomas. Mucinous material may be obtained by fine-needle aspiration.

Meningiomas arising in the sellar region may be difficult to distinguish from nonfunctioning pituitary adenomas. Meningiomas typically enhance on MRI and may show evidence of calcification or bony erosion. Meningiomas may cause compressive symptoms.

Histiocytosis X comprises a variety of syndromes associated with foci of eosinophilic granulomas. Diabetes insipidus, exophthalmos, and punched-out lytic bone lesions (*Hand-Schüller-Christian disease*) are associated with granulomatous lesions visible on MRI, as well as a characteristic axillary skin rash. Rarely, the pituitary stalk may be involved.

Pituitary metastases occur in ~3% of cancer patients. Bloodborne metastatic deposits are found almost exclusively in the posterior pituitary. Accordingly, diabetes insipidus can be a presenting feature of lung, gastrointestinal, breast, and other pituitary metastases. About half of pituitary metastases originate from breast cancer; about 25% of patients with metastatic breast cancer have such deposits. Rarely, pituitary stalk involvement results in anterior pituitary insufficiency. The MRI diagnosis of a metastatic lesion may be difficult to distinguish from an aggressive pituitary adenoma; the diagnosis may require histologic examination of excised tumor tissue. Primary or metastatic lymphoma, leukemias, and plasmacytomas also occur within the sella.

Hypothalamic hamartomas and *gangliocytomas* may arise from astrocytes, oligodendrocytes, and neurons with varying degrees of differentiation. These tumors may overexpress hypothalamic neuropeptides including GnRH, GHRH, or CRH. In GnRH-producing tumors, children present with precocious puberty, psychomotor delay, and laughing-associated seizures. Medical treatment of GnRH-producing hamartomas with long-acting GnRH analogues effectively suppresses gonadotropin secretion and controls premature pubertal development. Rarely, hamartomas are also associated with craniofacial abnormalities; imperforate anus; cardiac, renal, and lung disorders; and pituitary failure as features of *Pallister-Hall syndrome*, which is caused by mutations in the carboxy terminus of the *GLI3* gene. Hypothalamic hamartomas are often contiguous with the pituitary, and preoperative MRI diagnosis may not be possible. Histologic evidence of hypothalamic neurons in tissue resected at transsphenoidal surgery may be the first indication of a primary hypothalamic lesion.

Hypothalamic gliomas and *optic gliomas* occur mainly in childhood and usually present with visual loss. Adults have more aggressive tumors; about a third are associated with neurofibromatosis.

Brain germ cell tumors may arise within the sellar region. These include *dysgerminomas*, which are frequently associated with diabetes insipidus and visual loss. They rarely metastasize. *Germinomas*, *embryonal carcinomas*, *teratomas*, and *choriocarcinomas* may arise in the parasellar region and produce hCG. These germ cell tumors present with precocious puberty, diabetes insipidus, visual field defects, and thirst disorders. Many patients are GH-deficient with short stature.

METABOLIC EFFECTS OF HYPOTHALAMIC LESIONS

Lesions involving the anterior and preoptic hypothalamic regions cause paradoxical vasoconstriction, tachycardia, and hyperthermia. Acute hyperthermia is usually due to a hemorrhagic insult, but poikilothermia may also occur. Central disorders of thermoregulation result from posterior hypothalamic damage. The *periodic hypothermia syndrome* comprises episodic attacks of rectal temperatures <30°C, sweating, vasodilation, vomiting, and bradycardia. Damage to the ventromedial hypothalamic nuclei by craniopharyngiomas, hypothalamic trauma, or inflammatory disorders may be associated with *hyperphagia* and *obesity*.

This region appears to contain an energy-satiety center where melanocortin receptors are influenced by leptin, insulin, POMC products, and gastrointestinal peptides (Chap. 16). Polydipsia and hypodipsia are associated with damage to central osmoreceptors located in preoptic nuclei (Chap. 3). Slow-growing hypothalamic lesions can cause increased somnolence and disturbed sleep cycles as well as obesity, hypothermia, and emotional outbursts. Lesions of the central hypothalamus may stimulate sympathetic neurons, leading to elevated serum catecholamine and cortisol levels. These patients are predisposed to cardiac arrhythmias, hypertension, and gastric erosions.

EVALUATION

Local Mass Effects

Clinical manifestations of sellar lesions vary, depending on the anatomic location of the mass and direction of its extension (Table 2-6). The dorsal sellar diaphragm presents the least resistance to soft tissue expansion from the sella; consequently, pituitary adenomas frequently extend in a suprasellar direction. Bony invasion may occur as well.

Headaches are common features of small intrasellar tumors, even with no demonstrable suprasellar extension. Because of the confined nature of the pituitary, small changes in intrasellar pressure stretch the dural plate; however, headache severity correlates poorly with adenoma size or extension.

Suprasellar extension can lead to visual loss by several mechanisms, the most common being compression of the optic chiasm, but direct invasion of the optic nerves or obstruction of CSF flow leading to secondary visual disturbances also occurs. Pituitary stalk compression by a hormonally active or inactive intrasellar mass may compress the portal vessels, disrupting pituitary access to hypothalamic hormones and dopamine; this results in hyperprolactinemia and concurrent loss of other pituitary hormones. This "stalk section" phenomenon may also be caused by trauma, whiplash injury with posterior clinoid stalk compression, or skull base fractures. Lateral mass invasion may impinge on the cavernous sinus and compress its neural contents, leading to cranial nerve III, IV, and VI palsies as well as effects on the ophthalmic and maxillary branches of the fifth cranial nerve. Patients may present with diplopia, ptosis, ophthalmoplegia, and decreased facial sensation, depending on the extent of neural damage. Extension into the sphenoid sinus indicates that the pituitary mass has eroded through the sellar floor. Aggressive tumors rarely invade the palate roof and cause nasopharyngeal obstruction, infection, and CSF leakage. Temporal and frontal lobe involvement may lead to uncinate seizures, personality disorders, and anosmia. Direct hypothalamic encroachment by an invasive pituitary mass may cause important metabolic sequelae, including precocious puberty or hypogonadism, diabetes insipidus, sleep disturbances, dysthermia, and appetite disorders.

TABLE 2-6

FEATURES OF SELLAR MASS LESIONS[a]

IMPACTED STRUCTURE	CLINICAL IMPACT
Pituitary	Hypogonadism Hypothyroidism Growth failure and adult hyposomatotropism Hypoadrenalism
Optic chiasm	Loss of red perception Bitemporal hemianopia Superior or bitemporal field defect Scotoma Blindness
Hypothalamus	Temperature dysregulation Appetite and thirst disorders Obesity Diabetes insipidus Sleep disorders Behavioral dysfunction Autonomic dysfunction
Cavernous sinus	Ophthalmoplegia with or without ptosis or diplopia Facial numbness
Frontal lobe	Personality disorder Anosmia
Brain	Headache Hydrocephalus Psychosis Dementia Laughing seizures

[a]As the intrasellar mass expands, it first compresses intrasellar pituitary tissue, then usually invades dorsally through the dura to lift the optic chiasm or laterally to the cavernous sinuses. Bony erosion is rare, as is direct brain compression. Microadenomas may present with headache.

MRI

Sagittal and coronal T1-weighted MRI imaging, before and after administration of gadolinium, allow precise visualization of the pituitary gland with clear delineation of the hypothalamus, pituitary stalk, pituitary tissue and surrounding suprasellar cisterns, cavernous sinuses, sphenoid sinus, and optic chiasm. Pituitary gland height ranges from 6 mm in children to 8 mm in adults; during pregnancy and puberty, the height may reach 10–12 mm. The upper aspect of the adult pituitary is flat or slightly concave, but in adolescent and pregnant individuals, this surface may be convex, reflecting physiologic pituitary enlargement. The stalk should be midline and vertical. CT scan is indicated to define the extent of bony erosion or the presence of calcification.

Anterior pituitary gland soft tissue consistency is slightly heterogeneous on MRI, and signal intensity resembles that of brain matter on T1-weighted imaging

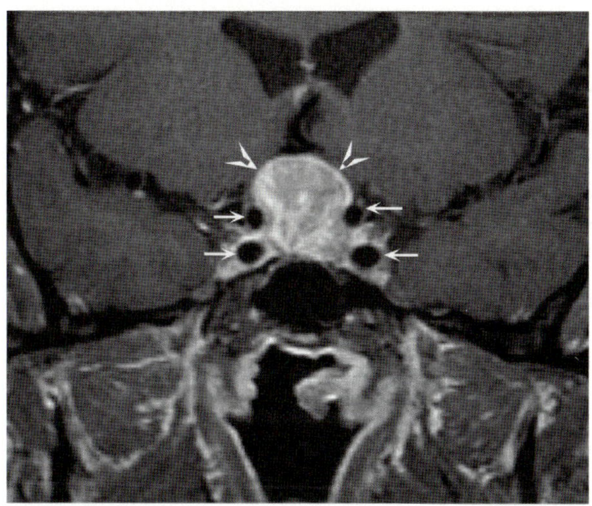

FIGURE 2-4

Pituitary adenoma. Coronal T1-weighted postcontrast magnetic resonance image shows a homogeneously enhancing mass (*arrowheads*) in the sella turcica and suprasellar region compatible with a pituitary adenoma; the small arrows outline the carotid arteries.

(Fig. 2-4). Adenoma density is usually lower than that of surrounding normal tissue on T1-weighted imaging, and the signal intensity increases with T2-weighted images. The high phospholipid content of the posterior pituitary results in a "pituitary bright spot."

Sellar masses are commonly encountered as incidental findings on MRI, and most of these are pituitary adenomas (incidentalomas). In the absence of hormone hypersecretion, these small lesions can be safely monitored by MRI, which is performed annually and then less often if there is no evidence of growth. Resection should be considered for incidentally discovered macroadenomas, as about one-third become invasive or cause local pressure effects. If hormone hypersecretion is evident, specific therapies are indicated. When larger masses (>1 cm) are encountered, they should also be distinguished from nonadenomatous lesions. Meningiomas are often associated with bony hyperostosis; craniopharyngiomas may be calcified and are usually hypodense, whereas gliomas are hyperdense on T2-weighted images.

Ophthalmologic Evaluation

Because optic tracts may be contiguous to an expanding pituitary mass, reproducible visual field assessment that uses perimetry techniques should be performed on all patients with sellar mass lesions that abut the optic chiasm. Bitemporal hemianopia or superior bitemporal defects are classically observed, reflecting the location of these tracts within the inferior and posterior part of the chiasm. Homonymous cuts reflect postchiasmal and monocular field cuts prechiasmal lesions. Loss of red perception is an early sign of optic tract pressure. Early diagnosis reduces the risk of blindness, scotomas, or other visual disturbances.

Laboratory Investigation

The presenting clinical features of functional pituitary adenomas (e.g., acromegaly, prolactinomas, or Cushing's syndrome) should guide the laboratory studies (Table 2-7). However, for a sellar mass with no obvious clinical features of hormone excess, laboratory studies are geared toward determining the nature of the tumor and assessing the possible presence of hypopituitarism. When a pituitary adenoma is suspected based on MRI, initial hormonal evaluation usually includes (1) basal PRL; (2) insulin-like growth factor (IGF) I; (3) 24-h urinary free cortisol and/or overnight oral dexamethasone (1 mg) suppression test; (4) α subunit, FSH, and LH; and (5) thyroid function tests. Additional hormonal evaluation may be indicated based on the results of these tests. Pending more detailed assessment of hypopituitarism, a menstrual history, testosterone and 8 A.M. cortisol levels, and thyroid function tests usually identify patients with pituitary hormone deficiencies that require hormone replacement before further testing or surgery.

TABLE 2-7

SCREENING TESTS FOR FUNCTIONAL PITUITARY ADENOMAS

	TEST	COMMENTS
Acromegaly	Serum IGF-I Oral glucose tolerance test with GH obtained at 0, 30, and 60 min	Interpret IGF-I relative to age- and gender-matched controls Normal subjects should suppress growth hormone to <1 μg/L
Prolactinoma	Serum PRL	Exclude medications MRI of the sella should be ordered if prolactin is elevated
Cushing's disease	24-h urinary free cortisol Dexamethasone (1 mg) at 11 P.M. and fasting plasma cortisol measured at 8 A.M. ACTH assay	Ensure urine collection is total and accurate Normal subjects suppress to <5 μg/dL Distinguishes adrenal adenoma (ACTH suppressed) from ectopic ACTH or Cushing's disease (ACTH normal or elevated)

Note: For abbreviations, see text.

Immunohistochemical staining of pituitary tumor specimens obtained at transsphenoidal surgery confirms clinical and laboratory studies and provides a histologic diagnosis when hormone studies are equivocal and in cases of clinically nonfunctioning tumors. Occasionally, ultrastructural assessment by electron microscopy is required for diagnosis.

Rx Treatment: HYPOTHALAMIC, PITUITARY, AND OTHER SELLAR MASSES

OVERVIEW Successful management of sellar masses requires accurate diagnosis as well as selection of optimal therapeutic modalities. Most pituitary tumors are benign and slow-growing. Clinical features result from local mass effects and hormonal hypo- or hypersecretion syndromes caused directly by the adenoma or as a consequence of treatment. Thus, lifelong management and follow-up are necessary for these patients.

MRI technology with gadolinium enhancement for pituitary visualization, new advances in transsphenoidal surgery and in stereotactic radiotherapy (including gamma-knife radiotherapy), and novel therapeutic agents have improved pituitary tumor management. The goals of pituitary tumor treatment include normalization of excess pituitary secretion, amelioration of symptoms and signs of hormonal hypersecretion syndromes, and shrinkage or ablation of large tumor masses with relief of adjacent structure compression. Residual anterior pituitary function should be preserved and can sometimes be restored by removing the tumor mass. Ideally, adenoma recurrence should be prevented.

TRANSSPHENOIDAL SURGERY Transsphenoidal rather than transfrontal resection is the desired surgical approach for pituitary tumors, except for the rare invasive suprasellar mass surrounding the frontal or middle fossa, surrounding the optic nerves, or invading posteriorly behind the clivus. Intraoperative microscopy facilitates visual distinction between adenomatous and normal pituitary tissue, as well as microdissection of small tumors that may not be visible by MRI (Fig. 2-5). Transsphenoidal surgery also avoids the cranial invasion and manipulation of brain tissue required by subfrontal surgical approaches. Endoscopic techniques with three-dimensional intraoperative localization have improved visualization and access to tumor tissue.

In addition to correction of hormonal hypersecretion, pituitary surgery is indicated for mass lesions that impinge on surrounding structures. Surgical decompression and resection are required for an expanding pituitary mass accompanied by persistent headache, progressive visual field defects, cranial nerve palsies, internal hydrocephalus, and, occasionally, intrapituitary hemorrhage and apoplexy. Transsphenoidal surgery is sometimes used for pituitary tissue biopsy to establish a histologic diagnosis.

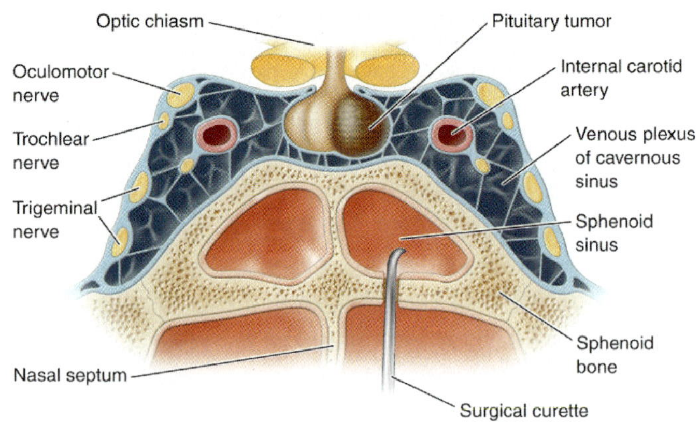

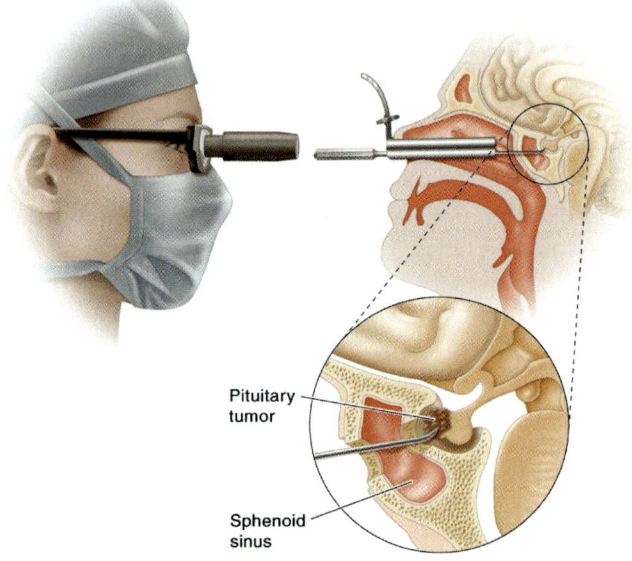

FIGURE 2-5
Transsphenoidal resection of pituitary mass via the endonasal approach. *(Adapted from R Fahlbusch: Endocrinol Metab Clin 21:669, 1992.)*

Whenever possible, the pituitary mass lesion should be selectively excised; normal tissue should be manipulated or resected only when critical for effective mass dissection. Nonselective hemihypophysectomy or total hypophysectomy may be indicated if no mass lesion is clearly discernible, multifocal lesions are present, or the remaining nontumorous pituitary tissue is obviously necrotic. This strategy, however, increases the likelihood of hypopituitarism and the need for lifelong hormonal replacement.

Preoperative mass effects, including visual field defects or compromised pituitary function, may be reversed by surgery, particularly when these deficits are not longstanding. For large and invasive tumors, it is necessary to determine the optimal balance between maximal tumor resection and preservation of anterior pituitary function, especially for preserving growth and reproductive function in younger patients. Similarly, tumor invasion outside of the sella is rarely amenable to surgical cure; the surgeon must judge the risk-versus-benefit ratio of extensive tumor resection.

Side Effects Tumor size, the degree of invasiveness, and experience of the surgeon largely determine the incidence of surgical complications. The operative mortality rate is about 1%. Transient diabetes insipidus and hypopituitarism occur in up to 20% of patients. Permanent diabetes insipidus, cranial nerve damage, nasal septal perforation, or visual disturbances may be encountered in up to 10% of patients. CSF leaks occur in 4% of patients. Less common complications include carotid artery injury, loss of vision, hypothalamic damage, and meningitis. Permanent side effects are rare after surgery for microadenomas.

RADIATION Radiation is used either as a primary therapy for pituitary or parasellar masses or, more commonly, as an adjunct to surgery or medical therapy. Focused megavoltage irradiation is achieved by precise MRI localization, using a high-voltage linear accelerator and accurate isocentric rotational arcing. A major determinant of accurate irradiation is reproduction of the patient's head position during multiple visits and maintenance of absolute head immobility. A total of <50 Gy (5000 rad) is given as 180-cGy (180-rad) fractions split over about 6 weeks. Stereotactic radiosurgery delivers a large, single, high-energy dose from a cobalt 60 source (gamma knife), linear accelerator, or cyclotron. Long-term effects of gamma-knife surgery are as yet unknown.

The role of radiation therapy in pituitary tumor management depends on multiple factors including the nature of the tumor, age of the patient, and availability of surgical and radiation expertise. Because of its relatively slow onset of action, radiation therapy is usually reserved for postsurgical management. As an adjuvant to surgery, radiation is used to treat residual tumor and in an attempt to prevent regrowth. Irradiation offers the only effective means for ablating significant postoperative residual nonfunctioning tumor tissue. In contrast, PRL-, GH-, and sometimes ACTH-secreting tumor tissues are amenable to medical therapy.

Side Effects In the short term, radiation may cause transient nausea and weakness. Alopecia and loss of taste and smell may be more long lasting. Failure of pituitary hormone synthesis is common in patients who have undergone head and neck or pituitary-directed irradiation. More than 50% of patients develop loss of GH, ACTH, TSH, and/or gonadotropin secretion within 10 years, usually due to hypothalamic damage. Lifelong follow-up with testing of anterior pituitary hormone reserve is therefore necessary after radiation treatment. Optic nerve damage with impaired vision due to optic neuritis is reported in about 2% of patients who undergo pituitary irradiation. Cranial nerve damage is uncommon now that radiation doses are ≤2 Gy (200 rad) at any one treatment session and the maximum dose is <50 Gy (5000 rad). The use of stereotactic radiotherapy may reduce damage to adjacent structures. Radiotherapy of pituitary tumors has been associated with an adverse mortality rate, mainly from cerebrovascular disease. The cumulative risk of developing a secondary tumor after conventional radiation is 1.3% after 10 years and 1.9% after 20 years.

MEDICAL Medical therapy for pituitary tumors is highly specific and depends on tumor type. For prolactinomas, dopamine agonists are the treatment of choice. For acromegaly and TSH-secreting tumors, somatostatin analogues and, occasionally, dopamine agonists are indicated. ACTH-secreting tumors and nonfunctioning tumors are generally not responsive to medications and require surgery and/or irradiation.

PROLACTIN

SYNTHESIS

PRL consists of 198 amino acids and has a molecular mass of 21,500 kDa; it is weakly homologous to GH and human placental lactogen (hPL), reflecting the duplication and divergence of a common GH-PRL-hPL precursor gene on chromosome 6. PRL is synthesized in lactotropes, which constitute about 20% of anterior pituitary cells. Lactotropes and somatotropes are derived from a common precursor cell that may give rise to a tumor secreting both PRL and GH. Marked lactotrope cell hyperplasia develops during the last two trimesters of pregnancy and the first few months of lactation. These transient functional changes in the lactotrope population are induced by estrogen.

SECRETION

Normal adult serum PRL levels are about 10–25 μg/L in women and 10–20 μg/L in men. PRL secretion is pulsatile, with the highest secretory peaks occurring during rapid eye movement sleep. Peak serum PRL levels (up to 30 μg/L) occur between 4:00 and 6:00 A.M. The circulating half-life of PRL is about 50 min.

PRL is unique among the pituitary hormones in that the predominant central control mechanism is inhibitory, reflecting dopamine-mediated suppression of PRL release. This regulatory pathway accounts for the spontaneous PRL hypersecretion that occurs after pituitary stalk section, often a consequence of compressive mass lesions at the skull base. Pituitary, dopamine type 2 (D_2) receptors mediate PRL inhibition. Targeted disruption (gene knockout) of the murine D_2 receptor in mice results in hyperprolactinemia and lactotrope proliferation. As discussed below, dopamine agonists play a central role in the management of hyperprolactinemic disorders.

Thyrotropin-releasing hormone (TRH) (pyro Glu-His-Pro-NH2) is a hypothalamic tripeptide that releases prolactin within 15–30 min after intravenous injection. The physiologic relevance of TRH for PRL regulation is unclear, and it appears primarily to regulate TSH (Chap. 4). *Vasoactive intestinal peptide* (VIP) also induces PRL release, whereas glucocorticoids and thyroid hormone weakly suppress PRL secretion.

Serum PRL levels rise transiently after exercise, meals, sexual intercourse, minor surgical procedures, general anesthesia, acute myocardial infarction, and other forms of acute stress. PRL levels increase significantly (about tenfold) during pregnancy and decline rapidly within 2 weeks of parturition. If breastfeeding is initiated, basal PRL levels remain elevated; suckling stimulates reflex increases in PRL levels that last for about 30–45 min. Breast suckling activates neural afferent pathways in the hypothalamus that induce PRL release. With time, the suckling-induced responses diminish and interfeeding PRL levels return to normal.

ACTION

The PRL receptor is a member of the type I cytokine receptor family that also includes GH and interleukin (IL) 6 receptors. Ligand binding induces receptor dimerization and intracellular signaling by Janus kinase (JAK), which stimulates translocation of the signal transduction and activators of transcription (STAT) family to activate target genes. In the breast, the lobuloalveolar epithelium proliferates in response to PRL, placental lactogens, estrogen, progesterone, and local paracrine growth factors, including IGF-I.

PRL acts to induce and maintain lactation, decrease reproductive function, and suppress sexual drive. These functions are geared toward ensuring that maternal lactation is sustained and not interrupted by pregnancy. PRL inhibits reproductive function by suppressing hypothalamic GnRH and pituitary gonadotropin secretion and by impairing gonadal steroidogenesis in both women and men. In the ovary, PRL blocks folliculogenesis and inhibits granulosa cell aromatase activity, leading to hypoestrogenism and anovulation. PRL also has a luteolytic effect, generating a shortened, or inadequate, luteal phase of the menstrual cycle. In men, attenuated LH secretion leads to low testosterone levels and decreased spermatogenesis. These hormonal changes decrease libido and reduce fertility in patients with hyperprolactinemia.

HYPERPROLACTINEMIA

Etiology

Hyperprolactinemia is the most common pituitary hormone hypersecretion syndrome in both men and women. PRL-secreting pituitary adenomas (prolactinomas) are the most common cause of PRL levels >100 μg/L. Less pronounced PRL elevation can also be seen with microprolactinomas but is more commonly caused by drugs, pituitary stalk compression, hypothyroidism, or renal failure (Table 2-8).

TABLE 2-8

ETIOLOGY OF HYPERPROLACTINEMIA[a]

I. **Physiologic hypersecretion**
- Pregnancy
- Lactation
- Chest wall stimulation
- Sleep
- Stress

II. **Hypothalamic-pituitary stalk damage**
- Tumors
  - Craniopharyngioma
  - Suprasellar pituitary mass extension
  - Meningioma
  - Dysgerminoma
  - Metastases
- Empty sella
- Lymphocytic hypophysitis
- Adenoma with stalk compression
- Granulomas
- Rathke's cyst
- Irradiation
- Trauma
  - Pituitary stalk section
  - Suprasellar surgery

III. **Pituitary hypersecretion**
- Prolactinoma
- Acromegaly

IV. **Systemic disorders**
- Chronic renal failure
- Hypothyroidism
- Cirrhosis
- Pseudocyesis
- Epileptic seizures

V. **Drug-induced hypersecretion**
- Dopamine receptor blockers
  - Phenothiazines: chlorpromazine, perphenazine
  - Butyrophenones: haloperidol
  - Thioxanthenes
  - Metoclopramide
- Dopamine synthesis inhibitors
  - α-Methyldopa
- Catecholamine depletors
  - Reserpine
- Opiates
- H_2 antagonists
  - Cimetidine, ranitidine
- Imipramines
  - Amitriptyline, amoxapine
- Serotonin reuptake inhibitors
  - Fluoxetine
- Calcium channel blockers
  - Verapamil
- Hormones
  - Estrogens
  - Antiandrogens
  - TRH

[a]Hyperprolactinemia >100 mg/L almost invariably is indicative of a prolactin-secreting pituitary adenoma. Physiologic causes, hypothyroidism, and drug-induced hyperprolactinemia should be excluded before extensive evaluation.

Pregnancy and lactation are the important physiologic causes of hyperprolactinemia. Sleep-associated hyperprolactinemia reverts to normal within an hour of awakening. Nipple stimulation and sexual orgasm may also increase PRL. Chest wall stimulation or trauma (including chest surgery and herpes zoster) invoke the reflex suckling arc with resultant hyperprolactinemia. Chronic renal failure elevates PRL by decreasing peripheral clearance. Primary hypothyroidism is associated with mild hyperprolactinemia, probably because of compensatory TRH secretion.

Lesions of the hypothalamic-pituitary region that disrupt hypothalamic dopamine synthesis, portal vessel delivery, or lactotrope responses are associated with hyperprolactinemia. Thus, hypothalamic tumors, cysts, infiltrative disorders, and radiation-induced damage cause elevated PRL levels, usually in the range of 30–100 μg/L. Plurihormonal adenomas (including GH and ACTH tumors) may directly hypersecrete PRL. Pituitary masses, including clinically nonfunctioning pituitary tumors, may compress the pituitary stalk to cause hyperprolactinemia.

Drug-induced inhibition or disruption of dopaminergic receptor function is a common cause of hyperprolactinemia (Table 2-8). Thus, antipsychotics and antidepressants are a relatively common cause of mild hyperprolactinemia. Methyldopa inhibits dopamine synthesis and verapamil blocks dopamine release, also leading to hyperprolactinemia. Hormonal agents that induce PRL include estrogens, antiandrogens, and TRH.

Presentation and Diagnosis

Amenorrhea, galactorrhea, and infertility are the hallmarks of hyperprolactinemia in women. If hyperprolactinemia develops prior to menarche, primary amenorrhea results. More commonly, hyperprolactinemia develops later in life and leads to oligomenorrhea and, ultimately, to amenorrhea. If hyperprolactinemia is sustained, vertebral bone mineral density can be reduced compared with age-matched controls, particularly when associated with pronounced hypoestrogenemia. Galactorrhea is present in up to 80% of hyperprolactinemic women. Although usually bilateral and spontaneous, it may be unilateral or only expressed manually. Patients may also complain of decreased libido, weight gain, and mild hirsutism.

In men with hyperprolactinemia, diminished libido, infertility, and visual loss (from optic nerve compression) are the usual presenting symptoms. Gonadotropin suppression leads to reduced testosterone, impotence, and oligospermia. True galactorrhea is uncommon in men with hyperprolactinemia. If the disorder is longstanding, secondary effects of hypogonadism are evident, including osteopenia, reduced muscle mass, and decreased beard growth.

The diagnosis of idiopathic hyperprolactinemia is made by exclusion of known causes of hyperprolactinemia in the setting of a normal pituitary MRI. Some of these patients may harbor small microadenomas below MRI sensitivity (~2 mm).

GALACTORRHEA

Galactorrhea, the inappropriate discharge of milk-containing fluid from the breast, is considered abnormal if it persists for longer than 6 months after childbirth or discontinuation of breast-feeding. Postpartum galactorrhea associated with amenorrhea is a self-limiting disorder usually associated with moderately elevated PRL levels. Galactorrhea may occur spontaneously, or it may be elicited by nipple pressure. In both men and women, galactorrhea may vary in color and consistency (transparent, milky, or bloody) and arise either unilaterally or bilaterally. Mammography or ultrasound is indicated for bloody discharges (particularly from a single duct), which may be caused by breast cancer. Galactorrhea is commonly associated with hyperprolactinemia caused by any of the conditions listed in Table 2-8. Acromegaly is associated with galactorrhea in about one-third of patients. Treatment of galactorrhea usually involves managing the underlying disorder [e.g., replacing L-thyroxine (T_4) for hypothyroidism; discontinuing a medication; treating prolactinoma].

Laboratory Investigation

Basal, fasting morning PRL levels (normally <20 μg/L) should be measured to assess hypersecretion. Because hormone secretion is pulsatile and levels vary widely in some individuals with hyperprolactinemia, it may be necessary to measure levels on several different occasions when clinical suspicion is high. Both false-positive and false-negative results may be encountered. In patients with markedly elevated PRL levels (>1000 μg/L), results may be falsely lowered because of assay artifacts; sample dilution is required to measure these high values accurately. Falsely elevated values may be caused by aggregated forms of circulating PRL, which are biologically inactive (macroprolactinemia). Hypothyroidism should be excluded by measuring TSH and T_4 levels.

Rx Treatment: HYPERPROLACTINEMIA

Treatment of hyperprolactinemia depends on the cause of elevated PRL levels. Regardless of the etiology, however, treatment should be aimed at normalizing PRL levels to alleviate suppressive effects on gonadal function, halt galactorrhea, and preserve bone mineral density. Dopamine agonists are effective for many different causes of hyperprolactinemia (see Treatment for "Prolactinoma" later in the chapter).

If the patient is taking a medication known to cause hyperprolactinemia, the drug should be withdrawn, if possible. For psychiatric patients who require neuroleptic agents, dose titration or the addition of a dopamine agonist can help restore normoprolactinemia and alleviate reproductive symptoms. However, dopamine agonists sometimes worsen the underlying psychiatric condition, especially at high doses. Hyperprolactinemia usually resolves after adequate thyroid hormone replacement in hypothyroid patients or after renal transplantation in patients undergoing dialysis. Resection of hypothalamic or sellar mass lesions can reverse hyperprolactinemia caused by reduced dopamine tone. Granulomatous infiltrates occasionally respond to glucocorticoid administration. In patients with irreversible hypothalamic damage, no treatment may be warranted. In up to 30% of patients with hyperprolactinemia—with or without a visible pituitary microadenoma—the condition resolves spontaneously.

PROLACTINOMA

Etiology and Prevalence

Tumors arising from lactotrope cells account for about half of all functioning pituitary tumors, with an annual incidence of ~3/100,000 population. Mixed tumors secreting combinations of GH and PRL, ACTH and PRL, and, rarely, TSH and PRL are also seen. These plurihormonal tumors are usually recognized by immunohistochemistry, often without apparent clinical manifestations from the production of additional hormones. Microadenomas are classified as <1 cm in diameter and do not usually invade the parasellar region. Macroadenomas are >1 cm in diameter and may be locally invasive and impinge on adjacent structures. The female/male ratio for microprolactinomas is 20:1, whereas the gender ratio is near 1:1 for macroadenomas. Tumor size generally correlates directly with PRL concentrations; values >100 μg/L are usually associated with macroadenomas. Men tend to present with larger tumors than women, possibly because the features of hypogonadism are less readily evident. PRL levels remain stable in most patients, reflecting the slow growth of these tumors. About 5% of microadenomas progress in the long term to macroadenomas. Hyperprolactinemia resolves spontaneously in about 30% of microadenomas.

Presentation and Diagnosis

Women usually present with amenorrhea, infertility, and galactorrhea. If the tumor extends outside of the sella, visual field defects or other mass effects may be seen. Men often present with impotence, loss of libido, infertility, or signs of central CNS compression including headaches and visual defects. Assuming that physiologic and medication-induced causes of hyperprolactinemia are excluded (Table 2-8), the diagnosis of prolactinoma is likely with a PRL level >100 μg/L. PRL levels <100 μg/L may be caused by microadenomas, other sellar lesions that decrease dopamine inhibition, or nonneoplastic causes of hyperprolactinemia. For this reason, an MRI should be performed in all patients with hyperprolactinemia. It is important to remember that hyperprolactinemia caused secondarily by the mass effects of nonlactotrope lesions is also corrected by treatment with dopamine agonists, despite failure to shrink the underlying mass. Consequently, PRL suppression by dopamine agonists does not necessarily indicate that the lesion is a prolactinoma.

℞ Treatment: PROLACTINOMA

As microadenomas rarely progress to become macroadenomas, no treatment may be needed if fertility is not desired. Estrogen replacement is indicated to prevent bone loss and other consequences of hypoestrogenemia and does not appear to increase the risk of tumor enlargement. These patients should be monitored by regular serial PRL and MRI measurements.

For symptomatic microadenomas, therapeutic goals include control of hyperprolactinemia, reduction of tumor size, restoration of menses and fertility, and resolution of galactorrhea. Dopamine agonist doses should be titrated to achieve maximal PRL suppression and restoration of reproductive function (Fig. 2-6). A normalized PRL level does not ensure reduced tumor size. However, tumor shrinkage is not usually seen in those who do not respond with lowered PRL levels. For macroadenomas, formal visual field testing should be performed before initiating dopamine agonists. MRI and visual fields should be assessed at 6- to 12-month intervals until the mass shrinks and annually thereafter until maximum size reduction has occurred.

MEDICAL Oral dopamine agonists (cabergoline or bromocriptine) are the mainstay of therapy for patients with micro- or macroprolactinomas. Dopamine agonists suppress PRL secretion and synthesis as well as lactotrope cell proliferation. About 20% of patients are resistant to dopaminergic treatment; these adenomas may exhibit decreased D_2 dopamine receptor numbers or a postreceptor defect. D_2 receptor gene mutations in the pituitary have not been reported.

Cabergoline An ergoline derivative, cabergoline is a long-acting dopamine agonist with high D_2 receptor affinity. The drug effectively suppresses PRL for >14 days after a single oral dose and induces prolactinoma shrinkage in most patients. Cabergoline (0.5 to 1.0 mg twice weekly) achieves normoprolactinemia and resumption of normal gonadal function in ~80% of patients with microadenomas; galactorrhea improves or resolves in 90% of patients. Cabergoline normalizes

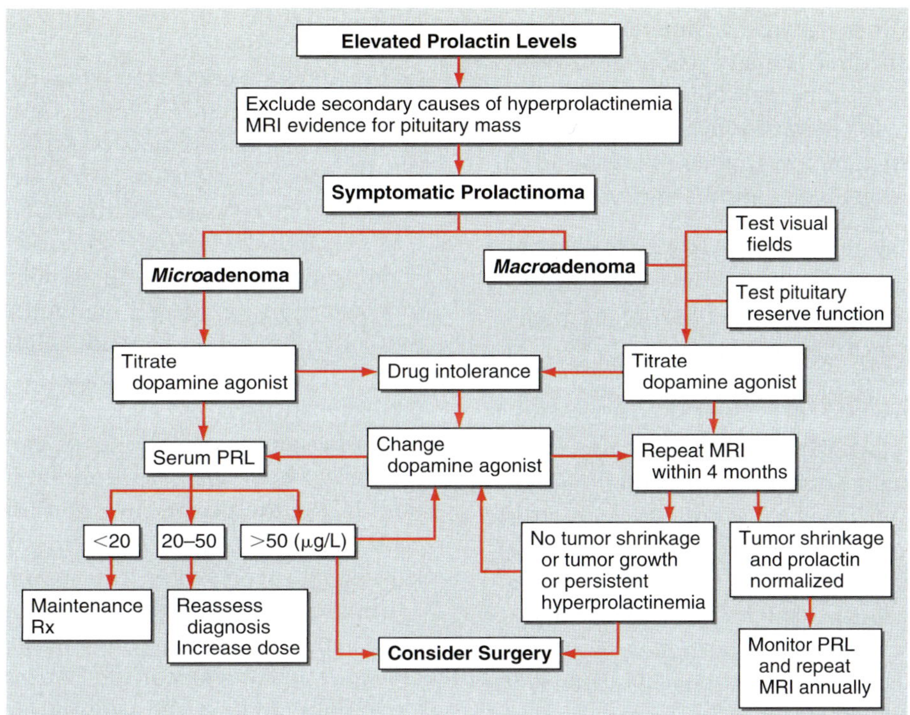

FIGURE 2-6
Management of prolactinoma. MRI, magnetic resonance imaging; PRL, prolactin.

PRL and shrinks ~70% of macroprolactinomas. Mass effect symptoms, including headaches and visual disorders, usually improve dramatically within days after cabergoline initiation; improvement of sexual function requires several weeks of treatment but may occur before complete normalization of prolactin levels. After initial control of PRL levels has been achieved, cabergoline should be reduced to the lowest effective maintenance dose. In ~5% of treated patients, hyperprolactinemia may resolve and not recur when dopamine agonists are discontinued after long-term treatment. Cabergoline may also be effective in patients resistant to bromocriptine. Adverse effects and drug intolerance are encountered less commonly than with bromocriptine.

Bromocriptine The ergot alkaloid bromocriptine mesylate is a dopamine receptor agonist that suppresses prolactin secretion. Because it is short-acting, the drug is preferred when pregnancy is desired. In patients with microadenomas, bromocriptine rapidly lowers serum prolactin levels to normal in up to 70% of patients, decreases tumor size, and restores gonadal function. In patients with macroadenomas, prolactin levels are also normalized in 70% of patients and tumor mass shrinkage (≥50%) is achieved in up to 40% of patients.

Therapy is initiated by administering a low bromocriptine dose (0.625–1.25 mg) at bedtime with a snack, followed by gradually increasing the dose. Most patients are successfully controlled with a daily dose of ≤7.5 mg (2.5 mg tid).

Other Dopamine Agonists These include *pergolide mesylate*, an ergot derivative with dopaminergic properties; *lisuride*, an ergot derivative; and *quinagolide* (CV 205-502, Norprolac), a nonergot oral dopamine agonist with specific D_2 receptor activity.

Side Effects Side effects of dopamine agonists include constipation, nasal stuffiness, dry mouth, nightmares, insomnia, and vertigo; decreasing the dose usually alleviates these problems. Nausea, vomiting, and postural hypotension with faintness may occur in ~25% of patients after the initial dose. These symptoms may persist in some patients. In general, fewer side effects are reported with cabergoline. For the approximately 15% of patients who are intolerant of oral bromocriptine, cabergoline may be better tolerated. Intravaginal administration of bromocriptine is often efficacious in patients with intractable gastrointestinal side effects. Auditory hallucinations, delusions, and mood swings have been reported in up to 5% of patients and may be due to the dopamine agonist properties or to the lysergic acid derivative of the compounds. Rare reports of leukopenia, thrombocytopenia, pleural fibrosis, cardiac arrhythmias, and hepatitis have been described.

Surgery Indications for surgical adenoma debulking include dopamine resistance or intolerance, or the presence of an invasive macroadenoma with compromised vision that fails to improve after drug treatment. Initial PRL normalization is achieved in about 70% of microprolactinomas after surgical resection, but only 30% of macroadenomas can be successfully resected. Follow-up studies have shown that hyperprolactinemia recurs in up to 20% of patients within the first year after surgery; long-term recurrence rates exceed 50% for macroadenomas. Radiotherapy for prolactinomas is reserved for patients with aggressive tumors that do not respond to maximally tolerated dopamine agonists and/or surgery.

PREGNANCY The pituitary increases in size during pregnancy, reflecting the stimulatory effects of estrogen and perhaps other growth factors. About 5% of microadenomas significantly increase in size, but 15–30% of macroadenomas grow during pregnancy. Bromocriptine has been used for more than 30 years to restore fertility in women with hyperprolactinemia, without evidence of teratogenic effects. Nonetheless, most authorities recommend strategies to minimize fetal exposure to the drug. For women taking bromocriptine who desire pregnancy, mechanical contraception should be used through three regular menstrual cycles to allow for conception timing. When pregnancy is confirmed, bromocriptine should be discontinued and PRL levels followed serially, especially if headaches or visual symptoms occur. For women harboring macroadenomas, regular visual field testing is recommended, and the drug should be reinstituted if tumor growth is apparent. Although pituitary MRI may be safe during pregnancy, this procedure should be reserved for symptomatic patients with severe headache and/or visual field defects. Surgical decompression may be indicated if vision is threatened. Although comprehensive data support the efficacy and relative safety of bromocriptine-facilitated fertility, patients should be advised of potential unknown deleterious effects and the risk of tumor growth during pregnancy. As cabergoline is long-acting with a high D_2-receptor affinity, it is not approved for use in women when fertility is desired.

GROWTH HORMONE

SYNTHESIS

GH is the most abundant anterior pituitary hormone, and GH-secreting somatotrope cells constitute up to 50% of the total anterior pituitary cell population. Mammosomatotrope cells, which co-express PRL with GH, can be identified using double immunostaining techniques. Somatotrope development and GH transcription are determined by expression of the cell-specific Pit-1 nuclear transcription factor. Five distinct genes on chromosome 17q22 encode GH and related proteins. The pituitary GH gene (*hGH-N*) produces two alternatively spliced products that give rise to 22-kDa GH (191 amino acids) and a less abundant 20-kDa GH molecule, with similar biologic activity. Placental syncytiotrophoblast cells express a GH variant (*hGH-V*) gene; the related hormone human chorionic somatotropin (hCS) is expressed by distinct members of the gene cluster.

SECRETION

GH secretion is controlled by complex hypothalamic and peripheral factors. *GHRH* is a 44-amino-acid hypothalamic peptide that stimulates GH synthesis and release. Ghrelin, an octanoylated gastric-derived peptide, as well as synthetic agonists of the *GHRP* receptor, induce GHRH and also directly stimulate GH release. *Somatostatin* [somatotropin-release inhibiting factor (SRIF)] is synthesized in the medial preoptic area of the hypothalamus and inhibits GH secretion. GHRH is secreted in discrete spikes that elicit GH pulses, whereas SRIF sets basal GH tone. SRIF is also expressed in many extrahypothalamic tissues, including the CNS, gastrointestinal tract, and pancreas, where it also acts to inhibit islet hormone secretion. *IGF-I*, the peripheral target hormone for GH, feeds back to inhibit GH; estrogen induces GH, whereas chronic glucocorticoid excess suppresses GH release.

Surface receptors on the somatotrope regulate GH synthesis and secretion. The GHRH receptor is a G protein–coupled receptor (GPCR) that signals through the intracellular cyclic AMP pathway to stimulate somatotrope cell proliferation as well as GH production. Inactivating mutations of the GHRH receptor cause profound dwarfism. A distinct surface receptor for ghrelin, a gastric-derived GH secretagogue, is expressed in the hypothalamus and pituitary. Somatostatin binds to five distinct receptor subtypes (SSTR1 to SSTR5); SSTR2 and SSTR5 subtypes preferentially suppress GH (and TSH) secretion.

GH secretion is pulsatile, with highest peak levels occurring at night, generally correlating with sleep onset. GH secretory rates decline markedly with age so that hormone levels in middle age are about 15% of pubertal levels. These changes are paralleled by an age-related decline in lean muscle mass. GH secretion is also reduced in obese individuals, though IGF-I levels may not be suppressed, suggesting a change in the setpoint for feedback control. Elevated GH levels occur within an hour of deep sleep onset as well as after exercise, physical stress, and trauma and during sepsis. Integrated 24-h GH secretion is higher in women and is also enhanced by estrogen replacement. Using standard assays, random GH measurements are undetectable in ~50% of daytime samples obtained from healthy subjects and are also undetectable in most obese and elderly subjects. Thus, single random GH measurements do not distinguish patients with adult GH deficiency from normal persons.

GH secretion is profoundly influenced by nutritional factors. Using newer ultrasensitive chemiluminescence-based GH assays with a sensitivity of 0.002 μg/L, a glucose load can be shown to suppress GH to <0.7 μg/L in women and to <0.07 μg/L in men. Increased GH pulse frequency and peak amplitudes occur with chronic malnutrition or prolonged fasting. GH is stimulated by intravenous L-arginine, dopamine, and apomorphine (a dopamine receptor agonist), as well as by α-adrenergic pathways. β-Adrenergic blockage induces basal GH and enhances GHRH- and insulin-evoked GH release.

ACTION

The pattern of GH secretion may affect tissue responses. The higher GH pulsatility observed in men, as compared to the relatively continuous GH secretion in women, may be an important biologic determinant of linear growth patterns and liver enzyme induction.

The 70-kDa peripheral GH receptor protein shares structural homology with the cytokine/hematopoietic superfamily. A fragment of the receptor extracellular domain generates a soluble GH-binding protein (GHBP) that interacts with GH in the circulation. The liver and cartilage contain the greatest number of GH receptors. GH binding to receptor dimers is followed by signaling through the JAK/STAT pathway. The activated STAT proteins translocate to the nucleus, where they modulate expression of GH-regulated target genes. GH analogues that bind to the receptor, but are incapable of mediating receptor signaling, are potent antagonists of GH action. A GH receptor antagonist (pegvisomant) has been approved for treatment of acromegaly.

GH induces protein synthesis and nitrogen retention and impairs glucose tolerance by antagonizing insulin action. GH also stimulates lipolysis, leading to increased circulating fatty acid levels, reduced omental fat mass, and enhanced lean body mass. GH promotes sodium, potassium, and water retention and elevates serum levels of inorganic phosphate. Linear bone growth occurs as a result of complex hormonal and growth factor actions, including those of IGF-I. GH stimulates epiphyseal prechondrocyte differentiation. These precursor cells produce IGF-I locally and are also responsive to the growth factor.

INSULIN-LIKE GROWTH FACTORS

Although GH exerts direct effects in target tissues, many of its physiologic effects are mediated indirectly through IGF-I, a potent growth and differentiation factor. The liver is the major source of circulating IGF-I. In peripheral tissues, IGF-I exerts local paracrine actions that appear to be both dependent on and independent of GH. Thus, GH administration induces circulating IGF-I as well as stimulating IGF-I production in multiple tissues.

Both IGF-I and -II are bound to high-affinity circulating IGF-binding proteins (IGFBPs) that regulate IGF bioactivity. Levels of IGFBP3 are GH-dependent, and it serves as the major carrier protein for circulating IGF-I. GH deficiency and malnutrition are usually associated with low IGFBP3 levels. IGFBP1 and -2 regulate local tissue IGF action but do not bind appreciable amounts of circulating IGF-I.

Serum IGF-I concentrations are profoundly affected by physiologic factors. Levels increase during puberty, peak at 16 years, and subsequently decline by >80% during the aging process. IGF-I concentrations are higher in women than in men. Because GH is the major determinant of hepatic IGF-I synthesis, abnormalities of GH synthesis or action (e.g., pituitary failure, GHRH receptor defect, or GH receptor defect) reduce IGF-I levels. Hypocaloric states are associated with GH resistance; IGF-I levels are therefore low with cachexia, malnutrition, and sepsis. In acromegaly, IGF-I levels are invariably high and reflect a log-linear relationship with GH concentrations.

IGF-I Physiology

IGF-I has been approved for use in patients with GH-resistance syndromes. Injected IGF-I (100 μg/kg) induces hypoglycemia, and lower doses improve insulin sensitivity in patients with severe insulin resistance and diabetes. In cachectic subjects, IGF-I infusion (12 μg/kg per hour) enhances nitrogen retention and lowers cholesterol levels. Longer-term subcutaneous IGF-I injections enhance protein synthesis and are anabolic. Although bone formation markers are induced, bone turnover may also be stimulated by IGF-I.

IGF-I side effects are dose-dependent, and overdose may result in hypoglycemia, hypotension, fluid retention, temporomandibular jaw pain, and increased intracranial pressure, all of which are reversible. Avascular femoral head necrosis has been reported. Chronic excess IGF-I would presumably result in features of acromegaly.

DISORDERS OF GROWTH AND DEVELOPMENT

Skeletal Maturation and Somatic Growth

The growth plate is dependent on a variety of hormonal stimuli including GH, IGF-I, sex steroids, thyroid hormones, paracrine growth factors, and cytokines. The growth-promoting process also requires caloric energy, amino acids, vitamins, and trace metals and consumes about 10% of normal energy production. Malnutrition impairs chondrocyte activity and reduces circulating IGF-I and IGFBP3 levels.

Linear bone growth rates are very high in infancy and are pituitary-dependent. Mean growth velocity is ~6 cm/year in later childhood and is usually maintained within a given range on a standardized percentile chart. Peak growth rates occur during midpuberty when bone age is 12 (girls) or 13 (boys). Secondary sexual development is associated with elevated sex steroids that cause progressive epiphyseal growth plate closure. *Bone age* is delayed in patients with all forms of true GH deficiency or GH receptor defects that result in attenuated GH action.

Short stature may occur as a result of constitutive intrinsic growth defects or because of acquired extrinsic factors that impair growth. In general, delayed bone age in a child with short stature is suggestive of a hormonal or systemic disorder, whereas normal bone age in a short child is more likely to be caused by a genetic cartilage dysplasia or growth plate disorder.

GH Deficiency in Children

GH Deficiency

Isolated GH deficiency is characterized by short stature, micropenis, increased fat, high-pitched voice, and a propensity to hypoglycemia due to relatively unopposed insulin action. Familial modes of inheritance are seen in one-third of these individuals and may be autosomal dominant, recessive, or X-linked. About 10% of children with GH deficiency have mutations in the *GH-N* gene, including gene deletions and a wide range of point mutations. Mutations in transcription factors Pit-1 and Prop-1, which control somatotrope development, cause GH deficiency in combination with other pituitary hormone deficiencies, which may become manifest only in adulthood. The diagnosis of *idiopathic GH deficiency* (IGHD) should be made only after known molecular defects have been excluded.

GHRH Receptor Mutations

Recessive mutations of the GHRH receptor gene in subjects with severe proportionate dwarfism are associated with low basal GH levels that cannot be stimulated by exogenous GHRH, GHRP, or insulin-induced hypoglycemia. The syndrome exemplifies the importance of the GHRH receptor for somatotrope cell proliferation and hormonal responsiveness.

Growth Hormone Insensitivity

This is caused by defects of GH receptor structure or signaling. Homozygous or heterozygous mutations of the GH receptor are associated with partial or complete GH insensitivity and growth failure (*Laron syndrome*). The diagnosis is based on normal or high GH levels, with decreased circulating GHBP, and low IGF-I levels. Very rarely, defective IGF-I, defective IGF-I receptor, or IGF-I signaling defects are also encountered. *STAT5B* mutations result in immunodeficiency with abrogated GH signaling, leading to short stature with normal or elevated GH levels and low IGF-I levels.

Nutritional Short Stature

Caloric deprivation and malnutrition, uncontrolled diabetes, and chronic renal failure represent secondary causes of abrogated GH receptor function. These conditions also stimulate production of proinflammatory cytokines, which act to further exacerbate the block of GH-mediated signal transduction. Children with these conditions typically exhibit features of acquired short stature with elevated GH and low IGF-I levels. Circulating GH receptor antibodies may rarely cause peripheral GH insensitivity.

Psychosocial Short Stature

Emotional and social deprivation lead to growth retardation accompanied by delayed speech, discordant hyperphagia, and attenuated response to administered GH. A nurturing environment restores growth rates.

Presentation and Diagnosis

Short stature is commonly encountered in clinical practice, and the decision to evaluate these children requires clinical judgment in association with auxologic data and family history. Short stature should be comprehensively evaluated if a patient's height is >3 SD below the mean for age or if the growth rate has decelerated. Skeletal maturation is best evaluated by measuring a radiologic bone age, which is based mainly on the degree of growth plate fusion. Final height can be predicted using standardized scales (Bayley-Pinneau or Tanner-Whitehouse) or estimated by adding 6.5 cm (boys) or subtracting 6.5 cm (girls) from the midparental height.

Laboratory Investigation

Because GH secretion is pulsatile, GH deficiency is best assessed by examining the response to provocative stimuli including exercise, insulin-induced hypoglycemia, and other pharmacologic tests that normally increase GH to >7 μg/L in children. Random GH measurements do not distinguish normal children from those with true GH deficiency. Adequate adrenal and thyroid hormone replacement should be ensured before testing. Age- and gender-matched IGF-I levels are not sufficiently sensitive or specific to make the diagnosis but can be useful to confirm GH deficiency. Pituitary MRI may reveal pituitary mass lesions or structural defects.

℞ Treatment: DISORDERS OF GROWTH AND DEVELOPMENT

Replacement therapy with recombinant GH (0.02–0.05 mg/kg per d subcutaneously) restores growth velocity in GH-deficient children to ~10 cm/year. If pituitary insufficiency is documented, other associated hormone deficits should be corrected—especially adrenal steroids. GH treatment is also moderately effective for accelerating growth rates in children with Turner syndrome and chronic renal failure.

In patients with GH insensitivity and growth retardation due to mutations of the GH receptor, treatment with IGF-I bypasses the dysfunctional GH receptor.

ADULT GH DEFICIENCY (AGHD)

This disorder is usually caused by hypothalamic or pituitary somatotrope damage. Acquired pituitary hormone deficiency follows a typical pattern whereby loss of adequate GH reserve foreshadows subsequent hormone deficits. The sequential order of hormone loss is usually GH → FSH/LH → TSH → ACTH.

Presentation and Diagnosis

The clinical features of AGHD include changes in body composition, lipid metabolism, and quality of life and cardiovascular dysfunction (Table 2-9). Body composition changes are common and include reduced lean body mass, increased fat mass with selective deposition of intraabdominal visceral fat, and increased waist-to-hip ratio. Hyperlipidemia, left ventricular dysfunction, hypertension, and increased plasma fibrinogen levels may also be present. Bone mineral content is reduced, with resultant increased fracture rates. Patients may experience social isolation, depression, and difficulty in maintaining gainful employment. Adult hypopituitarism is associated with a threefold increased cardiovascular mortality rate in comparison to age- and sex-matched controls, and this may be due to GH deficiency.

Laboratory Investigation

AGHD is rare, and in light of the nonspecific nature of associated clinical symptoms, patients appropriate for testing should be carefully selected on the basis of well-defined criteria. With few exceptions, testing should be restricted to patients with the following predisposing factors: (1) pituitary surgery, (2) pituitary or hypothalamic tumor or granulomas, (3) history of cranial irradiation, (4) radiologic evidence of a pituitary lesion, (5) childhood requirement for GH replacement therapy, or, rarely, (6) unexplained low age- and sex-matched IGF-I levels. The transition of the GH-deficient adolescent to adulthood requires retesting to document adult GH deficiency. Up to 20% of patients previously treated for childhood-onset GH deficiency are found to be GH-sufficient on repeat testing as adults.

A significant proportion (~25%) of truly GH-deficient adults have low-normal IGF-I levels. Thus, as in the evaluation of GH deficiency in children, valid age- and gender-matched IGF-I measurements provide a useful index of therapeutic responses but are not sufficiently sensitive for diagnostic purposes. The most validated test to distinguish pituitary-sufficient patients from those with AGHD is insulin-induced (0.05–0.1 U/kg) hypoglycemia. After glucose reduction to ~40 mg/dL, most individuals experience neuroglycopenic symptoms (Chap. 20), and peak GH release occurs at 60 min and remains elevated for up to 2 h. About 90% of healthy adults exhibit GH responses >5 μg/L; AGHD is defined by a peak GH response to hypoglycemia of <3 μg/L. Although insulin-induced hypoglycemia is safe when performed under appropriate supervision, it is contraindicated in patients with diabetes, ischemic heart disease, cerebrovascular disease, or epilepsy, and in elderly patients. Alternative stimulatory tests include intravenous arginine (30 g), GHRH (1 μg/kg), and GHRP-6 (90 μg). Combinations of these tests may evoke GH secretion in subjects not responsive to a single test.

TABLE 2-9

FEATURES OF ADULT GROWTH HORMONE DEFICIENCY

Clinical Impaired quality of life Decreased energy and drive Poor concentration Low self-esteem Social isolation Body composition changes Increased body fat mass Central fat deposition Increased waist-to-hip ratio Decreased lean body mass Reduced exercise capacity Reduced maximum O_2 uptake Impaired cardiac function Reduced muscle mass	Cardiovascular risk factors Impaired cardiac structure and function Abnormal lipid profile Decreased fibrinolytic activity Atherosclerosis Omental obesity **Imaging** Pituitary: Mass or structural damage Bone: Reduced bone mineral density Abdomen: Excess omental adiposity **Laboratory** Evoked GH <3 ng/mL IGF-I and IGFBP3 low or normal Increased LDL-cholesterol Concomitant gonadotropin, TSH, and/or ACTH reserve deficits may be present

Note: LDL, low-density lipoprotein. For other abbreviations, see text.

℞ Treatment: ADULT GH DEFICIENCY

Once the diagnosis of AGHD is unequivocally established, replacement of GH may be indicated. Contraindications to therapy include the presence of an active neoplasm, intracranial hypertension, or uncontrolled diabetes and retinopathy. The starting dose of 0.1–0.2 mg/d should be titrated (up to a maximum of 1.25 mg/d) to maintain IGF-I levels in the mid-normal range for age- and gender-matched controls (Fig. 2-7). Women require higher doses than men, and elderly patients require less GH. Long-term GH maintenance sustains normal IGF-I levels and is associated with persistent body composition changes (e.g., enhanced lean body mass and lower body fat). High-density lipoprotein cholesterol increases, but total cholesterol and insulin levels do not change significantly. Lumbar spine bone mineral density increases, but this response is gradual (>1 year). Many patients note significant improvement in quality of life when evaluated by standardized questionnaires. The effect of GH replacement on mortality rates in GH-deficient patients is currently the subject of long-term prospective investigation.

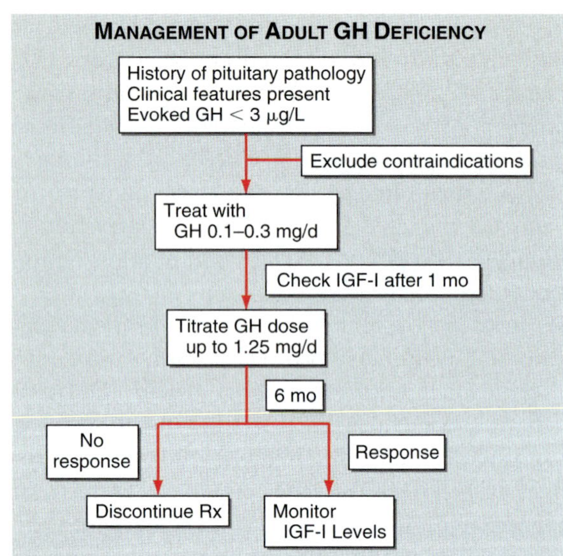

FIGURE 2-7

Management of adult growth hormone (GH) deficiency. IGF, insulin-like growth factor.

About 30% of patients exhibit reversible dose-related fluid retention, joint pain, and carpal tunnel syndrome, and up to 40% exhibit myalgias and paresthesia. Patients receiving insulin require careful monitoring for dosing adjustments, as GH is a potent counterregulatory hormone for insulin action. Patients with type 2 diabetes mellitus initially develop further insulin resistance. However, glycemic control improves with the sustained loss of abdominal fat associated with long-term GH replacement. Headache, increased intracranial pressure, hypertension, atrial fibrillation, and tinnitus occur rarely. Prevalence of pituitary tumor regrowth and potential progression of skin lesions are currently being assessed in long-term surveillance programs. To date, development of these potential side effects does not appear significant.

ACROMEGALY

Etiology

GH hypersecretion is usually the result of a somatotrope adenoma but may rarely be caused by extrapituitary lesions (Table 2-10). In addition to more common GH-secreting somatotrope adenomas, mixed mammosomatotrope tumors and acidophilic stem cell adenomas secrete both GH and PRL. In patients with acidophilic stem cell adenomas, features of hyperprolactinemia (hypogonadism and galactorrhea) predominate over the less clinically evident signs of acromegaly. Occasionally, mixed plurihormonal tumors are encountered that secrete ACTH, the glycoprotein hormone subunit, or TSH, in addition to GH. Patients with partially empty sellae may present with GH hypersecretion due to a small GH-secreting adenoma within the compressed rim of pituitary tissue; some of these may reflect the spontaneous necrosis of tumors that were previously larger. GH-secreting tumors rarely arise from ectopic pituitary tissue remnants in the nasopharynx or midline sinuses.

TABLE 2-10

CAUSES OF ACROMEGALY

	PREVALENCE, %
Excess Growth Hormone Secretion	
Pituitary	98
Densely or sparsely granulated GH cell adenoma	60
Mixed GH cell and PRL cell adenoma	25
Mammosomatrope cell adenoma	10
Plurihormonal adenoma	
GH cell carcinoma or metastases	
Multiple endocrine neoplasia type 1 (GH cell adenoma)	
McCune-Albright syndrome	
Ectopic sphenoid or parapharyngeal sinus pituitary adenoma	
Extrapituitary tumor	
Pancreatic islet cell tumor	<1
Lymphoma	
Excess Growth Hormone–Releasing Hormone Secretion	
Central	<1
Hypothalamic hamartoma, choristoma, ganglioneuroma	<1
Peripheral	<1
Bronchial carcinoid, pancreatic islet cell tumor, small cell lung cancer, adrenal adenoma, medullary thyroid carcinoma, pheochromocytoma	

Source: Adapted from S Melmed: N Engl J Med 322:966, 1990.

There are case reports of ectopic GH secretion by tumors of pancreatic, ovarian, lung, or hematopoietic origin. Excess GHRH production may cause acromegaly because of chronic stimulation of somatotropes. These patients present with classic features of acromegaly, elevated GH levels, pituitary enlargement on MRI, and pathologic characteristics of pituitary hyperplasia. The most common cause of GHRH-mediated acromegaly is a chest or abdominal carcinoid tumor. Although these tumors usually express positive GHRH immunoreactivity, clinical features of acromegaly are evident in only a minority of patients with carcinoid disease. Excessive GHRH may also be elaborated by hypothalamic tumors, usually choristomas or neuromas.

Presentation and Diagnosis

Protean manifestations of GH and IGF-I hypersecretion are indolent and often are not clinically diagnosed for 10 years or more. Acral bony overgrowth results in frontal bossing, increased hand and foot size, mandibular

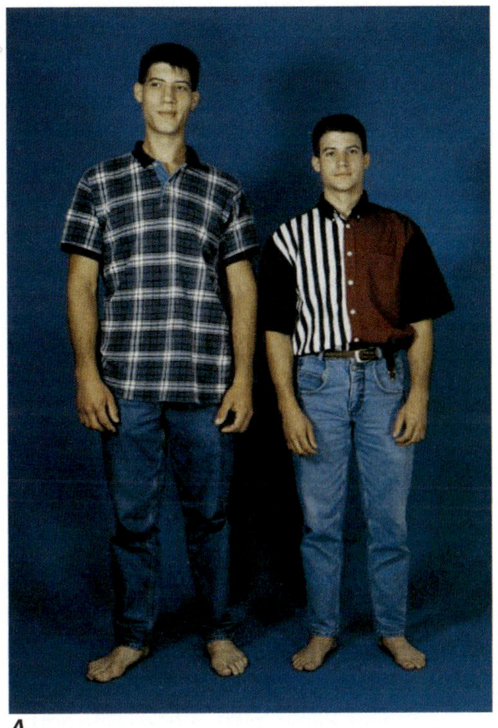

A

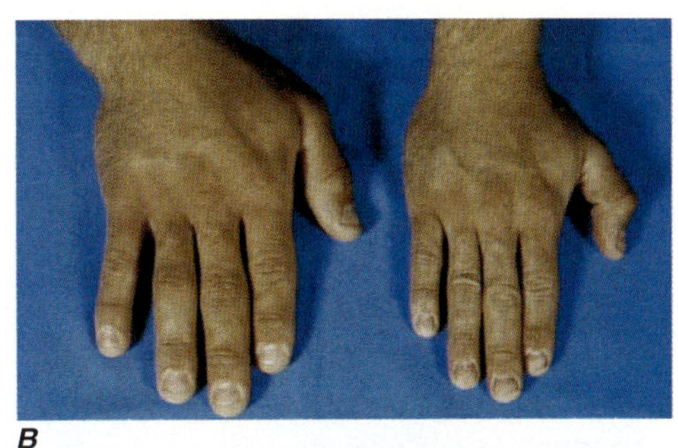

B

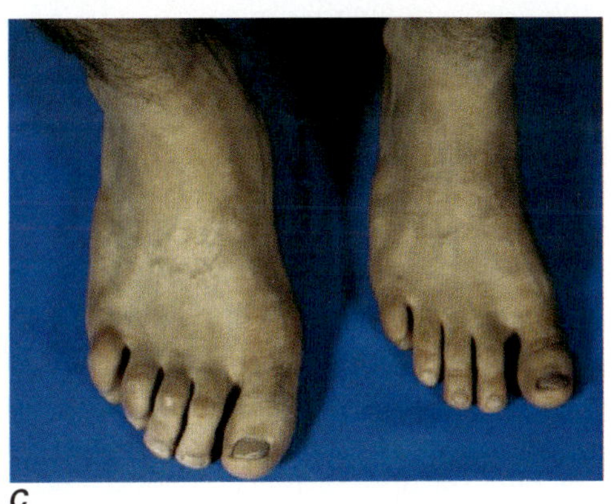

C

FIGURE 2-8

Features of acromegaly/gigantism. A 22-year-old man with gigantism due to excess growth hormone is shown to the left of his identical twin. The increased height and prognathism (***A***) and enlarged hand (***B***) and foot (***C***) of the affected twin are apparent. Their clinical features began to diverge at the age of approximately 13 years. (*Reproduced from R Gagel, IE McCutcheon: N Engl J Med 324:524, 1999; with permission.*)

enlargement with prognathism, and widened space between the lower incisor teeth. In children and adolescents, initiation of GH hypersecretion prior to epiphyseal long bone closure is associated with development of pituitary gigantism (Fig. 2-8). Soft tissue swelling results in increased heel pad thickness, increased shoe or glove size, ring tightening, characteristic coarse facial features, and a large fleshy nose. Other commonly encountered clinical features include hyperhidrosis, deep and hollow-sounding voice, oily skin, arthropathy, kyphosis, carpal tunnel syndrome, proximal muscle weakness and fatigue, acanthosis nigricans, and skin tags. Generalized visceromegaly occurs, including cardiomegaly, macroglossia, and thyroid gland enlargement.

The most significant clinical impact of GH excess occurs with respect to the cardiovascular system. Coronary heart disease, cardiomyopathy with arrhythmias, left ventricular hypertrophy, decreased diastolic function, and hypertension occur in about 30% of patients. Upper airway obstruction with sleep apnea occurs in more than 60% of patients and is associated with both soft tissue laryngeal airway obstruction and central sleep dysfunction. Diabetes mellitus develops in 25% of patients with acromegaly, and most patients are intolerant of a glucose load (as GH counteracts the action of insulin). Acromegaly is associated with an increased risk of colon polyps and mortality from colonic malignancy; polyps are diagnosed in up to one-third of patients. The overall mortality rate is increased about threefold and is due primarily to cardiovascular and cerebrovascular disorders and respiratory disease. Unless GH levels are controlled, survival is reduced by an average of 10 years compared with an age-matched control population.

Laboratory Investigation

Age- and gender-matched serum IGF-I levels are elevated in acromegaly. Consequently, an IGF-I level provides a useful laboratory screening measure when clinical features raise the possibility of acromegaly. Due to the pulsatility of GH secretion, measurement of a single random GH level is not useful for the diagnosis or exclusion of acromegaly and does not correlate with disease severity. The diagnosis of acromegaly is confirmed by demonstrating the failure of GH suppression to <1 μg/L within 1–2 h of an oral glucose load (75 g). Using newer ultrasensitive GH assays, normal nadir GH levels are even lower (<0.05 μg/L). About 20% of patients exhibit a paradoxical GH rise after glucose. PRL should be measured, as it is elevated in ~25% of patients with acromegaly. Thyroid function, gonadotropins, and sex steroids may be attenuated because of tumor mass effects. Because most patients will undergo surgery with glucocorticoid coverage, tests of ACTH reserve in asymptomatic patients are more efficiently deferred until after surgery.

℞ Treatment: ACROMEGALY

Surgical resection of GH-secreting adenomas is the initial treatment for most patients (**Fig. 2-9**). Somatostatin analogues are used as adjuvant treatment for preoperative shrinkage of large invasive macroadenomas, immediate relief of debilitating symptoms, and reduction of GH hypersecretion in frail patients experiencing morbidity, in patients who decline surgery, or, when surgery fails, to achieve biochemical control. Irradiation or repeat surgery may be required for patients who cannot tolerate or do not respond to adjunctive medical therapy. The high rate of late hypopituitarism and the slow rate (5–15 years) of biochemical response are the main disadvantages of radiotherapy. Irradiation is relatively ineffective in normalizing IGF-I levels. Stereotactic ablation of GH-secreting adenomas by gamma-knife radiotherapy is promising, but long-term results are not available and the side effects have not been clearly delineated. Somatostatin analogues may be given while awaiting the full benefits of radiotherapy. Systemic sequelae of acromegaly, including cardiovascular disease, diabetes, and arthritis, should also be managed aggressively. Maxillofacial surgery for mandibular repair may be indicated.

SURGERY Transsphenoidal surgical resection by an experienced surgeon is the preferred primary treatment for both microadenomas (cure rate ~70%) and macroadenomas (<50% cured). Soft tissue swelling improves immediately after tumor resection. GH levels return to normal within an hour, and IGF-I levels are normalized within 3–4 days. In ~10% of patients, acromegaly may recur several years after apparently successful surgery; hypopituitarism develops in up to 15% of patients.

SOMATOSTATIN ANALOGUES Somatostatin analogues exert their therapeutic effects through SSTR2 and -5 receptors, both of which are invariably expressed by GH-secreting tumors. Octreotide acetate is an eight-amino-acid synthetic somatostatin analogue. In contrast to native somatostatin, the analogue is relatively resistant to plasma degradation. It has a 2-h serum half-life and possesses fortyfold greater potency than native somatostatin to suppress GH. Octreotide is administered by subcutaneous injection, beginning with 50 μg tid; the dose can be gradually increased up to 1500 μg/d. Fewer than 10% of patients do not respond to the analogue. Octreotide suppresses integrated GH levels to <5 μg/L in ~70% of patients and to <2 μg/L in up to 60% of patients. It normalizes IGF-I levels in ~75% of treated patients. Prolonged use of the analogue is not associated with desensitization, even after ≥20 years of treatment. Rapid relief of headache and soft tissue swelling occurs in ~75% of patients within days to weeks of treatment initiation. Subjective clinical benefits of octreotide therapy occur more frequently than biochemical remission, and most patients report symptomatic improvement, including amelioration of headache, perspiration, obstructive apnea, and cardiac failure. Modest pituitary tumor size reduction occurs in about 40% of patients, but this effect is reversed when treatment is stopped.

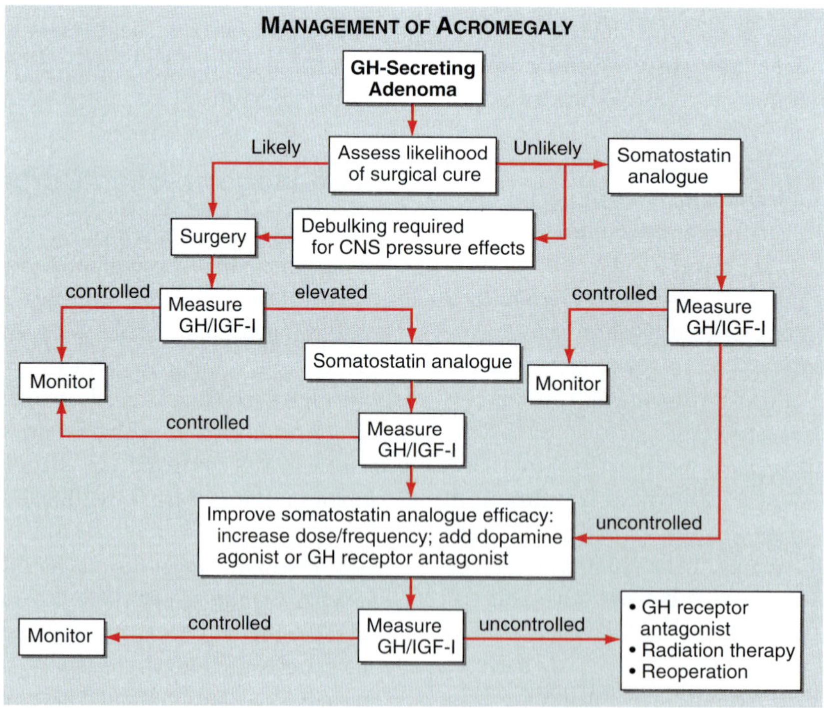

FIGURE 2-9

Management of acromegaly. GH, growth hormone; CNS, central nervous system; IGF, insulin-like growth factor. *(Adapted from S Melmed et al: J Clin Endocrinol Metab 83:2646, 1998; © The Endocrine Society.)*

The long-acting somatostatin depot formulations, octreotide and lanreotide, are the preferred medical treatment for patients with acromegaly. *Sandostatin-LAR* is a sustained-release, long-acting formulation of octreotide incorporated into microspheres that sustain drug levels for several weeks after intramuscular injection. GH suppression occurs for as long as 6 weeks after a 30-mg injection; long-term monthly treatment sustains GH and IGF-I suppression and also reduces pituitary tumor size in ~50% of patients. *Lanreotide*, a slow-release depot somatostatin preparation, is a cyclic somatostatin octapeptide analogue that suppresses GH and IGF-I hypersecretion for 10–14 days after a 30-mg intramuscular injection. Long-term administration controls GH hypersecretion in two-thirds of treated patients and improves patient compliance because of the long interval required between drug injections. A subcutaneous long-acting gel formulation is also available. Lanreotide is not currently approved in the United States.

Side Effects Somatostatin analogues are well tolerated in most patients. Adverse effects are short-lived and mostly relate to drug-induced suppression of gastrointestinal motility and secretion. Nausea, abdominal discomfort, fat malabsorption, diarrhea, and flatulence occur in one-third of patients, and these symptoms usually remit within 2 weeks. Octreotide suppresses postprandial gallbladder contractility and delays gallbladder emptying; up to 30% of patients develop long-term echogenic sludge or asymptomatic cholesterol gallstones. Other side effects include mild glucose intolerance due to transient insulin suppression, asymptomatic bradycardia, hypothyroxinemia, and local injection site discomfort.

GH RECEPTOR ANTAGONISTS Pegvisomant antagonizes endogenous GH action by blocking peripheral GH binding to its receptor. Consequently, serum IGF-I levels are suppressed, reducing the deleterious effects of excess endogenous GH. Pegvisomant is administered by daily subcutaneous injection (10–20 mg) and normalizes IGF-I in >90% of patients. GH levels, however, remain elevated as the drug does not have antitumor actions. Side effects include reversible liver enzyme elevation, lipodystrophy, and injection site pain. Tumor size should be monitored by MRI.

Combined treatment with monthly octreotide-LAR and weekly or biweekly pegvisomant injections has been effectively used for resistant patients.

DOPAMINE AGONISTS Bromocriptine and cabergoline may suppress GH secretion in some patients, particularly those with cosecretion of PRL. High bromocriptine doses (≥20 mg/d) are usually required to achieve modest GH therapeutic efficacy. Cabergoline also modestly suppresses GH when given at a relatively high dose of 0.5 mg/d. Combined treatment with octreotide and cabergoline may induce additive biochemical control compared to either drug alone.

RADIATION External radiation therapy or high-energy stereotactic techniques are used as adjuvant therapy for acromegaly. An advantage of radiation is that patient compliance with long-term treatment is not required. Tumor mass is reduced, and GH levels are attenuated over time. However, 50% of patients require at least 8 years for GH levels to be suppressed to <5 μg/L; this level of GH reduction is achieved in about 90% of patients after 18 years but represents suboptimal GH suppression. Patients may require interim medical therapy for several years prior to attaining maximal radiation benefits. Most patients also experience hypothalamic-pituitary damage, leading to gonadotropin, ACTH, and/or TSH deficiency within 10 years of therapy.

In summary, surgery is the preferred primary treatment for GH-secreting microadenomas (Fig. 2-9). The high frequency of GH hypersecretion after macroadenoma resection usually necessitates adjuvant or primary medical therapy for these larger tumors. Patients unable to receive or respond to unimodal medical treatment may benefit from combined treatments, or can be offered radiation.

ADRENOCORTICOTROPIN HORMONE

(See also Chap. 5)

SYNTHESIS

ACTH-secreting corticotrope cells constitute about 20% of the pituitary cell population. ACTH (39 amino acids) is derived from the POMC precursor protein (266 amino acids) that also generates several other peptides, including β-lipotropin, β-endorphin, met-enkephalin, α-melanocyte-stimulating hormone (α-MSH), and corticotropin-like intermediate lobe protein (CLIP). The POMC gene is potently suppressed by glucocorticoids and induced by CRH, arginine vasopressin (AVP), and proinflammatory cytokines, including IL-6, as well as leukemia inhibitory factor.

CRH, a 41-amino-acid hypothalamic peptide synthesized in the paraventricular nucleus as well as in higher brain centers, is the predominant stimulator of ACTH synthesis and release. The CRH receptor is a GPCR that is expressed on the corticotrope and induces POMC transcription.

SECRETION

ACTH secretion is pulsatile and exhibits a characteristic circadian rhythm, peaking at 6 A.M. and reaching a nadir at about midnight. Adrenal glucocorticoid secretion, which is driven by ACTH, follows a parallel diurnal pattern. ACTH circadian rhythmicity is determined by variations in secretory pulse amplitude rather than changes in pulse frequency. Superimposed on this endogenous rhythm, ACTH levels are increased by AVP, physical stress, exercise, acute illness, and insulin-induced hypoglycemia.

Loss of cortisol feedback inhibition, as occurs in primary adrenal failure, results in extremely high ACTH levels. Glucocorticoid-mediated negative regulation of the hypothalamic-pituitary-adrenal (HPA) axis occurs as a consequence of both hypothalamic CRH suppression and direct attenuation of pituitary POMC gene expression and ACTH release.

Acute inflammatory or septic insults activate the HPA axis through the integrated actions of proinflammatory cytokines, bacterial toxins, and neural signals. The overlapping cascade of ACTH-inducing cytokines [tumor necrosis factor (TNF); IL-1, -2, and -6; and leukemia inhibitory factor] activates hypothalamic CRH and AVP secretion, pituitary POMC gene expression, and local paracrine pituitary cytokine networks. The resulting cortisol elevation restrains the inflammatory response and enables host protection. Concomitantly, cytokine-mediated central glucocorticoid receptor resistance impairs glucocorticoid suppression of the HPA axis. Thus, the neuroendocrine stress response reflects the net result of highly integrated hypothalamic, intrapituitary, and peripheral hormone and cytokine signals.

ACTION

The major function of the HPA axis is to maintain metabolic homeostasis and to mediate the neuroendocrine stress response. ACTH induces adrenocortical steroidogenesis by maintaining adrenal cell proliferation and function. The receptor for ACTH, designated *melanocortin-2 receptor*, is a GPCR that induces steroidogenesis by stimulating a cascade of steroidogenic enzymes (Chap. 5).

ACTH DEFICIENCY

Presentation and Diagnosis

Secondary adrenal insufficiency occurs as a result of pituitary ACTH deficiency. It is characterized by fatigue, weakness, anorexia, nausea, vomiting, and, occasionally, hypoglycemia. In contrast to primary adrenal failure, hypocortisolism associated with pituitary failure is not usually accompanied by pigmentation changes or mineralocorticoid deficiency. *TPIT* mutations result in primary ACTH deficiency.

ACTH deficiency is commonly due to glucocorticoid withdrawal following treatment-associated suppression of the HPA axis. Isolated ACTH deficiency may occur after surgical resection of an ACTH-secreting pituitary adenoma that has suppressed the HPA axis; this phenomenon is suggestive of a surgical cure. The mass effects of other pituitary adenomas or sellar lesions may lead to ACTH deficiency, but usually in combination with other pituitary hormone deficiencies. Partial ACTH deficiency may be unmasked in the presence of an acute medical or surgical illness, when clinically significant hypocortisolism reflects diminished ACTH reserve.

Laboratory Diagnosis

Inappropriately low ACTH levels in the setting of low cortisol levels are characteristic of diminished ACTH reserve. Low basal serum cortisol levels are associated with blunted cortisol responses to ACTH stimulation and impaired cortisol response to insulin-induced hypoglycemia, or testing with metyrapone or CRH. For description of provocative ACTH tests, see "Tests of Pituitary-Adrenal Responsiveness" in Chap. 5.

℞ Treatment: ACTH DEFICIENCY

Glucocorticoid replacement therapy improves most features of ACTH deficiency. The total daily dose of hydrocortisone replacement should not exceed 30 mg daily, divided into two or three doses. Prednisone (5 mg each morning; 2.5 mg each evening) is longer-acting and has fewer mineralocorticoid effects than hydrocortisone. Some authorities advocate lower maintenance doses in an effort to avoid cushingoid side effects. Doses should be increased several-fold during periods of acute illness or stress.

CUSHING'S SYNDROME (ACTH-PRODUCING ADENOMA)

(See also Chap. 5)

Etiology and Prevalence

Pituitary corticotrope adenomas account for 70% of patients with endogenous causes of Cushing's syndrome. However, it should be emphasized that iatrogenic hypercortisolism is the most common cause of cushingoid features. Ectopic tumor ACTH production, cortisol-producing adrenal adenomas, adrenal carcinoma, and adrenal hyperplasia account for the other causes; rarely, ectopic tumor CRH production is encountered.

ACTH-producing adenomas account for about 10–15% of all pituitary tumors. Because the clinical features of Cushing's syndrome often lead to early diagnosis, most ACTH-producing pituitary tumors are relatively small microadenomas. However, macroadenomas are also seen, and some ACTH-secreting adenomas are clinically silent. Cushing's disease is 5–10 times more common in women than in men. These pituitary adenomas exhibit unrestrained ACTH secretion, with resultant hypercortisolemia. However, they retain partial suppressibility in the presence of high doses of administered glucocorticoids, providing the basis for dynamic testing to distinguish pituitary and nonpituitary causes of Cushing's syndrome.

Presentation and Diagnosis

The diagnosis of Cushing's syndrome presents two great challenges: (1) to distinguish patients with pathologic cortisol excess from those with physiologic or other disturbances of cortisol production and (2) to determine the etiology of cortisol excess.

Typical features of chronic cortisol excess include thin, fragile skin; central obesity; hypertension; plethoric moon facies; purple striae and easy bruisability; glucose intolerance or diabetes mellitus; gonadal dysfunction; osteoporosis; proximal muscle weakness; signs of hyperandrogenism (acne, hirsutism); and psychological disturbances (depression, mania, and psychoses) (Table 2-11). Hematopoietic features of hypercortisolism include leukocytosis, lymphopenia, and eosinopenia. Immune suppression includes delayed hypersensitivity. The protean manifestations of hypercortisolism make it challenging to decide which patients mandate formal laboratory evaluation. Certain features make pathologic causes of hypercortisolism more likely—these include characteristic central redistribution of fat, thin skin with striae and bruising, and proximal muscle weakness. In children and in young females, early osteoporosis may be particularly prominent. The primary cause of death is cardiovascular disease, but infections and risk of suicide are also increased.

TABLE 2-11

CLINICAL FEATURES OF CUSHING'S SYNDROME (ALL AGES)

SYMPTOMS/SIGNS	FREQUENCY, %
Obesity or weight gain (>115% ideal body weight)	80
Thin skin	80
Moon facies	75
Hypertension	75
Purple skin striae	65
Hirsutism	65
Abnormal glucose tolerance	55
Impotence	55
Menstrual disorders (usually amenorrhea)	60
Plethora	60
Proximal muscle weakness	50
Truncal obesity	50
Acne	45
Bruising	45
Mental changes	45
Osteoporosis	40
Edema of lower extremities	30
Hyperpigmentation	20
Hypokalemic alkalosis	15
Diabetes mellitus	15

Source: Adapted from MA Magiokou et al, in ME Wierman (ed), *Diseases of the Pituitary*. Totowa, NJ, Humana, 1997.

Rapid development of features of hypercortisolism associated with skin hyperpigmentation and severe myopathy suggests an ectopic source of ACTH. Hypertension, hypokalemic alkalosis, glucose intolerance, and edema are also more pronounced in these patients. Serum potassium levels <3.3 mmol/L are evident in ~70% of patients with ectopic ACTH secretion but are seen in <10% of patients with pituitary-dependent Cushing's syndrome.

Laboratory Investigation

The diagnosis of Cushing's syndrome is based on laboratory documentation of endogenous hypercortisolism. Measurement of 24-h urine free cortisol is a precise and cost-effective screening test. Alternatively, the failure to suppress plasma cortisol after an overnight 1-mg dexamethasone suppression test can be used to identify patients with hypercortisolism. As nadir levels of cortisol occur at night, elevated midnight samples of cortisol are suggestive of Cushing's syndrome. Basal plasma ACTH levels often distinguish patients with ACTH-independent (adrenal or exogenous glucocorticoid) from those with ACTH-dependent (pituitary, ectopic ACTH) Cushing's syndrome. Mean basal ACTH levels are about eightfold higher in patients with ectopic ACTH secretion compared to those with pituitary ACTH-secreting adenomas. However, extensive overlap of ACTH levels in these two disorders precludes using ACTH to make the distinction. Instead, dynamic testing, based on differential sensitivity to glucocorticoid feedback, or ACTH stimulation in response to CRH or cortisol reduction is used to discriminate ectopic versus pituitary sources of excess ACTH (Table 2-12). Very rarely, circulating CRH levels are elevated, reflecting ectopic tumor-derived secretion of CRH and often ACTH. For further discussion of dynamic testing for Cushing's syndrome, see Chap. 5.

Most ACTH-secreting pituitary tumors are <5 mm in diameter, and about half are undetectable by sensitive MRI. The high prevalence of incidental pituitary microadenomas diminishes the ability to distinguish ACTH-secreting pituitary tumors accurately by MRI.

Inferior Petrosal Venous Sampling

Because pituitary MRI with gadolinium enhancement is insufficiently sensitive to detect small (<2 mm) pituitary ACTH-secreting adenomas, bilateral inferior petrosal sinus ACTH sampling before and after CRH administration may be required to distinguish these lesions from ectopic ACTH-secreting tumors that may have similar clinical and biochemical characteristics. Simultaneous assessment of ACTH concentrations in each inferior petrosal vein and in the peripheral circulation provides a strategy for confirming and localizing pituitary ACTH production. Sampling is performed at baseline and 2, 5, and 10 min after intravenous bovine CRH (1 μg/kg)

TABLE 2-12

DIFFERENTIAL DIAGNOSIS OF ACTH-DEPENDENT CUSHING'S SYNDROME[a]

	ACTH-SECRETING PITUITARY TUMOR	ECTOPIC ACTH SECRETION
Etiology	Pituitary corticotrope adenoma Plurihormonal adenoma	Bronchial, abdominal carcinoid Small cell lung cancer Thymoma
Gender	F > M	M > F
Clinical features	Slow onset	Rapid onset Pigmentation Severe myopathy
Serum potassium <3.3 μg/L	<10%	75%
24-h urinary free cortisol (UFC)	High	High
Basal ACTH level	Inappropriately high	Very high
Dexamethasone suppression		
1 mg overnight		
Low dose (0.5 mg q6h)	Cortisol >5 μg/dL	Cortisol >5 μg/dL
High dose (2 mg q6h)	Cortisol <5 μg/dL	Cortisol >5 μg/dL
UFC > 80% suppressed	Microadenomas: 90% Macroadenomas: 50%	10%
Inferior petrosal sinus sampling (IPSS)		
Basal		
IPSS: peripheral	>2	<2
CRH-induced		
IPSS: peripheral	>3	<3

[a]ACTH-independent causes of Cushing's syndrome are diagnosed by suppressed ACTH levels and an adrenal mass in the setting of hypercortisolism. Iatrogenic Cushing's syndrome is excluded by history.

Note: ACTH, adrenocorticotropin hormone; F, female; M, male; CRH, corticotropin-releasing hormone.

injection. An increased ratio (>2) of inferior petrosal to peripheral vein ACTH confirms pituitary Cushing's syndrome. After CRH injection, peak petrosal-to-peripheral ACTH ratios of ≥3 confirm the presence of a pituitary ACTH-secreting tumor. The sensitivity of this test is >95%, with very rare false-positive results. False-negative results may be encountered in patients with aberrant venous drainage. Petrosal sinus catheterizations are technically difficult, and about 0.05% of patients develop neurovascular complications. The procedure should not be performed in patients with hypertension or in the presence of a well-visualized pituitary adenoma on MRI.

℞ Treatment: CUSHING'S SYNDROME

Selective transsphenoidal resection is the treatment of choice for Cushing's syndrome (**Fig. 2-10**). The remission rate for this procedure is ~80% for microadenomas but <50% for macroadenomas. After successful tumor resection, most patients experience a postoperative period of symptomatic ACTH deficiency that lasts for up to 12 months. This usually requires low-dose cortisol replacement, as patients experience steroid withdrawal symptoms as well as having a suppressed HPA axis. Biochemical recurrence occurs in approximately 5% of patients in whom surgery was initially successful.

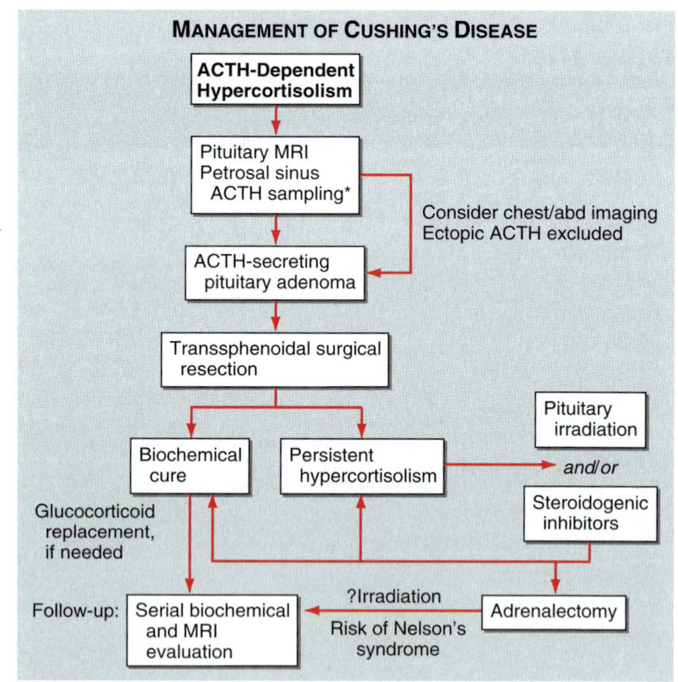

FIGURE 2-10

Management of Cushing's syndrome. ACTH, adrenocorticotropin hormone; MRI, magnetic resonance imaging.*, Not usually required.

When initial surgery is unsuccessful, repeat surgery is sometimes indicated, particularly when a pituitary source for ACTH is well documented. In older patients, in whom issues of growth and fertility are less important, hemi- or total hypophysectomy may be necessary if a discrete adenoma is not recognized. Pituitary irradiation may be used after unsuccessful surgery, but it cures only about 15% of patients. Because radiation is slow and only partially effective in adults, steroidogenic inhibitors are used in combination with pituitary irradiation to block the adrenal effects of persistently high ACTH levels.

Ketoconazole, an imidazole derivative antimycotic agent, inhibits several P450 enzymes and effectively lowers cortisol in most patients with Cushing's disease when administered twice daily (600–1200 mg/d). Elevated hepatic transaminases, gynecomastia, impotence, gastrointestinal upset, and edema are common side effects. *Metyrapone* (2–4 g/d) inhibits 11β-hydroxylase activity and normalizes plasma cortisol in up to 75% of patients. Side effects include nausea and vomiting, rash, and exacerbation of acne or hirsutism. *Mitotane* (*o*, *p*′-DDD; 3–6 g/d orally in four divided doses) suppresses cortisol hypersecretion by inhibiting 11β-hydroxylase and cholesterol side-chain cleavage enzymes and by destroying adrenocortical cells. Side effects of mitotane include gastrointestinal symptoms, dizziness, gynecomastia, hyperlipidemia, skin rash, and hepatic enzyme elevation. It may also lead to hypoaldosteronism. Other agents include *aminoglutethimide* (250 mg tid), *trilostane* (200–1000 mg/d), *cyproheptadine* (24 mg/d), and IV *etomidate* (0.3 mg/kg per hour). Glucocorticoid insufficiency is a potential side effect of agents used to block steroidogenesis.

The use of steroidogenic inhibitors has decreased the need for bilateral adrenalectomy. Removal of both adrenal glands corrects hypercortisolism but may be associated with a significant morbidity rate and necessitates permanent glucocorticoid and mineralocorticoid replacement. Adrenalectomy in the setting of residual corticotrope adenoma tissue predisposes to the development of *Nelson's syndrome*, a disorder characterized by rapid pituitary tumor enlargement and increased pigmentation secondary to high ACTH levels. Radiation therapy may be indicated to prevent the development of Nelson's syndrome after adrenalectomy.

GONADOTROPINS: FSH AND LH

SYNTHESIS AND SECRETION

Gonadotrope cells constitute about 10% of anterior pituitary cells and produce two gonadotropins—LH and FSH. Like TSH and hCG, LH and FSH are glycoprotein hormones consisting of α and β subunits. The α subunit is common to these glycoprotein hormones; specificity is conferred by the β subunits, which are expressed by separate genes.

Gonadotropin synthesis and release are dynamically regulated. This is particularly true in women, in whom the rapidly fluctuating gonadal steroid levels vary throughout the menstrual cycle. Hypothalamic GnRH, a 10-amino-acid peptide, regulates the synthesis and secretion of both LH and FSH. GnRH is secreted in discrete pulses every 60–120 min, which in turn elicit LH and FSH pulses (Fig. 2-3). The pulsatile mode of GnRH input is essential to its action; pulses prime gonadotrope responsiveness, whereas continuous GnRH exposure induces desensitization. Based on this phenomenon, long-acting GnRH agonists are used to suppress gonadotropin levels in children with precocious puberty and in men with prostate cancer and are used in some ovulation-induction protocols to reduce endogenous gonadotropins (Chap. 10). Estrogens act at the hypothalamic and pituitary levels to control gonadotropin secretion. Chronic estrogen exposure is inhibitory, whereas rising estrogen levels, as occur during the preovulatory surge, exert positive feedback to increase gonadotropin pulse frequency and amplitude. Progesterone slows GnRH pulse frequency but enhances gonadotropin responses to GnRH. Testosterone feedback in men also occurs at the hypothalamic and pituitary levels and is mediated in part by its conversion to estrogens.

Although GnRH is the main regulator of LH and FSH secretion, FSH synthesis is also under separate control by the gonadal peptides inhibin and activin, which are members of the transforming growth factor β (TGF-β) family. Inhibin selectively suppresses FSH, whereas activin stimulates FSH synthesis (Chap. 10).

ACTION

The gonadotropin hormones interact with their respective GPCRs expressed in the ovary and testis, evoking germ cell development and maturation and steroid hormone biosynthesis. In women, FSH regulates ovarian follicle development and stimulates ovarian estrogen production. LH mediates ovulation and maintenance of the corpus luteum. In men, LH induces Leydig cell testosterone synthesis and secretion and FSH stimulates seminiferous tubule development and regulates spermatogenesis.

GONADOTROPIN DEFICIENCY

Hypogonadism is the most common presenting feature of adult hypopituitarism, even when other pituitary hormones are also deficient. It is often a harbinger of hypothalamic or pituitary lesions that impair GnRH production or delivery through the pituitary stalk. As noted above, hypogonadotropic hypogonadism is a common presenting feature of hyperprolactinemia.

A variety of inherited and acquired disorders are associated with *isolated hypogonadotropic hypogonadism*

(IHH) (Chap. 8). Hypothalamic defects associated with GnRH deficiency include two X-linked disorders, Kallmann syndrome (see earlier) and mutations in the *DAX1* gene, as well as dominant mutations in *FGFR1*. Mutations in GPR54, the GnRH receptor, and the LH β or FSH β subunit genes are additional causes of selective gonadotropin deficiency. Acquired forms of GnRH deficiency leading to hypogonadotropism are seen in association with anorexia nervosa, stress, starvation, and extreme exercise, but may also be idiopathic. Hypogonadotropic hypogonadism in these disorders is reversed by removal of the stressful stimulus, or caloric replenishment.

Presentation and Diagnosis

In premenopausal women, hypogonadotropic hypogonadism presents as diminished ovarian function leading to oligomenorrhea or amenorrhea, infertility, decreased vaginal secretions, decreased libido, and breast atrophy. In hypogonadal adult men, secondary testicular failure is associated with decreased libido and potency, infertility, decreased muscle mass with weakness, reduced beard and body hair growth, soft testes, and characteristic fine facial wrinkles. Osteoporosis occurs in both untreated hypogonadal women and men.

Laboratory Investigation

Central hypogonadism is associated with low or inappropriately normal serum gonadotropin levels in the setting of low sex hormone concentrations (testosterone in men, estradiol in women). Because gonadotropin secretion is pulsatile, valid assessments may require repeated measurements or using pooled serum samples. Men have abnormal semen analysis.

Intravenous GnRH (100 μg) stimulates gonadotropes to secrete LH (which peaks within 30 min) and FSH (which plateaus during the ensuing 60 min). Normal responses vary according to menstrual cycle stage, age, and sex of the patient. Generally, LH levels increase about threefold, whereas FSH responses are less pronounced. In the setting of gonadotropin deficiency, a normal gonadotropin response to GnRH indicates intact gonadotrope function and suggests a hypothalamic abnormality. An absent response, however, cannot reliably distinguish pituitary from hypothalamic causes of hypogonadism. For this reason, GnRH testing usually adds little to the information gained from baseline evaluation of the hypothalamic-pituitary-gonadotrope axis, except in cases of isolated GnRH deficiency (e.g., Kallmann syndrome).

MRI examination of the sellar region and assessment of other pituitary functions are usually indicated in patients with documented central hypogonadism.

℞ Treatment: GONADOTROPIN DEFICIENCY

In males, testosterone replacement is necessary to achieve and maintain normal growth and development of the external genitalia, secondary sex characteristics, male sexual behavior, and androgenic anabolic effects including maintenance of muscle function and bone mass. Testosterone may be administered by intramuscular injections every 1–4 weeks or using patches that are replaced daily (Chap. 8). Testosterone gels are also available. Gonadotropin injections [hCG or human menopausal gonadotropin (hMG)] over 12–18 months are used to restore fertility. Pulsatile GnRH therapy (25–150 ng/kg every 2 h), administered by a subcutaneous infusion pump, is also effective for treatment of hypothalamic hypogonadism when fertility is desired.

In premenopausal women, cyclical replacement of estrogen and progesterone maintains secondary sexual characteristics and integrity of genitourinary tract mucosa and prevents premature osteoporosis (Chap. 10). Gonadotropin therapy is used for ovulation induction. Follicular growth and maturation are initiated using hMG or recombinant FSH; hCG is subsequently injected to induce ovulation. As in men, pulsatile GnRH therapy can be used to treat hypothalamic causes of gonadotropin deficiency.

NONFUNCTIONING AND GONADOTROPIN-PRODUCING PITUITARY ADENOMAS

Etiology and Prevalence

Nonfunctioning pituitary adenomas include those that secrete little or no pituitary hormones, as well as tumors that produce too little hormone to result in recognizable clinical features. They are the most common type of pituitary adenoma and are usually macroadenomas at the time of diagnosis because clinical features are inapparent until tumor mass effects occur. Based on immunohistochemistry, most clinically nonfunctioning adenomas can be shown to originate from gonadotrope cells. These tumors typically produce small amounts of intact gonadotropins (usually FSH) as well as uncombined α, LH β, and FSH β subunits. Tumor secretion may lead to elevated α- and FSH β-subunit and, rarely, to increased LH β-subunit levels. Some adenomas express α subunits without FSH or LH. TRH administration often induces an atypical increase of tumor-derived gonadotropins or subunits.

Presentation and Diagnosis

Clinically nonfunctioning tumors often present with optic chiasm pressure and other symptoms of local expansion or may be incidentally discovered on an MRI performed for another indication (incidentaloma). Menstrual disturbances or ovarian hyperstimulation rarely occur in women with large tumors that produce FSH and LH. More commonly, adenoma compression of the pituitary stalk or surrounding pituitary tissue leads to attenuated LH and features of hypogonadism. PRL levels are usually slightly increased, also because of stalk compression. It is important to distinguish this circumstance from true prolactinomas, as most nonfunctioning tumors respond poorly to treatment with dopamine agonists.

Laboratory Investigation

The goal of laboratory testing in clinically nonfunctioning tumors is to classify the type of tumor, to identify hormonal markers of tumor activity, and to detect possible hypopituitarism. Free α-subunit levels may be elevated in 10–15% of patients with nonfunctioning tumors. In female patients, peri- or postmenopausal basal FSH concentrations are difficult to distinguish from tumor-derived FSH elevation. Premenopausal women have cycling FSH levels, also preventing clear-cut diagnostic distinction from tumor-derived FSH. In men, gonadotropin-secreting tumors may be diagnosed because of slightly increased gonadotropins (FSH > LH) in the setting of a pituitary mass. Testosterone levels are usually low, despite the normal or increased LH level, perhaps reflecting reduced LH bioactivity or the loss of normal LH pulsatility. Because this pattern of hormone tests is also seen in primary gonadal failure and, to some extent, with aging (Chap. 8), the finding of increased gonadotropins alone is insufficient for the diagnosis of a gonadotropin-secreting tumor. In the majority of patients with gonadotrope adenomas, TRH administration stimulates LH β-subunit secretion; this response is not seen in normal individuals. GnRH testing, however, is not helpful for making the diagnosis. For nonfunctioning and gonadotropin-secreting tumors, the diagnosis usually rests on immunohistochemical analyses of resected tumor tissue, as the mass effects of these tumors usually necessitate resection.

Although acromegaly or Cushing's syndrome usually presents with unique clinical features, clinically inapparent somatotrope or corticotrope adenomas can be excluded by a normal IGF-I value and normal 24-h urinary free cortisol levels. If PRL levels are <100 μg/L in a patient harboring a pituitary mass, a nonfunctioning adenoma causing pituitary stalk compression should be considered.

Rx Treatment: NONFUNCTIONING AND GONADOTROPIN-PRODUCING PITUITARY ADENOMAS

Asymptomatic small nonfunctioning adenomas with no threat to vision may be followed with regular MRI and visual field testing without immediate intervention. However, for larger macroadenomas, transsphenoidal surgery reduces tumor size and relieves mass effects (Fig. 2-11). Although it is not usually possible to remove all adenoma tissue surgically, vision improves in 70% of patients with preoperative visual field defects. Preexisting hypopituitarism that results from tumor mass effects commonly improves or may resolve completely. Beginning about 6 months postoperatively, MRI scans should be performed yearly to detect tumor regrowth. Within 5–6 years following successful surgical resection, ~15% of nonfunctioning tumors recur. When substantial tumor remains after transsphenoidal surgery, adjuvant radiotherapy may be indicated to prevent tumor regrowth. Radiotherapy may be deferred if no postoperative residual mass is evident.

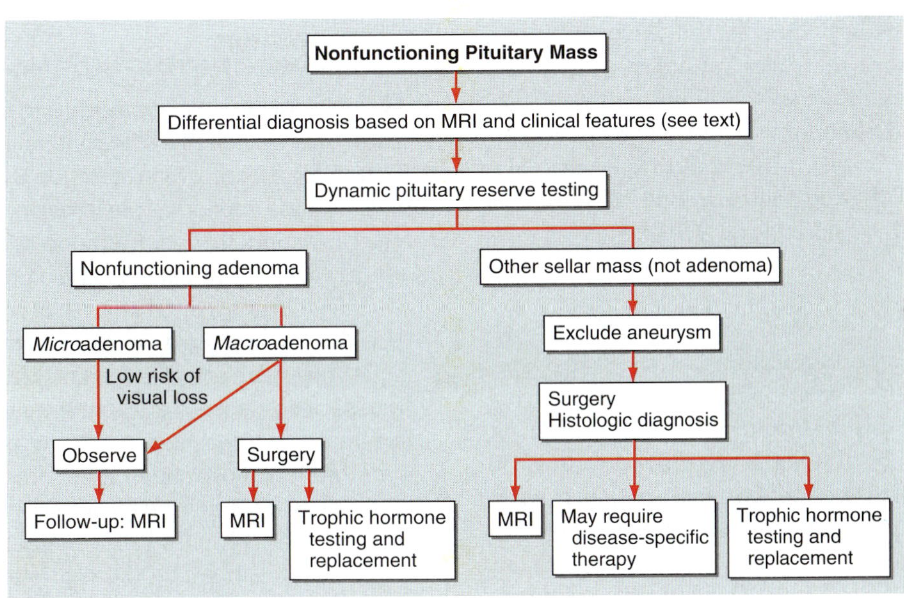

FIGURE 2-11
Management of a nonfunctioning pituitary mass.

Nonfunctioning pituitary tumors respond poorly to dopamine agonist treatment, with modest tumor shrinkage occurring in <10% of patients. Although SSTR subtypes 2 and 5 have been identified on nonfunctioning pituitary adenomas, octreotide is largely ineffective for shrinking these tumors. The selective GnRH antagonist, Nal-Glu GnRH, suppresses FSH hypersecretion but has no effect on adenoma size.

THYROID-STIMULATING HORMONE

SYNTHESIS AND SECRETION

TSH-secreting thyrotrope cells constitute 5% of the anterior pituitary cell population. TSH is structurally related to LH and FSH. It shares a common α subunit with these hormones but contains a specific TSH β subunit. TRH is a hypothalamic tripeptide (pyroglutamyl histidylprolinamide) that acts through a GPCR to stimulate TSH synthesis and secretion; it also stimulates the lactotrope cell to secrete PRL. TSH secretion is stimulated by TRH, whereas thyroid hormones, dopamine, somatostatin, and glucocorticoids suppress TSH by overriding TRH induction.

Thyrotrope growth and TSH secretion are both induced when negative feedback inhibition by thyroid hormones is removed. Thus, thyroid damage (including surgical thyroidectomy), radiation-induced hypothyroidism, chronic thyroiditis, or prolonged goitrogen exposure are associated with increased TSH. Longstanding untreated hypothyroidism can lead to thyrotrope hyperplasia and pituitary enlargement, which may be evident on MRI.

ACTION

TSH is secreted in pulses, though the excursions are modest in comparison to other pituitary hormones because of the low amplitude of the pulses and the relatively long half-life of TSH. Consequently, single determinations of TSH suffice to assess its circulating levels. TSH binds to a GPCR on thyroid follicular cells to stimulate thyroid hormone synthesis and release (Chap. 4).

TSH DEFICIENCY

Features of central hypothyroidism due to TSH deficiency mimic those seen with primary hypothyroidism but are generally less severe. Pituitary hypothyroidism is characterized by low basal TSH levels in the setting of low free thyroid hormone. In contrast, patients with hypothyroidism of hypothalamic origin (presumably due to a lack of endogenous TRH) may exhibit normal or even slightly elevated TSH levels. The TSH produced in this circumstance appears to have reduced biologic activity because of altered glycosylation.

TRH (200 μg) injected intravenously causes a two- to threefold increase in TSH (and PRL) levels within 30 min. Although TRH testing can be used to assess TSH reserve, abnormalities of the thyroid axis can usually be detected based on basal free T_4 and TSH levels, and TRH testing is rarely indicated.

Thyroid-replacement therapy should be initiated after establishing adequate adrenal function. Dose adjustment is based on thyroid hormone levels and clinical parameters rather than the TSH level.

TSH-SECRETING ADENOMAS

TSH-producing macroadenomas are rare but are often large and locally invasive when they occur. Patients usually present with thyroid goiter and hyperthyroidism, reflecting overproduction of TSH. Diagnosis is based on demonstrating elevated serum free T_4 levels, inappropriately normal or high TSH secretion, and MRI evidence of a pituitary adenoma.

It is important to exclude other causes of inappropriate TSH secretion, such as resistance to thyroid hormone, an autosomal dominant disorder caused by mutations in the thyroid hormone β receptor (Chap. 4). The presence of a pituitary mass and elevated α-subunit levels are suggestive of a TSH-secreting tumor. Dysalbuminemic hyperthyroxinemia syndromes, caused by mutations in serum thyroid hormone–binding proteins, are also characterized by elevated thyroid hormone levels, but with normal rather than suppressed TSH levels. Moreover, free thyroid hormone levels are normal in these disorders, most of which are familial.

℞ Treatment: TSH-SECRETING ADENOMAS

The initial therapeutic approach is to remove or debulk the tumor mass surgically, using either a transsphenoidal or subfrontal approach. Total resection is not often achieved as most of these adenomas are large and locally invasive. Normal circulating thyroid hormone levels are achieved in about two-thirds of patients after surgery. Thyroid ablation or antithyroid drugs (methimazole or propylthiouracil) can be used to reduce thyroid hormone levels. Somatostatin analogue treatment effectively normalizes TSH and α-subunit hypersecretion, shrinks the tumor mass in 50% of patients, and improves visual fields in 75% of patients; euthyroidism is restored in most patients. In some patients, octreotide markedly suppresses TSH, causing biochemical hypothyroidism that requires concomitant thyroid hormone replacement. Lanreotide (30 mg intramuscularly), a long-acting somatostatin analogue, effectively suppresses TSH and thyroid hormone in patients treated every 14 days.

DIABETES INSIPIDUS

See Chap. 3 for diagnosis and treatment of diabetes insipidus.

FURTHER READINGS

AIMARETTI G et al: Residual pituitary function after brain injury-induced hypopituitarism: A prospective 12-month study. J Clin Endocrinol Metab 90:6085, 2005

CATUREGLI P et al: Autoimmune hypophysitis. Endocr Rev 26:599, 2005

COLAO A et al: Predictors of remission of hyperprolactinaemia after long-term withdrawal of cabergoline therapy. Clin Endocrinol (Oxf) Sep;67(3):426, 2007

COZZI R et al: Primary treatment of acromegaly with octreotide LAR: A long-term (up to nine years) prospective study of its efficacy in the control of disease activity and tumor shrinkage. J Clin Endocrinol Metab 91:1397, 2006

ELAMIN MB et al.: Accuracy of diagnostic tests for Cushing's syndrome: A systematic review and metaanalyses. J Clin Endocrinol Metab 93:1553, 2008

GILLAM MP et al: Advances in the treatment of prolactinomas. Endocr Rev 27:485, 2006

ILIAS I et al: Cushing's syndrome due to ectopic corticotropin secretion: Twenty years' experience at the National Institutes of Health. J Clin Endocrinol Metab 90:4955, 2005

JALLAD RS et al: Does partial surgical tumour removal influence the response to octreotide-LAR in acromegalic patients previously resistant to the somatostatin analogue? Clin Endocrinol (Oxf) 67:310, 2007

LIEW A et al: Is hypopituitarism predictable after traumatic brain injury? Nat Clin Pract Endocrinol Metab 4:126, 2008

LIU H et al: Systematic review: The safety and efficacy of growth hormone in the healthy elderly. Ann Intern Med 146:104, 2007

MEHTA A et al: Congenital hypopituitarism: Clinical, molecular and neuroradiological correlates. Clin Endocrinol (Oxf), 2009[D2]

MELMED S: ACROMEGALY. N Engl J Med 355(24):2558, 2006

MINNITI G et al: Risk of second brain tumor after conservative surgery and radiotherapy for pituitary adenomas: Update after an additional 10 years. J Clin Endocrinol Metab 90:800, 2005

MOLITCH ME: Evaluation and treatment of adult growth hormone deficiency: An Endocrine Society Clinical Practice Guideline. J Clin Endocrinol Metab 91:1621, 2006

NIEMAN LK et al: The diagnosis of Cushing's syndrome: An Endocrine Society Clinical Practice Guideline. J Clin Endocrinol Metab 93:1526, 2008

SWEARINGEN B et al: Does radiosurgery have a role in the treatment of acromegaly? Nat Clin Pract Endocrinol Metab 4:592, 2008

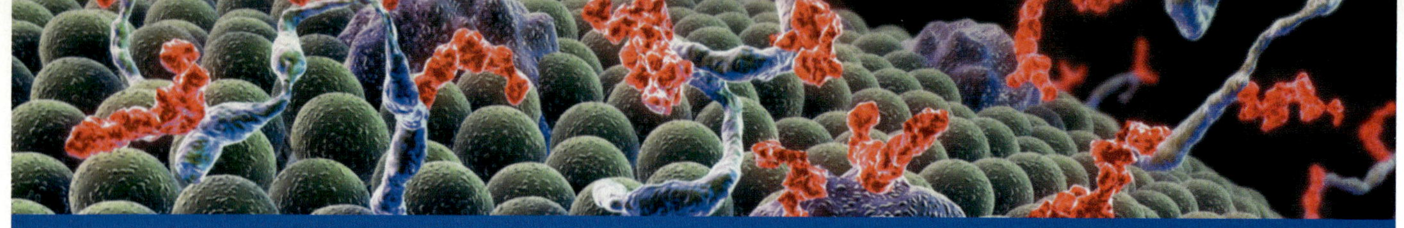

CHAPTER 3

DISORDERS OF THE NEUROHYPOPHYSIS

Gary L. Robertson

The neurohypophysis, or posterior pituitary gland, is formed by axons that originate in large cell bodies in the supraoptic and paraventricular nuclei of the hypothalamus. It produces two hormones: (1) arginine vasopressin (AVP), also known as antidiuretic hormone; and (2) oxytocin. AVP acts on the renal tubules to reduce water loss by concentrating the urine. Oxytocin stimulates postpartum milk letdown in response to suckling. AVP deficiency causes diabetes insipidus (DI), characterized by the production of large amounts of dilute urine. Excessive or inappropriate AVP production predisposes to hyponatremia if water intake is not reduced in parallel with urine output.

VASOPRESSIN

ACTION

AVP is a nonapeptide composed of a six-membered disulfide ring and a tripeptide tail (**Fig. 3-1**). The most important, if not the only, physiologic action of AVP is to reduce water excretion by promoting concentration of urine. This antidiuretic effect is achieved by increasing the hydroosmotic permeability of cells that line the distal tubule and medullary collecting ducts of the kidney (**Fig. 3-2**). In the absence of AVP, these cells are impermeable to water and reabsorb little, if any, of the relatively large volume of dilute filtrate that enters from the proximal nephron. This results in the excretion of very large volumes (as much as 0.2 mL/kg per min) of maximally dilute urine (specific gravity and osmolarity ~1.000 and 50 mosmol/L, respectively), a condition known as a *water diuresis*. In the presence of AVP, these cells become selectively permeable to water, allowing it to diffuse back down the osmotic gradient created by the hypertonic renal medulla. As a result, the dilute fluid passing through the tubules is concentrated and the rate of urine flow decreases. The magnitude of this effect varies in direct proportion to the plasma AVP concentration and, at maximum levels, approximates a urine flow rate as low as 0.35 mL/min and a urine osmolarity as high as 1200 mosmol/L. AVP action is mediated via binding to G protein–coupled V_2 receptors on the serosal surface of the cell, activation of adenyl cyclase, and insertion into the luminal surface of water channels composed of a protein known as *aquaporin 2*.

At high concentrations, AVP also causes contraction of smooth muscle in blood vessels and in the gastrointestinal tract, induces glycogenolysis in the liver, and potentiates adrenocorticotropic hormone (ACTH) release by corticotropin-releasing factor. These effects are mediated by V_{1a} or V_{1b} receptors that are coupled to phospholipase C. Their role, if any, in human physiology/pathophysiology is still uncertain.

SYNTHESIS AND SECRETION

AVP secretion is synthesized via a polypeptide precursor that includes AVP, neurophysin, and copeptin. After preliminary processing and folding, the precursor is

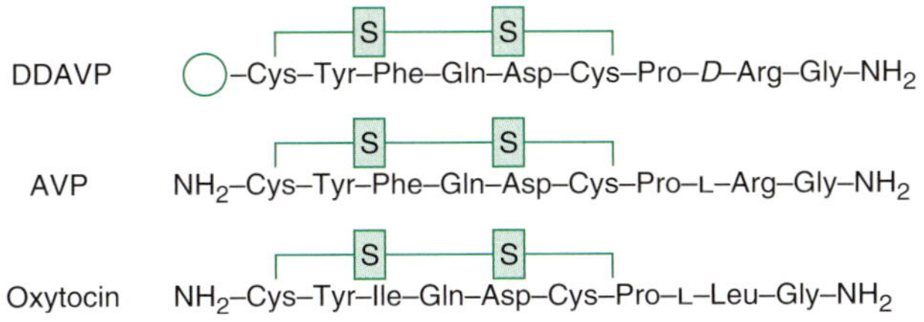

FIGURE 3-1

Primary structures of arginine vasopressin (AVP), oxytocin, and desmopressin.

packaged in neurosecretory vesicles where it is transported down the axon, further processed to AVP, and stored until the hormone and other components are released by exocytosis into peripheral blood.

AVP secretion is regulated primarily by the "effective" osmotic pressure of body fluids. This control is mediated by specialized hypothalamic cells, known as *osmoreceptors*, which are extremely sensitive to small changes in the plasma concentration of sodium and certain other solutes but are insensitive to other solutes such as urea or glucose. The osmoreceptors appear to include inhibitory as well as stimulatory components that function in concert to form a threshold, or set point, control system for AVP release. Below this threshold, plasma AVP is suppressed to levels that permit the development of a maximum water diuresis. Above it, plasma AVP rises steeply in direct proportion to plasma osmolarity, quickly reaching levels sufficient to effect a maximum antidiuresis. The absolute levels of plasma osmolarity/sodium at which minimally and maximally effective levels of plasma AVP occur vary appreciably from person to person, owing apparently to genetic influences on the set and sensitivity of the system. However, the average threshold, or set point, for AVP release corresponds to a plasma osmolarity or sodium of about 280 mosmol/L or 135 meq/L, respectively; levels only 2–4% higher normally result in maximum antidiuresis. Though relatively stable in a healthy adult, the set of the osmoregulatory system can also be lowered by pregnancy, the menstrual cycle, estrogen, and relatively large, acute reductions in blood pressure or volume.

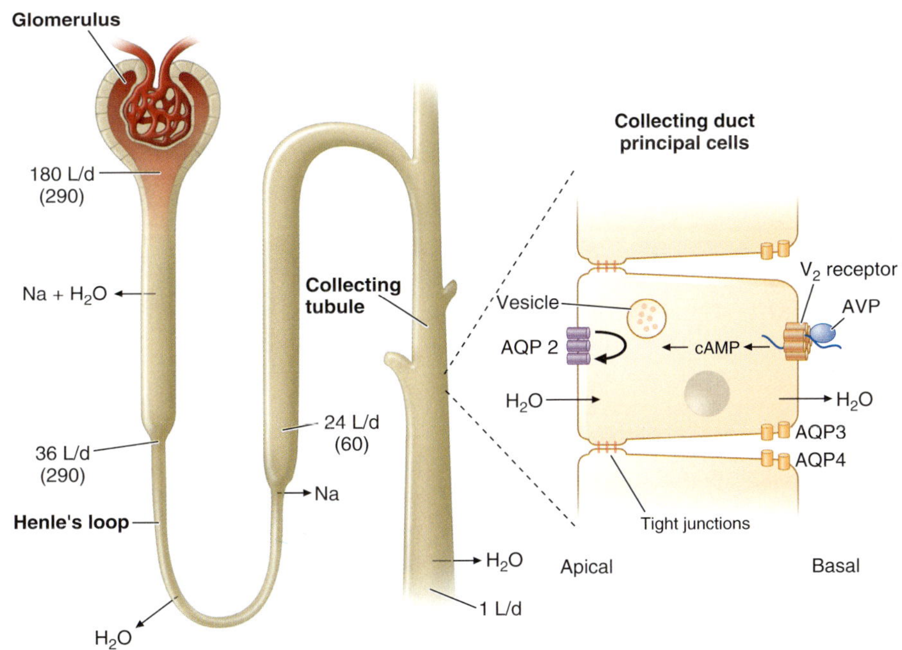

FIGURE 3-2

Antidiuretic effect of arginine vasopressin (AVP) in the regulation of urine volume. In a typical 70-kg adult, the kidney filters ~180 L/d of plasma. Of this, ~144 L (80%) is reabsorbed isosmotically in the proximal tubule and another 8 L (4–5%) is reabsorbed without solute in the descending limb of Henle's loop. The remainder is diluted to an osmolarity of ~60 mmol/kg by selective reabsorption of sodium and chloride in the ascending limb. In the absence of AVP, the urine issuing from the loop passes largely unmodified through the distal tubules and collecting ducts, resulting in a maximum water diuresis. In the presence of AVP, solute-free water is reabsorbed osmotically through the principal cells of the collecting ducts, resulting in the excretion of a much smaller volume of concentrated urine. This antidiuretic effect is mediated via a G protein–coupled V_2 receptor that increases intracellular cyclic AMP, thereby inducing translocation of aquaporin 2 (AQP 2) water channels into the apical membrane. The resultant increase in permeability permits an influx of water that diffuses out of the cell through AQP 3 and AQP 4 water channels on the basal-lateral surface. The net rate of flux across the cell is determined by the number of AQP 2 water channels in the apical membrane and the strength of the osmotic gradient between tubular fluid and the renal medulla. Tight junctions on the lateral surface of the cells serve to prevent unregulated water flow.

The effects of acute changes in blood volume or pressure are mediated largely by neuronal afferents that originate in transmural pressure receptors of the heart and large arteries and project via the vagus and glossopharyngeal nerves to the brainstem, from whence postsynaptic projections ascend to the hypothalamus. These pathways maintain a tonic inhibitory tone that decreases when blood volume or pressure falls by >10–20%. This baroregulatory system is probably of minor importance in the physiology of AVP secretion because the hemodynamic changes required to affect it do not usually occur during normal activities. However, the baroregulatory system undoubtedly plays an important role in AVP secretion in patients with large, acute disturbances of hemodynamic function.

AVP secretion can also be stimulated by nausea, acute hypoglycemia, glucocorticoid deficiency, smoking, and, possibly, hyperangiotensinemia. The emetic stimuli are extremely potent since they typically elicit immediate, 50- to 100-fold increases in plasma AVP, even when the nausea is transient and unassociated with vomiting or other symptoms. They appear to act via the emetic center in the medulla and can be completely blocked by treatment with antiemetics such as fluphenazine. There is no evidence that pain or other noxious stresses have any effect on AVP unless they elicit a vasovagal reaction with its associated nausea and hypotension.

METABOLISM

AVP distributes rapidly into a space roughly equal to the extracellular fluid volume. It is cleared irreversibly with a $t_{1/2}$ of 10–30 min. Most AVP clearance is due to degradation in the liver and kidneys. During pregnancy, the metabolic clearance of AVP is increased three- to fourfold due to placental production of an N-terminal peptidase.

THIRST

Because AVP cannot reduce water loss below a certain minimum level obligated by urinary solute load and evaporation from skin and lungs, a mechanism for ensuring adequate intake is essential for preventing dehydration. This vital function is performed by the thirst mechanism. Like AVP, thirst is regulated primarily by an osmostat that is located in the anteromedial hypothalamus and is able to detect very small changes in the plasma concentration of sodium and certain other effective solutes. The thirst osmostat appears to be "set" about 5% higher than the AVP osmostat. This arrangement ensures that thirst, polydipsia, and dilution of body fluids do not occur until plasma osmolarity/sodium start to exceed the defensive capacity of the antidiuretic mechanism.

OXYTOCIN

Oxytocin is also a nonapeptide and differs from AVP only at positions 3 and 8 (Fig. 3-1). However, it has relatively little antidiuretic effect and seems to act mainly on mammary ducts to facilitate milk letdown during nursing. It may also help to initiate or facilitate labor by stimulating contraction of uterine smooth muscle, but it is not yet clear if this action is physiologic or necessary for normal delivery.

DEFICIENCIES OF VASOPRESSIN SECRETION AND ACTION

DIABETES INSIPIDUS

Clinical Characteristics

Decreased secretion or action of AVP usually manifests as DI, a syndrome characterized by the production of abnormally large volumes of dilute urine. The 24-h urine volume is >50 mL/kg body weight and the osmolarity is <300 mosmol/L. The polyuria produces symptoms of urinary frequency, enuresis, and/or nocturia, which may disturb sleep and cause mild daytime fatigue or somnolence. It is also associated with thirst and a commensurate increase in fluid intake (polydipsia). Clinical signs of dehydration are uncommon unless fluid intake is impaired.

Etiology

Deficient secretion of AVP can be primary or secondary. The primary form usually results from agenesis or irreversible destruction of the neurohypophysis and is variously referred to as *neurohypophyseal DI*, *pituitary DI*, or *central DI*. It can be caused by a variety of congenital, acquired, or genetic disorders, but almost half the time it is idiopathic (**Table 3-1**). The genetic form of neurohypophyseal DI is usually transmitted in an autosomal dominant mode and is caused by diverse mutations in the coding region of the AVP–neurophysin II (or *AVP-NPII*) gene. All of the mutations alter one or more amino acids known to be critical for correct folding of the prohormone, thus interfering with its processing and trafficking through the endoplasmic reticulum. The AVP deficiency and DI develop several months to several years after birth and appear to result from selective degeneration of AVP-producing magnocellular neurons, probably caused by accumulation of misfolded precursor. An autosomal recessive form due to an inactivating mutation in the AVP portion of the gene, an X-linked recessive form due to an unidentified gene on Xq28, and an autosomal recessive form due to mutations of the *WFS 1* gene responsible for Wolfram's syndrome (diabetes insipidus, diabetes mellitus, optic atrophy, and neural deafness; DIDMOAD) have also been described.

TABLE 3-1

CAUSES OF DIABETES INSIPIDUS

Pituitary Diabetes Insipidus

- Acquired
    - Head trauma (closed and penetrating)
    - Neoplasms
        - Primary
            - Craniopharyngioma
            - Pituitary adenoma (suprasellar)
            - Dysgerminoma
            - Meningioma
        - Metastatic (lung, breast)
        - Hematologic (lymphoma, leukemia)
    - Granulomas
        - Neurosarcoid
        - Histiocytosis
        - Xanthoma disseminatum
    - Infectious
        - Chronic meningitis
        - Viral encephalitis
        - Toxoplasmosis
    - Inflammatory
        - Lymphocytic infundibuloneurohypophysitis
        - Wegener's granulomatosis
        - Lupus erythematosus
        - Scleroderma
    - Chemical toxins
        - Tetrodotoxin
        - Snake venom
    - Vascular
        - Sheehan's syndrome
        - Aneurysm (internal carotid)
        - Aortocoronary bypass
        - Hypoxic encephalopathy
    - Pregnancy (vasopressinase)
    - Idiopathic
- Congenital malformations
    - Septooptic dysplasia
    - Midline craniofacial defects
    - Holoprosencephaly
    - Hypogenesis, ectopia of pituitary
- Genetic
    - Autosomal dominant (AVP-neurophysin gene)
    - Autosomal recessive (AVP-neurophysin gene)
    - Autosomal recessive-Wolfram-(4p – WFS 1 gene)
    - X-linked recessive (Xq28)
    - Deletion chromosome 7q

Nephrogenic Diabetes Insipidus

- Acquired
    - Drugs
        - Lithium
        - Demeclocycline
        - Methoxyflurane
        - Amphotericin B
        - Aminoglycosides
        - Cisplatin
        - Rifampin
        - Foscarnet
    - Metabolic
        - Hypercalcemia, hypercalciuria
        - Hypokalemia
    - Obstruction (ureter or urethra)
    - Vascular
        - Sickle cell disease and trait
        - Ischemia (acute tubular necrosis)
    - Granulomas
        - Neurosarcoid
    - Neoplasms
        - Sarcoma
    - Infiltration
        - Amyloidosis
    - Pregnancy
    - Idiopathic
- Genetic
    - X-linked recessive (AVP receptor-2 gene)
    - Autosomal recessive (aquaporin-2 gene)
    - Autosomal dominant (aquaporin-2 gene)

Primary Polydipsia

- Acquired
    - Psychogenic
        - Schizophrenia
        - Obsessive-compulsive disorder
    - Dipsogenic (abnormal thirst)
        - Granulomas
            - Neurosarcoid
        - Infectious
            - Tuberculous meningitis
        - Head trauma (closed and penetrating)
        - Demyelination
            - Multiple sclerosis
        - Drugs
            - Lithium
            - Carbamazepine
        - Idiopathic
    - Iatrogenic

A primary deficiency of plasma AVP can also result from increased metabolism by an N-terminal aminopeptidase produced by the placenta. It is referred to as *gestational DI* since the signs and symptoms manifest during pregnancy and usually remit several weeks after delivery. However, a subclinical deficiency in AVP secretion can often be demonstrated in the nonpregnant state, indicating that damage to the neurohypophysis may also contribute to the AVP deficiency.

Secondary deficiencies of AVP result from inhibition of secretion by excessive intake of fluids. They are referred to as *primary polydipsia* and can be divided into three subcategories. One of them, called *dipsogenic DI*, is characterized by inappropriate thirst caused by a reduction in the "set" of the osmoregulatory mechanism. It sometimes occurs in association with multifocal diseases of the brain such as neurosarcoid, tuberculous meningitis, or multiple sclerosis but is often idiopathic. The second subtype, called *psychogenic polydipsia*, is not associated with thirst, and the polydipsia seems to be a feature of psychosis. The third subtype, which may be referred to as *iatrogenic polydipsia*, results from recommendations to increase fluid intake for its presumed health benefits.

Primary deficiencies in the antidiuretic action of AVP result in *nephrogenic DI* (Table 3-1). They can be genetic, acquired, or caused by exposure to various drugs. The genetic form is usually transmitted in an X-linked mode and is caused by mutations in the coding region of the V_2 receptor gene. Autosomal recessive or dominant forms result from mutations in the gene encoding the aquaporin protein that forms the water channels in the distal nephron.

Secondary deficiencies in the antidiuretic response to AVP result from polyuria per se. They are caused by washout of the medullary concentration gradient and/or suppression of aquaporin function. They usually resolve 24–48 h after the polyuria is corrected but often complicate interpretation of acute tests commonly used for differential diagnosis.

Pathophysiology

When the secretion or action of AVP is reduced below 80–85% of normal, urine concentration ceases and the rate of output increases to symptomatic levels. If the defect is primary (e.g., the patient has pituitary, gestational, or nephrogenic DI), the polyuria results in a small (1–2%) decrease in body water and a commensurate increase in plasma osmolarity and sodium concentration that stimulate thirst and a compensatory increase in water intake. As a result, *overt physical or laboratory signs of dehydration do not develop unless the patient also has a defect in thirst* (see below) *or fails to drink for some other reason.*

The severity of the antidiuretic defect varies markedly among patients with pituitary, gestational, or nephrogenic DI. In some, the deficiencies in AVP secretion or action are so severe that basal urine output approximates the maximum (10–15 mL/min); even an intense stimulus such as nausea or severe dehydration does not raise plasma AVP enough to concentrate the urine. In others, however, the deficiency in AVP secretion or action is incomplete, and a modest stimulus such as a few hours of fluid deprivation, smoking, or a vasovagal reaction increases plasma AVP sufficiently to produce a profound antidiuresis. The maximum urine osmolarity achieved in these patients is usually less than normal, largely because their maximal concentrating capacity is temporarily impaired by chronic polyuria. However, in a few patients with partial pituitary or nephrogenic DI, it can reach levels as high as 800 mosmol/L.

In primary polydipsia, the pathogenesis of the polydipsia and polyuria is the reverse of that in pituitary, nephrogenic, and gestational DI. Thus, the excessive intake of fluids slightly increases body water, thereby reducing plasma osmolarity, AVP secretion, and urinary concentration. The latter results in a compensatory increase in urinary free-water excretion that varies in direct proportion to intake. Therefore, clinically appreciable overhydration is uncommon unless the compensatory water diuresis is impaired by a drug or disease that stimulates or mimics endogenous AVP.

In the dipsogenic form of primary polydipsia, fluid intake is excessive because the osmotic threshold for thirst appears to be reset to the left, often well below that for AVP release. When deprived of fluids or subjected to some other acute osmotic or nonosmotic stimulus, these individuals invariably increase plasma AVP normally, but the resultant increase in urine concentration is usually subnormal because their renal capacity to concentrate the urine is also blunted by chronic polyuria. Thus, their antidiuretic response to these stimuli may be indistinguishable from that in patients with partial pituitary, partial gestational, or partial nephrogenic DI. Patients with psychogenic or iatrogenic polydipsia respond similarly to fluid restriction but do not complain of thirst and usually offer other explanations for their high fluid intake.

Differential Diagnosis

When symptoms of urinary frequency, enuresis, nocturia, and/or persistent thirst are present, a 24-h urine should be collected on an ad libitum fluid intake. If the volume exceeds 50 mL/kg per day (3500 mL in a 70-kg man), polyuria is present. If the osmolarity is >300 mosmol/L, the polyuria is due to a solute diuresis and the patient should be evaluated for glucosuria or other less common causes of excessive solute excretion. However, if the 24-h urine osmolarity is <300 mosmol/L, the patient has a water diuresis and should be evaluated further to determine which type of DI is present.

In differentiating between the various types of DI, the history, physical examination, and routine laboratory tests may be helpful but are rarely sufficient because few, if any, of the findings are pathognomonic. Except in the rare patient who is clearly dehydrated under basal conditions of ad libitum fluid intake, this evaluation should begin with a *fluid deprivation test*. To minimize patient discomfort, avoid excessive dehydration, and maximize the information obtained, the test should be started in the morning and water balance should be monitored closely with hourly measurements of body weight, plasma osmolarity and/or sodium concentration, and urine volume and osmolarity.

If fluid deprivation does not result in urine concentration (osmolarity >300 mosmol/L, specific gravity

>1.010) before body weight decreases by 5% or plasma osmolarity/sodium exceed the upper limit of normal, the patient has severe pituitary or severe nephrogenic DI. These disorders can usually be distinguished by administering desmopressin (DDAVP, 0.03 μg/kg SC or IV) and repeating the measurement of urine osmolarity 1–2 h later. An increase of >50% indicates severe pituitary DI, whereas a smaller or absent response is strongly suggestive of nephrogenic DI.

If fluid deprivation results in concentration of the urine, the differential diagnosis is more difficult because the patient can have either partial pituitary DI, partial nephrogenic DI, or a form of primary polydipsia. In this situation, the change in urine osmolarity after the administration of desmopressin does not differentiate the possible disorders because the responses are variable and overlap in the three types of DI. The best way to differentiate between them is to measure plasma or urine AVP before and during the fluid deprivation test and analyze the results in relation to the concurrent plasma or urine osmolarity (**Fig. 3-3**). This approach invariably differentiates partial nephrogenic DI from partial pituitary DI and primary polydipsia. It also differentiates partial pituitary DI from primary polydipsia if the hormone is measured when plasma osmolarity or sodium is clearly above the normal range. The requisite level of hypertonic dehydration may be difficult to produce by fluid deprivation alone when the urine is concentrated. Therefore, it is usually necessary to infuse hypertonic (3%) saline at a rate of 0.1 mL/kg per min while continuing the fluid deprivation and repeat the AVP measurements as soon as plasma osmolarity rises to >300 mosmol/L (Na^+ >145 mmol/L). This endpoint is usually reached within 30–120 min.

The differential diagnosis of DI may also be facilitated by MRI of the pituitary and hypothalamus. In most healthy adults and children, the posterior pituitary emits a hyperintense signal in T1-weighted mid-sagittal images. This "bright spot" is almost always present in patients with primary polydipsia but is invariably absent or abnormally small in patients with pituitary DI. It is usually also small or absent in nephrogenic DI, presumably because of high secretion and turnover of vasopressin. Thus, a normal bright spot virtually excludes pituitary DI, is against nephrogenic DI, and strongly suggests primary polydipsia. Lack of the bright spot is less helpful, however, because it is absent not only in pituitary and nephrogenic DI but also in some normal persons and in patients with empty sella who do not have DI.

The other way to distinguish between the three basic types of DI is to closely monitor the effects of antidiuretic therapy on changes in water balance.

℞ Treatment: DIABETES INSIPIDUS

The signs and symptoms of uncomplicated pituitary DI can be eliminated completely by treatment with desmopressin (DDAVP), a synthetic analogue of AVP (Fig. 3-1). It acts selectively at V_2 receptors to increase urine concentration and decrease urine flow in a dose-dependent manner (**Fig. 3-4**). It is also more resistant to degradation than AVP and has a three- to fourfold longer duration of action. Desmopressin (DDAVP) can be given by IV or SC injection, nasal inhalation, or oral tablet. The doses required to completely control pituitary DI vary widely, depending on the patient and the route of administration. However, they usually range from 1–2 μg qd or bid by injection, 10–20 μg bid or tid by nasal spray, or 100–400 μg bid or tid PO. The onset of action is rapid, ranging from as little as 15 min after injection to 60 min after oral administration. When given in doses sufficient to completely normalize urinary osmolarity and flow, desmopressin produces a slight (1–3%) increase in

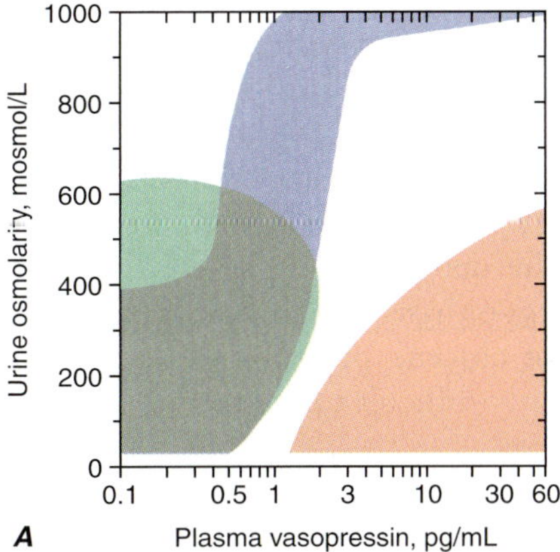

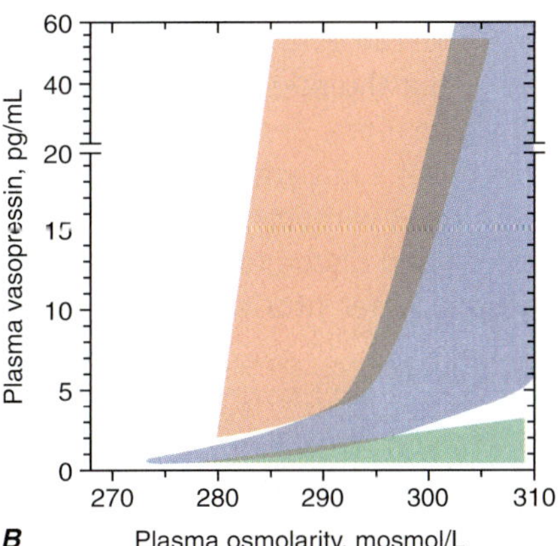

FIGURE 3-3

Relationship of plasma AVP to urine osmolarity (*A*) and plasma osmolarity (*B*) before and during fluid deprivation–hypertonic saline infusion test in patients who are normal (blue zones) or have primary polydipsia (blue zones), pituitary diabetes insipidus (green zones), or nephrogenic diabetes insipidus (pink zones).

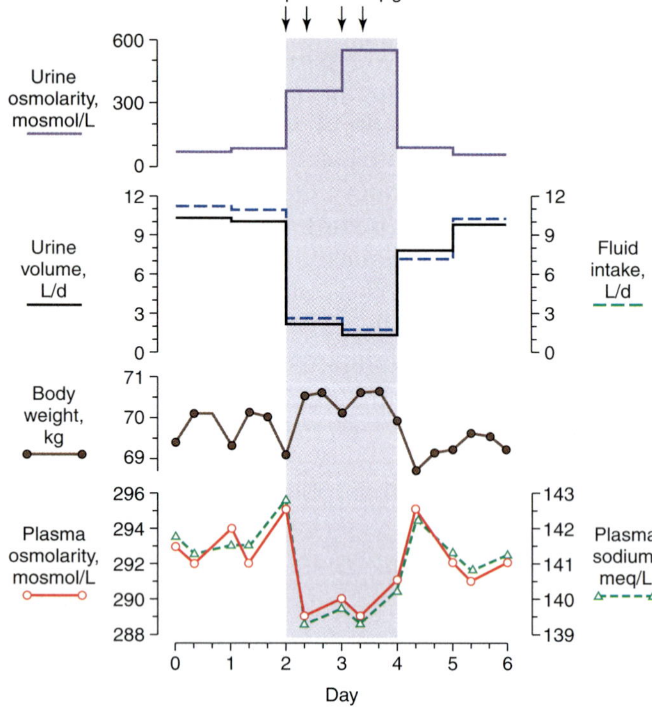

FIGURE 3-4

Effect of desmopressin therapy on water balance in patient with uncomplicated pituitary diabetes insipidus. Note that treatment rapidly reduces thirst and fluid intake as well as urine output to normal, with only a slight increase in body water (weight) and decrease in plasma osmolarity/sodium. [*From Endocrinology and Metabolism, 4th ed, P Felig, L Frohman (eds). New York, McGraw-Hill, 2001; with permission.*]

total-body water and a commensurate decrease in plasma osmolarity and sodium concentration that rapidly eliminate thirst and polydipsia. Consequently, water balance is maintained and hyponatremia does not develop unless the patient has an associated abnormality in the osmoregulation of thirst or ingests/ receives excessive amounts of fluid for some other reason. Fortunately, thirst is usually normal in patients with pituitary DI, and the other causes of excessive intake can usually be eliminated by educating the patient about the risks of drinking for reasons other than thirst. Therefore, desmopressin can usually be given safely in doses sufficient to maintain a completely normal urine output without subjecting the patient to the inconvenience and discomfort of allowing intermittent escape to prevent water intoxication.

Primary polydipsia cannot be treated safely with desmopressin. It inhibits the polyuria but, unlike pituitary DI, does not eliminate the urge to drink. Therefore, it almost always produces water intoxication within 24–48 h. Iatrogenic polydipsia can often be corrected by patient counseling, but there is no effective treatment for either psychogenic or dipsogenic DI.

The symptoms and signs of nephrogenic DI are not affected by treatment with desmopressin but may be reduced by treatment with a thiazide diuretic and/or amiloride in conjunction with a low-sodium diet. Inhibitors of prostaglandin synthesis (e.g., indomethacin) are also very effective in some patients.

ADIPSIC HYPERNATREMIA

Clinical Characteristics

Adipsic hypernatremia is a syndrome characterized by chronic or recurrent hypertonic dehydration caused by a deficiency in the osmoregulation of thirst. The hypernatremia varies widely in severity and is usually associated with signs of hypovolemia such as tachycardia, postural hypotension, azotemia, hyperuricemia, and hypokalemia. Muscle weakness, pain, rhabdomyolysis, hyperglycemia, hyperlipidemia, and acute renal failure may also occur. DI is usually not present at least at presentation.

Pathophysiology

Adipsic hypernatremia is caused by agenesis or destruction of the hypothalamic osmoreceptors that normally regulate thirst and AVP secretion (**Fig. 3-5**). The deficiency of osmoregulation is usually due to a congenital or acquired disease in the hypothalamus (**Table 3-2**). Whatever the cause, the lack of thirst results in a failure to drink enough water to replenish renal and extrarenal losses resulting in hypernatremic, hypertonic dehydration. In most patients, the osmoregulation of AVP secretion is also impaired partially or completely (Fig. 3-5). If the deficiency is partial, severe dehydration stimulates the release of enough AVP to concentrate the urine. However, as rehydration decreases the hypertonicity and hypovolemia, plasma AVP falls and polyuria develops. Patients with a complete lack of osmoregulation do not develop DI at any level of hydration because they cannot osmotically suppress or stimulate AVP secretion. Therefore, they have permanent inappropriate antidiuresis and develop hyponatremia if overhydrated during treatment. In most patients, the neurohypophysis and the AVP response to hemodynamic or emetic stimuli are normal. Consequently, hypovolemia and/or hypotension become the dominant influence on AVP release, especially when the dehydration is severe. In some, however, the neurohypophysis is also deficient, resulting in a combination of chronic pituitary DI and hypodipsia that is particularly difficult to manage.

Differential Diagnosis

Adipsic hypernatremia should be distinguished from hypernatremia caused by physical restrictions to drinking (e.g., coma, paralysis, restraints, absence of fresh water) or intake of large amounts of sodium. This distinction can

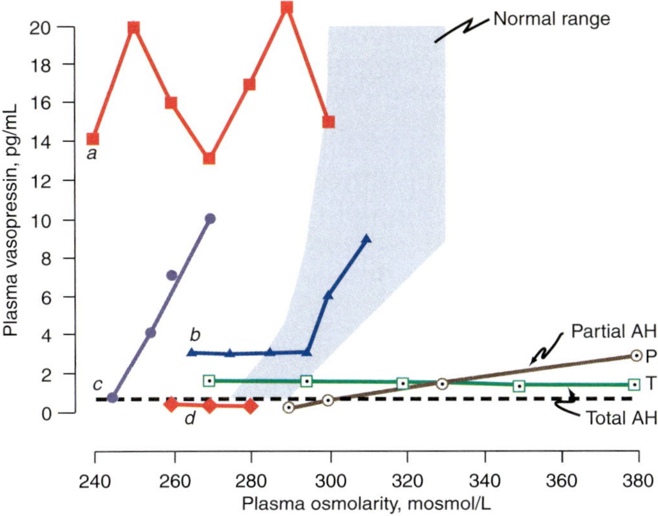

FIGURE 3-5

Heterogeneity of osmoregulatory dysfunction in adipsic hypernatremia (AH) and the syndrome of inappropriate antidiuresis (SIAD). Each line depicts schematically the relationship of plasma arginine vasopressin (AVP) to plasma osmolarity during water loading and/or infusion of 3% saline in a patient with either AH (open symbols) or SIAD (closed symbols). The shaded area indicates the normal range of the relationship. The horizontal broken line indicates the plasma AVP level below which the hormone is undetectable and urinary concentration usually does not occur. Lines P and T represent patients with a selective deficiency in the osmoregulation of thirst and AVP that is either partial (s) or total (h). In the latter, plasma AVP does not change in response to increases or decreases in plasma osmolarity but remains within a range sufficient to concentrate the urine even if overhydration produces hypotonic hyponatremia. In contrast, if the osmoregulatory deficiency is partial (s), rehydration of the patient suppresses plasma AVP to levels that result in urinary dilution and polyuria before plasma osmolarity and sodium are reduced to normal. Lines *a–d* represent different defects in the osmoregulation of plasma AVP observed in patients with SIAD. In *a* (■), plasma AVP is markedly elevated and fluctuates widely without relation to changes in plasma osmolarity, indicating complete loss of osmoregulation. In *b* (▲), plasma AVP remains fixed at a slightly elevated level until plasma osmolarity reaches the normal range, at which point it begins to rise appropriately, indicating a selective defect in the inhibitory component of the osmoregulatory mechanism. In *c* (●), plasma AVP rises in close correlation with plasma osmolarity before the latter reaches the normal range, indicating downward resetting of the osmostat. In *d* (◆), plasma AVP appears to be osmoregulated normally, suggesting that the inappropriate antidiuresis is caused by some other abnormality.

usually be made from the history, physical examination, and routine laboratory tests. If a conscious patient denies thirst and/or does not drink vigorously when hypernatremic, the diagnosis of hypodipsia or adipsia can be made with confidence irrespective of the volume status.

TABLE 3-2

CAUSES OF ADIPSIC HYPERNATREMIA
Acquired
Vascular: Occlusion anterior communicating artery
Tumors
Primary
Craniopharyngioma
Pinealoma, germinoma
Meningioma
Glioma
Metastatic (lung, breast)
Granulomas: Neurosarcoid
Histiocytosis
Trauma: Closed
Penetrating (pituitary-hypothalamic surgery)
Psychogenic: Psychotic depression
Other: Hydrocephalus
Neurodegenerative
AIDS, cytomegalovirus encephalitis
Idiopathic
Congenital
Midline malformation (septum and corpus callosum)
Microcephaly
Genetic: Autosomal recessive (Schinzel-Giedion syndrome)

If the patient is obtunded at the time of presentation, the possibility of adipsic hypernatremia can be evaluated after rehydration by assessing the thirst and plasma AVP response to a controlled fluid deprivation–hypertonic saline infusion test similar to that described for evaluation of DI. A history of one or more previous episodes of hypernatremia is also virtually diagnostic.

℞ Treatment: ADIPSIC HYPERNATREMIA

Severe dehydration in adipsic hypernatremia should be corrected by administering water PO, if the patient is alert, or 0.45% saline IV, if the patient is obtunded or uncooperative. The number of liters of free water required to correct the deficit (ΔFW) can be estimated from body weight in kg (BW) and the serum sodium concentration in mmol/L (S_{Na}) by the formula $\Delta FW = 0.5BW \times [(S_{Na} - 140)/140]$. If serum glucose ($S_{Glu}$) is elevated, the measured S_{Na} should be corrected (S_{Na}^*) by the formula $S_{Na}^* = S_{Na} + [(S_{Glu} - 90)/36]$. This amount plus an allowance for continuing insensible and urinary losses should be given over a 24- to 48-h period. Close monitoring of serum sodium as well as fluid intake and urinary output is essential because, depending on the extent of osmoreceptor deficiency (Fig. 3-5), some patients will develop AVP-deficient DI requiring desmopressin therapy to complete rehydration; others will develop hyponatremia and a syndrome of inappropriate antidiuresis (SIAD)-like picture if overhydrated. If hyperglycemia and/or hypokalemia are present, insulin and/or potassium supplements should be given with the expectation that both can be discontinued soon after rehydration is complete. Plasma urea/creatinine should be monitored closely for signs of acute renal failure.

Once the patient has been rehydrated, an MRI of the brain and tests of anterior pituitary function should be performed to look for the cause and collateral defects in other hypothalamic functions. A long-term management plan to prevent or minimize recurrence of the fluid and electrolyte imbalance should also be developed. This should include a practical method that the patient can use to regulate fluid intake in accordance with day-to-day variations in water balance. The most effective way to do this is to prescribe desmopressin to control DI, if it is present, and teach the patient how to use day-to-day changes in body weight as a guide for adjusting fluid intake. It may also be possible to adjust fluid intake by monitoring day-to-day changes in serum sodium using equipment recently developed for home use. Prescribing a constant fluid intake is ineffective and potentially dangerous because it does not take into account the large, uncontrolled variations in insensible loss that inevitably result from changes in ambient temperature and physical activity.

EXCESS VASOPRESSIN SECRETION AND ACTION

HYPONATREMIA

Clinical Characteristics

Excessive secretion or action of AVP results in the production of decreased volumes of more highly concentrated urine. If not accompanied by a commensurate reduction in fluid intake or an increase in insensible loss, the reduction in urine output results in excess water retention with expansion and dilution of all body fluids. In some patients, excessive intake results from inappropriate thirst. If the hyponatremia develops gradually or has been present for more than a few days, it may be largely asymptomatic. However, if it develops acutely, it is almost always accompanied by symptoms and signs of water intoxication that may include mild headache, confusion, anorexia, nausea, vomiting, coma, and convulsions. Severe hyponatremia may be lethal.

Etiology

Hyponatremia and impaired urinary dilution can be caused by a primary defect in the regulation of AVP secretion or action or can be secondary to a recognized nonosmotic stimulus such as hypovolemia, hypotension, nausea, or glucocorticoid deficiency. The primary forms are generally referred to as SIAD. They have many different causes, including ectopic production of AVP by lung cancer or other neoplasms; eutopic release by various diseases or drugs; and exogenous administration of AVP, desmopressin, or large doses of oxytocin (Table 3-3). The ectopic forms result from abnormal expression of the AVP-NPII gene by primary or metastatic malignancies. The eutopic forms occur most often in patients with acute infections or strokes but have also been associated with many other diseases and injuries. The mechanisms by which these diseases disrupt osmoregulation are not known. The defect in osmoregulation can take any of four distinct forms (Fig. 3-5). In one of the most common (reset osmostat), AVP secretion remains fully responsive to changes in plasma osmolarity/sodium, but the threshold, or set point, of the osmoregulatory system is abnormally low. These patients differ from those with the other types of osmoregulatory defect in that they are able to maximally suppress plasma AVP and dilute their urine if their fluid intake is high enough to reduce their plasma osmolarity/sodium to the new set point. Another, smaller subgroup (~10% of the total) has inappropriate antidiuresis without a demonstrable defect in the osmoregulation of plasma AVP (Fig. 3-5). These patients may have some intrarenal defect in the regulation of antidiuresis. In a few patients, this has been traced to a constitutively activating mutation of the V_2 receptor.

TABLE 3-3

CAUSES OF SYNDROME OF INAPPROPRIATE ANTIDIURESIS (SIAD)

Neoplasms	Neurologic
Carcinomas	Guillain-Barré syndrome
Lung	Multiple sclerosis
Duodenum	Delirium tremens
Pancreas	Amyotrophic lateral sclerosis
Ovary	Hydrocephalus
Bladder, ureter	Psychosis
Other neoplasms	Peripheral neuropathy
Thymoma	Congenital malformations
Mesothelioma	Agenesis corpus callosum
Bronchial adenoma	Cleft lip/palate
Carcinoid	Other midline defects
Gangliocytoma	Metabolic
Ewing's sarcoma	Acute intermittent porphyria
Head trauma (closed and penetrating)	Pulmonary
Infections	Asthma
Pneumonia, bacterial or viral	Pneumothorax
Abscess, lung or brain	Positive-pressure respiration
Cavitation (aspergillosis)	Drugs
Tuberculosis, lung or brain	Vasopressin or desmopressin
Meningitis, bacterial or viral	Chlorpropamide
Encephalitis	Oxytocin, high dose
AIDS	Vincristine
Vascular	Carbamazepine
Cerebrovascular occlusions, hemorrhage	Nicotine

The secondary forms of osmotically inappropriate antidiuresis also have multiple causes and are usually subdivided into three types, depending on the nature of the abnormal stimulus and the state of extracellular fluid volume. Type I occurs in sodium-retaining, edema-forming states such as congestive heart failure, cirrhosis, or nephrosis and is associated with marked hypervolemia of the extravascular compartment. The antidiuresis is thought to be due to stimulation of AVP secretion by a large reduction in "effective" blood volume caused by low cardiac output and/or redistribution of plasma from the intravascular to the interstitial space. Type II occurs in sodium-depleted states such as severe gastroenteritis, diuretic abuse, or mineralocorticoid deficiency and is due to stimulation of AVP by a large reduction in blood volume and/or pressure. In both types, the abnormal AVP secretion appears to be due to resetting of the osmostat similar to that in some patients with SIAD. Type IIIA results from stimulation of AVP secretion by nausea or isolated glucocorticoid deficiency. In this case, the hyponatremia is not associated with overt hyper- or hypovolemia and can closely resemble SIAD type IIIB, in which extracellular volume also appears to be normal (Table 3-4). However, they must be distinguished because their treatments differ. In type IIIA, the excess AVP secretion can be corrected quickly and completely by treatments (antiemetics or glucocorticoids) that are not useful in type IIIB SIAD.

Pathophysiology

When osmotic suppression of antidiuresis is impaired for any reason, significant expansion and dilution of body fluids occurs only if water intake exceeds the rate of insensible and urinary losses. The excess water intake is sometimes due to an associated defect in the osmoregulation of thirst but can also be psychogenic or iatrogenic, including the administration of IV fluids.

In SIAD, the excessive retention of water has two other effects. First, by increasing extracellular volume, it increases glomerular filtration and atrial natriuretic hormone, suppresses plasma renin activity, and increases urinary sodium excretion. This natriuresis serves to counteract the extracellular hypervolemia but aggravates the hyponatremia. Second, by producing hyponatremia, it increases intracellular volume in all organs including the brain. This swelling increases intracranial pressure, which is probably responsible for the symptoms of acute

TABLE 3-4

DIFFERENTIAL DIAGNOSIS OF HYPONATREMIA BASED ON CLINICAL ASSESSMENT OF EXTRACELLULAR FLUID VOLUME (ECFV)

CLINICAL FINDINGS	TYPE I, HYPERVOLEMIC	TYPE II, HYPOVOLEMIC	TYPE IIIA, EUVOLEMIC	TYPE IIIB, EUVOLEMIC (SIAD)
History				
CHF, cirrhosis, or nephrosis	Yes	No	No	No
Salt and water loss	No	Yes	No	No
ACTH–cortisol deficiency and/or nausea and vomiting	No	No	Yes	No
Physical examination				
Generalized edema, ascites	Yes	No	No	No
Postural hypotension	Maybe	Maybe	Maybe[a]	No
Laboratory				
BUN, creatinine	High-normal	High-normal	Low-normal	Low-normal
Uric acid	High-normal	High-normal	Low-normal	Low-normal
Serum potassium	Low-normal	Low-normal[b]	Normal[c]	Normal
Serum albumin	Low-normal	High-normal	Normal	Normal
Serum cortisol	Normal-high	Normal-high[d]	Low[e]	Normal
Plasma renin activity	High	High	Low[f]	Low
Urinary sodium (meq unit of time)[g]	Low	Low[h]	High[i]	High[i]

[a]Postural hypotension may occur in secondary (ACTH-dependent) adrenal insufficiency even though ECFV and aldosterone are usually normal.
[b]Serum potassium may be high if hypovolemia is due to aldosterone deficiency.
[c]Serum potassium may be low if vomiting causes alkalosis.
[d]Serum cortisol is low if hypovolemia is due to primary adrenal insufficiency (Addison's disease).
[e]Serum cortisol will be normal or high if the cause is nausea and vomiting rather than secondary (ACTH-dependent) adrenal insufficiency.
[f]Plasma renin activity may be high if the cause is secondary (ACTH) adrenal insufficiency.
[g]Urinary sodium should be expressed as the *rate of excretion* rather than the concentration. In a hyponatremic adult, an excretion rate >25 meq/d (or 25 μeq/mg of creatinine) could be considered high.
[h]The rate of urinary sodium excretion may be high if the hypovolemia is due to diuretic abuse, primary adrenal insufficiency, or other causes of renal sodium wasting.
[i]The rate of urinary sodium excretion may be low if intake is curtailed by symptoms or treatment.

Note: SIAD, syndrome of inappropriate antidiuresis; CHF, congestive heart failure; ACTH, adrenocorticotropic hormone; BUN, blood urea nitrogen.

water intoxication. Within a few days, this swelling may be counteracted by inactivation or elimination of intracellular solutes, resulting in the remission of symptoms even though the hyponatremia persists. The pathophysiology of type IIIA (euvolemic) hyponatremia is probably similar to SIAD.

In type I (edematous) or type II (hypovolemic) hyponatremia, the antidiuretic effect of hemodynamically induced AVP release is enhanced by decreased distal delivery of glomerular filtrate that results from increased reabsorption of sodium in proximal nephrons. Again, if the marked reduction in urine output that ensues is not associated with a commensurate reduction in water intake or an increase in insensible loss, body fluids are expanded and diluted, resulting in hyponatremia. Unlike SIAD, however, glomerular filtration is reduced and plasma renin activity and aldosterone are elevated due to the hypovolemic stimulus. Thus, urinary sodium is low (unless sodium reabsorption is impaired by a diuretic) and the hyponatremia is usually accompanied by hypokalemia, azotemia, and hyperuricemia. The sodium retention is an appropriate compensatory response to severe volume and sodium depletion present in type II but is inappropriate and deleterious in type I since body sodium and extracellular volume are already markedly increased.

Differential Diagnosis

SIAD is a diagnosis of exclusion that can usually be accomplished with routine historic, physical, and laboratory information. In a patient with hyponatremia, the possibility of simple dilution caused by an osmotically driven shift of water from the intracellular to the extracellular space should be excluded by measuring plasma glucose and/or plasma osmolarity. If the glucose is not elevated enough to account for the hyponatremia [serum sodium decreases ~1 meq/L for each rise in glucose of 2.0 mmol/L (36 mg/dL)] and/or plasma osmolarity is reduced in proportion to sodium (each decrease in serum sodium of 1 meq/L should reduce plasma osmolarity by ~2 mosmol/L), the hyponatremia is "true" and can be typed or classified by standard clinical indicators of the extracellular fluid volume (Table 3-4). If these findings are ambiguous or contradictory, measuring the rate of urinary sodium excretion or plasma renin activity may be helpful. These measurements can be misleading, however, if SIAD is stable or resolving or if the patient has type II hyponatremia due to a primary defect in renal conservation of sodium, surreptitious diuretic abuse, or hyporeninemic hypoaldosteronism. The latter may be suspected if serum potassium is elevated instead of low, as is usually seen in types I and II hyponatremia. Measurements of plasma AVP are currently of no diagnostic value since the abnormalities are similar in all three types of hyponatremia. In patients who fulfill the clinical criteria for type III (euvolemic) hyponatremia, plasma cortisol should also be measured to rule out secondary adrenal insufficiency. If cortisol is normal and there is no history of nausea/vomiting or other obvious cause for type III hyponatremia, a careful search for occult lung cancer should also be undertaken.

℞ Treatment: HYPONATREMIA

The management of patients with hyponatremia differs depending not only on the type but also on the severity and duration of symptoms. In a patient with SIAD type IIIB and few symptoms, the objective is to gradually reduce body water by restricting total fluid intake to less than the sum of urinary and insensible losses. Because the water derived from food (300–700 mL/d) usually approximates basal insensible losses in adults, total discretionary intake (all liquids) should be at least 500 mL less than urinary output. If achieved, this deficit usually reduces body water and increases serum sodium by about 1–2% per day. If more rapid correction of the hyponatremia is desired to eliminate severe symptoms or signs, the fluid restriction can be supplemented by IV infusion of hypertonic (3%) saline. This treatment has the advantage of correcting the sodium deficiency that is partly responsible for the hyponatremia and also produces a solute diuresis that serves to remove some of the excess water. However, if hypertonic saline is given too rapidly in a patient in whom hyponatremia has been present for >24–48 h, it also has the potential to produce central pontine myelinolysis, an acute, potentially fatal neurologic syndrome characterized by quadriparesis, ataxia, and abnormal extraocular movements. The risk of this complication can be minimized by observing several precautions: 3% saline should be infused at a rate ≤0.05 mL/kg body weight per min; the effect should be monitored continuously by STAT measurements of serum sodium at least once every 2 h; and the infusion should be stopped as soon as serum sodium increases by 12 mmol/L or to 130 mmol/L, whichever comes first. Urinary output should also be monitored continuously since SIAD can remit spontaneously at any time, resulting in an acute water diuresis that greatly accelerates the rate of rise in serum sodium produced by fluid restriction and 3% saline infusion.

In chronic, persistent SIAD, the hyponatremia can be corrected by treatment with demeclocycline, 150–300 mg PO three or four times a day, or fludrocortisone, 0.05–0.2 mg PO twice a day. The effect of the demeclocycline manifests in 7–14 days and is due to production of a reversible form of nephrogenic DI. Potential side effects include phototoxicity and azotemia. The effect of fludrocortisone also requires 1–2 weeks and is partly due to increased retention of sodium and possibly inhibition of thirst. It also increases urinary potassium excretion, which may require replacement through dietary adjustments or supplements. Fludrocortisone may induce hypertension, occasionally necessitating discontinuation of the treatment.

Nonpeptide AVP antagonists that block the antidiuretic effect of AVP have also been used experimentally in acute and chronic SIAD. They produce a dose-dependent increase in urinary free-water excretion, which, if combined with a modest restriction of fluid intake, gradually reduce body water and correct the hyponatremia. These studies have shown no adverse effect but, like hypertonic saline, the antagonists probably carry the risk of inducing osmotic demyelinization if the hyponatremia is corrected too rapidly. One of them, a combined V_2/V_{1a} antagonist (Conivaptan), has recently been approved for short-term in-hospital treatment of SIAD, and other antagonists are currently in phase 3 trials.

In euvolemic hyponatremia due to protracted nausea and vomiting or isolated glucocorticoid deficiency (type IIIA), all abnormalities can be corrected quickly and completely by giving an antiemetic or hydrocortisone. As with other treatments, care must be taken to ensure that serum sodium does not rise too quickly or too far.

In type I hyponatremia, fluid restriction is also appropriate and somewhat effective, if it can be maintained. However, infusion of hypertonic saline is contraindicated because it further increases total body sodium and edema and may precipitate cardiovascular decompensation. Preliminary studies with antagonists of V_2 receptors indicate that they are almost as effective in type I hyponatremia as they are in SIAD, but they have not yet been approved for this indication.

In type II hyponatremia, the defect in AVP secretion and water balance can usually be corrected easily and quickly by stopping the loss of sodium and water and/or replacing the deficits PO or IV infusion of normal or hypertonic saline. As with the treatment of other forms of hyponatremia, care must be taken to ensure that plasma sodium does not increase too rapidly. Fluid restriction and administration of AVP antagonists are contraindicated in type II as they would only aggravate the underlying volume depletion and could result in hemodynamic collapse.

FURTHER READINGS

BICHET DG: Hereditary polyuric disorders: New concepts and differential diagnosis. Semin Nephrol 26:224, 2006

CHITTURI S et al: Utility of AVP gene testing in familial neurohypophyseal diabetes insipidus. Clin Endocrinol (Oxf) 69:926, 2008

CHRISTENSEN JH, RITTIG S: Familial neurohypophyseal diabetes insipidus—an update. Semin Nephrol 26:209, 2006

DECAUX G et al: Non-peptide arginine-vasopressin antagonists: The vaptans. Lancet 371:1624, 2008

FELDMAN BJ et al: Nephrogenic syndrome of inappropriate antidiuresis. N Engl J Med 352:1884, 2005

LIAMIS G et al: A review of drug-induced hyponatremia. Am J Kidney Dis 52:144, 2008

ROBERTSON GL: Antidiuretic hormone: Normal and disordered function. Endocrinol Metab Clin North Am 30:671, 2001

SHARIF-NAEINI R et al: Contribution of TRPV channels to osmosensory transduction, thirst, and vasopressin release. Kidney Int 73:811, 2008

TORRES VE: Role of vasopressin antagonists. Clin J Am Soc Nephrol 3:1212, 2008

VERBALIS JG (ed): Hyponatremia: New understanding, new therapy. Am J Med 119(Suppl 1): 1, 2006

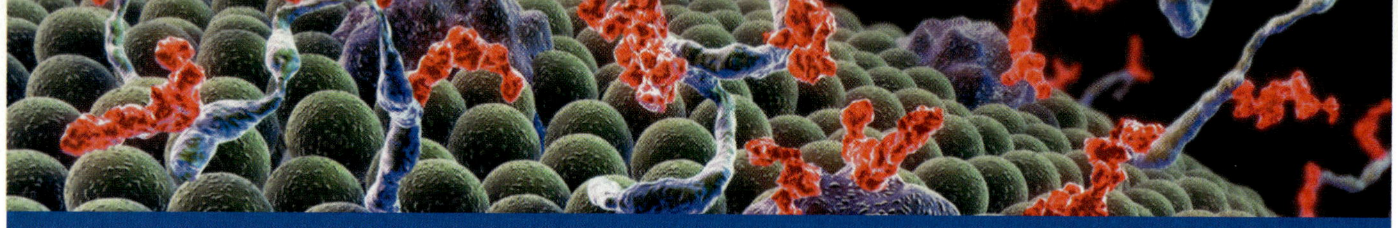

CHAPTER 4

DISORDERS OF THE THYROID GLAND

J. Larry Jameson ■ Anthony P. Weetman

The thyroid gland produces two related hormones, thyroxine (T_4) and triiodothyronine (T_3) (**Fig. 4-1**). Acting through nuclear receptors, these hormones play a critical role in cell differentiation during development and help maintain thermogenic and metabolic homeostasis in the adult. Autoimmune disorders of the thyroid gland can either stimulate the overproduction of thyroid hormones (*thyrotoxicosis*) or cause glandular destruction and hormone deficiency (*hypothyroidism*). In addition, benign nodules and various forms of thyroid cancer are relatively common and amenable to detection by physical examination.

ANATOMY AND DEVELOPMENT

The thyroid (Greek *thyreos*, "shield," plus *eidos*, "form") consists of two lobes that are connected by an isthmus. It is located anterior to the trachea between the cricoid cartilage and the suprasternal notch. The normal thyroid is 12–20 g in size, highly vascular, and soft in consistency. Four parathyroid glands, which produce parathyroid hormone (Chap. 27), are located posterior to each pole of the thyroid. The recurrent laryngeal nerves traverse the lateral borders of the thyroid gland and must be identified during thyroid surgery to avoid vocal cord paralysis.

The thyroid gland develops from the floor of the primitive pharynx during the third week of gestation. The developing gland migrates along the thyroglossal duct to reach its final location in the neck. This feature accounts for the rare ectopic location of thyroid tissue at the base of the tongue (lingual thyroid) as well as the occurrence of thyroglossal duct cysts along this developmental tract. Thyroid hormone synthesis normally begins at about 11 weeks' gestation.

Neural crest derivatives from the ultimobranchial body give rise to thyroid medullary C cells that produce calcitonin, a calcium-lowering hormone. The C cells are interspersed throughout the thyroid gland, although

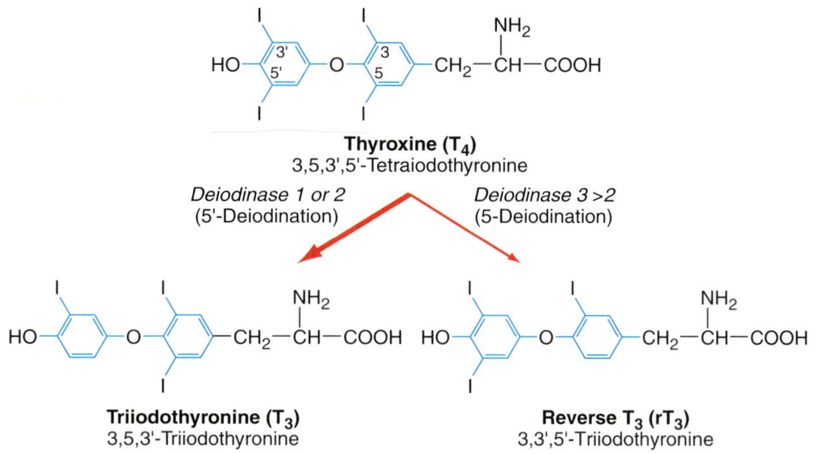

FIGURE 4-1

Structures of thyroid hormones. Thyroxine (T_4) contains four iodine atoms. Deiodination leads to production of the potent hormone triiodothyronine (T_3), or the inactive hormone reverse T_3.

their density is greatest in the juncture of the upper one-third and lower two-thirds of the gland.

Thyroid gland development is orchestrated by the coordinated expression of several developmental transcription factors. Thyroid transcription factor (TTF)-1, TTF-2, and paired homeobox-8 (PAX-8) are expressed selectively, but not exclusively, in the thyroid gland. In combination, they dictate thyroid cell development and the induction of thyroid-specific genes such as thyroglobulin (Tg), thyroid peroxidase (TPO), the sodium iodide symporter (NIS), and the thyroid-stimulating hormone receptor (TSH-R). Mutations in these developmental transcription factors or their downstream target genes are rare causes of thyroid agenesis or dyshormonogenesis, though the causes of most forms of congenital hypothyroidism remain unknown (Table 4-1). Because congenital hypothyroidism occurs in approximately 1 in 4000 newborns, neonatal screening is now performed in most industrialized countries. Transplacental passage of maternal thyroid hormone occurs before the fetal thyroid gland begins to function and provides partial support to a fetus with congenital hypothyroidism. Early thyroid hormone replacement in newborns with congenital hypothyroidism prevents potentially severe developmental abnormalities.

The thyroid gland consists of numerous spherical follicles composed of thyroid follicular cells that surround secreted colloid, a proteinaceous fluid containing large amounts of thyroglobulin, the protein precursor of thyroid hormones

TABLE 4-1

GENETIC CAUSES OF CONGENITAL HYPOTHYROIDISM

DEFECTIVE GENE PROTEIN	INHERITANCE	CONSEQUENCES
PROP-1	Autosomal recessive	Combined pituitary hormone deficiencies with preservation of adrenocorticotropic hormone
PIT-1	Autosomal recessive Autosomal dominant	Combined deficiencies of growth hormone, prolactin, thyroid-stimulating hormone (TSH)
TSHβ	Autosomal recessive	TSH deficiency
TTF-1 (TITF-1)	Autosomal dominant	Variable thyroid hypoplasia, choreoathetosis, pulmonary problems
TTF-2 (FOXE-1)	Autosomal recessive	Thyroid agenesis, choanal atresia, spiky hair
PAX-8	Autosomal dominant	Thyroid dysgenesis
TSH-receptor	Autosomal recessive	Resistance to TSH
$G_s\alpha$ (Albright hereditary osteodystrophy)	Autosomal dominant	Resistance to TSH
Na^+/I^- symporter	Autosomal recessive	Inability to transport iodide
THOX2	Autosomal dominant	Organification defect
Thyroid peroxidase	Autosomal recessive	Defective organification of iodide
Thyroglobulin	Autosomal recessive	Defective synthesis of thyroid hormone
Pendrin	Autosomal recessive	Pendred's syndrome: sensorineural deafness and partial organification defect in thyroid
Dehalogenase	Autosomal recessive	Loss of iodide reutilization

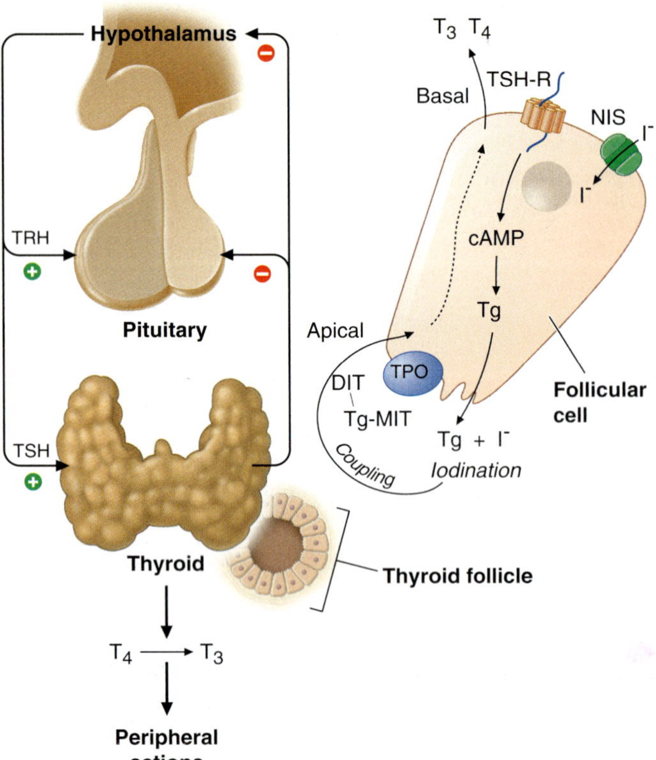

FIGURE 4-2

Regulation of thyroid hormone synthesis. ***Left***. Thyroid hormones thyroxine (T_4) and triiodothyronine (T_3) feed back to inhibit hypothalamic production of thyrotropin-releasing hormone (TRH) and pituitary production of thyroid-stimulating hormone (TSH). TSH stimulates thyroid gland production of T_4 and T_3. ***Right***. Thyroid follicles are formed by thyroid epithelial cells surrounding proteinaceous colloid, which contains thyroglobulin. Follicular cells, which are polarized, synthesize thyroglobulin and carry out thyroid hormone biosynthesis (see text for details). TSH-R, thyroid-stimulating hormone receptor; Tg, thyroglobulin; NIS, sodium-iodide symporter; TPO, thyroid peroxidase; DIT, diiodotyrosine; MIT, monoiodotyrosine.

(Fig. 4-2). The thyroid follicular cells are polarized—the basolateral surface is apposed to the bloodstream and an apical surface faces the follicular lumen. Increased demand for thyroid hormone is regulated by thyroid-stimulating hormone (TSH), which binds to its receptor on the basolateral surface of the follicular cells, leading to Tg reabsorption from the follicular lumen and proteolysis within the cell to yield thyroid hormones for secretion into the bloodstream.

REGULATION OF THE THYROID AXIS

TSH, secreted by the thyrotrope cells of the anterior pituitary, plays a pivotal role in control of the thyroid axis and serves as the most useful physiologic marker of thyroid hormone action. TSH is a 31-kDa hormone composed of α and β subunits; the α subunit is common to the other glycoprotein hormones [luteinizing hormone, follicle-stimulating hormone, human chorionic gonadotropin (hCG)], whereas the TSH β subunit is unique to TSH. The extent and nature of carbohydrate modification are modulated by thyrotropin-releasing hormone (TRH) stimulation and influence the biologic activity of the hormone.

The thyroid axis is a classic example of an endocrine feedback loop. Hypothalamic TRH stimulates pituitary production of TSH, which, in turn, stimulates thyroid hormone synthesis and secretion. Thyroid hormones feed back to inhibit TRH and TSH production (Fig. 4-2). The "set point" in this axis is established by TSH. TRH is the major positive regulator of TSH synthesis and secretion. Peak TSH secretion occurs ~15 min after administration of exogenous TRH. Dopamine, glucocorticoids, and somatostatin suppress TSH but are not of major physiologic importance except when these agents are administered in pharmacologic doses. Reduced levels of thyroid hormone increase basal TSH production and enhance TRH-mediated stimulation of TSH. High thyroid hormone levels rapidly and directly suppress TSH gene expression secretion and inhibit TRH stimulation of TSH, indicating that thyroid hormones are the dominant regulator of TSH production. Like other pituitary hormones, TSH is released in a pulsatile manner and exhibits a diurnal rhythm; its highest levels occur at night. However, these TSH excursions are modest in comparison to those of other pituitary hormones, in part because TSH has a relatively long plasma half-life (50 min). Consequently, single measurements of TSH are adequate for assessing its circulating level. TSH is measured using immunoradiometric assays that are highly sensitive and specific. These assays readily distinguish between normal and suppressed TSH values; thus, TSH can be used for the diagnosis of hyperthyroidism (low TSH) as well as hypothyroidism (high TSH).

THYROID HORMONE SYNTHESIS, METABOLISM, AND ACTION

THYROID HORMONE SYNTHESIS

Thyroid hormones are derived from Tg, a large iodinated glycoprotein. After secretion into the thyroid follicle, Tg is iodinated on tyrosine residues that are subsequently coupled via an ether linkage. Reuptake of Tg into the thyroid follicular cell allows proteolysis and the release of newly synthesized T_4 and T_3.

Iodine Metabolism and Transport

Iodide uptake is a critical first step in thyroid hormone synthesis. Ingested iodine is bound to serum proteins, particularly albumin. Unbound iodine is excreted in the urine. The thyroid gland extracts iodine from the circulation in a highly efficient manner. For example, 10–25% of radioactive tracer (e.g., ^{123}I) is taken up by the normal thyroid gland over 24 h; this value can rise to 70–90% in Graves' disease. Iodide uptake is mediated by the Na^+/I^- symporter (NIS), which is expressed at the basolateral membrane of thyroid follicular cells. NIS is most highly expressed in the thyroid gland, but low levels are present in the salivary glands, lactating breast, and placenta. The iodide transport mechanism is highly regulated, allowing adaptation to variations in dietary supply. Low iodine levels increase the amount of NIS and stimulate uptake, whereas high iodine levels suppress NIS expression and uptake. The selective expression of NIS in the thyroid allows isotopic scanning, treatment of hyperthyroidism, and ablation of thyroid cancer with radioisotopes of iodine, without significant effects on other organs. Mutation of the *NIS* gene is a rare cause of congenital hypothyroidism, underscoring its importance in thyroid hormone synthesis. Another iodine transporter, pendrin, is located on the apical surface of thyroid cells and mediates iodine efflux into the lumen. Mutation of the *PENDRIN* gene causes *Pendred syndrome*, a disorder characterized by defective organification of iodine, goiter, and sensorineural deafness.

Iodine deficiency is prevalent in many mountainous regions and in central Africa, central South America, and northern Asia (**Fig. 4-3**). The World Health Organization (WHO) estimates that about 2 billion people are iodine-deficient, based on urinary excretion data. In areas of relative iodine deficiency, there is an increased prevalence of goiter and, when deficiency is severe, hypothyroidism and cretinism. *Cretinism* is characterized by mental and growth retardation and occurs when children who live in iodine-deficient regions are not treated with iodine or thyroid hormone to restore normal thyroid hormone levels during early life. These children are often born to mothers with iodine deficiency, and it is likely that maternal thyroid hormone deficiency worsens the condition. Concomitant selenium deficiency may also contribute to the neurologic manifestations of cretinism. Iodine supplementation of salt, bread, and other food substances has markedly reduced the prevalence of cretinism. Unfortunately, however, iodine deficiency remains the most common cause of preventable mental deficiency, often because of societal resistance to food additives or the cost of supplementation. In addition to overt cretinism, mild iodine deficiency can lead to subtle reduction of IQ. Oversupply of iodine, through supplements or foods enriched in iodine (e.g., shellfish, kelp), is associated with an increased incidence of autoimmune thyroid disease. The recommended average daily intake of iodine is 150 μg/d for adults, 90–120 μg/d for children, and 200 μg/d for pregnant women. Urinary iodine is >10 μg/dL in iodine-sufficient populations.

Organification, Coupling, Storage, Release

After iodide enters the thyroid, it is trapped and transported to the apical membrane of thyroid follicular cells, where it is oxidized in an organification reaction that involves TPO and hydrogen peroxide. The reactive iodine atom is added to selected tyrosyl residues within Tg, a large (660 kDa) dimeric protein that consists of 2769 amino acids. The iodotyrosines in Tg are then coupled via an ether linkage in

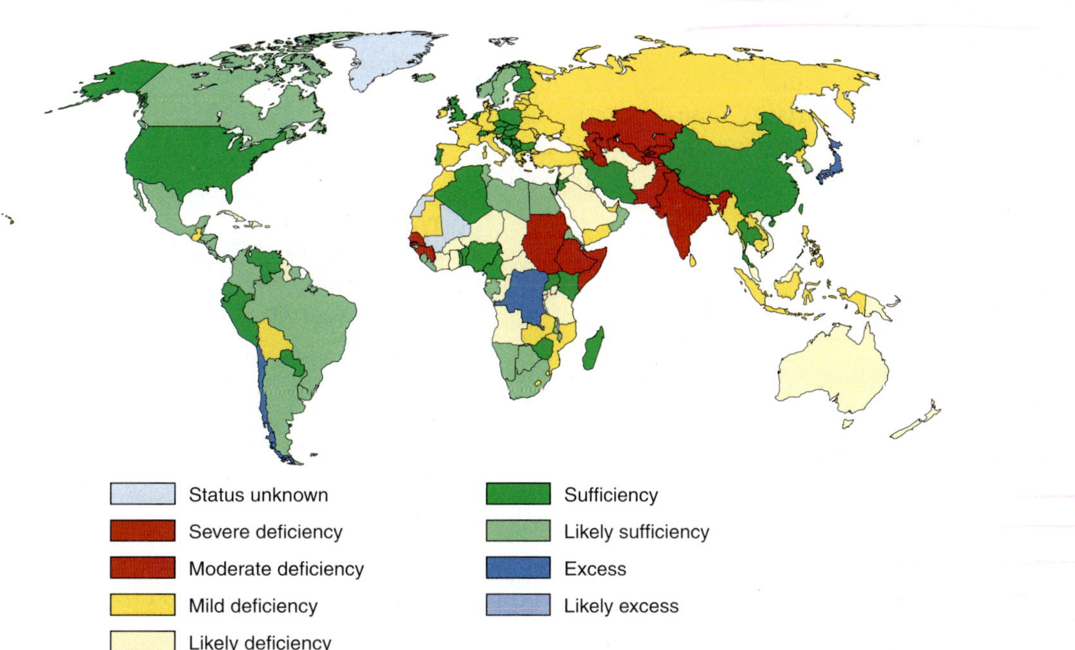

FIGURE 4-3

Worldwide iodine nutrition. Data are from the WHO and the International Council for the Control of Iodine Deficiency Disorders (*http://indorgs.virginia.edu/iccidd/mi/cidds.html*).

a reaction that is also catalyzed by TPO. Either T_4 or T_3 can be produced by this reaction, depending on the number of iodine atoms present in the iodotyrosines. After coupling, Tg is taken back into the thyroid cell, where it is processed in lysosomes to release T_4 and T_3. Uncoupled mono- and diiodotyrosines (MITs, DITs) are deiodinated by the enzyme dehalogenase, thereby recycling any iodide that is not converted into thyroid hormones.

Disorders of thyroid hormone synthesis are rare causes of congenital hypothyroidism. The vast majority of these disorders are due to recessive mutations in TPO or Tg, but defects have also been identified in the TSH-R, NIS, pendrin, hydrogen peroxide generation, and dehalogenase. Because of the biosynthetic defect, the gland is incapable of synthesizing adequate amounts of hormone, leading to increased TSH and a large goiter.

TSH Action

TSH regulates thyroid gland function through the TSH-R, a seven-transmembrane G protein–coupled receptor (GPCR). The TSH-R is coupled to the α subunit of stimulatory G protein ($G_s\alpha$), which activates adenylyl cyclase, leading to increased production of cyclic AMP. TSH also stimulates phosphatidylinositol turnover by activating phospholipase C. The functional role of the TSH-R is exemplified by the consequences of naturally occurring mutations. Recessive loss-of-function mutations cause thyroid hypoplasia and congenital hypothyroidism. Dominant gain-of-function mutations cause sporadic or familial hyperthyroidism that is characterized by goiter, thyroid cell hyperplasia, and autonomous function. Most of these activating mutations occur in the transmembrane domain of the receptor. They are thought to mimic the conformational changes induced by TSH binding or the interactions of thyroid-stimulating immunoglobulins (TSIs) in Graves' disease. Activating TSH-R mutations also occur as somatic events and lead to clonal selection and expansion of the affected thyroid follicular cell.

Other Factors That Influence Hormone Synthesis and Release

Although TSH is the dominant hormonal regulator of thyroid gland growth and function, a variety of growth factors, most produced locally in the thyroid gland, also influence thyroid hormone synthesis. These include insulin-like growth factor I (IGF-I), epidermal growth factor, transforming growth factor β (TGF-β), endothelins, and various cytokines. The quantitative roles of these factors are not well understood, but they are important in selected disease states. In acromegaly, for example, increased levels of growth hormone and IGF-I are associated with goiter and predisposition to multinodular goiter (MNG). Certain cytokines and interleukins (ILs) produced in association with autoimmune thyroid disease induce thyroid growth, whereas others lead to apoptosis. Iodine deficiency increases thyroid blood flow and upregulates the NIS, stimulating more efficient uptake. Excess iodide transiently inhibits thyroid iodide organification, a phenomenon known as the *Wolff-Chaikoff effect*. In individuals with a normal thyroid, the gland escapes from this inhibitory effect and iodide organification resumes; the suppressive action of high iodide may persist, however, in patients with underlying autoimmune thyroid disease.

THYROID HORMONE TRANSPORT AND METABOLISM

Serum Binding Proteins

T_4 is secreted from the thyroid gland in about twentyfold excess over T_3 (Table 4-2). Both hormones are bound to plasma proteins, including thyroxine-binding globulin (TBG); transthyretin (TTR, formerly known as thyroxine-binding prealbumin, or TBPA); and albumin. The plasma-binding proteins increase the pool of circulating hormone, delay hormone clearance, and may modulate hormone delivery to selected tissue sites. The concentration of TBG is relatively low (1–2 mg/dL), but because of its high affinity for thyroid hormones ($T_4 > T_3$), it carries about 80% of the bound hormones. Albumin has relatively low affinity for thyroid hormones but has a high plasma concentration (~3.5 g/dL), and it binds up to 10% of T_4 and 30% of T_3. TTR carries about 10% of T_4 but little T_3.

When the effects of the various binding proteins are combined, approximately 99.98% of T_4 and 99.7% of T_3 are protein-bound. Because T_3 is less tightly bound than T_4, the fraction of unbound T_3 is greater than unbound T_4, but there is less unbound T_3 in the circulation because it is produced in smaller amounts and cleared more rapidly than T_4. The unbound, or free, concentrations of the hormones are $\sim 2 \times 10^{-11}$ *M* for T_4 and $\sim 6 \times 10^{-12}$ *M* for T_3, which

TABLE 4-2

CHARACTERISTICS OF CIRCULATING T_4 AND T_3

HORMONE PROPERTY	T_4	T_3
Serum concentrations		
Total hormone	8 µg/dL	0.14 µg/dL
Fraction of total hormone in the free form	0.02%	0.3%
Free (unbound) hormone	21×10^{-12} *M*	6×10^{-12} *M*
Serum half-life	7 d	0.75 d
Fraction directly from the thyroid	100%	20%
Production rate, including peripheral conversion	90 µg/d	32 µg/d
Intracellular hormone fraction	~20%	~70%
Relative metabolic potency	0.3	1
Receptor binding	10^{-10} *M*	10^{-11} *M*

roughly correspond to the thyroid hormone receptor binding constants for these hormones (see below). The unbound hormone is thought to be biologically available to tissues, although the discovery of megalin as a cellular transporter of protein-bound steroids raises the possibility of distinct transport systems for bound and unbound hormones. Nonetheless, the homeostatic mechanisms that regulate the thyroid axis are directed toward maintenance of normal concentrations of unbound hormones.

Abnormalities of Thyroid Hormone–Binding Proteins

A number of inherited and acquired abnormalities affect thyroid hormone–binding proteins. X-linked TBG deficiency is associated with very low levels of total T_4 and T_3. However, because unbound hormone levels are normal, patients are euthyroid and TSH levels are normal. It is important to recognize this disorder to avoid efforts to normalize total T_4 levels, as this leads to thyrotoxicosis and is futile because of rapid hormone clearance in the absence of TBG. TBG levels are elevated by estrogen, which increases sialylation and delays TBG clearance. Consequently, in women who are pregnant or taking estrogen-containing contraceptives, elevated TBG increases total T_4 and T_3 levels; however, unbound T_4 and T_3 levels are normal. These features explain why women with hypothyroidism require increased amounts of L-thyroxine replacement when TBG levels are increased by pregnancy or estrogen treatment. Mutations in TBG, TTR, and albumin may increase the binding affinity for T_4 and/or T_3 and cause disorders known as *euthyroid hyperthyroxinemia* or *familial dysalbuminemic hyperthyroxinemia* (FDH) (Table 4-3). These disorders result in increased total T_4 and/or T_3, but unbound hormone levels are normal. The familial nature of the disorders, and the fact that TSH levels are normal rather than suppressed, should suggest this diagnosis. Unbound hormone levels (ideally measured by dialysis) are normal in FDH. The diagnosis can be confirmed by using tests that measure the affinities of radiolabeled hormone binding to specific transport proteins or by performing DNA sequence analyses of the abnormal transport protein genes.

Certain medications, such as salicylates and salsalate, can displace thyroid hormones from circulating binding proteins. Although these drugs transiently perturb the thyroid axis by increasing free thyroid hormone levels, TSH is suppressed until a new steady state is reached, thereby restoring euthyroidism. Circulating factors associated with acute illness may also displace thyroid hormone from binding proteins (see "Sick Euthyroid Syndrome," later).

Deiodinases

T_4 may be thought of as a precursor for the more potent T_3. T_4 is converted to T_3 by the deiodinase enzymes

TABLE 4-3

CONDITIONS ASSOCIATED WITH EUTHYROID HYPERTHYROXINEMIA

DISORDER	CAUSE	TRANSMISSION	CHARACTERISTICS
Familial dysalbuminemic hyperthyroxinemia (FDH)	Albumin mutations, usually R218H	AD	Increased T_4 Normal unbound T_4 Rarely increased T_3
TBG			
Familial excess	Increased TBG production	XL	Increased total T_4, T_3 Normal unbound T_4, T_3
Acquired excess	Medications (estrogen), pregnancy, cirrhosis, hepatitis	Acquired	Increased total T_4, T_3 Normal unbound T_4, T_3
Transthyretin[a]			
Excess	Islet tumors	Acquired	Usually normal T_4, T_3
Mutations	Increased affinity for T_4 or T_3	AD	Increased total T_4, T_3 Normal unbound T_4, T_3
Medications: propranolol, ipodate, iopanoic acid, amiodarone	Decreased $T_4 \rightarrow T_3$ conversion	Acquired	Increased T_4 Decreased T_3 Normal or increased TSH
Sick euthyroid syndrome	Acute illness, especially psychiatric disorders	Acquired	Transiently increased unbound T_4 Decreased TSH T_4 and T_3 may also be decreased (see text)
Resistance to thyroid hormone (RTH)	Thyroid hormone receptor β mutations	AD	Increased unbound T_4, T_3 Normal or increased TSH Some patients clinically thyrotoxic

[a]Also known as thyroxine-binding prealbumin, TBPA.

Note: AD, autosomal dominant; TBG, thyroxine-binding globulin; TSH, thyroid-stimulating hormone; XL, X-linked.

(Fig. 4-1). Type I deiodinase, which is located primarily in thyroid, liver, and kidney, has a relatively low affinity for T_4. Type II deiodinase has a higher affinity for T_4 and is found primarily in the pituitary gland, brain, brown fat, and thyroid gland. Expression of type II deiodinase allows it to regulate T_3 concentrations locally, a property that may be important in the context of levothyroxine (T_4) replacement. Type II deiodinase is also regulated by thyroid hormone; hypothyroidism induces the enzyme, resulting in enhanced $T_4 \rightarrow T_3$ conversion in tissues such as brain and pituitary. $T_4 \rightarrow T_3$ conversion is impaired by fasting, systemic illness or acute trauma, oral contrast agents, and a variety of medications (e.g., propylthiouracil, propranolol, amiodarone, glucocorticoids). Type III deiodinase inactivates T_4 and T_3 and is the most important source of reverse T_3 (rT_3). Massive hemangiomas that express type III deiodinase are a rare cause of hypothyroidism in infants.

THYROID HORMONE ACTION

Thyroid Hormone Transport

Circulating thyroid hormones enter cells by passive diffusion and via the monocarboxylate 8 (MCT8) transporter that was identified in patients with multiple neurologic deficits and thyroid function abnormalities (low T4, high T3, and high TSH). After entering cells, thyroid hormones act primarily through nuclear receptors, although they also stimulate plasma membrane and mitochondrial enzymatic responses.

Nuclear Thyroid Hormone Receptors

Thyroid hormones bind with high affinity to nuclear *thyroid hormone receptors* (TRs) α and β. Both TRα and TRβ are expressed in most tissues, but their relative expression levels vary among organs; TRα is particularly abundant in brain, kidney, gonads, muscle, and heart, whereas TRβ expression is relatively high in the pituitary and liver. Both receptors are variably spliced to form unique isoforms. The TRβ2 isoform, which has a unique amino terminus, is selectively expressed in the hypothalamus and pituitary, where it plays a role in feedback control of the thyroid axis. The TRα2 isoform contains a unique carboxy terminus that precludes thyroid hormone binding; it may function to block the action of other TR isoforms.

The TRs contain a central DNA-binding domain and a C-terminal ligand-binding domain. They bind to specific DNA sequences, termed *thyroid response elements* (TREs), in the promoter regions of target genes (Fig. 4-4). The receptors bind as homodimers or, more commonly, as heterodimers with retinoic acid X receptors (RXRs) (Chap. 1). The activated receptor can either stimulate gene transcription (e.g., myosin heavy chain α) or inhibit

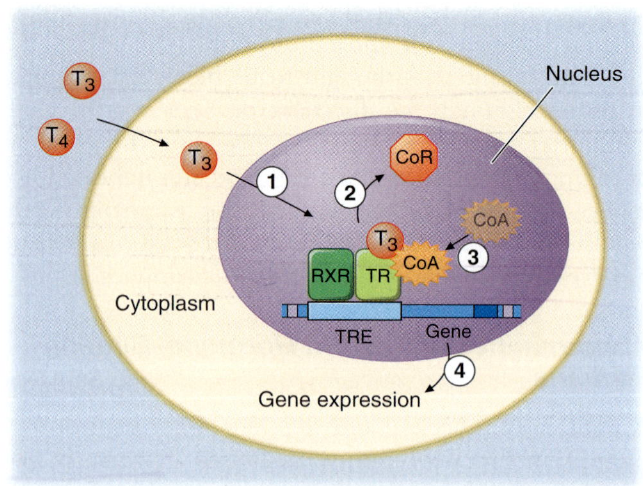

FIGURE 4-4

Mechanism of thyroid hormone receptor action. The thyroid hormone receptor (TR) and retinoid X receptor (RXR) form heterodimers that bind specifically to thyroid hormone response elements (TREs) in the promoter regions of target genes. In the absence of hormone, TR binds co-repressor (CoR) proteins that silence gene expression. The numbers refer to a series of ordered reactions that occur in response to thyroid hormone: (1) thyroxine (T_4) or triiodothyronine (T_3) enters the nucleus; (2) T_3 binding dissociates CoR from TR; (3) coactivators (CoA) are recruited to the T_3-bound receptor; (4) gene expression is altered.

transcription (e.g., TSH β-subunit gene), depending on the nature of the regulatory elements in the target gene.

Thyroid hormones (T_3 and T_4) bind with similar affinities to TRα and TRβ. However, structural differences in the ligand-binding domains provide the potential for developing receptor-selective agonists or antagonists. T_3 is bound with 10–15 times greater affinity than T_4, which explains its increased hormonal potency. Though T_4 is produced in excess of T_3, receptors are occupied mainly by T_3, reflecting $T_4 \rightarrow T_3$ conversion by peripheral tissues, greater T_3 bioavailability in the plasma, and receptors' greater affinity for T_3. After binding to TRs, thyroid hormone induces conformational changes in the receptors that modify its interactions with accessory transcription factors. In the absence of thyroid hormone binding, the aporeceptors bind to co-repressor proteins that inhibit gene transcription. Hormone binding dissociates the co-repressors and allows the recruitment of coactivators that enhance transcription. The discovery of TR interactions with co-repressors explains the fact that TR silences gene expression in the absence of hormone binding. Consequently, hormone deficiency has a profound effect on gene expression because it causes gene repression as well as loss of hormone-induced stimulation. This concept has been corroborated by the finding that targeted deletion of the TR genes in mice has a less pronounced phenotypic effect than hormone deficiency.

Thyroid Hormone Resistance

Resistance to thyroid hormone (RTH) is an autosomal dominant disorder characterized by elevated thyroid hormone levels and inappropriately normal or elevated TSH. Individuals with RTH do not, in general, exhibit signs and symptoms that are typical of hypothyroidism because hormone resistance is partial and is compensated by increased levels of thyroid hormone. The clinical features of RTH can include goiter, attention deficit disorder, mild reduction in IQ, delayed skeletal maturation, tachycardia, and impaired metabolic responses to thyroid hormone.

RTH is caused by mutations in the TRβ receptor gene. These mutations, located in restricted regions of the ligand-binding domain, cause loss of receptor function. However, because the mutant receptors retain the capacity to dimerize with RXRs, bind to DNA, and recruit co-repressor proteins, they function as antagonists of the remaining normal TRβ and TRα receptors. This property, referred to as "dominant negative" activity, explains the autosomal dominant mode of transmission. The diagnosis is suspected when unbound thyroid hormone levels are increased without suppression of TSH. Similar hormonal abnormalities are found in other affected family members, although the TRβ mutation arises de novo in about 20% of patients. DNA sequence analysis of the TRβ gene provides a definitive diagnosis. RTH must be distinguished from other causes of euthyroid hyperthyroxinemia (e.g., FDH) and inappropriate secretion of TSH by TSH-secreting pituitary adenomas (Chap. 2). In most patients, no treatment is indicated; the importance of making the diagnosis is to avoid inappropriate treatment of mistaken hyperthyroidism and to provide genetic counseling.

PHYSICAL EXAMINATION

In addition to the examination of the thyroid itself, the physical examination should include a search for signs of abnormal thyroid function and the extrathyroidal features of ophthalmopathy and dermopathy. Examination of the neck begins by inspecting the seated patient from the front and side and noting any surgical scars, obvious masses, or distended veins. The thyroid can be palpated with both hands from behind or while facing the patient, using the thumbs to palpate each lobe. It is best to use a combination of these methods, especially when nodules are small. The patient's neck should be slightly flexed to relax the neck muscles. After locating the cricoid cartilage, the isthmus can be identified and followed laterally to locate either lobe (normally the right lobe is slightly larger than the left). By asking the patient to swallow sips of water, thyroid consistency can be better appreciated as the gland moves beneath the examiner's fingers.

Features to be noted include thyroid size, consistency, nodularity, and any tenderness or fixation. An estimate of thyroid size (normally 12–20 g) should be made, and a drawing is often the best way to record findings. However, ultrasound is the method of choice when it is important to determine thyroid size accurately. The size, location, and consistency of any nodules should also be defined. A bruit over the gland indicates increased vascularity, as occurs in hyperthyroidism. If the lower borders of the thyroid lobes are not clearly felt, a goiter may be retrosternal. Large retrosternal goiters can cause venous distention over the neck and difficulty breathing, especially when the arms are raised (Pemberton's sign). With any central mass above the thyroid, the tongue should be extended, as thyroglossal cysts then move upward. The thyroid examination is not complete without assessment for lymphadenopathy in the supraclavicular and cervical regions of the neck.

LABORATORY EVALUATION

Measurement of Thyroid Hormones

The enhanced sensitivity and specificity of *TSH assays* have greatly improved laboratory assessment of thyroid function. Because TSH levels change dynamically in response to alterations of T_4 and T_3, a logical approach to thyroid testing is to first determine whether TSH is suppressed, normal, or elevated. With rare exceptions, a normal TSH level excludes a primary abnormality of thyroid function. This strategy depends on the use of immunochemiluminometric assays (ICMAs) for TSH that are sensitive enough to discriminate between the lower limit of the reference range and the suppressed values that occur with thyrotoxicosis. Extremely sensitive (fourth generation) assays can detect TSH levels ≤0.004 mU/L, but for practical purposes assays sensitive to ≤0.1 mU/L are sufficient. The widespread availability of the TSH ICMA has rendered the TRH stimulation test obsolete, as the failure of TSH to rise after an IV bolus of 200–400 μg TRH has the same implications as a suppressed basal TSH measured by ICMA.

The finding of an abnormal TSH level must be followed by measurements of circulating thyroid hormone levels to confirm the diagnosis of hyperthyroidism (suppressed TSH) or hypothyroidism (elevated TSH). Radioimmunoassays are widely available for serum *total* T_4 and *total* T_3. T_4 and T_3 are highly protein-bound, and numerous factors (illness, medications, genetic factors) can influence protein binding. It is useful, therefore, to measure the free, or unbound, hormone levels, which correspond to the biologically available hormone pool. Two direct methods are used to measure *unbound thyroid hormones*: (1) unbound thyroid hormone competition with radiolabeled T_4 (or an analogue) for binding to a solid-phase antibody, and (2) physical separation of the unbound hormone fraction by ultracentrifugation or equilibrium dialysis. Though early unbound hormone immunoassays suffered from artifacts, newer assays correlate well with the results of the more technically demanding and expensive physical separation methods. An indirect method to estimate unbound thyroid hormone levels is to calculate the free T_3 or free T_4 index from the total T_4 or T_3 concentration and the *thyroid hormone–binding ratio* (THBR). The latter is derived from the *T_3-resin uptake test*, which determines the distribution of radiolabeled T_3 between an absorbent resin and the unoccupied thyroid hormone-binding proteins in the sample. The binding of the labeled T_3 to the resin is increased when there is reduced unoccupied protein-binding sites (e.g., TBG deficiency) or increased total thyroid hormone in the sample; it is decreased under the opposite circumstances. The product of THBR and total T_3 or T_4 provides the *free T_3 or T_4 index*. In effect, the index corrects for anomalous total hormone values caused by abnormalities in hormone-protein binding.

Total thyroid hormone levels are *elevated* when TBG is increased due to estrogens (pregnancy, oral contraceptives, hormone therapy, tamoxifen) and *decreased* when TBG binding is reduced (androgens, nephrotic syndrome). Genetic disorders and acute illness can also cause abnormalities in thyroid hormone–binding proteins, and various drugs [phenytoin, carbamazepine, salicylates, and nonsteroidal anti-inflammatory drugs (NSAIDs)] can interfere with thyroid hormone binding. Because unbound thyroid hormone levels are normal and the patient is euthyroid in all of these circumstances, assays that measure unbound hormone are preferable to those for total thyroid hormones.

For most purposes, the unbound T_4 level is sufficient to confirm thyrotoxicosis, but 2–5% of patients have only an elevated T_3 level (T_3 toxicosis). Thus, unbound T_3 levels should be measured in patients with a suppressed TSH but normal unbound T_4 levels.

There are several clinical conditions in which the use of TSH as a screening test may be misleading, particularly without simultaneous unbound T_4 determinations. Any severe nonthyroidal illness can cause abnormal TSH levels (see below). Although hypothyroidism is the most common cause of an elevated TSH level, rare causes include a TSH-secreting pituitary tumor (Chap. 2), thyroid hormone resistance, and assay artifact. Conversely, a suppressed TSH level, particularly <0.1 mU/L, usually indicates thyrotoxicosis but may also be seen during the first trimester of pregnancy (due to hCG secretion), after treatment of hyperthyroidism (because TSH can remain suppressed for several months), and in response to certain medications (e.g., high doses of glucocorticoids or dopamine). Importantly, secondary hypothyroidism, caused by hypothalamic-pituitary disease, is associated with a variable (low to high-normal) TSH level, which is inappropriate for the low T_4 level. Thus, *TSH should not be used to assess thyroid function in patients with suspected or known pituitary disease.*

Tests for the end organ effects of thyroid hormone excess or depletion, such as estimation of basal metabolic rate, tendon reflex relaxation rates, or serum cholesterol, are not useful as clinical determinants of thyroid function.

Tests to Determine the Etiology of Thyroid Dysfunction

Autoimmune thyroid disease is detected most easily by measuring circulating antibodies against TPO and Tg. As antibodies to Tg alone are uncommon, it is reasonable to measure only TPO antibodies. About 5–15% of euthyroid women and up to 2% of euthyroid men have thyroid antibodies; such individuals are at increased risk of developing thyroid dysfunction. Almost all patients with autoimmune hypothyroidism, and up to 80% of those with Graves' disease, have TPO antibodies, usually at high levels.

TSIs are antibodies that stimulate the TSH-R in Graves' disease. They can be measured in bioassays or indirectly in assays that detect antibody binding to the receptor. The main use of these assays is to predict neonatal thyrotoxicosis caused by high maternal levels of TSIs in the last trimester of pregnancy.

Serum Tg levels are increased in all types of thyrotoxicosis except *thyrotoxicosis factitia* caused by self-administration of thyroid hormone. Tg levels are particularly increased in thyroiditis, reflecting thyroid tissue destruction and release of Tg. The main role for Tg measurement, however, is in the follow-up of thyroid cancer patients. After total thyroidectomy and radioablation, Tg levels should be undetectable; measurable levels indicate incomplete ablation or recurrent cancer.

Radioiodine Uptake and Thyroid Scanning

The thyroid gland selectively transports radioisotopes of iodine (^{123}I, ^{125}I, ^{131}I) and ^{99m}Tc pertechnetate, allowing thyroid imaging and quantitation of radioactive tracer fractional uptake.

Nuclear imaging of Graves' disease is characterized by an enlarged gland and increased tracer uptake that is distributed homogeneously. Toxic adenomas appear as focal areas of increased uptake, with suppressed tracer uptake in the remainder of the gland. In toxic MNG, the gland is enlarged—often with distorted architecture—and there are multiple areas of relatively increased or decreased tracer uptake. Subacute thyroiditis is associated with very low uptake because of follicular cell damage and TSH suppression. Thyrotoxicosis factitia is also associated with low uptake.

Although the use of fine-needle aspiration (FNA) biopsy has diminished the use of thyroid scans in the evaluation of solitary thyroid nodules, the functional features of thyroid nodules have some prognostic significance. So-called cold nodules, which have diminished tracer uptake, are usually benign. However, these nodules are more likely to be malignant (~5–10%) than so-called hot nodules, which are almost never malignant.

Thyroid scanning is also used in the follow-up of thyroid cancer. After thyroidectomy and ablation using ^{131}I, there is diminished radioiodine uptake in the thyroid bed, allowing the detection of metastatic thyroid cancer deposits that retain the ability to transport iodine. Whole-body scans using 111–185 MBq (3–5 mCi) ^{131}I are typically performed after thyroid hormone withdrawal to raise the TSH level or after the administration of recombinant human TSH.

Thyroid Ultrasound

Ultrasonography is used increasingly to assist in the diagnosis of nodular thyroid disease, a reflection of the limitations of the physical examination and improvements in ultrasound technology. Using 10-MHz instruments, spatial resolution and image quality are excellent, allowing the detection of nodules and cysts >3 mm. In addition to detecting thyroid nodules, ultrasound is useful for monitoring nodule size and for the aspiration of cystic lesions. Ultrasound-guided FNA biopsy of thyroid lesions lowers the rate of inadequate sampling. Ultrasonography is also used in the evaluation of recurrent thyroid cancer, including possible spread to cervical lymph nodes.

HYPOTHYROIDISM

Iodine deficiency remains the most common cause of hypothyroidism worldwide. In areas of iodine sufficiency, autoimmune disease (Hashimoto's thyroiditis) and iatrogenic causes (treatment of hyperthyroidism) are most common (Table 4-4).

TABLE 4-4

CAUSES OF HYPOTHYROIDISM

Primary
Autoimmune hypothyroidism: Hashimoto's thyroiditis, atrophic thyroiditis
Iatrogenic: ^{131}I treatment, subtotal or total thyroidectomy, external irradiation of neck for lymphoma or cancer
Drugs: iodine excess (including iodine-containing contrast media and amiodarone), lithium, antithyroid drugs, *p*-aminosalicylic acid, interferon-α and other cytokines, aminoglutethimide
Congenital hypothyroidism: absent or ectopic thyroid gland, dyshormonogenesis, TSH-R mutation
Iodine deficiency
Infiltrative disorders: amyloidosis, sarcoidosis, hemochromatosis, scleroderma, cystinosis, Riedel's thyroiditis
Overexpression of type III deiodinase in infantile hemangioma
Transient
Silent thyroiditis, including postpartum thyroiditis
Subacute thyroiditis
Withdrawal of thyroxine treatment in individuals with an intact thyroid
After ^{131}I treatment or subtotal thyroidectomy for Graves' disease
Secondary
Hypopituitarism: tumors, pituitary surgery or irradiation, infiltrative disorders, Sheehan's syndrome, trauma, genetic forms of combined pituitary hormone deficiencies
Isolated TSH deficiency or inactivity
Bexarotene treatment
Hypothalamic disease: tumors, trauma, infiltrative disorders, idiopathic

Note: TSH, thyroid-stimulating hormone; TSH-R, TSH receptor.

CONGENITAL HYPOTHYROIDISM

Prevalence

Hypothyroidism occurs in about 1 in 4000 newborns. It may be transient, especially if the mother has TSH-R–blocking antibodies or has received antithyroid drugs, but permanent hypothyroidism occurs in the majority. Neonatal hypothyroidism is due to thyroid gland dysgenesis in 80–85% and to inborn errors of thyroid hormone synthesis in 10–15%, and is TSH-R antibody-mediated in 5% of affected newborns. The developmental abnormalities are twice as common in girls. Mutations that cause congenital hypothyroidism are being increasingly recognized, but the vast majority remain idiopathic (Table 4-1).

Clinical Manifestations

The majority of infants appear normal at birth, and <10% are diagnosed based on clinical features, which include prolonged jaundice, feeding problems, hypotonia, enlarged tongue, delayed bone maturation, and umbilical hernia. Importantly, permanent neurologic damage results if treatment is delayed. Typical features of adult hypothyroidism may also be present (Table 4-5). Other congenital malformations, especially cardiac, are four times more common in congenital hypothyroidism.

Diagnosis and Treatment

Because of the severe neurologic consequences of untreated congenital hypothyroidism, neonatal screening programs have been established. These are generally based on measurement of TSH or T_4 levels in heel-prick blood specimens. When the diagnosis is confirmed, T_4 is instituted at a dose of 10–15 μg/kg per d, and the dose is adjusted by close monitoring of TSH levels. T_4 requirements are relatively great during the first year of life, and a high circulating T_4 level is usually needed to normalize TSH. Early treatment with T_4 results in normal IQ levels, but subtle neurodevelopmental abnormalities may occur in those with the most

TABLE 4-5

SIGNS AND SYMPTOMS OF HYPOTHYROIDISM (DESCENDING ORDER OF FREQUENCY)

SYMPTOMS	SIGNS
Tiredness, weakness	Dry, coarse skin; cool peripheral extremities
Dry skin	Puffy face, hands, and feet (myxedema)
Feeling cold	Diffuse alopecia
Hair loss	Bradycardia
Difficulty concentrating and poor memory	Peripheral edema
Constipation	Delayed tendon reflex relaxation
Weight gain with poor appetite	Carpal tunnel syndrome
Dyspnea	Serous cavity effusions
Hoarse voice	
Menorrhagia (later oligomenorrhea or amenorrhea)	
Paresthesia	
Impaired hearing	

severe hypothyroidism at diagnosis or when treatment is suboptimal.

AUTOIMMUNE HYPOTHYROIDISM

Classification

Autoimmune hypothyroidism may be associated with a goiter (Hashimoto's, or *goitrous thyroiditis*) or, at the later stages of the disease, minimal residual thyroid tissue (*atrophic thyroiditis*). Because the autoimmune process gradually reduces thyroid function, there is a phase of compensation when normal thyroid hormone levels are maintained by a rise in TSH. Though some patients may have minor symptoms, this state is called *subclinical hypothyroidism*. Later, unbound T_4 levels fall and TSH levels rise further; symptoms become more readily apparent at this stage (usually TSH >10 mU/L), which is referred to as *clinical hypothyroidism* or *overt hypothyroidism*.

Prevalence

The mean annual incidence rate of autoimmune hypothyroidism is up to 4 per 1000 women and 1 per 1000 men. It is more common in certain populations, such as the Japanese, probably because of genetic factors and chronic exposure to a high-iodine diet. The mean age at diagnosis is 60 years, and the prevalence of overt hypothyroidism increases with age. Subclinical hypothyroidism is found in 6–8% of women (10% over the age of 60) and 3% of men. The annual risk of developing clinical hypothyroidism is about 4% when subclinical hypothyroidism is associated with positive TPO antibodies.

Pathogenesis

In Hashimoto's thyroiditis, there is a marked lymphocytic infiltration of the thyroid with germinal center formation, atrophy of the thyroid follicles accompanied by oxyphil metaplasia, absence of colloid, and mild to moderate fibrosis. In atrophic thyroiditis, the fibrosis is much more extensive, lymphocyte infiltration is less pronounced, and thyroid follicles are almost completely absent. Atrophic thyroiditis likely represents the end stage of Hashimoto's thyroiditis rather than a distinct disorder.

As with most autoimmune disorders, susceptibility to autoimmune hypothyroidism is determined by a combination of genetic and environmental factors, and the risk of either autoimmune hypothyroidism or Graves' disease is increased among siblings. HLA-DR polymorphisms are the best documented genetic risk factors for autoimmune hypothyroidism, especially HLA-DR3, -DR4, and -DR5 in Caucasians. A weak association also exists between polymorphisms in *CTLA-4*, a T cell–regulatory gene, and autoimmune hypothyroidism. Both of these genetic associations are shared by other autoimmune diseases, which may explain the relationship between autoimmune hypothyroidism and other autoimmune diseases, especially type 1 diabetes mellitus, Addison's disease, pernicious anemia, and vitiligo (Chap. 23). HLA-DR and *CTLA*-4 polymorphisms account for approximately half of the genetic susceptibility to autoimmune hypothyroidism. The other contributory loci remain to be identified. A gene on chromosome 21 may be responsible for the association between autoimmune hypothyroidism and Down's syndrome. The female preponderance of thyroid autoimmunity is most likely due to sex steroid effects on the immune response, but an X chromosome–related genetic factor is also possible, which may account for the high frequency of autoimmune hypothyroidism in Turner syndrome. Environmental susceptibility factors are poorly defined at present. A high iodine intake may increase the risk of autoimmune hypothyroidism by immunologic effects or direct thyroid toxicity. There is no convincing evidence for a role of infection except for the congenital rubella syndrome, in which there is a high frequency of autoimmune hypothyroidism. Viral thyroiditis does not induce subsequent autoimmune thyroid disease.

The thyroid lymphocytic infiltrate in autoimmune hypothyroidism is composed of activated CD4+ and CD8+ T cells, as well as B cells. Thyroid cell destruction is primarily mediated by the CD8+ cytotoxic T cells, which destroy their targets by either perforin-induced cell necrosis or granzyme B–induced apoptosis. In addition, local T cell production of cytokines, such as tumor necrosis factor (TNF), IL-1, and interferon γ (IFN-γ), may render thyroid cells more susceptible to apoptosis mediated by death receptors, such as Fas, which are activated by their respective ligands on T cells. These cytokines also impair thyroid cell function directly and induce the expression of other proinflammatory molecules by the thyroid cells themselves, such as cytokines, HLA class I and class II molecules, adhesion molecules, CD40, and nitric oxide. Administration of high concentrations of cytokines for therapeutic purposes (especially IFN-α) is associated with increased autoimmune thyroid disease, possibly through mechanisms similar to those in sporadic disease.

Antibodies to Tg and TPO are clinically useful markers of thyroid autoimmunity, but any pathogenic effect is restricted to a secondary role in amplifying an ongoing autoimmune response. TPO antibodies fix complement, and complement membrane attack complexes are present in the thyroid in autoimmune hypothyroidism. However, transplacental passage of Tg or TPO antibodies has no effect on the fetal thyroid, which suggests that T cell–mediated injury is required to initiate autoimmune damage to the thyroid.

Up to 20% of patients with autoimmune hypothyroidism have antibodies against the TSH-R, which, in contrast to TSIs, do not stimulate the receptor but prevent the binding of TSH. These TSH-R-blocking antibodies therefore cause hypothyroidism and, especially in Asian patients, thyroid atrophy. Their transplacental passage may induce transient neonatal hypothyroidism. Rarely, patients have a mixture of TSI- and TSH-R-blocking antibodies, and thyroid function can oscillate between hyperthyroidism and hypothyroidism as one or the other antibody becomes dominant. Predicting the course of disease in such individuals is difficult, and they require close monitoring of thyroid function. Bioassays can be used to document that TSH-R-blocking antibodies reduce the cyclic AMP–inducing effect of TSH on cultured TSH-R-expressing cells, but these assays are difficult to perform. Assays that measure the binding of antibodies to the receptor by competition with radiolabeled TSH [TSH-binding inhibiting immunoglobulins (TBIIs)] do not distinguish between TSI- and TSH-R-blocking antibodies, but a positive result in a patient with spontaneous hypothyroidism is strong evidence for the presence of blocking antibodies. The use of these assays does not generally alter clinical management, although they may be useful to confirm the cause of transient neonatal hypothyroidism.

Clinical Manifestations

The main clinical features of hypothyroidism are summarized in Table 4-5. The onset is usually insidious, and the patient may become aware of symptoms only when euthyroidism is restored. Patients with Hashimoto's thyroiditis may present because of goiter rather than symptoms of hypothyroidism. The goiter may not be large but is usually irregular and firm in consistency. It is often possible to palpate a pyramidal lobe, normally a vestigial remnant of the thyroglossal duct. Rarely, uncomplicated Hashimoto's thyroiditis is associated with pain.

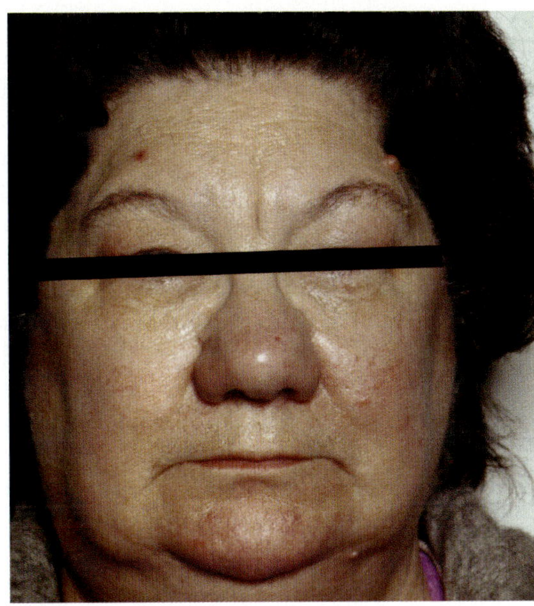

FIGURE 4-5
Facial appearance in hypothyroidism. Note puffy eyes and thickened, pale skin.

Patients with atrophic thyroiditis or the late stage of Hashimoto's thyroiditis present with symptoms and signs of hypothyroidism. The skin is dry, and there is decreased sweating, thinning of the epidermis, and hyperkeratosis of the stratum corneum. Increased dermal glycosaminoglycan content traps water, giving rise to skin thickening without pitting (*myxedema*). Typical features include a puffy face with edematous eyelids and nonpitting pretibial edema (Fig. 4-5). There is pallor, often with a yellow tinge to the skin due to carotene accumulation. Nail growth is retarded, and hair is dry, brittle, and difficult to manage and falls out easily. In addition to diffuse alopecia, there is thinning of the outer third of the eyebrows, although this is not a specific sign of hypothyroidism.

Other common features include constipation and weight gain (despite a poor appetite). In contrast to popular perception, the weight gain is usually modest and due mainly to fluid retention in the myxedematous tissues. Libido is decreased in both sexes, and there may be oligomenorrhea or amenorrhea in longstanding disease, but menorrhagia is also common. Fertility is reduced and the incidence of miscarriage is increased. Prolactin levels are often modestly increased (Chap. 2) and may contribute to alterations in libido and fertility and cause galactorrhea.

Myocardial contractility and pulse rate are reduced, leading to a reduced stroke volume and bradycardia. Increased peripheral resistance may be accompanied by hypertension, particularly diastolic. Blood flow is diverted from the skin, producing cool extremities. Pericardial effusions occur in up to 30% of patients but rarely compromise cardiac function. Though alterations in myosin heavy chain isoform expression have been documented, cardiomyopathy is unusual. Fluid may also accumulate in other serous cavities and in the middle ear, giving rise to conductive deafness. Pulmonary function is generally normal, but dyspnea may be caused by pleural effusion, impaired respiratory muscle function, diminished ventilatory drive, or sleep apnea.

Carpal tunnel and other entrapment syndromes are common, as is impairment of muscle function with stiffness, cramps, and pain. On examination, there may be slow relaxation of tendon reflexes and pseudomyotonia. Memory and concentration are impaired. Rare neurologic problems include reversible cerebellar ataxia, dementia, psychosis, and myxedema coma. *Hashimoto's encephalopathy* has been defined as a steroid-responsive syndrome associated with TPO antibodies, myoclonus, and slow-wave activity on electroencephalography, but the relationship with thyroid autoimmunity or hypothyroidism is not established. The hoarse voice and occasionally clumsy speech of hypothyroidism reflect fluid accumulation in the vocal cords and tongue.

The features described above are the consequence of thyroid hormone deficiency. However, autoimmune hypothyroidism may be associated with signs or symptoms of other autoimmune diseases, particularly vitiligo, pernicious anemia, Addison's disease, alopecia areata, and type 1 diabetes mellitus. Less-common associations include celiac disease, dermatitis herpetiformis, chronic active hepatitis, rheumatoid arthritis, systemic lupus erythematosus (SLE), and Sjögren's syndrome. Thyroid-associated ophthalmopathy, which usually occurs in Graves' disease, occurs in about 5% of patients with autoimmune hypothyroidism.

Autoimmune hypothyroidism is uncommon in children and usually presents with slow growth and delayed facial maturation. The appearance of permanent teeth is also delayed. Myopathy, with muscle swelling, is more common in children than in adults. In most cases, puberty is delayed, but precocious puberty sometimes occurs. There may be intellectual impairment if the onset is before 3 years and the hormone deficiency is severe.

Laboratory Evaluation

A summary of the investigations used to determine the existence and cause of hypothyroidism is provided in Fig. 4-6. A normal TSH level excludes primary (but not secondary) hypothyroidism. If the TSH is elevated, an unbound T_4 level is needed to confirm the presence of clinical hypothyroidism, but T_4 is inferior to TSH when used as a screening test, as it will not detect subclinical hypothyroidism. Circulating unbound T_3 levels are normal in about 25% of patients, reflecting adaptive deiodinase responses to hypothyroidism. T_3 measurements are therefore not indicated.

Once clinical or subclinical hypothyroidism is confirmed, the etiology is usually easily established by demonstrating the presence of TPO antibodies, which are present in >90% of patients with autoimmune hypothyroidism. TBIIs can be found in 10–20% of patients, but these determinations are not needed routinely. If there is any doubt about the cause of a goiter associated with hypothyroidism, FNA biopsy can be used to confirm the presence of autoimmune thyroiditis. Other abnormal laboratory findings in hypothyroidism may include increased creatine phosphokinase, elevated

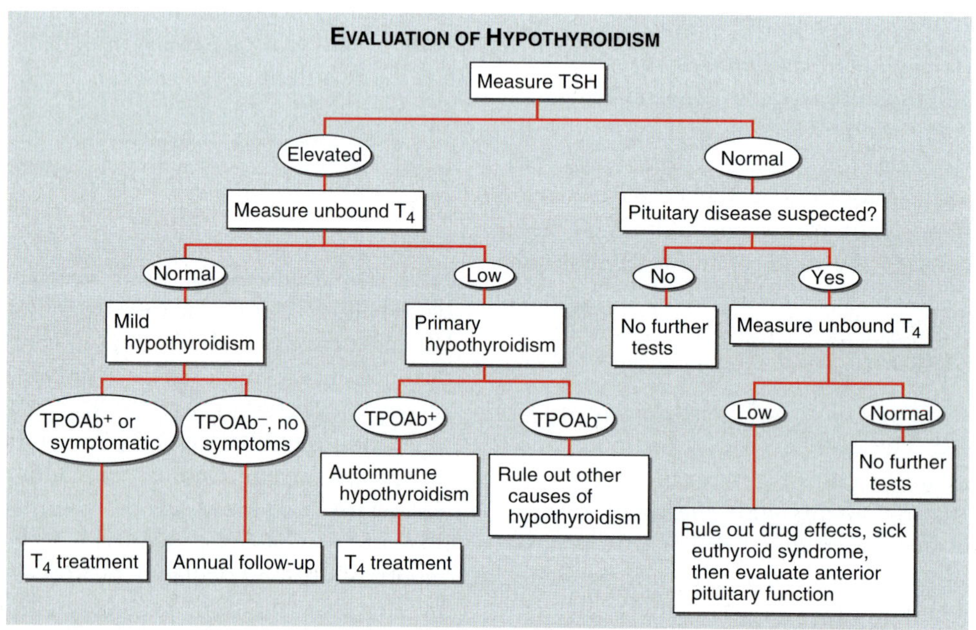

FIGURE 4-6

Evaluation of hypothyroidism. TPOAb+, thyroid peroxidase antibodies present; TPOAb−, thyroid peroxidase antibodies not present; TSH, thyroid-stimulating hormone.

cholesterol and triglycerides, and anemia (usually normocytic or macrocytic). Except when accompanied by iron deficiency, the anemia and other abnormalities gradually resolve with thyroxine replacement.

Differential Diagnosis

An asymmetric goiter in Hashimoto's thyroiditis may be confused with a multinodular goiter or thyroid carcinoma, in which thyroid antibodies may also be present. Ultrasound can be used to show the presence of a solitary lesion or a multinodular goiter rather than the heterogeneous thyroid enlargement typical of Hashimoto's thyroiditis. FNA biopsy is useful in the investigation of focal nodules. Other causes of hypothyroidism are discussed below but rarely cause diagnostic confusion (Table 4-4).

OTHER CAUSES OF HYPOTHYROIDISM

Iatrogenic hypothyroidism is a common cause of hypothyroidism and can often be detected by screening before symptoms develop. In the first 3–4 months after radioiodine treatment, transient hypothyroidism may occur due to reversible radiation damage. Low-dose thyroxine treatment can be withdrawn if recovery occurs. Because TSH levels are suppressed by hyperthyroidism, unbound T_4 levels are a better measure of thyroid function than TSH in the months following radioiodine treatment. Mild hypothyroidism after subtotal thyroidectomy may also resolve after several months, as the gland remnant is stimulated by increased TSH levels.

Iodine deficiency is responsible for endemic goiter and cretinism but is an uncommon cause of adult hypothyroidism unless the iodine intake is very low or there are complicating factors, such as the consumption of thiocyanates in cassava or selenium deficiency. Though hypothyroidism due to iodine deficiency can be treated with thyroxine, public health measures to improve iodine intake should be advocated to eliminate this problem. Iodized salt or bread or a single bolus of oral or IM iodized oil have all been used successfully.

Paradoxically, chronic iodine excess can also induce goiter and hypothyroidism. The intracellular events that account for this effect are unclear, but individuals with autoimmune thyroiditis are especially susceptible. Iodine excess is responsible for the hypothyroidism that occurs in up to 13% of patients treated with amiodarone. Other drugs, particularly lithium, may also cause hypothyroidism. Transient hypothyroidism caused by thyroiditis is discussed below.

Secondary hypothyroidism is usually diagnosed in the context of other anterior pituitary hormone deficiencies; isolated TSH deficiency is very rare (Chap. 2). TSH levels may be low, normal, or even slightly increased in secondary hypothyroidism; the latter is due to secretion of immunoactive but bioinactive forms of TSH. The diagnosis is confirmed by detecting a low unbound T_4 level. The goal of treatment is to maintain T_4 levels in the upper half of the reference range, as TSH levels cannot be used to monitor therapy.

℞ Treatment: HYPOTHYROIDISM

CLINICAL HYPOTHYROIDISM If there is no residual thyroid function, the daily replacement dose of levothyroxine is usually 1.6 μg/kg body weight (typically 100–150 μg). In many patients, however, lower doses suffice until residual thyroid tissue is destroyed. In patients who develop hypothyroidism after the treatment of Graves' disease, there is often underlying autonomous function, necessitating lower replacement doses (typically 75–125 μg/d).

Adult patients under 60 without evidence of heart disease may be started on 50–100 μg levothyroxine (T_4) daily. The dose is adjusted on the basis of TSH levels, with the goal of treatment being a normal TSH, ideally in the lower half of the reference range. TSH responses are gradual and should be measured about 2 months after instituting treatment or after any subsequent change in levothyroxine dosage. The clinical effects of levothyroxine replacement are often slow to appear. Patients may not experience full relief from symptoms until 3–6 months after normal TSH levels are restored. Adjustment of levothyroxine dosage is made in 12.5- or 25-μg increments if the TSH is high; decrements of the same magnitude should be made if the TSH is suppressed. Patients with a suppressed TSH of any cause, including T_4 overtreatment, have an increased risk of atrial fibrillation and reduced bone density.

Although desiccated animal thyroid preparations (thyroid extract USP) are available, they are not recommended as the ratio of T_3 to T_4 is nonphysiologic. The use of levothyroxine combined with liothyronine (triiodothyronine, T_3) has been advocated, but benefit has not been confirmed in several prospective studies. There is no place for liothyronine alone as long-term replacement, because the short half-life necessitates three or four daily doses and is associated with fluctuating T_3 levels.

Once full replacement is achieved and TSH levels are stable, follow-up measurement of TSH is recommended at annual intervals and may be extended to every 2–3 years if a normal TSH is maintained over several years. It is important to ensure ongoing adherence, however, as patients do not feel any symptomatic difference after missing a few doses of levothyroxine, and this sometimes leads to self-discontinuation.

In patients of normal body weight who are taking ≥200 μg of levothyroxine per day, an elevated TSH level is often a sign of poor adherence to treatment. This is also the likely explanation for fluctuating TSH levels, despite a constant levothyroxine dosage. Such patients often have normal or high unbound T_4 levels, despite an elevated TSH, because they remember to take medication for a few days before testing; this is sufficient to normalize T_4, but not TSH, levels. It is important to consider variable adherence, as this pattern of thyroid function tests is otherwise suggestive of disorders associated with inappropriate TSH secretion (Table 4-3). Because T_4 has a long half-life (7 days), patients who miss doses can be advised to take two or three doses of the skipped tablets at once. Other causes of increased levothyroxine requirements must be excluded, particularly malabsorption (e.g., celiac disease, small-bowel surgery), estrogen therapy, and drugs that interfere with T_4 absorption or clearance such as cholestyramine, ferrous sulfate, calcium supplements, lovastatin, aluminum hydroxide, rifampicin, amiodarone, carbamazepine, and phenytoin.

SUBCLINICAL HYPOTHYROIDISM By definition, subclinical hypothyroidism refers to biochemical evidence of thyroid hormone deficiency in patients who have few or no apparent clinical features of hypothyroidism. There are no universally accepted recommendations for the management of subclinical hypothyroidism, but the most recently published guidelines do not recommend treatment when TSH levels are below 10 mU/L. It is important to confirm that any elevation of TSH is sustained over a 3-month period before treatment is given. As long as excessive treatment is avoided, there is no risk in correcting a slightly increased TSH. Moreover, there is a risk that patients will progress to overt hypothyroidism, particularly when the TSH level is elevated and TPO antibodies are present. Treatment is administered by starting with a low dose of levothyroxine (25–50 μg/d) with the goal of normalizing TSH. If thyroxine is not given, thyroid function should be evaluated annually.

SPECIAL TREATMENT CONSIDERATIONS Rarely, levothyroxine replacement is associated with pseudotumor cerebri in children. Presentation appears to be idiosyncratic and occurs months after treatment has begun. Women with a history or high risk of hypothyroidism should ensure that they are euthyroid prior to conception and during early pregnancy as maternal hypothyroidism may adversely affect fetal neural development. Thyroid function should be evaluated immediately after pregnancy is confirmed and at the beginning of the second and third trimesters. The dose of levothyroxine may need to be increased by ≥50% during pregnancy and returned to previous levels after delivery. Elderly patients may require up to 20% less thyroxine than younger patients. In the elderly, especially patients with known coronary artery disease, the starting dose of levothyroxine is 12.5–25 μg/d with similar increments every 2–3 months until TSH is normalized. In some patients it may be impossible to achieve full replacement, despite optimal antianginal treatment. *Emergency surgery* is generally safe in patients with untreated hypothyroidism, although routine surgery in a hypothyroid patient should be deferred until euthyroidism is achieved.

Myxedema coma still has a high mortality rate, despite intensive treatment. Clinical manifestations include reduced level of consciousness, sometimes associated with seizures, as well as the other features of hypothyroidism (Table 4-5). Hypothermia can reach 23°C (74°F). There may be a history of treated hypothyroidism with poor compliance, or the patient may be previously undiagnosed. Myxedema coma almost always occurs in the elderly and is usually precipitated by factors that impair respiration, such as drugs (especially sedatives, anesthetics, and antidepressants), pneumonia, congestive heart failure, myocardial infarction, gastrointestinal bleeding, or cerebrovascular accidents. Sepsis should also be suspected. Exposure to cold may also be a risk factor. Hypoventilation, leading to hypoxia and hypercapnia, plays a major role in pathogenesis; hypoglycemia and dilutional hyponatremia also contribute to the development of myxedema coma.

Levothyroxine can initially be administered as a single IV bolus of 500 μg, which serves as a loading dose. Although further levothyroxine is not strictly necessary for several days, it is usually continued at a dose of 50–100 μg/d. If suitable IV preparation is not available, the same initial dose of levothyroxine can be given by nasogastric tube (though absorption may be impaired in myxedema). An alternative is to give liothyronine (T_3) IV or via nasogastric tube, in doses ranging from 10 to 25 μg every 8–12 h. This treatment has been advocated because $T_4 \rightarrow T_3$ conversion is impaired in myxedema coma. However, excess liothyronine has the potential to provoke arrhythmias. Another option is to combine levothyroxine (200 μg) and liothyronine (25 μg) as a single, initial IV bolus followed by daily treatment with levothyroxine (50–100 μg/d) and liothyronine (10 μg every 8 h).

Supportive therapy should be provided to correct any associated metabolic disturbances. External warming is indicated only if the temperature is <30°C, as it can result in cardiovascular collapse. Space blankets should be used to prevent further heat loss. Parenteral hydrocortisone (50 mg every 6 h) should be administered, as there is impaired adrenal reserve in profound hypothyroidism. Any precipitating factors should be treated, including the early use of broad-spectrum antibiotics, pending the exclusion of infection. Ventilatory support with regular blood gas analysis is usually needed during the first 48 h. Hypertonic saline or IV glucose may be needed if there is severe hyponatremia or hypoglycemia; hypotonic IV fluids should be avoided because they may exacerbate water retention secondary to reduced renal perfusion and inappropriate vasopressin secretion.

The metabolism of most medications is impaired, and sedatives should be avoided if possible or used in reduced doses. Medication blood levels should be monitored, when available, to guide dosage.

THYROTOXICOSIS

Thyrotoxicosis is defined as the state of thyroid hormone excess and is not synonymous with *hyperthyroidism*, which is the result of excessive thyroid function. However, the major etiologies of thyrotoxicosis are hyperthyroidism caused by Graves' disease, toxic MNG, and toxic adenomas. Other causes are listed in Table 4-6.

GRAVES' DISEASE

Epidemiology

Graves' disease accounts for 60–80% of thyrotoxicosis. The prevalence varies among populations, depending mainly on iodine intake (high iodine intake is associated with an increased prevalence of Graves' disease). Graves' disease occurs in up to 2% of women but is one-tenth as frequent in men. The disorder rarely begins before adolescence and typically occurs between 20 and 50 years of age, but it also occurs in the elderly.

TABLE 4-6

CAUSES OF THYROTOXICOSIS
Primary Hyperthyroidism
Graves' disease
Toxic multinodular goiter
Toxic adenoma
Functioning thyroid carcinoma metastases
Activating mutation of the TSH receptor
Activating mutation of $G_s\alpha$ (McCune-Albright syndrome)
Struma ovarii
Drugs: iodine excess (Jod-Basedow phenomenon)
Thyrotoxicosis without Hyperthyroidism
Subacute thyroiditis
Silent thyroiditis
Other causes of thyroid destruction: amiodarone, radiation, infarction of adenoma
Ingestion of excess thyroid hormone (thyrotoxicosis factitia) or thyroid tissue
Secondary Hyperthyroidism
TSH-secreting pituitary adenoma
Thyroid hormone resistance syndrome: occasional patients may have features of thyrotoxicosis
Chorionic gonadotropin-secreting tumors[a]
Gestational thyrotoxicosis[a]

[a]Circulating TSH levels are low in these forms of secondary hyperthyroidism.
Note: TSH, thyroid-stimulating hormone.

Pathogenesis

As in autoimmune hypothyroidism, a combination of environmental and genetic factors, including polymorphisms in HLA-DR, *CTLA-4*, and *PTPN22* (a T cell regulatory gene), contributes to Graves' disease susceptibility. The concordance for Graves' disease in monozygotic twins is 20–30%, compared to <5% in dizygotic twins. Indirect evidence suggests that stress is an important environmental factor, presumably operating through neuroendocrine effects on the immune system. Smoking is a minor risk factor for Graves' disease and a major risk factor for the development of ophthalmopathy. Sudden increases in iodine intake may precipitate Graves' disease, and there is a threefold increase in the occurrence of Graves' disease in the postpartum period.

The hyperthyroidism of Graves' disease is caused by TSIs that are synthesized in the thyroid gland as well as in bone marrow and lymph nodes. Such antibodies can be detected by bioassays or by using the more widely available TBII assays. The presence of TBIIs in a patient with thyrotoxicosis implies the existence of TSIs, and these assays are useful in monitoring pregnant Graves' patients in whom high levels of TSIs can cross the placenta and cause neonatal thyrotoxicosis. Other thyroid autoimmune responses, similar to those in autoimmune hypothyroidism, occur concurrently in patients with Graves' disease. In particular, TPO antibodies occur in up to 80% of cases and serve as a readily measurable marker of autoimmunity. Because the coexisting thyroiditis can also affect thyroid function, there is no direct correlation between the level of TSIs and thyroid hormone levels in Graves' disease. In the long term, spontaneous autoimmune hypothyroidism may develop in up to 15% of Graves' patients.

Cytokines appear to play a major role in thyroid-associated ophthalmopathy. There is infiltration of the extraocular muscles by activated T cells; the release of cytokines such as IFN-γ, TNF, and IL-1 results in fibroblast activation and increased synthesis of glycosaminoglycans that trap water, thereby leading to characteristic muscle swelling. Late in the disease, there is irreversible fibrosis of the muscles. Orbital fibroblasts may be particularly sensitive to cytokines, perhaps explaining the anatomic localization of the immune response. Though the pathogenesis of thyroid-associated ophthalmopathy remains unclear, there is mounting evidence that the TSH-R may be a shared autoantigen that is expressed in the orbit, and this would explain the close association with autoimmune thyroid disease. Increased fat is an additional cause of retrobulbar tissue expansion. The increase in intraorbital pressure can lead to proptosis, diplopia, and optic neuropathy.

Clinical Manifestations

Signs and symptoms include features that are common to any cause of thyrotoxicosis (Table 4-7) as well as

TABLE 4-7

SIGNS AND SYMPTOMS OF THYROTOXICOSIS (DESCENDING ORDER OF FREQUENCY)

SYMPTOMS	SIGNS[a]
Hyperactivity, irritability, dysphoria	Tachycardia; atrial fibrillation in the elderly
Heat intolerance and sweating	Tremor
Palpitations	Goiter
Fatigue and weakness	Warm, moist skin
Weight loss with increased appetite	Muscle weakness, proximal myopathy
Diarrhea	Lid retraction or lag
Polyuria	Gynecomastia
Oligomenorrhea, loss of libido	

[a]Excludes the signs of ophthalmopathy and dermopathy specific for Graves' disease.

those specific for Graves' disease. The clinical presentation depends on the severity of thyrotoxicosis, the duration of disease, individual susceptibility to excess thyroid hormone, and the patient's age. In the elderly, features of thyrotoxicosis may be subtle or masked, and patients may present mainly with fatigue and weight loss, a condition known as *apathetic thyrotoxicosis*.

Thyrotoxicosis may cause unexplained weight loss, despite an enhanced appetite, due to the increased metabolic rate. Weight gain occurs in 5% of patients, however, because of increased food intake. Other prominent features include hyperactivity, nervousness, and irritability, ultimately leading to a sense of easy fatigability in some patients. Insomnia and impaired concentration are common; apathetic thyrotoxicosis may be mistaken for depression in the elderly. Fine tremor is a frequent finding, best elicited by having patients stretch out their fingers while feeling the fingertips with the palm. Common neurologic manifestations include hyperreflexia, muscle wasting, and proximal myopathy without fasciculation. Chorea is a rare feature. Thyrotoxicosis is sometimes associated with a form of hypokalemic periodic paralysis; this disorder is particularly common in Asian males with thyrotoxicosis.

The most common cardiovascular manifestation is sinus tachycardia, often associated with palpitations, occasionally caused by supraventricular tachycardia. The high cardiac output produces a bounding pulse, widened pulse pressure, and an aortic systolic murmur and can lead to worsening of angina or heart failure in the elderly or those with preexisting heart disease. Atrial fibrillation is more common in patients >50 years of age. Treatment of the thyrotoxic state alone converts atrial fibrillation to normal sinus rhythm in about half of patients, suggesting the existence of an underlying cardiac problem in the remainder.

The skin is usually warm and moist, and the patient may complain of sweating and heat intolerance, particularly during warm weather. Palmar erythema, onycholysis, and, less commonly, pruritus, urticaria, and diffuse hyperpigmentation may be evident. Hair texture may become fine, and a diffuse alopecia occurs in up to 40% of patients, persisting for months after restoration of euthyroidism. Gastrointestinal transit time is decreased, leading to increased stool frequency, often with diarrhea and occasionally mild steatorrhea. Women frequently experience oligomenorrhea or amenorrhea; in men, there may be impaired sexual function and, rarely, gynecomastia. The direct effect of thyroid hormones on bone resorption leads to osteopenia in long-standing thyrotoxicosis; mild hypercalcemia occurs in up to 20% of patients, but hypercalciuria is more common. There is a small increase in fracture rate in patients with a previous history of thyrotoxicosis.

In Graves' disease the thyroid is usually diffusely enlarged to two to three times its normal size. The consistency is firm, but less so than in MNG. There may be a thrill or bruit due to the increased vascularity of the gland and the hyperdynamic circulation.

Lid retraction, causing a staring appearance, can occur in any form of thyrotoxicosis and is the result of sympathetic overactivity. However, Graves' disease is associated with specific eye signs that comprise *Graves' ophthalmopathy* (**Fig. 4-7*A***). This condition is also called *thyroid-associated*

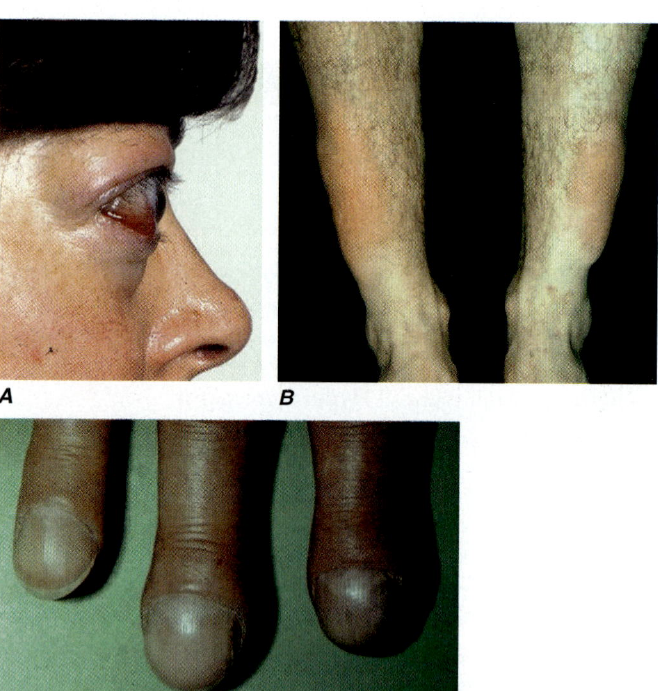

FIGURE 4-7

Features of Graves' disease. *A*. Ophthalmopathy in Graves' disease; lid retraction, periorbital edema, conjunctival injection, and proptosis are marked. ***B*.** Thyroid dermopathy over the lateral aspects of the shins. ***C*.** Thyroid acropachy.

ophthalmopathy, as it occurs in the absence of Graves' disease in 10% of patients. Most of these individuals have autoimmune hypothyroidism or thyroid antibodies. The onset of Graves' ophthalmopathy occurs within the year before or after the diagnosis of thyrotoxicosis in 75% of patients but can sometimes precede or follow thyrotoxicosis by several years, accounting for some cases of euthyroid ophthalmopathy.

Some patients with Graves' disease have little clinical evidence of ophthalmopathy. However, the enlarged extraocular muscles typical of the disease, and other subtle features, can be detected in almost all patients when investigated by ultrasound or CT imaging of the orbits. Unilateral signs are found in up to 10% of patients. The earliest manifestations of ophthalmopathy are usually a sensation of grittiness, eye discomfort, and excess tearing. About a third of patients have proptosis, best detected by visualization of the sclera between the lower border of the iris and the lower eyelid, with the eyes in the primary position. Proptosis can be measured using an exophthalmometer. In severe cases, proptosis may cause corneal exposure and damage, especially if the lids fail to close during sleep. Periorbital edema, scleral injection, and chemosis are also frequent. In 5–10% of patients, the muscle swelling is so severe that diplopia results, typically but not exclusively when the patient looks up and laterally. The most serious manifestation is compression of the optic nerve at the apex of the orbit, leading to papilledema, peripheral field defects, and, if left untreated, permanent loss of vision.

Many scoring systems have been used to gauge the extent and activity of the orbital changes in Graves' disease. The "NO SPECS" scheme is an acronym derived from the following eye changes:

0 = **N**o signs or symptoms
1 = **O**nly signs (lid retraction or lag), no symptoms
2 = **S**oft tissue involvement (periorbital edema)
3 = **P**roptosis (>22 mm)
4 = **E**xtraocular muscle involvement (diplopia)
5 = **C**orneal involvement
6 = **S**ight loss

Although useful as a mnemonic, the NO SPECS scheme is inadequate to describe the eye disease fully, and patients do not necessarily progress from one class to another. When Graves' eye disease is active and severe, referral to an ophthalmologist is indicated and objective measurements are needed, such as lid fissure width; corneal staining with fluorescein; and evaluation of extraocular muscle function (e.g., Hess chart), intraocular pressure and visual fields, acuity, and color vision.

Thyroid dermopathy occurs in <5% of patients with Graves' disease (**Fig. 4-7*B***), almost always in the presence of moderate or severe ophthalmopathy. Although most frequent over the anterior and lateral aspects of the lower leg (hence the term *pretibial myxedema*), skin changes can occur at other sites, particularly after trauma. The typical lesion is a noninflamed, indurated plaque with a deep pink or purple color and an "orange-skin" appearance. Nodular involvement can occur, and the condition can rarely extend over the whole lower leg and foot, mimicking elephantiasis. *Thyroid acropachy* refers to a form of clubbing found in <1% of patients with Graves' disease (**Fig. 4-7*C***). It is so strongly associated with thyroid dermopathy that an alternative cause of clubbing should be sought in a Graves' patient without coincident skin and orbital involvement.

Laboratory Evaluation

Investigations used to determine the existence and cause of thyrotoxicosis are summarized in **Fig. 4-8**. In Graves' disease, the TSH level is suppressed and total and unbound thyroid hormone levels are increased. In 2–5% of patients (and more in areas of borderline iodine intake), only T_3 is increased (T_3 toxicosis). The converse state of T_4 toxicosis, with elevated total and unbound T_4 and normal T_3 levels, is occasionally seen when hyperthyroidism is induced by excess iodine, providing surplus substrate for thyroid hormone synthesis. Measurement of TPO antibodies is useful in differential diagnosis. Measurement of TBIIs or TSIs will confirm the diagnosis but is not needed routinely. Associated abnormalities that may cause diagnostic confusion in thyrotoxicosis include elevation of bilirubin, liver enzymes, and ferritin. Microcytic anemia and thrombocytopenia may occur.

Differential Diagnosis

Diagnosis of Graves' disease is straightforward in a patient with biochemically confirmed thyrotoxicosis, diffuse goiter on palpation, ophthalmopathy, positive TPO or TSH-R antibodies, and often a personal or family history of autoimmune disorders. For patients with thyrotoxicosis who lack these features, the most reliable diagnostic method is a radionuclide (^{99m}Tc, ^{123}I, or ^{131}I) scan of the thyroid, which will distinguish the diffuse, high uptake of Graves' disease from nodular thyroid disease, destructive thyroiditis, ectopic thyroid tissue, and factitious thyrotoxicosis. In secondary hyperthyroidism due to a TSH-secreting pituitary tumor, there is also a diffuse goiter. The presence of a nonsuppressed TSH level and the finding of a pituitary tumor on CT or MRI scan readily identify such patients.

Clinical features of thyrotoxicosis can mimic certain aspects of other disorders, including panic attacks, mania, pheochromocytoma, and weight loss associated with malignancy. The diagnosis of thyrotoxicosis can be easily excluded if the TSH and unbound T_4 and T_3 levels are normal. A normal TSH also excludes Graves' disease as a cause of diffuse goiter.

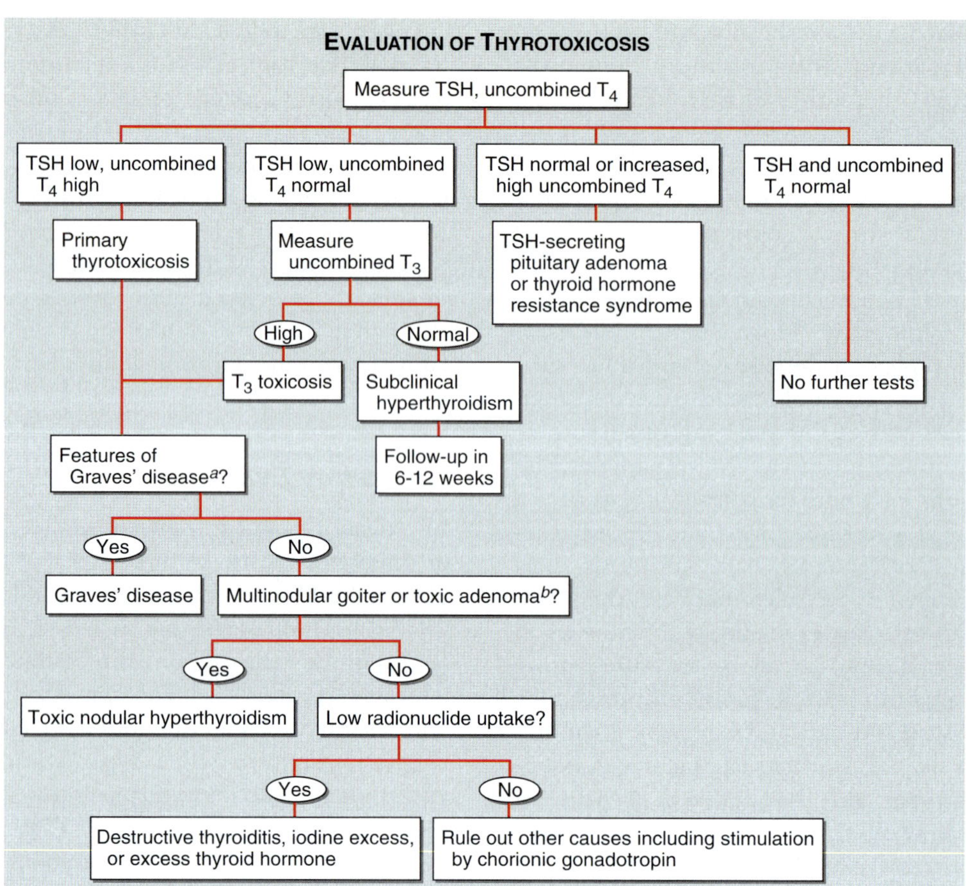

FIGURE 4-8

Evaluation of thyrotoxicosis. [a]Diffuse goiter, positive thyroid peroxidase (TPO) antibodies, ophthalmopathy, dermopathy; [b]can be confirmed by radionuclide scan. TSH, thyroid-stimulating hormone.

Clinical Course

Clinical features generally worsen without treatment; mortality was 10–30% before the introduction of satisfactory therapy. Some patients with mild Graves' disease experience spontaneous relapses and remissions. Rarely, there may be fluctuation between hypo- and hyperthyroidism due to changes in the functional activity of TSH-R antibodies. About 15% of patients who enter remission after treatment with antithyroid drugs develop hypothyroidism 10–15 years later as a result of the destructive autoimmune process.

The clinical course of ophthalmopathy does not follow that of the thyroid disease. Ophthalmopathy typically worsens over the initial 3–6 months, followed by a plateau phase over the next 12–18 months, with spontaneous improvement, particularly in the soft tissue changes. However, the course is more fulminant in up to 5% of patients, requiring intervention in the acute phase if there is optic nerve compression or corneal ulceration. Diplopia may appear late in the disease due to fibrosis of the extraocular muscles. Some studies suggest that radioiodine treatment for hyperthyroidism worsens the eye disease in a small proportion of patients (especially smokers). Antithyroid drugs or surgery have no adverse effects on the clinical course of ophthalmopathy. Thyroid dermopathy, when it occurs, usually appears 1–2 years after the development of Graves' hyperthyroidism; it may improve spontaneously.

℞ Treatment: GRAVES' DISEASE

The *hyperthyroidism* of Graves' disease is treated by reducing thyroid hormone synthesis, using antithyroid drugs, or reducing the amount of thyroid tissue with radioiodine (^{131}I) treatment or by thyroidectomy. Antithyroid drugs are the predominant therapy in many centers in Europe and Japan, whereas radioiodine is more often the first line of treatment in North America. These differences reflect the fact that no single approach is optimal and that patients may require multiple treatments to achieve remission.

The main *antithyroid drugs* are the thionamides, such as propylthiouracil, carbimazole, and the active metabolite of the latter, methimazole. All inhibit the function of

TPO, reducing oxidation and organification of iodide. These drugs also reduce thyroid antibody levels by mechanisms that remain unclear, and they appear to enhance rates of remission. Propylthiouracil inhibits deiodination of $T_4 \rightarrow T_3$. However, this effect is of minor benefit, except in the most severe thyrotoxicosis, and is offset by the much shorter half-life of this drug (90 min) compared to methimazole (6 h).

There are many variations of antithyroid drug regimens. The initial dose of carbimazole or methimazole is usually 10–20 mg every 8 or 12 h, but once-daily dosing is possible after euthyroidism is restored. Propylthiouracil is given at a dose of 100–200 mg every 6–8 h, and divided doses are usually given throughout the course. Lower doses of each drug may suffice in areas of low iodine intake. The starting dose of antithyroid drugs can be gradually reduced (titration regimen) as thyrotoxicosis improves. Alternatively, high doses may be given combined with levothyroxine supplementation (block-replace regimen) to avoid drug-induced hypothyroidism. Initial reports suggesting superior remission rates with the block-replace regimen have not been reproduced in several other trials. The titration regimen is often preferred to minimize the dose of antithyroid drug and provide an index of treatment response.

Thyroid function tests and clinical manifestations are reviewed 3–4 weeks after starting treatment, and the dose is titrated based on unbound T_4 levels. Most patients do not achieve euthyroidism until 6–8 weeks after treatment is initiated. TSH levels often remain suppressed for several months and therefore do not provide a sensitive index of treatment response. The usual daily maintenance doses of antithyroid drugs in the titration regimen are 2.5–10 mg of carbimazole or methimazole and 50–100 mg of propylthiouracil. In the block-replace regimen, the initial dose of antithyroid drug is held constant and the dose of levothyroxine is adjusted to maintain normal unbound T_4 levels. When TSH suppression is alleviated, TSH levels can also be used to monitor therapy.

Maximum remission rates (up to 30–50% in some populations) are achieved by 18–24 months for the titration regimen and by 6 months for the block-replace regimen. For unclear reasons, remission rates appear to vary in different geographic regions. Patients with severe hyperthyroidism and large goiters are most likely to relapse when treatment stops, but outcome is difficult to predict. All patients should be followed closely for relapse during the first year after treatment and at least annually thereafter.

The common side effects of antithyroid drugs are rash, urticaria, fever, and arthralgia (1–5% of patients). These may resolve spontaneously or after substituting an alternative antithyroid drug. Rare but major side effects include hepatitis, an SLE-like syndrome, and, most important, agranulocytosis (<1%). It is essential that antithyroid drugs are stopped and not restarted if a patient develops major side effects. Written instructions should be provided regarding the symptoms of possible agranulocytosis (e.g., sore throat, fever, mouth ulcers) and the need to stop treatment pending a complete blood count to confirm that agranulocytosis is not present. It is not useful to monitor blood counts prospectively, as the onset of agranulocytosis is idiosyncratic and abrupt.

Propranolol (20–40 mg every 6 h) or longer-acting beta blockers such as atenolol may be helpful to control adrenergic symptoms, especially in the early stages before antithyroid drugs take effect. The need for anticoagulation with Coumadin should be considered in all patients with atrial fibrillation. If digoxin is used, increased doses are often needed in the thyrotoxic state.

Radioiodine causes progressive destruction of thyroid cells and can be used as initial treatment or for relapses after a trial of antithyroid drugs. There is a small risk of thyrotoxic crisis after radioiodine, which can be minimized by pretreatment with antithyroid drugs for at least a month before treatment. Antecedent treatment with antithyroid drugs should be considered for all elderly patients or for those with cardiac problems, to deplete thyroid hormone stores before administration of radioiodine. Carbimazole or methimazole must be stopped at least 3 days before radioiodine administration to achieve optimum iodine uptake. Propylthiouracil has a prolonged radioprotective effect and should be stopped several weeks before radioiodine is given, or a larger dose of radioiodine will be necessary.

Efforts to calculate an optimal dose of radioiodine that achieves euthyroidism without a high incidence of relapse or progression to hypothyroidism have not been successful. Some patients inevitably relapse after a single dose because the biologic effects of radiation vary between individuals, and hypothyroidism cannot be uniformly avoided even using accurate dosimetry. A practical strategy is to give a fixed dose based on clinical features, such as the severity of thyrotoxicosis, the size of the goiter (increases the dose needed), and the level of radioiodine uptake (decreases the dose needed). ^{131}I dosage generally ranges between 185 MBq (5 mCi) and 555 MBq (15 mCi). Incomplete treatment or early relapse is more common in males and in patients <40 years of age. Many authorities favor an approach aimed at thyroid ablation (as opposed to euthyroidism), given that levothyroxine replacement is straightforward and most patients ultimately progress to hypothyroidism over 5–10 years, frequently with some delay in the diagnosis of hypothyroidism.

Certain radiation safety precautions are necessary in the first few days after radioiodine treatment, but the exact guidelines vary depending on local protocols.

In general, patients need to avoid close, prolonged contact with children and pregnant women for several days because of possible transmission of residual isotope and excessive exposure to radiation emanating from the gland. Rarely, there may be mild pain due to radiation thyroiditis 1–2 weeks after treatment. Hyperthyroidism can persist for 2–3 months before radioiodine takes full effect. For this reason, β-adrenergic blockers or antithyroid drugs can be used to control symptoms during this interval. Persistent hyperthyroidism can be treated with a second dose of radioiodine, usually 6 months after the first dose. The risk of hypothyroidism after radioiodine depends on the dosage but is at least 10–20% in the first year and 5% per year thereafter. Patients should be informed of this possibility before treatment and require close follow-up during the first year and annual thyroid function testing.

Pregnancy and breast-feeding are absolute contraindications to radioiodine treatment, but patients can conceive safely 6 months after treatment. The presence of severe ophthalmopathy requires caution, and some authorities advocate the use of prednisone, 40 mg/d, at the time of radioiodine treatment, tapered over 2–3 months to prevent exacerbation of ophthalmopathy. The overall risk of cancer after radioiodine treatment in adults is not increased. Although many physicians avoid radioiodine in children and adolescents because of the theoretical risks of malignancy, emerging evidence suggests that radioiodine can be used safely in older children.

Subtotal or near-total thyroidectomy is an option for patients who relapse after antithyroid drugs and prefer this treatment to radioiodine. Some experts recommend surgery in young individuals, particularly when the goiter is very large. Careful control of thyrotoxicosis with antithyroid drugs, followed by potassium iodide (3 drops SSKI PO tid), is needed prior to surgery to avoid thyrotoxic crisis and to reduce the vascularity of the gland. The major complications of surgery—bleeding, laryngeal edema, hypoparathyroidism, and damage to the recurrent laryngeal nerves—are unusual when the procedure is performed by highly experienced surgeons. Recurrence rates in the best series are <2%, but the rate of hypothyroidism is only slightly less than that following radioiodine treatment.

The titration regimen of antithyroid drugs should be used to manage Graves' disease in *pregnancy*, as blocking doses of these drugs produce fetal hypothyroidism. Propylthiouracil is usually used because of relatively low transplacental transfer and its ability to block $T_4 \rightarrow T_3$ conversion. Also, carbimazole and methimazole have been associated with rare cases of fetal *aplasia cutis* and other defects, such as choanal atresia. The lowest effective dose of propylthiouracil should be given, and it is often possible to stop treatment in the last trimester since TSIs tend to decline in pregnancy. Nonetheless, the transplacental transfer of these antibodies rarely causes *fetal* or *neonatal thyrotoxicosis*. Poor intrauterine growth, a fetal heart rate of >160 beats/min, and high levels of maternal TSIs in the last trimester may herald this complication. Antithyroid drugs given to the mother can be used to treat the fetus and may be needed for 1–3 months after delivery, until the maternal antibodies disappear from the baby's circulation. The postpartum period is a time of major risk for relapse of Graves' disease. Breast-feeding is safe with low doses of antithyroid drugs. Graves' disease in *children* is usually managed with antithyroid drugs, often given as a prolonged course of the titration regimen. Surgery or radioiodine may be indicated for severe disease.

Thyrotoxic crisis, or *thyroid storm*, is rare and presents as a life-threatening exacerbation of hyperthyroidism, accompanied by fever, delirium, seizures, coma, vomiting, diarrhea, and jaundice. The mortality rate due to cardiac failure, arrhythmia, or hyperthermia is as high as 30%, even with treatment. Thyrotoxic crisis is usually precipitated by acute illness (e.g., stroke, infection, trauma, diabetic ketoacidosis), surgery (especially on the thyroid), or radioiodine treatment of a patient with partially treated or untreated hyperthyroidism. Management requires intensive monitoring and supportive care, identification and treatment of the precipitating cause, and measures that reduce thyroid hormone synthesis. Large doses of propylthiouracil (600 mg loading dose and 200–300 mg every 6 h) should be given PO or by nasogastric tube or per rectum; the drug's inhibitory action on $T_4 \rightarrow T_3$ conversion makes it the antithyroid drug of choice. One hour after the first dose of propylthiouracil, stable iodide is given to block thyroid hormone synthesis via the Wolff-Chaikoff effect (the delay allows the antithyroid drug to prevent the excess iodine from being incorporated into new hormone). A saturated solution of potassium iodide (5 drops SSKI every 6 h), or ipodate or iopanoic acid (0.5 mg per 12 h), may be given PO. (Sodium iodide, 0.25 g IV every 6 h, is an alternative but is not generally available.) Propranolol should also be given to reduce tachycardia and other adrenergic manifestations (40–60 mg PO every 4 h, or 2 mg IV every 4 h). Although other β-adrenergic blockers can be used, high doses of propranolol decrease $T_4 \rightarrow T_3$ conversion, and the doses can be easily adjusted. Caution is needed to avoid acute negative inotropic effects, but controlling the heart rate is important, as some patients develop a form of high-output heart failure. Additional therapeutic measures include glucocorticoids (e.g., dexamethasone, 2 mg every 6 h), antibiotics if infection is present, cooling, oxygen, and IV fluids.

Ophthalmopathy requires no active treatment when it is mild or moderate, as there is usually spontaneous improvement. General measures include meticulous control of thyroid hormone levels, cessation of smoking, and an explanation of the natural history of ophthalmopathy. Discomfort can be relieved with artificial tears (e.g., 1% methylcellulose), eye ointment, and the use of dark glasses with side frames. Periorbital edema may respond to a more upright sleeping position or a diuretic. Corneal exposure during sleep can be avoided by using patches or taping the eyelids shut. Minor degrees of diplopia improve with prisms fitted to spectacles. Severe ophthalmopathy, with optic nerve involvement or chemosis resulting in corneal damage, is an emergency requiring joint management with an ophthalmologist. Short-term benefit can be gained in about two-thirds of patients by the use of high-dose glucocorticoids (e.g., prednisone, 40–80 mg daily), sometimes combined with cyclosporine. Glucocorticoid doses are tapered by 5 mg every 2 weeks, but the taper often results in reemergence of congestive symptoms. Pulse therapy with IV methylprednisolone (e.g., 1 g of methylprednisolone in 250 mL of saline infused over 2 h daily for 1 week) followed by an oral regimen is also used. When glucocorticoids are ineffective, orbital decompression can be achieved by removing bone from any wall of the orbit, thereby allowing displacement of fat and swollen extraocular muscles. The transantral route is used most often, as it requires no external incision. Proptosis recedes an average of 5 mm, but there may be residual or even worsened diplopia. Once the eye disease has stabilized, surgery may be indicated for relief of diplopia and correction of the appearance. External beam radiotherapy of the orbits has been used for many years, especially for ophthalmopathy of recent onset, but the objective evidence that this therapy is beneficial remains equivocal.

Thyroid dermopathy does not usually require treatment but can cause cosmetic problems or interfere with the fit of shoes. Surgical removal is not indicated. If necessary, treatment consists of topical, high-potency glucocorticoid ointment under an occlusive dressing. Octreotide may be beneficial in some cases.

OTHER CAUSES OF THYROTOXICOSIS

Destructive thyroiditis (subacute or silent thyroiditis) typically presents with a short thyrotoxic phase due to the release of preformed thyroid hormones and catabolism of Tg (see "Subacute Thyroiditis" later in the chapter). True hyperthyroidism is absent, as demonstrated by a low radionuclide uptake. Circulating Tg levels are usually increased. Other causes of thyrotoxicosis with low or absent thyroid radionuclide uptake include *thyrotoxicosis factitia*; iodine excess and, rarely, ectopic thyroid tissue, particularly teratomas of the ovary (*struma ovarii*); and functional metastatic follicular carcinoma. Whole-body radionuclide studies can demonstrate ectopic thyroid tissue, and thyrotoxicosis factitia can be distinguished from destructive thyroiditis by the clinical features and low levels of Tg. Amiodarone treatment is associated with thyrotoxicosis in up to 10% of patients, particularly in areas of low iodine intake.

TSH-secreting pituitary adenoma is a rare cause of thyrotoxicosis. It can be identified by the presence of an inappropriately normal or increased TSH level in a patient with hyperthyroidism, diffuse goiter, and elevated T_4 and T_3 levels (Chap. 2). Elevated levels of the subunit of TSH, released by the TSH-secreting adenoma, support this diagnosis, which can be confirmed by demonstrating the pituitary tumor on MRI or CT scan. A combination of transsphenoidal surgery, sella irradiation, and octreotide may be required to normalize TSH, as many of these tumors are large and locally invasive at the time of diagnosis. Radioiodine or antithyroid drugs can be used to control thyrotoxicosis.

Thyrotoxicosis caused by *toxic MNG* and *hyperfunctioning solitary nodules* is discussed below.

THYROIDITIS

A clinically useful classification of thyroiditis is based on the onset and duration of disease (Table 4-8).

ACUTE THYROIDITIS

Acute thyroiditis is rare and due to suppurative infection of the thyroid. In children and young adults, the most common cause is the presence of a piriform sinus, a remnant of the fourth branchial pouch that connects the oropharynx with the thyroid. Such sinuses are predominantly left-sided. A longstanding goiter and degeneration in a thyroid malignancy are risk factors in the elderly. The patient presents with thyroid pain, often

TABLE 4-8

CAUSES OF THYROIDITIS
Acute
Bacterial infection: especially *Staphylococcus*, *Streptococcus*, and *Enterobacter*
Fungal infection: *Aspergillus*, *Candida*, *Coccidioides*, *Histoplasma*, and *Pneumocystis*
Radiation thyroiditis after ^{131}I treatment
Amiodarone (may also be subacute or chronic)
Subacute
Viral (or granulomatous) thyroiditis
Silent thyroiditis (including postpartum thyroiditis)
Mycobacterial infection
Chronic
Autoimmunity: focal thyroiditis, Hashimoto's thyroiditis, atrophic thyroiditis
Riedel's thyroiditis
Parasitic thyroiditis: echinococcosis, strongyloidiasis, cysticercosis
Traumatic: after palpation

referred to the throat or ears, and a small, tender goiter that may be asymmetric. Fever, dysphagia, and erythema over the thyroid are common, as are systemic symptoms of a febrile illness and lymphadenopathy.

The differential diagnosis of *thyroid pain* includes subacute or, rarely, chronic thyroiditis, hemorrhage into a cyst, malignancy including lymphoma, and, rarely, amiodarone-induced thyroiditis or amyloidosis. However, the abrupt presentation and clinical features of acute thyroiditis rarely cause confusion. The erythrocyte sedimentation rate (ESR) and white blood cell count are usually increased, but thyroid function is normal. FNA biopsy shows infiltration by polymorphonuclear leukocytes; culture of the sample can identify the organism. Caution is needed in immunocompromised patients as fungal, mycobacterial, or *Pneumocystis* thyroiditis can occur in this setting. Antibiotic treatment is guided initially by Gram stain and subsequently by cultures of the FNA biopsy. Surgery may be needed to drain an abscess, which can be localized by CT scan or ultrasound. Tracheal obstruction, septicemia, retropharyngeal abscess, mediastinitis, and jugular venous thrombosis may complicate acute thyroiditis but are uncommon with prompt use of antibiotics.

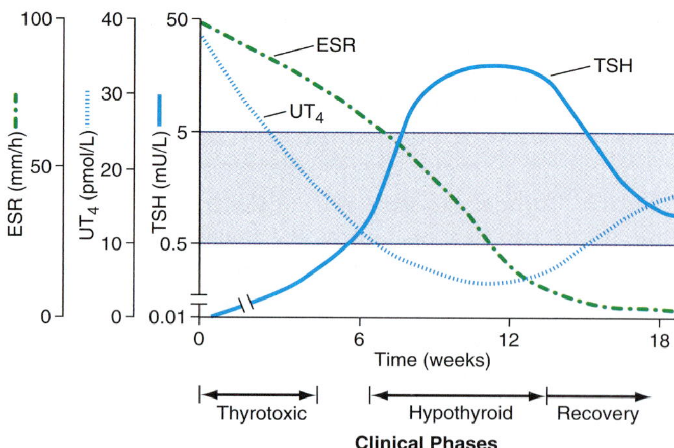

FIGURE 4-9

Clinical course of subacute thyroiditis. The release of thyroid hormones is initially associated with a thyrotoxic phase and suppressed thyroid-stimulating hormone (TSH). A hypothyroid phase then ensues, with low thyroxine (T_4) and TSH levels that are initially low but gradually increase. During the recovery phase, increased TSH levels combined with resolution of thyroid follicular injury leads to normalization of thyroid function, often several months after the beginning of the illness. ESR, erythrocyte sedimentation rate; UT_4, unbound T_4.

SUBACUTE THYROIDITIS

This is also termed *de Quervain's thyroiditis, granulomatous thyroiditis*, or *viral thyroiditis*. Many viruses have been implicated, including mumps, coxsackie, influenza, adenoviruses, and echoviruses, but attempts to identify the virus in an individual patient are often unsuccessful and do not influence management. The diagnosis of subacute thyroiditis is often overlooked because the symptoms can mimic pharyngitis. The peak incidence occurs at 30–50 years, and women are affected three times more frequently than men.

Pathophysiology

The thyroid shows a characteristic patchy inflammatory infiltrate with disruption of the thyroid follicles and multinucleated giant cells within some follicles. The follicular changes progress to granulomas accompanied by fibrosis. Finally, the thyroid returns to normal, usually several months after onset. During the initial phase of follicular destruction, there is release of Tg and thyroid hormones, leading to increased circulating T_4 and T_3 and suppression of TSH (Fig. 4-9). During this destructive phase, radioactive iodine uptake is low or undetectable. After several weeks, the thyroid is depleted of stored thyroid hormone and a phase of hypothyroidism typically occurs, with low unbound T_4 (and sometimes T_3) and moderately increased TSH levels. Radioactive iodine uptake returns to normal or is even increased as a result of the rise in TSH. Finally, thyroid hormone and TSH levels return to normal as the disease subsides.

Clinical Manifestations

The patient usually presents with a painful and enlarged thyroid, sometimes accompanied by fever. There may be features of thyrotoxicosis or hypothyroidism, depending on the phase of the illness. Malaise and symptoms of an upper respiratory tract infection may precede the thyroid-related features by several weeks. In other patients, the onset is acute, severe, and without obvious antecedent. The patient typically complains of a sore throat, and examination reveals a small goiter that is exquisitely tender. Pain is often referred to the jaw or ear. Complete resolution is the usual outcome, but permanent hypothyroidism can occur, particularly in those with coincidental thyroid autoimmunity. A prolonged course over many months, with one or more relapses, occurs in a small percentage of patients.

Laboratory Evaluation

As depicted in Fig. 4-9, thyroid function tests characteristically evolve through three distinct phases over about 6 months: (1) thyrotoxic phase, (2) hypothyroid phase, and (3) recovery phase. In the thyrotoxic phase, T_4 and T_3 levels are increased, reflecting their discharge from the damaged thyroid cells, and TSH is suppressed. The T_4/T_3 ratio is greater than in Graves' disease or thyroid autonomy, in which T_3 is often disproportionately increased. The diagnosis is confirmed by a high ESR and low radioiodine uptake. The white blood cell count may be increased, and thyroid antibodies are negative. If the diagnosis is in doubt, FNA biopsy may be useful, particularly to distinguish unilateral involvement from bleeding into a cyst or neoplasm.

℞ Treatment: SUBACUTE THYROIDITIS

Relatively large doses of aspirin (e.g., 600 mg every 4–6 h) or NSAIDs are sufficient to control symptoms in many cases. If this treatment is inadequate, or if the patient has marked local or systemic symptoms, glucocorticoids should be given. The usual starting dose is 40–60 mg prednisone, depending on severity. The dose is gradually tapered over 6–8 weeks, in response to improvement in symptoms and the ESR. If a relapse occurs during glucocorticoid withdrawal, treatment should be started again and withdrawn more gradually. In these patients, it is useful to wait until the radioactive iodine uptake normalizes before stopping treatment. Thyroid function should be monitored every 2–4 weeks using TSH and unbound T_4 levels. Symptoms of thyrotoxicosis improve spontaneously but may be ameliorated by β-adrenergic blockers; antithyroid drugs play no role in treatment of the thyrotoxic phase. Levothyroxine replacement may be needed if the hypothyroid phase is prolonged, but doses should be low enough (50 to 100 μg daily) to allow TSH-mediated recovery.

SILENT THYROIDITIS

Painless thyroiditis, or *"silent" thyroiditis*, occurs in patients with underlying autoimmune thyroid disease. It has a clinical course similar to that of subacute thyroiditis, except that there is little or no thyroid tenderness. The condition occurs in up to 5% of women 3–6 months after pregnancy and is then termed *postpartum thyroiditis*. Typically, patients have a brief phase of thyrotoxicosis lasting 2–4 weeks, followed by hypothyroidism for 4–12 weeks, and then resolution; often, however, only one phase is apparent. The condition is associated with the presence of TPO antibodies antepartum, and it is three times more common in women with type 1 diabetes mellitus. As in subacute thyroiditis, the radioactive iodine uptake is initially suppressed. In addition to the painless goiter, silent thyroiditis can be distinguished from subacute thyroiditis by a normal ESR and the presence of TPO antibodies. Glucocorticoid treatment is not indicated for silent thyroiditis. Severe thyrotoxic symptoms can be managed with a brief course of propranolol, 20–40 mg three or four times daily. Thyroxine replacement may be needed for the hypothyroid phase but should be withdrawn after 6–9 months, as recovery is the rule. Annual follow-up thereafter is recommended, as a proportion of these individuals develop permanent hypothyroidism.

DRUG-INDUCED THYROIDITIS

Patients receiving cytokines such as IFN-α or IL-2 may develop painless thyroiditis. IFN-α, which is used to treat chronic hepatitis B or C and hematologic and skin malignancies, causes thyroid dysfunction in up to 5% of treated patients. It has been associated with painless thyroiditis, hypothyroidism, and Graves' disease, and is most common in women with TPO antibodies prior to treatment. For discussion of amiodarone, see "Amiodarone Effects on Thyroid Function" later in the chapter.

CHRONIC THYROIDITIS

Focal thyroiditis is present in 20–40% of euthyroid autopsy cases and is associated with serologic evidence of autoimmunity, particularly the presence of TPO antibodies. These antibodies are 4–10 times more common in otherwise healthy women than men. The most common clinically apparent cause of chronic thyroiditis is *Hashimoto's thyroiditis*, an autoimmune disorder that often presents as a firm or hard goiter of variable size. *Riedel's thyroiditis* is a rare disorder that typically occurs in middle-aged women. It presents with an insidious, painless goiter with local symptoms due to compression of the esophagus, trachea, neck veins, or recurrent laryngeal nerves. Dense fibrosis disrupts normal gland architecture and can extend outside the thyroid capsule. Despite these extensive histologic changes, thyroid dysfunction is uncommon. The goiter is hard, nontender, often asymmetric, and fixed, leading to suspicion of a malignancy. Diagnosis requires open biopsy as FNA biopsy is usually inadequate. Treatment is directed to surgical relief of compressive symptoms. Tamoxifen may also be beneficial. There is an association between Riedel's thyroiditis and idiopathic fibrosis at other sites (retroperitoneum, mediastinum, biliary tree, lung, and orbit).

SICK EUTHYROID SYNDROME

Any acute, severe illness can cause abnormalities of circulating TSH or thyroid hormone levels in the absence of underlying thyroid disease, making these measurements potentially misleading. The major cause of these hormonal changes is the release of cytokines such as IL-6. Unless a thyroid disorder is strongly suspected, the routine testing of thyroid function should be avoided in acutely ill patients.

The most common hormone pattern in sick euthyroid syndrome (SES) is a decrease in total and unbound T_3 levels (low T_3 syndrome) with normal levels of T_4 and TSH. The magnitude of the fall in T_3 correlates with the severity of the illness. T_4 conversion to T_3 via peripheral deiodination is impaired, leading to increased rT_3. Despite this effect, decreased clearance rather than increased production is the major basis for increased rT_3. Also, T_4 is alternately metabolized to the hormonally inactive T_3 sulfate. It is generally assumed that this low T_3 state is adaptive, as it can be induced in normal individuals by fasting. Teleologically, the fall in T_3 may limit catabolism in starved or ill patients.

Very sick patients may exhibit a dramatic fall in total T_4 and T_3 levels (low T_4 syndrome). This state has a poor prognosis. A key factor in the fall in T_4 levels is altered binding to TBG. T_4 assays usually demonstrate a normal unbound T_4 level in such patients, depending on the assay method used. Fluctuation in TSH levels also creates challenges in the interpretation of thyroid function in sick patients. TSH levels may range from <0.1 to >20 mU/L; these alterations reverse after recovery, confirming the absence of underlying thyroid disease. A rise in cortisol or administration of glucocorticoids may provide a partial explanation for decreased TSH levels. The exact mechanisms underlying the subnormal TSH seen in 10% of sick patients and the increased TSH seen in 5% remain unclear but may be mediated by cytokines including IL-12 and IL-18.

Any severe illness can induce changes in thyroid hormone levels, but certain disorders exhibit a distinctive pattern of abnormalities. Acute liver disease is associated with an initial rise in total (but not unbound) T_3 and T_4 levels, due to TBG release; these levels become subnormal with progression to liver failure. A transient increase in total and unbound T_4 levels, usually with a normal T_3 level, is seen in 5–30% of acutely ill psychiatric patients. TSH values may be transiently low, normal, or high in these patients. In the early stage of HIV infection, T_3 and T_4 levels rise, even if there is weight loss. T_3 levels fall with progression to AIDS, but TSH usually remains normal. Renal disease is often accompanied by low T_3 concentrations, but with normal rather than increased rT_3 levels, due to an unknown factor that increases uptake of rT_3 into the liver.

The diagnosis of SES is challenging. Historic information may be limited, and patients often have multiple metabolic derangements. Useful features to consider include previous history of thyroid disease and thyroid function tests, evaluation of the severity and time course of the patient's acute illness, documentation of medications that may affect thyroid function or thyroid hormone levels, and measurements of rT_3 together with unbound thyroid hormones and TSH. The diagnosis of SES is frequently presumptive, given the clinical context and pattern of laboratory values; only resolution of the test results with clinical recovery can clearly establish this disorder. Treatment of SES with thyroid hormone (T_4 and/or T_3) is controversial, but most authorities recommend monitoring the patient's thyroid function tests during recovery, without administering thyroid hormone, unless there is historic or clinical evidence suggestive of hypothyroidism. Sufficiently large randomized controlled trials using thyroid hormone are unlikely to resolve this therapeutic controversy in the near future, because clinical presentations and outcomes are highly variable.

AMIODARONE EFFECTS ON THYROID FUNCTION

Amiodarone is a commonly used type III antiarrhythmic agent. It is structurally related to thyroid hormone and contains 39% iodine by weight. Thus, typical doses of amiodarone (200 mg/d) are associated with very high iodine intake, leading to greater than fortyfold increase in plasma and urinary iodine levels. Moreover, because amiodarone is stored in adipose tissue, high iodine levels persist for >6 months after discontinuation of the drug. Amiodarone inhibits deiodinase activity, and its metabolites function as weak antagonists of thyroid hormone action. Amiodarone has the following effects on thyroid function: (1) acute, transient suppression of thyroid function; (2) hypothyroidism in patients susceptible to the inhibitory effects of a high iodine load; and (3) thyrotoxicosis that may be caused by a Jod-Basedow effect from the iodine load in the setting of MNG, a thyroiditis-like condition, or possibly induction of autoimmune Graves' disease.

The initiation of amiodarone treatment is associated with a transient decrease of T_4 levels, reflecting the inhibitory effect of iodine on T_4 release. Soon thereafter, most individuals escape from iodide-dependent suppression of the thyroid (Wolff-Chaikoff effect), and the inhibitory effects on deiodinase activity and thyroid hormone receptor action become predominant. These events lead to the following pattern of thyroid function tests: increased T_4, decreased T_3, increased rT_3, and a transient increase of TSH (up to 20 mU/L). TSH levels normalize or are slightly suppressed by 1–3 months.

The incidence of hypothyroidism from amiodarone varies geographically, apparently correlating with iodine intake. Hypothyroidism occurs in up to 13% of amiodarone-treated patients in iodine-replete countries, such as the United States, but is less common (<6% incidence) in areas of lower iodine intake, such as Italy or Spain. The pathogenesis appears to involve an inability of the thyroid gland to escape from the Wolff-Chaikoff effect in autoimmune thyroiditis. Consequently, amiodarone-associated hypothyroidism is more common in women and individuals with positive TPO antibodies. It is usually unnecessary to discontinue amiodarone for this side effect, as levothyroxine can be used to normalize thyroid function. TSH levels should be monitored, because T_4 levels are often increased for the reasons described above.

The management of amiodarone-induced thyrotoxicosis (AIT) is complicated by the fact that there are several causes of thyrotoxicosis and because the increased thyroid hormone levels exacerbate underlying arrhythmias and coronary artery disease. Amiodarone treatment causes thyrotoxicosis in 10% of patients living in areas of low iodine intake and in 2% of patients in regions of high iodine intake. There are two major forms of AIT, although some patients have features of both. Type 1 AIT is associated with an underlying thyroid abnormality (preclinical Graves' disease or nodular goiter). Thyroid hormone synthesis becomes excessive as a result of increased iodine exposure (Jod-Basedow phenomenon). Type 2 AIT occurs in individuals with no intrinsic thyroid abnormalities and is the result of drug-induced lysosomal activation leading to destructive thyroiditis with histiocyte accumulation in the thyroid. Mild forms of type 2 AIT can resolve spontaneously or can occasionally lead to hypothyroidism. Color-flow Doppler thyroid scanning shows increased vascularity in type 1 AIT but decreased vascularity in type 2 AIT. Thyroid scintiscans are difficult to interpret in this setting, because the high endogenous iodine levels diminish tracer uptake. However, the presence of normal or increased uptake favors type 1 AIT.

In AIT the drug should be stopped, if possible, although this is often impractical because of the underlying cardiac disorder. Discontinuation of amiodarone will not have an acute effect because of its storage and prolonged half-life. High doses of antithyroid drugs can be used in type 1 AIT but are often ineffective. In type 2 AIT, oral contrast agents, such as sodium ipodate (500 mg/d) or sodium tyropanoate (500 mg, 1–2 doses/d), rapidly reduce T_4 and T_3 levels, decrease $T_4 \rightarrow T_3$ conversion, and may block tissue uptake of thyroid hormones. Potassium perchlorate, 200 mg every 6 h, has been used to reduce thyroidal iodide content. Perchlorate treatment has been associated with agranulocytosis, though the risk appears relatively low with short-term use. Glucocorticoids, administered as for subacute thyroiditis, are of variable benefit in type 2 AIT. Lithium blocks thyroid hormone release and can provide modest benefit. Near-total thyroidectomy rapidly decreases thyroid hormone levels and may be the most effective long-term solution, if the patient can undergo the procedure safely.

THYROID FUNCTION IN PREGNANCY

Five factors alter thyroid function in pregnancy: (1) the transient increase in hCG during the first trimester, which stimulates the TSH-R; (2) the estrogen-induced rise in TBG during the first trimester, which is sustained during pregnancy; (3) alterations in the immune system, leading to the onset, exacerbation, or amelioration of an underlying autoimmune thyroid disease; (4) increased thyroid hormone metabolism by the placenta; and (5) increased urinary iodide excretion, which can cause impaired thyroid hormone production in areas of marginal iodine sufficiency. Women with a precarious iodine intake (<50 μg/d) are most at risk of developing a goiter during pregnancy, and iodine supplementation should be considered to prevent maternal and fetal hypothyroidism and the development of neonatal goiter.

The rise in circulating hCG levels during the first trimester is accompanied by a reciprocal fall in TSH that persists into the middle of pregnancy. This appears to reflect weak binding of hCG, which is present at very high levels, to the TSH-R. Rare individuals have been described with variant TSH-R sequences that enhance hCG binding and TSH-R activation. hCG-induced changes in thyroid function can result in transient gestational hyperthyroidism and/or *hyperemesis gravidarum*, a condition characterized by severe nausea and vomiting and risk of volume depletion. Antithyroid drugs are rarely needed, and parenteral fluid replacement usually suffices until the condition resolves.

Maternal hypothyroidism occurs in 2–3% of women of childbearing age and is associated with increased risk of developmental delay in the offspring. Consequently, TSH screening for hypothyroidism is indicated in early pregnancy and should be considered in women who are planning pregnancy, particularly if they have a goiter or strong family history of autoimmune thyroid disease. Thyroid hormone requirements are increased by 25–50 μg/d during pregnancy.

GOITER AND NODULAR THYROID DISEASE

Goiter refers to an enlarged thyroid gland. Biosynthetic defects, iodine deficiency, autoimmune disease, and nodular diseases can each lead to goiter, though by different mechanisms. Biosynthetic defects and iodine deficiency are associated with reduced efficiency of thyroid hormone synthesis, leading to increased TSH, which stimulates thyroid growth as a compensatory mechanism to overcome the block in hormone synthesis. Graves' disease and Hashimoto's thyroiditis are also associated with goiter. In Graves' disease, the goiter results mainly from the TSH-R-mediated effects of TSI. The goitrous form of Hashimoto's thyroiditis occurs because of acquired defects in hormone synthesis, leading to elevated levels of TSH and its consequent growth effects. Lymphocytic infiltration and immune system induced growth factors also contribute to thyroid enlargement in Hashimoto's thyroiditis. Nodular disease is characterized by the disordered growth of thyroid cells, often combined with the gradual development of fibrosis. Because the management of goiter depends on the etiology, the detection of thyroid enlargement on physical examination should prompt further evaluation to identify its cause.

Nodular thyroid disease is common, occurring in about 3–7% of adults when assessed by physical examination. Using more sensitive techniques, such as ultrasound, it is present in >25% of adults. Thyroid nodules may be solitary or multiple, and they may be functional or nonfunctional.

DIFFUSE NONTOXIC (SIMPLE) GOITER

Etiology and Pathogenesis

When diffuse enlargement of the thyroid occurs in the absence of nodules and hyperthyroidism, it is referred to as a *diffuse nontoxic goiter*. This is sometimes called *simple goiter*, because of the absence of nodules, or *colloid goiter*, because of the presence of uniform follicles that are filled with colloid. Worldwide, diffuse goiter is most commonly caused by iodine deficiency and is termed *endemic goiter* when it affects >5% of the population. In nonendemic regions, *sporadic goiter* occurs, and the cause is usually unknown. Thyroid enlargement in teenagers is sometimes referred to as *juvenile goiter*. In general, goiter is more common in women than men, probably because of the greater prevalence of underlying autoimmune disease and the increased iodine demands associated with pregnancy.

In *iodine-deficient areas*, thyroid enlargement reflects a compensatory effort to trap iodide and produce sufficient hormone under conditions in which hormone synthesis is relatively inefficient. Somewhat surprisingly, TSH levels are usually normal or only slightly increased, suggesting increased sensitivity to TSH or activation of other pathways that lead to thyroid growth. Iodide appears to have direct actions on thyroid vasculature and may indirectly affect growth through vasoactive substances such as endothelins and nitric oxide. Endemic goiter is also caused by exposure to environmental *goitrogens* such as cassava root, which contains a thiocyanate; vegetables of the Cruciferae family (e.g., brussels sprouts, cabbage, and cauliflower); and milk from regions where goitrogens are present in grass. Though relatively rare, inherited defects in thyroid hormone synthesis lead to a diffuse nontoxic goiter. Abnormalities at each step in hormone synthesis, including iodide transport (NIS), Tg synthesis, organification and coupling (TPO), and the regeneration of iodide (dehalogenase), have been described.

CLINICAL MANIFESTATIONS AND DIAGNOSIS

If thyroid function is preserved, most goiters are asymptomatic. Spontaneous hemorrhage into a cyst or nodule may cause the sudden onset of localized pain and swelling. Examination of a diffuse goiter reveals a symmetrically enlarged, nontender, generally soft gland without palpable nodules. Goiter is defined, somewhat arbitrarily, as a lateral lobe with a volume greater than the thumb of the individual being examined. If the thyroid is markedly enlarged, it can cause tracheal or esophageal compression. These features are unusual, however, in the absence of nodular disease and fibrosis. *Substernal goiter* may obstruct the thoracic inlet. *Pemberton's sign* refers to symptoms of faintness with evidence of facial congestion and external jugular venous obstruction when the arms are raised above the head, a maneuver that draws the thyroid into the thoracic inlet. Respiratory flow measurements and CT or MRI should be used to evaluate substernal goiter in patients with obstructive signs or symptoms.

Thyroid function tests should be performed in all patients with goiter to exclude thyrotoxicosis or hypothyroidism. It is not unusual, particularly in iodine deficiency, to find a low total T_4, with normal T_3 and TSH, reflecting enhanced $T_4 \rightarrow T_3$ conversion. A low TSH, particularly in older patients, suggests the possibility of thyroid autonomy or undiagnosed Graves' disease, causing subclinical thyrotoxicosis. TPO antibodies may be useful to identify patients at increased risk of autoimmune thyroid disease. Low urinary iodine levels (<10 μg/dL) support a diagnosis of iodine deficiency. Thyroid scanning is not generally necessary but will reveal increased uptake in iodine deficiency and most cases of dyshormonogenesis. Ultrasound is not generally indicated in the evaluation of diffuse goiter unless a nodule is palpable on physical examination.

℞ Treatment:
DIFFUSE NONTOXIC (SIMPLE) GOITER

Iodine or thyroid hormone replacement induces variable regression of goiter in iodine deficiency, depending on how long it has been present and the degree of fibrosis that has developed. Because of the possibility of underlying thyroid autonomy, caution should be exercised when instituting suppressive thyroxine therapy in patients with goiter, particularly if the baseline TSH is in the low-normal range. In younger patients, the dose of levothyroxine can be started at 100 μg/d and adjusted to suppress the TSH into the low-normal but detectable range. Treatment of elderly patients should be initiated at 50 μg/d. The efficacy of suppressive treatment is greater in younger patients and for those with soft goiters. Significant regression is usually seen within 3–6 months of treatment; after this time it is unlikely to occur. In older patients, and in those with some degree of nodular disease or fibrosis, fewer than one-third demonstrate significant shrinkage of the goiter. Surgery is rarely indicated for diffuse goiter. Exceptions include documented evidence of tracheal compression or obstruction of the thoracic inlet, which are more likely to be associated with substernal multinodular goiters. Subtotal or near-total thyroidectomy for these or cosmetic reasons should be performed by an experienced surgeon to minimize complication rates, which occur in up to 10% of cases. Surgery should be followed by mild suppressive treatment with levothyroxine to prevent regrowth of the goiter. Radioiodine reduces goiter size by about 50% in the majority of patients. It is rarely associated with transient acute swelling of the thyroid, which is usually inconsequential unless there is severe tracheal narrowing. If not treated with levothyroxine, patients should be followed after radioiodine treatment for the possible development of hypothyroidism.

NONTOXIC MULTINODULAR GOITER

Etiology and Pathogenesis

Depending on the population studied, MNG occurs in up to 12% of adults. MNG is more common in women than men and increases in prevalence with age. It is more common in iodine-deficient regions but also occurs in regions of iodine sufficiency, reflecting multiple genetic, autoimmune, and environmental influences on the pathogenesis.

There is typically wide variation in nodule size. Histology reveals a spectrum of morphologies ranging from hypercellular regions to cystic areas filled with colloid. Fibrosis is often extensive, and areas of hemorrhage or lymphocytic infiltration may be seen. Using molecular techniques, most nodules within a MNG are polyclonal in origin, suggesting a hyperplastic response to locally produced growth factors and cytokines. TSH, which is usually not elevated, may play a permissive or contributory role. Monoclonal lesions also occur within a MNG, reflecting mutations in genes that confer a selective growth advantage to the progenitor cell.

Clinical Manifestations

Most patients with nontoxic MNG are asymptomatic and, by definition, euthyroid. MNG typically develops over many years and is detected on routine physical examination or when an individual notices an enlargement in the neck. If the goiter is large enough, it can ultimately lead to compressive symptoms including difficulty swallowing, respiratory distress (tracheal compression), or plethora (venous congestion), but these symptoms are uncommon. Symptomatic MNGs are usually extraordinarily large and/or develop fibrotic areas that cause compression. Sudden pain in a MNG is usually caused by hemorrhage into a nodule but should raise the possibility of invasive malignancy. Hoarseness, reflecting laryngeal nerve involvement, also suggests malignancy.

Diagnosis

On examination, thyroid architecture is distorted, and multiple nodules of varying size can be appreciated. Because many nodules are deeply embedded in thyroid tissue or reside in posterior or substernal locations, it is not possible to palpate all nodules. A TSH level should be measured to exclude subclinical hyper- or hypothyroidism, but thyroid function is usually normal. Tracheal deviation is common, but compression must usually exceed 70% of the tracheal diameter before there is significant airway compromise. Pulmonary function testing can be used to assess the functional effects of compression and to detect tracheomalacia, which characteristically causes inspiratory stridor. CT or MRI can be used to evaluate the anatomy of the goiter and the extent of substernal extension, which is often much greater than is apparent on physical examination. A barium swallow may reveal the extent of esophageal compression. The risk of malignancy in MNG is similar to that in solitary nodules. Ultrasonography can be used to identify which nodules should be biopsied, including large, dominant nodules or those with sonographic characteristics suggestive of malignancy (e.g., microcalcifications, hypoechogenicity, increased vascularity).

Rx Treatment: NONTOXIC MULTINODULAR GOITER

Most nontoxic MNGs can be managed conservatively. T_4 suppression is rarely effective for reducing goiter size and introduces the risk of thyrotoxicosis, particularly if there is underlying autonomy or if it develops during treatment. If levothyroxine is used, it should be started at low doses (50 μg) and advanced gradually while monitoring the TSH level to avoid excessive suppression. Contrast agents and other iodine-containing substances should be avoided because of the risk of inducing the *Jod-Basedow effect*, characterized by enhanced thyroid hormone production by autonomous nodules. Radioiodine is being used with increasing frequency because it often decreases goiter size and may selectively ablate regions of autonomy. Dosage of ^{131}I depends on the size of the goiter and radioiodine uptake but is usually about 3.7 MBq (0.1 mCi) per gram of tissue, corrected for uptake [typical dose 370–1070 Mbq (10 to 29 mCi)]. Repeat treatment may be needed. It is possible to achieve a 40–50% reduction in goiter size in most patients. Earlier concerns about radiation-induced thyroid swelling and tracheal compression have diminished as recent studies have shown this complication to be rare. When acute compression occurs, glucocorticoid treatment or surgery may be needed. Radiation-induced hypothyroidism is less common than after treatment for Graves' disease. However, posttreatment autoimmune thyrotoxicosis may occur in up to 5% of patients treated for nontoxic MNG. Surgery remains highly effective but is not without risk, particularly in older patients with underlying cardiopulmonary disease.

TOXIC MULTINODULAR GOITER

The pathogenesis of toxic MNG appears to be similar to that of nontoxic MNG; the major difference is the presence of functional autonomy in toxic MNG. The molecular basis for autonomy in toxic MNG remains unknown. As in nontoxic goiters, many nodules are polyclonal, while others are monoclonal and vary in their clonal origins. Genetic abnormalities known to confer functional autonomy, such as activating TSH-R or $G_s\alpha$ mutations, are not usually found in the autonomous regions of toxic MNG goiter.

In addition to features of goiter, the clinical presentation of toxic MNG includes subclinical hyperthyroidism or mild thyrotoxicosis. The patient is usually elderly and may present with atrial fibrillation or palpitations, tachycardia, nervousness, tremor, or weight loss. Recent exposure to iodine, from contrast dyes or other sources, may precipitate or exacerbate thyrotoxicosis. The TSH level is low. The T_4 level may be normal or minimally increased; T_3 is often elevated to a greater degree than T_4. Thyroid scan shows heterogeneous uptake with multiple regions of increased and decreased uptake; 24-h uptake of radioiodine may not be increased.

Rx Treatment: TOXIC MULTINODULAR GOITER

The management of toxic MNG is challenging. Antithyroid drugs, often in combination with beta blockers, can normalize thyroid function and address clinical features of thyrotoxicosis. This treatment, however, often stimulates the growth of the goiter, and in contrast to Graves' disease, spontaneous remission does not occur. Radioiodine can be used to treat areas of autonomy as well as to decrease the mass of the goiter. Usually, however, some degree of autonomy remains, presumably because multiple autonomous regions emerge as soon as others are treated. Nonetheless, a trial of radioiodine should be considered before subjecting patients, many of whom are elderly, to surgery. Surgery provides definitive treatment of underlying thyrotoxicosis as well as goiter. Patients should be rendered euthyroid using antithyroid drugs before operation.

HYPERFUNCTIONING SOLITARY NODULE

A solitary, autonomously functioning thyroid nodule is referred to as *toxic adenoma*. The pathogenesis of this disorder has been unraveled by demonstrating the functional effects of mutations that stimulate the TSH-R signaling pathway. Most patients with solitary hyperfunctioning nodules have acquired somatic, activating mutations in the TSH-R (**Fig. 4-10**). These mutations, located primarily in the receptor transmembrane domain, induce constitutive receptor coupling to $G_s\alpha$, increasing cyclic AMP levels and leading to enhanced thyroid follicular cell proliferation and function. Less commonly, somatic mutations are identified in $G_s\alpha$. These mutations, which are similar to those seen in McCune-Albright syndrome (Chap. 29) or in a subset of somatotrope adenomas (Chap. 2), impair GTP hydrolysis, also causing constitutive activation of the cyclic AMP signaling pathway. In most series, activating mutations in either the TSH-R or the $G_s\alpha$ subunit genes are identified in >90% of patients with solitary hyperfunctioning nodules.

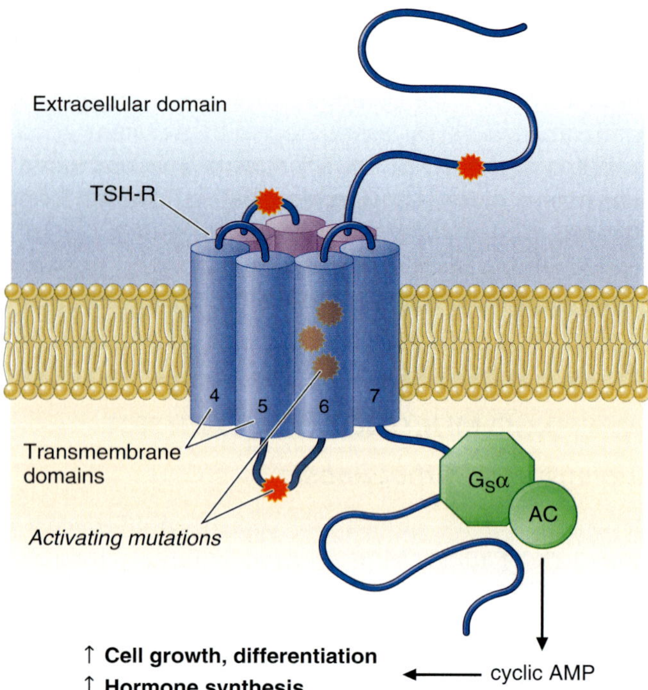

FIGURE 4-10

Activating mutations of the TSH-R. Mutations (*) that activate the thyroid-stimulating hormone receptor (TSH-R) reside mainly in transmembrane 5 and intracellular loop 3, though mutations have occurred in a variety of different locations. The effect of these mutations is to induce conformational changes that mimic TSH binding, thereby leading to coupling to stimulatory G protein ($G_s\alpha$) and activation of adenylate cyclase (AC), an enzyme that generates cyclic AMP.

Thyrotoxicosis is usually mild. The disorder is suggested by the presence of the thyroid nodule, which is generally large enough to be palpable, and by the absence of clinical features suggestive of Graves' disease or other causes of thyrotoxicosis. A thyroid scan provides a definitive diagnostic test, demonstrating focal uptake in the hyperfunctioning nodule and diminished uptake in the remainder of the gland, as activity of the normal thyroid is suppressed.

Rx Treatment: HYPERFUNCTIONING SOLITARY NODULE

Radioiodine ablation is usually the treatment of choice. Because normal thyroid function is suppressed, ^{131}I is concentrated in the hyperfunctioning nodule with minimal uptake and damage to normal thyroid tissue. Relatively large radioiodine doses [e.g., 370–1110 MBq (10–29.9 mCi) ^{131}I] have been shown to correct thyrotoxicosis in about 75% of patients within 3 months. Hypothyroidism occurs in <10% of patients over the next 5 years. Surgical resection is also effective and is usually limited to enucleation of the adenoma or lobectomy, thereby preserving thyroid function and minimizing risk of hypoparathyroidism or damage to the recurrent laryngeal nerves. Medical therapy using antithyroid drugs and beta blockers can normalize thyroid function but is not an optimal long-term treatment. Ethanol injection under ultrasound guidance has been used successfully in some centers to ablate hyperfunctioning nodules. Repeated injections (often more than five sessions) are required to reduce nodule size. Normal thyroid function can be achieved in most patients using this technique.

BENIGN NEOPLASMS

The various types of benign thyroid nodules are listed in Table 4-9. These lesions are common (5–10% adults), particularly when assessed by sensitive techniques such as ultrasound. The risk of malignancy is very low for *macrofollicular adenomas* and *normofollicular adenomas*. *Microfollicular, trabecular, and Hürthle cell variants* raise greater concern, and the histology is more difficult to interpret. About one-third of palpable nodules are *thyroid cysts*. These may be recognized by their ultrasound appearance or based on aspiration of large amounts of pink or straw-colored fluid (colloid). Many are mixed cystic/solid lesions, in which case it is desirable to aspirate cellular components under ultrasound or harvest cells after cytospin of cyst fluid. Cysts frequently recur, even after repeated aspiration, and may require surgical excision if they are large or if the cytology is suspicious. Sclerosis has been used with variable success but is often painful and may be complicated by infiltration of the sclerosing agent.

The treatment approach for benign nodules is similar to that for MNG. TSH suppression with levothyroxine decreases the size of about 30% of nodules and may prevent further growth. The TSH level should be suppressed into the low-normal range, assuming there are no contraindications; alternatively, nodule size can be monitored without suppression. If a nodule has not decreased in size after 6–12 months of suppressive therapy, treatment should be discontinued since little benefit is likely to accrue from long-term treatment.

TABLE 4-9

CLASSIFICATION OF THYROID NEOPLASMS

BENIGN	
Follicular epithelial cell adenomas	
Macrofollicular (colloid)	
Normofollicular (simple)	
Microfollicular (fetal)	
Trabecular (embryonal)	
Hürthle cell variant (oncocytic)	
MALIGNANT	**APPROXIMATE PREVALENCE, %**
Follicular epithelial cell	
Well-differentiated carcinomas	
Papillary carcinomas	80–90
Pure papillary	
Follicular variant	
Diffuse sclerosing variant	
Tall cell, columnar cell variants	
Follicular carcinomas	5–10
Minimally invasive	
Widely invasive	
Hürthle cell carcinoma (oncocytic)	
Insular carcinoma	
Undifferentiated (anaplastic) carcinomas	
C cell (calcitonin-producing)	
Medullary thyroid cancer	10
Sporadic	
Familial	
MEN 2	
Other malignancies	
Lymphomas	1–2
Sarcomas	
Metastases	
Others	

Note: MEN, multiple endocrine neoplasia.

THYROID CANCER

Thyroid carcinoma is the most common malignancy of the endocrine system. Malignant tumors derived from the follicular epithelium are classified according to histologic features. Differentiated tumors, such as papillary thyroid cancer (PTC) or follicular thyroid cancer (FTC), are often curable, and the prognosis is good for patients identified with early-stage disease. In contrast, anaplastic thyroid cancer (ATC) is aggressive, responds poorly to treatment, and is associated with a bleak prognosis.

The incidence of thyroid cancer (~9/100,000 per year) increases with age, plateauing after about age 50 (Fig. 4-11). Age is also an important prognostic factor—thyroid cancer at a young age (<20) or in older persons (>45) is associated with a worse prognosis. Thyroid cancer is twice as common in women as men, but male sex is associated with a worse prognosis. Additional important risk factors include a history of childhood head or neck irradiation, large nodule size (≥4 cm), evidence for local

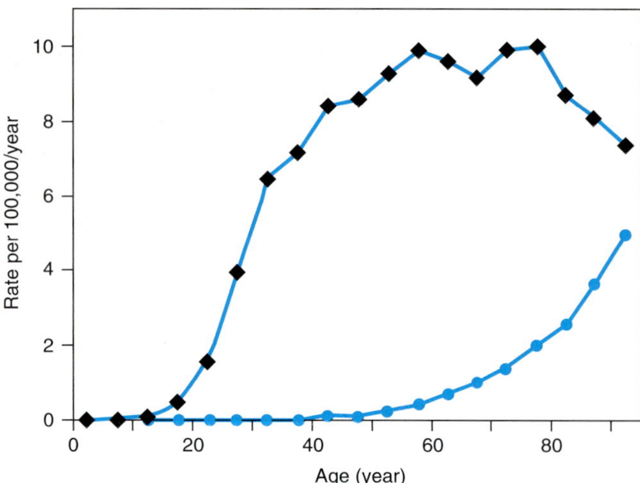

FIGURE 4-11

Age-associated incidence (—◆—) and mortality (—●—) rates for invasive thyroid cancer. [*Adapted from LAG Ries et al (eds): SEER Cancer Statistics Review, 1973–1996, Bethesda, National Cancer Institute, 1999.*]

tumor fixation or invasion into lymph nodes, and the presence of metastases (Table 4-10).

Several unique features of thyroid cancer facilitate its management: (1) thyroid nodules are readily palpable, allowing early detection and biopsy by FNA; (2) iodine radioisotopes can be used to diagnose (^{123}I) and treat (^{131}I) differentiated thyroid cancer, reflecting the unique uptake of this anion by the thyroid gland; and (3) serum markers allow the detection of residual or recurrent disease, including the use of Tg levels for PTC and FTC and calcitonin for medullary thyroid cancer (MTC).

CLASSIFICATION

Thyroid neoplasms can arise in each of the cell types that populate the gland, including thyroid follicular cells, calcitonin-producing C cells, lymphocytes, and stromal and vascular elements, as well as metastases from other sites (Table 4-9). The American Joint Committee on Cancer (AJCC) has designated a staging system using the TNM classification (Table 4-11). Several other classification and staging systems are also widely used, some of which place greater emphasis on histologic features or risk factors such as age or gender.

TABLE 4-10

RISK FACTORS FOR THYROID CARCINOMA IN PATIENTS WITH THYROID NODULE

History of head and neck irradiation	Family history of thyroid cancer or MEN 2
Age <20 or >45 years	Vocal cord paralysis, hoarse voice
Bilateral disease	Nodule fixed to adjacent structures
Increased nodule size (>4 cm)	Extrathyroidal extension
New or enlarging neck mass	Suspected lymph node involvement
Male sex	Iodine deficiency (follicular cancer)

Note: MEN, multiple endocrine neoplasia.

TABLE 4-11

THYROID CANCER CLASSIFICATION[a]

Papillary or Follicular Thyroid Cancers		
	< 45 years	> 45 years
Stage I	Any T, any N, M0	T1, N0, M0
Stage II	Any T, any N, M1	T2 or T3, N0, M0
Stage III	—	T4, N0, M0 Any T, N1, M0
Stage IV	—	Any T, any N, M1
Anaplastic Thyroid Cancer		
Stage IV	All cases are stage IV	
Medullary Thyroid Cancer		
Stage I	T1, N0, M0	
Stage II	T2–T4, N0, M0	
Stage III	Any T, N1, M0	
Stage IV	Any T, any N, M1	

[a]Criteria include T, the size and extent of the primary tumor (T1, ≤1 cm; T2, >1 cm and ≤ 4 cm; T3, >4 cm; T4, direct invasion through the thyroid capsule); N, the absence (N0) or presence (N1) of regional node involvement; M, the absence (M0) or presence (M1) of metastases.
Source: American Joint Committee on Cancer staging system for thyroid cancers using the TNM classification.

PATHOGENESIS AND GENETIC BASIS

Radiation

Early studies of the pathogenesis of thyroid cancer focused on the role of external radiation, which predisposes to chromosomal breaks, presumably leading to genetic rearrangements and loss of tumor-suppressor genes. External radiation of the mediastinum, face, head, and neck region was administered in the past to treat an array of conditions, including acne and enlargement of the thymus, tonsils, and adenoids. Radiation exposure increases the risk of benign and malignant thyroid nodules, is associated with multicentric cancers, and shifts the incidence of thyroid cancer to an earlier age group. Radiation from nuclear fallout also increases the risk of thyroid cancer. Children seem more predisposed to the effects of radiation than adults. Of note, radiation derived from ^{131}I therapy appears to contribute minimal increased risk of thyroid cancer.

TSH and Growth Factors

Many differentiated thyroid cancers express TSH receptors and, therefore, remain responsive to TSH. This observation provides the rationale for T_4 suppression of TSH in patients with thyroid cancer. Residual expression of TSH receptors also allows TSH-stimulated uptake of ^{131}I therapy.

Oncogenes and Tumor-Suppressor Genes

Thyroid cancers are monoclonal in origin, consistent with the idea that they originate as a consequence of mutations that confer a growth advantage to a single cell. In addition to increased rates of proliferation, some thyroid cancers exhibit impaired apoptosis and features that enhance invasion, angiogenesis, and metastasis. By analogy with the model of multistep carcinogenesis proposed for colon cancer, thyroid neoplasms have been analyzed for a variety of genetic alterations, but without clear evidence of an ordered acquisition of somatic mutations as they progress from the benign to the malignant state. On the other hand, certain mutations are relatively specific for thyroid neoplasia, some of which correlate with histologic classification (Table 4-12).

TABLE 4-12

GENETIC ALTERATIONS IN THYROID NEOPLASIA

GENE/PROTEIN	TYPE OF GENE	CHROMOSOMAL LOCATION	GENETIC ABNORMALITY	TUMOR
TSH receptor	GPCR receptor	14q31	Point mutations	Toxic adenoma, differentiated carcinomas
$G_s\alpha$	G protein	20q13.2	Point mutations	Toxic adenoma, differentiated carcinomas
RET/PTC	Receptor tyrosine kinase	10q11.2	Rearrangements PTC1: (inv(10)q11.2q21) PTC2: (t(10;17)(q11.2;q23)) PTC3: ELE1/TK	PTC
RET	Receptor tyrosine kinase	10q11.2	Point mutations	MEN 2, medullary thyroid cancer
BRAF	MEK kinase	7q24	Point mutations, rearrangements	PTC
TRK	Receptor tyrosine kinase	1q23-24	Rearrangements	Multinodular goiter, papillary thyroid cancer
RAS	Signal transducing p21	Hras 11p15.5 Kras 12p12.1; Nras 1p13.2	Point mutations	Differentiated thyroid carcinoma, adenomas
p53	Tumor suppressor, cell cycle control, apoptosis	17p13	Point mutations Deletion, insertion	Anaplastic cancer
APC	Tumor suppressor, adenomatous polyposis coli gene	5q21-q22	Point mutations	Anaplastic cancer, also associated with familial polyposis coli
p16 (MTS1, CDKN2A)	Tumor suppressor, cell cycle control	9p21	Deletions	Differentiated carcinomas
p21/WAF	Tumor suppressor, cell cycle control	6p21.2	Overexpression	Anaplastic cancer
MET	Receptor tyrosine kinase	7q31	Overexpression	Follicular thyroid cancer
c-MYC	Receptor tyrosine kinase	8q24.12-13	Overexpression	Differentiated carcinoma
PTEN	Phosphatase	10q23	Point mutations	PTC in Cowden's syndrome (multiple hamartomas, breast tumors, gastrointestinal polyps, thyroid tumors)
CTNNB1	β-Catenin	3p22	Point mutations	Anaplastic cancer
Loss of heterozygosity (LOH)	?Tumor suppressors	3p; 11q13 Other loci	Deletions	Differentiated thyroid carcinomas, anaplastic cancer
PAX8-PPARγ1	Transcription factor Nuclear receptor fusion	t(2;3)(q13;p25)	Translocation	Follicular adenoma or carcinoma

Note: TSH, thyroid-stimulating hormone; $G_s\alpha$, G-protein stimulating (-subunit; RET, rearranged during transfection proto-oncogene; PTC, papillary thyroid cancer; TRK, tyrosine kinase receptor; RAS, rat sarcoma proto-oncogene; p53, p53 tumor suppressor gene; MET, met proto-oncogene (hepatocyte growth factor receptor); c-MYC, cellular homologue of myelocytomatosis virus proto-oncogene; PTEN, phosphatase and tensin homologue; APC, adenomatous polyposis coli; MTS, multiple tumor suppressor; CDKN2A, cyclin-dependent kinase inhibitor 2A; P21, p21 tumor suppressor; WAF, wild-type p53 activated fragment; GPCR, G protein–coupled receptor; ELE1/TK, ret-activating geneele1/tyrosine kinase; MEN 2, multiple endocrine neoplasia-2; PAX8, paired domain transcription factor; PPARγ1, peroxisome-proliferator activated receptor γ1; BRAF, v-raf homologue, B1; MEK, mitogen extracellular signal-regulated kinase.

Source: Adapted with permission from P Kopp, JL Jameson, in JL Jameson (ed): Principles of Molecular Medicine. Totowa, NJ, Humana Press, 1998.

Activating mutations of the TSH-R and the $G_s\alpha$ subunit are associated with autonomously functioning nodules. Though these mutations induce thyroid cell growth, this type of nodule is almost always benign.

Activation of the RET-RAS-BRAF signaling pathway is seen in most PTCs, though the types of mutations are heterogeneous. A variety of rearrangements involving the *RET* gene on chromosome 10 brings this receptor tyrosine kinase under the control of other promoters, leading to receptor overexpression. *RET* rearrangements occur in 20–40% of PTCs in different series and were observed with increased frequency in tumors developing after the Chernobyl radiation accident. Rearrangements in PTC have also been observed for another tyrosine kinase gene, *TRK1*, which is located on chromosome 1. To date, the identification of PTC with *RET* or *TRK1* rearrangements has not proven useful for predicting prognosis or treatment responses. *BRAF* mutations appear to be the most common genetic alteration in PTC. These mutations activate the kinase, which stimulates the mitogen-activated protein MAP kinase (MAPK) cascade. *RAS* mutations, which also stimulate the MAPK cascade, are found in about 20–30% of thyroid neoplasms, including both PTC and FTC. Of note, simultaneous *RET*, *BRAF*, and *RAS* mutations do not occur in the same tumor, suggesting that activation of the MAPK cascade is critical for tumor development, independent of the step that initiates the cascade.

As noted above, *RAS* mutations also occur in FTCs. In addition, a rearrangement of the thyroid developmental transcription factor PAX8 with the nuclear receptor PPARγ is identified in a significant fraction of FTCs. Loss of heterozygosity of 3p or 11q, consistent with deletions of tumor-suppressor genes, is also common in FTCs.

Most of the mutations seen in differentiated thyroid cancers have also been detected in ATCs. Mutations in CTNNB1, which encodes β-catenin, occur in about two-thirds of ATCs, but not in PTC or FTC. Mutations of the tumor suppressor p53 also play an important role in the development of ATC. Because p53 plays a role in cell cycle surveillance, DNA repair, and apoptosis, its loss may contribute to the rapid acquisition of genetic instability as well as poor treatment responses (Table 4-12).

MTC, when associated with multiple endocrine neoplasia (MEN) type 2, harbors an inherited mutation of the *RET* gene. Unlike the rearrangements of *RET* seen in PTC, the mutations in MEN 2 are point mutations that induce constitutive activity of the tyrosine kinase (Chap. 23). MTC is preceded by hyperplasia of the C cells, raising the likelihood that as-yet-unidentified "second hits" lead to cellular transformation. A subset of sporadic MTC contains somatic mutations that activate *RET*.

WELL-DIFFERENTIATED THYROID CANCER

Papillary

PTC is the most common type of thyroid cancer, accounting for 70–90% of well-differentiated thyroid malignancies. Microscopic PTC is present in up to 25% of thyroid glands at autopsy, but most of these lesions are very small (several millimeters) and are not clinically significant. Characteristic cytologic features of PTC help make the diagnosis by FNA or after surgical resection; these include psammoma bodies, cleaved nuclei with an "orphan Annie" appearance caused by large nucleoli, and the formation of papillary structures.

PTC tends to be multifocal and to invade locally within the thyroid gland as well as through the thyroid capsule and into adjacent structures in the neck. It has a propensity to spread via the lymphatic system but can metastasize hematogenously as well, particularly to bone and lung. Because of the relatively slow growth of the tumor, a significant burden of pulmonary metastases may accumulate, sometimes with remarkably few symptoms. The prognostic implication of lymph node spread is debated. Lymph node involvement by thyroid cancer can be remarkably well tolerated but appears to increase the risk of recurrence and mortality, particularly in older patients. The staging of PTC by the TNM system is outlined in Table 4-11. Most papillary cancers are identified in the early stages (>80% stages I or II) and have an excellent prognosis, with survival curves similar to expected survival (Fig. 4-12*A*). Mortality is markedly increased in stage IV disease (distant metastases), but this group comprises only about 1% of patients. The treatment of PTC is described below.

Follicular

The incidence of FTC varies widely in different parts of the world; it is more common in iodine-deficient regions. FTC is difficult to diagnose by FNA because the distinction between benign and malignant follicular neoplasms rests largely on evidence of invasion into vessels, nerves, or adjacent structures. FTC tends to spread by hematogenous routes leading to bone, lung, and central nervous system metastases. Mortality rates associated with FTC are less favorable than for PTC, in part because a larger proportion of patients present with stage IV disease (Fig. 4-12*B*). Poor prognostic features include distant metastases, age >50 years, primary tumor size >4 cm, Hürthle cell histology, and the presence of marked vascular invasion.

Rx Treatment: WELL-DIFFERENTIATED THYROID CANCER

SURGERY All well-differentiated thyroid cancers should be surgically excised. In addition to removing the primary lesion, surgery allows accurate histologic diagnosis and staging, and multicentric disease is commonly found in the contralateral thyroid lobe. Lymph node

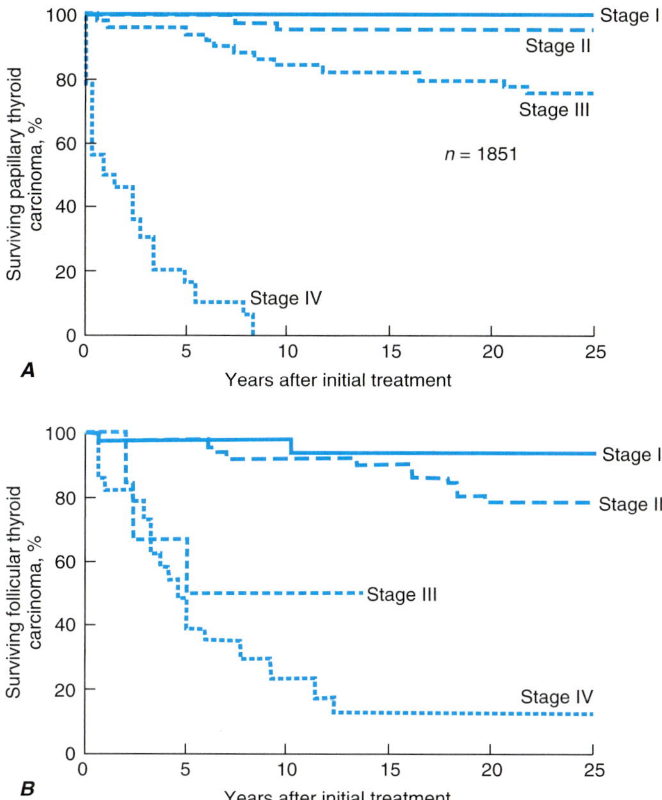

FIGURE 4-12

Survival rates in patients with differentiated thyroid cancer. ***A.*** Papillary cancer, cohort of 1851 patients. I, 1107 (60%); II, 408 (22%); III, 312 (17%); IV, 24 (1%); $n = 1185$. ***B.*** Follicular cancer, cohort of 153 patients. I, 42 (27%); II, 82 (54%); III, 6 (4%); IV, 23 (15%); $n = 153$. [*Adapted from PR Larsen et al: Williams Textbook of Endocrinology, 9th ed, JD Wilson et al (eds). Philadelphia, Saunders, 1998, pp 389–575, with permission.*]

spread can also be assessed at the time of surgery, and involved nodes can be removed. Recommendations about the extent of surgery vary for stage I disease, as survival rates are similar for lobectomy and near-total thyroidectomy. Lobectomy is associated with a lower incidence of hypoparathyroidism and injury to the recurrent laryngeal nerves. However, it is not possible to monitor Tg levels or to perform whole-body ^{131}I scans in the presence of the residual lobe. Moreover, if final staging or subsequent follow-up indicates the need for radioiodine scanning or treatment, repeat surgery is necessary to remove the remaining thyroid tissue. Therefore, near-total thyroidectomy is preferable in almost all patients; complication rates are acceptably low if the surgeon is highly experienced in the procedure. Postsurgical radioablation of the remnant thyroid tissue is increasingly being used as it may destroy remaining or multifocal thyroid carcinoma, and it facilitates the use of Tg determinations and radioiodine scanning for long-term follow-up by eliminating residual normal or neoplastic tissue.

TSH SUPPRESSION THERAPY As most tumors are still TSH-responsive, levothyroxine suppression of TSH is a mainstay of thyroid cancer treatment. Though TSH suppression clearly provides therapeutic benefit, there are no prospective studies that identify the optimal level of TSH suppression. A reasonable goal is to suppress TSH as much as possible without subjecting the patient to unnecessary side effects from excess thyroid hormone, such as atrial fibrillation, osteopenia, anxiety, and other manifestations of thyrotoxicosis. For patients at low risk of recurrence, TSH should be suppressed into the low but detectable range (0.1–0.5 IU/L). For patients at high risk of recurrence or with known metastatic disease, complete TSH suppression is indicated if there are no strong contraindications to mild thyrotoxicosis. In this instance, unbound T_4 must also be monitored to avoid excessive treatment.

RADIOIODINE TREATMENT Well-differentiated thyroid cancer still incorporates radioiodine, though less efficiently than normal thyroid follicular cells. Radioiodine uptake is determined primarily by expression of the NIS and is stimulated by TSH, requiring expression of the TSH-R. The retention time for radioactivity is influenced by the extent to which the tumor retains differentiated functions such as iodide trapping and organification. After near-total thyroidectomy, substantial thyroid tissue often remains, particularly in the thyroid bed and surrounding the parathyroid glands. Consequently, ^{131}I ablation is necessary to eliminate remaining normal thyroid tissue and to treat residual tumor cells.

Indications The use of therapeutic doses of radioiodine remains an area of controversy in thyroid cancer management. However, postoperative thyroid ablation and radioiodine treatment of known residual PTC or FTC clearly reduce recurrence rates but have a smaller impact on mortality, particularly in patients at relatively low risk. This low-risk group includes most patients with stage I PTC with primary tumors <1.5 cm in size. For patients with larger papillary tumors, spread to the adjacent lymph nodes, FTC, or evidence of metastases, thyroid ablation and radioiodine treatment are generally indicated.

^{131}I Thyroid Ablation and Treatment As noted above, the decision to use ^{131}I for thyroid ablation should be coordinated with the surgical approach, as radioablation is much more effective when there is minimal remaining normal thyroid tissue. A typical strategy is to treat the patient for several weeks postoperatively with liothyronine (25 μg bid or tid), followed by thyroid hormone withdrawal. Ideally, the TSH level should increase to >50 IU/L over 3–4 weeks. The level to which TSH rises is dictated largely by the amount of normal thyroid tissue remaining postoperatively. Recombinant human TSH (rhTSH) has also been used to enhance ^{131}I uptake for postsurgical ablation. It appears to be at least as effective as thyroid hormone withdrawal and should be particularly useful as residual thyroid tissue prevents an adequate endogenous TSH rise. rhTSH is currently approved for postoperative ablation in Europe but not in the United States.

A pretreatment scanning dose of ^{131}I [usually 111–185 MBq (3–5 mCi)] can reveal the amount of residual tissue and provides guidance about the dose needed to accomplish ablation. However, because of concerns about radioactive "stunning" that impairs subsequent treatment, there is a trend to avoid pretreatment scanning and to proceed directly to ablation, unless there is suspicion that the amount of residual tissue will alter therapy. A maximum outpatient ^{131}I dose is 1110 MBq (29.9 mCi) in the United States, though ablation is often more complete using greater doses [1850–3700 MBq (50–100 mCi)]. Patients should be placed on a low-iodine diet (<50 μg/d urinary iodine) to increase radioiodine uptake. In patients with known residual cancer, the larger doses ensure thyroid ablation and may destroy remaining tumor cells. A whole-body scan following the high-dose radioiodine treatment is useful to identify possible metastatic disease.

Follow-Up Whole-Body Thyroid Scanning and Thyroglobulin Determinations An initial whole-body scan should be performed about 6 months after thyroid ablation. The strategy for follow-up management of thyroid cancer has been altered by the availability of rhTSH to stimulate ^{131}I uptake and by the improved sensitivity of Tg assays to detect residual or recurrent disease. A scheme for using either rhTSH or thyroid hormone withdrawal for thyroid scanning is summarized in Fig. 4-13. After thyroid ablation, rhTSH can be used in follow-up to stimulate Tg and ^{131}I uptake without subjecting patients to thyroid hormone withdrawal and its associated symptoms of hypothyroidism as well as the risk of tumor growth after prolonged TSH stimulation. Alternatively, in patients who are likely to require ^{131}I treatment, the traditional approach of thyroid hormone withdrawal can be used to increase TSH. This involves switching patients from levothyroxine (T_4) to the more rapidly cleared hormone liothyronine (T_3), thereby allowing TSH to increase more quickly. Because TSH stimulates Tg levels, Tg measurements should be obtained after administration of rhTSH or when TSH levels have risen after thyroid hormone withdrawal.

In low-risk patients who have no clinical evidence of residual disease after ablation and a basal Tg <1 ng/mL, increasing evidence supports the use of rhTSH-stimulated Tg levels 1 year after ablation, without the need for radioiodine scanning. If stimulated Tg levels are low (<2 ng/mL) and, ideally, undetectable, these patients can be managed with suppressive therapy and

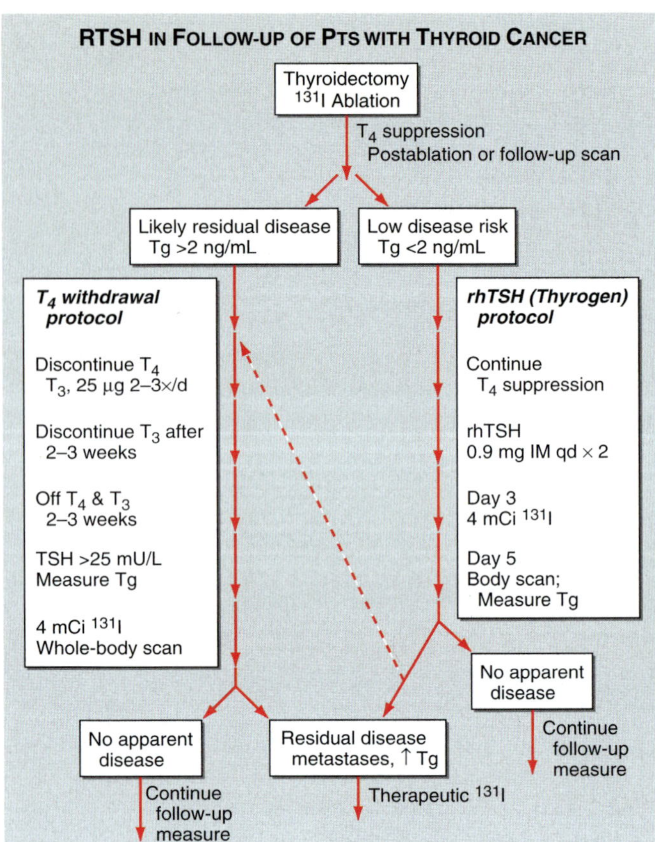

FIGURE 4-13

Use of recombinant thyroid-stimulating hormone (TSH) in the follow-up of patients with thyroid cancer. Tg, thyroglobulin; rhTSH, recombinant human TSH.

measurements of unstimulated Tg every 6–12 months. The absence of Tg antibodies should be confirmed in these patients. On the other hand, patients with residual disease on whole-body scanning or those with elevated Tg levels require additional ^{131}I therapy. In addition, most authorities advocate radioiodine treatment for scan-negative, Tg-positive (Tg >5–10 ng/mL) patients, as many derive therapeutic benefit from a large dose of ^{131}I.

In addition to radioiodine, external beam radiotherapy is also used to treat specific metastatic lesions, particularly when they cause bone pain or threaten neurologic injury (e.g., vertebral metastases).

ANAPLASTIC AND OTHER FORMS OF THYROID CANCER

Anaplastic Thyroid Cancer

As noted above, ATC is a poorly differentiated and aggressive cancer. The prognosis is poor, and most patients die within 6 months of diagnosis. Because of the undifferentiated state of these tumors, the uptake of radioiodine is usually negligible, but it can be used therapeutically if there is residual uptake. Chemotherapy has been attempted with multiple agents, including anthracyclines and paclitaxel, but it is usually ineffective. External beam radiation therapy can be attempted and continued if tumors are responsive.

Thyroid Lymphoma

Lymphoma in the thyroid gland often arises in the background of Hashimoto's thyroiditis. A rapidly expanding thyroid mass suggests the possibility of this diagnosis. Diffuse large-cell lymphoma is the most common type in the thyroid. Biopsies reveal sheets of lymphoid cells that can be difficult to distinguish from small cell lung cancer or ATC. These tumors are often highly sensitive to external radiation. Surgical resection should be avoided as initial therapy because it may spread disease that is otherwise localized to the thyroid. If staging indicates disease outside of the thyroid, treatment should follow guidelines used for other forms of lymphoma.

MEDULLARY THYROID CARCINOMA

MTC can be sporadic or familial and accounts for about 5–10% of thyroid cancers. There are three familial forms of MTC: MEN 2A, MEN 2B, and familial MTC without other features of MEN (Chap. 23). In general, MTC is more aggressive in MEN 2B than in MEN 2A, and familial MTC is more aggressive than sporadic MTC. Elevated serum calcitonin provides a marker of residual or recurrent disease. It is reasonable to test all patients with MTC for *RET* mutations, as genetic counseling and testing of family members can be offered to those individuals who test positive for mutations.

The management of MTC is primarily surgical. Unlike tumors derived from thyroid follicular cells, these tumors do not take up radioiodine. External radiation treatment and chemotherapy may provide palliation in patients with advanced disease (Chap. 23).

Approach to the Patient: A THYROID NODULE

Palpable thyroid nodules are found in about 5% of adults, but the prevalence varies considerably worldwide. Given this high prevalence rate, it is common for the practitioner to identify thyroid nodules. The main goal of this evaluation is to identify, in a cost-effective manner, the small subgroup of individuals with malignant lesions.

As described above, nodules are more common in iodine-deficient areas, in women, and with aging. Most palpable nodules are >1 cm in diameter, but the ability to feel a nodule is influenced by its location within the gland (superficial versus deeply embedded), the anatomy of the patient's neck, and the experience of the examiner. More sensitive methods of detection, such as CT, thyroid ultrasound, and pathologic studies, reveal thyroid nodules in >20% of glands. The presence of these thyroid incidentalomas has led to much debate about how to detect nodules and which nodules to investigate further. Most authorities still rely on physical examination to detect thyroid nodules, reserving ultrasound for monitoring nodule size or as an aid in thyroid biopsy.

An approach to the evaluation of a solitary nodule is outlined in Fig. 4-14. Most patients with thyroid nodules have normal thyroid function tests. Nonetheless, thyroid function should be assessed by measuring a TSH level, which may be suppressed by one or more autonomously functioning nodules. If the TSH is suppressed, a radionuclide scan is indicated to determine if the identified nodule is "hot," as lesions with increased uptake are almost never malignant and FNA is unnecessary. Otherwise, FNA biopsy should be the first step in the evaluation of a thyroid nodule. FNA has good sensitivity and specificity when performed by physicians familiar with the procedure and when the results are interpreted by experienced cytopathologists. The technique is particularly good for detecting PTC. The distinction of benign and malignant follicular lesions is often not possible using cytology alone.

In several large studies, FNA biopsies yielded the following findings: 70% benign, 10% malignant or suspicious for malignancy, and 20% nondiagnostic or yielding insufficient material for diagnosis. Characteristic features of malignancy mandate surgery. A diagnosis of follicular neoplasm also warrants surgery, as benign and malignant lesions cannot be distinguished based on cytopathology or frozen section. The management of patients with benign lesions is more variable. Many authorities advocate TSH suppression, whereas others monitor nodule size without suppression. With either approach, thyroid nodule size should be monitored, ideally using ultrasound. Repeat FNA is indicated if a nodule enlarges, and a second biopsy should be performed within 2–5 years to confirm the benign status of the nodule.

Nondiagnostic biopsies occur for many reasons, including a fibrotic reaction with relatively few cells available for aspiration, a cystic lesion in which cellular components reside along the cyst margin, or a nodule that may be too small for accurate aspiration. For these reasons, ultrasound-guided FNA is indicated when the FNA is repeated. Ultrasound is also increasingly used for initial biopsies in an effort to enhance nodule localization and the accuracy of sampling. Ultrasound characteristics are also useful for deciding which nodules to biopsy when multiple nodules are present.

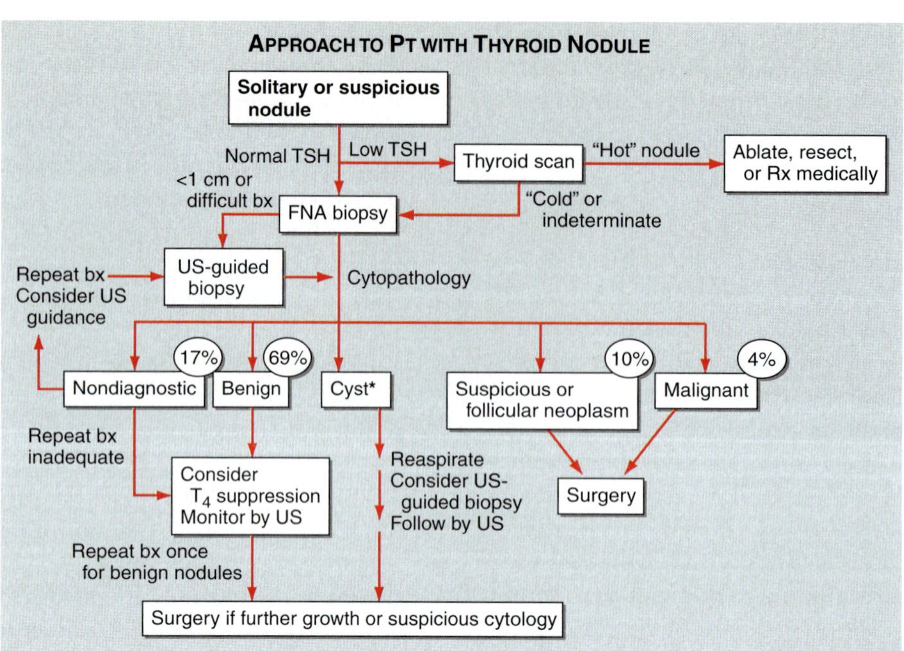

FIGURE 4-14

Approach to the patient with a thyroid nodule. See text and references for details. *About one-third of nodules are cystic or mixed solid-cystic. US, ultrasound; TSH, thyroid-stimulating hormone; FNA, fine-needle aspiration.

Sonographic characteristics suggestive of malignancy include microcalcifications, increased vascularity, and hypoechogenicity within the nodule.

The evaluation of a thyroid nodule is stressful for most patients. They are concerned about the possibility of thyroid cancer, whether verbalized or not. It is constructive, therefore, to review the diagnostic approach and to reassure patients when no malignancy is found. When a suspicious lesion or thyroid cancer is identified, an explanation of the generally favorable prognosis and available treatment options should be provided.

FURTHER READINGS

ABALOVICH M et al: Management of thyroid dysfunction during pregnancy and postpartum: An Endocrine Society Clinical Practice Guideline. J Clin Endocrinol Metab 92(Suppl):S1, 2007

ACHARYA SH et al: Radioiodine therapy (RAI) for Graves' disease (GD) and the effect on ophthalmopathy: A systematic review. Clin Endocrinol (Oxf) 69:943, 2008

BAUER M et al: Brain glucose metabolism in hypothyroidism: A positron emission tomography study before and after thyroid hormone replacement therapy. J Clin Endocrinol Metab 94:2922, 2009

BRENT GA: Clinical practice. Graves' disease. N Engl J Med 358:2594, 2008

CARLE A et al: Thyroid volume in hypothyroidism due to autoimmune disease follows a unimodal distribution: Evidence against primary thyroid atrophy and autoimmune thyroiditis being distinct diseases. J Clin Endocrinol Metab 94:833, 2009

COOPER DS: Antithyroid drugs. N Engl J Med 352:905, 2005

DE FELICE M, DI LAURO R: Thyroid development and its disorders: Genetics and molecular mechanisms. Endo Rev 25:722, 2004

DEGROOT LJ et al: Thyroid gland (Part 10, Vol 2), in *Endocrinology*, 5th ed, LJ DeGroot, JL Jameson (eds). Philadelphia, Elsevier Saunders, 2006

ESCOBAR-MORREALE HF et al: Treatment of hypothyroidism with combinations of levothyroxine plus liothyronine. J Clin Endocrinol Metab 90:4946, 2005

GHARIB H et al: Subclinical thyroid dysfunction: A joint statement on management from the American Association of Clinical Endocrinologists, the American Thyroid Association, and the Endocrine Society. J Clin Endocrinol Metab 90:581, 2005

KONDO T et al: Pathogenetic mechanisms in thyroid follicular cell neoplasia. Nat Rev Cancer 6:292, 2006

MORENO JC et al: Mutations in the iodotyrosine deiodinase gene and hypothyroidism. N Engl J Med 358:1811, 2008

PEARCE EN: Diagnosis and management of thyrotoxicosis. BMJ 332(7554):1369, 2006

ROBERTS CGP, Ladenson PW: Hypothyroidism. Lancet 363:793, 2004

SHERMAN SI et al: Motesanib diphosphate in progressive differentiated thyroid cancer. N Engl J Med 359:31, 2008

WEETMAN AP: Cellular immune responses in autoimmune thyroid disease. Clin Endocrinol 61:405, 2004

ZIMMERMANN MB: Iodine deficiency. Endocr Rev 30:376, 2009

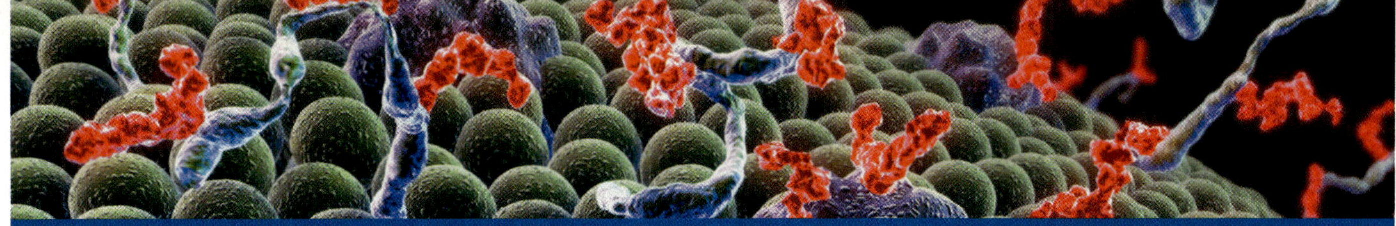

CHAPTER 5

DISORDERS OF THE ADRENAL CORTEX

Gordon H. Williams ■ Robert G. Dluhy

BIOCHEMISTRY AND PHYSIOLOGY

The adrenal cortex produces three major classes of steroids: (1) glucocorticoids, (2) mineralocorticoids, and (3) adrenal androgens. Consequently, normal adrenal function is important for modulating intermediary metabolism and immune responses through glucocorticoids; blood pressure, vascular volume, and electrolytes through mineralocorticoids; and secondary sexual characteristics (in females) through androgens. The adrenal axis plays an important role in the stress response by rapidly increasing cortisol levels. Adrenal disorders include hyperfunction (Cushing's syndrome) and hypofunction (adrenal insufficiency), as well as a variety of genetic abnormalities of steroidogenesis.

STEROID NOMENCLATURE

The basic structure of steroids is built upon a five-ring nucleus (**Fig. 5-1**). The carbon atoms are numbered in a sequence beginning with ring A. Adrenal steroids contain either 19 or 21 carbon atoms. The C_{19} steroids have methyl groups at C-18 and C-19. C_{19} steroids with a ketone group at C-17 are termed *17-ketosteroids*; C_{19} steroids have predominantly androgenic activity. The C_{21} steroids have a 2-carbon side chain (C-20 and C-21) attached at position 17 and methyl groups at C-18 and C-19; C_{21} steroids with a hydroxyl group at position 17 are termed *17-hydroxycorticosteroids*. The C_{21} steroids have either glucocorticoid or mineralocorticoid properties.

BIOSYNTHESIS OF ADRENAL STEROIDS

Cholesterol, derived from the diet and from endogenous synthesis, is the substrate for steroidogenesis. Uptake of cholesterol by the adrenal cortex is mediated by the low-density lipoprotein (LDL) receptor. With long-term stimulation of the adrenal cortex by adrenocorticotropic hormone (ACTH), the number of LDL receptors increases. The three major adrenal biosynthetic pathways lead to the production of glucocorticoids (cortisol), mineralocorticoids (aldosterone), and adrenal androgens (dehydroepiandrosterone). Separate zones of the adrenal

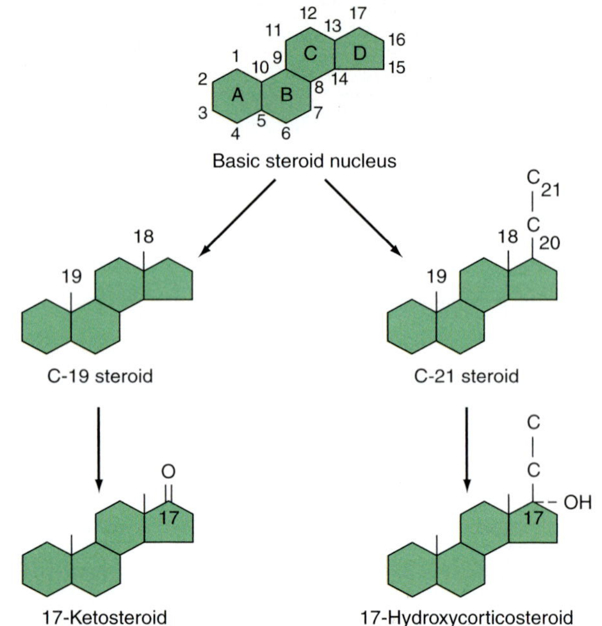

FIGURE 5-1

Basic steroid structure and nomenclature.

cortex synthesize specific hormones (**Fig. 5-2**). This zonation is accompanied by the selective expression of the genes encoding the enzymes unique to the formation of each type of steroid: aldosterone synthase is normally expressed only in the outer (glomerulosa) cell layer, whereas 21- and 17-hydroxylase are expressed in the (inner) fasciculata-reticularis cell layers, which are the sites of cortisol and androgen biosynthesis, respectively.

STEROID TRANSPORT

Cortisol circulates in the plasma as free cortisol, protein-bound cortisol, and cortisol metabolites. *Free cortisol* is a physiologically active hormone that is not protein-bound and therefore can act directly on tissue sites. Normally, <5% of circulating cortisol is free. Only the unbound cortisol and its metabolites are filterable at the glomerulus. Increased quantities of free steroid are excreted in the urine in states characterized by hypersecretion of cortisol, because the unbound fraction of plasma cortisol rises. Plasma has two cortisol-binding systems. One is a high-affinity, low-capacity α_2-globulin termed *transcortin* or *cortisol-binding globulin* (CBG), and the other is a low-affinity, high-capacity protein, *albumin*. Cortisol binding to CBG is reduced in areas of inflammation, thus increasing the local concentration of free cortisol. When the concentration of cortisol is >700 nmol/L (25 μg/dL), part of the excess binds to albumin, and a greater proportion than usual circulates unbound. CBG is increased in high-estrogen states (e.g., pregnancy, oral contraceptive administration). The rise in CBG is accompanied by a parallel rise in *protein-bound cortisol*, with the result that the total plasma cortisol concentration is elevated. However, the free cortisol level probably remains normal, and manifestations of glucocorticoid excess are absent. Most synthetic glucocorticoid analogues bind less efficiently to CBG (~70% binding). This may explain the propensity of some synthetic analogues to produce cushingoid effects at low doses. *Cortisol metabolites* are biologically inactive and bind only weakly to circulating plasma proteins.

Aldosterone is bound to proteins to a smaller extent than cortisol, and an ultrafiltrate of plasma contains as much as 50% of circulating aldosterone.

STEROID METABOLISM AND EXCRETION

Glucocorticoids

The daily secretion of cortisol ranges between 40 and 80 μmol (15 and 30 mg; 8–10 mg/m^2), with a pronounced circadian cycle. The plasma concentration of cortisol is determined by the rate of secretion, the rate of inactivation, and the rate of excretion of free cortisol. The liver is the major organ responsible for steroid inactivation. A major enzyme regulating cortisol metabolism is 11β-hydroxysteroid dehydrogenase (11β-HSD). There are two isoforms: 11β-HSD 1 is primarily expressed in the liver and acts as a reductase, converting the inactive cortisone to the active glucocorticoid, cortisol; the 11β-HSD 2 isoform is expressed in a number of tissues and converts cortisol to the inactive metabolite, cortisone. Mutations in the *HSD11β1* gene are associated with rapid cortisol turnover, leading to activation of the hypothalamic-pituitary-adrenal (HPA) axis and excessive adrenal androgen production in women. In animal models, excess omental expression of 11β-HSD 1 increases local glucocorticoid production and is associated with central obesity and insulin resistance. The oxidative reaction of 11β-HSD 1 is increased in hypothyroidism. Mutations in the *HSD11β2* gene cause the syndrome of *apparent mineralocorticoid excess*, reflecting insufficient inactivation of cortisol in the kidney, allowing inappropriate cortisol activation of the mineralocorticoid receptor (see below).

Mineralocorticoids

In individuals with normal salt intake, the average daily secretion of aldosterone ranges between 0.1 and 0.7 μmol (50 and 250 μg). During a single passage through the liver, >75% of circulating aldosterone is normally inactivated by conjugation with glucuronic acid. However, under certain conditions, such as congestive failure, this rate of inactivation is reduced.

Adrenal Androgens

The major androgen secreted by the adrenal is dehydroepiandrosterone (DHEA) and its sulfuric acid ester (DHEAS). Approximately 15–30 mg of these compounds

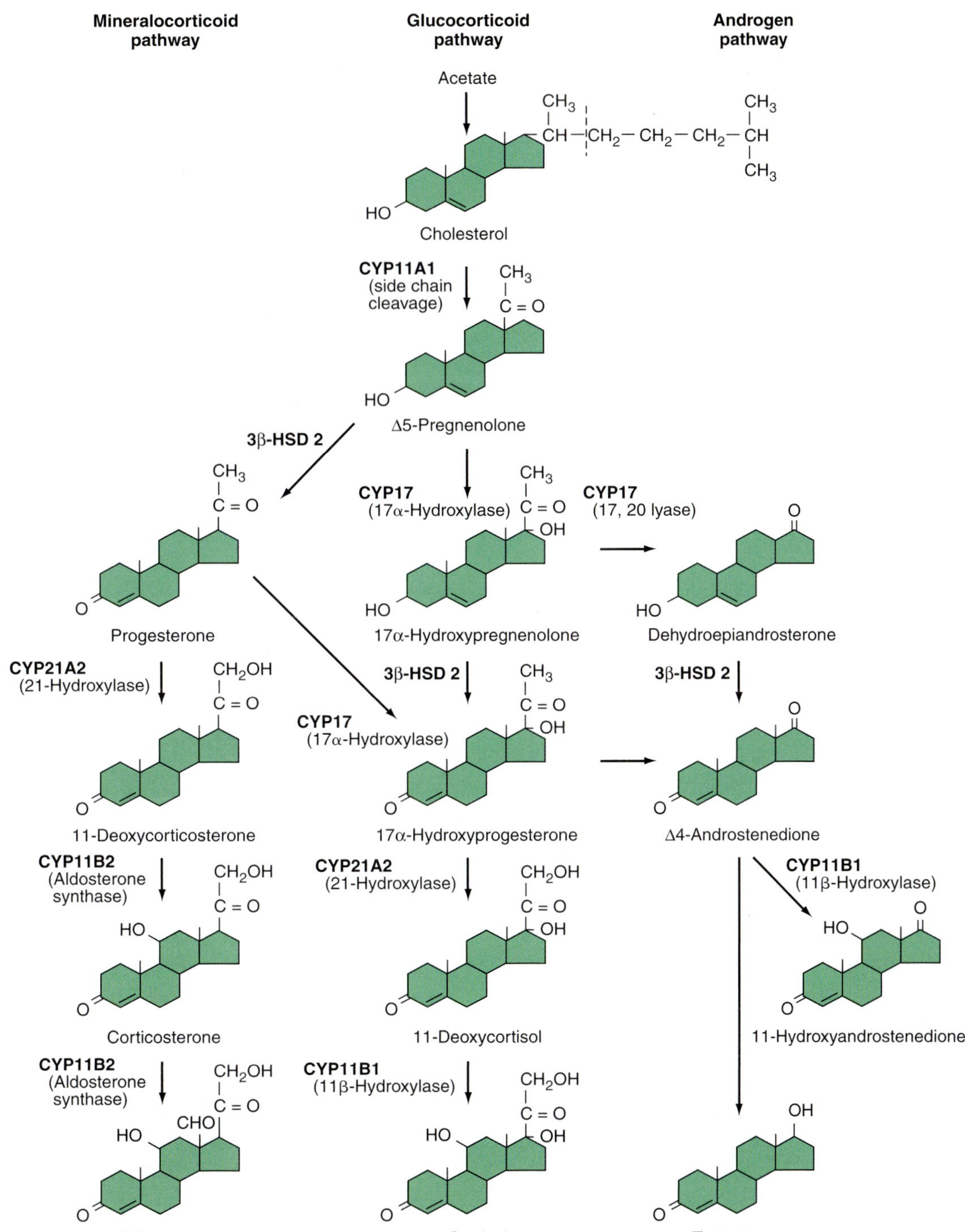

FIGURE 5-2

Biosynthetic pathways for adrenal steroid production; major pathways to mineralocorticoids, glucocorticoids, and androgens. 3β-HSD, 3β-hydroxysteroid dehydrogenase.

is secreted daily. Smaller amounts of androstenedione, 11β-hydroxyandrostenedione, and testosterone are secreted. DHEA is the major precursor of the urinary 17-ketosteroids. Two-thirds of the urine 17-ketosteroids in the male are derived from adrenal metabolites, and the remaining one-third comes from testicular androgens. In the female, almost all urine 17-ketosteroids are derived from the adrenal.

Steroids diffuse passively through the cell membrane and bind to intracellular receptors (Chap. 1[D1]). Glucocorticoids and mineralocorticoids bind with nearly equal affinity to the mineralocorticoid receptor (MR). However, only glucocorticoids bind to the glucocorticoid receptor (GR). After the steroid binds to the receptor, the steroid-receptor complex is transported to the nucleus, where it binds to specific sites on steroid-regulated genes, altering levels of transcription. Some actions of glucocorticoids (e.g., anti-inflammatory effects) are mediated by GR-mediated inhibition of other transcription factors, such as activating protein-1 (AP-1) or nuclear factor kappa B (NFκB), which normally stimulate the activity of various cytokine genes. Because cortisol binds to the MR with the same affinity as aldosterone, mineralocorticoid specificity is achieved by local metabolism of cortisol to the inactive compound cortisone by 11β-HSD 2. The glucocorticoid effects of other steroids, such as high-dose progesterone, correlate with their relative binding affinities for the GR. Inherited defects in the GR cause glucocorticoid resistance states. Individuals with GR defects have high levels of cortisol but do not have manifestations of hypercortisolism.

ACTH PHYSIOLOGY

ACTH and a number of other peptides (lipotropins, endorphins, and melanocyte-stimulating hormones) are processed from a larger precursor molecule of 31,000 mol wt—proopiomelanocortin (POMC) (Chap. 2). POMC is made in a variety of tissues, including brain, anterior and posterior pituitary, and lymphocytes. The constellation of POMC-derived peptides secreted depends on the tissue. ACTH, a 39-amino-acid peptide, is synthesized and stored in basophilic cells of the anterior pituitary. The N-terminal 18-amino-acid fragment of ACTH has full biologic potency, and shorter N-terminal fragments have partial biologic activity. Release of ACTH and related peptides from the anterior pituitary gland is stimulated by corticotropin-releasing hormone (CRH), a 41-amino-acid peptide produced in the median eminence of the hypothalamus (Fig. 5-3). Urocortin, a neuropeptide related to CRH, mimics many of the central effects of CRH (e.g., appetite suppression, anxiety), but its role in ACTH regulation is unclear. Some related peptides such as β-lipotropin (β-LPT) are released in equimolar concentrations with ACTH, suggesting that they are cleaved enzymatically from the parent POMC before or during the secretory process. However, β-endorphin levels may or may not correlate with circulating levels of ACTH, depending on the nature of the stimulus.

The major factors controlling ACTH release include CRH, the free cortisol concentration in plasma, stress, and the sleep-wake cycle (Fig. 5-3). Plasma ACTH varies during the day as a result of its pulsatile secretion and follows a circadian pattern, with a peak just prior to waking and a nadir before sleeping. If a new sleep-wake cycle is adopted, the pattern changes over several days to conform to it. ACTH and cortisol levels also increase in response to eating. Stress (e.g., pyrogens, surgery, hypoglycemia, exercise, and severe emotional trauma) causes the release of CRH and arginine vasopressin (AVP) and activation of the sympathetic nervous system. These

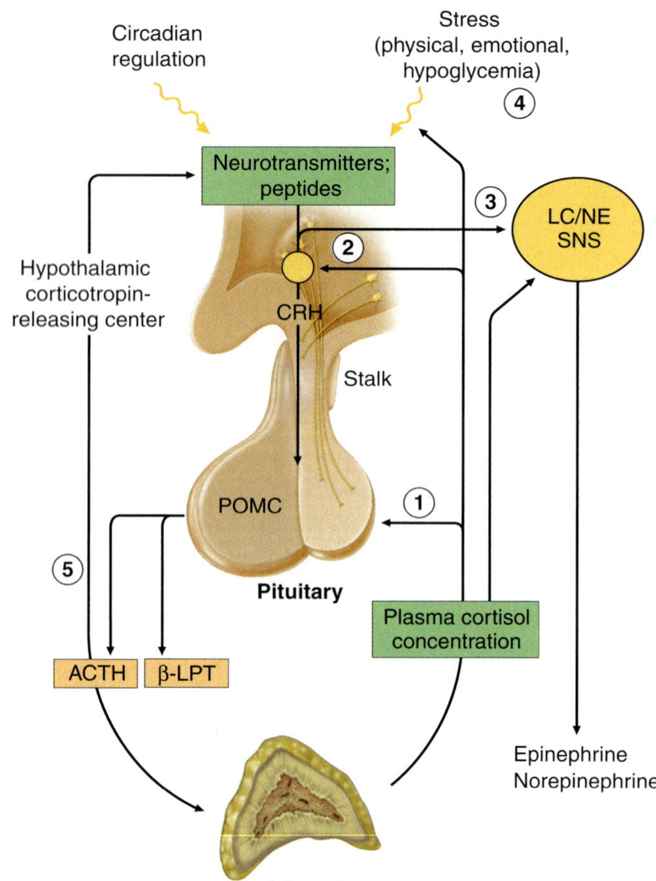

FIGURE 5-3

The hypothalamic-pituitary-adrenal axis. The main sites for feedback control by plasma cortisol are the pituitary gland (1) and the hypothalamic corticotropin-releasing center (2). Feedback control by plasma cortisol also occurs at the locus coeruleus/sympathetic system (3) and may involve higher nerve centers (4) as well. There may also be a short feedback loop involving inhibition of corticotropin-releasing hormone (CRH) by adrenocorticotropic hormone (ACTH) (5). Hypothalamic neurotransmitters influence CRH release; serotoninergic and cholinergic systems stimulate the secretion of CRH and ACTH; adrenergic agonists and γ-aminobutyric acid (GABA) probably inhibit CRH release. The opioid peptides β-endorphin and enkephalin inhibit, and vasopressin and angiotensin II augment, the secretion of CRH and ACTH. β-LPT, β-lipotropin; POMC, pro-opiomelanocortin; LC, locus coeruleus; NE, norepinephrine.

changes in turn enhance ACTH release, acting individually or in concert. For example, AVP release acts synergistically with CRH to amplify ACTH secretion; CRH also stimulates the locus coeruleus/sympathetic system. Stress-related secretion of ACTH abolishes the circadian periodicity of ACTH levels but is, in turn, suppressed by prior high-dose glucocorticoid administration. The normal pulsatile, circadian pattern of ACTH release is regulated by CRH; this mechanism is the so-called open feedback loop. CRH secretion, in turn, is influenced by

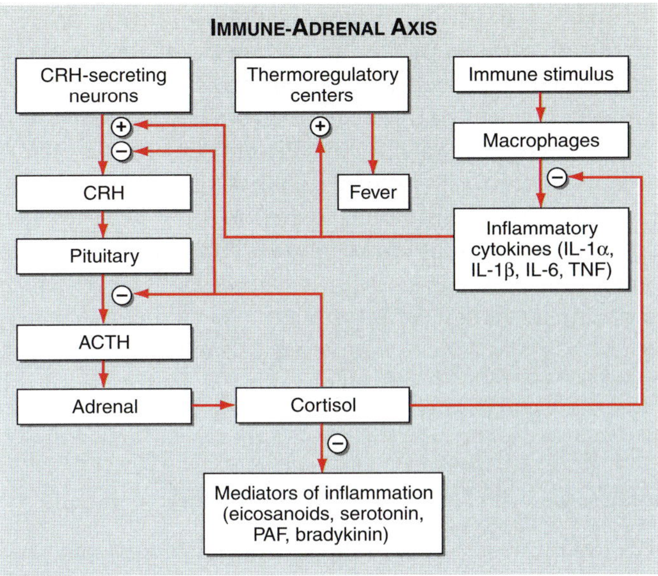

FIGURE 5-4

The immune-adrenal axis. Cortisol has anti-inflammatory properties that include effects on the microvasculature, cellular actions, and the suppression of inflammatory cytokines (the so-called immune-adrenal axis). A stress such as sepsis increases adrenal secretion, and cortisol in turn suppresses the immune response via this system. –, suppression; +, stimulation; CRH, corticotropin-releasing hormone; ACTH, adrenocorticotropic hormone; IL, interleukin; TNF, tumor necrosis factor; PAF, platelet activating factor.

hypothalamic neurotransmitters including the serotoninergic and cholinergic pathways. The immune system also influences the HPA axis (Fig. 5-4). For example, inflammatory cytokines [tumor necrosis factor α (TNF-α), interleukin (IL) 1α, IL-1β, and IL-6] produced by monocytes increase ACTH release by stimulating secretion of CRH and/or AVP. Finally, ACTH release is regulated by the level of free cortisol in plasma. Cortisol decreases the responsiveness of pituitary corticotropic cells to CRH; the response of the POMC mRNA to CRH is also inhibited by glucocorticoids. In addition, glucocorticoids inhibit the locus coeruleus/sympathetic system and CRH release. The latter servomechanism establishes the primacy of cortisol in the control of ACTH secretion. The suppression of ACTH secretion that results in adrenal atrophy following *prolonged* glucocorticoid therapy is caused primarily by suppression of hypothalamic CRH release, as exogenous CRH administration in this circumstance produces a rise in plasma ACTH. Cortisol also exerts feedback effects on higher brain centers (hippocampus, reticular system, and septum) and perhaps on the adrenal cortex.

The biologic half-life of ACTH in the circulation is <10 min. The action of ACTH is also rapid; within minutes of its release, the concentration of steroids in the adrenal venous blood increases. ACTH stimulates steroidogenesis via activation of adenyl cyclase. Cyclic AMP, in turn, stimulates the synthesis of protein kinase enzymes, thereby resulting in the phosphorylation of proteins that activate steroid biosynthesis.

RENIN-ANGIOTENSIN PHYSIOLOGY

Renin is a proteolytic enzyme that is produced and stored in the granules of the juxtaglomerular cells surrounding the afferent arterioles of glomeruli in the kidney. Renin acts on the basic substrate angiotensinogen (a circulating α_2-globulin made in the liver) to form the decapeptide angiotensin I (Fig. 5-5). Angiotensin I is then enzymatically transformed by angiotensin-converting enzyme (ACE), which is present in many tissues (particularly the pulmonary vascular endothelium), to the octapeptide angiotensin II by the removal of the two C-terminal amino acids. Angiotensin II is a potent pressor agent and exerts its action by a direct effect on arteriolar smooth muscle. In addition, angiotensin II stimulates

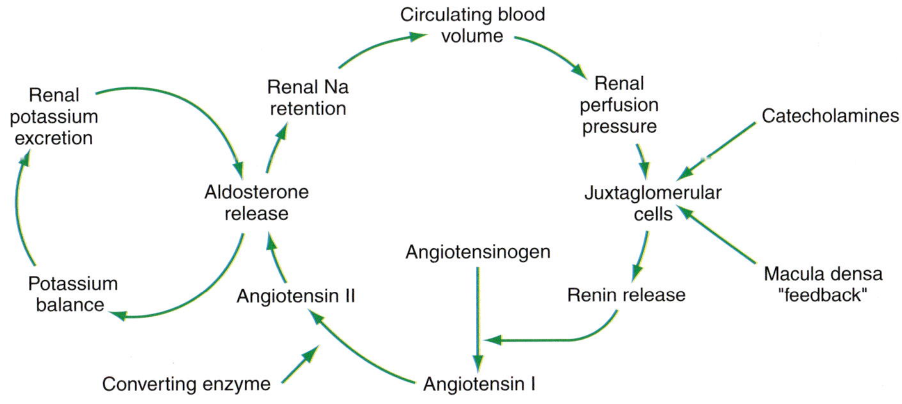

FIGURE 5-5

The interrelationship of the volume and potassium feedback loops on aldosterone secretion. Integration of signals from each loop determines the level of aldosterone secretion.

production of aldosterone by the zona glomerulosa of the adrenal cortex; the heptapeptide angiotensin III may also stimulate aldosterone production. The two major classes of angiotensin receptors are termed *AT1* and *AT2*; AT1 may exist as two subtypes α and β. Most of the effects of angiotensins II and III are mediated by the AT1 receptor. Angiotensinases rapidly destroy angiotensin II (half-life, 1 min), while the half-life of renin is more prolonged (10–20 min). In addition to circulating renin-angiotensin, many tissues have a local renin-angiotensin system and the ability to produce angiotensin II. These tissues include the uterus, placenta, vascular tissue, heart, brain, and, particularly, adrenal cortex and kidney. Although the role of locally generated angiotensin II is not established, it may modulate the growth and function of the adrenal cortex and vascular smooth muscle.

The amount of renin released reflects the combined effects of four interdependent factors. The *juxtaglomerular cells*, which are specialized myoepithelial cells that cuff the afferent arterioles, act as miniature pressure transducers, sensing renal perfusion pressure and corresponding changes in afferent arteriolar perfusion pressures. For example, a reduction in circulating blood volume leads to a corresponding reduction in renal perfusion pressure and afferent arteriolar pressure (Fig. 5-5). This change is perceived by the juxtaglomerular cells as a decreased stretch exerted on the afferent arteriolar walls, and the juxtaglomerular cells release more renin into the renal circulation. This results in the formation of angiotensin I, which is converted in the kidney and peripherally to angiotensin II by ACE. Angiotensin II influences sodium homeostasis via two major mechanisms: it changes renal blood flow so as to maintain a constant glomerular filtration rate, thereby changing the filtration fraction of sodium, and it stimulates the adrenal cortex to release aldosterone. Increasing plasma levels of aldosterone enhance renal sodium retention and thus result in expansion of the extracellular fluid volume (ECFV), which, in turn, dampens the stimulus for renin release. In this context, the renin-angiotensin-aldosterone system regulates volume by modifying renal hemodynamics and tubular sodium transport.

A second control mechanism for renin release is centered in the *macula densa cells*, a group of distal convoluted tubular epithelial cells directly opposed to the juxtaglomerular cells. They may function as chemoreceptors, monitoring the sodium (or chloride) load presented to the distal tubule. Under conditions of increased delivery of filtered sodium to the macula densa, a signal is conveyed to decrease juxtaglomerular cell release of renin, thereby modulating the glomerular filtration rate and the filtered load of sodium.

The *sympathetic nervous system* regulates the release of renin in response to assumption of the upright posture. The mechanism is either a direct effect on the juxtaglomerular cell to increase adenyl cyclase activity or an indirect effect on either the juxtaglomerular or the macula densa cells via vasoconstriction of the afferent arteriole.

Finally, circulating factors influence renin release. Increased dietary intake of potassium decreases renin release, whereas decreased potassium intake increases it. The significance of these effects is unclear. *Angiotensin II* exerts negative feedback control on renin release that is independent of alterations in renal blood flow, blood pressure, or aldosterone secretion. *Atrial natriuretic peptides* also inhibit renin release. Thus, the control of renin release involves both *intrarenal* (pressor receptor and macula densa) and *extrarenal* (sympathetic nervous system, potassium, angiotensin, etc.) mechanisms. Steady-state renin levels reflect all these factors, with the intrarenal mechanism predominating.

GLUCOCORTICOID PHYSIOLOGY

The division of adrenal steroids into glucocorticoids and mineralocorticoids is arbitrary in that most glucocorticoids have some mineralocorticoid-like properties. The descriptive term *glucocorticoid* is used for adrenal steroids whose predominant action is on intermediary metabolism. Their overall actions are directed at enhancing the production of the high-energy fuel, glucose, and reducing all other metabolic activity not directly involved in that process. Sustained activation, however, results in a pathophysiologic state, e.g., Cushing's syndrome. The principal glucocorticoid is cortisol (hydrocortisone). The effect of glucocorticoids on intermediary metabolism is mediated by the GR. Physiologic effects of glucocorticoids include the regulation of protein, carbohydrate, lipid, and nucleic acid metabolism. Glucocorticoids raise the blood glucose level by antagonizing the secretion and actions of insulin, thereby inhibiting peripheral glucose uptake, which promotes hepatic glucose synthesis (gluconeogenesis) and hepatic glycogen content. The actions on protein metabolism are mainly catabolic, resulting in an increase in protein breakdown and nitrogen excretion. In large part, these actions reflect a mobilization of glycogenic amino acid precursors from peripheral supporting structures, such as bone, skin, muscle, and connective tissue, due to protein breakdown and inhibition of protein synthesis and amino acid uptake. Hyperaminoacidemia also facilitates gluconeogenesis by stimulating glucagon secretion. Glucocorticoids act directly on the liver to stimulate the synthesis of certain enzymes, such as tyrosine aminotransferase and tryptophan pyrrolase. Glucocorticoids regulate fatty acid mobilization by enhancing the activation of cellular lipase by lipid-mobilizing hormones (e.g., catecholamines and pituitary peptides).

The actions of cortisol on protein and adipose tissue vary in different parts of the body. For example, pharmacologic doses of cortisol can deplete the protein matrix of the vertebral column (trabecular bone), whereas long bones (which are primarily compact bone) are affected only minimally; similarly, peripheral adipose tissue mass decreases, whereas abdominal and interscapular fat expand.

Glucocorticoids have anti-inflammatory properties, which are probably related to effects on the microvasculature and to suppression of inflammatory cytokines. In this sense, glucocorticoids modulate the immune response via the so-called immune-adrenal axis (Fig. 5-4). This "loop" is one mechanism by which a stress, such as sepsis, increases adrenal hormone secretion, and the elevated cortisol level in turn suppresses the immune response. For example, cortisol maintains vascular responsiveness to circulating vasoconstrictors and opposes the increase in capillary permeability during acute inflammation. Glucocorticoids cause a leukocytosis that reflects release from the bone marrow of mature cells as well as inhibition of their egress through the capillary wall. Glucocorticoids produce a depletion of circulating eosinophils and lymphoid tissue, specifically T cells, by causing a redistribution from the circulation into other compartments. Thus, cortisol impairs cell-mediated immunity. Glucocorticoids also inhibit the production and action of the mediators of inflammation, such as the lymphokines and prostaglandins. Glucocorticoids inhibit the production and action of interferon by T lymphocytes and the production of IL-1 and IL-6 by macrophages. The antipyretic action of glucocorticoids may be explained by an effect on IL-1, which appears to be an endogenous pyrogen. Glucocorticoids also inhibit the production of T cell growth factor (IL-2) by T lymphocytes. Glucocorticoids reverse macrophage activation and antagonize the action of migration-inhibiting factor (MIF), leading to reduced adherence of macrophages to vascular endothelium. Glucocorticoids reduce prostaglandin and leukotriene production by inhibiting the activity of phospholipase A_2, thus blocking release of arachidonic acid from phospholipids. Finally, glucocorticoids inhibit the production and inflammatory effects of bradykinin, platelet-activating factor, and serotonin. It is probably only at pharmacologic dosages that antibody production is reduced and lysosomal membranes are stabilized, the latter effect suppressing the release of acid hydrolases.

Cortisol levels respond within minutes to stress, whether physical (trauma, surgery, exercise), psychological (anxiety, depression), or physiologic (hypoglycemia, fever). The reasons why elevated glucocorticoid levels protect the organism under stress are not understood, but in conditions of glucocorticoid deficiency, such stresses may cause hypotension, shock, and death. Consequently, in individuals with adrenal insufficiency, glucocorticoid administration should be increased during stress.

Cortisol has major effects on body water. It helps regulate the ECFV by retarding the migration of water into cells and by promoting renal water excretion, the latter effect mediated by suppression of vasopressin secretion, by an increase in the rate of glomerular filtration, and by a direct action on the renal tubule. The consequence is to prevent water intoxication by increasing solute-free water clearance. Glucocorticoids also have weak mineralocorticoid-like properties, and high doses promote renal tubular sodium reabsorption and increased urine potassium excretion. Glucocorticoids can also influence behavior; emotional disorders may occur with either an excess or a deficit of cortisol. Finally, cortisol suppresses the secretion of pituitary POMC and its derivative peptides (ACTH, β-endorphin, and β-LPT) and the secretion of hypothalamic CRH and vasopressin.

MINERALOCORTICOID PHYSIOLOGY

Mineralocorticoids modify function in two classes of cells—epithelial and nonepithelial.

Effects on Epithelia

Classically, mineralocorticoids are considered major regulators of ECFV and are the major determinants of potassium metabolism. These effects are mediated by the binding of aldosterone to the MR in epithelial cells, primarily the principal cells in the renal cortical collecting duct. Because of its electrochemical gradient, sodium passively enters these cells from the urine via epithelial sodium channels located on the luminal membrane and is actively extruded from the cell via the Na/K-activated ATPase ("sodium pump") located on the basolateral membrane. The sodium pump also provides the driving force of potassium loss into the urine through potassium-selective luminal channels, again assisted by the electrochemical gradient for potassium in these cells. Aldosterone stimulates all three of these processes by increasing gene expression directly (for the sodium pump and the potassium channels) or via a complex process (for epithelial sodium channels) to increase both the number and activity of the sodium channels. Water passively follows the transported sodium, thus expanding intra- and extravascular volume.

Because the concentration of hydrogen ion is greater in the lumen than in the cell, hydrogen ion is also actively secreted. Mineralocorticoids also act on the epithelium of the salivary ducts, sweat glands, and gastrointestinal tract to cause reabsorption of sodium in exchange for potassium.

When normal individuals are given aldosterone, an initial period of sodium retention is followed by natriuresis, and sodium balance is reestablished after 3–5 days. As a result, edema does not develop. This process is referred to as the *escape phenomenon*, signifying an "escape" by the renal tubules from the sodium-retaining action of aldosterone. While renal hemodynamic factors may play a role in the escape, the level of atrial natriuretic peptide also increases. However, it is important to realize that there is no escape from the potassium-losing effects of mineralocorticoids.

Effect on Nonepithelial Cells

The MR has been identified in a number of nonepithelial cells, e.g., neurons in the brain, myocytes, endothelial cells, and vascular smooth-muscle cells. In these cells, the actions of aldosterone differ from those in epithelial cells in several ways:

1. They do not modify sodium-potassium homeostasis.
2. The groups of regulated genes differ, although only a few are known; for example, in nonepithelial cells, aldosterone modifies the expression of several collagen genes controlling tissue growth factors, e.g., transforming growth factor (TGF) β, plasminogen activator inhibitor type 1 (PAI-1), adiponectin, and leptin.
3. In some of these tissues (e.g., myocardium and brain), the MR is not protected by the 11-HSD 2 enzyme. Thus, cortisol rather than aldosterone may be activating the MR. In other tissues (e.g., the vasculature), 11-HSD 2 is expressed in a manner similar to that of the kidney. Therefore, aldosterone is activating the MR.
4. Some effects on nonepithelial cells may be via nongenomic mechanisms. These actions are too rapid—occurring within 1–2 min and peaking within 5–10 min—to be considered genomic, suggesting that they are secondary to activation of a cell-surface receptor. However, no cell-surface MR has been identified, raising the possibility that the same MR is mediating both genomic and nongenomic effects. In the vasculature, the nongenomic effects mediated by aldosterone include an increase in the phosphorylation of protein kinase C and extracellular regulated kinase (ERK), and a reduction in the phosphorylation of epithelial nitric oxide synthase. In the intact organism, some, if not all, of both nongenomic and genomic effects are mediated via an interaction between the MR, aldosterone, and proteins in specialized areas in the target cell's surface membrane termed *caveolae*. However, caveolin proteins are not always required as aldosterone still produces adverse cardiovascular effects in caveolin-knockout animals. Rapid, nongenomic effects have also been described for other steroids including estradiol, progesterone, thyroxine, and vitamin D.
5. Some of these tissues—the myocardium and vasculature—may also produce aldosterone, although this theory is controversial and may be both species- and condition-specific.

Regulation of Aldosterone Secretion

Three primary mechanisms control adrenal aldosterone secretion: the renin-angiotensin system, potassium, and ACTH (Table 5-1). Whether these are also the primary regulatory mechanisms modifying nonadrenal production is uncertain. The renin-angiotensin system controls ECFV via regulation of aldosterone secretion (Fig. 5-5). In effect, the renin-angiotensin system maintains the circulating blood volume constant by causing aldosterone-induced sodium retention during volume deficiency and by decreasing aldosterone-dependent sodium retention when volume is ample. There is an increasing body of evidence indicating that some tissues, in addition to the kidney, produce angiotensin II and may participate in the regulation of aldosterone secretion either from the adrenal or extraadrenal sources. Intriguingly, the adrenal itself is capable of synthesizing angiotensin II. What role the extrarenal production of angiotensin II plays in normal physiology is still largely unknown. However, the tissue renin-angiotensin system is activated in utero in response to growth and development and/or later in life in response to injury.

TABLE 5-1

FACTORS REGULATING ALDOSTERONE BIOSYNTHESIS

FACTOR	EFFECT
Renin-angiotensin system	Stimulation
Sodium ion	Inhibition (?physiologic)
Potassium ion	Stimulation
Neurotransmitters	
Dopamine	Inhibition
Serotonin	Stimulation
Pituitary hormones	
ACTH	Stimulation
Non-ACTH pituitary hormones (e.g., growth hormone)	Permissive (for optimal response to sodium restriction)
β-Endorphin	Stimulation
γ-Melanocyte-stimulating hormone	Permissive
Atrial natriuretic peptide	Inhibition
Ouabain-like factors	Inhibition
Endothelin	Stimulation

Note: ACTH, adrenocorticotropic hormone.

Potassium ion directly stimulates aldosterone secretion, independent of the circulating renin-angiotensin system, which it suppresses (Fig. 5-5). In addition to a direct effect, potassium also modifies aldosterone secretion indirectly by activating the local renin-angiotensin system in the zona glomerulosa. This effect can be blocked by the administration of ACE inhibitors that reduce the local production of angiotensin II and thereby reduce the acute aldosterone response to potassium. An increase in serum potassium of as little as 0.1 mmol/L increases plasma aldosterone levels under certain circumstances. Oral potassium loading therefore increases aldosterone secretion, plasma levels, and excretion.

Physiologic amounts of ACTH stimulate aldosterone secretion acutely, but this action is not sustained unless ACTH is administered in a pulsatile fashion. Most studies relegate ACTH to a minor role in the control of aldosterone. For example, subjects receiving high-dose glucocorticoid therapy, and with presumed complete suppression of ACTH, have normal aldosterone secretion in response to sodium restriction.

Prior dietary intake of both potassium and sodium can alter the magnitude of the aldosterone response to acute stimulation. This effect results from a change in the expression and activity of aldosterone synthase. Increasing potassium intake or decreasing sodium intake sensitizes the response of the glomerulosa cells to acute stimulation by ACTH, angiotensin II, and/or potassium.

Neurotransmitters (dopamine and serotonin) and some peptides, such as atrial natriuretic peptide, γ-melanocyte-stimulating hormone (γ-MSH), and β-endorphin, also participate in the regulation of aldosterone secretion (Table 5-1). Thus, the control of aldosterone secretion involves both stimulatory and inhibitory factors.

ANDROGEN PHYSIOLOGY

Androgens regulate male secondary sexual characteristics and can cause virilizing symptoms in women (Chap. 13). Adrenal androgens have a minimal effect in males, whose sexual characteristics are predominately determined by gonadal steroids (testosterone). In females, however, several androgen-like effects, e.g., sexual hair, are largely mediated by adrenal androgens. The principal adrenal androgens are DHEA, androstenedione, and 11-hydroxyandrostenedione. DHEA and androstenedione are weak androgens and exert their effects via conversion to the potent androgen testosterone in extraglandular tissues. DHEA also has poorly understood effects on the immune and cardiovascular systems. Adrenal androgen formation is regulated by ACTH, not by gonadotropins. Adrenal androgens are suppressed by exogenous glucocorticoid administration.

LABORATORY EVALUATION OF ADRENOCORTICAL FUNCTION

A basic assumption is that measurements of the plasma or urinary level of a given steroid reflect the rate of adrenal *secretion* of that steroid. However, urine *excretion* values may not truly reflect the secretion rate because of improper collection or altered metabolism. Plasma levels reflect the level of secretion only at the time of measurement. The plasma level (*PL*) depends on two factors: the secretion rate (*SR*) of the hormone and the rate at which it is metabolized, i.e., its metabolic clearance rate (*MCR*). These three factors can be related as follows:

$$PL = \frac{SR}{MCR} \quad \text{or} \quad SR = MCR \times PL$$

BLOOD LEVELS

Peptides

The plasma levels of ACTH and angiotensin II can be measured by immunoassay techniques. Basal ACTH secretion shows a circadian rhythm, with lower levels in the early evening than in the morning. However, ACTH is secreted in a pulsatile manner, leading to rapid fluctuations superimposed on this circadian rhythm. Angiotensin II levels also vary diurnally and are influenced by dietary sodium and potassium intakes and posture. Both upright posture and sodium restriction elevate angiotensin II levels.

Most clinical determinations of the renin-angiotensin system, however, involve measurements of peripheral *plasma renin activity* (PRA) in which the renin activity is gauged by the generation of angiotensin I during a standardized incubation period. This method depends on the presence of sufficient angiotensinogen in the plasma as substrate. The generated angiotensin I is measured by radioimmunoassay. The PRA depends on the dietary sodium intake and on whether the patient is ambulatory. In normal humans, the PRA shows a diurnal rhythm characterized by peak values in the morning and a nadir in the afternoon. An alternative approach is to measure plasma active renin, which is easier and not dependent on endogenous substrate concentration. PRA and active renin correlate very well on low-sodium diets but less well on high-sodium diets.

Steroids

Cortisol and aldosterone are both secreted episodically, and levels vary during the day, with peak values in the morning and low levels in the evening. In addition, the plasma level of aldosterone, but not of cortisol, is increased by dietary potassium loading, by sodium restriction, or by assumption of the upright posture. Measurement of the sulfate conjugate of DHEA may be a useful index of adrenal androgen secretion, as little DHEA sulfate is formed in the gonads and because the half-life of DHEA sulfate is 7–9 h. However, DHEA sulfate levels reflect both DHEA production and sulfatase activity.

URINE LEVELS

For the assessment of glucocorticoid secretion, the urine 17-hydroxycorticosteroid assay has been replaced by measurement of urinary free cortisol. Elevated levels of urinary free cortisol correlate with states of hypercortisolism, reflecting changes in the levels of unbound, physiologically active circulating cortisol. Normally, the rate of excretion is higher in the daytime (7 A.M.–7 P.M.) than at night (7 P.M.–7 A.M.).

Urinary 17-ketosteroids originate in either the adrenal gland or the gonad. In normal women, 90% of urinary 17-ketosteroids is derived from the adrenal, and in men 60–70% is of adrenal origin. Urine 17-ketosteroid values are highest in young adults and decline with age.

A carefully timed urine collection is a prerequisite for all excretory determinations. Urinary creatinine should be measured simultaneously to determine the accuracy and adequacy of the collection procedure.

STIMULATION TESTS

Stimulation tests are useful in the diagnosis of hormone deficiency states.

Tests of Glucocorticoid Reserve

Within minutes after administration of ACTH, cortisol levels increase. This responsiveness can be used as an index of the functional reserve of the adrenal gland for production of cortisol. Under maximal ACTH stimulation, cortisol secretion increases tenfold, to 800 μmol/d (300 mg/d), but maximal stimulation can be achieved only with prolonged ACTH infusions.

A screening test (the so-called rapid ACTH stimulation test) involves the administration of 25 units (0.25 mg) of cosyntropin IV or IM and measurement of plasma cortisol levels before administration and 30 and 60 min after administration; the test can be performed at any time of the day. The most clear-cut criterion for a normal response is a stimulated cortisol level of >500 nmol/L (>18 μg/dL), and the minimal stimulated normal increment of cortisol is >200 nmol/L (>7 μg/dL) above baseline. Severely ill patients with elevated basal cortisol levels may show no further increases following acute ACTH administration.

Tests of Mineralocorticoid Reserve and Stimulation of the Renin-Angiotensin System

Stimulation tests use protocols designed to create a programmed volume depletion, such as sodium restriction, diuretic administration, or upright posture. A simple, potent test consists of severe sodium restriction and upright posture. After 3–5 days of a 10-mmol/d sodium intake, rates of aldosterone secretion or excretion should increase two- to threefold over the control values. Supine morning plasma aldosterone levels are usually increased three- to sixfold, and they increase a further two- to fourfold in response to 2–3 h of upright posture.

When the dietary sodium intake is normal, stimulation testing requires the administration of a potent diuretic, such as 40–80 mg furosemide, followed by 2–3 h of upright posture. The normal response is a two- to fourfold rise in plasma aldosterone levels.

SUPPRESSION TESTS

Suppression tests to document hypersecretion of adrenal hormones involve measurement of the target hormone response after standardized suppression of its tropic hormone.

Tests of Pituitary-Adrenal Suppressibility

The ACTH release mechanism is sensitive to the circulating glucocorticoid level. When blood levels of glucocorticoid are increased in normal individuals, less ACTH is released from the anterior pituitary and less steroid is produced by the adrenal gland. The integrity of this feedback mechanism can be tested clinically by giving a glucocorticoid and judging the suppression of ACTH secretion by analysis of urine steroid levels and/or plasma cortisol and ACTH levels. A potent glucocorticoid such as dexamethasone is used, so that the agent can be given in an amount small enough not to contribute significantly to the pool of steroids to be analyzed.

The best *screening* procedure is the overnight dexamethasone suppression test. This involves the measurement of plasma cortisol levels at 8 A.M. following the oral administration of 1 mg dexamethasone the previous midnight. The 8 A.M. value for plasma cortisol in normal individuals should be <140 nmol/L (5 μg/dL).

The definitive test of adrenal suppressibility involves administering 0.5 mg dexamethasone every 6 h for two successive days while collecting urine over a 24-h period for determination of creatinine and free cortisol and/or measuring plasma cortisol levels. In a patient with a normal hypothalamic-pituitary ACTH release mechanism, a fall in the urine free cortisol to <25 nmol/d (10 μg/d) or of plasma cortisol to <140 nmol/L (5 μg/dL) is seen on the second day of administration.

A normal response to either suppression test implies that the glucocorticoid regulation of ACTH and its control of the adrenal glands are physiologically normal. However, an isolated abnormal result, particularly to the overnight suppression test, does not in itself demonstrate pituitary and/or adrenal disease.

Tests of Mineralocorticoid Suppressibility

These tests rely on an expansion of ECFV, which should decrease circulating plasma renin activity and decrease the secretion and/or excretion of aldosterone. Various tests differ in the rate at which ECFV is expanded. One convenient suppression test involves the IV infusion of 500 mL/h of normal saline solution for 4 h, which normally suppresses plasma aldosterone levels to <220 pmol/L (<8 ng/dL) from a sodium-restricted diet or to <140 pmol/L (<5 ng/dL) from a normal sodium intake. Alternatively, a high-sodium diet can be administered for 3 days with 0.2 mg fludrocortisone twice daily. Aldosterone excretion is measured on the third day and should be <28 nmol/d (10 μg/d). These tests should not be performed in potassium-depleted individuals since they carry a risk of precipitating hypokalemia.

TESTS OF PITUITARY-ADRENAL RESPONSIVENESS

Stimuli such as insulin-induced hypoglycemia, AVP, and pyrogens induce the release of ACTH from the pituitary by an action on higher neural centers or on the pituitary itself. Insulin-induced hypoglycemia is particularly useful, because it stimulates the release of both growth hormone and ACTH. In this test, regular insulin (0.05–0.1 U/kg body weight) is given IV as a bolus to reduce the fasting glucose level to at least 50% below basal. The normal cortisol response is a rise to >500 nmol/L (18 μg/dL). Glucose levels must be monitored during insulin-induced hypoglycemia, and it should be terminated by feeding or IV glucose, if subjects develop symptoms of hypoglycemia. This test is contraindicated in individuals with coronary artery disease or a seizure disorder.

Metyrapone inhibits 11β-hydroxylase in the adrenal. As a result, the conversion of 11-deoxycortisol (compound S) to cortisol is impaired, causing 11-deoxycortisol to accumulate in the blood and the blood level of cortisol to decrease (Fig. 5-2). The hypothalamic-pituitary axis responds to the declining cortisol blood levels by releasing more ACTH. Note that assessment of the response depends on both an intact hypothalamic-pituitary axis and an intact adrenal gland.

Although modifications of the original metyrapone test have been described, a commonly used protocol involves administering 750 mg of the drug PO every 4 h over a 24-h period and comparing the control and postmetyrapone plasma levels of 11-deoxycortisol, cortisol, and ACTH. In normal individuals, plasma 11-deoxycortisol levels should be >210 nmol/L (7 μg/dL) and ACTH levels should be >17 pmol/L (75 pg/mL) following metyrapone administration. The metyrapone test does not accurately reflect ACTH reserve if subjects are ingesting exogenous glucocorticoids or drugs that accelerate the metabolism of metyrapone (e.g., phenytoin).

A direct and selective test of the pituitary corticotrophs can be achieved with CRH. The bolus injection of ovine CRH (corticorelin ovine triflutate; 1 μg/kg body weight) stimulates secretion of ACTH and β-LPT in normal human subjects within 15–60 min. In normal individuals, the mean increment in ACTH is 9 pmol/L (40 pg/mL). However, the magnitude of the ACTH response is less than that produced by insulin-induced hypoglycemia, implying that additional factors (such as vasopressin) augment stress-induced increases in ACTH secretion.

The rapid ACTH test can often distinguish between primary and secondary adrenal insufficiency, because aldosterone secretion is preserved in secondary adrenal failure by the renin-angiotensin system and potassium. Cosyntropin (25 units) is given IV or IM, and plasma cortisol and aldosterone levels are measured before and at 30 and 60 min after administration. The cortisol response is abnormal in both groups, but patients with secondary insufficiency show an increase in aldosterone levels of at least 140 pmol/L (5 ng/dL). No aldosterone response is seen in patients in whom the adrenal cortex is destroyed. Alternatively, ACTH at a physiologic dose (1 μg), the so-called low-dose ACTH test, may be used to detect secondary adrenal insufficiency. An abnormal response is similar to that in the rapid ACTH test. However, levels need to be measured at 30 min, and the ACTH needs to be directly injected IV because it can be absorbed by plastic tubing. Because the use of a bolus of exogenous ACTH does not invariably exclude a diagnosis of secondary adrenocortical insufficiency, direct tests of pituitary ACTH reserve (metyrapone test, insulin-induced hypoglycemia) may be required in the appropriate clinical setting.

HYPERFUNCTION OF THE ADRENAL CORTEX

Excess cortisol is associated with Cushing's syndrome; excess aldosterone causes aldosteronism; and excess adrenal androgens cause adrenal virilism. These syndromes do not always occur in the "pure" form but may have overlapping features.

CUSHING'S SYNDROME

Etiology

Cushing described a syndrome characterized by truncal obesity, hypertension, fatigability and weakness, amenorrhea, hirsutism, purplish abdominal striae, edema, glucosuria, osteoporosis, and a basophilic tumor of the pituitary. As awareness of this syndrome has increased, the diagnosis of Cushing's syndrome has been broadened into the classification shown in Table 5-2. Regardless of etiology, all cases of endogenous Cushing's syndrome are due to increased production of cortisol by the adrenal. In most cases, the cause is *bilateral adrenal hyperplasia* due to hypersecretion of pituitary ACTH or ectopic production of ACTH by a nonpituitary source. The incidence of pituitary-dependent adrenal hyperplasia is three times greater in women than in men, and the most frequent age of onset is the third or fourth decade. Most evidence indicates that the primary defect is the de novo development of a pituitary adenoma, as tumors are found in >90% of patients with pituitary-dependent adrenal hyperplasia. Alternatively, the defect may occasionally reside in the hypothalamus or in higher neural centers, leading to release of CRH inappropriate to the level of circulating cortisol. This primary defect leads to hyperstimulation of the pituitary, resulting in hyperplasia or tumor formation. In surgical series, most individuals with hypersecretion of pituitary ACTH are found to have a microadenoma (<10 mm in diameter; 50% are ≤5 mm in diameter), but a pituitary macroadenoma (>10 mm) or

TABLE 5-2

CAUSES OF CUSHING'S SYNDROME

Adrenal hyperplasia
Secondary to pituitary ACTH overproduction
Pituitary-hypothalamic dysfunction
Pituitary ACTH-producing micro- or macroadenomas
Secondary to ACTH- or CRH-producing nonendocrine tumors (bronchogenic carcinoma, carcinoid of the thymus, pancreatic carcinoma, bronchial adenoma)
Adrenal macronodular hyperplasia (including ectopic expression of GIP receptors in the adrenal cortex)
Adrenal micronodular dysplasia
Sporadic
Familial (Carney's syndrome)
Adrenal neoplasia
Adenoma
Carcinoma
Exogenous, iatrogenic causes
Prolonged use of glucocorticoids
Prolonged use of ACTH

Note: ACTH, adrenocorticotropic hormone; CRH, corticotropin-releasing hormone; GIP, gastric inhibitory peptide.

diffuse hyperplasia of the corticotrope cells may be found. Traditionally, only an individual who has an ACTH-producing pituitary tumor is defined as having Cushing's *disease*, whereas Cushing's *syndrome* refers to all causes of excess cortisol: exogenous ACTH tumor, adrenal tumor, pituitary ACTH-secreting tumor, or excessive glucocorticoid treatment.

The *ectopic ACTH syndrome* is caused by nonpituitary tumors that secrete ACTH and/or CRH and cause bilateral adrenal hyperplasia (Chap. 24). The ectopic production of CRH results in clinical, biochemical, and radiologic features indistinguishable from those caused by hypersecretion of pituitary ACTH. The typical signs and symptoms of Cushing's syndrome may be absent or minimal with ectopic ACTH production, and hypokalemic alkalosis is a prominent manifestation. Most of these cases are associated with the primitive small cell (oat cell) type of bronchogenic carcinoma or with carcinoid tumors of the thymus, pancreas, or ovary; medullary carcinoma of the thyroid; or bronchial adenomas. The onset of Cushing's syndrome may be sudden, particularly in patients with carcinoma of the lung, and this feature accounts in part for the failure of these patients to exhibit the classic manifestations. On the other hand, patients with carcinoid tumors or pheochromocytomas have longer clinical courses and usually exhibit the typical cushingoid features. The ectopic secretion of ACTH is also accompanied by the accumulation of ACTH fragments in plasma and by elevated plasma levels of ACTH precursor molecules. Because such tumors may produce large amounts of ACTH, baseline steroid values are usually very high and increased skin pigmentation may be present.

Approximately 20–25% of patients with Cushing's syndrome have an adrenal neoplasm. These tumors are usually unilateral, and about half are malignant. Occasionally, patients have biochemical features both of pituitary ACTH excess and of an adrenal adenoma. These individuals may have *nodular hyperplasia* of both adrenal glands, often the result of prolonged ACTH stimulation in the absence of a pituitary adenoma. Two additional entities cause nodular hyperplasia: a familial disorder in children or young adults (so-called pigmented micronodular dysplasia) and an abnormal cortisol response to gastric inhibitory polypeptide or luteinizing hormone, secondary to ectopic expression of receptors for these hormones in the adrenal cortex.

The most common cause of Cushing's syndrome is *iatrogenic* administration of steroids for a variety of reasons. Although the clinical features bear some resemblance to those seen with adrenal tumors, these patients are usually distinguishable on the basis of history and laboratory studies.

Clinical Signs, Symptoms, and Laboratory Findings

Many of the signs and symptoms of Cushing's syndrome follow logically from the known action of glucocorticoids (Table 5-3). Catabolic responses in peripheral supportive tissue cause muscle weakness and fatigability, osteoporosis, broad violaceous cutaneous striae (Fig. 5-6), and easy bruisability. The latter signs are secondary to weakening and rupture of collagen fibers in the dermis. Osteoporosis may cause collapse of vertebral bodies and pathologic fractures of other bones. Decreased bone mineralization is particularly

TABLE 5-3

FREQUENCY OF SIGNS AND SYMPTOMS IN CUSHING'S SYNDROME

SIGN OR SYMPTOM	PERCENT OF PATIENTS
Typical habitus (centripetal obesity)[a]	97
Increased body weight	94
Fatigability and weakness	87
Hypertension (blood pressure >150/90)	82
Hirsutism[a]	80
Amenorrhea	77
Broad violaceous cutaneous striae[a]	67
Personality changes	66
Ecchymoses[a]	65
Proximal myopathy[a]	62
Edema	62
Polyuria, polydipsia	23
Hypertrophy of clitoris	19

[a]Features more specific for Cushing's syndrome.

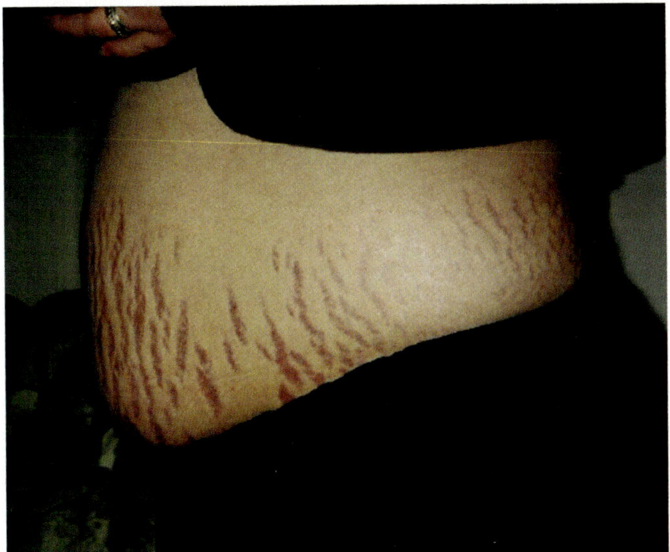

FIGURE 5-6
Clinical features of Cushing's syndrome. Note the central obesity and wide, violaceous striae.

pronounced in children. Increased hepatic gluconeogenesis and insulin resistance can cause impaired glucose tolerance. Overt diabetes mellitus occurs in <20% of patients, who probably are individuals with a predisposition to this disorder. Hypercortisolism promotes the deposition of adipose tissue in characteristic sites, notably the upper face (producing the typical "moon" facies), the interscapular area (producing the "buffalo hump"), supraclavicular fat pads, and the mesenteric bed (producing "truncal" obesity) (Fig. 5-6). Rarely, episternal fatty tumors and mediastinal widening secondary to fat accumulation occur. The reason for this peculiar distribution of adipose tissue is not known, but it is associated with insulin resistance and/or elevated insulin levels. The face appears plethoric, even in the absence of any increase in red blood cell concentration. Hypertension is common, and emotional changes may be profound, ranging from irritability and emotional lability to severe depression, confusion, or even frank psychosis. In women, increased levels of adrenal androgens can cause acne, hirsutism, and oligomenorrhea or amenorrhea. Some signs and symptoms in patients with hypercortisolism—i.e., obesity, hypertension, osteoporosis, and diabetes—are nonspecific and therefore are less helpful in diagnosing the condition. On the other hand, easy bruising, typical striae, myopathy, and virilizing signs (although less frequent) are, if present, more suggestive of Cushing's syndrome (Table 5-3).

Except in iatrogenic Cushing's syndrome, plasma and urine cortisol levels are elevated. Occasionally, hypokalemia, hypochloremia, and metabolic alkalosis are present, particularly with ectopic production of ACTH.

Diagnosis

The diagnosis of Cushing's syndrome depends on the demonstration of increased cortisol production and failure to suppress cortisol secretion normally when dexamethasone is administered (Chap. 2). Once the diagnosis is established, further testing is designed to determine the etiology (Fig. 5-7 and Table 5-4).

For initial screening, the overnight dexamethasone suppression test is recommended (see above). In difficult cases (e.g., in obese or depressed patients), measurement of a 24-h urine free cortisol can also be used as a screening test. A level >140 nmol/d (50 μg/d) is suggestive of Cushing's syndrome. The definitive diagnosis is then established by failure of urinary cortisol to fall to <25 nmol/d (10 μg/d) or of plasma cortisol to fall to <140 nmol/L (5 μg/dL) after a standard low-dose dexamethasone suppression test (0.5 mg every 6 h for 48 h). Owing to circadian variability,

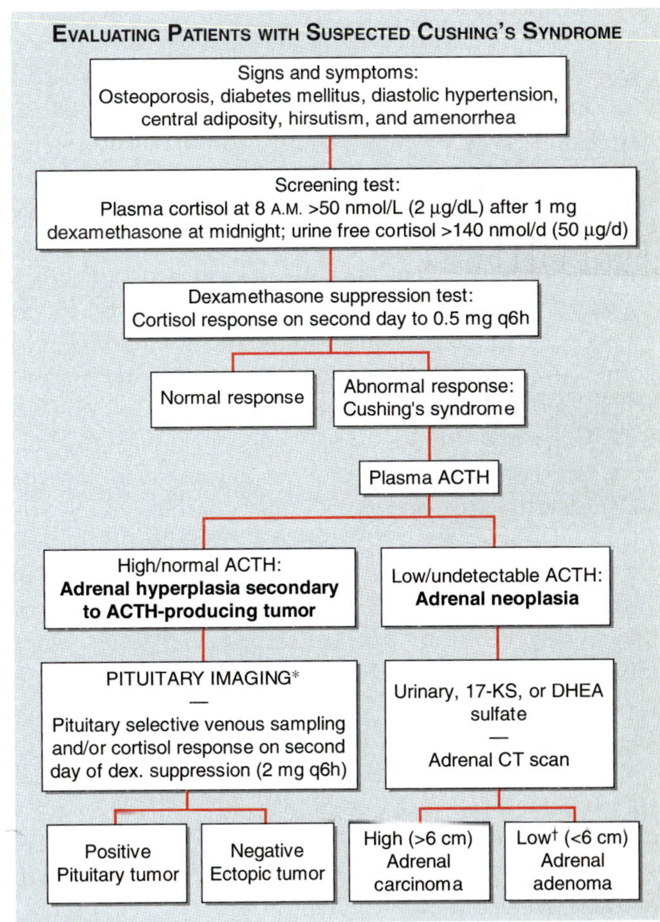

FIGURE 5-7
Evaluating patients suspected of having Cushing's syndrome. *A microadenoma or macroadenoma may be visualized by pituitary magnetic resonance scanning. †Risk of carcinoma in adrenal tumors 4–6 cm is 6%. Radiographic clues include tumor heterogeneity and irregular borders (see Fig. 5-8). 17-KS, 17-ketosteroids; DHEA, dehydroepiandrosterone; ACTH, adrenocorticotropic hormone; CT, computed tomography.

TABLE 5-4

DIAGNOSTIC TESTS TO DETERMINE THE TYPE OF CUSHING'S SYNDROME

TEST	PITUITARY MACROADENOMA	PITUITARY MICROADENOMA	ECTOPIC ACTH OR CRH PRODUCTION	ADRENAL TUMOR
Plasma ACTH level	↑ to ↑↑	N to ↑	↑ to↑↑↑	↓
Percent who respond to high-dose dexamethasone	<10	95	<10	<10
Percent who respond to CRH	>90	>90	<10	<10

Note: ACTH, adrenocorticotropic hormone; CRH, corticotropin-releasing hormone; N, normal; ↑, elevated; ↓, decreased. See text for definition of a response.

plasma cortisol and, to a certain extent, ACTH determinations are not meaningful when performed in isolation, but the absence of the normal fall of plasma cortisol at midnight is consistent with Cushing's syndrome because there is loss of the diurnal cortisol rhythm.

The task of determining the etiology of Cushing's syndrome is complicated by the fact that all the available tests lack specificity and by the fact that the tumors producing this syndrome are prone to spontaneous and often dramatic changes in hormone secretion (periodic hormonogenesis). No test has a specificity >95%, and it may be necessary to use a combination of tests to arrive at the correct diagnosis.

Plasma ACTH levels can be useful in distinguishing the various causes of Cushing's syndrome, particularly in separating ACTH-dependent from ACTH-independent causes. In general, measurement of plasma ACTH is useful in the diagnosis of ACTH-independent etiologies of the syndrome, since most adrenal tumors cause low or undetectable ACTH levels [<2 pmol/L (10 pg/mL)]. Furthermore, ACTH-secreting pituitary macroadenomas and ACTH-producing nonendocrine tumors usually result in elevated ACTH levels. In the ectopic ACTH syndrome, ACTH levels may be elevated to >110 pmol/L (500 pg/mL), and in most patients the level is >40 pmol/L (200 pg/mL). In Cushing's syndrome as the result of a microadenoma or pituitary-hypothalamic dysfunction, ACTH levels range from 6–30 pmol/L (30–150 pg/mL) [normal, <14 pmol/L (<60 pg/mL)], with half of values falling in the normal range. However, the main problem with the use of ACTH levels in the differential diagnosis of Cushing's syndrome is that ACTH levels may be similar in individuals with hypothalamic-pituitary dysfunction, pituitary microadenomas, ectopic CRH production, and ectopic ACTH production (especially carcinoid tumors) (Table 5-4).

A useful step to distinguish patients with an ACTH-secreting pituitary microadenoma or hypothalamic-pituitary dysfunction from those with other forms of Cushing's syndrome is to determine the response of cortisol output to administration of high-dose dexamethasone (2 mg every 6 h for 2 days). An alternative 8-mg, overnight high-dose dexamethasone test has been developed; however, this test has a lower sensitivity and specificity than the standard test. When the diagnosis of Cushing's syndrome is clear-cut on the basis of baseline urinary and plasma assays, the high-dose dexamethasone suppression test may be used without performing the preliminary low-dose suppression test. The high-dose suppression test provides close to 100% specificity if the criterion used is suppression of urinary free cortisol by >90%. Occasionally, in individuals with bilateral nodular hyperplasia and/or ectopic CRH production, steroid output is also suppressed. Failure of low- and high-dose dexamethasone administration to suppress cortisol production (Table 5-4) can occur in patients with adrenal hyperplasia secondary to an ACTH-secreting pituitary macroadenoma or an ACTH-producing tumor of nonendocrine origin and in those with adrenal neoplasms.

Because of these difficulties, several additional tests have been advocated, such as the metyrapone and CRH infusion tests. The rationale underlying these tests is that steroid hypersecretion by an adrenal tumor or the ectopic production of ACTH will suppress the hypothalamic-pituitary axis so that inhibition of pituitary ACTH release can be demonstrated by either test. Thus, most patients with pituitary-hypothalamic dysfunction and/or a microadenoma have an increase in steroid or ACTH secretion in response to metyrapone or CRH administration, whereas most patients with ectopic ACTH-producing tumors do not. Most pituitary macroadenomas also respond to CRH, but their response to metyrapone is variable. However, false-positive and false-negative CRH tests can occur in patients with ectopic ACTH and pituitary tumors.

The main diagnostic dilemma in Cushing's syndrome is to distinguish those instances due to microadenomas of the pituitary from those due to ectopic sources (e.g., carcinoids or pheochromocytoma) that produce CRH and/or ACTH. The clinical manifestations are similar unless the ectopic tumor produces other symptoms, such as diarrhea and flushing from a carcinoid tumor or episodic hypertension from a pheochromocytoma. Sometimes, one can distinguish between ectopic and pituitary ACTH production by using metyrapone or CRH tests, as noted above. In these situations, CT of the pituitary gland is usually normal. MRI with the enhancing agent gadolinium may be better than CT for this purpose but demonstrates pituitary microadenomas in only half of patients with Cushing's disease. Because microadenomas can be detected in up to 10–20% of individuals without known pituitary disease, a positive imaging study does not prove that the pituitary is the source of ACTH excess. In those with negative imaging studies, selective petrosal sinus venous sampling for ACTH is now used in many referral centers. ACTH levels are measured at baseline and 2, 5, and 10 min after ovine CRH (1 μg/kg IV) injections. Peak petrosal/peripheral ACTH ratios of >3:1 confirm the presence of a pituitary ACTH-secreting tumor. In centers where petrosal sinus sampling is performed frequently, it has proved highly sensitive for distinguishing pituitary and nonpituitary sources of ACTH excess. However, the catheterization procedure is technically difficult, and complications have occurred.

The diagnosis of a *cortisol-producing adrenal adenoma* is suggested by low ACTH and disproportionate elevations in baseline urine free cortisol levels with only modest changes in urinary 17-ketosteroids or plasma DHEA sulfate. Adrenal androgen secretion is usually reduced in these patients owing to the cortisol-induced suppression of ACTH and subsequent involution of the androgen-producing zona reticularis.

The diagnosis of *adrenal carcinoma* is suggested by a palpable abdominal mass and by markedly elevated baseline values of both urine 17-ketosteroids and plasma DHEA sulfate. Plasma and urine cortisol levels are variably elevated. Adrenal carcinoma is usually resistant to both ACTH stimulation and dexamethasone suppression. Elevated adrenal androgen secretion often leads to virilization in the female. Estrogen-producing adrenocortical carcinoma usually presents with gynecomastia in men and dysfunctional uterine bleeding in women. These adrenal tumors secrete increased amounts of androstenedione, which is converted peripherally to the estrogens estrone and estradiol. Adrenal carcinomas that produce Cushing's syndrome are often associated with elevated levels of the intermediates of steroid biosynthesis (especially 11-deoxycortisol), suggesting inefficient conversion of the intermediates to the final product. This feature also accounts for the characteristic increase in 17-ketosteroids. Approximately 20% of adrenal carcinomas are not associated with endocrine syndromes and are presumed to be nonfunctioning or to produce biologically inactive steroid precursors. In addition, the excessive production of steroids is not always clinically evident (e.g., androgens in adult men).

Differential Diagnosis

Pseudo-Cushing's Syndrome

Problems in diagnosis include patients with obesity, chronic alcoholism, depression, and acute illness of any type. Extreme *obesity* is uncommon in Cushing's syndrome; furthermore, with exogenous obesity, the adiposity is generalized, not truncal. On adrenocortical testing, abnormalities in patients with exogenous obesity are usually modest. Basal urine steroid excretion levels in obese patients are also either normal or slightly elevated, and the diurnal pattern in blood and urine levels is normal. Patients with *chronic alcoholism* and those with *depression* share similar abnormalities in steroid output: modestly elevated urine cortisol, blunted circadian rhythm of cortisol levels, and resistance to suppression using the overnight dexamethasone test. In contrast to alcoholic subjects, depressed patients do not have signs and symptoms of Cushing's syndrome. Following discontinuation of alcohol and/or improvement in the emotional status, results of steroid testing usually return to normal. One or more of three tests have been used to differentiate mild Cushing's syndrome and pseudo-Cushing's syndrome. The serum cortisol level following the standard 2-day low-dose dexamethasone test has very high sensitivity and specificity. Although the CRH test alone is less useful, in combination with the low-dose dexamethasone test, there is nearly complete discrimination between these two conditions. Finally, a midnight cortisol level obtained in awake patients may have similar predictive value as the low-dose dexamethasone test if a cut-off of 210 nmol/L (7.5 μg/dL) is used. Patients with *acute illness* often have abnormal results on laboratory tests and fail to exhibit pituitary-adrenal suppression in response to dexamethasone, since major stress (such as pain or fever) interrupts the normal regulation of ACTH secretion. *Iatrogenic Cushing's syndrome*, induced by the administration of glucocorticoids or other steroids such as megestrol that bind to the glucocorticoid receptor, is indistinguishable by physical findings from endogenous adrenocortical hyperfunction. The distinction can be made, however, by measuring blood or urine cortisol levels in a basal state; in the iatrogenic syndrome these levels are low secondary to suppression of the pituitary-adrenal axis. The severity of iatrogenic Cushing's syndrome is related to the total steroid dose, the biologic half-life of the steroid, and the duration of therapy. Also, individuals taking afternoon and evening doses of glucocorticoids develop Cushing's syndrome more readily and with a smaller total daily dose than do patients taking morning doses only.

Radiologic Evaluation for Cushing's Syndrome

The preferred radiologic study for visualizing the adrenals is a CT scan of the abdomen (**Fig. 5-8**). CT is of value both for localizing adrenal tumors and for diagnosing bilateral hyperplasia. All patients believed to have hypersecretion of pituitary ACTH should have a pituitary MRI scan with gadolinium contrast. Even with this technique, small microadenomas may be undetectable; alternatively, false-positive masses due to cysts

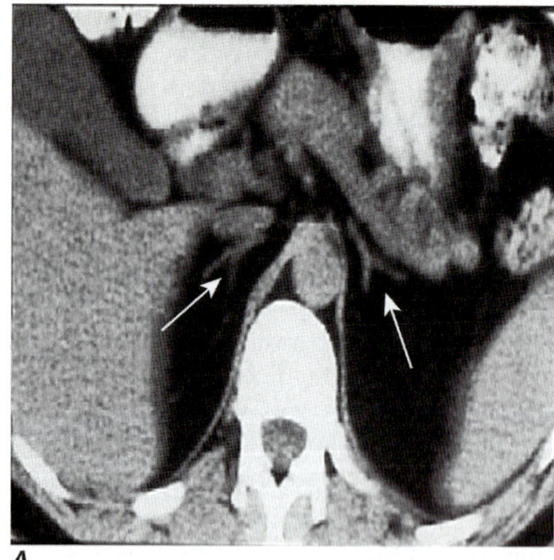

A

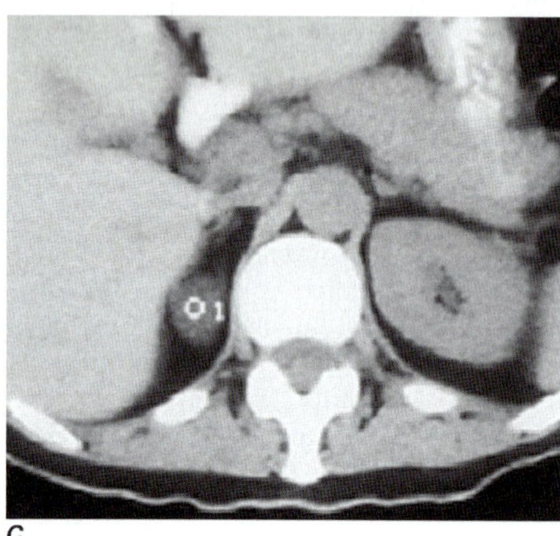

C

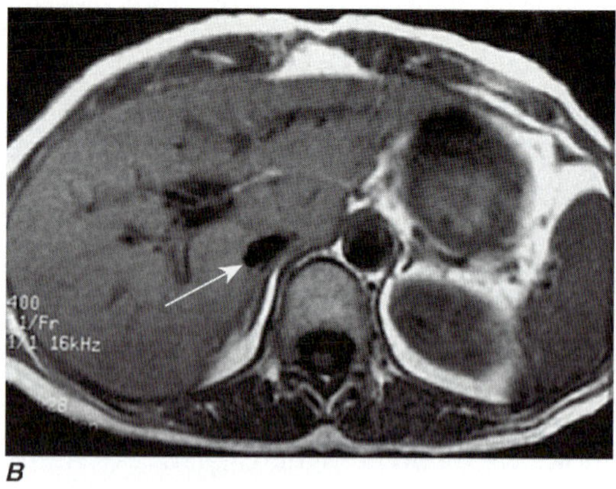

B

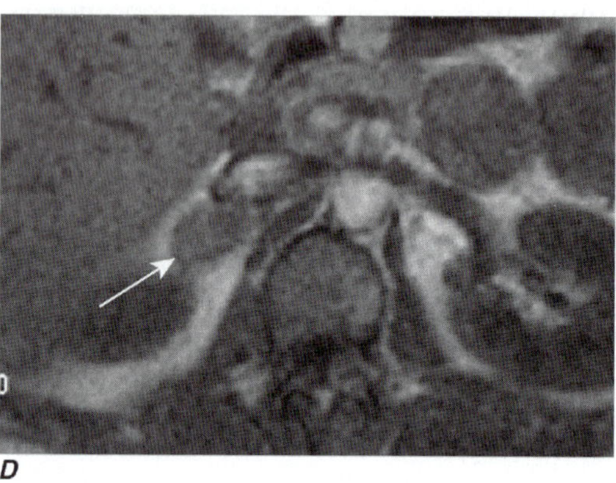

D

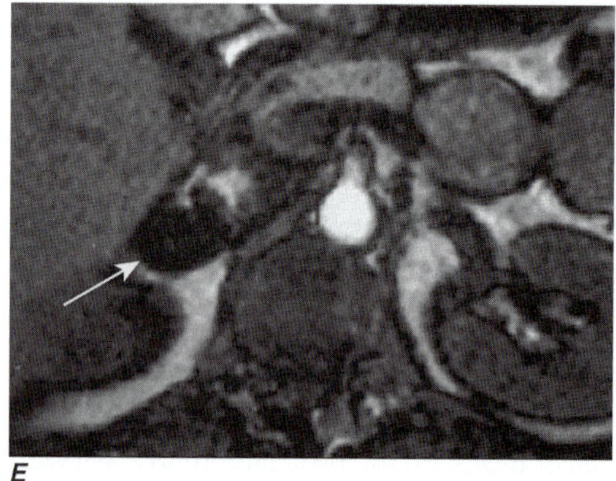

E

FIGURE 5-8

CT and MRI of the adrenal glands. *A.* Normal adrenal on CT. ***B.*** Normal adrenal on T1-weighted MRI. ***C.*** CT of benign adrenal adenoma. Right adrenal mass with 1.5 cm homogeneous attenuation (–5 Hounsfield units). ***D.*** Right adrenal mass (2 cm) showing homogeneous intermediate signal intensity on MRI in-phase gradient echo sequence. ***E.*** There is homogeneous loss of signal on the corresponding out-of-phase sequence, consistent with a diagnosis of adrenal adenoma.

or nonsecretory lesions of the normal pituitary may be imaged. In patients with ectopic ACTH production, high-resolution chest CT is a useful first step.

Evaluation of Asymptomatic Adrenal Masses

Many incidental masses (so-called incidentalomas) are discovered during radiographic testing for another condition, rather than testing performed because of a suspected adrenal disorder. This is not surprising since ~6% of adult/elderly subjects at autopsy have adrenocortical adenomas. However, the prevalence of incidental adenomas is age-dependent, i.e., cortical adenomas are very uncommon in individuals <30 years of age.

An important early step in the evaluation of adrenal incidentalomas is to determine whether the patient has a history of prior malignancy. In this circumstance, the adrenal mass will be a metastasis in about one-half of the patients. If the primary tumor is being treated and there are no other metastases, it may be prudent to obtain a biopsy of the mass. A CT-guided fine-needle aspiration (FNA) can usually identify nonadrenal or metastatic tissue. However, pheochromocytoma should always be excluded before a FNA is performed.

The next step is to determine whether the tumor is functioning, although the great majority (70–80%) are nonsecretory. Overt clinical symptoms are usually absent in incidentally discovered adrenal masses, but the clinician should search for subtle signs and symptoms of hormonal overproduction, such as cushingoid features and paroxysmal symptomatology. All patients with incidentally discovered masses should be screened for pheochromocytoma (Chap. 6), regardless of radiographic features that are considered typical for cortical adenomas (see below). Measurement of plasma free metanephrines is the recommended test due to its high sensitivity, and a negative test essentially rules out this disorder. All patients should also be screened with an overnight dexamethasone suppression test since autonomous cortisol production in patients without typical features of hypercortisolism (so-called preclinical or subclinical Cushing's syndrome) is the most common hypersecretory syndrome in incidentally discovered adrenal masses (**Fig. 5-9**). Such patients may experience side effects of mild overproduction of cortisol (such as hypertension, glucose intolerance, and osteoporosis) and may benefit from excision of the mass. Patients with hypertension should also be screened for primary aldosteronism by measurement of plasma aldosterone and plasma renin activity. Finally, females with signs of androgen excess or males with feminization should be tested for the overproduction of the appropriate sex steroids.

A major consideration is whether the incidentally discovered mass is an adrenocortical carcinoma (ACC). Although the probability of ACC is very low (<0.01%), and the vast majority of adrenal masses are benign adenomas, ACC is associated with a poor prognosis, especially if discovered at a late stage. Radiographic characterization of the adrenal mass has been crucial in this decision-making process; size and imaging phenotype are the best predictors of possible malignancy. Features suggestive of malignancy include large size (>4–6 cm), irregular margins and tumor inhomogeneity, soft tissue calcifications visible on CT, and high unenhanced CT attenuation values (>10 HU). Similar findings characteristic of malignancy are seen on chemical-shift MRI. In contrast, the common benign adrenocortical adenoma is characterized by diameter <4 cm and tumor homogeneity with sharp margins and low unenhanced CT values (<10 HU). FNA is not useful to distinguish between benign and malignant primary adrenal tumors. If the radiographic criteria favor a benign adrenocortical neoplasm, reassurance is gained if the mass remains unchanged in size at follow-up scanning in 3–6 months. On the other hand, benign cortical adenomas may increase in size (up to 1–2 cm) over several years of follow-up.

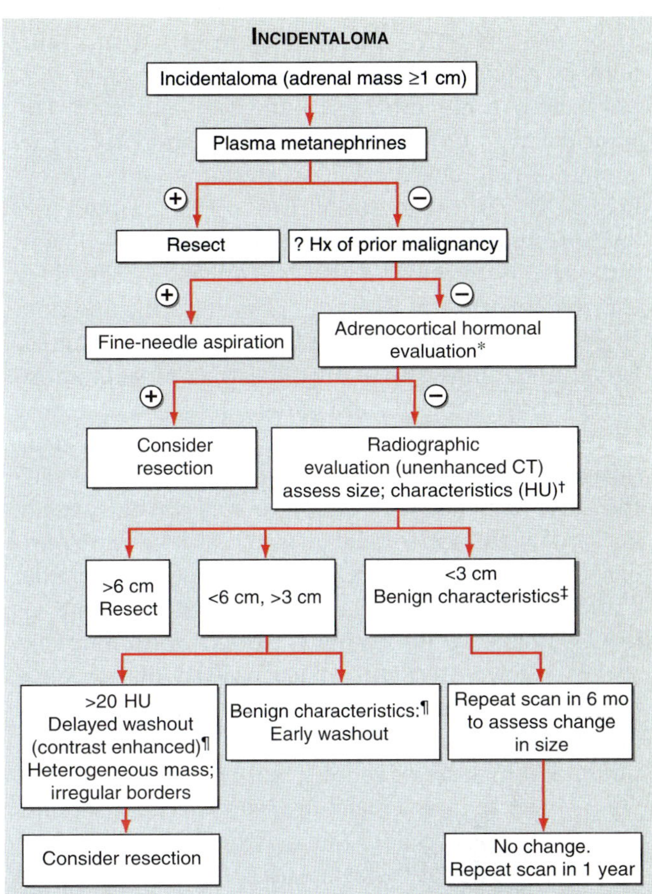

FIGURE 5-9

Incidentaloma. *Adrenocortical hormonal evaluation: Dexamethasone suppression test in all patients; plasma renin activity/aldosterone ratio for hypertensives; sex steroid (DHEA sulfate, estradiol) for clinical signs in females and males, respectively. †Hounsfield units (HU): a measurement of x-ray attenuation or lipid content of neoplasms. A lipid-rich mass (<10 HU) is diagnostic of a benign cortical adenoma. ‡Benign characteristics: homogeneous mass, smooth borders, HU <10. ¶Benign adrenal adenomas are also characterized by earlier washout of contrast enhancement than other neoplasms.

℞ Treatment: CUSHING'S SYNDROME

ADRENAL NEOPLASM Adrenal adenomas may be resected using laparoscopic techniques. Because of the possibility of atrophy of the contralateral adrenal, the patient should be treated with glucocorticoids and mineralocorticoids pre- and postoperatively as if for total adrenalectomy, even when a unilateral lesion is suspected, the routine being similar to that for an Addisonian patient undergoing elective surgery.

Despite operative intervention, most patients with adrenal carcinoma die within 3 years of diagnosis. Metastases occur most often to liver and lung. The principal drug for the treatment of adrenocortical carcinoma is mitotane (*o,p′*-DDD), an isomer of the insecticide DDT. Mitotane suppresses cortisol production and decreases plasma and urine steroid levels. Although its cytotoxic action is relatively selective for the glucocorticoid-secreting zone of the adrenal cortex, the zona glomerulosa may also be inhibited. Because mitotane also alters the extraadrenal metabolism of cortisol, plasma and urinary cortisol levels must be assessed to titrate the effect. The drug is usually given in divided doses three to four times a day, with the dose increased gradually to tolerability (usually <6 g daily). At higher doses, almost all patients experience side effects, which may be gastrointestinal (anorexia, diarrhea, vomiting) or neuromuscular (lethargy, somnolence, dizziness). All patients treated with mitotane should receive long-term glucocorticoid maintenance therapy, and, in some, mineralocorticoid replacement is appropriate. In approximately one-third of patients, both tumor and metastases regress, but long-term survival is not altered. In many patients, mitotane only inhibits steroidogenesis and does not cause regression of tumor metastases. Osseous metastases are usually refractory to the drug and should be treated with radiation therapy. Mitotane can also be given as adjunctive therapy after surgical resection of an adrenal carcinoma, although there is no evidence that this improves survival. Because of the absence of a long-term benefit with mitotane, alternative chemotherapeutic approaches based on platinum therapy have been used. However, there are no data presently available indicating a prolongation of life.

BILATERAL HYPERPLASIA Patients with hyperplasia usually have a relative or absolute increase in ACTH levels. Since therapy would logically be directed at reducing ACTH levels, the ideal primary treatment for ACTH- or CRH-producing tumors, whether pituitary or ectopic, is surgical removal. Occasionally (particularly with ectopic ACTH production) surgical excision is not possible because the disease is far advanced. In this situation, "medical" or surgical adrenalectomy may correct the hypercortisolism.

Controversy exists as to the proper treatment for bilateral adrenal hyperplasia when the source of the ACTH overproduction is not apparent. In some centers, these patients (especially those who suppress after the administration of a high-dose dexamethasone test) undergo surgical exploration of the pituitary via a transsphenoidal approach in the expectation that a microadenoma will be found (Chap. 2). However, in most circumstances selective petrosal sinus venous sampling is recommended, and the patient is referred to an appropriate center if the procedure is not available locally. If a microadenoma is not found at the time of exploration, total hypophysectomy may be needed. Complications of transsphenoidal surgery include cerebrospinal fluid rhinorrhea, diabetes insipidus, panhypopituitarism, and optic or cranial nerve injuries.

In other centers, total adrenalectomy is the treatment of choice. The cure rate with this procedure is close to 100%. The adverse effects include the certain need for lifelong mineralocorticoid and glucocorticoid replacement and a 10–20% probability of a pituitary tumor developing over the next 10 years (Nelson's syndrome; Chap. 2). It is uncertain whether these tumors arise de novo or if they were present prior to adrenalectomy but were too small to be detected. Periodic radiologic evaluation of the pituitary gland by MRI as well as serial ACTH measurements should be performed in all individuals after bilateral adrenalectomy for Cushing's disease. Such pituitary tumors may become locally invasive and impinge on the optic chiasm or extend into the cavernous or sphenoid sinuses.

Except in children, pituitary irradiation is rarely used as primary treatment, being reserved rather for postoperative tumor recurrences. In some centers, high levels of gamma radiation can be focused on the desired site with less scattering to surrounding tissues by using stereotactic techniques. Side effects of radiation include ocular motor palsy and hypopituitarism. There is a long lag time between treatment and remission, and the remission rate is usually <50%.

Finally, in occasional patients in whom a surgical approach is not feasible, "medical" adrenalectomy may be indicated (**Table 5-5**). Inhibition of steroidogenesis may also be indicated in severely cushingoid patients prior to surgical intervention. Chemical adrenalectomy may be accomplished by the administration of the inhibitor of steroidogenesis ketoconazole (600–1200 mg/d). In addition, mitotane (2 or 3 g/d) and/or the blockers of steroid

TABLE 5-5

TREATMENT MODALITIES FOR PATIENTS WITH ADRENAL HYPERPLASIA SECONDARY TO PITUITARY ACTH HYPERSECRETION

Treatments
Treatments to reduce pituitary ACTH production
Transsphenoidal resection of microadenoma
Radiation therapy
Treatments to reduce or eliminate adrenocortical cortisol secretion
Bilateral adrenalectomy
Medical adrenalectomy (metyrapone, mitotane, aminoglutethimide, ketoconazole)[a]

[a]Not curative but effective as long as chronically administered in selected patients.

Note: ACTH, adrenocorticotropic hormone.

synthesis, aminoglutethimide (1 g/d) and metyrapone (2 or 3 g/d), may be effective either alone or in combination. Mitotane is slow to take effect (weeks). Mifepristone, a competitive inhibitor of the binding of glucocorticoid to its receptor, may be a treatment option. Adrenal insufficiency is a risk with all these agents, and replacement steroids may be required.

ALDOSTERONISM

Aldosteronism is a syndrome associated with hypersecretion of the mineralocorticoid aldosterone. In *primary* aldosteronism the cause for the excessive aldosterone production resides within the adrenal gland; in *secondary* aldosteronism the stimulus is extraadrenal.

Primary Aldosteronism with an Adrenal Tumor

In the original descriptions of excessive and inappropriate aldosterone production, the disease was the result of an *aldosterone-producing adrenal adenoma* (Conn's syndrome). Most cases involve a unilateral adenoma, which is usually small and may occur on either side. Rarely, primary aldosteronism is due to an adrenal carcinoma. Aldosteronism is twice as common in women as in men, usually occurs between the ages of 30 and 50, and is present in ~1% of unselected hypertensive patients.

Primary Aldosteronism without an Adrenal Tumor

In many patients with clinical and biochemical features of primary aldosteronism, a solitary adenoma is not found at surgery. Instead, these patients have *bilateral cortical nodular hyperplasia*. In the literature, this disease is also termed *idiopathic hyperaldosteronism* and *nodular hyperplasia*. The cause is unknown. Often it is difficult to distinguish these patients from those with low renin essential hypertension. In contrast to patients with an aldosteronoma, those with bilateral hyperplasia are unlikely to have hypokalemia and usually have lower levels of aldosterone and less radiologic evidence for adrenal pathology. They constitute perhaps as many as 80% of patients with primary aldosteronism and largely contribute to the increased prevalence of primary aldosteronism reported during the past few years. Although the prevalence of the tumor form of primary aldosteronism in the general hypertension population remains in the ≤1% range, the prevalence of the bilateral hyperplasia form has been reported to range as high as 10%, depending on the criteria used and the study population.

Signs and Symptoms

Hypersecretion of aldosterone increases the renal distal tubular exchange of intratubular sodium for secreted potassium and hydrogen ions, with progressive depletion of body potassium and development of hypokalemia. Most patients have diastolic hypertension, which may be very severe, and headaches. The hypertension is probably due to the increased sodium reabsorption and extracellular volume expansion. *Potassium depletion* is responsible for the muscle weakness and fatigue and is due to the effect of potassium depletion on the muscle cell membrane. The polyuria results from impairment of urinary concentrating ability and is often associated with polydipsia. However, some individuals with mild disease, particularly most with the bilateral hyperplasia type, may have potassium levels in the low-normal range and therefore have no symptoms associated with hypokalemia.

Electrocardiographic and roentgenographic signs of left ventricular enlargement are, in part, secondary to the hypertension. However, the left ventricular hypertrophy is disproportionate to the level of blood pressure when compared to individuals with essential hypertension, and regression of the hypertrophy occurs even if blood pressure is not reduced after removal of an aldosteronoma. If potassium depletion is present, there may be electrocardiographic signs of hypokalemia including prominent U waves, cardiac arrhythmias, and premature contractions. In the absence of associated congestive heart failure, renal disease, or preexisting abnormalities (such as thrombophlebitis), edema is characteristically absent. However, structural damage to the cerebral circulation, retinal vasculature, and kidney occurs more frequently than would be predicted based on the level and duration of the hypertension. Proteinuria may occur in as many as 50% of patients with primary aldosteronism, and renal failure occurs in up to 15%. Thus, it is probable that excess aldosterone production induces cardiovascular damage independent of its effect on blood pressure.

Laboratory Findings

Laboratory findings depend on both the duration and the severity of potassium depletion. An overnight concentration test often reveals impaired ability to concentrate the urine, probably secondary to the hypokalemia. Urine pH is neutral to alkaline because of excessive secretion of ammonium and bicarbonate ions to compensate for the metabolic alkalosis. Again these findings are infrequent in patients with bilateral hyperplasia.

Hypokalemia may be severe (<3 mmol/L) and reflects body potassium depletion, usually >300 mmol. In mild forms of primary aldosteronism, potassium levels may be normal. *Hypernatremia* is infrequent but may be caused by sodium retention, concomitant water loss from polyuria, and resetting of the osmostat. Metabolic alkalosis and elevation of serum bicarbonate are caused by hydrogen ion loss into the urine and migration into potassium-depleted cells. The alkalosis is perpetuated by potassium deficiency, which increases the capacity of the proximal convoluted tubule to reabsorb filtered bicarbonate. If hypokalemia is severe, serum magnesium levels are also reduced.

Diagnosis

Moderate to severe hyperaldosteronism is suggested by persistent hypokalemia in a nonedematous patient with a normal sodium intake who is not receiving potassium-wasting diuretics (furosemide, ethacrynic acid, thiazides). If hypokalemia occurs in a hypertensive patient taking a potassium-wasting diuretic, the diuretic should be discontinued and the patient should be given potassium supplements. After 1–2 weeks, the potassium level should be remeasured, and if hypokalemia persists, the patient should be evaluated for a mineralocorticoid excess syndrome (**Fig. 5-10**). Milder forms of the disease, particularly those with bilateral hyperplasia, are suggested by having hypertension resistant to two or more antihypertensives.

The criteria for the diagnosis of primary aldosteronism are (1) diastolic hypertension without edema, (2) hyposecretion of renin (as judged by low plasma renin activity levels) that fails to increase appropriately during volume depletion (upright posture, sodium depletion), and (3) hypersecretion of aldosterone that does not suppress appropriately in response to volume expansion.

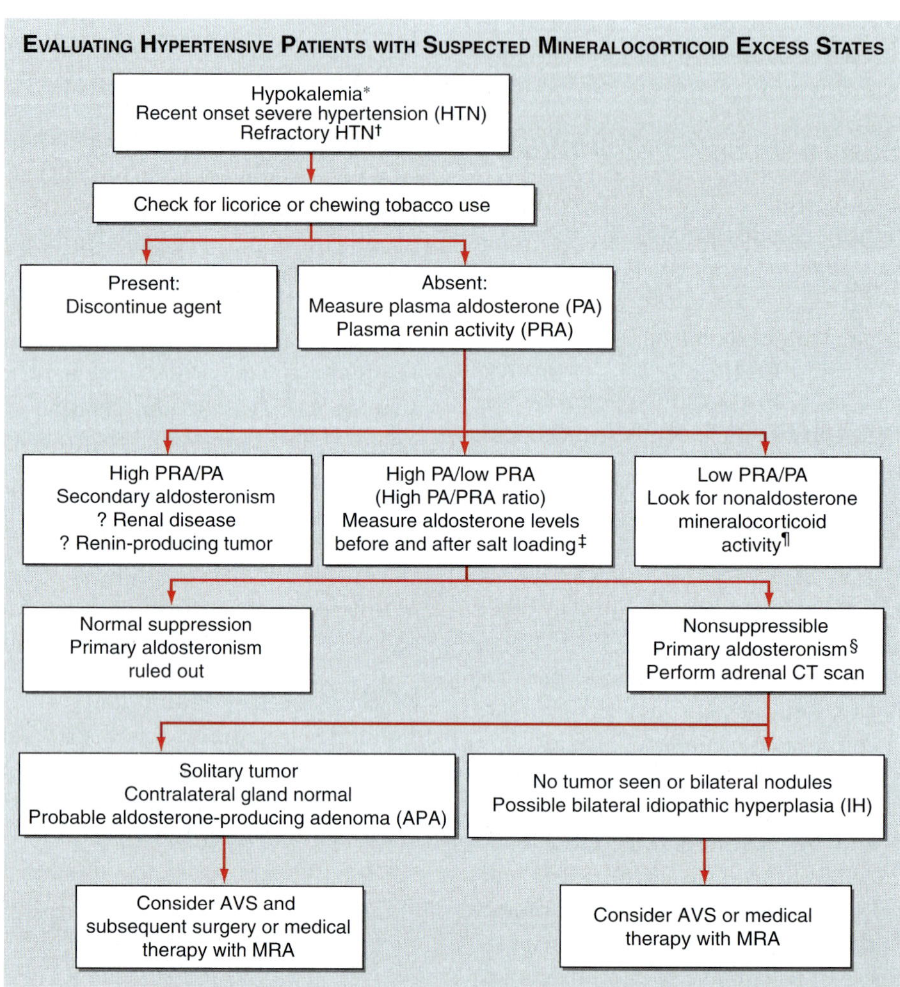

FIGURE 5-10

Diagnostic flowchart for evaluating patients with possible mineralocorticoid excess states, including primary aldosteronism (PA). *Serum K may be normal in some patients with mild mineralocorticoid excess states or those who are taking potassium-sparing diuretics (spironolactone, triamterene) or those who ingest low sodium and high potassium intakes. †Inadequate control of hypertension (HTN) on three antihypertensives (including a diuretic). ‡This step should not be taken if hypertension is severe (diastolic pressure >115 mmHg) or if cardiac failure is present. Also, serum potassium levels should be corrected before the infusion of a saline solution. Alternative methods that produce comparable suppression of aldosterone secretion include oral sodium loading (200 mmol/d) and the administration of fludrocortisone, 0.2 mg bid, for 3–4 days. ¶For example, Liddle's syndrome, apparent mineralocorticoid excess syndrome, or a deoxycorticosterone-secreting tumor. §Consider diagnosis of glucocorticoid-remediable aldosteronism (GRA) in patients with early-onset HTN (<20 years old) or those with a positive family history of early-onset HTN or primary aldosteronism. See text. AVS, bilateral adrenal vein sampling, to lateralize aldosterone production in APA or confirm bilateral secretion in IH; CT, computed tomography; MRA, mineralocorticoid receptor antagonist.

Patients with primary aldosteronism characteristically *do not have edema*, since they exhibit an "escape" phenomenon from the sodium-retaining aspects of mineralocorticoids. Rarely, pretibial edema is present in patients with associated nephropathy and azotemia.

The estimation of plasma renin activity is of limited value in separating patients with primary aldosteronism from those with hypertension of other causes. Although failure of plasma renin activity to rise normally during volume-depletion maneuvers is a criterion for the diagnosis of primary aldosteronism, suppressed renin activity also occurs in 25% of patients with essential hypertension.

Although a renin measurement alone lacks specificity, the ratio of serum aldosterone to plasma renin activity is a very useful screening test. A high ratio (>30), when aldosterone is expressed as ng/dL and plasma renin activity as ng/mL per hour, strongly suggests autonomy of aldosterone secretion. Aldosterone levels need to be >500 pmol/L (>15 ng/dL) when salt intake is not restricted. In some centers, the aldosterone/plasma renin activity ratio is used as a primary screen test in all normokalemic, difficult-to-control hypertensive patients, in addition to those with hypokalemia. Ultimately, it is necessary to demonstrate a lack of aldosterone suppression to diagnose primary aldosteronism (Fig. 5-10). The autonomy exhibited in these patients refers only to the resistance to suppression of secretion during volume expansion; aldosterone can and does respond in a normal or above-normal fashion to the stimulus of potassium loading or ACTH infusion.

Once hyposecretion of renin and failure of aldosterone secretion suppression are demonstrated, aldosterone-producing adenomas should be localized by abdominal CT scan, using a high-resolution scanner as many aldosteronomas are <1 cm in size. If the CT scan is negative, percutaneous transfemoral bilateral adrenal vein catheterization with adrenal vein sampling may demonstrate a two- to threefold increase in plasma aldosterone concentration on the involved side. In cases of hyperaldosteronism secondary to cortical nodular hyperplasia, no lateralization is found. It is important for samples to be obtained simultaneously, if possible, and for cortisol levels to be measured to ensure that false localization does not reflect dilution or an ACTH- or stress-induced rise in aldosterone levels. In a patient with an adenoma, the aldosterone/cortisol ratio lateralizes to the side of the lesion.

Differential Diagnosis

Patients with hypertension and hypokalemia may have either primary or secondary hyperaldosteronism (Fig. 5-11). A useful maneuver to distinguish between these conditions is the measurement of plasma renin activity. Secondary hyperaldosteronism in patients with accelerated hypertension is due to elevated plasma renin levels; in contrast, patients with primary aldosteronism have suppressed plasma renin levels. Indeed, in patients with a serum potassium concentration <2.5 mmol/L, a high ratio of plasma aldosterone to plasma renin activity in a random sample is usually sufficient to establish the diagnosis of primary aldosteronism without additional testing. Ectopic ACTH production should also be considered in patients with hypertension and severe hypokalemia.

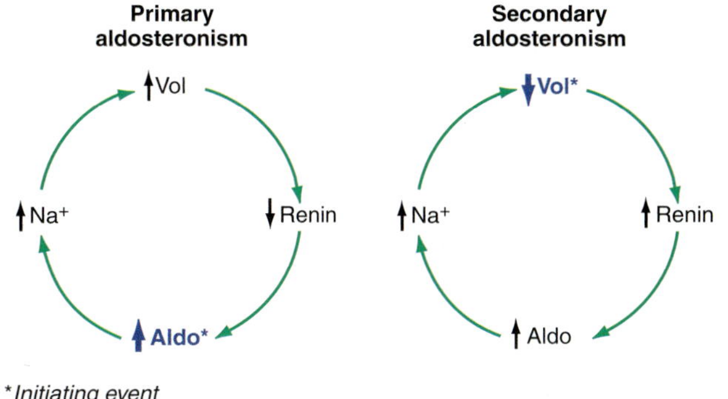

FIGURE 5-11
Responses of the renin-aldosterone volume control loop in primary versus secondary aldosteronism.

The most common problem is to distinguish between hyperaldosteronism due to an adenoma and that due to idiopathic bilateral nodular hyperplasia. This distinction is important because hypertension associated with idiopathic hyperplasia does not usually benefit from bilateral adrenalectomy, whereas hypertension associated with aldosterone-producing tumors is usually improved or cured by removal of the adenoma. Although patients with idiopathic bilateral nodular hyperplasia tend to have higher potassium levels (many in the normal range), lower aldosterone secretion, and higher plasma renin activity than do patients with primary aldosteronism, differentiation is impossible solely on clinical and/or biochemical grounds. An anomalous postural decrease in plasma aldosterone and elevated plasma 18-hydroxycorticosterone levels are present in most patients with a unilateral lesion. However, these tests are also of limited diagnostic value in the individual patient, because some adenoma patients have an increase in plasma aldosterone with upright posture, so-called renin-responsive aldosteronoma. A definitive diagnosis is best made by radiographic studies, including bilateral adrenal vein catheterization, as noted above.

Primary aldosteronism must also be distinguished from other *hypermineralocorticoid states*. In a few instances, hypertensive patients with hypokalemic alkalosis have adenomas that secrete deoxycorticosterone. Such patients have reduced plasma renin activity levels, but aldosterone levels are either normal or reduced, suggesting the diagnosis of mineralocorticoid excess due to a hormone other than aldosterone. Several inherited disorders have clinical features similar to those of primary aldosteronism.

Rx Treatment: PRIMARY ALDOSTERONISM

Primary aldosteronism due to an adenoma is usually treated by surgical excision of the adenoma. Where possible, a laparoscopic approach is favored. However, dietary sodium restriction and the administration of an aldosterone antagonist—e.g., spironolactone—are effective in many cases. Hypertension and hypokalemia are usually controlled by doses of 25–100 mg of spironolactone every 8 h. In some patients, medical management has been successful for years, but chronic therapy in men is usually limited by side effects of spironolactone such as gynecomastia, decreased libido, and impotence. Eplerenone, a less potent but more specific MR antagonist with minimal, if any, antiandrogen effect, is also useful in doses of 50–150 mg every 8 h.

When idiopathic bilateral hyperplasia is suspected, surgery is indicated only when significant, symptomatic hypokalemia cannot be controlled with medical therapy, i.e., by spironolactone, eplerenone, triamterene, or amiloride. Hypertension associated with idiopathic hyperplasia is usually not benefited by bilateral adrenalectomy.

Secondary Aldosteronism

Secondary aldosteronism refers to an appropriately increased production of aldosterone in response to activation of the renin-angiotensin system (Fig. 5-11). The production rate of aldosterone is often higher in patients with secondary aldosteronism than in those with primary aldosteronism. Secondary aldosteronism usually occurs in association with the accelerated phase of hypertension or on the basis of an underlying edema disorder. Secondary aldosteronism in pregnancy is a normal physiologic response to estrogen-induced increases in circulating levels of renin substrate and plasma renin activity and to the antialdosterone actions of progestogens.

Secondary aldosteronism in hypertensive states is due either to a primary overproduction of renin (primary reninism) or to an overproduction of renin secondary to a decrease in renal blood flow and/or perfusion pressure (Fig. 5-11). Secondary hypersecretion of renin can be due to a narrowing of one or both of the major renal arteries by atherosclerosis or by fibromuscular hyperplasia. Overproduction of renin from both kidneys also occurs in severe arteriolar nephrosclerosis (malignant hypertension) or with profound renal vasoconstriction (the accelerated phase of hypertension). The secondary aldosteronism is characterized by hypokalemic alkalosis, moderate to severe increases in plasma renin activity, and moderate to marked increases in aldosterone levels.

Secondary aldosteronism with hypertension can also be caused by rare renin-producing tumors (primary reninism). In these patients, the biochemical characteristics are of renal vascular hypertension, but the primary defect is renin secretion by a juxtaglomerular cell tumor. The diagnosis can be made by demonstration of normal renal vasculature and/or demonstration of a space-occupying lesion in the kidney by radiographic techniques and documentation of a unilateral increase in renal vein renin activity. Rarely, these tumors arise in tissues such as the ovary.

Secondary aldosteronism is present in many forms of *edema*. The rate of aldosterone secretion is usually increased in patients with edema caused by either cirrhosis or the nephrotic syndrome. In congestive heart failure, elevated aldosterone secretion varies depending on the severity of cardiac failure. The stimulus for aldosterone release in these conditions appears to be *arterial hypovolemia* and/or hypotension. Thiazides and furosemide often exaggerate secondary aldosteronism via volume depletion; hypokalemia and, on occasion, alkalosis can then become prominent features. On occasion, secondary hyperaldosteronism occurs without edema or hypertension (Bartter and Gitelman syndromes, see later in the chapter).

Aldosterone and Cardiovascular Damage

Although many studies have investigated the role of angiotensin II in mediating cardiovascular damage, additional evidence indicates that aldosterone has an important role that is independent of angiotensin II. Patients with primary aldosteronism (in which angiotensin II levels are usually very low) have a higher incidence of left ventricular hypertrophy (LVH), albuminuria, and stroke than do patients with essential hypertension. Experimental animal models mimicking secondary aldosteronism (angiotensin infusion) or primary aldosteronism (aldosterone infusion) reveal a common pathophysiologic sequence. Within the first few days there is activation of proinflammatory molecules with a histologic picture of perivascular macrophage infiltrate and inflammation, followed by cellular death, fibrosis, and ventricular hypertrophy. These events are prevented if a MR antagonist is used or if adrenalectomy is performed initially. The same pathophysiologic sequence is seen in animals with average aldosterone levels and cardiovascular damage, i.e., diabetes mellitus, or genetic hypertensive rats. There are two important additional observations. First, the level of sodium intake is a critical co-factor. If salt intake is severely restricted, no damage occurs even though the aldosterone levels are markedly elevated. Thus, it is not the level of aldosterone per se that is responsible for the damage, but its level relative to the volume or sodium status of the individual. Second, the dose of an MR antagonist required to prevent cardiovascular damage in these experimental models is much lower than that required to induce substantial volume depletion.

Several clinical trials support these experimental results. In the RALES trial, patients with class II/IV heart failure were randomized to standard care or a low dose of the MR antagonist, spironolactone. There was a 30% reduction in all-cause mortality and cardiovascular mortality and hospitalizations after 36 months. Two studies in hypertensive subjects addressed the question of the relative importance of a reduction of angiotensin II formation versus blockade of the MR in mediating cardiovascular damage. Subjects were randomized to eplerenone (an MR antagonist), enalapril (an ACE inhibitor), or both agents. In the first study, the subjects had LVH, with the endpoint being a reduction in LVH. In the second, the subjects had diabetes mellitus and proteinuria, with the endpoint being a reduction in proteinuria. In both studies, all three treatment arms substantially reduced the primary endpoint; however, the most potent effect occurred in the combination arms of the studies. In the monotherapy LVH arms, the reduction in LVH was similar, while in the proteinuria study, eplerenone produced a greater reduction than did enalapril. A follow-up study in diabetics with proteinuria provided insight into the maximally effective therapeutic dose. In this study, all subjects were treated with enalapril and randomized to treatment with placebo or 50 mg or 100 mg of eplerenone. The two doses reduced proteinuria to the same extent. These results, coupled with the low dose of spironolactone that was highly effective in the RALES trial, suggest that the maximally effective dose necessary to reduce cardiovascular damage is much lower than that required to reduce blood pressure maximally. The final study was the EPHESUS trial, where individuals who developed congestive heart failure after an acute myocardial infarction were randomized to standard-of-care treatment with or without a small dose of eplerenone. Eplerenone administration produced a significantly greater reduction in mortality (15–17%) and in cardiovascular-related hospitalizations than the placebo arm. These clinical studies provide strong support to the hypothesis that MR blockade has a significant added advantage over standard-of-care therapy in reducing cardiovascular mortality and surrogate adverse cardiovascular endpoints.

SYNDROMES OF ADRENAL ANDROGEN EXCESS

Adrenal androgen excess results from excess production of DHEA and androstenedione, which are converted to testosterone in extraglandular tissues; elevated testosterone levels account for most of the virilization. Adrenal androgen excess may be associated with the secretion of greater or smaller amounts of other adrenal hormones and may, therefore, present as "pure" syndromes of virilization or as "mixed" syndromes associated with excessive glucocorticoids and Cushing's syndrome. For further discussion of hirsutism and virilization, see Chap. 13.

HYPOFUNCTION OF THE ADRENAL CORTEX

Cases of adrenal insufficiency can be divided into two general categories: (1) those associated with primary inability of the adrenal to elaborate sufficient quantities of hormone, and (2) those associated with a secondary failure due to inadequate ACTH formation or release (Table 5-6).

PRIMARY ADRENOCORTICAL DEFICIENCY (ADDISON'S DISEASE)

The original description of Addison's disease—"general languor and debility, feebleness of the heart's action, irritability of the stomach, and a peculiar change of the color of the skin"—summarizes the dominant clinical features. Advanced cases are usually easy to diagnose, but recognition of the early phases can be challenging.

Incidence

Acquired forms of primary insufficiency are relatively rare, may occur at any age, and affect both sexes equally. Because of the common therapeutic use of steroids, secondary adrenal insufficiency is relatively common.

Etiology and Pathogenesis

Addison's disease results from progressive destruction of the adrenals, which must involve >90% of the glands

TABLE 5-6

CLASSIFICATION OF ADRENAL INSUFFICIENCY
Primary Adrenal Insufficiency
Anatomic destruction of gland (chronic or acute)
"Idiopathic" atrophy (autoimmune, adrenoleukodystrophy)
Surgical removal
Infection (tuberculous, fungal, viral—especially in AIDS patients)
Hemorrhage
Invasion: metastatic
Metabolic failure in hormone production
Congenital adrenal hyperplasia
Enzyme inhibitors (metyrapone, ketoconazole, aminoglutethimide)
Cytotoxic agents (mitotane)
ACTH-blocking antibodies
Mutation in ACTH receptor gene
Adrenal hypoplasia congenita
Secondary Adrenal Insufficiency
Hypopituitarism due to hypothalamic-pituitary disease
Suppression of hypothalamic-pituitary axis
By exogenous steroid
By endogenous steroid from tumor

Note: ACTH, adrenocorticotropic hormone.

before adrenal insufficiency appears. The adrenal is a frequent site for chronic granulomatous diseases, predominantly tuberculosis but also histoplasmosis, coccidioidomycosis, and cryptococcosis. In early series, tuberculosis was responsible for 70–90% of cases, but the most frequent cause now is *idiopathic* atrophy, and an autoimmune mechanism is probably responsible. Rarely, other lesions are encountered, such as adrenoleukodystrophy, bilateral hemorrhage, tumor metastases, HIV, cytomegalovirus (CMV), amyloidosis, adrenomyeloneuropathy, familial adrenal insufficiency, or sarcoidosis.

Although half of patients with idiopathic atrophy have circulating adrenal antibodies, autoimmune destruction is probably secondary to cytotoxic T lymphocytes. Specific adrenal antigens to which autoantibodies may be directed include 21-hydroxylase (CYP21A2) and side chain cleavage enzyme, but the significance of these antibodies in the pathogenesis of adrenal insufficiency is unknown. Some antibodies cause adrenal insufficiency by blocking the binding of ACTH to its receptors. Some patients also have antibodies to thyroid, parathyroid, and/or gonadal tissue (Chap. 23). There is also an increased incidence of chronic lymphocytic thyroiditis, premature ovarian failure, type 1 diabetes mellitus, and hypo- or hyperthyroidism. The presence of two or more of these autoimmune endocrine disorders in the same person defines the polyglandular autoimmune syndrome type II. Additional features include pernicious anemia, vitiligo, alopecia, nontropical sprue, and myasthenia gravis. Within families, multiple generations are affected by one or more of the above diseases. Type II polyglandular syndrome is associated with a mutant gene on chromosome 6 as well as with HLA alleles B8 and DR3.

The combination of parathyroid and adrenal insufficiency and chronic mucocutaneous candidiasis constitutes type I polyglandular autoimmune syndrome. Other autoimmune diseases in this disorder include pernicious anemia, chronic active hepatitis, alopecia, primary hypothyroidism, and premature gonadal failure. There is no HLA association; this syndrome is inherited as an autosomal recessive trait. It is caused by mutations in the *a*utoimmune *p*oly*e*ndocrinopathy *c*andidiasis *e*ctodermal *d*ystrophy (APECED) gene located on chromosome 21q22.3. The gene encodes a transcription factor thought to be involved in lymphocyte function. The type I syndrome usually presents during childhood, whereas the type II syndrome is usually manifested in adulthood.

Clinical suspicion of adrenal insufficiency should be high in patients with AIDS. CMV regularly involves the adrenal glands (so-called CMV necrotizing adrenalitis), and involvement with *Mycobacterium avium-intracellulare*, *Cryptococcus*, and Kaposi's sarcoma has been reported. Adrenal insufficiency in AIDS patients may not be manifest clinically, but tests of adrenal reserve frequently give abnormal results. When interpreting tests of adrenocortical function, it is important to remember that medications such as rifampin, phenytoin, ketoconazole, megestrol, and opiates may cause or potentiate adrenal insufficiency. Adrenal hemorrhage and infarction occur in patients on anticoagulants and in those with circulating anticoagulants and hypercoagulable states, such as the antiphospholipid syndrome.

There are several rare genetic causes of adrenal insufficiency that present primarily in infancy and childhood.

Clinical Signs and Symptoms

Adrenocortical insufficiency caused by gradual adrenal destruction is characterized by an insidious onset of fatigability, weakness, anorexia, nausea and vomiting, weight loss, cutaneous and mucosal pigmentation, hypotension, and occasionally hypoglycemia (Table 5-7). Depending on the duration and degree of adrenal hypofunction, the manifestations vary from mild chronic fatigue to fulminating shock associated with acute destruction of the glands, as described by Waterhouse and Friderichsen.

Asthenia is the cardinal symptom. Early it may be sporadic, usually most evident at times of stress; as adrenal function becomes more impaired, the patient is continuously fatigued, and bed rest is necessary.

Hyperpigmentation may be striking or absent. It commonly appears as a diffuse brown, tan, or bronze darkening of parts such as the elbows or creases of the hand and of areas that normally are pigmented such as the areolae about the nipples. Bluish-black patches may appear on the mucous membranes. Some patients develop dark freckles, and irregular areas of vitiligo may paradoxically be present. As an early sign, tanning following sun exposure may be persistent.

Arterial hypotension with postural accentuation is frequent, and blood pressure may be in the range of 80/50 or less.

Abnormalities of gastrointestinal function are often the presenting complaint. Symptoms vary from mild anorexia

TABLE 5-7

FREQUENCY OF SYMPTOMS AND SIGNS IN ADRENAL INSUFFICIENCY

SIGN OR SYMPTOM	PERCENT OF PATIENTS
Weakness	99
Pigmentation of skin	98
Weight loss	97
Anorexia, nausea, and vomiting	90
Hypotension (<110/70)	87
Pigmentation of mucous membranes	82
Abdominal pain	34
Salt craving	22
Diarrhea	20
Constipation	19
Syncope	16
Vitiligo	9

with weight loss to fulminating nausea, vomiting, diarrhea, and ill-defined abdominal pain, which may be so severe as to be confused with an acute abdomen. Patients may have personality changes, usually consisting of excessive irritability and restlessness. Enhancement of the sensory modalities of taste, olfaction, and hearing is reversible with therapy. Axillary and pubic hair may be decreased in women due to loss of adrenal androgens.

Laboratory Findings

In the early phase of gradual adrenal destruction, there may be no demonstrable abnormalities in the routine laboratory parameters, but adrenal reserve is decreased—i.e., while basal steroid output may be normal, a subnormal increase occurs after stress. Adrenal stimulation with ACTH uncovers abnormalities in this stage of the disease, eliciting a subnormal increase of cortisol levels or no increase at all. In more advanced stages of adrenal destruction, serum sodium, chloride, and bicarbonate levels are reduced, and the serum potassium level is elevated. The hyponatremia is due both to loss of sodium into the urine (due to aldosterone deficiency) and to movement into the intracellular compartment. This extravascular sodium loss depletes ECFV and accentuates hypotension. Elevated plasma vasopressin and angiotensin II levels may contribute to the hyponatremia by impairing free-water clearance. Hyperkalemia is due to a combination of aldosterone deficiency, impaired glomerular filtration, and acidosis. Basal levels of cortisol and aldosterone are subnormal and fail to increase following ACTH administration. Mild to moderate hypercalcemia occurs in 10–20% of patients for unclear reasons. The electrocardiogram may show nonspecific changes, and the electroencephalogram exhibits a generalized reduction and slowing. There may be a normocytic anemia, a relative lymphocytosis, and a moderate eosinophilia.

Diagnosis

The diagnosis of adrenal insufficiency should be made only with ACTH stimulation testing to assess adrenal reserve capacity for steroid production (see above for ACTH test protocols). In brief, the best screening test is the cortisol response 60 min after 250 μg of cosyntropin given IM or IV. Cortisol levels should be >495 nmol/L (18 μg/dL). If the response is abnormal, then primary and secondary adrenal insufficiency can be distinguished by measuring aldosterone levels from the same blood samples. In secondary, but not primary, adrenal insufficiency, the aldosterone increment will be normal [≥150 pmol/L (5 ng/dL)]. Furthermore, in primary adrenal insufficiency, plasma ACTH and associated peptides (β-LPT) are elevated because of loss of the usual cortisol-hypothalamic-pituitary feedback relationship, whereas in secondary adrenal insufficiency, plasma ACTH values are low or "inappropriately" normal (Fig. 5-12).

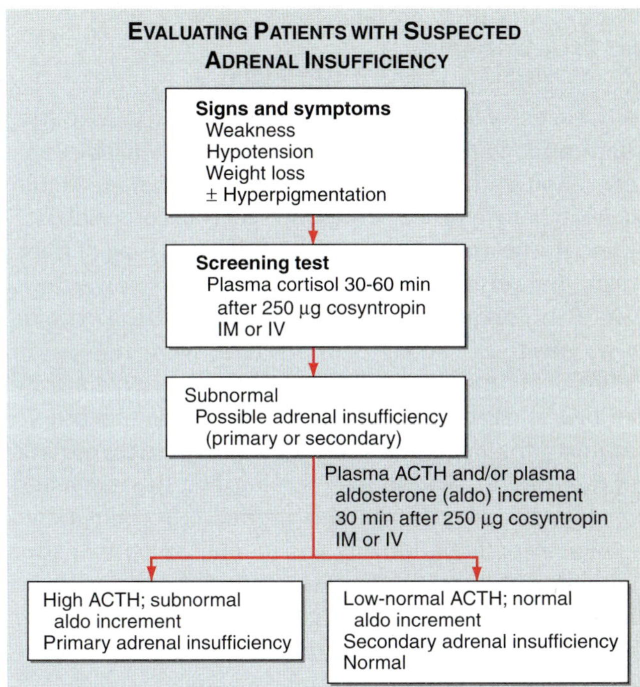

FIGURE 5-12

Diagnostic flowchart for evaluating patients with suspected adrenal insufficiency. Plasma adrenocorticotropic hormone (ACTH) levels are low in secondary adrenal insufficiency. In adrenal insufficiency secondary to pituitary tumors or idiopathic panhypopituitarism, other pituitary hormone deficiencies are present. On the other hand, ACTH deficiency may be isolated, as seen following prolonged use of exogenous glucocorticoids. Because the isolated blood levels obtained in these screening tests may not be definitive, the diagnosis may need to be confirmed by a continuous 24-h ACTH infusion. Normal subjects and patients with secondary adrenal insufficiency may be distinguished by insulin tolerance or metyrapone testing.

Differential Diagnosis

Because weakness and fatigue are common, diagnosis of early adrenocortical insufficiency may be difficult. However, the combination of mild gastrointestinal distress, weight loss, anorexia, and a suggestion of increased pigmentation makes it mandatory to perform ACTH stimulation testing to rule out adrenal insufficiency, particularly before steroid treatment is begun. Weight loss is useful in evaluating the significance of weakness and malaise. Racial pigmentation may be a confounding feature, but a *recent* and progressive *increase* in pigmentation is usually reported by the patient with gradual adrenal destruction. Hyperpigmentation is usually absent when adrenal destruction is rapid, as in bilateral adrenal hemorrhage. The fact that hyperpigmentation occurs with other diseases may also present a problem, but the appearance and distribution of pigment in adrenal insufficiency are usually characteristic. When doubt exists, measurement of ACTH levels and testing of adrenal reserve with the infusion of ACTH provide clear-cut differentiation.

℞ Treatment: ADRENAL INSUFFICIENCY

All patients with adrenal insufficiency should receive specific hormone replacement. These patients require careful education about the disease. Replacement therapy should correct both glucocorticoid and mineralocorticoid deficiencies. Hydrocortisone (cortisol) is the mainstay of treatment. The dose for most adults (depending on size) is 20–30 mg/d. Patients are advised to take glucocorticoids with meals or, if that is impractical, with milk or an antacid, because the drugs may increase gastric acidity and exert direct toxic effects on the gastric mucosa. To simulate the normal diurnal adrenal rhythm, two-thirds of the dose is taken in the morning, and the remaining one-third is taken in the late afternoon. Some patients exhibit insomnia, irritability, and mental excitement after initiation of therapy; in these, the dosage should be reduced. Other situations that may necessitate smaller doses are hypertension and diabetes mellitus. Obese individuals and those on anticonvulsive medications may require increased dosages. Measurements of plasma ACTH or cortisol or of urine cortisol levels do not appear to be useful in determining optimal glucocorticoid dosages.

Since the replacement dosage of hydrocortisone does not replace the mineralocorticoid component of the adrenal hormones, mineralocorticoid supplementation is usually needed. This is accomplished by the administration of 0.05–0.1 mg fludrocortisone per day PO. Patients should also be instructed to maintain an ample intake of sodium (3–4 g/d).

The adequacy of mineralocorticoid therapy can be assessed by measurement of blood pressure and serum electrolytes. Blood pressure should be normal and without postural changes; serum sodium, potassium, creatinine, and urea nitrogen levels should also be normal. Measurement of plasma renin levels may also be useful in titrating the dose.

In female patients with adrenal insufficiency, androgen levels are also low. Thus, some physicians believe that daily replacement with 25–50 mg of DHEA PO may improve quality of life and bone mineral density.

Complications of glucocorticoid therapy, with the exception of gastritis, are *rare* at the dosages recommended for treatment of adrenal insufficiency. Complications of mineralocorticoid therapy include hypokalemia, hypertension, cardiac enlargement, and even congestive heart failure due to sodium retention. Periodic measurements of body weight, serum potassium level, and blood pressure are useful. All patients with adrenal insufficiency should carry medical identification, should be instructed in the parenteral self-administration of steroids, and should be registered with a medical alerting system.

SPECIAL THERAPEUTIC PROBLEMS During periods of intercurrent illness, especially in the setting of fever, the dose of hydrocortisone should be doubled. With severe illness it should be increased to 75–150 mg/d. When oral administration is not possible, parenteral routes should be employed. Likewise, before surgery or dental extractions, supplemental glucocorticoids should be administered. Patients should also be advised to increase the dose of fludrocortisone and to add salt to their otherwise normal diet during periods of strenuous exercise with sweating, during extremely hot weather, and with gastrointestinal upsets such as diarrhea. A simple strategy is to supplement the diet one to three times daily with salty broth [250 mL (1 cup) of beef or chicken bouillon contains 35 mmol of sodium]. For a representative program of steroid therapy for the patient with adrenal insufficiency who is undergoing major surgery, see **Table 5-8**. This schedule is designed so that on the day of surgery it will mimic the output of cortisol in normal individuals undergoing prolonged major stress (10 mg/h, 250–300 mg/d). Thereafter, if the patient is improving and is afebrile, the dose of hydrocortisone is tapered by 20–30% daily. Mineralocorticoid administration is unnecessary at hydrocortisone doses >100 mg/d because of the mineralocorticoid effects of hydrocortisone at such dosages.

SECONDARY ADRENOCORTICAL INSUFFICIENCY

ACTH deficiency causes *secondary* adrenocortical insufficiency; it may be a selective deficiency, as is seen following prolonged administration of excess glucocorticoids, or it may occur in association with deficiencies of multiple pituitary hormones (panhypopituitarism) (Chap. 2). Patients with secondary adrenocortical hypofunction have many symptoms and signs in common with those having primary disease but are *not hyperpigmented*, since ACTH and related peptide levels are low. In fact, plasma ACTH levels distinguish between primary and secondary adrenal insufficiency, since they are elevated in the former and decreased to absent in the latter. Patients with total pituitary insufficiency have manifestations of multiple hormone deficiencies. An additional feature distinguishing primary adrenocortical insufficiency is the *near-normal level of aldosterone secretion* seen in pituitary and/or isolated ACTH deficiencies (Fig. 5-12). Patients with pituitary insufficiency may have hyponatremia, which can be dilutional or secondary to a subnormal increase in aldosterone secretion in response to severe sodium restriction. However, severe *dehydration*, *hyponatremia*, and *hyperkalemia* are characteristic of severe mineralocorticoid insufficiency and favor a diagnosis of primary adrenocortical insufficiency.

TABLE 5-8

STEROID THERAPY SCHEDULE FOR A PATIENT WITH ADRENAL INSUFFICIENCY UNDERGOING SURGERY[a]

	HYDROCORTISONE INFUSION, CONTINUOUS, mg/h		HYDROCORTISONE (ORALLY)		FLUDROCORTISONE (ORALLY), 8 A.M.
			8 A.M.	4 P.M.	
Routine daily medication			20	10	0.1
Day before operation			20	10	0.1
Day of operation	10				
Day 1	5–7.5				
Day 2	2.5–5				
Day 3	2.5–5	*or*	40	20	0.1
Day 4	2.5–5	*or*	40	20	0.1
Day 5			40	20	0.1
Day 6			20	20	0.1
Day 7			20	10	0.1

[a]All steroid doses are given in milligrams. An alternative approach is to give 100 mg hydrocortisone as an IV bolus injection every 8 h on the day of the operation (see text).

Patients receiving long-term steroid therapy, despite physical findings of Cushing's syndrome, may develop adrenal insufficiency because of prolonged pituitary-hypothalamic suppression and adrenal atrophy secondary to the loss of endogenous ACTH. These patients have two deficits, a loss of adrenal responsiveness to ACTH and a failure of pituitary ACTH release. They are characterized by low blood cortisol and ACTH levels, a low baseline rate of steroid excretion, and abnormal ACTH and metyrapone responses. Most patients with steroid-induced adrenal insufficiency eventually recover normal HPA responsiveness, but recovery time varies from days to months. The rapid ACTH test provides a convenient assessment of recovery of HPA function. Because the plasma cortisol concentrations after injection of cosyntropin and during insulin-induced hypoglycemia are usually similar, the rapid ACTH test assesses the integrated HPA function (see "Tests of Pituitary-Adrenal Responsiveness" earlier in the chapter). Some investigators suggest using the low-dose (1 μg) ACTH test for suspected secondary ACTH deficiency. Additional tests to assess pituitary ACTH reserve include the standard metyrapone and insulin-induced hypoglycemia tests.

Glucocorticoid therapy in patients with secondary adrenocortical insufficiency does not differ from that for the primary disorder. Mineralocorticoid therapy is usually not necessary, as aldosterone secretion is preserved.

ACUTE ADRENOCORTICAL INSUFFICIENCY

Acute adrenocortical insufficiency may result from several processes. On the one hand, *adrenal crisis* may be a rapid and overwhelming intensification of chronic adrenal insufficiency, usually precipitated by sepsis or surgical stress. Alternatively, acute hemorrhagic destruction of both adrenal glands can occur in previously well individuals. In children, this event is usually associated with septicemia with *Pseudomonas* or meningococcemia (Waterhouse-Friderichsen syndrome). In adults, anticoagulant therapy or a coagulation disorder may result in bilateral adrenal hemorrhage. Occasionally, bilateral adrenal hemorrhage in the newborn results from birth trauma. Hemorrhage has been observed during pregnancy, following idiopathic adrenal vein thrombosis, and as a complication of venography (e.g., infarction of an adenoma). The third and most frequent cause of acute insufficiency is the rapid withdrawal of steroids from patients with adrenal atrophy owing to chronic steroid administration. Acute adrenocortical insufficiency may also occur in patients with congenital adrenal hyperplasia or those with decreased adrenocortical reserve when they are given drugs capable of inhibiting steroid synthesis (mitotane, ketoconazole) or of increasing steroid metabolism (phenytoin, rifampin).

Adrenal Crisis

The long-term survival of patients with adrenocortical insufficiency depends largely on the prevention and treatment of adrenal crisis. Consequently, the occurrence of infection, trauma (including surgery), gastrointestinal upsets, or other stresses necessitates an immediate increase in hormone. In untreated patients, preexisting symptoms are intensified. Nausea, vomiting, and abdominal pain may become intractable. Fever may be severe or absent. Lethargy deepens into somnolence, and hypovolemic vascular collapse ensues. In contrast, patients previously maintained on chronic glucocorticoid therapy may not exhibit dehydration or hypotension until they are in a preterminal state, since mineralocorticoid secretion is usually preserved. In all patients in crisis, a precipitating cause should be sought.

℞ Treatment: ADRENAL CRISIS

Treatment is directed primarily toward repletion of circulating glucocorticoids and replacement of the sodium and water deficits. Hence, an IV infusion of 5% glucose in normal saline solution should be started with a bolus IV infusion of 100 mg hydrocortisone followed by a continuous infusion of hydrocortisone at a rate of 10 mg/h. An alternative approach is to administer a 100-mg bolus of hydrocortisone IV every 6 h. However, only continuous infusion maintains the plasma cortisol constantly at stress levels [>830 nmol/L (30 μg/dL)]. Effective treatment of hypotension requires glucocorticoid replacement and repletion of sodium and water deficits. If the crisis was preceded by prolonged nausea, vomiting, and dehydration, several liters of saline solution may be required in the first few hours. Vasoconstrictive agents (such as dopamine) may be indicated in extreme conditions as adjuncts to volume replacement. With large doses of steroid, i.e., 100–200 mg hydrocortisone, the patient receives a maximal mineralocorticoid effect, and supplementary mineralocorticoid is superfluous. Following improvement, the steroid dosage is tapered over the next few days to maintenance levels, and mineralocorticoid therapy is reinstituted if needed (Table 5-8).

ADRENAL CORTISOL INSUFFICIENCY IN ACUTELY ILL PATIENTS

The physiology of the HPA axis is dramatically altered during critical illnesses such as trauma, surgery, sepsis, and shock. In such situations cortisol levels rise four- to sixfold, diurnal variation is abolished, and the unbound fractions of cortisol rise in the circulation and in target tissues. Inadequate cortisol production during critical illness can result in hypotension, reduced systemic vascular resistance, shock, and death.

A major area of controversy in presumably normal individuals is the correlation of clinical outcomes with the cortisol levels measured during critical illness. Subnormal cortisol production during acute severe illness has been termed "functional" or "relative" adrenal insufficiency. Conceptually, the elevated cortisol levels that are observed are viewed as insufficient to control the inflammatory response and maintain blood pressure. Observational and experimental data in acute illness support this concept since routine stress doses of hydrocortisone reduce inflammatory markers and improve blood pressure and blood flow without impairing immune responses. Thus, if such patients can be identified, treatment with supplementary cortisol could be beneficial.

Clinical trial data support the concept that most patients with septic shock have relative adrenal insufficiency, defined as a <255-μmol/L (<9-μg/dL) increment between peak and baseline cortisol levels following administration of 250 μg of cosyntropin as an IV bolus. If patients with relative adrenal insufficiency are treated for 7 days with standard stress doses of hydrocortisone, 50 mg every 6 h, and 50 μg of 9α-fludrocortisone, 28-day survival is increased and steroid-treated subjects are more likely to have pressor agents withdrawn than placebo-treated subjects. No differences in adverse events have been reported between placebo- and steroid-treated subjects, and responders to cosyntropin receive no benefit from steroid treatment.

Thus, experimental and clinical trial data strongly support treating patients with relative adrenal insufficiency for a week. However, it has been difficult to establish a level of cortisol in a critically ill patient below which replacement glucocorticoids may improve prognosis. In most circumstances the cortisol level obtained, either randomly or following a cosyntropin test, needs to be interpreted in the context of the clinical picture. Many have accepted that a random cortisol level of ≤441 nmol/L (15 μg/dL) is indicative of relative adrenal insufficiency and a random cortisol level >938 nmol/L (34 μg/dL) usually excludes that diagnosis. In patients who have random cortisol levels between 441 and 938 nmol/L (15 and 34 μg/dL), a cosyntropin stimulation test may identify patients with diminished adrenal reserve [increment <255 nmol/L (9 μg/dL)] who may benefit from supplementary cortisol treatment. However, many acutely ill subjects who are hemodynamically stable without pressor treatment have values below this level. Thus, the clinical state is still an important factor to be considered before initiating steroid therapy.

One approach is to assume that an acutely ill patient with hemodynamic instability not secondary to blood loss, particularly if septic shock is present, has relative adrenal insufficiency until proven otherwise. Treatment with supplementary cortisol should be initiated promptly following the measurement of a random cortisol level and/or performing a cosyntropin stimulation test. Such patients should be treated with 50–75 mg of hydrocortisone IV every 6 h as bolus treatment or the same amount as a continuous infusion. This dose of hydrocortisone is sufficient to saturate the MR, and additional treatment with 9α-fludrocortisone is not necessary. Treatment can be terminated if the cortisol levels obtained at the outset are appropriately elevated. On the other hand, those patients with abnormal testing should be treated for 1 week and then tapered. In surviving patients, pituitary-adrenal function should be reevaluated after resolution of the critical illness.

HYPOALDOSTERONISM

Isolated aldosterone deficiency accompanied by normal cortisol production occurs in association with hyporeninism, as an inherited biosynthetic defect, postoperatively following removal of aldosterone-secreting adenomas, during protracted heparin administration, in pretectal disease of the nervous system, and in severe postural hypotension.

The feature common to all forms of hypoaldosteronism is the inability to increase aldosterone secretion appropriately in response to salt restriction. Most patients have unexplained hyperkalemia, which is often exacerbated by restriction of dietary sodium intake. In severe cases, urine sodium wastage occurs at a normal salt intake, whereas in milder forms, excessive loss of urine sodium occurs only with salt restriction.

Most cases of isolated hypoaldosteronism occur in patients with a deficiency in renin production (so-called hyporeninemic hypoaldosteronism), most commonly in adults with diabetes mellitus and mild renal failure and in whom hyperkalemia and metabolic acidosis are out of proportion to the degree of renal impairment. Plasma renin levels fail to rise normally following sodium restriction and postural changes. The pathogenesis is uncertain. Possibilities include renal disease (the most likely), autonomic neuropathy, ECFV expansion, and defective conversion of renin precursors to active renin. Aldosterone levels also fail to rise normally after salt restriction and volume contraction; this effect is probably related to the hyporeninism, since biosynthetic defects in aldosterone secretion usually cannot be demonstrated. In these patients, aldosterone secretion increases promptly after ACTH stimulation, but it is uncertain whether the magnitude of the response is normal. On the other hand, the level of aldosterone appears to be subnormal in relationship to the hyperkalemia.

Hypoaldosteronism can also be associated with high renin levels and low or elevated levels of aldosterone (see below). Severely ill patients may also have hyperreninemic hypoaldosteronism; such patients have a high mortality rate (80%). Hyperkalemia is not present. Possible explanations for the hypoaldosteronism include adrenal necrosis (uncommon) or a shift in steroidogenesis from mineralocorticoids to glucocorticoids, possibly related to prolonged ACTH stimulation.

Before the diagnosis of isolated hypoaldosteronism is considered for a patient with hyperkalemia, "pseudohyperkalemia" (e.g., hemolysis, thrombocytosis) should be excluded by measuring the *plasma* potassium level. The next step is to demonstrate a normal cortisol response to ACTH stimulation. Then, the response of renin and aldosterone levels to stimulation (upright posture, sodium restriction) should be measured. Low renin and aldosterone levels establish the diagnosis of hyporeninemic hypoaldosteronism. A combination of high renin levels and low aldosterone levels is consistent with an aldosterone biosynthetic defect or a selective unresponsiveness to angiotensin II. Finally, there is a condition that clinically and biochemically mimics hypoaldosteronism with elevated renin levels. However, the aldosterone levels are not low but high—so-called pseudohypoaldosteronism. This inherited condition is caused by a mutation in the epithelial sodium channel.

℞ Treatment: HYPOALDOSTERONISM

The treatment is to replace the mineralocorticoid deficiency. For practical purposes, the administration of 0.05–0.15 mg fludrocortisone PO daily should restore electrolyte balance if salt intake is adequate (e.g., 150–200 mmol/d). However, patients with hyporeninemic hypoaldosteronism may require higher doses of mineralocorticoid to correct hyperkalemia. This need poses a potential risk in patients with hypertension, mild renal insufficiency, or congestive heart failure. An alternative approach is to reduce salt intake and to administer furosemide, which can ameliorate acidosis and hyperkalemia. Occasionally, a combination of these two approaches is efficacious.

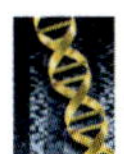

GENETIC CONSIDERATIONS

Glucocorticoid Diseases

Congenital Adrenal Hyperplasia

Congenital adrenal hyperplasia (CAH) is the consequence of recessive mutations that cause one of several distinct enzymatic defects (see below). Because cortisol is the principal adrenal steroid regulating ACTH elaboration and because ACTH stimulates adrenal growth and function, a block in cortisol synthesis may result in the enhanced secretion of adrenal androgens and/or mineralocorticoids depending on the site of the enzyme block. In severe congenital virilizing hyperplasia, the adrenal output of cortisol may be so compromised as to cause adrenal deficiency despite adrenal hyperplasia.

CAH is the most common adrenal disorder of infancy and childhood (Chap. 7). Partial enzyme deficiencies can be expressed after adolescence, predominantly in women with hirsutism and oligomenorrhea but minimal virilization. Late-onset adrenal hyperplasia may account for 5–25% of cases of hirsutism and oligomenorrhea in women, depending on the population.

Etiology

Enzymatic defects have been described in 21-hydroxylase (CYP21A2), 17α-hydroxylase/17,20-lyase (CYP17), 11β-hydroxylase (CYP11B1), and 3β-HSD 2 (Fig. 5-2). Although the genes encoding these enzymes have been cloned, the diagnosis of specific enzyme deficiencies with genetic techniques is not practical because of the large number of different deletions and missense mutations. CYP21A2 deficiency is closely linked to the HLA-B locus of chromosome 6 so that HLA typing and/or DNA polymorphism can be used to detect the heterozygous carriers and to diagnose affected individuals in some families. The clinical expression in the different disorders is variable, ranging from virilization of the female (CYP2/A2) to feminization of the male (3β-HSD 2) (Chap. 7).

Adrenal virilization in the female at birth is associated with ambiguous external genitalia (*female pseudohermaphroditism*). Virilization begins after the fifth month of intrauterine development. At birth, there may be enlargement of the clitoris, partial or complete fusion of the labia, and sometimes a urogenital sinus in the female. If the labial fusion is nearly complete, the female infant has external genitalia resembling a penis with hypospadias. In the *postnatal* period, CAH is associated with virilization in the female and isosexual precocity in the male. The excessive androgen levels result in accelerated growth, so that bone age exceeds chronologic age. Because epiphyseal closure occurs early, growth stops, but truncal development continues, the characteristic appearance being a short child with a well-developed trunk.

The most common form of CAH (95% of cases) is a result of impairment of CYP21A2. In addition to cortisol deficiency, aldosterone secretion is decreased in approximately one-third of the patients. Thus, with CYP21A2 deficiency, adrenal virilization occurs with or without a salt-losing tendency due to aldosterone deficiency (Fig. 5-2).

CYP11B1 deficiency causes a "hypertensive" variant of CAH. Hypertension and hypokalemia occur because of the impaired conversion of 11-deoxycorticosterone to corticosterone, resulting in the accumulation of 11-deoxycorticosterone, a potent mineralocorticoid. The degree of hypertension is variable. Steroid precursors are shunted into the androgen pathway.

CYP17 deficiency is characterized by hypogonadism, hypokalemia, and hypertension. This rare disorder causes decreased production of cortisol and shunting of precursors into the mineralocorticoid pathway with hypokalemic alkalosis, hypertension, and suppressed plasma renin activity. Usually, 11-deoxycorticosterone production is elevated. Because CYP17 hydroxylation is required for biosynthesis of both adrenal androgens and gonadal testosterone and estrogen, this defect is associated with sexual immaturity, high gonadotropin levels, and low urinary 17-ketosteroid excretion. Female patients have primary amenorrhea and lack of development of secondary sexual characteristics. Because of deficient androgen production, male patients have either ambiguous external genitalia or a female phenotype (*underandrogenization*). Exogenous glucocorticoids can correct the hypertensive syndrome, and treatment with appropriate gonadal steroids results in sexual maturation.

With 3β-HSD 2 deficiency, conversion of pregnenolone to progesterone is impaired, so that the synthesis of both cortisol and aldosterone is blocked, with shunting into the adrenal androgen pathway via 17α-hydroxypregnenolone and DHEA. Because DHEA is a weak androgen, and because this enzyme deficiency is also present in the gonad, the genitalia of the male fetus may be incompletely virilized or feminized. Conversely, in the female, overproduction of DHEA may produce partial virilization.

Diagnosis

The diagnosis of CAH should be considered in infants having episodes of acute adrenal insufficiency or salt wasting or hypertension. The diagnosis is further suggested by the finding of hypertrophy of the clitoris, fused labia, or a urogenital sinus in the female or of isosexual precocity in the male. In infants and children with a CYP21A2 defect, increased urine 17-ketosteroid excretion and increased plasma DHEA sulfate levels are typically associated with an increase in the blood levels of 17-hydroxyprogesterone and the excretion of its urinary metabolite pregnanetriol. Demonstration of elevated levels of 17-hydroxyprogesterone in amniotic fluid at 14–16 weeks of gestation allows prenatal detection of affected female infants. Prenatal genetic testing is also possible in families in whom the specific genetic defect is known.

The diagnosis of a *salt-losing form* of CAH due to defects in CYP21A2 is suggested by episodes of acute adrenal insufficiency with hyponatremia, hyperkalemia, dehydration, and vomiting. These infants and children often crave salt and have laboratory findings indicating deficits in both cortisol and aldosterone secretion.

With the *hypertensive form* of CAH due to CYP11B1 deficiency, 11-deoxycorticosterone and 11-deoxycortisol accumulate. The diagnosis is confirmed by demonstrating increased levels of 11-deoxycortisol in the blood or increased amounts of tetrahydro-11-deoxycortisol in the urine. Elevation of 17-hydroxyprogesterone levels does not imply a coexisting CYP21A2 deficiency.

Very high levels of urine DHEA with low levels of pregnanetriol and of cortisol metabolites in urine are characteristic of children with 3β-HSD 2 deficiency. Marked salt wasting may also occur.

Adults with *late-onset adrenal hyperplasia* (partial deficiency of CYP21A2, CYP11B1, or 3β-HSD 2) are characterized by normal or moderately elevated levels of urinary 17-ketosteroids and plasma DHEA sulfate. A high basal level of a precursor of cortisol biosynthesis (such as 17-hydroxyprogesterone, 17-hydroxypregnenolone, or 11-deoxycortisol), or elevation of such a precursor after ACTH stimulation, confirms the diagnosis of a partial deficiency. Measurement of steroid precursors 60 min after bolus administration of ACTH is usually sufficient. Adrenal androgen output is easily suppressed by the standard low-dose (2 mg) dexamethasone test.

℞ Treatment: CONGENITAL ADRENAL HYPERPLASIA

Therapy in CAH patients consists of daily administration of glucocorticoids to suppress pituitary ACTH secretion. Because of its low cost and intermediate half-life, prednisone is the drug of choice except in infants, in whom hydrocortisone is usually used. In adults with late-onset adrenal hyperplasia, the smallest single bedtime dose of a long- or intermediate-acting glucocorticoid that suppresses pituitary ACTH secretion should be administered. The amount of steroid required by children with CAH is ~1–1.5 times the normal cortisol production rate of 27–35 μmol (10–13 mg) of cortisol per square meter of body surface per day and is given in divided doses two or three times per day. The dosage schedule is governed by repetitive analysis of the urinary 17-ketosteroids, plasma DHEA sulfate, and/or precursors of cortisol biosynthesis. Skeletal growth and maturation must also be monitored closely, as overtreatment with glucocorticoid replacement therapy retards linear growth.

Receptor Mutations

Isolated glucocorticoid deficiency is a rare autosomal recessive disease secondary to a mutation in the ACTH receptor. Usually mineralocorticoid function is normal. Adrenal insufficiency is manifest within the first 2 years of life as hyperpigmentation, convulsions, and/or frequent episodes of hypoglycemia. In some patients, the adrenal insufficiency is associated with achalasia and alacrima—Allgrove's, or triple A, syndrome. However, in some triple A syndrome patients, no mutation in the ACTH receptor has been identified, suggesting that a distinct genetic abnormality causes this syndrome. *Adrenal hypoplasia congenita* is a rare X-linked disorder caused by a mutation in the *DAX1* gene. This gene encodes an orphan nuclear receptor that plays an important role in the development of the adrenal cortex and also the hypothalamic-pituitary-gonadal axis. Thus, patients present with signs and symptoms secondary to deficiencies of all three major adrenal steroids—cortisol, aldosterone, and adrenal androgens—as well as gonadotropin deficiency. Finally, a rare cause of hypercortisolism without cushingoid stigmata is *primary cortisol resistance* due to mutations in the glucocorticoid receptor. The resistance is incomplete because patients do not exhibit signs of adrenal insufficiency.

Miscellaneous Conditions

Adrenoleukodystrophy causes severe demyelination and early death in children, and adrenomyeloneuropathy is associated with a mixed motor and sensory neuropathy with spastic paraplegia in adults; both disorders are associated with elevated circulating levels of very long chain fatty acids and cause adrenal insufficiency. Autosomal recessive mutations in the *st*eroidogenic *a*cute *r*egulatory (STAR) protein gene cause congenital lipoid adrenal hyperplasia (Chap. 7), which is characterized by adrenal insufficiency and defective gonadal steroidogenesis. In genetic males, this leads to female phenotype. In genetic females, sexual differentiation is normal but there is premature ovarian failure. Because STAR mediates cholesterol transport into the mitochondrion, mutations in the protein cause massive lipid accumulation in steroidogenic cells, ultimately leading to cell toxicity.

MINERALOCORTICOID DISEASES

Some forms of CAH have a mineralocorticoid component. Others are caused by a mutation in other enzymes or ion channels important in mediating or mimicking aldosterone's action.

Hypermineralocorticoidism

Low Plasma Renin Activity

Rarely, hypermineralocorticoidism is due to a defect in cortisol biosynthesis, specifically 11- or 17-hydroxylation. ACTH levels are increased, with a resultant increase in the production of the mineralocorticoid 11-deoxycorticosterone. Hypertension and hypokalemia can be corrected by glucocorticoid administration. The definitive diagnosis is made by demonstrating an elevation of precursors of cortisol biosynthesis in the blood or urine or by direct demonstration of the genetic defect.

Glucocorticoid administration can also ameliorate hypertension or produce normotension even though a hydroxylase deficiency cannot be identified. These patients have normal to slightly elevated aldosterone levels that do not suppress in response to saline but do suppress in response to 2 days of dexamethasone (2 mg/d). The condition is inherited as an autosomal dominant trait and is termed *glucocorticoid-remediable aldosteronism* (GRA). This entity is secondary to a chimeric gene duplication whereby the 11β-hydroxylase gene promoter (which is under the control of ACTH) is fused to the aldosterone synthase coding sequence. Thus, aldosterone synthase activity is ectopically expressed in the zona fasciculata and is regulated by ACTH, in a fashion similar to the regulation of cortisol secretion. Screening for this defect is best performed by assessing the presence or absence of the chimeric gene. Because the abnormal gene may be present in the absence of hypokalemia, its frequency as a cause of hypertension is unknown. Individuals with suppressed plasma renin levels and juvenile-onset hypertension or a history of early-onset hypertension in first-degree relatives should be screened for this disorder. Early hemorrhagic stroke also occurs in GRA-affected individuals.

GRA documented by genetic analysis may be treated with glucocorticoid administration or antimineralocorticoids, i.e., spironolactone, triamterene, or amiloride. Glucocorticoids should be used only in small doses to avoid inducing iatrogenic Cushing's syndrome. A combination approach is often necessary.

High Plasma Renin Activity

Bartter syndrome is characterized by severe hyperaldosteronism (hypokalemic alkalosis) with moderate to marked increases in renin activity and hypercalciuria, but normal blood pressure and no edema; this disorder usually begins in childhood. Renal biopsy shows juxtaglomerular hyperplasia. Bartter syndrome is caused by a mutation in the renal Na-K-2Cl co-transporter gene. The pathogenesis involves a defect in the renal conservation of sodium or chloride. The renal loss of sodium is thought to stimulate renin secretion and aldosterone production. Hyperaldosteronism produces potassium depletion, and hypokalemia further elevates prostaglandin production and plasma renin activity. In some cases, the hypokalemia may be potentiated by a defect in renal conservation of potassium.

Gitelman syndrome is an autosomal recessive trait characterized by renal salt wasting and, as a result, as in Bartter syndrome, activation of the renin-angiotensin-aldosterone system. As a consequence, affected individuals have low blood pressure, low serum potassium, low serum magnesium, and high serum bicarbonate. In contrast to Bartter's syndrome, urinary calcium excretion is reduced. Gitelman syndrome results from loss-of-function mutations of the renal thiazide-sensitive Na-Cl co-transporter.

Increased Mineralocorticoid Action

Liddle's syndrome is a rare autosomal dominant disorder that mimics hyperaldosteronism. The defect is in the genes encoding the β or η subunits of the epithelial sodium channel. Both renin and aldosterone levels are low, owing to the constitutively activated sodium channel and the resulting excess sodium reabsorption in the renal tubule.

A rare autosomal recessive cause of hypokalemia and hypertension is 11β-HSD 2 deficiency, in which cortisol cannot be converted to cortisone and hence binds to the MR and acts as a mineralocorticoid. This condition, also termed *apparent mineralocorticoid excess syndrome*, is caused by a defect in the gene encoding the renal isoform of this enzyme, 11β-HSD 2. Patients can be identified either by documenting an increased ratio of cortisol to cortisone in the urine or by genetic analysis. Patients with the 11β-HSD deficiency syndrome can be treated with small doses of dexamethasone, which suppresses ACTH and endogenous cortisol production but binds less well to the mineralocorticoid receptor than does cortisol.

The ingestion of candies or chewing tobacco containing certain forms of licorice produces a syndrome that mimics primary aldosteronism. The component of such agents that causes sodium retention is glycyrrhizinic acid, which inhibits 11β-HSD 2 and hence allows cortisol to act as a mineralocorticoid. The diagnosis is established or excluded by a careful history.

Decreased Mineralocorticoid Production or Action

In patients with a deficiency in aldosterone biosynthesis, the transformation of corticosterone into aldosterone is impaired, owing to a mutation in the aldosterone synthase (CYP11B2) gene. These patients have low to absent aldosterone secretion, elevated plasma renin levels, and elevated levels of the intermediates of aldosterone biosynthesis (corticosterone and 18-hydroxycorticosterone).

Pseudohypoaldosteronism type I (PHA-I) is an autosomal recessive disorder that is seen in the neonatal period and is characterized by salt wasting, hypotension, hyperkalemia, and high renin and aldosterone levels. In contrast to the gain-of-function mutations in the epithelial sodium channel in Liddle's syndrome, mutations in PHA-I result in loss of epithelial sodium channel function.

PHARMACOLOGIC CLINICAL USES OF ADRENAL STEROIDS

The widespread use of glucocorticoids emphasizes the need for a thorough understanding of the metabolic effects of these agents. Before adrenal hormone therapy is instituted, the expected gains should be weighed against undesirable effects. Several important questions should be addressed before initiating therapy. First, how serious is the disorder (the more serious, the greater the likelihood that the risk-versus-benefit ratio will be positive)? Second, how long will therapy be required (the longer the therapy, the greater the risk of adverse side effects)? Third, does the individual have preexisting conditions that glucocorticoids may exacerbate (**Table 5-9**)? If so, then a careful risk-versus-benefit assessment is required to ensure that the ratio is favorable given the increased likelihood of harm by steroids in these patients. Supplementary measures to minimize undesirable metabolic effects are shown in **Table 5-10**. Fourth, which preparation is best?

The following considerations should be taken into account in deciding which steroid preparation to use:

TABLE 5-9

A CHECKLIST PRIOR TO THE ADMINISTRATION OF GLUCOCORTICOIDS IN PHARMACOLOGIC DOSES
Presence of tuberculosis or other chronic infection (chest x-ray, tuberculin test)
Evidence of impaired glucose intolerance, history of gestational diabetes, or strong family history of type 2 diabetes mellitus in first-degree relative
Evidence of preexisting (or high risk for) osteoporosis (bone density assessment in organ transplant recipients or postmenopausal patients)
History of peptic ulcer, gastritis, or esophagitis (stool guaiac test)
Evidence of hypertension, cardiovascular disease, or hyperlipidemia (triglyceride level)
History of psychological disorders

TABLE 5-10

SUPPLEMENTARY MEASURES TO MINIMIZE UNDESIRABLE METABOLIC EFFECTS OF GLUCOCORTICOIDS

Diet
- Monitor caloric intake to prevent weight gain.
- Diabetic diet if glucose intolerant.
- Restrict sodium intake to prevent edema and minimize hypertension.
- Provide supplementary potassium if necessary.

Consider antacid, H_2 receptor antagonist, and/or H+, K+,- ATPase inhibitor therapy

Institute all-day steroid schedule, if possible
- Patients receiving steroid therapy over a prolonged period (months) should have an appropriate increase in hormone level during periods of acute stress. A rule of thumb is to *double* the maintenance dose.

Minimize loss of bone mineral density
- Consider administering gonadal hormone replacement therapy in postmenopausal women:
  - 0.625–1.25 mg conjugated estrogens given cyclically with progesterone, unless the uterus is absent (testosterone replacement in hypogonadal men).
- Ensure adequate calcium intake (should be ~1200 mg/d elemental calcium).
- Administer a minimum of 800–1000 IU/d supplemental vitamin D.
- Measure blood levels of calciferol and 1,25(OH)$_2$ vitamin D. Supplement as needed.
- Consider administering bisphosphonate prophylactically, orally, or parenterally in high-risk patients.

1. *The biologic half-life.* The rationale behind alternate-day therapy is to decrease the metabolic effects of the steroids for a significant part of each 48-h period while still producing a pharmacologic effect durable enough to be effective. Too long a half-life would defeat the first purpose, and too short a half-life would defeat the second. In general, the more potent the steroid, the longer its biologic half-life.
2. *The mineralocorticoid effects of the steroid.* Most synthetic steroids have less mineralocorticoid effect than hydrocortisone (**Table 5-11**).
3. *The biologically active form of the steroid.* Cortisone and prednisone have to be converted to biologically active metabolites before anti-inflammatory effects can occur. Because of this, in a condition for which steroids are known to be effective and when an adequate dose has been given without response, one should consider substituting hydrocortisone or prednisolone for cortisone or prednisone.
4. *The cost of the medication.* This is a serious consideration if chronic administration is planned. Prednisone is the least expensive of available steroid preparations.
5. *The type of formulation.* Topical steroids have the distinct advantage over oral steroids in reducing the likelihood of systemic side effects. In addition, some inhaled steroids have been designed to minimize side effects by increasing their hepatic inactivation if they are swallowed. However, all topical steroids can be absorbed into the systemic circulation.

TABLE 5-11

GLUCOCORTICOID PREPARATIONS

	ESTIMATED POTENCY[b]	
COMMONLY USED NAME[a]	GLUCOCORTICOID	MINERALOCORTICOID
Short-Acting		
Hydrocortisone	1	1
Cortisone	0.8	0.8
Intermediate-Acting		
Prednisone	4	0.25
Prednisolone	4	0.25
Methylprednisolone	5	<0.01
Triamcinolone	5	<0.01
Long-Acting		
Paramethasone	10	<0.01
Betamethasone	25	<0.01
Dexamethasone	30–40	<0.01

[a]The steroids are divided into three groups according to the duration of biologic activity. Short-acting preparations have a biologic half-life <12 h; long-acting, >48 h; and intermediate-acting, between 12 and 36 h. Triamcinolone has the longest half-life of the intermediate-acting preparations.

[b]Relative milligram comparisons with hydrocortisone, setting the glucocorticoid and mineralocorticoid properties of hydrocortisone as 1. Sodium retention is insignificant for commonly employed doses of methylprednisolone, triamcinolone, paramethasone, betamethasone, and dexamethasone.

FURTHER READINGS

ALLEN DB: Effects of inhaled steroids on growth, bone metabolism, and adrenal function. Adv Periatr 53:101, 2006

ARLT W: The approach to the adult with newly diagnosed adrenal insufficiency. J Clin Endocrinol Metab 94:1059, 2009

BILLER BM et al: Treatment of adrenocorticotropin-dependent Cushing's syndrome: a consensus statement. J Clin Endocrinol Metab 93:2454, 2008

BORNSTEIN SR: Predisposing factors for adrenal insufficiency. N Engl J Med 360:2328, 2009

DLUHY RG, WILLIAMS GH: Aldosterone: Villain or bystander? N Engl J Med 351:8, 2004

EPSTEIN M et al: Selective aldosterone blockade with eplerenone produces albuminuria in patients with type 2 diabetes. Clin J Am Soc Nephrol 1:940, 2006

FINDLING JW, RAFF H: Cushing's syndrome: Important issues in diagnosis and management. J Clin Endocrinol Metab 91:3746, 2006

FUNDER JW et al: Case detection, diagnosis, and treatment of patients with primary aldosteronism: An Endocrine Society clinical practice guideline. J Clin Endocrinol Metab 93:3266, 2008

GANNON TA et al: Adrenal insufficiency in the critically ill trauma population. Am Surg 72:373, 2006

HOOD SJ et al: The spironolactone, amiloride, losartan, and thiazide (SALT) double-blind crossover trial in patients with low-renin hypertension and elevated aldosterone-renin ratio. Circulation 116:268, 2007

MATTSSON C, YOUNG WF JR: Primary aldosteronism: Diagnostic and treatment strategies. Nat Clin Pract Nephrol 2:198, 2006

MOTTA-RAMIREZ GA et al: Comparison of CT findings in symptomatic and incidentally discovered pheochromocytomas. Am J Roentgenol 185:684, 2005

NEWELL-PRICE J: Diagnosis of Cushing's syndrome: Comparison of the specificity of first-line biochemical tests. Nat Clin Pract Endocrinol Metab 4:192, 2008

NIEMAN LK et al: The diagnosis of Cushing's syndrome: An Endocrine Society clinical practice guideline. J Clin Endocrinol Metab 93:1526, 2008

NIEMAN LK, Ilias I: Evaluation and treatment of Cushing's syndrome. Am J Med 118:1340, 2005

YOUNG WF JR: Clinical practice: The incidentally discovered adrenal mass. N Engl J Med 356:601, 2007

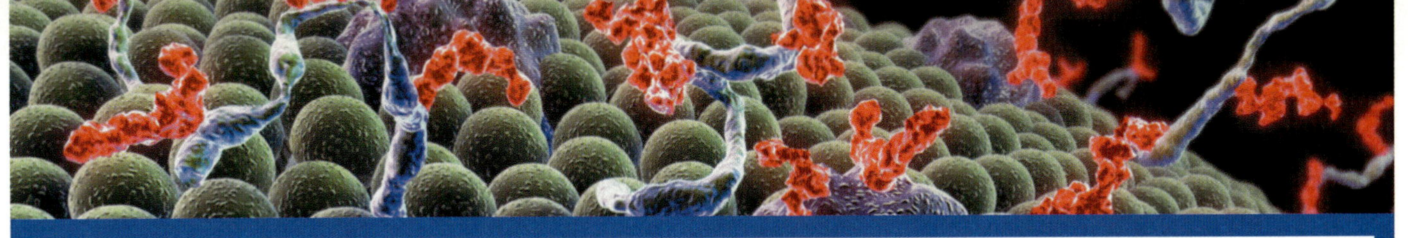

CHAPTER 6

PHEOCHROMOCYTOMA

Hartmut P. H. Neumann

Pheochromocytomas and paragangliomas are catecholamine-producing tumors derived from the sympathetic or parasympathetic nervous system. These tumors may arise sporadically or be inherited as features of multiple endocrine neoplasia type 2 or several other pheochromocytoma-associated syndromes. The diagnosis of pheochromocytomas provides a potentially correctable cause of hypertension, and their removal can prevent hypertensive crises that can be lethal. The clinical presentation is variable, ranging from an adrenal incidentaloma to a patient in hypertensive crisis with associated cerebrovascular or cardiac complications.

EPIDEMIOLOGY

Pheochromocytoma is estimated to occur in 2–8 out of 1 million persons per year, and about 0.1% of hypertensive patients harbor a pheochromocytoma. Autopsy series reveal prevalence figures of 0.2%. The mean age at diagnosis is about 40 years, although the tumors can occur from early childhood until late in life. The "rule of tens" for pheochromocytomas states that about 10% are bilateral, 10% are extraadrenal, and 10% are malignant. However, these percentages are higher in the inherited syndromes.

ETIOLOGY AND PATHOGENESIS

Pheochromocytomas and paragangliomas are well-vascularized tumors that arise from cells derived from the sympathetic (e.g., adrenal medulla) or parasympathetic (e.g., carotid body, glomus vagale) paraganglia (**Fig. 6-1**). The name *pheochromocytoma* reflects the black-colored staining caused by chromaffin oxidation of catecholamines. Although a variety of nomenclatures have been used to describe these tumors, most clinicians use the term *pheochromocytoma* to describe symptomatic catecholamine-producing tumors, including those located in extraadrenal retroperitoneal, pelvic, and thoracic sites. The term *paraganglioma* is used to describe catecholamine-producing tumors in the head and neck, as well as tumors that arise from the parasympathetic nervous system, which may secrete little or no catecholamines.

The etiology of most sporadic pheochromocytomas and paragangliomas is unknown. However, about 25% of patients have an inherited condition, including germ-line mutations in the *RET*, *VHL*, *NF1*, *SDHB*, *SDHC*, or *SDHD* genes. Biallelic gene inactivation has been demonstrated for the *VHL*, *NF1*, and *SDH* genes, whereas *RET* mutations activate the receptor tyrosine kinase activity. SDH is an enzyme of the Krebs cycle and the mitochondrial respiratory chain. The VHL protein is a component of a

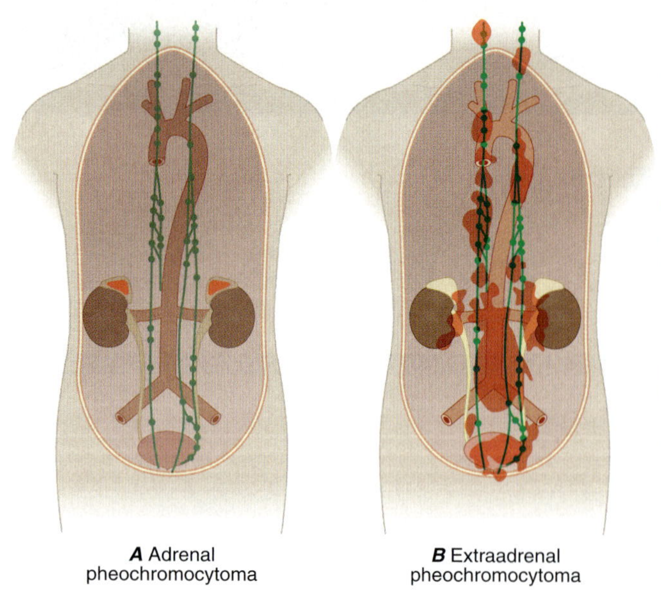

FIGURE 6-1

The paraganglial system and topographic sites (in red) of pheochromocytomas and paragangliomas. [***A, B,*** *from WM Manger, RW Gifford, Clinical and Experimental Pheochromocytoma. Cambridge, Blackwell Science, 1996.* ***C,*** *from GG Glenner, PM Grimley, Tumors of the extra-adrenal paraganglion system (including chemoreceptors), Atlas of Tumor Pathology, 2d Series, Fascicle 9. Washington, DC, AFIP, 1974.*]

ubiquitin E3 ligase. *VHL* mutations reduce protein degradation, resulting in upregulation of components involved in cell cycle progression, glucose metabolism, and oxygen sensing.

CLINICAL FEATURES

The clinical presentation is so variable that pheochromocytoma has been termed "the great masquerader" (Table 6-1). Among the presenting symptoms, episodes of palpitations, headaches, and profuse sweating are typical and constitute a classic triad. The presence of all three of these symptoms, in association with hypertension, makes pheochromocytoma a likely diagnosis. On the other hand, a pheochromocytoma can be asymptomatic for years, and some tumors have grown to a considerable size before patients noted symptoms.

The dominant sign is hypertension. Classically, patients have episodic hypertension, but sustained hypertension is also frequent. Catecholamine crises can lead to heart failure, pulmonary edema, arrhythmias, and intracranial hemorrhage. During episodes of hormone release, which can occur at very divergent intervals, patients are anxious and pale, and they experience tachycardia and palpitations. These paroxysms generally last less than an hour and may be precipitated by surgery, positional changes, exercise, pregnancy, urination (particularly bladder pheochromocytomas), and various medications (e.g., tricyclic antidepressants, opiates, metoclopramide).

TABLE 6-1

CLINICAL FEATURES ASSOCIATED WITH PHEOCHROMOCYTOMA

Headaches	Weight loss
Sweating attacks	Paradoxical response to antihypertensive drugs
Palpitation and tachycardia	Polyuria and polydipsia
Hypertension, sustained or paroxysmal	Constipation
Anxiety and panic attacks	Orthostatic hypotension
Pallor	Dilated cardiomyopathy
Nausea	Erythrocytosis
Abdominal pain	Elevated blood sugar
Weakness	Hypercalcemia

DIAGNOSIS

The diagnosis is based on documentation of catecholamine excess by biochemical testing and localization of the tumor by imaging. Both are of equal importance, although measurement of catecholamines is traditionally the first step.

Biochemical Testing

Pheochromocytomas and paragangliomas synthesize and store catecholamines, which include norepinephrine (noradrenaline), epinephrine (adrenaline), and dopamine. Elevated plasma and urinary levels of catecholamines and the methylated metabolites, metanephrines, are the cornerstone for the diagnosis. The hormonal activity of tumors fluctuates, resulting in considerable variation in serial catecholamine measurements. Thus, there is some value in obtaining tests during or soon after a symptomatic crisis. On the other hand, most tumors continuously leak O-methylated metabolites, which are detected by metanephrine measurements.

Catecholamines and metanephrines can be measured using many different methods (e.g., high-performance liquid chromatography, enzyme-linked immunosorbent assay, other immunoassays). In a clinical context suspicious for pheochromocytoma, when values are increased two to three times the upper limit of normal, a pheochromocytoma is highly likely, regardless of the assay used, assuming an appropriate clinical context. However, as summarized in Table 6-2, the sensitivity and specificity of available biochemical tests varies greatly, and these differences are important when assessing patients with borderline catecholamine elevation. Urinary tests for VMA, metanephrines (total or fractionated), and catecholamines are widely available and commonly used for initial testing. Among these tests, the fractionated metanephrines and catecholamines are the most sensitive. Plasma tests are more convenient and include measurements of catecholamines, metanephrines, and chromogranin A, a secretory product of endocrine cells. Plasma metanephrine measurements are most sensitive and are less susceptible to false-positive elevations from stress, including venipuncture. Although the incidence of false-positive test results has been reduced by the introduction of newer assays, physiologic stress responses and medications (e.g., levodopa, labetalol, sympathomimetics) that increase catecholamines can still confound testing. Because the tumors are relatively rare, borderline elevations are likely to be false positives. In this circumstance, repeated testing, often using different assays, may clarify the diagnosis. If possible, physiologic (e.g., heart failure, shock, hypertension) or pharmacologic (clonidine withdrawal, tricyclic antidepressants) factors that might cause false positives should be eliminated. The pattern of catecholamines can help in localizing the tumor, as epinephrine is virtually never increased in extraadrenal pheochromocytomas.

Pharmacologic tests, such as the phentolamine test, the glucagon provocation test, and the clonidine suppression test, are of relatively low sensitivity and are rarely used.

TABLE 6-2

BIOCHEMICAL AND IMAGING METHODS USED FOR PHEOCHROMOCYTOMA AND PARAGANGLIOMA DIAGNOSIS

DIAGNOSTIC METHOD	SENSITIVITY	SPECIFICITY
24-h urinary tests		
Vanillylmandelic acid	++	++++
Catecholamines	+++	+++
Fractionated metanephrines	++++	++
Total metanephrines	+++	++++
Plasma tests		
Catecholamines	+++	++
Free metanephrines	++++	+++
Chromogranin A	+++	++
CT	++++	+++
MRI	++++	+++
MIBG scintigraphy	+++	++++
Somatostatin receptor scintigraphy[a]	++	++
Dopa (dopamine) PET (preliminary data)	++++	++++

[a]Particularly high in head and neck paragangliomas.

Note: MIBG, metaiodobenzylguanidine; PET, positron emission tomography.

Diagnostic Imaging

A variety of methods have been used to localize pheochromocytomas and paragangliomas (Table 6-2). CT and MRI are similar in sensitivity. CT should be performed with contrast. T2-weighted MRI with gadolinium contrast is optimal for detecting pheochromocytomas and is somewhat better than CT for imaging extraadrenal pheochromocytomas and paragangliomas. About 5% of adrenal incidentalomas, usually detected by CT or MRI, prove to be pheochromocytomas after endocrinologic evaluation.

Tumors can also be localized using radioactive tracers including ^{131}I- or ^{123}I-metaiodobenzylguanidine (MIBG), ^{111}In-somatostatin analogues, or ^{18}F-dopa (or dopamine) positron emission tomography (PET). Because these agents exhibit selective uptake in paragangliomas, nuclear imaging is particularly useful in the hereditary syndromes.

Differential Diagnosis

When entertaining the possibility of a pheochromocytoma, other disorders to consider include essential hypertension, anxiety attacks, use of cocaine or amphetamines, mastocytosis or carcinoid syndrome (usually lacking hypertension), intracranial lesions, clonidine withdrawal, autonomic epilepsy, and factitious crises (usually from sympathomimetic amines). When an asymptomatic adrenal mass is identified, likely diagnoses other than pheochromocytoma include a nonfunctioning adrenal adenoma, aldosteronoma, and cortisol-producing adenoma (Cushing's syndrome).

℞ Treatment: PHEOCHROMOCYTOMA

Complete tumor removal is the ultimate therapeutic goal. Preoperative patient preparation is essential for safe surgery. α-Adrenergic blockers (phenoxybenzamine) should be initiated at relatively low doses (e.g., 5–10 mg PO three times per day) and increased as tolerated every few days. Because patients are volume constricted, liberal salt intake and hydration are necessary to avoid orthostasis. Adequate alpha blockade generally requires 10–14 days, with a typical final dose of 20–30 mg phenoxybenzamine three times per day. Prazosin PO or phentolamine IV can be used to manage paroxysms while awaiting adequate alpha blockade. Before surgery, the blood pressure should be consistently below 160/90 mmHg, with moderate orthostasis. Beta blockers (e.g., 10 mg propranolol three to four times per day) can be added after starting alpha blockers, and increased as needed, if tachycardia persists. Because beta blockers can induce a paradoxical increase in blood pressure in the absence of alpha blockade, they should be administered only after effective alpha blockade. Other antihypertensives, such as calcium channel blockers or angiotensin-converting enzyme inhibitors, have also been used when blood pressure is difficult to control with phenoxybenzamine alone.

Surgery should be performed by teams of anesthesiologists and surgeons with experience in the management of pheochromocytomas. Blood pressure can be labile during surgery, particularly at the onset of intubation or when manipulating the tumor. Nitroprusside infusion is useful for intraoperative hypertensive crises, and hypotension usually responds to volume infusion. Although laparotomy was the traditional surgical approach, laparoscopy, using either a transperitoneal or retroperitoneal (for bilateral adrenalectomy) approach, is associated with fewer complications and a faster recovery. Atraumatic endoscopic surgery was introduced in the early 1990s and has now become the method of choice. It may be possible to preserve the normal adrenal cortex, particularly in hereditary disorders in which bilateral pheochromocytomas are more likely. Extraadrenal abdominal pheochromocytomas can also be removed endoscopically. Postoperatively, catecholamine normalization should be documented. An adrenocorticotropic hormone test should be used to exclude cortisol deficiency when bilateral adrenal cortex–sparing surgery is performed.

MALIGNANT PHEOCHROMOCYTOMA

About 5–10% of pheochromocytomas and paragangliomas are malignant. The diagnosis of malignant pheochromocytoma is problematic. Typical histologic criteria of cellular atypia, presence of mitoses, and invasion of vessels or adjacent tissues do not reliably identify which tumors have the capacity to metastasize. Thus, the term *malignant pheochromocytoma* is generally restricted to tumors with distant metastases, most commonly found in lungs, bone, or liver, suggesting a vascular pathway of spread. Because hereditary syndromes are associated with multifocal tumor sites, these features should be anticipated in patients with germ-line mutations of *RET*, *VHL*, *SDHD*, or *SDHB*. However, distant metastases also occur in these syndromes, especially carriers of *SDHB* mutations.

Treatment of malignant pheochromocytoma or paraganglioma is challenging. Options include tumor mass reduction; alpha blockers for symptoms; chemotherapy; and nuclear medicine radiotherapy. Averbuch's chemotherapy protocol includes dacarbazine (600 mg/m^2 days 1 and 2), cyclophosphamide (750 mg/m^2 day 1), and vincristine (1.4 mg/m^2 day 1), repeated every 21 days for three to six cycles. Palliation (stable disease to shrinkage) is achieved in about half of patients. An alternative is ^{131}I-MIBG treatment using 200-mCi doses at monthly intervals, over three to six cycles. The prognosis of metastatic pheochromocytoma or paraganglioma is variable, with a 5-year survival of 30–60%.

PHEOCHROMOCYTOMA IN PREGNANCY

Pheochromocytomas are occasionally diagnosed in pregnancy. Endoscopic removal, preferably in the fourth to sixth month of gestation, is possible and can be followed by uneventful childbirth. Regular screening in families with inherited pheochromocytomas provides an opportunity to identify and remove asymptomatic tumors in women of reproductive age.

PHEOCHROMOCYTOMA-ASSOCIATED SYNDROMES

About 25–33% of patients with pheochromocytoma or paraganglioma have an inherited syndrome (Table 6-3). The mean age at diagnosis is about 15 years lower in patients with inherited syndromes compared to those with sporadic tumors.

Neurofibromatosis type 1 (NF 1) was the first described pheochromocytoma-associated syndrome. The *NF1* gene functions as a tumor suppressor by regulating the ras signaling cascade. Classic features of neurofibromatosis include multiple neurofibromas, café au lait spots, axillary freckling of the skin, and Lisch nodules of the iris (Fig. 6-2). Pheochromocytomas occur in only about 1% of these patients and are located predominantly in the adrenals. Malignant pheochromocytoma is not infrequent.

The most well-known pheochromocytoma-associated syndrome is the autosomal dominant *disorder multiple endocrine neoplasia type 2A and type 2B (MEN 2A, MEN 2B)* (Chap. 23). Both types of MEN 2 are caused by mutations in *RET* (*re*arranged in *t*ransfection), which encodes a tyrosine kinase. The locations of *RET* mutations correlate with the severity of disease and the type of MEN 2 (Chap. 23). MEN 2A is characterized by medullary thyroid carcinoma (MTC), pheochromocytoma, and hyperparathyroidism; MEN 2B also includes MTC and pheochromocytoma, as well as multiple mucosal neuromas, though it typically lacks hyperparathyroidism. Although

TABLE 6-3

PHEOCHROMOCYTOMA- AND PARAGANGLIOMA-ASSOCIATED SYNDROMES

	MEN 2	VHL	PGL4	PGL3	PGL1	NF 1
Mean age at diagnosis	34	16	34	41	26	43
Multifocal	65%	55%	12%	11%	48%	20%
Adrenal/abdominal extraadrenal	97%/3%	92%/17%	42%/58%	0	86%/57%	94%/6%
Thoracic	0	5%	12%	0	29%	0
Head and neck paraganglioma	0	0	6%	100%	48%	0
Malignancy	3%	4%	24%	0	0	12%
Associated tumors	Medullary thyroid carcinoma, primary hyperparathyroidism	Eye hemangiomas, hemangioblastomas of the CNS, clear cell renal carcinoma, pancreatic islet cell tumors, endolymphatic sac tumors of the inner ear	Renal cell carcinoma in a minority	No regular association with other tumors		Neurofibromas, café au lait spots, axillary freckling, optic pathway tumors, iris hamartomas
Inheritance	Autosomal dominant	Autosomal dominant	Autosomal dominant	Autosomal dominant, no manifestation in offspring of mothers	Autosomal dominant	Autosomal dominant
Gene name	*RET*	*VHL*	*SDHB*	*SDHC*	*SDHD*	*NF1*
Gene location	10q11.2	3p25–26	1p36	1q23	11q23	17q11.2
No. of exons	21	3	8	6	4	57

Note: CNS, central nervous system; MEN 2, multiple endocrine neoplasia type 2; NF 1, neurofibromatosis type 1; PGL, paraganglioma syndrome; VHL, von Hippel-Lindau syndrome.
Source: Adapted from the Freiburg International Pheochromocytoma and Paraganglioma Registry.

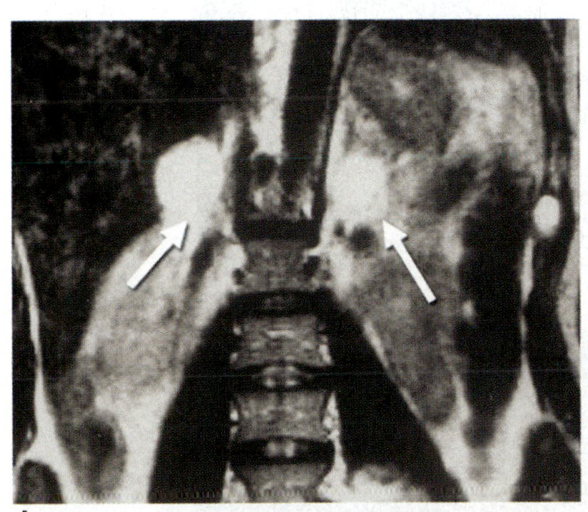

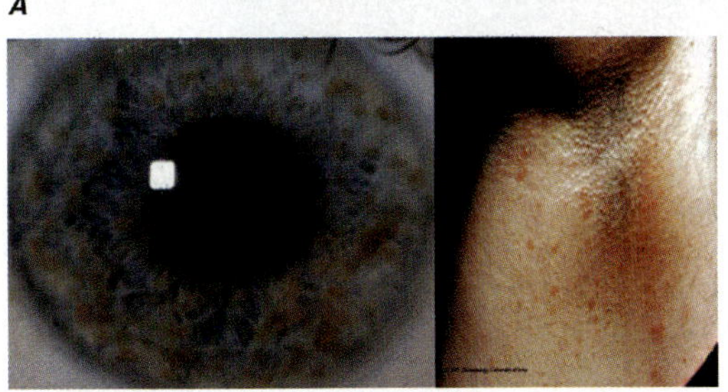

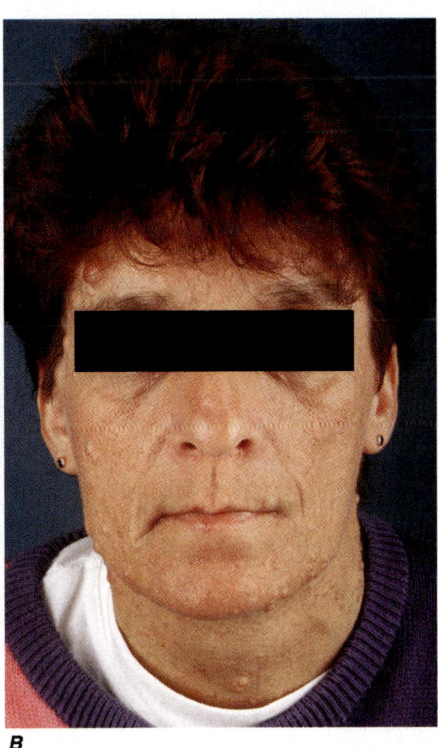

FIGURE 6-2

Neurofibromatosis. *A.* MRI of bilateral adrenal pheochromocytoma. ***B.*** Cutaneous neurofibromas. ***C.*** Lisch nodules of the iris. ***D.*** Axillary freckling. [***A,*** *from HPH Neumann et al: The Keio J Med 54(1):15, 2005; with permission.*]

MTC is seen in virtually all patients with MEN 2, pheochromocytoma occurs in only about 50% of patients. Most pheochromocytomas are benign, located in the adrenals, and bilateral (**Fig. 6-3**). Pheochromocytoma may be symptomatic before MTC. Prophylactic thyroidectomy is being performed in many carriers of *RET* mutations; pheochromocytomas should be excluded before surgery in these patients.

Von Hippel-Lindau syndrome (VHL) is an autosomal dominant disorder that predisposes to retinal and cerebellar hemangioblastomas, which also occur in the brainstem and spinal cord (**Fig. 6-4**). Other important features of VHL are clear cell renal carcinomas, pancreatic islet cell tumors, endolymphatic sac tumors (ELSTs) of the inner ear, cystadenomas of the epididymis and broad ligament, and multiple pancreatic or renal cysts.

The *VHL* gene encodes an E3 ubiquitin ligase that regulates expression of hypoxia-inducible factor-1 (HIF-1), among other genes. Loss of *VHL* is associated with increased expression of vascular endothelial growth factor (VEGF), which induces angiogenesis. Although the *VHL* gene can be inactivated by all types of mutations, patients with pheochromocytoma predominantly have missense mutations. About 20–30% of patients with VHL have pheochromocytomas, but in some families, the incidence can reach 90%. The recognition of pheochromocytoma as a VHL-associated feature provides an opportunity to diagnose retinal, renal, and central nervous system tumors at an earlier stage.

The *paraganglioma syndromes (PGLs)* have been classified by genetic analyses of families with head and neck paragangliomas. The susceptibility genes encode subunits

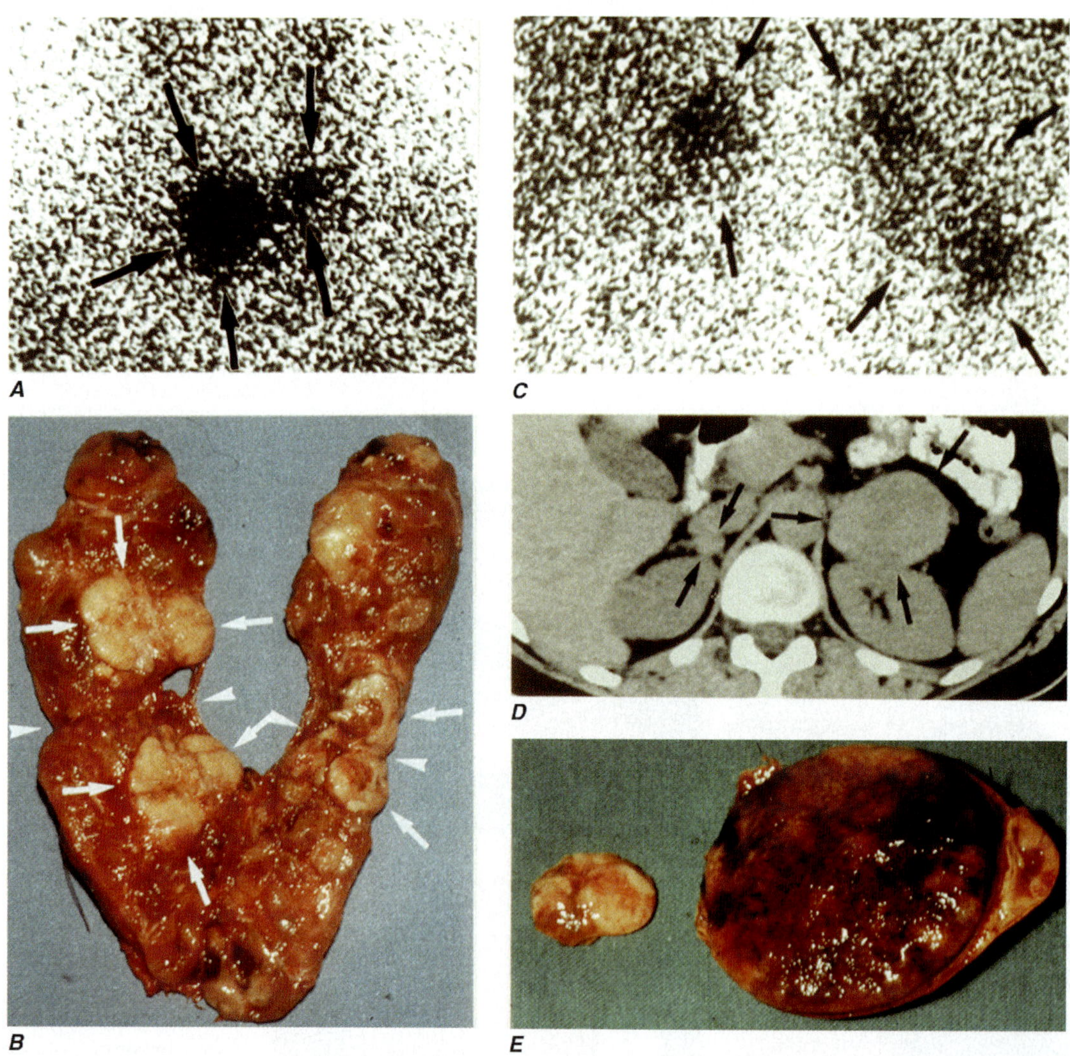

FIGURE 6-3

Multiple endocrine neoplasia type 2. Multifocal medullary thyroid carcinoma shown by (***A***) MIBG scintigraphy and (***B***) operative specimen; arrows demonstrate the tumors; arrowheads show the tissue bridge of the cut specimen. Bilateral adrenal pheochromocytoma shown by (***C***) MIBG scintigraphy, (***D***) CT imaging, and (***E***) operative specimens. [*From HPH Neumann et al: The Keio J Med 54(1):15, 2005; with permission.*]

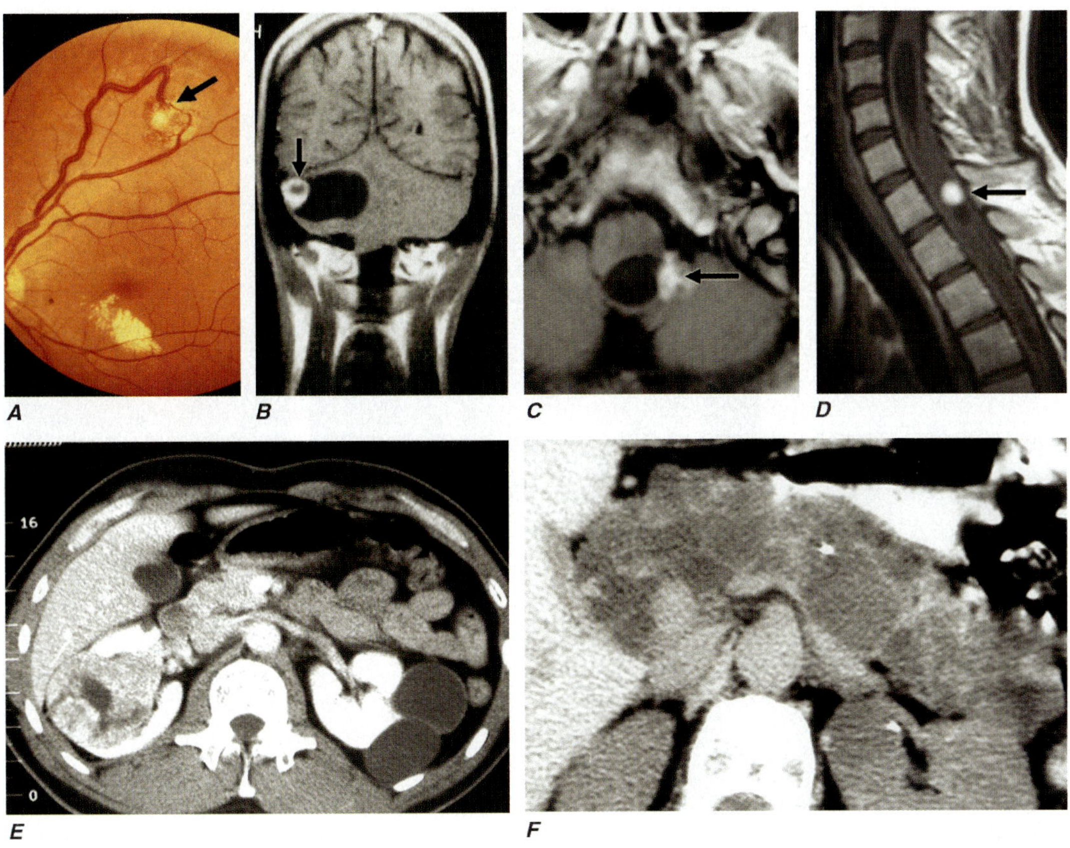

FIGURE 6-4

Von Hippel-Lindau disease with extraparaganglial features. Retinal angioma (***A***); hemangioblastomas of cerebellum are shown by MRI in (***B***) brainstem; (***C*** and ***D***) spinal cord; (***E***) carcinoma of the right kidney, cysts of the left kidney; and (***F***) multiple pancreatic cysts. [***A, D,*** *from HPH Neumann et al: Adv Nephrol Necker Hosp 27:361, 1997. Copyright Elsevier.* ***B,*** *from Inherited Disorders of the Kidney, SH Morgan, J-P Grunfeld (eds). Oxford, Oxford Univ Press, 1998.* ***E, F,*** *from HPH Neumann et al: Contrib Nephrol 136:193, 2001. Copyright S. Karger AG, Basel.*]

of the enzyme succinate dehydrogenase (SDH), a component in the Krebs cycle and the mitochondrial electron transport chain. SDH is formed by four subunits (A–D). Mutations of *SDHB* (PGL4), *SDHC* (PGL3), and *SDHD* (PGL1) predispose to three of the paraganglioma syndromes (Table 6-3). The gene for PGL2 has not been identified yet. Mutations of SDHA do not predispose to paraganglioma tumors but instead cause Leigh disease, a form of encephalopathy. The transmission of *SDHC* and *SDHB* mutations is autosomal dominant. In contrast, SDHD families exhibit a gene imprinting effect: only the offspring of affected fathers develop tumors. In a small number of patients with familial pheochromocytoma, a mutation has not yet been identified.

PGL1 is most frequent, followed by PGL4, and PGL3 is rare. Adrenal, extraadrenal abdominal, and thoracic pheochromocytomas are components of PGL1 and PGL4, but not of PGL3 (**Fig. 6-5**). About one-third of the patients develop metastases.

GUIDELINES FOR GENETIC SCREENING IN PATIENTS WITH PHEOCHROMOCYTOMA OR PARAGANGLIOMA

In addition to family history, general features suggesting an inherited syndrome include young age, multifocal tumors, extraadrenal tumors, or malignant tumors (**Fig. 6-6**). Given the relatively high prevalence of familial syndromes among patients who present with pheochromocytoma or paraganglioma, it is useful to identify germ-line mutations, even in patients without a known family history. A first step is to search for clinical features of inherited syndromes and to perform an in-depth, multigenerational family history. Each of these syndromes exhibits autosomal dominant transmission with variable penetrance (Table 6-3). Cutaneous neurofibromas, café au lait spots, and axillary freckling suggest neurofibromatosis. Germ-line mutations in *NF1* have not been reported in patients with sporadic pheochromocytomas. Thus, *NF1* testing does not need to be performed in the absence of

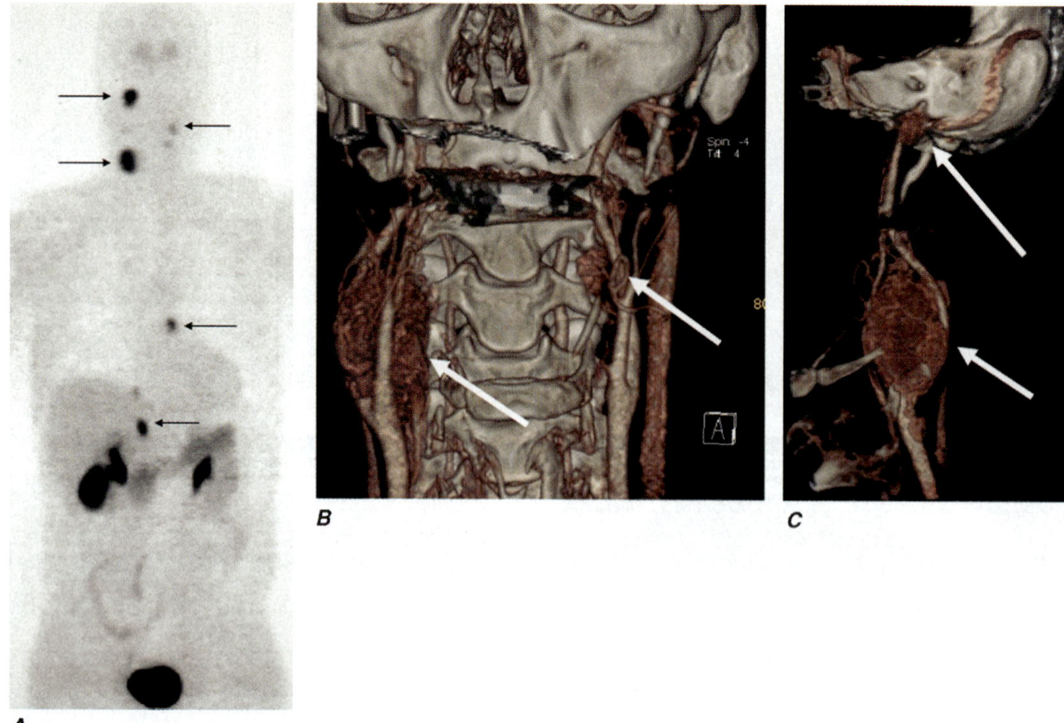

FIGURE 6-5

Paraganglioma syndrome. PGL1, a patient with incomplete resection of a left carotid body tumor and the SDHD W5X mutation. ***A.*** ^{18}F-dopa positron emission tomography demonstrating tumor uptake in the right jugular glomus, the right carotid body, the left carotid body, the left coronary glomus, and the right adrenal gland. Note the physiologic accumulation of the radiopharmaceutical agent in the kidneys, liver, gallbladder, renal pelvis, and urinary bladder. ***B*** and ***C.*** CT angiography with 3D reconstruction. Arrows point to the paraganglial tumors. [*From S Hoegerle et al: Eur J Nucl Med Mol Imaging 30(5):689, 2003; with permission.*]

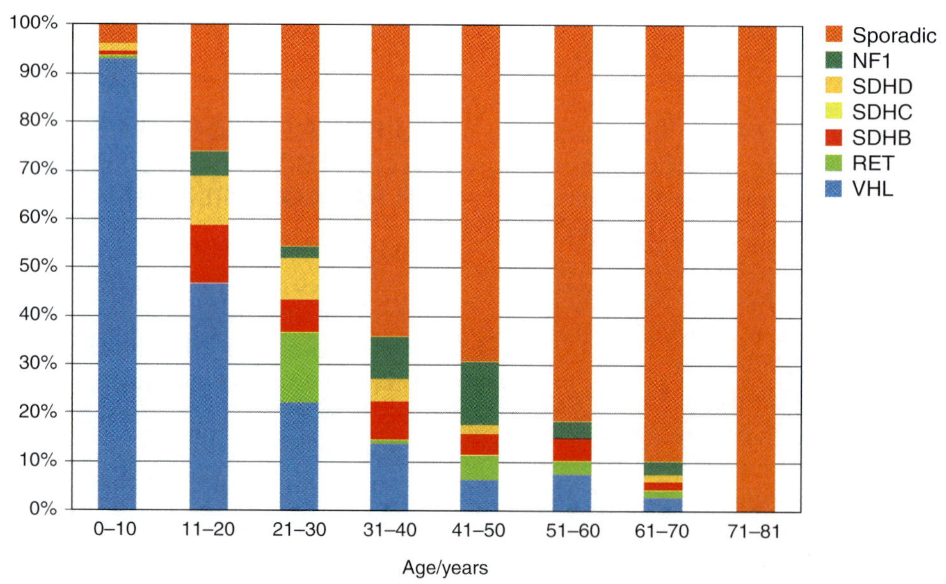

FIGURE 6-6

Mutation distribution in the *RET, VHL, NF1, SDHB, SDHC,* and *SDHD* genes. The bars depict the frequency of sporadic or various inherited forms of pheochromocytoma in different age groups. The inherited disorders are much more common among younger individuals presenting with pheochromocytoma. (*Data from the Freiburg International Pheochromocytoma and Paraganglioma Registry.*)

other clinical features of neurofibromatosis. A personal or family history of medullary thyroid cancer or parathyroid tumors strongly suggests MEN 2 and should prompt testing for *RET* mutations. A history of visual impairment, or tumors of the cerebellum, kidney, brainstem, or spinal cord, suggests the possibility of VHL.

A single adrenal pheochromocytoma in a patient with an otherwise unremarkable history may still be associated with mutations of *VHL*, *RET*, *SDHB*, or *SDHD* (in decreasing order of frequency). Two-thirds of extraadrenal tumors are associated with one of these syndromes, and multifocal tumors occur with decreasing frequency in carriers of *RET*, *SDHD*, *VHL*, and *SDHB* mutations. About 25% of head and neck paragangliomas are associated with germ-line mutations of one of the SDH subunit genes (particularly *SDHD*) and are rare in carriers of *VHL* or *RET* mutations.

Once the underlying syndrome is diagnosed, the benefit of genetic testing can be extended to relatives. For this purpose, it is necessary to identify the germ-line mutation in the proband and, after genetic counseling, perform DNA sequence analyses of the responsible gene in relatives to determine if they are affected. Other family members may benefit from biochemical screening for tumors in individuals who carry a germ-line mutation.

FURTHER READINGS

BAUSCH B et al: Clinical and genetic characteristics of patients with neurofibromatosis type 1 and pheochromocytoma. N Engl J Med 354:2729, 2006

——— et al: Germline NF1 mutational spectra and loss-of-heterozygosity analyses in patients with pheochromocytoma and neurofibromatosis type 1. J Clin Endocrinol Metab 92:2784, 2007

JOSHUA AM et al: Rationale and evidence for sunitinib in the treatment of malignant paraganglioma/pheochromocytoma. J Clin Endocrinol Metab 94:5, 2009

LENDERS JW et al: Phaeochromocytoma. Lancet 366:665, 2005

NEUMANN HP et al: Distinct clinical features of paraganglioma syndromes associated with *SDHB* and *SDHD* gene mutations. JAMA 292:943, 2004

——— et al: Evidence of MEN-2 in the original description of classic pheochromocytoma. N Engl J Med 357:1311, 2007

NOMURA K et al: Survival of patients with metastatic malignant pheochromocytoma and efficacy of combined cyclophosphamide, vincristine and dacarbazine chemotherapy. J Clin Endocrinol Metab 94:2850, 2009

SCHOLZ T et al: Clinical review: Current treatment of malignant pheochromocytoma. J Clin Endocrinol Metab 92:1217, 2007

WALZ MK et al: Laparoscopic and retroperitoneoscopic treatment of pheochromocytomas and retroperitoneal paragangliomas: Results of 161 tumors in 126 patients. World J Surg 30:899, 2006

SECTION II

REPRODUCTIVE ENDOCRINOLOGY

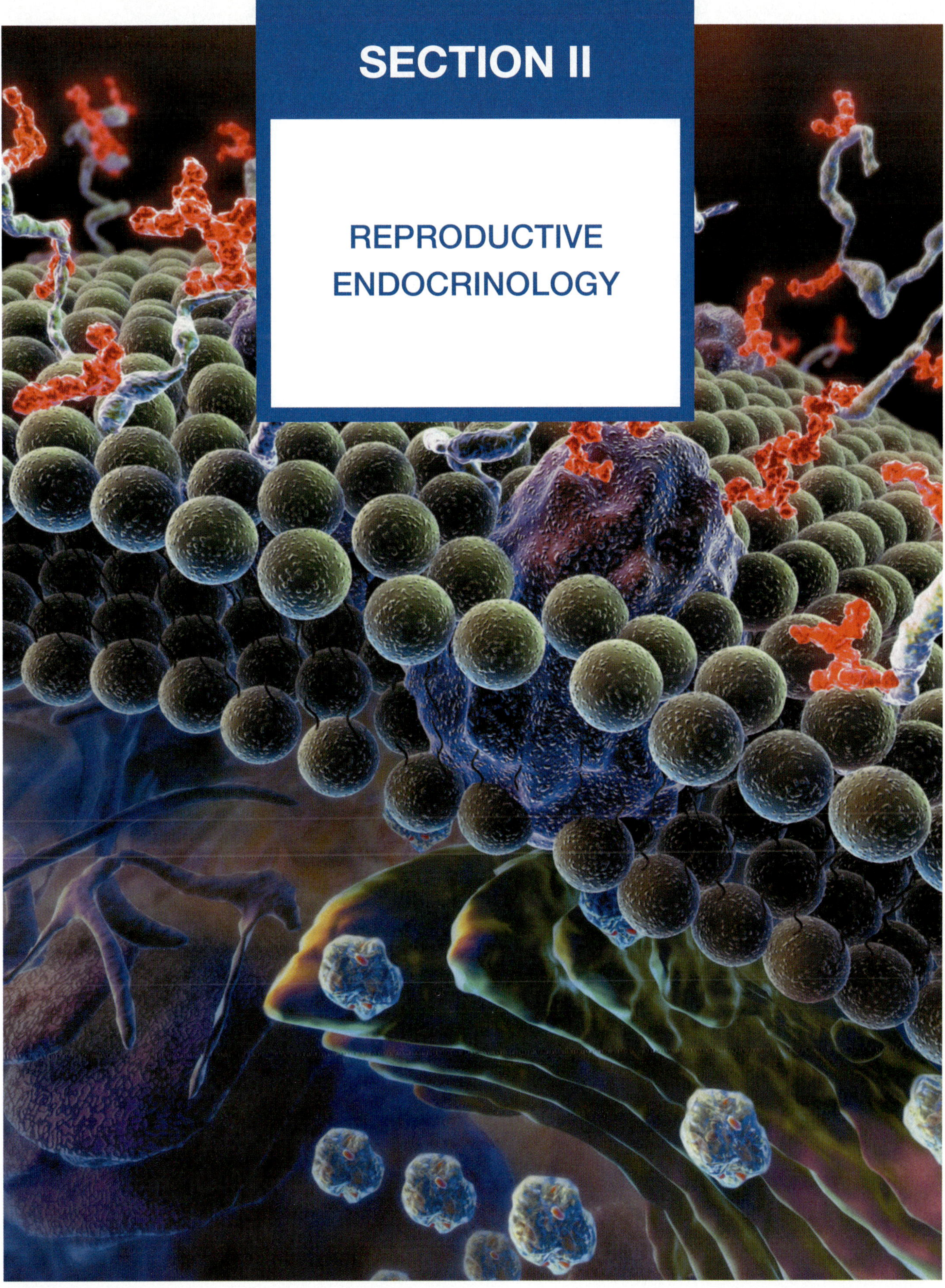

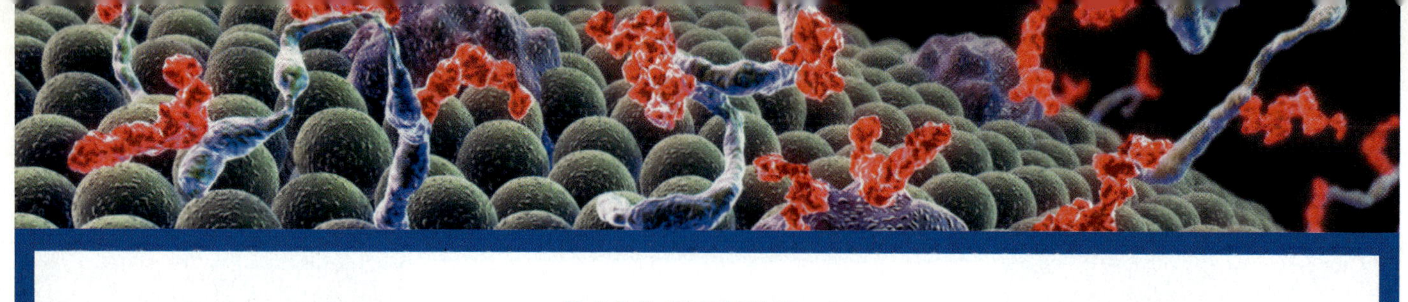

CHAPTER 7

DISORDERS OF SEX DEVELOPMENT

John C. Achermann ■ J. Larry Jameson

Sex development begins in utero but continues into young adulthood with the achievement of sexual maturity and reproductive capability. The early stages of sex development can be divided into three major components: chromosomal sex, gonadal sex (sex determination), and phenotypic sex (sex differentiation) (**Fig. 7-1**). Abnormalities at each of these stages can result in disorders of sex development (DSDs). The child born with ambiguous genitalia requires urgent assessment, as some causes, such as congenital adrenal hyperplasia (CAH), can be associated with life-threatening adrenal crises. Early gender assignment and clear communication with parents about the diagnosis and treatment options are essential. The involvement of an experienced multidisciplinary team is crucial for planning surgical intervention (if needed), medical management, and counseling. DSDs can also manifest later in life due to subtler forms of gonadal dysfunction [e.g., Klinefelter syndrome (KS)] and are often diagnosed by internists. Because DSDs are associated with a variety of psychological, reproductive, and metabolic consequences, an open dialogue must be established between the patient and health care providers to ensure continuity and attention to these issues.

NORMAL SEX DEVELOPMENT

Chromosomal sex describes the X and/or Y chromosome complement (46,XY male; 46,XX female) that is established at the time of fertilization. The presence of a normal Y chromosome determines that testis development will occur, even in the presence of multiple X chromosomes (e.g., 47,XXY or 48,XXXY). The loss of an X chromosome impairs gonad development (45,X or 45,X/46,XY mosaicism). Fetuses with no X chromosome (45,Y) are not viable.

Gonadal sex refers to the assignment of gonadal tissue as testis or ovary. The embryonic gonad is bipotential and can develop (from ~40 days' gestation) into either a testis or ovary, depending on which genes are expressed (**Fig. 7-2**). Testis development is initiated by expression of the Y chromosome gene *SRY* (sex-determining region on the Y chromosome), which encodes an HMG-box transcription factor. *SRY* is transiently expressed in cells destined to become Sertoli cells and serves as a pivotal switch to establish the testis lineage. Mutation of *SRY* prevents testis development in chromosomal 46, XY males, whereas translocation of *SRY* in 46,XX females is sufficient to induce testis development and a male phenotype. Other genes are necessary to continue testis development. *SOX9* (*SRY*-related HMG-box gene 9) is upregulated in the developing male gonad but is suppressed in the female gonad. Transgenic expression of *SOX9* is sufficient to initiate testis formation in mice, and mutations that disrupt *SOX9* impair testis development. *WT1* (Wilms' tumor– related gene 1) acts early in the genetic pathway and regulates the transcription of several genes including *SF1*, *DAX1*, and *AMH* (encoding *MIS*, müllerian-inhibiting substance). *SF1* (steroidogenic factor 1) encodes a nuclear receptor that functions in cooperation with other transcription

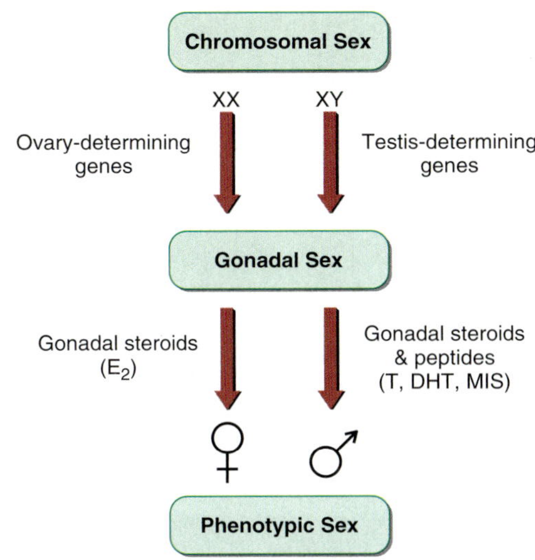

FIGURE 7-1

Sex development can be divided into three major components: chromosomal sex, gonadal sex, and phenotypic sex. T, testosterone; DHT, dihydrotestosterone; MIS, müllerian-inhibiting substance.

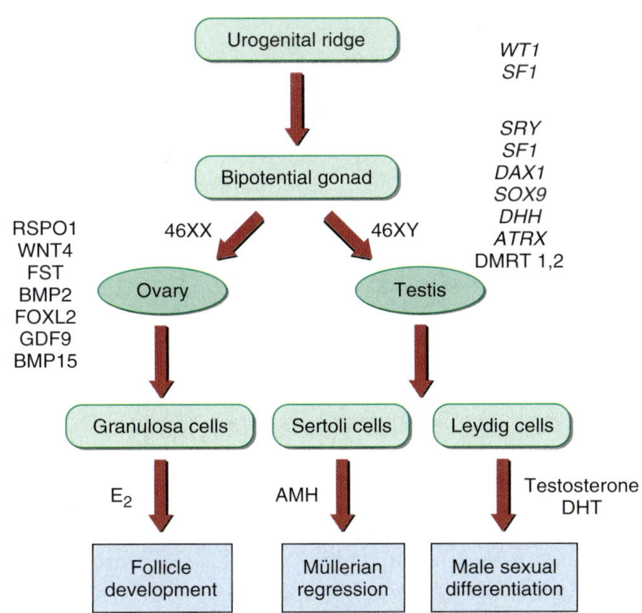

FIGURE 7-2

The genetic regulation of gonadal development. *WT1*, Wilms' tumor–related gene 1; *SF1*, steroidogenic factor 1; *SRY*, sex-determining region on the Y chromosome; *SOX9*, SRY-related HMG-box gene 9; *DHH*, desert hedgehog; *ATRX*, α-thalassemia, mental retardation on the X chromosome; *DAX1*, dosage-sensitive sex reversal, adrenal hypoplasia congenita on the X chromosome, gene 1; DMRT 1/2, double-sex MAB3-related transcription factor 1/2; WNT4, wingless-type MMTV integration site 4; FST, follistatin; BMP2 and 15, bone morpho factors 2 and 15; FOXL2, forkhead transcription factor L2; GDF9, growth differentiation factor 9; AMH, anti-müllerian hormone (müllerian-inhibiting substance); DHT, dihydrotestosterone; RSPO1, R-spondin 1.

factors to regulate a large array of adrenal and gonadal genes, including many genes involved in steroidogenesis. Heterozygous *SF1* mutations account for ~10% of XY patients with gonadal dysgenesis and impaired androgenization, indicating the sensitivity of the testis to *SF1* gene dosage. The early expression pattern of *SF1* in the gonad parallels that of another orphan nuclear receptor, *DAX1* (dosage-sensitive sex reversal, adrenal hypoplasia congenita on the X chromosome, gene 1). *DAX1* is downregulated as the testis develops. Duplication of *DAX1* impairs testis development, possibly by antagonizing the function of *SRY* and *SF1*. Deletions or mutations of *DAX1*, on the other hand, lead to disordered formation of testis cords, again revealing the exquisite sensitivity of the male sex–determining pathway to gene dosage effects. In addition to the genes mentioned above, studies of human and murine mutations indicate that at least 15 other genes are also involved in gonadal differentiation, development, and final positioning of the gonad (Fig. 7-2). These genes encode an array of signaling molecules and paracrine growth factors, in addition to transcription factors.

Although ovarian development was once considered to be a "default" process, it is now clear that specific genes are expressed during the earliest stages of ovary development (e.g., follistatin) (Fig. 7-2). Once the ovary has formed, additional genes are required for normal follicular development [e.g., follicle-stimulating hormone (FSH) receptor, *GDF9*]. Steroidogenesis in the ovary requires the development of follicles containing granulosa cells and theca cells surrounding the oocytes (Chap. 10). Thus, there is relatively limited ovarian steroidogenesis until gonadotropins are produced at puberty.

Germ cells also develop in a sex dimorphic manner. In the developing ovary, primordial germ cells (PGCs) enter meiosis, whereas they proliferate and then undergo mitotic arrest in the developing testis. PGC entry into meiosis is initiated by retinoic acid, which activates *STRA8* (*stimulated by retinoic acid 8*) and other genes involved in meiosis. The developing testis produces high levels of CYP26B1, an enzyme that degrades retinoic acid, thereby preventing PGC entry into meiosis.

Phenotypic sex refers to the structures of the external and internal genitalia and secondary sex characteristics. The male phenotype requires the secretion of anti-müllerian hormone (AMH, müllerian-inhibiting substance) from Sertoli cells and testosterone from testicular Leydig cells. AMH is a member of the transforming growth factor (TGF) β family and acts through specific receptors to cause regression of the müllerian structures (60–80 days' gestation). At ~60–140 days' gestation, testosterone supports the development of wolffian structures, including the epididymides, vasa deferentia, and seminal vesicles. Testosterone is the precursor for dihydrotestosterone (DHT), a potent androgen that promotes development

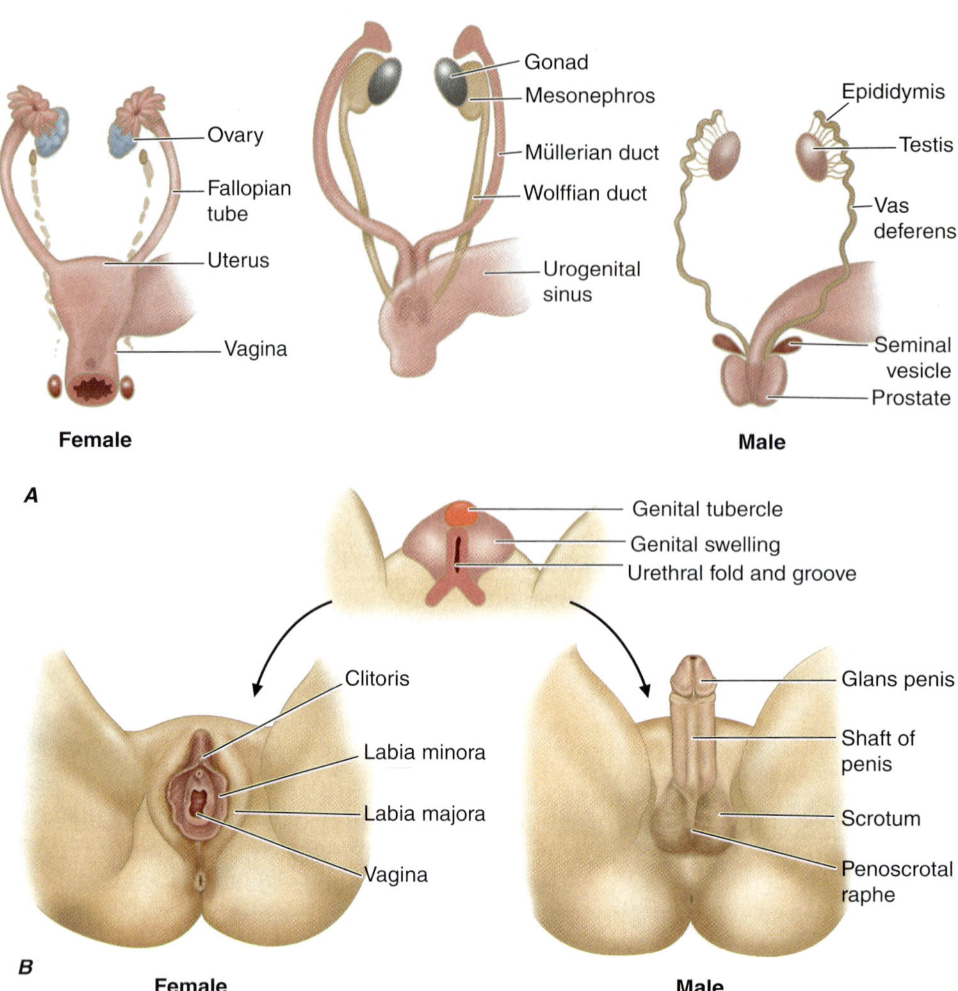

FIGURE 7-3

Normal sex development. *A.* Internal urogenital tract. ***B.*** External genitalia. [*After JD Wilson, JE Griffin, in E Braunwald et al (eds): Harrison's Principles of Internal Medicine, 15th ed. New York, McGraw-Hill, 2001.*]

of the external genitalia, including the penis and scrotum (65–100 days, and thereafter) (Fig. 7-3). The urogenital sinus develops into the prostate and prostatic urethra in the male and into the urethra and lower portion of the vagina in the female. The genital tubercle becomes the glans penis in the male and the clitoris in the female. The urogenital swellings form the scrotum or the labia majora, and the urethral folds fuse to form the shaft of the penis and the male urethra or the labia minora. In the female, wolffian ducts regress and the müllerian ducts form the fallopian tubes, uterus, and upper segment of the vagina. A normal female phenotype will develop in the absence of the gonad, but estrogen is needed for maturation of the uterus and breast at puberty.

DISORDERS OF CHROMOSOMAL SEX

Disorders of chromosomal sex result from abnormalities in the number or structure of the X or Y chromosomes (Table 7-1).

KLINEFELTER SYNDROME (47,XXY)

Pathophysiology

The classic form of KS (47,XXY) occurs following meiotic nondisjunction of the sex chromosomes during gametogenesis (40% during spermatogenesis, 60% during oogenesis). Mosaic forms of KS (46,XY/47,XXY) are thought to result from chromosomal mitotic nondisjunction within the zygote, and occur in at least 10% of individuals with this condition. Other chromosomal variants of KS (e.g., 48,XXYY; 48,XXXY) have been reported but are less common.

Clinical Features

KS is characterized by small testes, infertility, gynecomastia, eunuchoid proportions, and poor virilization in phenotypic males. It has an incidence of at least 1 in 1000 men, but many are not diagnosed. In severe cases, individuals present prepubertally with small testes, or with impaired

TABLE 7-1

CLINICAL FEATURES OF CHROMOSOMAL DISORDERS OF SEX DEVELOPMENT (DSDs)

DISORDER	COMMON CHROMOSOMAL COMPLEMENT	GONAD	GENITALIA		BREAST DEVELOPMENT	CLINICAL FEATURES
			EXTERNAL	INTERNAL		
Klinefelter syndrome	47,XXY or 46,XY/ 47,XXY	Hyalinized testes	Male	Male	Gynecomastia	Small testes, azoospermia, decreased facial and axillary hair, decreased libido, tall stature and increased leg length, decreased penile length, increased risk of breast tumors, thromboembolic disease, learning difficulties, obesity, diabetes mellitus, varicose veins
Turner syndrome	45,X or 45,X/ 46,XX	Streak gonad or immature ovary	Female	Hypoplastic female	Immature female	Infancy: lymphedema, web neck, shield chest, low-set hairline, cardiac defects and coarctation of the aorta, urinary tract malformations and horseshoe kidney Childhood: short stature, cubitus valgus, short neck, short 4th metacarpals, hypoplastic nails, micrognathia, scoliosis, otitis media and sensorineural hearing loss, ptosis and amblyopia, multiple nevi and keloid formation, autoimmune thyroid disease, visuospatial learning difficulties Adulthood: pubertal failure and primary amenorrhea, hypertension, obesity, dyslipidemia, impaired glucose tolerance and insulin resistance, autoimmune thyroid disease, cardiovascular disease, aortic root dilatation, osteoporosis, inflammatory bowel disease, chronic hepatic dysfunction, increased risk of colon cancer, hearing loss
Mixed gonadal dysgenesis	45,X/46,XY	Testis or streak gonad	Variable	Variable	Usually male	Short stature, increased risk of gonadal tumors, some Turner syndrome features
True hermaphroditism (ovotesticular DSD)	46,XX/46,XY	Testis and ovary or ovotestis	Variable	Variable	Gynecomastia	Possible increased risk of gonadal tumors

androgenization and gynecomastia at the time of puberty. Developmental delay and learning disabilities may be a feature. Later in life, eunuchoid features or infertility lead to the diagnosis. Testes are small and firm [median length 2.5 cm (4 mL volume); almost always <3.5 cm (12 mL)], and typically seem inappropriately small for the degree of androgenization. Biopsies are not usually necessary but reveal seminiferous tubule hyalinization and azoospermia. Other clinical features of KS are listed in Table 7-1. Plasma concentrations of FSH and luteinizing hormone (LH) are increased in most patients with 47,XXY (90 and 80%, respectively) and plasma testosterone is decreased (50–75%), reflecting primary gonadal failure. Estradiol is often increased because of chronic Leydig cell stimulation by LH and because of aromatization of androstenedione by adipose tissue; the increased ratio of estradiol/testosterone results in gynecomastia. Patients with mosaic forms of KS have less severe clinical features and larger testes, and sometimes achieve spontaneous fertility.

Rx Treatment: KLINEFELTER SYNDROME

Gynecomastia should be treated by surgical reduction if it causes concern (Chap. 8). Androgen supplementation improves virilization, libido, energy, hypofibrinolysis, and bone mineralization in underandrogenized men but may occasionally worsen gynecomastia (Chap. 8). Fertility has been achieved using in vitro fertilization in men with oligospermia or with intracytoplasmic sperm injection (ICSI) following retrieval of spermatozoa by testicular sperm extraction techniques. In specialized centers, successful spermatozoa retrieval using this technique is possible in >50% of men with nonmosaic KS. Following ICSI and embryo transfer, successful pregnancies can be achieved in ~50% of these cases. The risk of transmission of this chromosomal abnormality needs to be considered, and preimplantation screening may be desired.

TURNER SYNDROME (GONADAL DYSGENESIS; 45,X)

Pathophysiology

Approximately one-half of individuals with Turner syndrome (TS) have a 45,X karyotype, about 20% have 45,X/46,XX mosaicism, and the remainder have structural abnormalities of the X chromosome such as X fragments, isochromosomes, or rings. The clinical features of TS result from haploinsufficiency of multiple X chromosomal genes (e.g., short stature homeobox, *SHOX*). However, imprinted genes may also be affected when the inherited X has different parental origins.

Clinical Features

TS is characterized by bilateral streak gonads, primary amenorrhea, short stature, and multiple congenital anomalies in phenotypic females. It affects ~1 in 2500 women and is diagnosed at different ages depending on the dominant clinical features (Table 7-1). Prenatally, a diagnosis of TS is usually made incidentally after chorionic villous sampling or amniocentesis for unrelated reasons, such as advanced maternal age. Prenatal ultrasound findings include increased nuchal translucency and reduced fetal growth in some cases. The postnatal diagnosis of TS should be considered in female neonates or infants with lymphedema, nuchal folds, low hairline, or left-sided cardiac defects, and in girls with unexplained growth failure or pubertal delay. Although limited spontaneous pubertal development occurs in up to 30% of girls with TS (10%, 45,X; 30–40%, 45,X/46,XX), and ~2% reach menarche, the vast majority of women with TS develop complete ovarian failure. This diagnosis should be considered, therefore, in all women who present with primary or secondary amenorrhea and elevated gonadotropin levels.

Rx Treatment: TURNER SYNDROME

The management of girls and women with TS requires a multidisciplinary approach because of the number of potentially involved organ systems. Detailed cardiac and renal evaluation should be performed at the time of diagnosis. Individuals with congenital heart defects (CHDs) (30%) (bicuspid aortic valve, 30–50%; coarctation of the aorta, 30%; aortic root dilatation, 5%) require long-term follow-up by an experienced cardiologist, antibiotic prophylaxis for dental or surgical procedures, and serial imaging of aortic root dimensions, as progressive aortic root dilatation is associated with increased risk of aortic dissection. Individuals found to have congenital renal and urinary tract malformations (30%) are at risk for urinary tract infections, hypertension, and nephrocalcinosis. Hypertension can occur independent of cardiac and renal malformations and should be monitored and treated as in other patients with essential hypertension. Clitoral enlargement or other evidence of virilization suggests the presence of covert, translocated Y chromosomal material and is associated with increased risk of gonadoblastoma, apparently the consequence of Y chromosomal genes distinct from *SRY*. Regular assessment of thyroid function, weight, dentition, hearing, speech, vision, and educational issues should be performed during childhood. Otitis media and middle ear disease are prevalent in childhood (50–85%), and sensorineural hearing loss becomes progressively frequent with age (70–90%). Autoimmune hypothyroidism (15–30%) can occur in childhood but has a mean age of onset in the third decade. Counseling about long-term growth and fertility issues should be provided. Patient support groups are active throughout the world.

The treatment of short stature in children with TS remains a challenge, as untreated final height rarely exceeds 150 cm. High-dose recombinant growth hormone stimulates growth rate in children with TS and may be used alone or in combination with low doses of the nonaromatizable anabolic steroid oxandrolone (up to 0.05 mg/kg per d) in the older child (>8 years). However, final height increments are often modest (5–10 cm), and individualization of treatment regimens to response may be beneficial. Girls with evidence of gonadal failure require estrogen replacement to induce breast and uterine development, to support growth, and to maintain bone mineralization. Most physicians now choose to initiate low-dose estrogen therapy (one-tenth to one-eighth of the adult replacement dose) to induce puberty at an age-appropriate time (~12 years). Doses of estrogen are increased gradually to allow feminization over a 2–3-year period. Progestins are later added to regulate withdrawal bleeds, and some women with TS have now achieved successful pregnancy after ovum donation and in vitro fertilization. Long-term follow-up of women with TS involves careful surveillance of sex hormone replacement and reproductive function, bone mineralization, cardiac function and aortic root dimensions, blood pressure, weight and glucose tolerance, hepatic and lipid profiles, thyroid function, and hearing.

MIXED GONADAL DYSGENESIS (45,X/46,XY)

Mixed gonadal dysgenesis typically results from 45,X/46, XY mosaicism. The phenotype of patients with this condition varies considerably. Although some patients have a predominantly female phenotype with somatic features of TS, streak gonads, and müllerian structures, most 45,X/46,XY individuals have a male phenotype and testes, and the diagnosis is made incidentally after amniocentesis or during investigation of infertility. In practice, most children referred for assessment have ambiguous genitalia and variable somatic features. A female sex-of-rearing is often chosen (60%) if phallic development is poor and uterine structures are present. However, gonadectomy is indicated to prevent further androgen secretion and to prevent development of gonadoblastoma (up to 25%). Individuals raised as males may require reconstructive surgery for hypospadias and removal of dysgenetic gonads. Scrotal testes can be preserved but need regular examination for tumor development. Biopsy for carcinoma in situ is recommended in adolescence, and testosterone supplementation may be required for virilization in puberty. Height potential is usually limited.

OVOTESTICULAR DSD

Ovotesticular DSD (formerly called *true hermaphroditism*) occurs when both an ovary and testis, or when an ovotestis, are found in one individual. For unclear reasons, gonadal asymmetry most often occurs with a testis on the right and an ovary on the left. Most individuals with this diagnosis have a 46,XX karyotype, especially in Sub-Sahara Africa. A 46,XX/46,XY chimeric karyotype is less common and has a variable phenotype depending on the proportion of each cell line. Fluorescence in situ hybridization (FISH) or polymerase chain reaction (PCR) for *SRY* may detect translocations of this region of the Y chromosome in a subset of patients.

DISORDERS OF GONADAL AND PHENOTYPIC SEX

The clinical features of patients with disorders of gonadal and phenotypic sex are divided into the underandrogenization of 46,XY males (46,XY DSD) or excess androgenization of 46,XX females (46,XX DSD). These disorders comprise a spectrum of phenotypes ranging from "46,XY phenotypic females" or "46,XX males" to individuals with ambiguous genitalia.

46,XY DSD (UNDERANDROGENIZED MALES)

Underandrogenization of the 46,XY fetus (formerly called *male pseudohermaphroditism*) reflects defects in androgen production or action. It can result from disorders of testis development, defects of androgen synthesis, or resistance to testosterone and DHT (Table 7-2).

Disorders of Testis Development

Testicular Dysgenesis

Patients with *pure* (or *complete*) *gonadal dysgenesis* (*Swyer syndrome*) have streak gonads, müllerian structures [due to insufficient AMH/müllerian-inhibiting substance (MIS) secretion], and a complete absence of androgenization.

TABLE 7-2

DISORDERS CAUSING UNDERANDROGENIZATION IN KARYOTYPIC MALES (46,XY DSD)
Disorders of testis development
True hermaphroditism (46,XY)
Gonadal dysgenesis
Absent testis syndrome
Disorders of androgen synthesis
LH receptor mutations
Smith-Lemli-Opitz syndrome
Steroidogenic acute regulatory protein mutations
Cholesterol side chain cleavage (*CYP11A1*) deficiency
3β-Hydroxysteroid dehydrogenase 2 (*HSD3B2*) deficiency
17α-Hydroxylase/17,20-lyase (*CYP17*) deficiency
P450 oxidoreductase deficiency (*POR*)
17β-Hydroxysteroid dehydrogenase 3 (*HSD17B3*) deficiency
5α-Reductase 2 deficiency (*SRD5A2*)
Disorders of androgen action
Androgen insensitivity syndrome
Androgen receptor cofactor defects
Other disorders of male reproductive tract
Persistent müllerian duct syndrome
Isolated hypospadias
Cryptorchidism or undescended testes

Note: DSD, disorder of sex development; LH, luteinizing hormone.

Patients with *partial gonadal dysgenesis* (*dysgenetic testes*) produce enough MIS to regress the uterus and, sometimes, sufficient testosterone for partial androgenization. Gonadal dysgenesis can result from mutations or deletions of testis-promoting genes (*WT1*, *SF1*, *SRY*, *SOX9*, *DHH*, *ATRX*, *ARX*, *DMRT*) or duplication of chromosomal loci containing *WNT4* or *DAX1* (Table 7-3). Among these, deletions or mutations of *SRY* and heterozygous mutations of *SF1* appear to be most common but still account for <25% of cases. Associated clinical features

TABLE 7-3

GENETIC CAUSES OF UNDERANDROGENIZATION OF KARYOTYPIC MALES (46,XY DSD)

GENE	INHERITANCE	GONAD	UTERUS	EXTERNAL GENITALIA	ASSOCIATED FEATURES
Disorders of Testis Development					
WT1	AD	Dysgenetic testis	+/–	Female or ambiguous	Wilms' tumor, renal abnormalities, gonadal tumors (WAGR, Denys-Drash and Frasier syndromes)
SF1	AR/AD	Dysgenetic testis	+/–	Female or ambiguous	Primary adrenal failure
SRY	Y	Dysgenetic testis or ovotestis	+/–	Female or ambiguous	
SOX9	AD	Dysgenetic testis or ovotestis	+/–	Female or ambiguous	Campomelic dysplasia
DHH	AR	Dysgenetic testis	+	Female	Minifascicular neuropathy
ATRX	X	Dysgenetic testis	–	Female or ambiguous	α-Thalassemia, developmental delay
ARX	X	Dysgenetic testis	–	Male or ambiguous	Mental retardation; X-linked lissencephaly
DAX1	dupXp21	Dysgenetic testis	+/–	Female or ambiguous	
WNT4	dup1p35	Dysgenetic testis	+	Ambiguous	
Disorders of Androgen Synthesis					
LHR	AR	Testis	–	Female, ambiguous or micropenis	Leydig cell hypoplasia
DHCR7	AR	Testis	–	Variable	Smith-Lemli-Opitz syndrome: coarse facies, second-third toe syndactyly, failure to thrive, developmental delay, cardiac and visceral abnormalities
StAR	AR	Testis	–	Female or ambiguous	Congenital lipoid adrenal hyperplasia (primary adrenal failure)
CYP11A1	AR	Testis	–	Ambiguous	Primary adrenal failure
HSD3B2	AR	Testis	–	Ambiguous	CAH, primary adrenal failure, partial androgenization due to ↑ DHEA
CYP17	AR	Testis	–	Female or ambiguous	CAH, hypertension due to ↑ corticosterone and 11-deoxycorticosterone, except in isolated 17,20-lyase deficiency
POR	AR	Testis	–	Ambiguous or male	Mixed features of 21-hydroxylase deficiency and 17α-hydroxylase/17, 20-lyase deficiency, sometimes associated with Antley-Bixler craniosynostosis
HSD17B3	AR	Testis	–	Female or ambiguous	Partial androgenization at puberty, ↑ androstenedione/testosterone ratio
SRD5A2	AR	Testis	–	Ambiguous or micropenis	Partial androgenization at puberty, ↑ testosterone/dihydrotestosterone ratio
Disorders of Androgen Action					
Androgen receptor	X	Testis	–	Female, ambiguous, micropenis or normal male	Phenotypic spectrum from complete androgen insensitivity syndrome (female external genitalia) and partial androgen insensitivity (ambiguous) to normal male genitalia and infertility

Note: DSD, disorder of sex development; AR, autosomal recessive; AD, autosomal dominant; *WT1*, Wilms' tumor–related gene 1; WAGR, Wilms' tumor, aniridia, genitourinary anomalies, and mental retardation; *SF1*, steroidogenic factor 1; *SRY*, sex-related gene on the Y chromosome; *SOX9*, *SRY*-related HMG-box gene 9; *DHH*, desert hedgehog; *ATRX*, α-thalassemia, mental retardation on the X chromosome; *ARX*, aristaless related homeobox, X-linked; *DAX1*, dosage-sensitive sex reversal, adrenal hypoplasia congenita on the X chromosome, gene 1; *WNT4*, wingless-type mouse mammary tumor virus integration site, 4; *LHR*, LH receptor; *DHCR7*, sterol 7δ reductase; *StAR*, steroidogenic acute regulatory protein; *CYP11A1*, P450 cholesterol side chain cleavage; *HSD3B2*, 3β-hydroxysteroid dehydrogenase type 2; *CYP17*, 17α-hydroxylase and 17,20-lyase; *POR*, P450 oxidoreductase deficiency; *HSD17B3*, 17β-hydroxysteroid dehydrogenase type 3; *SRD5A2*, 5α-reductase type 2.

may be present, reflecting additional functional roles for these genes. For example, renal dysfunction occurs in patients with specific *WT1* mutations (Denys-Drash and Frasier syndromes), primary adrenal failure occurs with some patients with *SF1* mutations, and severe cartilage abnormalities (campomelic dysplasia) are the predominant clinical feature of *SOX9* mutations. Dysgenetic testes should be removed to prevent malignancy, and estrogens can be used to induce secondary sex characteristics in 46,XY individuals raised as females. *Absent (vanishing) testis syndrome (bilateral anorchia)* reflects regression of the testis during development. The etiology is unknown, but the absence of müllerian structures indicates adequate secretion of MIS in utero. Early testicular regression causes impaired androgenization in utero and, in most cases, androgenization of the external genitalia is either normal or slightly impaired (e.g., micropenis, hypospadias). These individuals can be offered testicular prostheses and should receive androgen replacement in adolescence.

Disorders of Androgen Synthesis

Defects in the pathway that regulates androgen synthesis (Fig. 7-4) cause underandrogenization of the male fetus (Table 7-3). Müllerian regression is unaffected because Sertoli cell function is preserved.

LH Receptor

Mutations in the LH receptor cause Leydig cell hypoplasia and androgen deficiency. Defects of LH receptor synthesis or function preclude human chorionic gonadotropin (hCG) stimulation of Leydig cells in utero, as well as LH stimulation of Leydig cells late in gestation and during the neonatal period. As a result, testosterone and DHT synthesis are insufficient for normal androgenization of the internal and external genitalia, causing a spectrum of phenotypes that range from complete underandrogenization to micropenis, depending on the severity of the mutation.

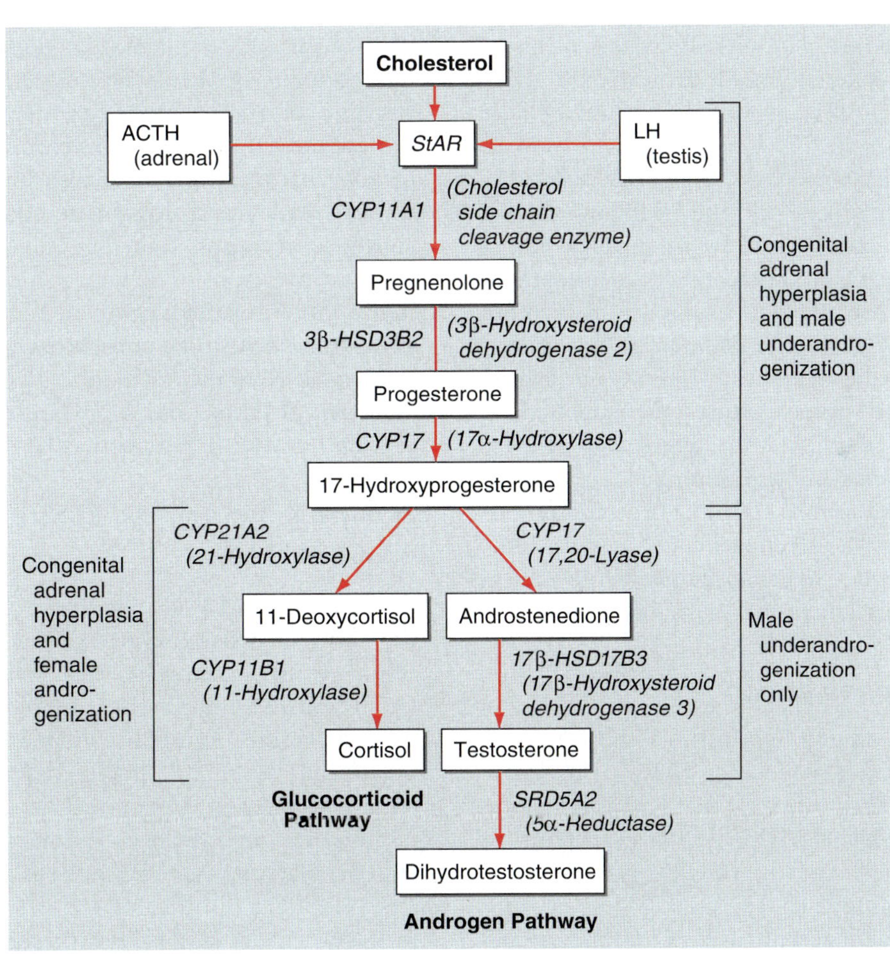

FIGURE 7-4

Simplified overview of glucocorticoid and androgen synthesis pathways. Defects in CYP21A2 and CYP11B1 shunt steroid precursors into the androgen pathway and cause androgenization of 46,XX females. Testosterone and dihydrotestosterone are synthesized in the testicular Leydig cells. Defects in enzymes involved in androgen synthesis result in underandrogenization of 46,XY males. StAR, steroidogenic acute regulatory protein. [*After JD Wilson, JE Griffin, in E Braunwald et al (eds): Harrison's Principles of Internal Medicine, 15th ed. New York, McGraw-Hill, 2001.*]

Steroidogenic Enzyme Pathways

Mutations in *steroidogenic acute regulatory protein* (*StAR*) and *CYP11A1* affect both adrenal and gonadal steroidogenesis (Chap. 5). Affected individuals (46,XY) usually have severe early-onset salt-losing adrenal failure and a female phenotype. Defects in *3β-hydroxysteroid dehydrogenase type 2* (*HSD3B2*) also cause adrenal insufficiency in severe cases, but the accumulation of dehydroepiandrosterone (DHEA) has a mild androgenizing effect resulting in ambiguous genitalia or hypospadias. Patients with congenital adrenal hyperplasia due to *17α-hydroxylase* (*CYP17*) *deficiency* have variable underandrogenization and develop hypertension and hypokalemia due to the potent salt-retaining effects of corticosterone and 11-deoxycorticosterone. Patients with complete loss of *17α-hydroxylase* function often present as phenotypic females who fail to enter puberty and are found to have inguinal testes and hypertension in adolescence. Some mutations in *CYP17* selectively impair 17,20-lyase activity, without altering 17α-hydroxylase activity, leading to underandrogenization without mineralocorticoid excess and hypertension. Mutations in *P450 oxidoreductase* (*POR*) affect multiple steroidogenic enzymes leading to impaired androgenization and a biochemical pattern of apparent combined 21-hydroxylase and 17α-hydroxylase deficiency, sometimes with skeletal abnormalities (Antley-Bixler craniosynostosis). Defects in *17β-hydroxysteroid dehydrogenase type 3* (*HSD17B3*) and *5α-reductase type 2* (*SRD5A2*) interfere with the synthesis of testosterone and DHT, respectively. These conditions are characterized by minimal or absent androgenization in utero, but some phallic development can occur during adolescence due to the action of other enzyme isoforms. Individuals with *5α-reductase type 2* deficiency have normal wolffian structures and do not usually develop breast tissue. In some cultures, these individuals change gender role behavior from female to male at puberty, because the increase in testosterone induces muscle mass and other virilizing features. DHT cream can improve prepubertal phallic growth in patients raised as male. Individuals raised as female require gonadectomy before adolescence and estrogen replacement at puberty.

Disorders of Androgen Action

Androgen Insensitivity Syndrome

Mutations in the androgen receptor (AR) cause resistance to androgen (testosterone, DHT) action or the *androgen insensitivity syndrome* (AIS). AIS is a spectrum of disorders that affects at least 1 in 100,000 chromosomal males. Because the androgen receptor is X-linked, only males are affected and maternal carriers are phenotypically normal. XY individuals with *complete AIS (formerly called testicular feminization syndrome)* have a female phenotype, normal breast development (due to aromatization of testosterone), a short vagina but no uterus (because MIS production is normal), scanty pubic and axillary hair, and female psychosexual orientation. Gonadotropins and testosterone levels can be low, normal, or elevated, depending on the degree of androgen resistance and the contribution of estradiol to feedback inhibition of the hypothalamic-pituitary gonadal axis. Most patients present with inguinal herniae (containing testes) in childhood or with primary amenorrhea in adulthood. Gonadectomy is usually performed, as there is a low risk of malignancy, and estrogen replacement is prescribed. Alternatively, the gonads can be left in situ until breast development is complete. The use of graded dilators in adolescence is usually sufficient to dilate the vagina and permit sexual intercourse.

Partial AIS (*Reifenstein syndrome*) results from less severe AR mutations. Patients often present in infancy with perineoscrotal hypospadias and small undescended testes, and with gynecomastia at the time of puberty. Those individuals raised as males require hypospadias repair in childhood and breast reduction in adolescence. Supplemental testosterone rarely enhances androgenization significantly, as endogenous testosterone is already increased. More severely underandrogenized patients present with clitoral enlargement and labial fusion and may be raised as females. The surgical and psychosexual management of these patients is complex and requires active involvement of the parents and the patient during the appropriate stages of development. *Azoospermia* and male-factor infertility have also been described in association with mild loss-of-function mutations in the androgen receptor. Trinucleotide (CAG) repeat expansion, from a mean of 22 repeats to >40 repeats, within a highly polymorphic region of the androgen receptor is associated with spinal and bulbar muscular atrophy (also known as Kennedy disease). These patients may show evidence of partial androgen insensitivity in adolescence or adulthood (e.g., gynecomastia).

OTHER DISORDERS AFFECTING 46,XY MALES

Persistent müllerian duct syndrome is the presence of a uterus in an otherwise normal male. This condition can result from mutations in AMH or its receptor (AMHR2). The uterus may be removed, but damage to vasa deferentia must be avoided. *Isolated hypospadias* occurs in ~1 in 200 males and is treated by surgical repair. Most cases are idiopathic, although evidence of penoscrotal hypospadias, poor phallic development, and/or bilateral cryptorchidism requires investigation for an underlying disorder of sex development (e.g., defect in testosterone action). Unilateral undescended testes (cryptorchidism) affects more than 3% of boys at birth. Orchidopexy should be considered if the testis has not descended by 6–12 months of age. Bilateral cryptorchidism occurs less frequently and should raise suspicion of gonadotropin deficiency or DSD. A subset of patients with cryptorchidism have mutations in the insulin-like 3 (*INSL3*) gene or its receptor LGR8 (also known as *GREAT*), which mediates normal testicular descent. Ascending testis is being increasingly recognized as a distinct condition for which management is currently unclear. *Syndromic associations* and *intrauterine growth retardation* also occur relatively frequently in association with impaired testicular function or target-tissue responsiveness, but the underlying etiology of many of these conditions is unknown.

46,XX DSD (ANDROGENIZED FEMALES)

Inappropriate androgenization of females (formerly called *female pseudohermaphroditism*) occurs when the gonad (ovary) contains androgen-secreting testicular material or after increased androgen exposure (Table 7-4).

Gonadal Transdifferentiation

Testicular tissue can develop in 46,XX testicular DSD (46,XX males) following translocation of *SRY* or duplication of *SOX9* or defects in *RSPO1* (Table 7-5).

TABLE 7-4

DISORDERS CAUSING ANDROGENIZATION IN KARYOTYPIC FEMALES (46,XX DSD)

Ovarian transdifferentiation
True hermaphroditism (46,XX)
XX male (46,XX testicular DSD)
Increased androgen synthesis
3β-Hydroxysteroid dehydrogenase 2 (*HSD3B2*) deficiency (mild)
21-Hydroxylase (*CYP21A2*) deficiency
P450 oxidoreductase (*POR*) deficiency
11β-Hydroxylase (*CYP11B1*) deficiency
Aromatase (*CYP19*) deficiency
Glucocorticoid receptor mutations
Increased androgen exposure
Maternal virilizing tumors (e.g., luteomas of pregnancy)
Androgenic drugs
Nonvirilizing disorders of the female reproductive tract
Ovarian dysgenesis
Müllerian agenesis
Vaginal agenesis

Note: DSD, disorder of sex development.

TABLE 7-5

GENETIC CAUSES OF ANDROGENIZATION OF KARYOTYPIC FEMALES (46,XX DSD)

GENE	INHERITANCE	GONAD	UTERUS	EXTERNAL GENITALIA	ASSOCIATED FEATURES
Ovarian Transdifferentiation					
SRY	Translocation	Testis or ovotestis	–	Male or ambiguous	
SOX9	dup17q24	Unknown	–	Male or ambiguous	
RSPO1	AR	Testis or ovotestis	±	Male or ambiguous	Palmar-plantar hyperkeratosis, squamous cell skin carcinoma
Increased Androgen Synthesis					
HSD3B2	AR	Ovary	+	Clitoromegaly	CAH, primary adrenal failure, mild androgenization due to ↑ DHEA
CYP21A2	AR	Ovary	+	Ambiguous	CAH, phenotypic spectrum from severe salt-losing forms associated with adrenal failure to simple virilizing forms with compensated adrenal function, ↑ 17-hydroxyprogesterone
POR	AR	Ovary	+	Ambiguous or female	Mixed features of 21-hydroxylase deficiency and 17α-hydroxylase/17, 20-lyase deficiency, sometimes associated with Antley-Bixler craniosynostosis
CYP11B1	AR	Ovary	+	Ambiguous	CAH, hypertension due to ↑ 11-deoxycortisol and 11-deoxycorticosterone
CYP19	AR	Ovary	+	Ambiguous	Maternal virilization during pregnancy, absent breast development at puberty
Glucocorticoid receptor	AR	Ovary	+	Ambiguous	↑ ACTH, 17-hydroxyprogesterone and cortisol; failure of dexamethasone suppression

Note: DSD, disorder of sex development; AR, autosomal recessive; *SRY*, sex-related gene on the Y chromosome; *SOX9, SRY*-related HMG-box gene 9; CAH, congenital adrenal hyperplasia; *HSD3B2*, 3β-hydroxysteroid dehydrogenase type 2; *CYP21A2*, 21-hydroxylase; POR, P450 oxidoreductase deficiency; *CYP11B1*, 11β-hydroxylase; *CYP19*, aromatase; ACTH, adrenocorticotropin; *RSPO1*, R-spondin 1.

21-Hydroxylase Deficiency (Congenital Adrenal Hyperplasia)

The *classic form* of 21-hydroxylase deficiency (21-OHD) is the most common cause of CAH (Chap. 5). It has an incidence of between 1 in 10,000 and 15,000 and is the most frequent cause of androgenization in chromosomal 46,XX females (Table 7-5). Affected individuals are homozygous or compound heterozygous for severe mutations in the enzyme 21-hydroxylase (*CYP21A2*). This mutation causes a block in adrenal glucocorticoid and mineralocorticoid synthesis, increasing 17-hydroxyprogesterone and shunting steroid precursors into the androgen synthesis pathway (Fig. 7-4). Glucocorticoid insufficiency causes a compensatory elevation of adrenocorticotropic hormone (ACTH), resulting in adrenal hyperplasia and additional synthesis of steroid precursors proximal to the enzymatic block. Increased androgen synthesis in utero causes androgenization of the female fetus in the first trimester. Ambiguous genitalia are seen at birth, with varying degrees of clitoral enlargement and labial fusion. Excess androgen production causes gonadotropin-independent precocious puberty in males with 21-OHD.

The *salt-wasting* form of 21-OHD results from severe combined glucocorticoid and mineralocorticoid deficiency. A salt-wasting crisis usually manifests between 7 and 21 days of life and is a potentially life-threatening event requiring urgent fluid resuscitation and steroid treatment. Thus, a diagnosis of 21-OHD should be considered in any baby with ambiguous genitalia with bilateral nonpalpable gonads. Males (46,XY) with 21-OHD have no genital abnormalities at birth but are equally susceptible to adrenal insufficiency and salt-losing crises.

Females with the *classic simple virilizing* form of 21-OHD also present with genital ambiguity. They have impaired cortisol biosynthesis but do not develop salt loss. Patients with *nonclassic 21-OHD* produce normal amounts of cortisol and aldosterone, but at the expense of producing excess androgens. Hirsutism (60%), oligomenorrhea (50%), and acne (30%) are the most frequent presenting features. This is one of the most frequent recessive disorders in humans, with an incidence as high as 1 in 100–500 in many populations and 1 in 27 in Ashkenazi Jews of Eastern European origin.

Biochemical features of acute salt-wasting 21-OHD are hypoglycemia, hyponatremia, hyperkalemia, low cortisol and aldosterone, and elevated 17-hydroxyprogesterone, ACTH, and plasma renin activity. Presymptomatic diagnosis of classic 21-OHD is now made by neonatal screening tests for increased 17-hydroxyprogesterone in many centers. In most cases, 17-hydroxyprogesterone is markedly increased. In adults, ACTH stimulation (0.25 mg cosyntropin IV) with assays for 17-hydroxyprogesterone at 0 and 30 min can be useful for detecting nonclassic 21-OHD and heterozygotes (Chap. 5).

℞ Treatment: CONGENITAL ADRENAL HYPERPLASIA

Acute salt-wasting crises require fluid resuscitation, IV hydrocortisone, and correction of hypoglycemia. Once stabilized, glucocorticoids must be given to correct the cortisol insufficiency and to suppress ACTH stimulation, thereby preventing further virilization, rapid skeletal maturation, and the development of polycystic ovaries. Typically, hydrocortisone (10–20 mg/m^2 per d in three divided doses) is used with a goal of partially suppressing 17-hydroxyprogesterone (100–<1000 ng/dL). The aim of treatment is to use the lowest glucocorticoid dose that adequately suppresses adrenal androgen production without causing signs of glucocorticoid excess, such as impaired growth and obesity. Salt-wasting conditions are treated with mineralocorticoid replacement. Infants usually need salt supplements up to the first year of life. Plasma renin activity and electrolytes are used to monitor mineralocorticoid replacement. Some patients with simple virilizing 21-OHD also benefit from mineralocorticoid supplements. Newer therapeutic approaches, such as antiandrogens and aromatase inhibitors (to block premature epiphyseal closure), are under evaluation. Parents and patients should be aware of the need for increased doses of steroids during sickness, and patients should carry medic alert systems.

Older adolescents and adults are often treated with prednisolone, or dexamethasone at night, to provide more complete ACTH suppression. Steroid doses should be adjusted to individual requirements as overtreatment results in weight gain and hypertension and can affect bone turnover. Androstenedione and testosterone may be useful measurements of long-term control with less fluctuation than 17-hydroxyprogesterone. Mineralocorticoid requirements often decrease in adulthood, and doses should be reduced to avoid hypertension. In very severe cases, adrenalectomy has been advocated but incurs the risks of major surgery and total adrenal insufficiency.

Girls with significant genital androgenization due to classic 21-OHD usually undergo vaginal reconstruction and clitoral reduction (maintaining the glans and nerve supply), but the optimal timing of these procedures is debated. There is a higher threshold for undertaking clitoral surgery in some centers as long-term sensation and ability to achieve orgasm can be affected, but the long-term results of newer techniques are not yet known. If surgery is performed in infancy, surgical revision or regular vaginal dilatation may be needed in adolescence or adulthood, and long-term psychological support and psychosexual counseling may be appropriate. Women with 21-OHD frequently develop polycystic ovaries and have reduced fertility, especially when control is poor. Fecundity is achieved in 50–90% of women, but ovulation induction (or even adrenalectomy) is frequently required.

Dexamethasone should be avoided in pregnancy. Men with poorly controlled 21-OHD may develop testicular adrenal rests and are at risk for reduced fertility. Prenatal treatment of 21-OHD by the administration of dexamethasone to mothers has been shown to reduce the degree of androgenization in affected female fetuses. However, treatment of the mother and child must be started ideally before 6–7 weeks; long-term effects of prenatal dexamethasone exposure on fetal development are still under evaluation.

The treatment of other forms of CAH includes mineralocorticoid and glucocorticoid replacement for salt-losing conditions (e.g., *StAR, CYP11A1, HSD3B2*), suppression of ACTH drive with glucocorticoids in disorders associated with hypertension (e.g., *CYP17, CYP11B1*), and appropriate sex-hormone replacement in adolescence and adulthood, where necessary.

Other Causes

Increased androgen synthesis can also occur in CAH due to defects in *POR*, *11β-hydroxylase* (*CYP11B1*), and *3β-hydroxysteroid dehydrogenase type 2* (*HSD3B2*), and with mutations in the genes encoding *aromatase* (*CYP19*) and the glucocorticoid receptor. Increased androgen exposure in utero can occur with maternal virilizing tumors and with ingestion of androgenic compounds.

OTHER DISORDERS AFFECTING 46,XX FEMALES

Congenital absence of the vagina occurs in association with *müllerian agenesis* or *hypoplasia* as part of the Mayer-Rokitansky-Kuster-Hauser syndrome (*WNT4* mutations). This diagnosis should be considered in otherwise phenotypically normal females with primary amenorrhea. Rarer associated features include renal (agenesis) and cervical spinal abnormalities.

GLOBAL CONSIDERATIONS

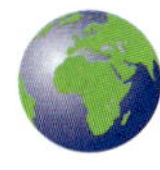

The approach to the child or adolescent with ambiguous genitalia or other DSDs requires cultural sensitivity, as the concepts of sex and gender vary widely. Rare genetic DSDs can occur more frequently in specific populations (e.g., 5β-*reductase type 2* in the Dominican Republic). Different forms of CAH also show ethnic and geographic variability. In many countries, appropriate biochemical tests may not be readily available, and access to appropriate forms of surgery or treatment may be limited.

FURTHER READINGS

Bojesen A, Gravholt CH: Klinefelter syndrome in clinical practice. Nat Clin Pract Urol 4:192, 2007

Bondy CA for the Turner Syndrome Consensus Study Group: Care of girls and women with Turner syndrome: A guideline of the Turner Syndrome Study Group. J Clin Endocrinol Metab 92:10, 2007

Cool J et al: Mixed signals: Development of the testis. Semin Reprod Med 27:5, 2009

Cools M et al: Germ cell tumors in the intersex gonad: Old paths, new directions, moving frontiers. Endocrinol Rev 27:468, 2006

Hiorta O et al: Disorders of sex development in developmental syndromes. Endocr Dev 14:174, 2009

Hughes IA: Disorders of sex development: A new definition and classification. Best Pract Res Clin Endocrinol Metab 22:119, 2008

Lee PA et al: Consensus statement of management of intersex disorders. Pediatrics 118:e488, 2006

MacLaughlin DT, Donahoe PK: Sex determination and differentiation. N Engl J Med 350:367, 2004

Ogilvie CM et al: Congenital adrenal hyperplasia in adults: A review of medical, surgical and psychological issues. Clin Endocrinol 64:2, 2006

Wilson CA, Davies DC: The control of sexual differentiation of the reproductive system and brain. Reproduction 133:331, 2007

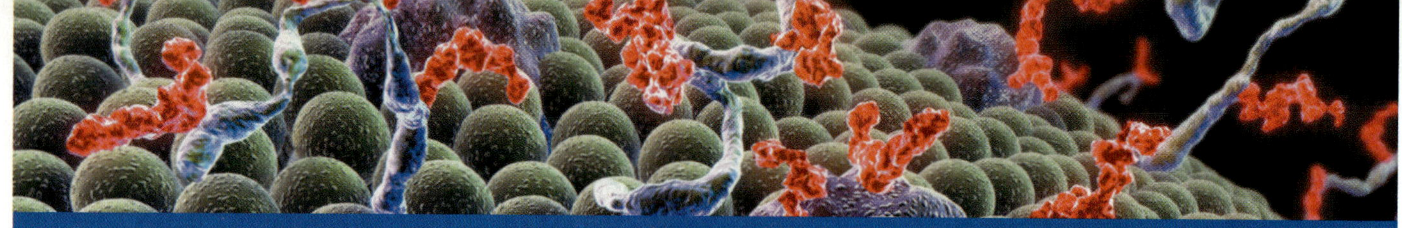

CHAPTER 8

DISORDERS OF THE TESTES AND MALE REPRODUCTIVE SYSTEM

Shalender Bhasin ■ J. Larry Jameson

The male reproductive system regulates sex differentiation, virilization, and the hormonal changes that accompany puberty, ultimately leading to spermatogenesis and fertility. Under the control of the pituitary hormones—luteinizing hormone (LH) and follicle-stimulating hormone (FSH)—the Leydig cells of the testes produce testosterone and germ cells are nurtured by Sertoli cells to divide, differentiate, and mature into sperm. During embryonic development, testosterone and dihydrotestosterone (DHT) induce the wolffian duct and virilization of the external genitalia. During puberty, testosterone promotes somatic growth and the development of secondary sex characteristics. In the adult, testosterone is necessary for spermatogenesis and stimulation of libido and normal sexual function. This chapter focuses on the physiology of the testes and disorders associated with decreased androgen production, which may be caused by gonadotropin deficiency or by primary testis dysfunction. A variety of testosterone formulations now allow more physiologic androgen replacement. Infertility occurs in ~5% of men and is increasingly amenable to treatment by hormone replacement or by using sperm transfer techniques. For further discussion of sexual dysfunction and testicular cancer, see Chaps. 15 and 9, respectively.

DEVELOPMENT AND STRUCTURE OF THE TESTIS

The fetal testis develops from the undifferentiated gonad after expression of a genetic cascade that is initiated by the SRY (sex-related gene on the Y chromosome) (Chap. 7). SRY induces differentiation of Sertoli cells, which surround germ cells and, together with peritubular myoid cells, form testis cords that will later develop into seminiferous tubules. Fetal Leydig cells and endothelial cells migrate into the gonad from the adjacent mesonephros but may also arise from interstitial cells that reside between testis cords. Leydig cells produce testosterone, which supports the growth and differentiation of wolffian duct structures that develop into the epididymis, vas deferens, and seminal vesicles. Testosterone is also converted to DHT, which induces formation of the prostate and the external male genitalia, including the penis, urethra, and scrotum. Testicular descent through the inguinal canal is controlled in part by Leydig cell production of insulin-like factor 3 (INSL3), which acts via a receptor termed *Great* (*G* protein–coupled *re*ceptor *a*ffecting *t*estis descent).

Sertoli cells produce müllerian-inhibiting substance (MIS), which causes regression of the müllerian structures, including the fallopian tube, uterus, and upper segment of the vagina.

NORMAL MALE PUBERTAL DEVELOPMENT

Although *puberty* commonly refers to the maturation of the reproductive axis and the development of secondary sex characteristics, it involves a coordinated response of multiple hormonal systems including the adrenal gland and the growth hormone (GH) axis (**Fig. 8-1**). The development of secondary sex characteristics is initiated by *adrenarche*, which usually occurs between 6 and 8 years of age when the adrenal gland begins to produce greater amounts of androgens from the zona reticularis, the principal site of dehydroepiandrosterone (DHEA) production. The sex maturation process is greatly accelerated by the activation of the hypothalamic-pituitary axis and the production of gonadotropin-releasing hormone (GnRH). The GnRH pulse generator in the hypothalamus is active during fetal life and early infancy but is quiescent until the early stages of puberty, when the sensitivity to steroid inhibition is gradually lost, causing reactivation of GnRH secretion. Although the pathways that initiate reactivation of the GnRH pulse generator have been elusive, mounting evidence supports involvement of GPR54, a G protein–coupled receptor that binds an endogenous ligand, metastin. Individuals with mutations of GPR54 fail to enter puberty, and experiments in primates demonstrate that infusion of the ligand is sufficient to induce premature puberty. Leptin, a hormone produced by adipose cells, may play a permissive role in the onset of puberty, as leptin-deficient individuals also fail to enter puberty (Chap. 16).

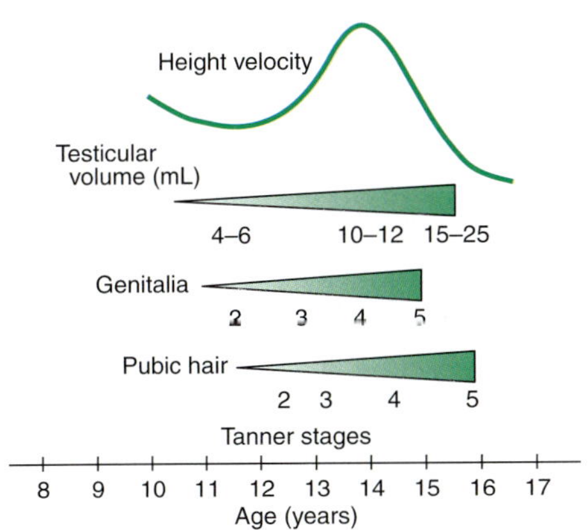

FIGURE 8-1

Pubertal events in males. Sexual maturity ratings for genitalia and pubic hair and divided into five stages. (*From WA Marshall, JM Tanner: Variations in the pattern of pubertal changes in boys. Arch Dis Child 45:13, 1970.*)

The early stages of puberty are characterized by nocturnal surges of LH and FSH. Growth of the testes is usually the first sign of puberty, reflecting an increase in seminiferous tubule volume. Increasing levels of testosterone deepen the voice and increase muscle growth. Conversion of testosterone to DHT leads to growth of the external genitalia and pubic hair. DHT also stimulates prostate and facial hair growth and initiates recession of the temporal hairline. The growth spurt occurs at a testicular volume of about 10–12 mL. GH increases early in puberty and is stimulated in part by the rise in gonadal steroids. GH increases the level of insulin-like growth factor I (IGF-I), which enhances linear bone growth. The prolonged pubertal exposure to gonadal steroids (mainly estradiol) ultimately causes epiphyseal closure and limits further bone growth.

REGULATION OF TESTICULAR FUNCTION

REGULATION OF THE HYPOTHALAMIC-PITUITARY-TESTIS AXIS IN ADULT MAN

Hypothalamic GnRH regulates the production of the pituitary gonadotropins, LH and FSH (**Fig. 8-2**). GnRH is released in discrete pulses approximately every 2 h, resulting in corresponding pulses of LH and FSH. These dynamic hormone pulses account in part for the wide variations in LH and testosterone, even within the same individual. LH acts primarily on the Leydig cell to stimulate testosterone synthesis. The regulatory control of androgen synthesis is mediated by testosterone and estrogen feedback on both the hypothalamus and the pituitary. FSH acts on the Sertoli cell to regulate spermatogenesis and the production of Sertoli products such as inhibin B, which acts to selectively suppress pituitary FSH. Despite these somewhat distinct Leydig and Sertoli cell–regulated pathways, testis function is integrated at several levels: GnRH regulates both gonadotropins; spermatogenesis requires high levels of testosterone; and numerous paracrine interactions between Leydig and Sertoli cells are necessary for normal testis function.

THE LEYDIG CELL: ANDROGEN SYNTHESIS

LH binds to its seven transmembrane, G protein–coupled receptor to activate the cyclic AMP pathway. Stimulation of the LH receptor induces *s*teroid *a*cute *r*egulatory (StAR) protein, along with several steroidogenic enzymes involved in androgen synthesis. LH receptor mutations cause Leydig cell hypoplasia or agenesis, underscoring the importance of this pathway for Leydig cell development and function. The rate-limiting process in testosterone synthesis is the delivery of cholesterol by the StAR protein to the inner mitochondrial membrane. Peripheral benzodiazepine receptor, a mitochondrial cholesterol-binding

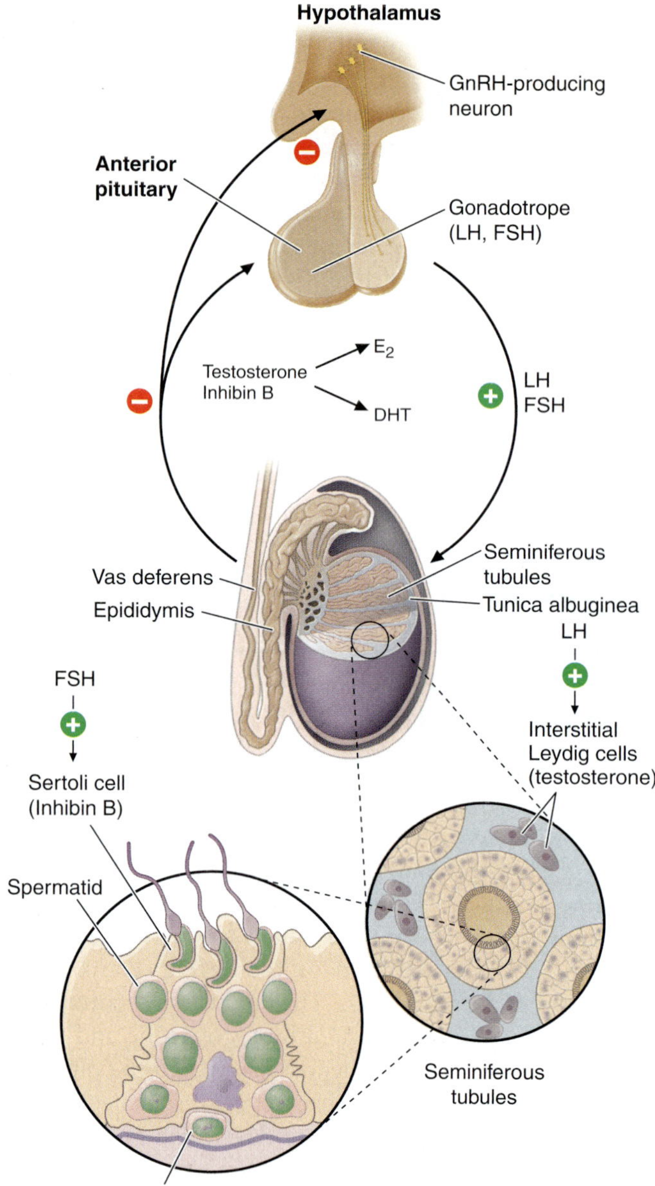

FIGURE 8-2

Human pituitary gonadotropin axis, structure of testis, seminiferous tubule. E_2, 17β-estradiol; DHT, dihydrotestosterone.

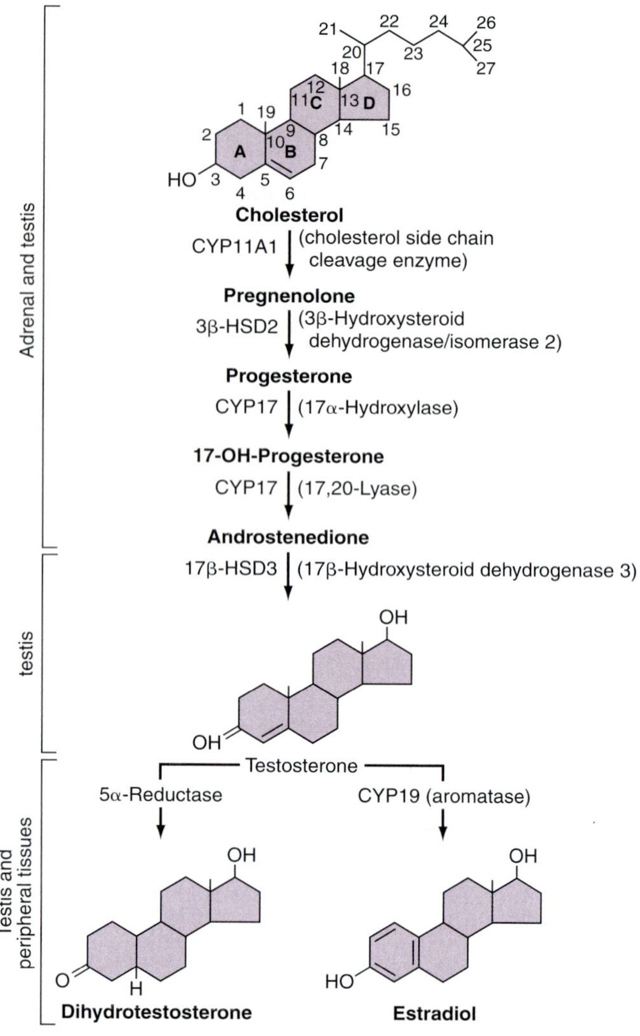

FIGURE 8-3

The biochemical pathway in the conversion of 27-carbon sterol cholesterol to androgens and estrogens.

protein, is also an acute regulator of Leydig cell steroidogenesis. The five major enzymatic steps involved in testosterone synthesis are summarized in Fig. 8-3. After cholesterol transport into the mitochondrion, the formation of pregnenolone by CYP11A1 (side chain cleavage enzyme) is a limiting enzymatic step. The 17α-hydroxylase and the 17,20-lyase reactions are catalyzed by a single enzyme, CYP17; posttranslational modification (phosphorylation) of this enzyme and the presence of specific enzyme cofactors confer 17,20-lyase activity selectively in the testis and zona reticularis of the adrenal gland. Testosterone can be converted to the more potent DHT by 5α-reductase, or it can be aromatized to estradiol by CYP19 (aromatase).

Testosterone Transport and Metabolism

In males, 95% of circulating testosterone is derived from testicular production (3–10 mg/d). Direct secretion of testosterone by the adrenal and the peripheral conversion of androstenedione to testosterone collectively account for another 0.5 mg/d of testosterone. Only a small amount of DHT (70 μg/d) is secreted directly by the testis; most circulating DHT is derived from peripheral conversion of testosterone. Most of the daily production of estradiol (approximately 45 μg/d) in men is derived from aromatase-mediated peripheral conversion of testosterone and androstenedione.

Circulating testosterone is bound to two plasma proteins: sex hormone–binding globulin (SHBG) and albumin (Fig. 8-4). SHBG binds testosterone with much greater affinity than albumin. Only 0.5–3% of testosterone is unbound. According to the "free hormone" hypothesis, only the unbound fraction is biologically active; however, albumin-bound hormone dissociates readily in the capillaries

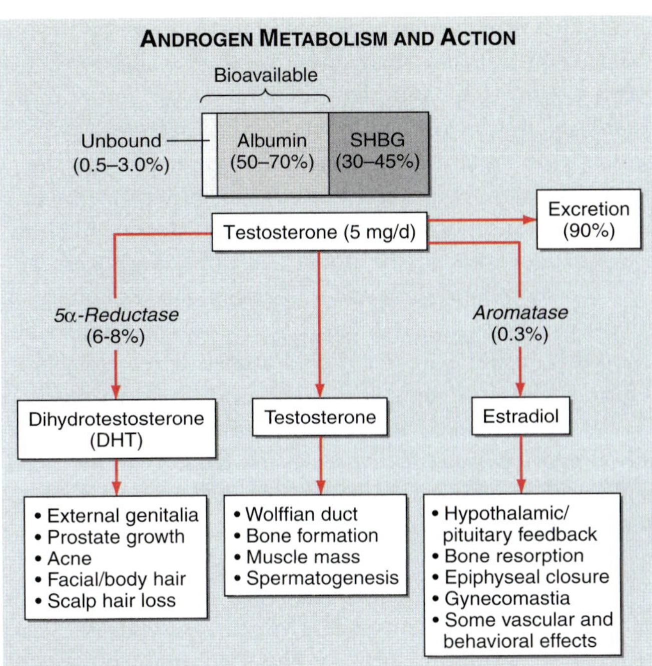

FIGURE 8-4

Androgen metabolism and actions. SHBG, sex hormone–binding globulin.

and may be bioavailable. The finding that SHBG-bound testosterone may be internalized through endocytic pits by binding to a protein called megalin have challenged the "free hormone" hypothesis. SHBG concentrations are decreased by androgens, obesity, insulin, and nephrotic syndrome. Conversely, estrogen administration, hyperthyroidism, many chronic inflammatory illnesses, and aging are associated with high SHBG concentrations.

Testosterone is metabolized predominantly in the liver, although some degradation occurs in peripheral tissues, particularly the prostate and the skin. In the liver, testosterone is converted by a series of enzymatic steps that involve 5α- and 5β-reductases, 3α- and 3β-hydroxysteroid dehydrogenases, and 17β-hydroxysteroid dehydrogenase into androsterone, etiocholanolone, DHT, and 3α-androstanediol. These compounds undergo glucuronidation or sulfation before being excreted by the kidneys.

Mechanism of Androgen Action

The androgen receptor (AR) is structurally related to the nuclear receptors for estrogen, glucocorticoids, and progesterone (Chap. 1). The AR is encoded by a gene on the long arm of the X chromosome and has a molecular mass of about 110 kDa. A polymorphic region in the amino terminus of the receptor, which contains a variable number of glutamine repeats, modifies the transcriptional activity of the receptor. The AR protein is distributed in both the cytoplasm and the nucleus. Androgen binding to the AR causes it to translocate into the nucleus, where it binds to DNA or other transcription factors already bound to DNA. The ligand also induces conformational changes that allow the recruitment and assembly of tissue-specific cofactors. Thus, the AR is a ligand-regulated transcription factor. Some androgen effects may be mediated by nongenomic AR signal transduction pathways. Testosterone binds to AR with half the affinity of DHT. The DHT-AR complex also has greater thermostability and a slower dissociation rate than the testosterone-AR complex. However, the molecular basis for selective testosterone versus DHT actions remains incompletely explained.

THE SEMINIFEROUS TUBULES: SPERMATOGENESIS

The seminiferous tubules are convoluted, closed loops with both ends emptying into the rete testis, a network of progressively larger efferent ducts that ultimately form the epididymis (Fig. 8-2). The seminiferous tubules total about 600 m in length and comprise about two-thirds of testis volume. The walls of the tubules are formed by polarized Sertoli cells that are apposed to peritubular myoid cells. Tight junctions between Sertoli cells create a blood-testis barrier. Germ cells comprise the majority of the seminiferous epithelium (~60%) and are intimately embedded within the cytoplasmic extensions of the Sertoli cells, which function as "nurse cells." Germ cells progress through characteristic stages of mitotic and meiotic divisions. A pool of type A spermatogonia serve as stem cells capable of self-renewal. Primary spermatocytes are derived from type B spermatogonia and undergo meiosis before progressing to spermatids that undergo spermiogenesis (a differentiation process involving chromatin condensation, acquisition of an acrosome, elongation of cytoplasm, and formation of a tail) and are released from Sertoli cells as mature spermatozoa. The complete differentiation process into mature sperm requires 74 days. Peristaltic-type action by peritubular myoid cells transports sperm into the efferent ducts. The spermatozoa spend an additional 21 days in the epididymis, where they undergo further maturation and capacitation. The normal adult testes produce >100 million sperm per day.

Naturally occurring mutations in the *FSH*β gene and in the FSH receptor confirm an important, but not essential, role for this pathway in spermatogenesis. Females with these mutations are hypogonadal and infertile because ovarian follicles do not mature; males exhibit variable degrees of reduced spermatogenesis, presumably because of impaired Sertoli cell function. Because Sertoli cells produce inhibin B, an inhibitor of FSH, seminiferous tubule damage (e.g., by radiation) causes a selective increase of FSH. Testosterone reaches very high concentrations locally in the testis and is essential for spermatogenesis. Several cytokines and growth factors are also involved in the regulation of spermatogenesis by paracrine and autocrine mechanisms. A number of knockout mouse models exhibit impaired germ cell development or spermatogenesis, presaging possible mutations associated with male infertility. The human Y chromosome contains a small pseudoautosomal region that can recombine with homologous regions of the X chromosome. Most of the Y chromosome does not recombine with the X chromosome and is referred to as the male-specific region of the Y (MSY). The MSY contains 156 transcription units that encode for 26 proteins, including nine families of Y-specific multicopy genes; many of these Y-specific genes are also testis-specific and necessary for spermatogenesis. Microdeletions of several Y chromosome azoospermia factor (*AZF*) genes (e.g., RNA-binding motif, *RBM*; deleted in azoospermia, *DAZ*) are associated with oligospermia or azoospermia.

Rx Treatment: MALE FACTOR INFERTILITY

Treatment options for male factor infertility have expanded greatly in recent years. Secondary hypogonadism is highly amenable to treatment with pulsatile GnRH or gonadotropins (see below). In vitro techniques have provided new opportunities for patients with primary testicular failure and disorders of sperm transport. Choice of initial treatment options depends on sperm concentration and motility. Expectant management should be attempted initially in men with mild male factor infertility (sperm count of 15–20 × 10^6/mL and normal motility). Moderate male factor infertility (10–15 × 10^6/mL and 20–40% motility) should begin with intrauterine insemination alone or in combination with treatment of the female partner with clomiphene or gonadotropins, but it may require in vitro fertilization (IVF) with or without intracytoplasmic sperm injection (ICSI). For men with a severe defect (sperm count of <10 × 10^6/mL, 10% motility), IVF with ICSI or donor sperm should be used.

CLINICAL AND LABORATORY EVALUATION OF MALE REPRODUCTIVE FUNCTION

HISTORY AND PHYSICAL EXAMINATION

The history should focus on developmental stages such as puberty and growth spurts, as well as androgen-dependent events such as early morning erections, frequency and intensity of sexual thoughts, and frequency of masturbation or intercourse. Although libido and the overall frequency of sexual acts are decreased in androgen-deficient men, young hypogonadal men may achieve erections in response to visual erotic stimuli. Men with acquired androgen deficiency often report decreased energy and increased irritability.

The physical examination should focus on secondary sex characteristics such as hair growth, gynecomastia, testicular volume, prostate, and height and body proportions. *Eunuchoid proportions* are defined as an arm span >2 cm greater than height and suggest that androgen deficiency occurred before epiphyseal fusion. Hair growth in the face, axilla, chest, and pubic regions is androgen-dependent; however, changes may not be noticeable unless androgen deficiency is severe and prolonged. Ethnicity also influences the intensity of hair growth (Chap. 13). Testicular volume is best assessed by using a Prader orchidometer. Testes range from 3.5 to 5.5 cm in length, which corresponds to a volume of 12–25 mL. Advanced age does not influence testicular size, although the consistency becomes less firm. Asian men generally have smaller testes than western Europeans, independent of differences in body size. Because of its possible role in infertility, the presence of varicocele should be sought by palpation while the patient is standing; it is more common on the left side. Patients with Klinefelter syndrome have markedly reduced testicular volumes (1–2 mL). In congenital hypogonadotropic hypogonadism, testicular volumes provide a good index for the degree of gonadotropin deficiency and the likelihood of response to therapy.

GONADOTROPIN AND INHIBIN MEASUREMENTS

LH and FSH are measured using two-site immunoradiometric, immunofluorometric, or chemiluminescent assays, which have very low cross-reactivity with other pituitary glycoprotein hormones and human chorionic gonadotropin (hCG) and have sufficient sensitivity to measure the low levels present in patients with hypogonadotropic hypogonadism. In men with a low testosterone level, an LH level can distinguish primary (high LH) versus secondary (low or inappropriately normal LH) hypogonadism. An elevated LH level indicates a primary defect at the testicular level, whereas a low or inappropriately normal LH level suggests a defect at the hypothalamic-pituitary level. LH pulses occur about every 1–3 h in normal men. Thus, gonadotropin levels fluctuate, and samples should be pooled or repeated when results are equivocal. FSH is less pulsatile than LH because it has a longer half-life. Increased FSH suggests damage to the seminiferous tubules. Inhibin B, a Sertoli cell product that suppresses FSH, is reduced with seminiferous tubule damage. Inhibin B is a dimer with α-β_B subunits and is measured by two-site immunoassays.

GnRH Stimulation Testing

The GnRH test is performed by measuring LH and FSH concentrations at baseline and at 30 and 60 min after IV administration of 100 μg of GnRH. A minimally acceptable response is a twofold LH increase and a 50% FSH increase. In the prepubertal period or with severe GnRH deficiency, the gonadotrope may not respond to a single bolus of GnRH because it has not been primed by endogenous hypothalamic GnRH; in these patients, GnRH responsiveness may be restored by chronic, pulsatile GnRH administration. With the availability of sensitive and specific LH assays, GnRH stimulation testing is used rarely except to evaluate gonadotrope function in patients who have undergone pituitary surgery or have a space-occupying lesion in the hypothalamic-pituitary region.

TESTOSTERONE ASSAYS

Total Testosterone

Total testosterone includes both unbound and protein-bound testosterone and is measured by radioimmunoassays, immunometric assays, or liquid chromatography tandem mass spectrometry (LC-MS/MS). LC-MS/MS involves extraction of serum by organic solvents, separation of testosterone from other steroids by high-performance liquid chromatography and mass spectrometry, and quantitation of unique testosterone fragments by mass spectrometry. LC-MS/MS provides accurate and sensitive measurements of testosterone levels even in the low range and is emerging as the method of choice for testosterone measurement. A single random sample provides a good approximation of the average testosterone concentration with the realization that testosterone levels fluctuate in response to pulsatile LH. Testosterone is generally lower in the late afternoon and is reduced by acute illness. The testosterone concentration in healthy young men ranges from 300 to 1000 ng/dL in most laboratories, although these reference ranges are not derived from population-based random samples. Alterations in SHBG levels due to aging, obesity, some types of medications, or chronic illness, or on a congenital basis, can affect total testosterone levels.

Measurement of Unbound Testosterone Levels

Most circulating testosterone is bound to SHBG and to albumin; only 0.5–3% of circulating testosterone is unbound, or "free." The unbound testosterone concentration can be measured by equilibrium dialysis or calculated from total testosterone, SHBG, and albumin concentrations by using published mass-action equations. Tracer analogue methods are relatively inexpensive and convenient, but they are inaccurate. *Bioavailable testosterone* refers to unbound testosterone plus testosterone that is loosely bound to albumin; it can be estimated by the ammonium sulfate precipitation method.

hCG Stimulation Test

The hCG stimulation test is performed by administering a single injection of 1500–4000 IU of hCG IM and measuring testosterone levels at baseline and 24, 48, 72, and 120 h after hCG injection. An alternative regimen involves three injections of 1500 units of hCG on successive days and measuring testosterone levels 24 h after the last dose. An acceptable response to hCG is a doubling of the testosterone concentration in adult men. In prepubertal boys, an increase in testosterone to >150 ng/dL indicates the presence of testicular tissue. No response may indicate an absence of testicular tissue or marked impairment of Leydig cell function. Measurement of MIS, a Sertoli cell product, is also used to detect the presence of testes in prepubertal boys with cryptorchidism.

SEMEN ANALYSIS

Semen analysis is the most important step in the evaluation of male infertility. Samples are collected by masturbation following a period of abstinence for 2–3 days. Semen volumes and sperm concentrations vary considerably among fertile men, and several samples may be needed before concluding that the results are abnormal. Analysis should be performed within an hour of collection. The normal ejaculate volume is 2–6 mL and contains sperm counts of >20 million/mL, with a motility of >50% and >15% normal morphology. Some men with low sperm counts are nevertheless fertile. A variety of tests for sperm function can be performed in specialized laboratories, but these add relatively little to the treatment options.

TESTICULAR BIOPSY

Testicular biopsy is useful in some patients with oligospermia or azoospermia as an aid in diagnosis and indication for the feasibility of treatment. Using local anesthesia, fine-needle aspiration biopsy is performed to aspirate tissue for histology. Alternatively, open biopsies can be performed under local or general anesthesia when more tissue is required. A normal biopsy in an azoospermic man with a normal FSH level suggests obstruction of the vas deferens, which may be correctable surgically. Biopsies are also used to harvest sperm for ICSI and to classify disorders such as hypospermatogenesis (all stages present but in reduced numbers), germ cell arrest (usually at primary spermatocyte stage), and Sertoli cell–only syndrome (absent germ cells) or hyalinization (sclerosis with absent cellular elements).

DISORDERS OF SEXUAL DIFFERENTIATION

See Chap. 7.

DISORDERS OF PUBERTY

PRECOCIOUS PUBERTY

Puberty in boys before age 9 is considered precocious. *Isosexual precocity* refers to premature sexual development consistent with phenotypic sex and includes features such as the development of facial hair and phallic growth. Isosexual precocity is divided into gonadotropin-dependent and gonadotropin-independent causes of androgen excess (Table 8-1). *Heterosexual precocity* refers to the premature development of estrogenic features in boys, such as breast development.

Gonadotropin-Dependent Precocious Puberty

This disorder, called *central precocious puberty* (CPP), is less common in boys than in girls. It is caused by premature activation of the GnRH pulse generator, sometimes because of central nervous system (CNS) lesions such as hypothalamic hamartomas, but it is often idiopathic. CPP is characterized by gonadotropin levels that are inappropriately elevated for age. Because pituitary priming has occurred, GnRH elicits LH and FSH responses typical of those seen in puberty or in adults. MRI should be performed to exclude a mass, structural defect, infection, or inflammatory process.

TABLE 8-1

CAUSES OF PRECOCIOUS OR DELAYED PUBERTY IN BOYS

I. Precocious puberty
- A. Gonadotropin-dependent
  - 1. Idiopathic
  - 2. Hypothalamic hamartoma or other lesions
  - 3. CNS tumor or inflammatory state
- B. Gonadotropin-independent
  - 1. Congenital adrenal hyperplasia
  - 2. hCG-secreting tumor
  - 3. McCune-Albright syndrome
  - 4. Activating LH receptor mutation
  - 5. Exogenous androgens

II. Delayed puberty
- A. Constitutional delay of growth and puberty
- B. Systemic disorders
  - 1. Chronic disease
  - 2. Malnutrition
  - 3. Anorexia nervosa
- C. CNS tumors and their treatment (radiotherapy and surgery)
- D. Hypothalamic-pituitary causes of pubertal failure (low gonadotropins)
  - 1. Congenital disorders (Table 8-2)
    - a. Hypothalamic syndromes (e.g., Prader-Willi)
    - b. Idiopathic hypogonadotropic hypogonadism
    - c. Kallmann syndrome
    - d. GnRH receptor mutations
    - e. Adrenal hypoplasia congenita
    - f. PROP1 mutations
    - g. Other mutations affecting pituitary development/function
  - 2. Acquired disorders
    - a. Pituitary tumors
    - b. Hyperprolactinemia
- E. Gonadal causes of pubertal failure (elevated gonadotropins)
  - 1. Klinefelter syndrome
  - 2. Bilateral undescended testes or anorchia
  - 3. Orchitis
  - 4. Chemotherapy or radiotherapy
- F. Androgen insensitivity

Note: CNS, central nervous system; hCG, human chronic gonadotropin; LH, luteinizing hormone; GnRH, gonadotropin-releasing hormone.

Gonadotropin-Independent Precocious Puberty

Androgens from the testis or the adrenal are increased but gonadotropins are low. This group of disorders includes hCG-secreting tumors; congenital adrenal hyperplasia; sex steroid–producing tumors of the testis, adrenal, and ovary; accidental or deliberate exogenous sex steroid administration; hypothyroidism; and activating mutations of the LH receptor or $G_s\alpha$ subunit.

Familial Male-Limited Precocious Puberty

Also called *testotoxicosis*, familial male-limited precocious puberty is an autosomal dominant disorder caused by activating mutations in the LH receptor, leading to constitutive stimulation of the cyclic AMP pathway and testosterone production. Clinical features include premature androgenization in boys, growth acceleration in early childhood, and advanced bone age followed by premature epiphyseal fusion. Testosterone is elevated, and LH is suppressed. Treatment options include inhibitors of testosterone synthesis (e.g., ketoconazole), androgen receptor antagonists (e.g., flutamide), and aromatase inhibitors (e.g., anastrazole).

McCune-Albright Syndrome

This is a sporadic disorder caused by somatic (postzygotic) activating mutations in the $G_s\alpha$ subunit that links G protein–coupled receptors to intracellular signaling pathways (Chap. 29). The mutations impair the guanosine triphosphatase activity of the $G_s\alpha$ protein, leading to constitutive activation of adenylyl cyclase. Like activating LH receptor mutations, this stimulates testosterone production and causes gonadotropin-independent precocious puberty. In addition to sexual precocity, affected individuals may have autonomy in the adrenals, pituitary, and thyroid glands. Café au lait spots are characteristic skin lesions that reflect the onset of the somatic mutations in melanocytes during embryonic development. Polyostotic fibrous dysplasia is caused by activation of the parathyroid hormone receptor pathway in bone. Treatment is similar to that in patients with activating LH receptor mutations. Bisphosphonates have been used to treat bone lesions.

Congenital Adrenal Hyperplasia

Boys with congenital adrenal hyperplasia (CAH) who are not well controlled with glucocorticoid suppression of adrenocorticotropic hormone (ACTH) can develop premature virilization because of excessive androgen production by the adrenal gland (Chaps. 5 and 7). LH is low, and the testes are small. Rarely, adrenal rests may develop within the testis because of chronic ACTH stimulation.

Heterosexual Sexual Precocity

Breast enlargement in prepubertal boys can result from familial aromatase excess, estrogen-producing tumors in the adrenal gland, Sertoli cell tumors in the testis, marijuana smoking, or exogenous estrogens or androgens. Occasionally, germ cell tumors that secrete hCG can be associated with breast enlargement due to excessive stimulation of estrogen production (see "Gynecomastia" later in the chapter).

Approach to the Patient: PRECOCIOUS PUBERTY

After verification of precocious development, serum LH and FSH levels should be measured to determine whether gonadotropins are increased in relation to chronologic age (gonadotropin-dependent) or whether sex steroid secretion is occurring independent of LH and FSH (gonadotropin-independent). In children with gonadotropin-dependent precocious puberty, CNS lesions should be excluded by history, neurologic examination, and MRI scan of the head. If organic causes are not found, one is left with the diagnosis of idiopathic central precocity. Patients with high testosterone but suppressed LH concentrations have gonadotropin-independent sexual precocity; in these patients, DHEA sulfate (DHEAS) and 17α-hydroxyprogesterone should be measured. High levels of testosterone and 17α-hydroxyprogesterone suggest the possibility of CAH due to 21α-hydroxylase or 11β-hydroxylase deficiency. If testosterone and DHEAS are elevated, adrenal tumors should be excluded by obtaining a CT scan of the adrenal glands. Patients with elevated testosterone but without increased 17α-hydroxyprogesterone or DHEAS should undergo careful evaluation of the testis by palpation and ultrasound to exclude a Leydig cell neoplasm. Activating mutations of the LH receptor should be considered in children with gonadotropin-independent precocious puberty in whom CAH, androgen abuse, and adrenal and testicular neoplasms have been excluded.

℞ Treatment: PRECOCIOUS PUBERTY

In patients with a known cause (e.g., a CNS lesion or a testicular tumor), therapy should be directed toward the underlying disorder. In patients with idiopathic CPP, long-acting GnRH analogues can be used to suppress gonadotropins and decrease testosterone, halt early pubertal development, delay accelerated bone maturation, and prevent early epiphyseal closure, without causing osteoporosis. The treatment is most effective for increasing final adult height if it is initiated before age 6. Puberty resumes after discontinuation of the GnRH analogue. Counseling is an important aspect of the overall treatment strategy.

In children with gonadotropin-independent precocious puberty, inhibitors of steroidogenesis, such as ketoconazole, and AR antagonists have been used empirically. Long-term treatment with spironolactone (a weak androgen antagonist), testolactone (aromatase inhibitor), and ketoconazole has been reported to normalize growth rate and bone maturation and to improve predicted height in small, nonrandomized trials in boys with familial male-limited precocious puberty.

DELAYED PUBERTY

Puberty is delayed in boys if it has not ensued by age 14, an age that is 2–2.5 standard deviations above the mean for healthy children. Delayed puberty is more common in boys than in girls. There are four main categories of delayed puberty: (1) constitutional delay of growth and puberty (~60% of cases), (2) functional hypogonadotropic hypogonadism caused by systemic illness or malnutrition (~20% of cases), (3) hypogonadotropic hypogonadism caused by genetic or acquired defects in the hypothalamic-pituitary region (~10% of cases), and (4) hypergonadotropic hypogonadism secondary to primary gonadal failure (~15% of cases) (Table 8-1). Functional hypogonadotropic hypogonadism is more common in girls than in boys. Permanent causes of hypogonadotropic or hypergonadotropic hypogonadism are identified in <25% of boys with delayed puberty.

Approach to the Patient: DELAYED PUBERTY

Any history of systemic illness, eating disorders, excessive exercise, social and psychological problems, and abnormal patterns of linear growth during childhood should be verified. Boys with pubertal delay may have accompanying emotional and physical immaturity relative to their peers, which can be a source of anxiety. Physical examination should focus on height; arm span; weight; visual fields; and secondary sex characteristics, including hair growth, testicular volume, phallic size, and scrotal reddening and thinning. Testicular size >2.5 cm generally indicates that the child has entered puberty.

The main diagnostic challenge is to distinguish those with constitutional delay, who will progress through puberty at a later age, from those with an underlying pathologic process. Constitutional delay should be suspected when there is a family history and when there are delayed bone age and short stature. Pituitary priming by pulsatile GnRH is required before LH and FSH are synthesized and secreted normally. Thus, blunted responses to exogenous GnRH can be seen in patients with constitutional delay, GnRH deficiency, or pituitary disorders (see "GnRH Stimulation Testing" earlier in the chapter). On the other hand, low-normal basal gonadotropin levels or a normal response to exogenous GnRH is consistent with an early stage of puberty, which is often heralded by nocturnal GnRH secretion. Thus, constitutional delay is a diagnosis of exclusion that requires ongoing evaluation until the onset of puberty and the growth spurt.

℞ Treatment: DELAYED PUBERTY

If therapy is considered appropriate, it can begin with 25–50 mg testosterone enanthate or testosterone cypionate every 2 weeks, or by using a 2.5-mg testosterone patch or 25-mg testosterone gel. Because aromatization of testosterone to estrogen is obligatory for mediating androgen effects on epiphyseal fusion, concomitant treatment with aromatase inhibitors may allow attainment of greater final adult height. Testosterone treatment should be interrupted after 6 months to determine if endogenous LH and FSH secretion have ensued. Other causes of delayed puberty should be considered when there are associated clinical features or when boys do not enter puberty spontaneously after a year of observation or treatment.

Reassurance without hormonal treatment is appropriate for many individuals with presumed constitutional delay of puberty. However, the impact of delayed growth and pubertal progression on a child's social relationships and school performance should be weighed. Also, boys with constitutional delay of puberty are less likely to achieve their full genetic height potential and have reduced total body bone mass as adults, mainly due to narrow limb bones and vertebrae as a result of impaired periosteal expansion during puberty. Administration of androgen therapy to boys with constitutional delay does not affect final height, and when administered with an aromatase inhibitor, it may improve final height.

DISORDERS OF THE MALE REPRODUCTIVE AXIS DURING ADULTHOOD

HYPOGONADOTROPIC HYPOGONADISM

Because LH and FSH are trophic hormones for the testes, impaired secretion of these pituitary gonadotropins results in secondary hypogonadism, which is characterized by low testosterone in the setting of low LH and FSH. Those with the most severe deficiency have complete absence of pubertal development, sexual infantilism, and, in some cases, hypospadias and undescended testes. Patients with partial gonadotropin deficiency have delayed or arrested sex development. The 24-h LH secretory profiles are heterogeneous in patients with hypogonadotropic hypogonadism, reflecting variable abnormalities of LH pulse frequency or amplitude. In severe cases, basal LH is low and there are no LH pulses. A smaller subset of patients have low-amplitude LH pulses or markedly reduced pulse frequency. Occasionally, only sleep-entrained LH pulses occur, reminiscent of the pattern seen in the early stages of puberty. Hypogonadotropic hypogonadism can be classified into congenital and acquired disorders. Congenital disorders most commonly involve GnRH deficiency, which leads to gonadotropin deficiency. Acquired disorders are much more common than congenital disorders and may result from a variety of sellar mass lesions or infiltrative diseases of the hypothalamus or pituitary.

Congenital Disorders Associated with Gonadotropin Deficiency

Most cases of congenital hypogonadotropic hypogonadism are idiopathic, despite extensive endocrine testing and imaging studies of the sellar region. Among known causes, familial hypogonadotropic hypogonadism can be transmitted as an X-linked (20%), autosomal recessive (30%), or autosomal dominant (50%) trait. Some individuals with idiopathic hypogonadotropic hypogonadism (IHH) have sporadic mutations in the same genes that cause inherited forms of the disorder. *Kallmann syndrome* is an X-linked disorder caused by mutations in the *KAL1* gene, which encodes anosmin, a protein that mediates the migration of neural progenitors of the olfactory bulb and GnRH-producing neurons. These individuals have GnRH deficiency and variable combinations of anosmia or hyposmia, renal defects, and neurologic abnormalities including mirror movements. Gonadotropin secretion and fertility can be restored by administration of pulsatile GnRH or by gonadotropin replacement. Mutations in the *FGFR1* gene cause an autosomal dominant form of hypogonadotropic hypogonadism that clinically resembles Kallmann syndrome. Prokineticin 2 (PROK2) also encodes a protein involved in migration and development of olfactory and GnRH neurons. Recessive mutations in PROK2 cause anosmia and hypogonadotropic hypogonadism. The *FGFR1* gene product may be the receptor for the *KAL1* gene product, anosmin, thereby explaining the similarity in clinical features. Other autosomal dominant causes remain unexplained. X-linked hypogonadotropic hypogonadism also occurs in *adrenal hypoplasia congenita*, a disorder caused by mutations in the *DAX1* gene, which encodes a nuclear receptor in the adrenal gland and reproductive axis. Adrenal hypoplasia congenita is characterized by absent development of the adult zone of the adrenal cortex, leading to neonatal adrenal insufficiency. Puberty usually does not occur or is arrested, reflecting variable degrees of gonadotropin deficiency. Although sexual differentiation is normal, some patients have testicular dysgenesis and impaired spermatogenesis despite gonadotropin replacement. Less commonly, adrenal hypoplasia congenita, sex reversal, and hypogonadotropic hypogonadism can be caused by mutations of steroidogenic factor 1 (SF1). *GnRH receptor mutations* account for ~40% of autosomal recessive and 10% of sporadic cases of hypogonadotropic hypogonadism. These patients have decreased LH response to exogenous GnRH. Some receptor mutations alter GnRH binding affinity, allowing apparently normal responses to pharmacologic doses of exogenous GnRH, whereas other mutations may alter signal transduction downstream of hormone binding. Recessive mutations in the G protein–coupled receptor GPR54 cause gonadotropin deficiency without anosmia. Patients retain responsiveness to exogenous GnRH, suggesting an abnormality in the neural pathways controlling GnRH release. Rarely, recessive mutations in the *LH*β or *FSH*β genes have been described in patients with selective deficiencies of these gonadotropins. Deletions or mutations of the *GnRH* gene have not been found in patients with hypogonadotropic hypogonadism.

A number of homeodomain transcription factors are involved in the development and differentiation of the specialized hormone-producing cells within the pituitary gland (**Table 8-2**). Patients with mutations of *PROP1* have combined pituitary hormone deficiency that includes GH, prolactin (PRL) thyroid-stimulating hormone (TSH), LH, and FSH, but not ACTH. *LHX3* mutations cause combined pituitary hormone deficiency in association with cervical spine rigidity. *HESX1* mutations cause septooptic dysplasia and combined pituitary hormone deficiency.

Prader-Willi syndrome is characterized by obesity, hypotonic musculature, mental retardation, hypogonadism, short stature, and small hands and feet. Prader-Willi syndrome is a genomic imprinting disorder caused by deletions of the proximal portion of paternally derived chromosome 15q, uniparental disomy of the maternal alleles, or mutations of the genes/loci involved in imprinting. *Laurence-Moon syndrome* is an autosomal recessive disorder characterized by obesity, hypogonadism, mental retardation, polydactyly, and retinitis pigmentosa. Recessive mutations of leptin, or its receptor, cause severe obesity and pubertal arrest, apparently because of hypothalamic GnRH deficiency (Chap. 16).

TABLE 8-2

CAUSES OF CONGENITAL HYPOGONADOTROPIC HYPOGONADISM

GENE	LOCUS	INHERITANCE	ASSOCIATED FEATURES
KAL1	Xp22	X-linked	Anosmia, renal agenesis, synkinesia, cleft lip/palate, oculomotor/visuospatial defects, gut malrotations
NELF	9q34.3	AR	Anosmia, hypogonadotropic hypogonadism
FGFR1	8p11-p12	AD	Anosmia, cleft lip/palate, synkinesia, syndactyly
PROK2	20p13	AR	Anosmia, hypogonadotropic hypogonadism
LEP	7q31	AR	Obesity
LEPR	1p31	AR	Obesity
PC1	5q15-21	AR	Obesity, diabetes mellitus, ACTH deficiency
HESX1	3p21	AR	Septooptic dysplasia, CPHD
		AD	Isolated GH insufficiency
LHX3	9q34	AR	CPHD (ACTH spared), cervical spine rigidity
PROP1	5q35	AR	CPHD (ACTH usually spared)
GPR54	19p13	AR	None
GNRHR	4q21	AR	None
*FSH*β	11p13	AR	↑ LH
*LH*β	19q13	AR	↑ FSH
SF1 (*NR5A1*)	9p33	AD/AR	Primary adrenal failure, XY sex reversal
DAX1 (*NR0B1*)	Xp21	X-linked	Primary adrenal failure, impaired spermatogenesis

Note: ACTH, adrenocorticotropic hormone; AD, autosomal dominant; AR, autosomal recessive; CPHD, combined pituitary hormone deficiency; KAL1, Interval-1 gene; NELF, nasal embryonic LHRH factor; FGFR1, fibroblast growth factor receptor 1; PROK2, prokineticin 2; LEP, leptin; LEPR, leptin receptor; PC1, prohormone convertase 1; HESX1, homeobox gene expressed in embryonic stem cells 1; LHX3, LIM homeobox gene 3; PROP1, Prophet of Pit 1; GPR54, G protein–coupled receptor 54; GNRHR, gonadotropin-releasing hormone receptor; FSHβ, follicle-stimulating hormone β subunit; LHβ, luteinizing hormone β subunit; SF1, steroidogenic factor 1; DAX1, *d*osage-sensitive sex reversal, *a*drenal hypoplasia congenita, *X* chromosome.

Severe Illness, Stress, Malnutrition, and Exercise

These may cause reversible gonadotropin deficiency. Although gonadotropin deficiency and reproductive dysfunction are well documented in these conditions in women, men exhibit similar but less-pronounced responses. Unlike women, most male runners and other endurance athletes have normal gonadotropin and sex steroid levels, despite low body fat and frequent intensive exercise. Testosterone levels fall at the onset of illness and recover during recuperation. The magnitude of gonadotropin suppression generally correlates with the severity of illness. Although hypogonadotropic hypogonadism is the most common cause of androgen deficiency in patients with acute illness, some have elevated levels of LH and FSH, which suggest primary gonadal dysfunction. The pathophysiology of reproductive dysfunction during acute illness is unknown but likely involves a combination of cytokine and/or glucocorticoid effects. There is a high frequency of low testosterone levels in patients with chronic illnesses such as HIV infection, end-stage renal disease, chronic obstructive lung disease, and many types of cancer and in patients receiving glucocorticoids. About 20% of HIV-infected men with low testosterone levels have elevated LH and FSH levels; these patients presumably have primary testicular dysfunction. The remaining 80% have either normal or low LH and FSH levels; these men have a central hypothalamic-pituitary defect or a dual defect involving both the testis and the hypothalamic-pituitary centers. Muscle wasting is common in chronic diseases associated with hypogonadism, which also leads to debility, poor quality of life, and adverse outcome of disease. There is great interest in exploring strategies that can reverse androgen deficiency or attenuate the sarcopenia associated with chronic illness.

Men using opioids for relief of cancer or noncancerous pain or because of addiction often have suppressed testosterone and LH levels; the degree of suppression is dose-related. Opioids suppress GnRH secretion and alter the sensitivity to feedback inhibition by gonadal steroids. Men who are heavy users of marijuana have decreased testosterone secretion and sperm production. The mechanism of marijuana-induced hypogonadism is decreased GnRH secretion. Gynecomastia observed in marijuana users can also be caused by plant estrogens in crude preparations.

Obesity

In men with mild to moderate obesity, SHBG levels decrease in proportion to the degree of obesity, resulting in lower total testosterone levels. However, free testosterone levels usually remain within the normal range. The decrease in SHBG levels is caused by increased circulating insulin, which inhibits SHBG production. Estradiol levels are higher in obese men compared to healthy, nonobese controls, because of aromatization of testosterone to estradiol in adipose tissue. Weight loss is associated with reversal of these abnormalities including an increase in total and free testosterone levels and a decrease in estradiol levels. A subset of massively obese men may have a defect in the hypothalamic-pituitary axis as suggested by low free testosterone in the absence of elevated gonadotropins. Weight gain in adult men can accelerate the rate of age-related decline in testosterone levels.

Hyperprolactinemia

(See also Chap. 2.) Elevated PRL levels are associated with hypogonadotropic hypogonadism. PRL inhibits hypothalamic GnRH secretion either directly or through modulation of tuberoinfundibular dopaminergic pathways. A PRL-secreting tumor may also destroy the surrounding gonadotropes by invasion or compression of the pituitary stalk. Treatment with dopamine agonists reverses gonadotropin deficiency, although there may be a delay relative to PRL suppression.

Sellar Mass Lesions

Neoplastic and nonneoplastic lesions in the hypothalamus or pituitary can directly or indirectly affect gonadotrope function. In adults, pituitary adenomas constitute the largest category of space-occupying lesions affecting gonadotropin and other pituitary hormone production. Pituitary adenomas that extend into the suprasellar region can impair GnRH secretion and mildly increase PRL secretion (usually <50 μg/L) because of impaired tonic inhibition by dopaminergic pathways. These tumors should be distinguished from prolactinomas, which typically secrete higher PRL levels. The presence of diabetes insipidus suggests the possibility of a craniopharyngioma, infiltrative disorder, or other hypothalamic lesions (Chap. 3).

Hemochromatosis

Both the pituitary and testis can be affected by excessive iron deposition. However, the pituitary defect is the predominant lesion in most patients with hemochromatosis and hypogonadism. The diagnosis of hemochromatosis is suggested by the association of characteristic skin discoloration, hepatic enlargement or dysfunction, diabetes mellitus, arthritis, cardiac conduction defects, and hypogonadism.

PRIMARY TESTICULAR CAUSES OF HYPOGONADISM

Common causes of primary testicular dysfunction include Klinefelter syndrome, uncorrected cryptorchidism, cancer chemotherapy, radiation to the testes, trauma, torsion, infectious orchitis, HIV infection, anorchia syndrome, and myotonic dystrophy. Primary testicular disorders may be associated with impaired spermatogenesis, decreased androgen production, or both. See Chap. 7 for disorders of testis development, androgen synthesis, and androgen action.

Klinefelter Syndrome

(See also Chap. 7.) Klinefelter syndrome is the most common chromosomal disorder associated with testicular dysfunction and male infertility. It occurs in about 1 in 1000 live-born males. Azoospermia is the rule in men with Klinefelter syndrome who have the 47,XXY karyotype; however, men with mosaicism may have germ cells, especially at a younger age. Testicular histology shows hyalinization of seminiferous tubules and absence of spermatogenesis. Although their function is impaired, the number of Leydig cells appears to increase. Testosterone is decreased and estradiol is increased, leading to clinical features of undervirilization and gynecomastia. Men with Klinefelter syndrome are at increased risk of breast cancer, non-Hodgkin's lymphoma, and lung cancer, and reduced risk of prostate cancer. Periodic mammography for breast cancer surveillance is recommended for men with Klinefelter syndrome.

Cryptorchidism

Cryptorchidism occurs when there is incomplete descent of the testis from the abdominal cavity into the scrotum. About 3% of full-term and 30% of premature male infants have at least one cryptorchid testis at birth, but descent is usually complete by the first few weeks of life. The incidence of cryptorchidism is <1% by 9 months of age. Cryptorchidism is associated with increased risk of malignancy and infertility. Unilateral cryptorchidism, even when corrected before puberty, is associated with decreased sperm count, possibly reflecting unrecognized damage to the fully descended testis or other genetic factors. Epidemiologic, clinical, and molecular evidence supports the idea that cryptorchidism, hypospadias, impaired spermatogenesis, and testicular cancer may be causally related to common genetic and environment perturbations, and are components of the testicular dysgenesis syndrome.

Acquired Testicular Defects

Viral orchitis may be caused by the mumps virus, echovirus, lymphocytic choriomeningitis virus, and group B arboviruses. Orchitis occurs in as many as one-fourth of adult men with mumps; the orchitis is unilateral in about two-thirds and bilateral in the remainder. Orchitis usually develops a few days after the onset of parotitis but may precede it. The testis may return to normal size and function or undergo atrophy. Semen analysis returns to normal for three-fourths of men with unilateral involvement but normal for only one-third of men with bilateral orchitis. *Trauma*, including testicular torsion, can also cause secondary atrophy of the testes. The exposed position of the testes in the scrotum renders them susceptible to both thermal and physical trauma, particularly in men with hazardous occupations.

The testes are sensitive to *radiation damage*. Doses >200 mGy (20 rad) are associated with increased FSH and LH levels and damage to the spermatogonia. After ~800 mGy (80 rad), oligospermia or azoospermia develops, and higher doses may obliterate the germinal epithelium. Permanent androgen deficiency in adult men is uncommon after therapeutic radiation; however, most boys given direct testicular radiation therapy for acute lymphoblastic leukemia have permanently low testosterone levels. Sperm banking should be considered before patients undergo radiation treatment or chemotherapy.

Drugs interfere with testicular function by several mechanisms, including inhibition of testosterone synthesis (e.g., ketoconazole), blockade of androgen action (e.g., spironolactone), increased estrogen (e.g., marijuana), or direct inhibition of spermatogenesis (e.g., chemotherapy).

Combination chemotherapy for acute leukemia, Hodgkin's disease, and testicular and other cancers may impair Leydig cell function and cause infertility. The degree of gonadal dysfunction depends on the type of chemotherapeutic agent and the dose and duration of therapy. Because of high response rates and the young age of these men, infertility and androgen deficiency have emerged as important long-term complications of cancer chemotherapy. Cyclophosphamide and combination regimens containing procarbazine are particularly toxic to germ cells. Thus, 90% of men with Hodgkin's lymphoma receiving MOPP (mechlorethamine, Oncovin, procarbazine, prednisone) therapy develop azoospermia or extreme oligozoospermia; newer regimens that do not include procarbazine, such as ABVD (Adriamycin, bleomycin, vinblastine, dacarbazine), are less toxic to germ cells.

Alcohol, when consumed in excess for prolonged periods, decreases testosterone, independent of liver disease or malnutrition. Elevated estradiol and decreased testosterone levels may occur in men taking digitalis.

The occupational and recreational history should be carefully evaluated in all men with infertility because of the toxic effects of many *chemical agents* on spermatogenesis. Known environmental hazards include microwaves and ultrasound and chemicals such as nematocide dibromochloropropane, cadmium, phthalates, and lead. In some populations, sperm density is said to have declined by as much as 40% in the past 50 years. Environmental estrogens or antiandrogens may be partly responsible.

Testicular failure also occurs as a part of *polyglandular autoimmune insufficiency* (Chap. 23). Sperm antibodies can cause isolated male infertility. In some instances, these antibodies are secondary phenomena resulting from duct obstruction or vasectomy. Granulomatous diseases can affect the testes, and testicular atrophy occurs in 10–20% of men with lepromatous leprosy because of direct tissue invasion by the mycobacteria. The tubules are involved initially, followed by endarteritis and destruction of Leydig cells.

Systemic disease can cause primary testis dysfunction in addition to suppressing gonadotropin production. In cirrhosis, a combined testicular and pituitary abnormality leads to decreased testosterone production independent of the direct toxic effects of ethanol. Impaired hepatic extraction of adrenal androstenedione leads to extraglandular conversion to estrone and estradiol, which partially suppresses LH. Testicular atrophy and gynecomastia are present in approximately one-half of men with cirrhosis. In chronic renal failure, androgen synthesis and sperm production decrease despite elevated gonadotropins. The elevated LH level is due to reduced clearance, but it does not restore normal testosterone production. About one-fourth of men with renal failure have hyperprolactinemia. Improvement in testosterone production with hemodialysis is incomplete, but successful renal transplantation may return testicular function to normal. Testicular atrophy is present in one-third of men with sickle cell anemia. The defect may be at either the testicular or the hypothalamic-pituitary level. Sperm density can decrease temporarily after acute febrile illness in the absence of a change in testosterone production. Infertility in men with celiac disease is associated with a hormonal pattern typical of androgen resistance, namely, elevated testosterone and LH levels.

Neurologic diseases associated with altered testicular function include myotonic dystrophy, spinobulbar muscular atrophy, and paraplegia. In myotonic dystrophy, small testes may be associated with impairment of both spermatogenesis and Leydig cell function. Spinobulbar muscular atrophy is caused by an expansion of the glutamine repeat sequences in the amino-terminal region of the AR; this expansion impairs function of the AR, but it is unclear how the alteration is related to the neurologic manifestations. Men with spinobulbar muscular atrophy often have undervirilization and infertility as a late manifestation. Spinal cord lesions that cause paraplegia can lead to a temporary decrease in testosterone levels and may cause persistent defects in spermatogenesis; some patients retain the capacity for penile erection and ejaculation.

ANDROGEN INSENSITIVITY SYNDROMES

Mutations in the AR cause resistance to the action of testosterone and DHT. These X-linked mutations are associated with variable degrees of defective male phenotypic development and undervirilization (Chap. 7). Although not technically hormone-insensitivity syndromes, two genetic disorders impair testosterone conversion to active sex steroids. Mutations in the *SRD5A2* gene, which encodes 5α-reductase type 2, prevent the conversion of testosterone to DHT, which is necessary for the normal development of the male external genitalia. Mutations in the *CYP19* gene, which encodes aromatase, prevent testosterone conversion to estradiol. Males with *CYP19* mutations have delayed epiphyseal fusion, tall stature, eunuchoid proportions, and osteoporosis, consistent with evidence from an estrogen receptor–deficient individual that these testosterone actions are mediated indirectly via estrogen.

GYNECOMASTIA

Gynecomastia refers to enlargement of the male breast. It is caused by excess estrogen action and is usually the result of an increased estrogen/androgen ratio. True gynecomastia is associated with glandular breast tissue that is >4 cm in diameter and often tender. Glandular tissue enlargement should be distinguished from excess adipose tissue: glandular tissue is firmer and contains fibrous-like cords. Gynecomastia occurs as a normal physiologic phenomenon in the newborn (due to transplacental transfer of maternal and placental estrogens), during puberty (high estrogen/androgen ratio in early stages of puberty), and with aging (increased fat tissue and increased aromatase activity), but it can also result from pathologic conditions associated with androgen deficiency or estrogen excess. The prevalence of gynecomastia increases with age and body mass index (BMI), likely because of increased aromatase activity in adipose tissue. Medications that alter androgen metabolism or action may also cause gynecomastia. The relative risk of breast cancer is increased in men with gynecomastia, although the absolute risk is relatively small.

PATHOLOGIC GYNECOMASTIA

Any cause of *androgen deficiency* can lead to gynecomastia, reflecting an increased estrogen/androgen ratio, as estrogen synthesis still occurs by aromatization of residual adrenal and gonadal androgens. Gynecomastia is a characteristic feature of Klinefelter syndrome (Chap. 7). *Androgen insensitivity* disorders also cause gynecomastia. *Excess estrogen production* may be caused by tumors, including Sertoli cell tumors in isolation or in association with Peutz-Jeghers syndrome or Carney complex. Tumors that produce hCG, including some testicular tumors, stimulate Leydig cell estrogen synthesis. *Increased conversion of androgens to estrogens* can be a result of increased availability of substrate (androstenedione) for extraglandular estrogen formation (CAH, hyperthyroidism, and most feminizing adrenal tumors) or to diminished catabolism of androstenedione (liver disease) so that estrogen precursors are shunted to aromatase in peripheral sites. Obesity is associated with increased aromatization of androgen precursors to estrogens. Extraglandular aromatase activity can also be increased in tumors of the liver or adrenal gland or rarely as an inherited disorder. Several families with *increased peripheral aromatase activity* inherited as an autosomal dominant or as an X-linked disorder have been described. In some families with this disorder, an inversion in chromosome 15q21.2-3 causes the CYP19 gene to be activated by the regulatory elements of contiguous genes resulting in excessive estrogen production in the fat and other extragonadal tissues. *Drugs* can cause gynecomastia by acting directly as estrogenic substances (e.g., oral contraceptives, phytoestrogens, digitalis), inhibiting androgen synthesis (e.g., ketoconazole), or action (e.g., spironolactone).

Because up to two-thirds of pubertal boys and half of hospitalized men have palpable glandular tissue that is benign, detailed investigation or intervention is not indicated in all men presenting with gynecomastia (**Fig. 8-5**). In addition to the extent of gynecomastia, recent onset, rapid growth, tender tissue, and occurrence in a lean subject should prompt more extensive evaluation. This should include a careful drug history, measurement and examination of the testes, assessment of virilization, evaluation of liver function, and hormonal measurements including testosterone, estradiol, and androstenedione, LH, and hCG. A karyotype should be obtained in men with very small testes to exclude Klinefelter syndrome.

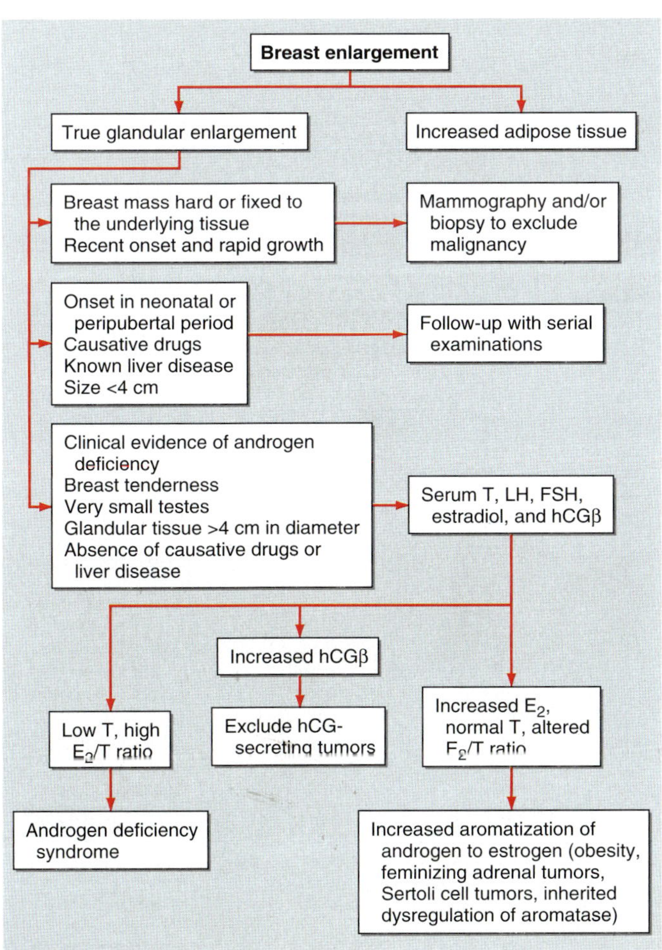

FIGURE 8-5

Evaluation of gynecomastia. T, testosterone; LH, luteinizing hormone; FSH, follicle-stimulating hormone; hCGβ, human chorionic gonadotropin β; E_2, 17β-estradiol.

In spite of extensive evaluation, the etiology is established in fewer than one-half of patients.

Rx Treatment: GYNECOMASTIA

When the primary cause can be identified and corrected, breast enlargement usually subsides over several months. However, if gynecomastia is of long duration, surgery is the most effective therapy. Indications for surgery include severe psychological and/or cosmetic problems, continued growth or tenderness, or suspected malignancy. In patients who have painful gynecomastia and in whom surgery cannot be performed, treatment with antiestrogens such as tamoxifen (20 mg/d) can reduce pain and breast tissue size in over half the patients. Aromatase inhibitors can be effective in the early proliferative phase of the disorder, although the experience is largely based on the use of testolactone, a relatively weak aromatase inhibitor; placebo-controlled trials with more potent aromatase inhibitors such as anastrozole, fadrozole, letrozole, or formestane are needed. In a randomized trial in men with established gynecomastia, anastrozole proved no more effective than placebo in reducing breast size.

AGING-RELATED CHANGES IN MALE REPRODUCTIVE FUNCTION

A number of cross-sectional and longitudinal studies (e.g., the Baltimore Longitudinal Study of Aging and the Massachusetts Male Aging Study) have established that testosterone concentrations decrease with advancing age. This age-related decline starts in the third decade of life and progresses slowly; the rate of decline in testosterone concentrations is greater for men with chronic illness and for those taking medications than in healthy older men. Because SHBG concentrations are higher in older men than in younger men, free or bioavailable testosterone concentrations decline with aging to a greater extent than total testosterone concentrations. The age-related decline in testosterone is due to defects at all levels of the hypothalamic-pituitary-testicular axis: pulsatile GnRH secretion is attenuated, LH response to GnRH is reduced, and testicular response to LH is impaired. However, the gradual rise of LH with aging suggests that testis dysfunction is the main cause of declining androgen levels. The term *andropause* has been used to denote age-related decline in testosterone concentrations; this term is a misnomer because there is no discrete time when testosterone concentrations decline abruptly.

In epidemiologic surveys, low total and bioavailable testosterone concentrations have been associated with decreased appendicular skeletal muscle mass and strength, decreased self-reported physical function, higher visceral fat mass, insulin resistance, and increased risk of coronary artery disease and mortality. In systematic reviews of randomized controlled trials, testosterone therapy of healthy older men with low or low-normal testosterone levels was associated with greater increments in lean body mass, grip strength, and self-reported physical function than that associated with placebo. Testosterone therapy also induced greater improvement in vertebral but not femoral bone mineral density. Testosterone therapy of older men with sexual dysfunction and unequivocally low testosterone levels improves libido, but testosterone effects on erectile function and response to selective phosphodiesterase inhibitors have been inconsistent. Testosterone therapy has not been shown to improve depression scores, fracture risk, cognitive function, or clinical outcomes in older men. Furthermore, the long-term risks of testosterone supplementation in older men remain largely unknown. In particular, physiologic testosterone replacement might increase the risk of prostate cancer or exacerbate cardiovascular disease. Population screening of all older men for low testosterone levels is not recommended, and testing should be restricted to men who have symptoms or physical features attributable to androgen deficiency. Testosterone therapy is not recommended for all older men with low testosterone levels. In older men with significant symptoms of androgen deficiency who have testosterone levels below 200 ng/dL, testosterone therapy may be considered on an individualized basis and should be instituted after careful discussion of the risks and benefits (see "Testosterone Replacement" later in the chapter).

Testicular morphology, semen production, and fertility are maintained up to a very old age in men. Although concern has been expressed about age-related increases in germ cell mutations and impairment of DNA repair mechanisms, the frequency of chromosomal aneuploidy or structural abnormalities does not increase in the sperm of older men. However, the incidence of autosomal dominant diseases, such as achondroplasia, polyposis coli, Marfan syndrome, and Apert's syndrome, increases in the offspring of men who are advanced in age, consistent with transmission of sporadic missense mutations.

Approach to the Patient: ANDROGEN DEFICIENCY

Hypogonadism is often heralded by decreased sex drive, reduced frequency of sexual intercourse or inability to maintain erections, reduced beard growth, loss of muscle mass, decreased testicular size, and gynecomastia. Less than 10% of patients with erectile dysfunction alone have testosterone deficiency. Thus, it is useful to look for a constellation of symptoms and signs suggestive of androgen deficiency. Except when extreme, these clinical features may be difficult to distinguish from changes that occur with normal aging. Moreover, androgen deficiency may develop gradually. Population studies, such as the Massachusetts Male Aging Study, suggest that about 4% of men between the ages of 40 and 70 have testosterone levels <150 ng/dL. Thus, androgen deficiency is not uncommon.

When symptoms or clinical features suggest possible androgen deficiency, the laboratory evaluation is initiated by the measurement of total testosterone, preferably in the morning (**Fig. 8-6**). A total testosterone level <200 ng/dL measured by a reliable assay, in association with symptoms, is evidence of testosterone deficiency. An early-morning testosterone level >350 ng/dL makes the diagnosis of androgen deficiency unlikely. In men with testosterone levels between 200 and 350 ng/dL, the total testosterone level should be repeated and a free testosterone level should be measured. In older men and in patients with other clinical states that are associated with

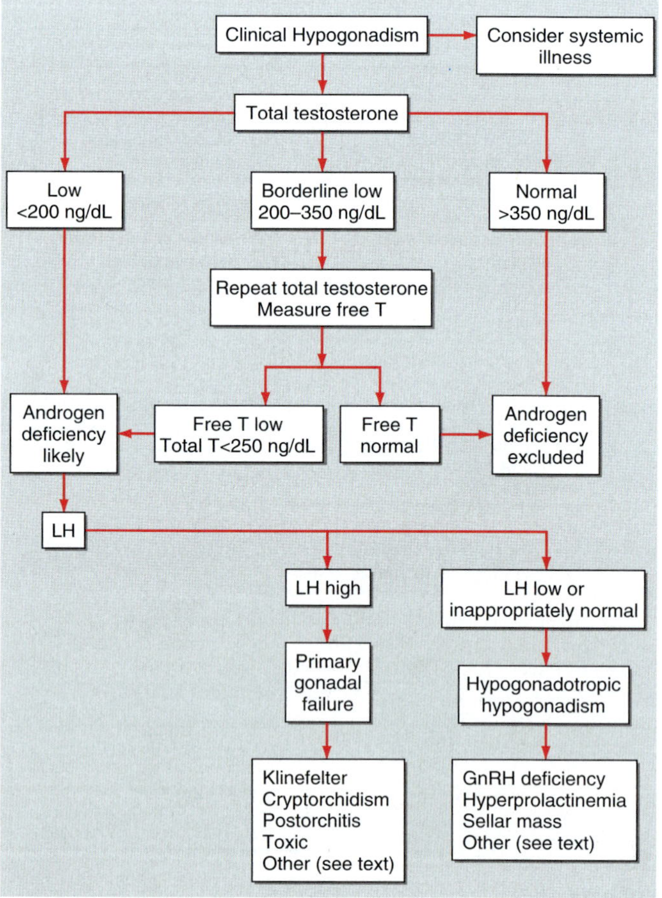

FIGURE 8-6

Evaluation of hypogonadism. T, testosterone; LH, luteinizing hormone; GnRH, gonadotropin-releasing hormone.

alterations in SHBG levels, a direct measurement of free testosterone level by equilibrium dialysis can be useful in unmasking testosterone deficiency.

When androgen deficiency has been confirmed by low testosterone concentrations, LH should be measured to classify the patient as having primary (high LH) or secondary (low or inappropriately normal LH) hypogonadism. An elevated LH level indicates that the defect is at the testicular level. Common causes of primary testicular failure include Klinefelter syndrome, HIV infection, uncorrected cryptorchidism, cancer chemotherapeutic agents, radiation, surgical orchiectomy, or prior infectious orchitis. Unless causes of primary testicular failure are known, a karyotype should be performed in men with low testosterone and elevated LH to exclude Klinefelter syndrome. Men who have a low testosterone but "inappropriately normal" or low LH levels have secondary hypogonadism; their defect resides at the hypothalamic-pituitary level. Common causes of acquired secondary hypogonadism include space-occupying lesions of the sella, hyperprolactinemia, chronic illness, hemochromatosis, excessive exercise, and substance abuse. Measurement of PRL and MRI scan of the hypothalamic-pituitary region can help exclude the presence of a space-occupying lesion. Patients in whom known causes of hypogonadotropic hypogonadism have been excluded are classified as having IHH. It is not unusual for congenital causes of hypogonadotropic hypogonadism, such as Kallmann syndrome, to be diagnosed in young adults.

℞ Treatment: AGE-RELATED REPRODUCTIVE DYSFUNCTION

GONADOTROPINS Gonadotropin therapy is used to establish or restore fertility in patients with gonadotropin deficiency of any cause. Several gonadotropin preparations are available. Human menopausal gonadotropin (hMG; purified from the urine of postmenopausal women) contains 75 IU FSH and 75 IU LH per vial. hCG (purified from the urine of pregnant women) has little FSH activity and resembles LH in its ability to stimulate testosterone production by Leydig cells. Recombinant hCG is now available. Because of the expense of hMG, treatment is usually begun with hCG alone, and hMG is added later to promote the FSH-dependent stages of spermatid development. Recombinant human FSH (hFSH) is now available and is indistinguishable from purified urinary hFSH in its biologic activity and pharmacokinetics in vitro and in vivo, although the mature β subunit of recombinant hFSH has seven fewer amino acids. Recombinant hFSH is available in ampoules containing 75 IU (~7.5 μg FSH), which accounts for >99% of protein content. Once spermatogenesis is restored using combined FSH and LH therapy, hCG alone is often sufficient to maintain spermatogenesis.

Although a variety of treatment regimens are used, 1500–2000 IU of hCG or recombinant human LH (rhLH) administered IM three times weekly is a reasonable starting dose. Testosterone levels should be measured 6–8 weeks later and 48–72 h after the hCG or rhLH injection; the hCG/rhLH dose should be adjusted to achieve testosterone levels in the mid-normal range. Sperm counts should be monitored on a monthly basis. It may take several months for spermatogenesis to be restored; therefore, it is important to forewarn patients about the potential length and expense of the treatment and to provide conservative estimates of success rates. If testosterone levels are in the mid-normal range but the sperm concentrations are low after 6 months of therapy with hCG alone, FSH should be added. This can be done by using hMG, highly purified urinary hFSH, or recombinant hFSH. The selection of FSH dose is empirical. A common practice is to start with the addition of 75 IU FSH three times each week in conjunction with the hCG/rhLH injections. If sperm densities are still low after 3 months of combined treatment, the FSH dose should be increased to 150 IU. Occasionally, it may take ≥18–24 months for spermatogenesis to be restored.

The two best predictors of success using gonadotropin therapy in hypogonadotropic men are testicular volume at presentation and time of onset. In general, men with testicular volumes >8 mL have better response rates than those who have testicular volumes <4 mL. Patients who became hypogonadotropic after puberty experience higher success rates than those who have never undergone pubertal changes. Spermatogenesis can usually be reinitiated by hCG alone, with high rates of success for men with postpubertal onset of hypogonadotropism. The presence of a primary testicular abnormality, such as cryptorchidism, will attenuate testicular response to gonadotropin therapy. Prior androgen therapy does not affect subsequent response to gonadotropin therapy.

GNRH In patients with documented GnRH deficiency, both pubertal development and spermatogenesis can be successfully induced by pulsatile administration of low doses of GnRH. This response requires normal pituitary and testicular function. Therapy usually begins with an initial dose of 25 ng/kg per pulse administered subcutaneously every 2 h by a portable infusion pump. Testosterone, LH, and FSH levels should be monitored. The dose of GnRH is increased until testosterone levels reach the mid-normal range. Doses ranging from 25 to 200 ng/kg may be required to induce virilization. Once pubertal changes have been initiated, the dose of GnRH can often be reduced. Increased sperm counts and testicular volume have been reported in >70% of treated men, and improvements in sexual function and virilization can be induced in >90% of patients. Cutaneous infections occur but are infrequent and minor. Carrying a portable infusion device can be cumbersome, and follow-up of these patients requires physician supervision and laboratory monitoring. Some patients with IHH have cryptorchidism; men with this additional testicular defect may not respond to GnRH or gonadotropin therapy.

Comparative studies of gonadotropin therapy and pulsatile GnRH administration demonstrate that these two therapies are similar in terms of the time to first appearance of sperm or pregnancy rates; both approaches are equally effective in inducing spermatogenesis in men with hypogonadotropic hypogonadism caused by GnRH deficiency. However, most patients find intermittent gonadotropin injections preferable to wearing a continuous infusion pump.

TESTOSTERONE REPLACEMENT Androgen therapy is indicated to restore testosterone levels to normal to correct features of androgen deficiency. Testosterone replacement improves libido and overall sexual activity; increases energy, lean muscle mass, and bone density; and gives the patient a better sense of well-being. The benefits of testosterone replacement therapy have only been proven in men who have documented androgen deficiency, as demonstrated by testosterone levels that are well below the lower limit of normal (<250 ng/dL).

Testosterone is available in a variety of formulations with distinct pharmacokinetics (Table 8-3). Testosterone serves as a prohormone and is converted to 17β-estradiol by aromatase and to 5α-dihydrotestosterone by 5α-reductase. Therefore, when evaluating testosterone formulations, it is important to consider whether the formulation being used can achieve physiologic estradiol and DHT concentrations, in addition to normal testosterone concentrations. Although testosterone concentrations at the lower end of the normal male range can restore sexual function, it is not clear whether low-normal testosterone levels can maintain bone mineral density and muscle mass. The current recommendation is to restore testosterone levels to the mid-normal range.

Oral Derivatives of Testosterone Testosterone is well absorbed after oral administration but quickly degrades during the first pass through the liver. Therefore, it is not possible to achieve sustained blood levels of testosterone after oral administration of crystalline testosterone. 17α-Alkylated derivatives of testosterone (e.g., 17α-methyl testosterone, oxandrolone, fluoxymesterone) are relatively resistant to hepatic degradation and can be administered orally; however, because of the potential for hepatotoxicity, including cholestatic jaundice, peliosis, and hepatoma, these formulations should not be used for testosterone replacement. Hereditary angioedema due to C1 esterase deficiency is the only exception to this general recommendation; in this condition, oral 17α-alkylated androgens are useful because they stimulate hepatic synthesis of the C1 esterase inhibitor.

Injectable Forms of Testosterone The esterification of testosterone at the 17β-hydroxy position makes the molecule hydrophobic and extends its duration of action. The slow release of testosterone ester from an oily depot in the muscle accounts for its extended duration of action. The longer the side chain, the greater the hydrophobicity of the ester and longer the duration of action. Thus, testosterone enanthate and cypionate with longer side chains have longer duration of action than testosterone propionate. Within 24 h after intramuscular administration of 200 mg testosterone enanthate or cypionate, testosterone levels rise into the high-normal or supraphysiologic range and then gradually decline into the hypogonadal range over the next 2 weeks. A bimonthly regimen of testosterone enanthate or cypionate therefore results in peaks and troughs in testosterone levels that are accompanied by changes in a patient's mood, sexual desire, and energy level. The kinetics of testosterone enanthate and cypionate are similar. Estradiol and DHT levels are normal if testosterone replacement is physiologic.

TRANSDERMAL TESTOSTERONE PATCH The nongenital testosterone patch, when applied in an appropriate dose, can normalize testosterone, DHT, and estradiol levels 4–12 h after application. Sexual function and a sense of well-being are restored in androgen-deficient men treated with the nongenital patch. One 5-mg patch may not be sufficient to increase testosterone into the mid-normal male range in all hypogonadal men; some patients may need daily administration of two 5-mg patches to achieve the targeted testosterone concentrations. The transdermal patches are more expensive than testosterone esters. The use of testosterone patches may be associated with skin irritation in some individuals.

TESTOSTERONE GEL Two testosterone gels, AndroGel and Testim, are available in 2.5- and 5-g unit doses that nominally deliver 25 and 50 mg of testosterone to the application site. Initial pharmacokinetic studies have demonstrated that 5-, 7.5-, and 10-g doses applied daily to the skin can maintain total and free testosterone concentrations in the mid- to high-normal range in hypogonadal men. Total and free testosterone concentrations are uniform throughout the 24-h period. The current recommendations are to begin with a 50-mg dose and adjust the dose based on testosterone levels. The advantages of the testosterone gel include the ease of application, its invisibility after application, and

TABLE 8-3

CLINICAL PHARMACOLOGY OF SOME TESTOSTERONE FORMULATIONS

FORMULATION	REGIMEN	PHARMACOKINETIC PROFILE	DHT AND ESTRADIOL	ADVANTAGES	DISADVANTAGES
Testosterone enanthate or cypionate	100 mg IM weekly or 200 mg IM every 2 weeks	After a single IM injection, serum testosterone levels rise into the supraphysiologic range and then decline gradually into the hypogonadal range by the end of the dosing interval	DHT and estradiol levels rise in proportion to the increase in testosterone levels; T:DHT and T:E_2 ratios do not change	Corrects symptoms of androgen deficiency Relatively inexpensive, if self-administered Flexibility of dosing	Requires IM injection Peaks and troughs in serum testosterone levels
Scrotal testosterone patch[a]	One scrotal patch designed to nominally deliver 6 mg over 24 h applied daily	Normalizes serum testosterone levels in many but not all androgen-deficient men	Serum estradiol levels are in the physiologic male range, but DHT levels rise into the supraphysiologic range; T:DHT ratio is significantly lower than in healthy men	Corrects symptoms of androgen deficiency	To promote optimum adherence of the patch, scrotal skin needs to be shaved High DHT levels
Nongenital transdermal system	1 or 2 patches, designed to nominally deliver 5–10 mg testosterone over 24 h applied daily on nonpressure areas	Restores serum testosterone, DHT, and estradiol levels into the physiologic male range	T:DHT and T:estradiol levels are in the physiologic male range	Ease of application, corrects symptoms of androgen deficiency, and mimics the normal diurnal rhythm of testosterone secretion Lesser increase in hemoglobin than injectable esters	Serum testosterone levels in some androgen-deficient men maybe in the low-normal range; these men may need application of 2 patches daily Skin irritation at the application site may be a problem for some patients
Testosterone gel	5–10 g testosterone gel containing 50–100 mg testosterone applied daily	Restores serum testosterone and estradiol levels into the physiologic male range	Serum DHT levels are higher and T:DHT ratios are lower in hypogonadal men treated with the testosterone gel than in healthy eugonadal men	Corrects symptoms of androgen deficiency, provides flexibility of dosing, ease of application, good skin tolerability	Potential of transfer to a female partner or child by direct skin-to-skin contact; moderately high DHT levels
17α-methyl testosterone	17α-alkylated compound that should not be used because of potential for liver toxicity	Orally active			Clinical responses are variable; potential for liver toxicity; should not be used for treatment of androgen deficiency

(Continued)

TABLE 8-3 (*CONTINUED*)

CLINICAL PHARMACOLOGY OF SOME TESTOSTERONE FORMULATIONS

FORMULATION	REGIMEN	PHARMACOKINETIC PROFILE	DHT AND ESTRADIOL	ADVANTAGES	DISADVANTAGES
Buccal, bioadhesive, testosterone tablets	30 mg controlled release, bioadhesive tablets used twice daily	Absorbed from the buccal mucosa	Normalizes serum testosterone and DHT levels in hypogonadal men	Corrects symptoms of androgen deficiency in healthy, hypogonadal men	Gum-related adverse events in 16% of treated men
Oral testosterone undecanoate[b]	40–80 mg orally 2 or 3 times daily with meals	When administered in oleic acid, testosterone undecanoate is absorbed through the lymphatics, bypassing the portal system; considerable variability in the same individual on different days and among individuals	High DHT:T ratio	Convenience of oral administration	Not approved in the U.S. Variable clinical responses, variable serum testosterone levels, high DHT:T ratio
Injectable long-acting testosterone undecanoate in oil[b]	1000 mg injected IM followed by 1000 mg at 6 weeks, then 1000 mg every 12 weeks	When administered at a dose of 1000 mg IM, serum testosterone levels are maintained in the normal range in a majority of treated men	DHT and estradiol levels rise in proportion to the increase in testosterone levels; T:DHT and T:E_2 ratios do not change	Corrects symptoms of androgen deficiency Requires infrequent administration	Requires IM injection of a large volume (4 mL)
Testosterone pellets	4–6 200-mg pellets implanted SC	Serum testosterone peaks at 1 month and then sustained in normal range for 4–6 months	T:DHT and T:E_2 ratios do not change	Corrects symptoms of androgen deficiency	Requires surgical incision for insertions; pellets may extrude spontaneously

[a]Not currently available in the United States.
[b]Formulation available outside the United States but not currently approved by the U.S. Food and Drug Administration.
Note: IM, intramuscular; DHT, dihydrotestosterone; T, testosterone; E2, 17®-estradiol; SC, subcutaneously.
Source: Reproduced from the Endocrine Society Guideline for Testosterone Therapy of Androgen Deficiency Syndromes in Adult Men (Bhasin et al).

its flexibility of dosing. A major concern is the potential for inadvertent transfer of the gel to a sexual partner or to children who may come in close contact with the patient. The ratio of DHT to testosterone concentrations is higher in men treated with the testosterone gel.

A buccal adhesive testosterone tablet, which adheres to the buccal mucosa and releases testosterone as it is slowly dissolved, has been approved. After twice-daily application of 30-mg tablets, serum testosterone levels are maintained within the normal male range in a majority of treated hypogonadal men. The adverse effects include buccal ulceration and gum problems in a few subjects. The clinical experience with this formulation is limited, and the effects of food and brushing on absorption have not been studied in detail.

TESTOSTERONE FORMULATIONS NOT AVAILABLE IN THE UNITED STATES Testosterone undecanoate, when administered orally in oleic acid, is absorbed preferentially through the lymphatics into the systemic circulation and is spared the first-pass degradation in the liver. Doses of 40–80 mg PO, two or three times daily, are typically used. However, the clinical responses are variable and suboptimal. DHT-to-testosterone ratios are higher in hypogonadal men treated with oral testosterone undecanoate, as compared to eugonadal men.

Implants of crystalline testosterone can be inserted in the subcutaneous tissue by means of a trocar through a small skin incision. Testosterone is released by surface erosion of the implant and absorbed into the systemic circulation. Four to six 200-mg implants can maintain testosterone in the mid- to high-normal range for up to 6 months. Potential drawbacks include incising the skin for insertion and removal, and spontaneous extrusions and fibrosis at the site of the implant.

After initial priming, long-acting testosterone undecanoate in oil, when administered IM every 12 weeks, maintains serum testosterone, estradiol, and DHT in the normal male range and corrects symptoms of androgen deficiency in a majority of treated men. However, large injection volume (4 mL) is its relative drawback.

NOVEL ANDROGEN FORMULATIONS A number of androgen formulations with better pharmacokinetics or more selective activity profiles are under development. A biodegradable testosterone microsphere formulation provides physiologic testosterone levels for 10–11 weeks. Two long-acting esters, testosterone buciclate and testosterone undecanoate, when injected IM, can maintain circulating testosterone concentrations in the male range for 7–12 weeks. Initial clinical trials have demonstrated the feasibility of administering testosterone by the sublingual or buccal routes. 7α-Methyl-19-nortestosterone is an androgen that cannot be 5α-reduced; therefore, compared to testosterone, it has relatively greater agonist activity in muscle and gonadotropin suppression but lesser activity on the prostate.

Analogous to the selective estrogen receptor modulators, such as raloxifene, it may be possible to develop selective androgen receptor modulators (SARMs) that exert the desired physiologic effects on muscle, bone, or sexual function but without adversely affecting the prostate and the cardiovascular system.

PHARMACOLOGIC USES OF ANDROGENS
Androgens and selective androgen receptor modulators are being evaluated as anabolic therapies for functional limitations associated with aging and chronic illness. Testosterone supplementation increases skeletal muscle mass, maximal voluntary strength, and muscle power in healthy men, hypogonadal men, older men with low testosterone levels, HIV-infected men with weight loss, and men receiving glucocorticoids. These anabolic effects of testosterone are related to testosterone dose and circulating concentrations. Systematic reviews have confirmed that testosterone therapy of HIV-infected men with weight loss promotes improvements in body weight, lean body mass, muscle strength, and depression indices, leading to recommendations that testosterone be considered as an adjunctive therapy in HIV-infected men who are experiencing unexplained weight loss and who have low testosterone levels. Similarly, in glucocorticoid-treated men, testosterone therapy should be considered to maintain muscle mass and strength, and vertebral bone mineral density. It is unknown whether testosterone therapy of older men with functional limitations can improve physical function, reduce disability, and improve health-related quality of life. Concerns about potential adverse effects of testosterone on prostate and cardiovascular event rates have encouraged the development of selective androgen receptor modulators that are preferentially anabolic and spare the prostate.

Testosterone administration induces hypertrophy of both type 1 and 2 fibers and increases satellite cell (muscle progenitor cells) and myonuclear number. Androgens promote the differentiation of mesenchymal, multipotent progenitor cells into the myogenic lineage and inhibit their differentiation into the adipogenic lineage. Testosterone may have additional effects on satellite cell replication and muscle protein synthesis, which may contribute to an increase in muscle mass.

Other indications for androgen therapy are in selected patients with anemia due to bone marrow failure (an indication largely supplanted by erythropoietin) or for hereditary angioedema.

MALE HORMONAL CONTRACEPTION BASED ON COMBINED ADMINISTRATION OF TESTOSTERONE AND GONADOTROPIN INHIBITORS Supraphysiologic doses of testosterone (200 mg testosterone enanthate weekly) act by suppressing LH and FSH secretion and induce azoospermia in 50% of Caucasian men and >95% of Chinese men. Because of concern about long-term adverse effects of supraphysiologic testosterone doses, regimens that combine other gonadotropin inhibitors, such as GnRH antagonists and progestins with replacement doses of testosterone, are being investigated. Oral etonogestrel daily in combination with IM testosterone decanoate every 4–6 weeks induced azoospermia or severe oligozoospermia (sperm density <1 million/mL) in 99% of treated men over a 1-year period. This regimen was associated with weight gain, deceased testicular volume, and decreased plasma high-density lipoprotein (HDL) cholesterol; the long-term safety has not been demonstrated. Selective androgen receptor modulators that are more potent inhibitors of gonadotropins than testosterone and spare the prostate hold promise for their contraceptive potential.

RECOMMENDED REGIMENS FOR ANDROGEN REPLACEMENT Testosterone esters are administered weekly at doses of 75–100 mg IM, or 150–200 mg every 2 weeks. One or two 5-mg nongenital testosterone patches can be applied daily over the skin of the back, thigh, or upper arm away from pressure areas. Testosterone gel is typically applied over a covered area of skin at a dose of 5–10 g daily; patients should wash their hands after gel application. Bioadhesive buccal testosterone tablets at a dose of 30 mg are typically applied twice daily on the buccal mucosa.

ESTABLISHING EFFICACY OF TESTOSTERONE REPLACEMENT THERAPY Because a clinically useful marker of androgen action is not available, restoration of testosterone levels into the mid-normal range remains the goal of therapy. Measurements of LH and FSH are not useful in assessing the adequacy of testosterone replacement. Testosterone should be measured 3 months after initiating therapy to assess adequacy of therapy. In patients who are treated with testosterone enanthate or cypionate, testosterone levels should be 350–600 ng/dL 1 week after the injection. If testosterone levels are outside this range, adjustments should be made to either the dose or the interval between injections. In men on transdermal patch or gel, or buccal testosterone therapy, testosterone levels should be in the mid-normal range (500–700 ng/dL) 4–12 h after application. If testosterone levels are outside this range, the dose should be adjusted.

Restoration of sexual function, secondary sex characteristics, and energy level and sense of well-being are important objectives of testosterone replacement therapy. The patient should also be asked about sexual desire and activity, the presence of early morning erections, and the ability to achieve and maintain erections adequate for sexual intercourse. Some hypogonadal men continue to complain about sexual dysfunction even after testosterone replacement has been instituted; these patients may benefit from counseling. The hair growth in response to androgen replacement is variable and depends on ethnicity. Hypogonadal men with prepubertal onset of androgen deficiency who begin testosterone therapy in their late 20s or 30s may find it difficult to adjust to their newly found sexuality and may benefit from counseling. If the patient has a sexual partner, the partner should be included in counseling because of the dramatic physical and sexual changes that occur with androgen treatment.

CONTRAINDICATIONS FOR ANDROGEN ADMINISTRATION Testosterone administration is contraindicated in men with a history of prostate or breast cancer (Table 8-4). Testosterone should not be prescribed to men with severe symptoms of benign prostatic hypertrophy (American Urological Association symptom score >19) or with baseline prostate-specific antigen (PSA) >3 ng/mL without a urologic evaluation. Testosterone replacement should not be administered to men with baseline hematocrit ≥50%. Testosterone can induce and exacerbate sleep apnea because of its neuromuscular effects on the upper airway. Testosterone should not be administered to men with congestive heart failure with class III or IV symptoms.

MONITORING POTENTIAL ADVERSE EXPERIENCES The clinical effectiveness and safety of testosterone replacement therapy should be performed 3 and 6 months after initiating testosterone therapy and annually thereafter (Table 8-5). Potential adverse

TABLE 8-4

CONDITIONS IN WHICH TESTOSTERONE ADMINISTRATION IS ASSOCIATED WITH A RISK OF ADVERSE OUTCOME

Conditions in which testosterone administration is associated with very high risk of serious adverse outcomes:
Metastatic prostate cancer
Breast cancer
Conditions in which testosterone administration is associated with moderate to high risk of adverse outcomes
Undiagnosed prostate nodule or induration
Unexplained PSA elevation
Erythrocytosis (hematocrit >50%)
Severe lower urinary tract symptoms associated with benign prostatic hypertrophy as indicated by American Urological Association/International prostate symptom score >19
Unstable severe congestive heart failure (class III or IV)

Note: PSA, prostate-specific antigen.

Source: Reproduced from the Endocrine Society Guideline for Testosterone Therapy of Androgen Deficiency Syndromes in Adult Men (Bhasin et al).

TABLE 8-5

MONITORING OF MEN RECEIVING TESTOSTERONE THERAPY
1. Evaluate the patient 3 months after treatment starts and then annually to assess whether symptoms have responded to treatment and whether the patient is suffering from any adverse effects.
2. Monitor testosterone levels 2 or 3 months after initiation of testosterone therapy.
The therapy should aim to raise serum testosterone levels into the mid-normal range.
Injectable testosterone enanthate or cypionate: Measure serum testosterone levels midway between injections. If testosterone is >700 ng/dL (24.5 nmol/L) or <350 ng/dL (12.3 nmol/L), adjust dose or frequency.
Transdermal patch: Assess testosterone levels 3–12 hours after application of the patch; adjust dose to achieve testosterone levels in the mid-normal range.
Buccal testosterone bioadhesive tablet: Assess levels immediately before or after application of fresh system.
Transdermal gel: Assess testosterone level any time after patient has been on treatment for at least 1 week; adjust dose to achieve serum testosterone levels in the mid-normal range.
Oral testosterone undecanoate[a]*:* Monitor serum testosterone levels 3–5 h after ingestion.
Injectable testosterone undecanoate[a]*:* Measure serum testosterone level just prior to each subsequent injection and adjust the dosing interval to maintain serum testosterone in mid-normal range.
3. Check hematocrit at baseline, at 3 months, and then annually. If hematocrit is >54%, stop therapy until hematocrit decreases to a safe level; evaluate the patient for hypoxia and sleep apnea; reinitiate therapy with a reduced dose.
4. Measure bone mineral density of lumbar spine and/or femoral neck after 1–2 years of testosterone therapy in hypogonadal men with osteoporosis or low trauma fracture, consistent with regional standard of care.
5. Perform digital rectal examination and check PSA level before initiating treatment, at 3 months, and then in accordance with guidelines for prostate cancer screening depending on the age and race of the patient.
6. Obtain urologic consultation if there is:
Verified serum PSA concentration >4.0 ng/mL
An increase in serum PSA concentration >1.4 ng/mL within any 12-month period of testosterone treatment
A PSA velocity of >0.4 ng/mL per year using the PSA level after 6 months of testosterone administration as the reference (only applicable if PSA data are available for a period exceeding 2 years)
Detection of a prostatic abnormality on digital rectal examination
An AUA/IPSS of >19
7. Evaluate formulation-specific adverse effects at each visit.
Buccal testosterone tablets: Inquire about alterations in taste and examine the gums and oral mucosa for irritation.
Injectable testosterone esters (enanthate and cypionate): Ask about fluctuations in mood or libido.
Testosterone patches: Look for skin reaction at the application site.
Testosterone gels: Advise patients to cover the application sites with a shirt and to wash the skin with soap and water before having skin-to-skin contact, as testosterone gels leave a testosterone residue on the skin that can be transferred to a woman or child who might come in close contact. Serum testosterone levels are maintained when the application site is washed 4–6 hours after application of the testosterone gel.

[a]Not approved for clinical use in the United States.

Note: PSA, prostate-specific antigen; AUA, American Urological Association; IPSS, International Prostate Symptom Score.

Source: Reproduced from the Endocrine Society Guideline for Testosterone Therapy of Androgen Deficiency Syndromes in Adult Men (Bhasin et al).

effects include acne, oiliness of skin, erythrocytosis, breast tenderness and enlargement, leg edema, induction and exacerbation of obstructive sleep apnea, and increased risk of prostate cancer, though it may increase the incidence of detection rather than the actual occurrence rate. In addition, there may be formulation-specific adverse effects such as skin irritation with transdermal patch, risk of gel transfer to a sexual partner with testosterone gels, buccal ulceration and gum problems with buccal testosterone, and pain and mood fluctuation with injectable testosterone esters.

Hemoglobin Levels Administration of testosterone to androgen-deficient men is typically associated with a 3–5% increase in hemoglobin levels, but the magnitude of hemoglobin increase may be greater in men who have sleep apnea, a significant smoking history, or chronic obstructive lung disease. Erythrocytosis is the most frequent adverse event reported in testosterone trials in middle-aged and older men and is also the most frequent cause of treatment discontinuation in these trials. The frequency of erythrocytosis is higher in older men than younger men and higher in hypogonadal men treated with injectable testosterone esters than in those treated with transdermal formulations, presumably due to the higher testosterone dose delivered by the typical regimens of testosterone esters. If hematocrit rises above 54%, testosterone therapy should be stopped until hematocrit has fallen to <50%. After evaluation of the patient for hypoxia and sleep apnea, testosterone therapy may be reinitiated at a lower dose.

Digital Examination of the Prostate and Serum PSA Levels Testosterone replacement therapy increases prostate volume to the size seen in age-matched controls but should not increase prostate volume beyond that expected for age. There is no evidence that testosterone replacement causes prostate cancer. However, androgen administration can exacerbate preexisting prostate cancer. Many older men harbor microscopic foci of cancer in their prostates. It is not known whether long-term testosterone administration will induce these microscopic foci to grow into clinically significant cancers.

PSA levels are lower in testosterone-deficient men and are restored to normal after testosterone replacement. There is considerable test-retest variability in PSA measurements; the average interassay coefficient of variation of PSA assays is 15%. The 95% confidence interval for the change in PSA values, measured 3–6 months apart, is 1.4 ng/mL. Increments in PSA levels after testosterone supplementation in androgen-deficient men are generally <0.5 ng/mL, and increments >1.0 ng/mL over a 3–6-month period are unusual. Nevertheless, administration of testosterone to men with baseline PSA levels between 2.5 and 4.0 ng/mL will cause PSA levels to exceed 4.0 ng/mL for some, and many of these men may undergo prostate biopsies. PSA velocity criterion can be used for patients who have sequential PSA measurements for >2 years; a change of >0.40 ng/mL per year merits closer urologic follow-up.

Cardiovascular Risk Assessment The long-term effects of testosterone supplementation on cardiovascular risk are unknown. Testosterone effects on lipids depend on the dose (physiologic or supraphysiologic), the route of administration (oral or parenteral), and the formulation (whether aromatizable or not). Physiologic testosterone replacement by an aromatizable androgen has a modest effect on HDL or no effect at all. In middle-aged men with low testosterone levels, physiologic testosterone replacement has been shown to improve insulin sensitivity and reduce visceral obesity. In epidemiologic studies, testosterone concentrations are inversely related to waist-to-hip ratio and directly correlated with HDL cholesterol levels. These data suggest that physiologic testosterone concentration is correlated with factors associated with reduced cardiovascular risk. However, no prospective studies have examined the effect on testosterone replacement on cardiovascular risk.

ANDROGEN ABUSE BY ATHLETES AND RECREATIONAL BODYBUILDERS The illicit use of androgenic steroids to enhance athletic performance is widespread among professional and high school athletes and recreational bodybuilders. Although androgen supplementation increases skeletal muscle mass and strength, whether and how androgens improve athletic performance is unknown. The most commonly used androgenic steroids include testosterone esters, nandrolone, stanozolol, methandienone, and methenolol. Athletes generally use increasing doses of multiple steroids in a practice known as stacking. A majority of athletes who abuse androgenic steroids also use other drugs that are perceived to be muscle-building or performance-enhancing, such as growth hormone; IGF-I; insulin; stimulants such as amphetamine, clenbuterol, ephedrine, and thyroxine; and drugs perceived to reduce adverse effects such as hCG, aromatase inhibitors, or estrogen antagonists.

The adverse effects of androgen abuse include a marked decrease in plasma HDL cholesterol and an increase in low-density lipoprotein (LDL) cholesterol, changes in clotting factors, suppression of spermatogenesis resulting in reduced fertility, and increase in liver enzymes. Elevations of liver enzymes, hepatic neoplasms, and peliosis hepatis have been reported, mostly with the use of oral, 17α-alkylated androgenic steroids but not with parenterally administered testosterone or its esters. There are anecdotal reports of the association of androgenic steroid use with "rage reactions." Breast tenderness and enlargement are not uncommon among athletes abusing aromatizable androgens. Oral 17α-alkylated androgens also can induce insulin resistance and glucose intolerance. A serious, underappreciated adverse effect of androgen use is the suppression of the hypothalamic-pituitary-testicular axis. Upon discontinuation of exogenous androgen use, the suppressed hypothalamic-pituitary axis may take weeks to months to recover. During this period when testosterone levels are low, the athletes may experience sexual dysfunction, hot flushes, fatigue, and depressed mood, causing some athletes to resume androgen use and thus perpetuating the cycle of abuse, withdrawal symptoms, and dependence. Also, the use of nonsterile needles confers the risk of local infection, sepsis, hepatitis, and HIV infection. Disproportionate gains in muscle mass and strength without commensurate adaptations in tendons and other connective tissues may predispose to the risk of tendon injuries.

Accredited laboratories use gas chromatography-mass spectrometry or liquid chromatography-mass spectrometry to detect anabolic steroid abuse. In recent years, the availability of high-resolution mass spectrometry and tandem mass spectrometry has further improved the sensitivity of detecting androgen abuse. Illicit testosterone use is detected generally by the application of the measurement of the urinary testosterone-to-epitestosterone ratio and further confirmed by the use of the $^{13}C:^{12}C$ ratio in testosterone by the use of isotope ratio combustion mass spectrometry. Exogenous testosterone administration increases urinary testosterone glucuronide excretion and consequently the testosterone-to-epitestosterone ratio. Ratios above 6 suggest exogenous testosterone use but can also reflect genetic variation. Synthetic testosterone has a lower ^{13}C:^{12}C ratio than endogenously produced testosterone and these differences in the ^{13}C:^{12}C ratio can be detected by isotope ratio combustion mass spectrometry, which is used to confirm exogenous testosterone use in individuals with a high testosterone-to-epitestosterone ratio.

FURTHER READINGS

ACHERMANN JC et al: Inherited disorders of the gonadotropin hormones. Mol Cell Endocrinol 179:89, 2001

BHASIN S: An approach to infertile men. J Clin Endocrinol Metab 92:1995, 2007

——— et al: Testosterone therapy in adult men with androgen deficiency syndromes: An Endocrine Society clinical practice guideline. J Clin Endocrinol Metab 91:1995, 2006

BOLONA ER et al: Testosterone use in men with sexual dysfunction: A systematic review and meta-analysis of randomized placebo-controlled trials. Mayo Clin Proc 82:20, 2007

BOULIGAND J et al: Isolated familial hypogonadotropic hypogonadism and a GNRH1 mutation. N Engl J Med 360:2742, 2009

FERLIN A et al: Molecular and clinical characterizations of Y chromosome microdeletions in infertile men: A 10-year experience in Italy. J Clin Endocrinol Metab 92:762, 2007

MAURAS N et al: Pharmacokinetics and pharmacodynamics of anastrozole in pubertal boys with recent onset gynecomastia. J Clin Endocrinol Metab, 2009

SEGAL TY et al: Role of gonadotropin-releasing hormone and human chorionic gonadotropin stimulation tests in differentiating patients with hypogonadotropic hypogonadism from those with constitutional delay of growth and puberty. J Clin Endocrinol Metab 94:780, 2009

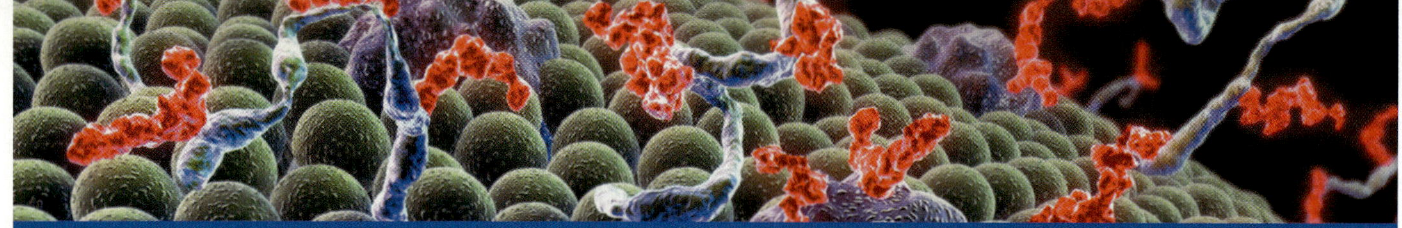

CHAPTER 9
TESTICULAR CANCER

Robert J. Motzer ■ George J. Bosl

Primary germ cell tumors (GCTs) of the testis, arising by the malignant transformation of primordial germ cells, constitute 95% of all testicular neoplasms. Infrequently, GCTs arise from an extragonadal site, including the mediastinum, the retroperitoneum, and, very rarely, the pineal gland. This disease is notable for the young age of the afflicted patients, the totipotent capacity for differentiation of the tumor cells, and its curability; about 95% of newly diagnosed patients are cured. Experience in the management of GCTs leads to improved outcome.

INCIDENCE AND EPIDEMIOLOGY

In 2007, 7920 new cases of testicular GCT were diagnosed in the United States; the incidence is decreasing after having increased slowly over the past 40 years. The tumor occurs most frequently in men between the ages of 20 and 40. A testicular mass in a male ≥50 years should be regarded as a lymphoma until proved otherwise. GCT is at least four to five times more common in white than in African-American males, and a higher incidence has been observed in Scandinavia and New Zealand than in the United States.

ETIOLOGY AND GENETICS

Cryptorchidism is associated with a severalfold higher risk of GCT. Abdominal cryptorchid testes are at a higher risk than inguinal cryptorchid testes. Orchiopexy should be performed before puberty, if possible. Early orchiopexy reduces the risk of GCT and improves the ability to save the testis. An abdominal cryptorchid testis that cannot be brought into the scrotum should be removed. About 2% of men with GCTs of one testis will develop a primary tumor in the other testis. Testicular feminization syndromes increase the risk of testicular GCT, and Klinefelter syndrome is associated with mediastinal GCT.

An isochromosome of the short arm of chromosome 12 [i(12p)] is pathognomonic for GCT of all histologic types. Excess 12p copy number, either in the form of i(12p) or as increased 12p on aberrantly banded marker chromosomes, occurs in nearly all GCTs, but the genes on 12p involved in the pathogenesis are not yet defined.

CLINICAL PRESENTATION

A painless testicular mass is pathognomonic for a testicular malignancy. More commonly, patients present with testicular discomfort or swelling suggestive of epididymitis and/or orchitis. In this circumstance, a trial of antibiotics is reasonable. However, if symptoms persist or a residual abnormality remains, then testicular ultrasound examination is indicated.

Ultrasound of the testis is indicated whenever a testicular malignancy is considered and for persistent or painful testicular swelling. If a testicular mass is detected, a radical inguinal orchiectomy should be performed. Because the testis develops from the gonadal ridge, its blood supply and lymphatic drainage originate in the abdomen and descend with the testis into the scrotum. An inguinal approach is taken to avoid breaching anatomic barriers and permitting additional pathways of spread.

Back pain from retroperitoneal metastases is common and must be distinguished from musculoskeletal pain. Dyspnea from pulmonary metastases occurs infrequently. Patients with increased serum levels of human chorionic gonadotropin (hCG) may present with gynecomastia. A delay in diagnosis is associated with a more advanced stage and possibly worse survival.

The staging evaluation for GCT includes a determination of serum levels of α-fetoprotein (AFP), hCG, and lactate dehydrogenase (LDH). After orchiectomy, a chest radiograph and a CT scan of the abdomen and pelvis should be performed. A chest CT scan is required if pulmonary nodules or mediastinal or hilar disease is suspected. Stage I disease is limited to the testis, epididymis, or spermatic cord. Stage II disease is limited to retroperitoneal (regional) lymph nodes. Stage III disease is disease outside the retroperitoneum, involving supradiaphragmatic nodal sites or viscera. The staging may be "clinical"—defined solely by physical examination, blood marker evaluation, and radiographs—or "pathologic"—defined by an operative procedure.

The regional draining lymph nodes for the testis are in the retroperitoneum, and the vascular supply originates from the great vessels (for the right testis) or the renal vessels (for the left testis). As a result, the lymph nodes that are involved first by a right testicular tumor are the interaortocaval lymph nodes just below the renal vessels. For a left testicular tumor, the first involved lymph nodes are lateral to the aorta (para-aortic) and below the left renal vessels. In both cases, further nodal spread is inferior, contralateral, and, less commonly, above the renal hilum. Lymphatic involvement can extend cephalad to the retrocrural, posterior mediastinal, and supraclavicular lymph nodes. Treatment is determined by tumor histology (seminoma versus nonseminoma) and clinical stage (Table 9-1).

PATHOLOGY

GCTs are divided into nonseminoma and seminoma subtypes. Nonseminomatous GCTs are most frequent in the third decade of life and can display the full spectrum of embryonic and adult cellular differentiation. This entity is composed of four histologies: embryonal carcinoma, teratoma, choriocarcinoma, and endodermal sinus (yolk sac) tumor. Choriocarcinoma, consisting of both cytotrophoblasts and syncytiophoblasts, represents malignant trophoblastic differentiation and is invariably associated with secretion of hCG. Endodermal sinus tumor is the malignant counterpart of the fetal yolk sac and is associated with secretion of AFP. Pure embryonal carcinoma may secrete AFP or hCG, or both; this pattern is biochemical evidence of differentiation. Teratoma is composed of somatic cell types derived from two or more germ layers (ectoderm, mesoderm, or endoderm). Each of these histologies may be present alone or in combination with others. Nonseminomatous GCTs tend to metastasize early to sites such as the retroperitoneal lymph nodes and lung parenchyma. One-third of patients present with disease limited to the testis (stage I), one-third with retroperitoneal metastases (stage II), and one-third with more extensive supradiaphragmatic nodal or visceral metastases (stage III).

TABLE 9-1

GERM CELL TUMOR STAGING AND TREATMENT

		TREATMENT	
STAGE	**EXTENT OF DISEASE**	**SEMINOMA**	**NONSEMINOMA**
IA	Testis only, no vascular/lymphatic invasion (T1)	Radiation therapy	RPLND or observation
IB	Testis only, with vascular/lymphatic invasion (T2), or extension through tunica albuginea (T2), or involvement of spermatic cord (T3) or scrotum (T4)	Radiation therapy	RPLND
IIA	Nodes <2 cm	Radiation therapy	RPLND or chemotherapy often followed by RPLND
IIB	Nodes 2–5 cm	Radiation therapy	RPLND ± adjuvant chemotherapy or chemotherapy followed by RPLND
IIC	Nodes >5 cm	Chemotherapy	Chemotherapy, often followed by RPLND
III	Distant metastases	Chemotherapy	Chemotherapy, often followed by surgery (biopsy or resection)

Note: RPLND, retroperitoneal lymph node dissection.

Seminoma represents about 50% of all GCTs, has a median age in the fourth decade, and generally follows a more indolent clinical course. Most patients (70%) present with stage I disease, about 20% with stage II disease, and 10% with stage III disease; lung or other visceral metastases are rare. Radiation therapy is the treatment of choice in patients with stage I disease and stage II disease where the nodes are <5 cm in maximum diameter. When a tumor contains both seminoma and nonseminoma components, patient management is directed by the more aggressive nonseminoma component.

TUMOR MARKERS

Careful monitoring of the serum tumor markers AFP and hCG is essential in the management of patients with GCT, as these markers are important for diagnosis, as prognostic indicators, in monitoring treatment response, and in detecting early relapse. Approximately 70% of patients presenting with disseminated nonseminomatous GCT have increased serum concentrations of AFP and/or hCG. While hCG concentrations may be increased in patients with either nonseminoma or seminoma histology, the AFP concentration is increased only in patients with nonseminoma. The presence of an increased AFP level in a patient whose tumor shows only seminoma indicates that an occult nonseminomatous component exists and the patient should be treated for nonseminomatous GCT. LDH levels are not as specific as AFP or hCG but are increased in 50–60% patients with metastatic nonseminoma and in up to 80% of patients with advanced seminoma.

AFP, hCG, and LDH levels should be determined before and after orchiectomy. Increased serum AFP and hCG concentrations decay according to first-order kinetics; the half-life is 24–36 h for hCG and 5–7 days for AFP. AFP and hCG should be assayed serially during and after treatment. The reappearance of hCG and/or AFP or the failure of these markers to decline according to the predicted half-life is an indicator of persistent or recurrent tumor.

℞ Treatment: TESTICULAR CANCER

STAGE I NONSEMINOMA If, after an orchiectomy (for clinical stage I disease), radiographs and physical examination show no evidence of disease and serum AFP and hCG concentrations are either normal or declining to normal according to the known half-life, patients may be managed by either a nerve-sparing retroperitoneal lymph node dissection (RPLND) or surveillance. The retroperitoneal lymph nodes are involved by GCT (pathologic stage II) in 20–50% of these patients. The choice of surveillance or RPLND is based on the pathology of the primary tumor. If the primary tumor shows no evidence for lymphatic or vascular invasion and is limited to the testis (T1), then either option is reasonable. If lymphatic or vascular invasion is present or the tumor extends into the tunica, spermatic cord, or scrotum (T2 through T4), then surveillance should not be offered. Either approach should cure >95% of patients.

RPLND is the standard operation for removal of the regional lymph nodes of the testis (retroperitoneal nodes). The operation removes the lymph nodes ipsilateral to the primary site and the nodal groups adjacent to the primary landing zone. The standard (modified bilateral) RPLND removes all node-bearing tissue down to the bifurcation of the great vessels, including the ipsilateral iliac nodes. The major long-term effect of this operation is retrograde ejaculation and infertility. Nerve-sparing RPLND, usually accomplished by identification and dissection of individual nerve fibers, may avoid injury to the sympathetic nerves responsible for ejaculation. Normal ejaculation is preserved in ~90% of patients. Patients with pathologic stage I disease are observed, and only the <10% who relapse require additional therapy. If retroperitoneal nodes are found to be involved at RPLND, then a decision regarding adjuvant chemotherapy is made on the basis of the extent of retroperitoneal disease.

Surveillance is an option in the management of clinical stage I disease when no vascular/lymphatic invasion is found (T1). Only 20–30% of patients have pathologic stage II disease, implying that most RPLNDs in this situation are not therapeutic. Surveillance and RPLND lead to equivalent long-term survival rates. Patient compliance is essential if surveillance is to be successful. Patients must be carefully followed with periodic chest radiography, physical examination, CT scan of the abdomen, and serum tumor marker determinations. The median time to relapse is about 7 months, and late relapses (>2 years) are rare. The 70–80% of patients who do not relapse require no intervention after orchiectomy; treatment is reserved for those who do relapse. When the primary tumor is classified as T2 through T4 (extension beyond testis and epididymis or lymphatic/vascular invasion is identified), nerve-sparing RPLND is preferred. About 50% of these patients have pathologic stage II disease and are destined to relapse without the RPLND.

STAGE II NONSEMINOMA Patients with limited, ipsilateral retroperitoneal adenopathy (nodes usually ≤3 cm in largest diameter) and normal levels of AFP and hCG generally undergo a modified bilateral RPLND as primary management. Increased levels of either AFP or hCG or both imply metastatic disease outside the retroperitoneum; chemotherapy is used in this setting. The local recurrence rate after a properly performed RPLND is very low. Depending on the extent of disease, the postoperative management options include either surveillance or two cycles of adjuvant chemotherapy. Surveillance is the preferred approach for patients with resected "low-volume" metastases (tumor nodes ≤2 cm in diameter *and* <6 nodes involved) because the probability of relapse is one-third or less. For those who relapse, risk-directed chemotherapy is indicated. Because relapse occurs in ≥50% of patients with "high-volume" metastases (>6 nodes involved, *or* any involved node >2 cm in largest diameter, *or* extranodal tumor extension), two cycles of adjuvant chemotherapy should be considered, as it results in cure in ≥98% of patients. Regimens consisting of etoposide (100 mg/m^2 daily on days 1–5) plus cisplatin (20 mg/m^2 daily on days 1–5) with or without bleomycin (30 units per day on days 2, 9, and 16) given at 3-week intervals are effective and well tolerated.

STAGES I AND II SEMINOMA Inguinal orchiectomy followed by retroperitoneal radiation therapy cures ~98% of patients with stage I seminoma. The dose of radiation therapy (2500–3000 cGy) is low and well tolerated, and the in-field recurrence rate is negligible. About 2% of patients relapse with supradiaphragmatic or systemic disease. Surveillance has been proposed as an option, and studies have shown that about 15% of patients relapse. The median time to relapse is 12–15 months, and late relapses (>5 years) may be more frequent than with nonseminoma. The relapse is usually treated with chemotherapy. Surveillance for clinical stage I seminoma is not recommended.

Nonbulky retroperitoneal disease (stage IIA and IIB) is also treated with radiation therapy. Prophylactic supradiaphragmatic fields are not used. Relapses in the anterior mediastinum are unusual. Approximately 90% of patients achieve relapse-free survival with retroperitoneal masses <5 cm in diameter. Because at least one-third of patients with bulkier disease relapse, initial chemotherapy is preferred for stage IIC disease.

CHEMOTHERAPY FOR ADVANCED GCT Regardless of histology, patients with stage IIC and stage III GCT are treated with chemotherapy. Combination chemotherapy programs based on cisplatin at doses of 100 mg/m^2 plus etoposide at doses of 500 mg/m^2 per cycle cure 70–80% of such patients, with or without bleomycin, depending on risk stratification. A complete response (the complete disappearance of all clinical evidence of tumor on physical examination and radiography plus normal serum levels of AFP and hCG for ≥1 month) occurs after chemotherapy alone in ~60% of patients, and another 10–20% become disease-free with surgical resection of residual masses containing viable GCT. Lower doses of cisplatin result in inferior survival rates.

The toxicity of four cycles of the cisplatin/bleomycin/etoposide (BEP) regimen is substantial. Nausea, vomiting, and hair loss occur in most patients, although nausea and vomiting have been markedly ameliorated by modern antiemetic regimens. Myelosuppression is frequent, and symptomatic bleomycin pulmonary toxicity occurs in ~5% of patients. Treatment-induced mortality due to neutropenia with septicemia or bleomycin-induced pulmonary failure occurs in 1–3% of patients. Dose reductions for myelosuppression are rarely indicated. Long-term permanent toxicities include nephrotoxicity (reduced glomerular filtration and persistent magnesium wasting), ototoxicity, and peripheral neuropathy. When bleomycin is administered by weekly bolus injection, Raynaud's phenomenon appears in 5–10% of patients. Other evidence of small blood vessel damage is seen less often, including transient ischemic attacks and myocardial infarction.

RISK-DIRECTED CHEMOTHERAPY Because not all patients are cured and treatment may cause significant toxicities, patients are stratified into "good-risk" and "poor-risk" groups according to pretreatment clinical features. For good-risk patients, the goal is to achieve maximum efficacy with minimal toxicity. For poor-risk patients, the goal is to identify more effective therapy with tolerable toxicity.

The International Germ Cell Cancer Consensus Group developed criteria to assign patients to three risk groups (good, intermediate, and poor) (**Table 9-2**). The marker cut-offs have been incorporated into the revised TNM (primary tumor, regional nodes, metastasis) staging of GCT. Hence, TNM stage groupings are now based on both anatomy (site and extent of disease) and biology (marker status and histology). Seminoma is either good or intermediate risk, based on the absence or presence of nonpulmonary visceral metastases. No poor-risk category exists for seminoma. Marker levels play no role in defining risk for seminoma. Nonseminomas have good-, intermediate-, and poor-risk categories based on the site of the primary tumor, the presence or absence of nonpulmonary visceral metastases, and marker levels.

For ~90% of patients with good-risk GCTs, four cycles of etoposide plus cisplatin (EP) or three cycles of BEP produce durable complete responses, with minimal acute and chronic toxicity. Pulmonary toxicity is absent when bleomycin is not used and is rare when therapy is limited to 9 weeks; myelosuppression with neutropenic fever is less frequent; and the treatment mortality rate is negligible. About 75% of intermediate-risk patients and 45% of poor-risk patients achieve durable complete remission with four cycles of BEP, and no regimen has proved superior. More effective therapy is needed.

POSTCHEMOTHERAPY SURGERY Resection of residual metastases after the completion of chemotherapy is an integral part of therapy. If the

TABLE 9-2

IGCCCG RISK CLASSIFICATION FOR ADVANCED GERM CELL TUMORS

RISK	NONSEMINOMA	SEMINOMA
Good	Gonadal or retroperitoneal primary site Absent nonpulmonary visceral metastases AFP <1000 ng/mL β-hCG <5000 mIU/mL LDH <1.5 × upper limit or normal (ULN)	Any primary site Absent nonpulmonary visceral metastases Any LDH, hCG
Intermediate	Gonadal or retroperitoneal primary site Absent nonpulmonary visceral metastases AFP 1000–10,000 ng/mL β-hCG 5000–50,000 mIU/mL LDH 1.5–10 × ULN	Any primary site Presence of nonpulmonary visceral metastases Any LDH, hCG
Poor	Mediastinal primary site Presence of nonpulmonary visceral metastases AFP ≥10,000 ng/ML β-hCG > 50,000 mIU/mL LDH >10 × ULN	No patients classified as poor prognosis

Note: AFP, α-fetoprotein; hCG, human chorionic gonadotropin; LDH, lactate dehydrogenase.
Source: From International Germ Cell Cancer Consensus Group.

initial histology is nonseminoma and the marker values have normalized, all sites of residual disease should be resected. In general, residual retroperitoneal disease requires a modified bilateral RPLND. Thoracotomy (unilateral or bilateral) and neck dissection are less frequently required to remove residual mediastinal, pulmonary parenchymal, or cervical nodal disease. Viable tumor (seminoma, embryonal carcinoma, yolk sac tumor, or choriocarcinoma) will be present in 15%, mature teratoma in 40%, and necrotic debris and fibrosis in 45% of resected specimens. The frequency of teratoma or viable disease is highest in residual mediastinal tumors. If necrotic debris or mature teratoma is present, no further chemotherapy is necessary. If viable tumor is present but is completely excised, two additional cycles of chemotherapy are given.

If the initial histology is pure seminoma, mature teratoma is rarely present, and the most frequent finding is necrotic debris. For residual retroperitoneal disease, a complete RPLND is technically difficult owing to extensive postchemotherapy fibrosis. Observation is recommended when no radiographic abnormality exists on CT scan. Positive findings on a positron emission tomography (PET) scan correlate with viable seminoma in residua and mandate surgical excision or biopsy.

SALVAGE CHEMOTHERAPY Of patients with advanced GCT, 20–30% fail to achieve a durable complete response to first-line chemotherapy. A combination of cisplatin, ifosfamide, and vinblastine (VeIP) will cure about 25% of patients as a second-line therapy. Substitution of paclitaxel for vinblastine may be more effective in this setting. Patients are more likely to achieve a durable complete response if they had a testicular primary tumor and relapsed from a prior complete remission to first-line cisplatin-containing chemotherapy. In contrast, if the patient failed to achieve a complete response or has a primary mediastinal nonseminoma, then standard-dose salvage therapy is rarely beneficial. Treatment options for such patients include dose-intensive treatment, experimental therapies, and surgical resection.

Chemotherapy consisting of dose-intensive, high-dose carboplatin (≥1500 mg/m^2) plus etoposide (≥1200 mg/m^2), with or without cyclophosphamide, or ifosfamide, with peripheral blood stem cell support, induces a complete response in 25–40% of patients who have progressed after ifosfamide-containing salvage chemotherapy. About one-half of the complete responses will be durable. High-dose therapy is the treatment of choice and standard of care for this patient population. Paclitaxel is also active in previously treated patients and shows promise in high-dose combination programs. Cure is still possible in some relapsed patients.

EXTRAGONADAL GCT AND MIDLINE CARCINOMA OF UNCERTAIN HISTOGENESIS

The prognosis and management of patients with extragonadal GCT depend on the tumor histology and site of origin. All patients with a diagnosis of extragonadal GCT should have a testicular ultrasound examination. Nearly all patients with retroperitoneal or mediastinal seminoma achieve a durable complete response to BEP or EP. The clinical features of patients with primary retroperitoneal nonseminoma GCT are similar to those of patients with a primary of testis origin, and careful evaluation will find evidence of a primary testicular GCT in about two-thirds of cases. In contrast, a primary mediastinal nonseminomatous GCT is associated with a poor prognosis; one-third of patients are cured with standard therapy (four cycles of BEP). Patients with newly diagnosed mediastinal nonseminoma are considered to have poor-risk disease and should be considered for clinical trials testing regimens of possibly greater efficacy. In addition, mediastinal nonseminoma is associated with hematologic disorders, including acute myelogenous leukemia, myelodysplastic syndrome, and essential thrombocytosis unrelated to previous chemotherapy. These hematologic disorders are very refractory to treatment. Nonseminoma of any primary site may change into other malignant histologies such as embryonal rhabdomyosarcoma or adenocarcinoma. This is called malignant transformation. i(12p) has been identified in the transformed cell type, indicating GCT clonal origin.

A group of patients with poorly differentiated tumors of unknown histogenesis, midline in distribution, and not associated with secretion of AFP or hCG has been described; a few (10–20%) are cured by standard cisplatin-containing chemotherapy. i(12p) is present in ~25% of such tumors (the fraction that are cisplatin-responsive), confirming their origin from primitive germ cells. This finding is also predictive of the response to cisplatin-based chemotherapy and resulting long-term survival. These tumors are heterogeneous; neuroepithelial tumors and lymphoma may also present in this fashion.

FERTILITY

Infertility is an important consequence of the treatment of GCTs. Preexisting infertility or impaired fertility is often present. Azoospermia and/or oligospermia are present at diagnosis in at least 50% of patients with testicular GCTs. Ejaculatory dysfunction is associated with RPLND, and germ cell damage may result from cisplatin-containing chemotherapy. Nerve-sparing techniques to preserve the retroperitoneal sympathetic nerves have made retrograde ejaculation less likely in the subgroups of patients who are candidates for this operation. Spermatogenesis does recur in some patients after chemotherapy. However, because of the significant risk of impaired reproductive capacity, semen analysis and cryopreservation of sperm in a sperm bank should be recommended to all patients before treatment.

FURTHER READINGS

Bosl GJ et al: Testicular germ-cell cancer. N Engl J Med 337:242, 1997

——— et al: Cancer of the testis, in *Cancer: Principles and Practice of Oncology*, 7th ed, VT DeVita et al (eds). Philadelphia, Lippincott Williams & Wilkins, 2005, pp 1269–1294

Chaganti RSK, Houldsworth J: Genetics and biology of human male germ cell tumors. Cancer Res 60:1475, 2000

Feldman DR et al: Medical treatment of advanced testicular cancer. JAMA 299:672, 2008

International Germ Cell Cancer Consensus Group: International Germ Cell Consensus Classification: A prognostic factor-based staging system for metastatic germ cell cancers. J Clin Oncol 15:594, 1997

Kondagunta GV et al: Etoposide and cisplatin chemotherapy for metastatic good-risk germ cell tumors. J Clin Oncol 23:9290, 2005

Moore CJ et al: Management of difficult germ-cell tumors. Oncology 20:1565, 2006

Motzer R et al: Sequential dose-intensive paclitaxel, ifosfamide, carboplatin, and etoposide salvage therapy for germ cell tumor patients. J Clin Oncol 18:1173, 2000

Sonpaude G et al: Management of recurrent testicular germ cell tumors. Oncologist 12:51, 2007

Torpy JM et al: JAMA patient page. Testicular cancer. JAMA 299:718, 2008

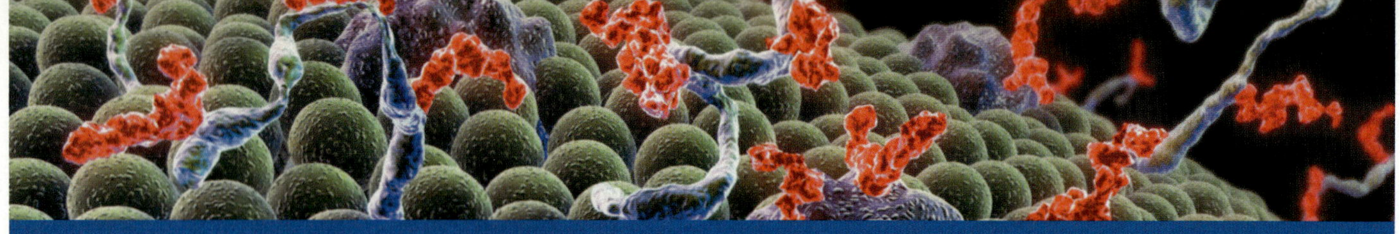

CHAPTER 10

THE FEMALE REPRODUCTIVE SYSTEM: INFERTILITY AND CONTRACEPTION

Janet E. Hall

The female reproductive system regulates the hormonal changes responsible for puberty and adult reproductive function. Normal reproductive function in women requires the dynamic integration of hormonal signals from the hypothalamus, pituitary, and ovary, resulting in repetitive cycles of follicle development, ovulation, and preparation of the endometrial lining of the uterus for implantation should conception occur.

For further discussion of related topics, see the following chapters: menstrual cycle disorders (Chap. 11), hyperandrogenic disorders (Chap. 13), sexual differentiation (Chap. 7), menopause (Chap. 12), gynecologic malignancies (Chap. 14), and male hormonal contraception (Chap. 8).

DEVELOPMENT OF THE OVARY AND EARLY FOLLICULAR GROWTH

The ovary orchestrates the development and release of a mature oocyte and also elaborates hormones (e.g., estrogen, progesterone, inhibin) that are critical for pubertal development and preparation of the uterus for conception, implantation, and the early stages of pregnancy. To achieve these functions in repeated monthly cycles, the ovary undergoes some of the most dynamic changes of any organ in the body.

Primordial germ cells can be identified by the third week of gestation and their migration to the genital ridge is complete by 6 weeks' gestation. Germ cells can only persist within the genital ridge and are then referred to as *oogonia*. In contrast to testis development, germ cells are essential for induction of normal ovarian development, reflecting a key role of oogonia in the formation of primordial follicles. Although one X chromosome undergoes X inactivation in somatic cells, it is reactivated in oogonia and genes on both X chromosomes are required for normal ovarian development. A streak ovary containing only stromal cells is found in patients with 45,X Turner syndrome (Chap. 7).

Starting at ~8 weeks' gestation, oogonia begin to enter prophase of the first meiotic division and become primary oocytes. This allows the oocyte to be surrounded by a single layer of flattened granulosa cells to form a primordial follicle. Granulosa cells are derived from mesonephric cells that invade the ovary early in its development, pushing the germ cells to the periphery or ovarian cortex. Although recent studies have reopened the debate, the weight of evidence supports the concept that the ovary contains a nonrenewable pool of germ cells. Through the combined processes of mitosis, meiosis, and atresia, the population of oogonia reaches its maximum of 6–7 million by 20 weeks' gestation, after which there is inexorable loss of both oogonia and primordial follicles through the process of atresia. At birth, oogonia are no longer present in the ovary, and only 1–2 million germ cells remain (Fig. 10-1).

The oocyte persists in prophase of the first meiotic division until just before ovulation, when meiosis resumes. The quiescent primordial follicles are recruited to further growth and differentiation through a highly regulated process that limits the size of the developing cohort to ensure that folliculogenesis can continue throughout the reproductive life span. This initial recruitment of primordial follicles to form primary follicles is characterized by growth of the oocyte and the transition from squamous to cuboidal granulosa cells (Fig. 10-2). The theca interna cells that surround the developing follicle begin to form as the primary follicle grows. Acquisition of a zona pellucida by the oocyte and the presence of several layers of surrounding cuboidal granulosa cells mark the development of secondary follicles. It is at this stage that granulosa cells develop follicle-stimulating hormone (FSH), estradiol, and androgen receptors and communicate with one another through the development of gap junctions.

In murine models, genes that regulate ovarian development and follicle formation have been identified (Fig. 10-3). Bidirectional signals between the oocyte and its surrounding somatic cells are essential for normal follicular development. For example, the oocyte-derived factor in the germline α (FIGα) is required for initial follicle formation. Anti-müllerian hormone (AMH) and activins derived from somatic cells induce the development of primary follicles from primordial follicles. Oocyte- derived growth differentiation factor 9 (GDF-9) is required for migration of pre-theca cells to the outer surface of the developing follicle (Fig. 10-2). GDF-9 is also required for formation of secondary follicles, as are granulosa cell–derived KIT ligand (KITL) and the forkhead transcription factor (Foxl2). All of these genes are potential candidates for premature ovarian failure in women, and mutations in the human *FOXL2* gene have already been shown to cause the syndrome of blepharophimosis/ptosis/epicanthus inversus, which is associated with ovarian failure.

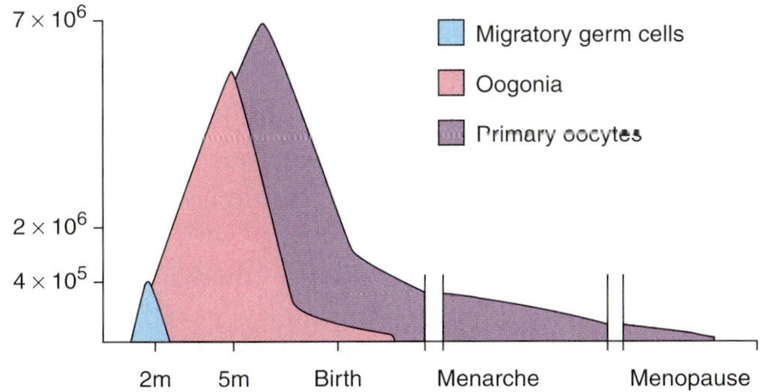

FIGURE 10-1
Ovarian germ cell number is maximal at mid-gestation, then decreases precipitously.

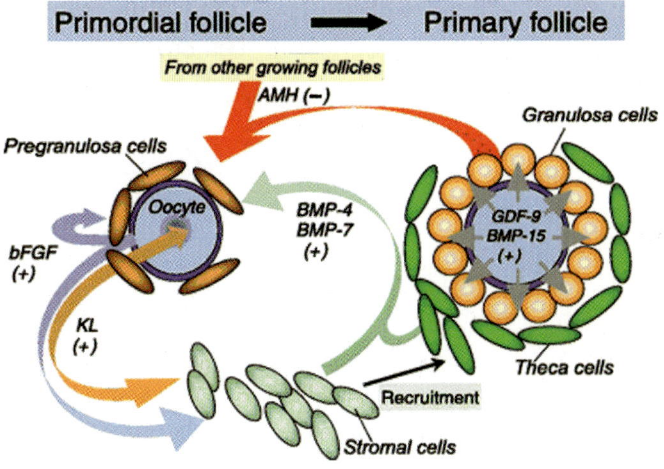

FIGURE 10-2
The primordial to primary follicle transition involves somatic cell differentiation to cuboidal granulosa cells and the formation of a theca cell layer from the surrounding stromal cells. These steps require the cooperative interaction of signals from the oocyte and the somatic cells. AMH, anti-müllerian hormone; bFGF, basic fibroblast growth factor; KL, kit ligand; BMP, bone morphogenic protein. (*From Knight and Glister, 2006; with permission.*)

DEVELOPMENT OF A MATURE FOLLICLE

The early stages of follicle growth are primarily driven by intraovarian factors, whereas maturation to the state required for ovulation, including the resumption of meiosis in the oocyte, requires the combined stimulus of FSH and luteinizing hormone (LH). Recruitment of secondary follicles from the resting follicle pool requires the direct action of FSH. Accumulation of follicular fluid between the layers of granulosa cells creates an antrum that divides the granulosa cells into two functionally distinct groups: mural cells that line the follicle wall and cumulus cells that surround the oocyte (Fig. 10-4). A single dominant follicle emerges from the growing follicle pool within the first 5–7 days after the onset of menses, and the majority of follicles fall off their growth trajectory and become atretic. Autocrine actions of activin and bone morphogenic protein 6 (BMP-6), derived from the

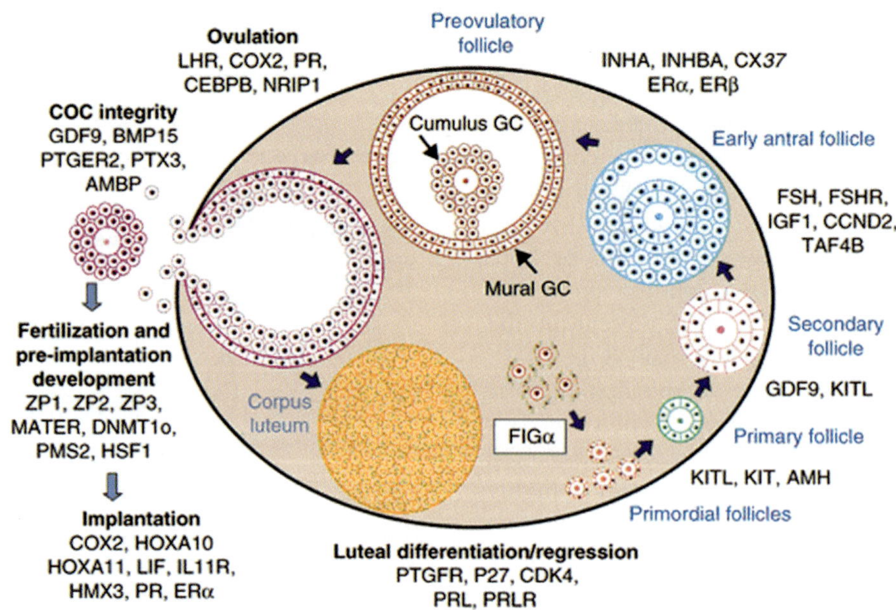

FIGURE 10-3

Specific genes control the orderly development of ovarian development and follicle formation. (*From MM Matzuk, DJ Lamb: Nat Cell Biol 4:Suppl S41–9, 2002; with permission.*)

granulosa cells, and paracrine actions of GDF-9, BMP-15, and BMP-6, derived from the oocyte, are involved in granulosa cell proliferation and modulation of FSH responsiveness. Differential exposure to these factors may explain why one follicle is selected for continued growth to the preovulatory stage. The dominant follicle can be distinguished by its size, evidence of granulosa cell proliferation, large number of FSH receptors, high aromatase activity, and elevated concentrations of estradiol and inhibin A in follicular fluid.

The dominant follicle undergoes rapid expansion during the 5–6 days prior to ovulation, reflecting granulosa cell proliferation and accumulation of follicular fluid. FSH induces LH receptors on the granulosa cells, and the preovulatory, or Graafian, follicle moves to the outer ovarian surface in preparation for ovulation. The LH surge triggers the resumption of meiosis, the suppression of granulosa cell proliferation, and the induction of cyclooxygenase 2 (COX-2), prostaglandins, and the progesterone receptor, each of which are required for ovulation, which involves cumulus expansion and the controlled expulsion of the egg and follicular fluid. The process of luteinization is induced by LH in conjunction with the loss of oocyte-derived luteinization inhibitors including GDF-9, BMP-15, and BMP-6.

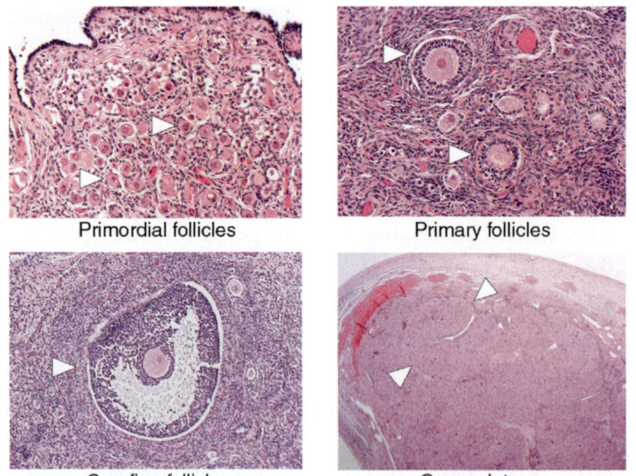

FIGURE 10-4

Development of ovarian follicles. (*Courtesy of JH Eichhorn and D Roberts, Massachusetts General Hospital; with permission.*)

REGULATION OF OVARIAN FUNCTION

HYPOTHALAMIC AND PITUITARY SECRETION

Gonadotropin-releasing hormone (GnRH) neurons develop from epithelial cells outside the central nervous system and migrate, initially alongside the olfactory neurons, to the medial basal hypothalamus. Approximately 7000 GnRH neurons, scattered throughout the medial basal hypothalamus, establish contacts with capillaries of the pituitary portal system in the median eminence. GnRH is secreted into the pituitary portal system in discrete pulses to stimulate synthesis and secretion of LH and FSH from pituitary gonadotropes, which comprise ~10% of cells in the pituitary (Chap. 2). Functional connections of GnRH neurons with the portal system are established by the end of the first trimester, coinciding

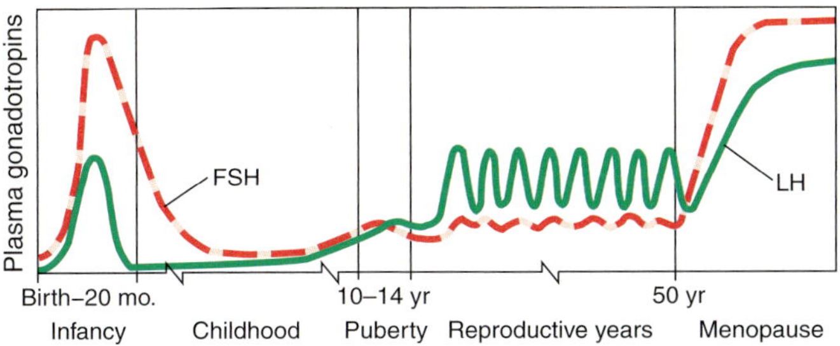

FIGURE 10-5

Follicle-stimulating hormone (FSH) and luteinizing hormone (LH) are increased during the neonatal years but go through a period of childhood quiescence before increasing again during puberty. Gonadotropin levels are cyclic during the reproductive years and increase dramatically with the loss of negative feedback that accompanies menopause.

with the production of pituitary gonadotropins. Thus, like the ovary, the hypothalamic and pituitary components of the reproductive system are present before birth. However, the high levels of estradiol and progesterone produced by the placenta suppress hormonal secretion in the fetus.

After birth, and the removal of placental steroids, gonadotropin levels rise. FSH levels are much higher in girls than in boys. This rise in FSH is associated with ovarian activation (evident on ultrasound) and increased inhibin B and estradiol levels. By 12–20 months of age, the reproductive axis is again suppressed, and a period of relative quiescence persists until puberty (Fig. 10-5). At the onset of puberty, pulsatile GnRH secretion induces pituitary gonadotropin production. In the early stages of puberty, LH and FSH secretion are apparent only during sleep, but as puberty develops, pulsatile gonadotropin secretion occurs throughout the day and night.

The mechanisms responsible for the childhood quiescence and pubertal reactivation of the reproductive axis remain incompletely understood. GnRH neurons in the hypothalamus respond to both excitatory and inhibitory factors. Increased sensitivity to the inhibitory influence of gonadal steroids has long been implicated in the inhibition of GnRH secretion during childhood. Metabolic signals, such as adipocyte-derived leptin, also play a permissive role in reproductive function (Chap. 16). Studies of patients with isolated GnRH deficiency reveal that mutations in the G protein–coupled receptor 54 (*GPR54*) gene preclude the onset of puberty. The ligand for this receptor, metastin, is derived from the parent peptide, kisspeptin-1 (KISS1), and is a powerful stimulant for GnRH release. A potential role for metastin in the onset of puberty has been suggested by upregulation of KISS1 and GPR54 transcripts in the hypothalamus at the time of puberty. The KISS/GPR54 system may also be involved in estrogen feedback regulation of GnRH secretion.

OVARIAN STEROIDS

Ovarian steroid–producing cells do not store hormones but produce them in response to LH and FSH during the normal menstrual cycle. The sequence of steps and the enzymes involved in the synthesis of steroid hormones are similar in the ovary, adrenal, and testes. However, the specific enzymes required to catalyze specific steps are compartmentalized and may not be abundant or even present in all cell types. Within the developing ovarian follicle, estrogen synthesis from cholesterol requires close integration between theca and granulosa cells—sometimes called the *two-cell model for steroidogenesis* (Fig. 10-6). FSH receptors are confined to the granulosa cells, whereas LH receptors are restricted to the theca cells until the late stages of follicular development, when they are also found on granulosa cells. The theca cells surrounding the follicle are highly vascularized and use cholesterol, derived primarily from circulating lipoproteins, as the starting point for the synthesis of androstenedione and testosterone under the control of LH. Androstenedione and testosterone are transferred across the basal lamina to the granulosa cells, which receive no direct blood supply. The mural granulosa cells are particularly rich in aromatase and, under the control of FSH, produce estradiol, the primary steroid secreted from the follicular phase ovary and the most potent estrogen. Theca cell–produced androstenedione and, to a lesser extent, testosterone are also secreted into peripheral blood, where they can be converted to dihydrotestosterone in skin and to estrogens in adipose tissue. The hilar interstitial cells of the ovary are functionally similar to Leydig cells and are also capable of secreting androgens. Although stromal

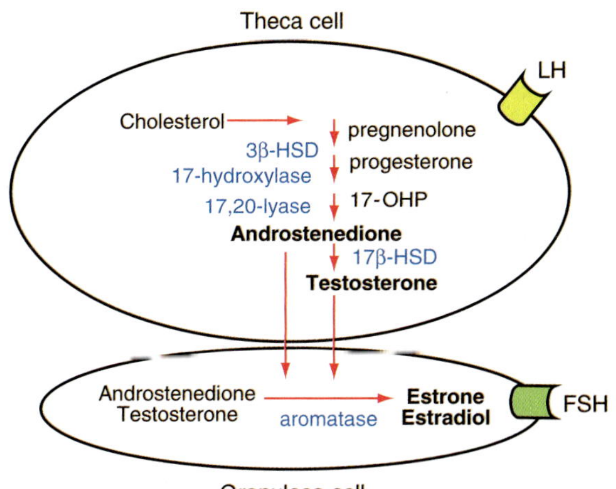

FIGURE 10-6

Estrogen production in the ovary requires the cooperative function of the theca and granulosa cells under the control of luteinizing hormone (LH) and follicle-stimulating hormone (FSH). HSD, hydroxysteroid dehydrogenase; OHP, hydroxyprogesterone.

cells proliferate in response to androgens [as in polycystic ovarian syndrome (PCOS)], they do not secrete androgens.

Rupture of the follicle at the time of ovulation is accompanied by the development of a rich capillary network induced by angiogenic factors such as granulosa cell–derived vascular endothelial growth factor (VEGF), making it possible for large molecules such as low-density lipoproteins (LDLs) to reach the luteinized granulosa and theca lutein cells. Luteinized granulosa cells express genes involved in progestin synthesis. Theca lutein cells produce 17-hydroxyprogesterone, a substrate for aromatization by the luteinized granulosa cells. While the major secretory product of the corpus luteum is progesterone, estradiol and 17-hydroxyprogesterone are also produced. LH is critical for normal structure and function of the corpus luteum. Because LH and human chorionic gonadotropin (hCG) bind to a common receptor, the role of LH in support of the corpus luteum can be replaced by hCG in the first 10 weeks after conception, and hCG is commonly used for luteal phase support in the treatment of infertility.

Steroid Hormone Actions

(See Chap. 1.) Both estrogen and progesterone play critical roles in the expression of secondary sexual characteristics in women. Estrogen promotes development of the ductule system in the breast, whereas progesterone is responsible for glandular development. In the reproductive tract, estrogens create a receptive environment for fertilization and support pregnancy and parturition through carefully coordinated changes in the endometrium, thickening of the vaginal mucosa, thinning of the cervical mucus, and uterine growth and contractions. Progesterone induces secretory activity in the estrogen-primed endometrium, increases the viscosity of cervical mucus, and inhibits uterine contractions. Both gonadal steroids play critical roles in the negative and positive feedback controls of gonadotropin secretion. Progesterone also increases basal body temperature and has therefore been used clinically as a marker of ovulation.

The vast majority of circulating estrogens and androgens are carried in the blood bound to carrier proteins, which restrain their free diffusion into cells and prolong their clearance, serving as a reservoir. High-affinity binding proteins include sex hormone–binding globulin (SHBG), which binds androgens with somewhat greater affinity than estrogens, and corticosteroid-binding globulin (CBG), which also binds progesterone. Modulations in binding protein levels by insulin, androgens, and estrogens contribute to high bioavailable testosterone levels in PCOS and to high circulating estrogen and progesterone levels during pregnancy.

Estrogens act primarily through binding to the nuclear receptors, estrogen receptor (ER) α and β. Transcriptional coactivators and co-repressors modulate ER action (Chap. 1). Both ER subtypes are present in the hypothalamus, pituitary, ovary, and reproductive tract. Although ERα and -β exhibit some functional redundancy, there is also a high degree of specificity, particularly in cell type expression. For example, ERα functions in the ovarian theca cells, whereas ERβ is critical for granulosa cell function. There is also evidence for membrane-initiated signaling by estrogen. Similar signaling mechanisms pertain for progesterone with evidence of transcriptional regulation through progesterone receptor (PR) A and B protein isoforms, as well as rapid membrane signaling.

OVARIAN PEPTIDES

Inhibin was initially isolated from gonadal fluids based on its ability to selectively inhibit FSH secretion from pituitary cells. Inhibin is a heterodimer composed of an α subunit and a βA or βB subunit to form inhibin A or inhibin B, both of which are secreted from the ovary. Activin is a homodimer of inhibin β subunits with the capacity to stimulate the synthesis and secretion of FSH. Inhibins and activins are members of the transforming growth factor β (TGF-β) superfamily of growth and differentiation factors. During the purification of inhibin, follistatin, an unrelated monomeric protein that inhibits FSH secretion, was discovered. Follistatin inhibits FSH secretion indirectly through binding and neutralizing activin.

Inhibin B is secreted from the granulosa cells of small antral follicles, whereas inhibin A is present in both granulosa and theca cells and is secreted by dominant follicles. Inhibin A is also present in luteinized granulosa cells and is a major secretory product of the corpus luteum. Inhibin B increases in serum in response to FSH and is used clinically as a marker of ovarian reserve. Inhibin B also plays an important negative feedback role on FSH, independent of estradiol, during the menstrual cycle. Although activin is also secreted from the ovary, the excess of follistatin in serum, combined with its nearly irreversible binding of activin, make it unlikely that ovarian activin plays an endocrine role in FSH regulation. However, as indicated above, there is evidence that activin plays an autocrine/paracrine role in the ovary, and it may also act locally in the pituitary to modulate FSH production.

Müllerian-inhibiting substance (MIS) (also known as anti-müllerian hormone) plays an important role in ovarian biology in addition to its traditional role in the degeneration of the müllerian ducts in the male. MIS is produced by granulosa cells and, like inhibin B, is a marker of ovarian reserve. MIS may also inhibit the recruitment of primordial follicles into the follicle pool by inhibiting aromatase expression.

HORMONAL INTEGRATION OF THE NORMAL MENSTRUAL CYCLE

The sequence of changes responsible for mature reproductive function is coordinated through a series of negative and positive feedback loops that alter pulsatile GnRH secretion, the pituitary response to GnRH, and the relative secretion of LH and FSH from the gonadotrope. The frequency and amplitude of pulsatile GnRH secretion influence the differential synthesis and secretion of LH and FSH, with slow frequencies favoring FSH synthesis and increased amplitudes favoring LH synthesis. Activin is produced in both pituitary gonadotropes and folliculostellate cells and stimulates the synthesis and secretion of FSH. Inhibins function as potent antagonists of activins through sequestration of the activin receptors. Although inhibin is expressed in the pituitary, gonadal inhibin is the principal source of feedback inhibition of FSH.

For the majority of the cycle, the reproductive system functions in a classic endocrine negative feedback mode. Estradiol and progesterone inhibit GnRH secretion, and the inhibins act at the pituitary to selectively inhibit FSH synthesis and secretion (Fig. 10-7). This negative feedback control of FSH is critical to development of the single mature oocyte that characterizes normal reproductive function in women. In addition to these negative feedback controls, the menstrual cycle is uniquely dependent on estrogen-induced positive feedback to produce an LH surge that is essential for ovulation of a mature follicle. The neural signaling pathways that distinguish estrogen-negative versus estrogen-positive feedback are incompletely understood.

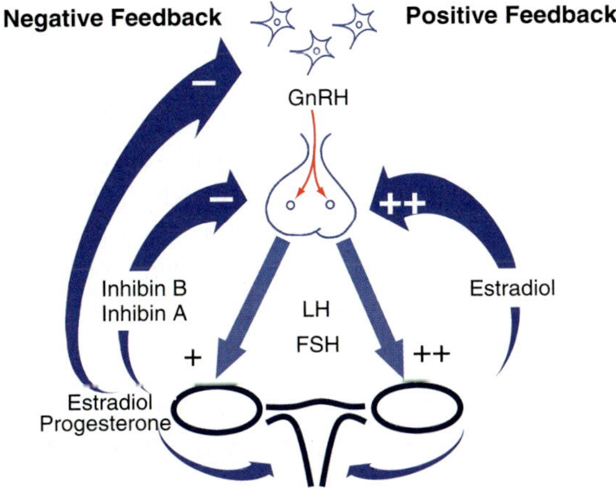

FIGURE 10-7

The reproductive system in women is critically dependent on both negative feedback of gonadal steroids and inhibin to modulate follicle-stimulating hormone (FSH) secretion and on estrogen positive feedback to generate the preovulatory luteinizing hormone (LH) surge. GnRH, gonadotropin-releasing hormone.

THE FOLLICULAR PHASE

This phase is characterized by recruitment of a cohort of secondary follicles and the ultimate selection of a dominant preovulatory follicle (Fig. 10-8). The follicular phase begins, by convention, on the first day of menses. However, follicular recruitment is initiated by the rise in FSH that begins in the late luteal phase in conjunction with the loss of negative feedback of gonadal steroids and likely inhibin A. The fact that a 20–30% increase in FSH is adequate for follicular recruitment speaks to the marked sensitivity of the resting follicle pool to FSH. The resultant granulosa cell proliferation is responsible for stimulating early follicular phase levels of inhibin B. Inhibin B in conjunction with rising levels of estradiol, and probably inhibin A, restrain FSH secretion during this critical period such that only a single follicle matures in the vast majority of cycles. The increased risk of multiple gestation associated with the increased levels of FSH characteristic of advanced maternal age, or with exogenous gonadotropin administration in the treatment of infertility, attests to the importance of the negative feedback regulation of FSH. With further growth of the dominant follicle, estradiol and inhibin A increase exponentially and the follicle acquires LH receptors. Increasing levels of estradiol are responsible for proliferative changes in the endometrium. The exponential rise in estradiol results in positive feedback on the pituitary, leading to the generation of an LH surge (and a smaller FSH surge), thereby triggering ovulation and luteinization of the granulosa cells.

THE LUTEAL PHASE

This phase begins with the formation of the corpus luteum from the ruptured follicle in response to ovulation signals. Progesterone and inhibin A are produced

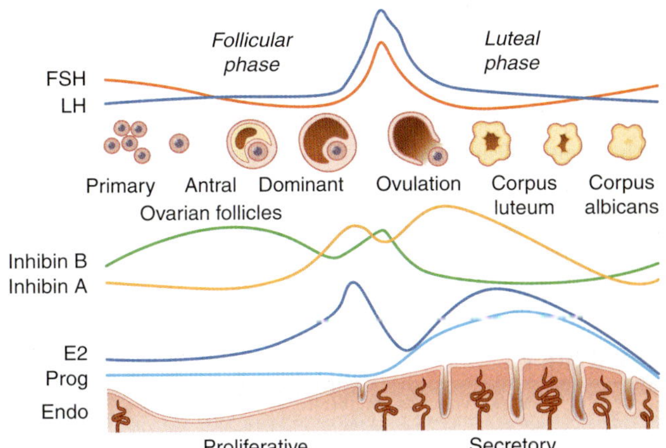

FIGURE 10-8

Relationship between gonadotropins, follicle development, gonadal secretion, and endometrial changes during the normal menstrual cycle. FSH, follicle-stimulating hormone; LH, luteinizing hormone; E_2, estradiol; Prog, progesterone; Endo, endometrium.

from the luteinized granulosa cells, which continue to aromatize theca-derived androgen precursors, producing estradiol. The combined actions of estrogen and progesterone are responsible for the secretory changes in the endometrium that are necessary for implantation. The corpus luteum is supported by LH but has a finite life span because of diminished sensitivity to LH. The demise of the corpus luteum results in a progressive decline in hormonal support of the endometrium. Inflammation or local hypoxia and ischemia result in vascular changes in the endometrium leading to the release of cytokines, cell death, and shedding of the endometrium.

If conception occurs, hCG produced by the trophoblast binds to LH receptors on the corpus luteum, maintaining steroid hormone production and preventing involution of the corpus luteum. The corpus luteum is essential for the hormonal maintenance of the endometrium during the first 6–10 weeks of pregnancy until this function is taken over by the placenta.

CLINICAL ASSESSMENT OF OVARIAN FUNCTION

Menstrual bleeding should become regular within 2 to 4 years of menarche, although anovulatory and irregular cycles are common before that. For the remainder of adult reproductive life, the cycle length, counted from the first day of menses to the first day of subsequent menses, is ~28 days, with a range of 25–35 days. However, cycle-to-cycle variability for an individual woman is ±2 days. Luteal phase length is relatively constant between 12 and 14 days in normal cycles; thus, the major variability in cycle length is due to variations in the follicular phase. The duration of menstrual bleeding in ovulatory cycles varies between 4 and 6 days. There is a gradual shortening of cycle length with age such that women over the age of 35 have cycles that are shorter than during their younger reproductive years. Anovulatory cycles increase as women approach the menopause, and bleeding patterns may be erratic.

Women who report regular monthly bleeding with cycles that do not vary by >4 days generally have ovulatory cycles, but several other clinical signs can be used to assess the likelihood of ovulation. Some women experience *mittelschmerz*, described as mid-cycle pelvic discomfort that is thought to be caused by the rapid expansion of the dominant follicle at the time of ovulation. A constellation of premenstrual moliminal symptoms such as bloating, breast tenderness, and food cravings often occur several days before menses in ovulatory cycles, but their absence cannot be used as evidence of anovulation. Methods that can be used to determine whether ovulation is likely include a serum progesterone level >5 ng/mL ~7 days before expected menses, an increase in basal body temperature of >0.5°F (0.24°C) in the second half of the cycle due to the thermoregulatory effect of progesterone, or the detection of the urinary LH surge using ovulation predictor kits. Because ovulation occurs ~36 h after the LH surge, urinary LH can be helpful in timing intercourse to coincide with ovulation.

Ultrasound can be used to detect the growth of the fluid-filled antrum of the developing follicle and to assess endometrial proliferation in response to increasing estradiol levels in the follicular phase, as well as the characteristic echogenicity of the secretory endometrium of the luteal phase.

PUBERTY

NORMAL PUBERTAL DEVELOPMENT IN GIRLS

The first menstrual period (*menarche*) occurs relatively late in the series of developmental milestones that characterize normal pubertal development (Table 10-1). Menarche is preceded by the appearance of pubic and then axillary hair as a result of maturation of the zona reticularis in the adrenal gland and increased adrenal androgen secretion, particularly dehydroepiandrosterone (DHEA). The triggers for adrenarche remain unknown but may involve increase in body mass index as well as in utero and neonatal factors. Menarche is also preceded by breast development (*thelarche*), which is exquisitely sensitive to the very low levels of estrogens that result from peripheral conversion of adrenal androgens and the low levels of estrogen secreted from the ovary early in pubertal maturation. Breast development precedes the appearance of pubic and axillary hair in ~60% of girls. The interval between the onset of breast development

TABLE 10-1

MEAN AGE (YEARS) OF PUBERTAL MILESTONES IN GIRLS, WITH 95% CONFIDENCE INTERVALS

	ONSET OF BREAST/ PUBIC HAIR DEVELOPMENT	AGE OF PEAK HEIGHT VELOCITY	MENARCHE	FINAL BREAST/PUBIC HAIR DEVELOPMENT	ADULT HEIGHT
Caucasian	10.2	11.9	12.6	14.3	17.1
African-American	9.6	11.5	12	13.6	16.5

Source: From FM Biro et al: J Pediatr 148:234, 2006.

and menarche is ~2 years. There has been a gradual decline in the age of menarche over the past century, attributed in large part to improvement in nutrition, and there is a relationship between adiposity and earlier sexual maturation in girls. In the United States, menarche occurs at an average age of 12.5 years (Table 10-1). Much of the variation in the timing of puberty is due to genetic factors, with heritability estimates of 50–80%. Both adrenarche and breast development occur ~1 year earlier in African-American compared with Caucasian girls, although the timing of menarche differs by only 6 months between these ethnic groups.

Other important hormonal changes also occur in conjunction with puberty. Growth hormone (GH) levels increase early in puberty, stimulated in part by the pubertal increases in estrogen secretion. GH increases IGF-I, which enhances linear growth. The growth spurt is generally less pronounced in girls than in boys, with a peak growth velocity of ~7 cm/year. Linear growth is ultimately limited by closure of epiphyses in the long bones as a result of prolonged exposure to estrogen. Puberty is also associated with mild insulin resistance.

DISORDERS OF PUBERTY

The differential diagnosis of precocious and delayed puberty is similar in boys and girls. However, there are differences in the timing of normal puberty and differences in the relative frequency of specific disorders in girls compared with boys.

Precocious Puberty

Traditionally, precocious puberty has been defined as the development of secondary sexual characteristics before the age of 8 in girls based on data from Marshall and Tanner in British girls studied in the 1960s. More recent studies led to recommendations that girls be evaluated for precocious puberty if breast development or pubic hair were present at <7 years of age for Caucasian girls or <6 years for African-American girls.

Precocious puberty is most often centrally mediated (Table 10-2), resulting from early activation of the hypothalamic-pituitary-ovarian axis. It is characterized by pulsatile LH secretion and an enhanced LH and FSH response to exogenous GnRH (two- to threefold stimulation) (Table 10-3). True precocity is marked by advancement in bone age of >2 SD, a recent history of growth acceleration, and progression of secondary sexual characteristics. In girls, centrally mediated precocious puberty is idiopathic in ~85% of cases; however, neurogenic causes must also be considered. GnRH agonists that induce pituitary desensitization are the mainstay of treatment to prevent premature epiphyseal closure and preserve adult height, as well to manage psychosocial repercussions of precocious puberty.

TABLE 10-2

DIFFERENTIAL DIAGNOSIS OF PRECOCIOUS PUBERTY

CENTRAL (GnRH DEPENDENT)	PERIPHERAL (GnRH INDEPENDENT)
Idiopathic	Congenital adrenal hyperplasia
CNS tumors	Estrogen-producing tumors
Hamartomas	Adrenal tumors
Astrocytomas	Ovarian tumors
Adenomyomas	Gonadotropin/hCG-producing tumors
Gliomas	Exogenous exposure to estrogen or androgen
Germinomas	McCune-Albright syndrome
CNS infection	Aromatase excess syndrome
Head trauma	
Iatrogenic	
Radiation	
Chemotherapy	
Surgical	
CNS malformation	
Arachnoid or suprasellar cysts	
Septo-optic dysplasia	
Hydrocephalus	

Note: GnRH, gonadotropin-releasing hormone; CNS, central nervous system; hCG, human chorionic gonadotropin.

TABLE 10-3

EVALUATION OF PRECOCIOUS AND DELAYED PUBERTY

	PRECOCIOUS	DELAYED
Initial screening tests		
History and physical	x	x
Assessment of growth velocity	x	x
Bone age	x	x
LH, FSH	x	x
Estradiol, testosterone	x	x
DHEAS	x	x
17-Hydroxyprogesterone	x	
TSH, T_4	x	x
Complete blood count		x
Sedimentation rate, C-reactive protein		x
Electrolytes, renal function		x
Liver enzymes		x
IGF-I, IGFBP-3		x
Urinalysis		x
Secondary tests		
Pelvic ultrasound	x	x
Cranial MRI	x	x
β-hCG	x	
GnRH/agonist stimulation test	x	x
ACTH stimulation test	x	
Inflammatory bowel disease panel	x	x
Celiac disease panel		x
Prolactin		x
Karyotype		x

Note: LH, luteinizing hormone; FSH, follicle-stimulating hormone; DHEAS, dehydroepiandrosterone sulfate; TSH, thyroid-stimulating hormone; T_4, thyroxine; IGF, insulin-like growth factor; IGFBP-3, IGF-binding protein 3; hCG, human chorionic gonadotropin; ACTH, adrenocorticotropic hormone.

Peripherally mediated precocious puberty does not involve activation of the hypothalamic-pituitary-ovarian axis and is characterized by suppressed gonadotropins in the presence of elevated estradiol. Management of peripheral precocious puberty involves treating the underlying disorder (Table 10-2) and limiting the effects of gonadal steroids using aromatase inhibitors, inhibitors of steroidogenesis, and estrogen receptor blockers. It is important to be aware that central precocious puberty can also develop in girls whose precocity was initially peripherally mediated, as in McCune-Albright syndrome and congenital adrenal hyperplasia.

Incomplete and intermittent forms of precocious puberty may also occur. For example, premature breast development may occur in girls before the age of 2 years, with no further progression and without significant advancement in bone age, androgen production, or compromised height. Premature adrenarche can also occur in the absence of progressive pubertal development, but it must be distinguished from late-onset congenital adrenal hyperplasia and androgen-secreting tumors, in which case it may be termed *heterosexual precocity*. Premature adrenarche may be associated with obesity, hyperinsulinemia, and subsequent predisposition to PCOS.

Delayed Puberty

Delayed puberty (**Table 10-4**) is defined as the absence of secondary sexual characteristics by age 13 in girls. The diagnostic considerations are very similar to those for primary amenorrhea (Chap. 11). Between 25 and 40% of delayed puberty in girls is of ovarian origin, with Turner syndrome constituting a majority of such patients. Functional hypogonadotropic hypogonadism encompasses diverse etiologies such as systemic illnesses, including celiac disease and chronic renal disease, and endocrinopathies, such as diabetes and hypothyroidism. In addition, girls appear to be particularly susceptible to the adverse effects of abnormalities in energy balance that result from exercise, dieting, and/or eating disorders. Together, these reversible conditions account for ~25% of delayed puberty in girls. Congenital hypogonadotropic hypogonadism in girls or boys can be caused by mutations in several different genes or combinations of genes (Chap. 8, Table 8-2). Family studies suggest that genes identified in association with absent puberty may cause delayed puberty and that there may be a genetic susceptibility to environmental stresses such as diet and exercise. Although neuroanatomic causes of delayed puberty are considerably less common in girls than in boys, it is always important to rule these out in the setting of hypogonadotropic hypogonadism.

TABLE 10-4

DIFFERENTIAL DIAGNOSIS OF DELAYED PUBERTY
Hypergonadotropic
Ovarian
Turner syndrome
Gonadal dysgenesis
Chemotherapy/radiation therapy
Galactosemia
Autoimmune oophoritis
Congenital lipoid hyperplasia
Steroidogenic enzyme abnormalities
17α-hydroxylase deficiency
Aromatase deficiency
Gonadotropin/receptor mutations
FSHβ, LHR, FSHR
Androgen resistance syndrome
Hypogonadotropic
Genetic
Hypothalamic syndromes
Leptin/leptin receptor
HESX1 (septo-optic dysplasia)
PC1 (prohormone convertase)
IHH and Kallmann syndrome
KAL, FGFR1
GnRHR, GPR54
Abnormalities of pituitary development/ function PROP1
CNS tumors/infiltrative disorders
Craniopharyngioma
Astrocytoma, germinoma, glioma
Prolactinomas, other pituitary tumors
Histiocytosis X
Chemotherapy/radiation
Functional
Chronic diseases
Malnutrition
Excessive exercise
Eating disorders

Note: FSHβ, follicle-stimulating hormone β chain; FSHR, FSH receptor; LHR, luteinizing hormone receptor; HESX1, homeobox, embryonic stem cell expressed 1; IHH, idiopathic hypogonadotropic hypogonadism; KAL, Kallmann; FGFR1, fibroblast growth factor 1; GnRHR, gonadotropin-releasing hormone receptor; GPR54, G protein–coupled receptor 54; PROP1, prophet of Pit1, paired-like homeodomain transcription factor; CNS, central nervous system.

INFERTILITY

DEFINITION AND PREVALENCE

Infertility is defined as the inability to conceive after 12 months of unprotected sexual intercourse. In a study of 5574 English and American women who ultimately conceived, pregnancy occurred in 50% within 3 months, 72% within 6 months, and 85% within 12 months. These findings are consistent with predictions based on *fecundability*, the probability of achieving pregnancy in one menstrual cycle (approximately 20–25% in healthy young couples). Assuming a fecundability of 0.25, 98% of couples should conceive within 13 months. Based on this definition, the National Survey of Family Growth reports a 14% rate of infertility in the United States in married women aged 15–44. The infertility rate has remained relatively stable over the past 30 years, although the proportion of couples without children has risen, reflecting a trend to delay childbearing. This trend has important implications because of an age-related decrease in fecundability, which begins at age 35 and decreases markedly after age 40.

CAUSES OF INFERTILITY

The spectrum of infertility ranges from reduced conception rates or the need for medical intervention to irreversible causes of infertility. Infertility can be attributed primarily to male factors in 25% and female factors in 58%, and is unexplained in about 17% of couples (Fig. 10-9). Not uncommonly, both male and female factors contribute to infertility.

Approach to the Patient: INFERTILITY

INITIAL EVALUATION In all couples presenting with infertility, the initial evaluation includes discussion of the appropriate timing of intercourse and discussion of modifiable risk factors such as smoking, alcohol, caffeine, and obesity. A description of the range of investigations that may be required and a brief description of infertility treatment options, including adoption, should be reviewed. Initial investigations are focused on determining whether the primary cause of the infertility is male, female, or both. These investigations include a semen analysis in the male, confirmation of ovulation in the female, and, in the majority of situations, documentation of tubal patency in the female. In some cases, after an extensive workup excluding all male and female factors, a specific cause cannot be identified and infertility may ultimately be classified as unexplained.

PSYCHOLOGICAL ASPECTS OF INFERTILITY Infertility is invariably associated with psychological stress related not only to the diagnostic and therapeutic procedures themselves but also to repeated cycles of hope and loss associated with each new procedure or cycle of treatment that does not result in the birth of a child. These feelings are often combined with a sense of isolation from friends and family. Counseling and stress-management techniques should be introduced early in the evaluation of infertility. Infertility and its treatment do not appear to be associated with long-term psychological sequelae.

FEMALE CAUSES Abnormalities in menstrual function constitute the most common cause of female infertility. These disorders, which include ovulatory dysfunction and abnormalities of the uterus or outflow tract, may present as amenorrhea or as irregular or short menstrual cycles. A careful history and physical examination and a limited number of laboratory tests will help to determine whether the abnormality is (1) hypothalamic or pituitary (low FSH, LH, and estradiol with or without an increase in prolactin), (2) PCOS (irregular cycles and hyperandrogenism in the absence of other causes of androgen excess), (3) ovarian (low estradiol with increased FSH), or (4) uterine or outflow tract abnormality. The frequency of these diagnoses depends on whether the amenorrhea is primary or occurs after normal puberty and menarche (see Fig. 11-2).

The approach to further evaluation of these disorders is described in detail in Chap. 11.

OVULATORY DYSFUNCTION In women with a history of regular menstrual cycles, *evidence of ovulation* should be sought as described above. An endometrial biopsy to exclude luteal phase insufficiency is no longer considered an essential part of the infertility workup for most patients. Even in the presence of ovulatory cycles, evaluation of *ovarian reserve* is recommended for women over 35 by measurement of FSH on day 3 of the cycle or in response to clomiphene, an estrogen antagonist. An FSH level <10 IU/mL on cycle day 3 predicts adequate ovarian oocyte reserve. Antral follicle count, inhibin B,

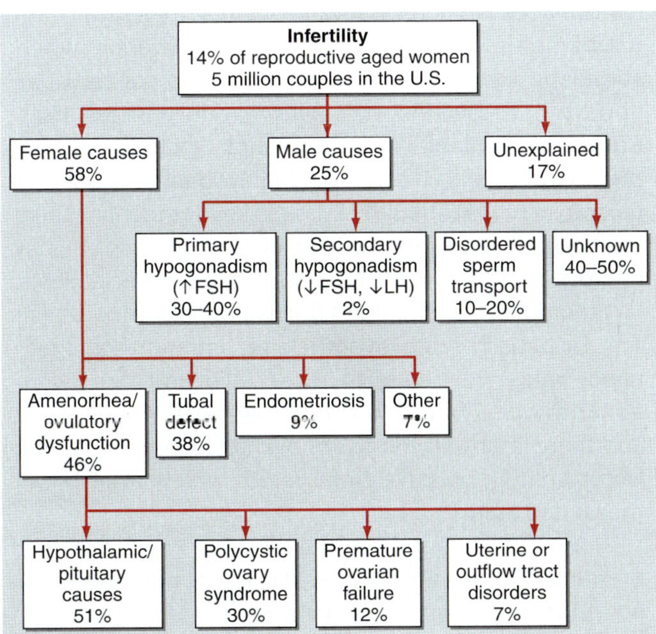

FIGURE 10-9
Causes of infertility. FSH, follicle-stimulating hormone; LH, luteinizing hormone.

and MIS are also being investigated as indicators of ovarian reserve.

TUBAL DISEASE This may result from pelvic inflammatory disease (PID), appendicitis, endometriosis, pelvic adhesions, tubal surgery, and previous use of an intrauterine device (IUD). However, a cause is not identified in up to 50% of patients with documented tubal factor infertility. Because of the high prevalence of tubal disease, evaluation of tubal patency by hysterosalpingogram (HSG) or laparoscopy should occur early in the majority of couples with infertility. Subclinical infections with *Chlamydia trachomatis* may be an underdiagnosed cause of tubal infertility and requires the treatment of both partners.

ENDOMETRIOSIS *Endometriosis* is defined as the presence of endometrial glands or stroma outside the endometrial cavity and uterine musculature. Its presence is suggested by a history of dyspareunia (painful intercourse), worsening dysmenorrhea that often begins before menses, or a thickened rectovaginal septum or deviation of the cervix on pelvic examination. The pathogenesis of the infertility associated with endometriosis is unclear but may involve effects on the normal endometrium as well as adhesions. Endometriosis is often clinically silent, however, and can only be excluded definitively by laparoscopy.

MALE CAUSES (See also Chap. 8.) Known causes of male infertility include primary testicular disease, disorders of sperm transport, and hypothalamic-pituitary disease resulting in secondary hypogonadism. However, the etiology is not ascertained in up to half of men with suspected male factor infertility. The key initial diagnostic test is a *semen analysis*. Testosterone levels should be measured if the sperm count is low on repeated examination or if there is clinical evidence of hypogonadism.

℞ Treatment: INFERTILITY

The treatment of infertility should be tailored to the problems unique to each couple. In many situations, including unexplained infertility, mild to moderate endometriosis, and/or borderline semen parameters, a stepwise approach to infertility is optimal, beginning with low-risk interventions and moving to more invasive, higher-risk interventions only if necessary. After determination of all infertility factors and their correction, if possible, this approach might include, in increasing order of complexity, (1) expectant management, (2) clomiphene citrate with or without intrauterine insemination (IUI), (3) gonadotropins with or without IUI, and (4) in vitro fertilization (IVF). The time used to complete the evaluation, correction, and expectant management can be longer in women <30 years of age, but this process should be advanced rapidly in women >35. In some situations expectant management will not be appropriate.

OVULATORY DYSFUNCTION Treatment of ovulatory dysfunction should first be directed at identification of the etiology of the disorder to allow specific management when possible. Dopamine agonists, for example, may be indicated in patients with hyperprolactinemia (Chap. 2); lifestyle modification may be successful in women with low body weight or a history of intensive exercise.

Medications used for ovulation induction include *clomiphene citrate*, gonadotropins, and pulsatile GnRH. Clomiphene citrate is a nonsteroidal estrogen antagonist that increases FSH and LH levels by blocking estrogen negative feedback at the hypothalamus. The efficacy of clomiphene for ovulation induction is highly dependent on patient selection. It induces ovulation in ~60% of women with PCOS and is the initial treatment of choice. It may be combined with agents that modify insulin levels, such as metformin. Clomiphene citrate is less successful in patients with hypogonadotropic hypogonadism. Aromatase inhibitors have also been investigated for the treatment of infertility. Initial studies are promising, but these medications have not been approved for this indication.

Gonadotropins are highly effective for ovulation induction in women with hypogonadotropic hypogonadism and PCOS and are used to induce multiple follicular recruitment in unexplained infertility and in older reproductive-aged women. Disadvantages include a significant risk of multiple gestation and the risk of ovarian hyperstimulation, but careful monitoring and a conservative approach to ovarian stimulation reduce these risks. Currently available gonadotropins include urinary preparations of LH and FSH, highly purified FSH, and recombinant FSH. Though FSH is the key component, there is growing data that the addition of some LH (or hCG) may improve results, particularly in hypogonadotropic patients.

Pulsatile GnRH is highly effective for restoring ovulation in patients with hypothalamic amenorrhea. Pregnancy rates are similar to those following the use of gonadotropins, but rates of multiple gestation are lower and there is virtually no risk of ovarian hyperstimulation. Unfortunately, pulsatile GnRH is not widely available in the United States.

None of these methods are effective in women with premature ovarian failure in whom donor oocyte or adoption are the methods of choice.

TUBAL DISEASE If hysterosalpingography suggests a tubal or uterine cavity abnormality, or if a patient is ≥35 at the time of initial evaluation, laparoscopy with tubal lavage is recommended, often with a hysteroscopy. Although tubal reconstruction may be attempted if tubal disease is identified, it is generally being replaced by the use of IVF. These patients are at increased risk of developing an ectopic pregnancy.

ENDOMETRIOSIS Though 60% of women with minimal or mild endometriosis may conceive within 1 year without treatment, laparoscopic resection or ablation appears to improve conception rates. Medical management of advanced stages of endometriosis is widely used for symptom control but has not been shown to enhance fertility. In moderate to severe endometriosis, conservative surgery is associated with pregnancy rates of 50 and 39%, respectively, compared with rates of 25 and 5% with expectant management alone. In some patients, IVF may be the treatment of choice.

MALE FACTOR INFERTILITY The treatment options for male factor infertility have expanded greatly in recent years (Chap. 8). Secondary hypogonadism is highly amenable to treatment with pulsatile GnRH or gonadotropins. In vitro techniques have provided new opportunities for patients with primary testicular failure and disorders of sperm transport. Choice of initial treatment options depends on sperm concentration and motility. Expectant management should be attempted initially in men with mild male factor infertility (sperm count of 15 to 20 $\times$ 10^6/mL and normal motility). Moderate male factor infertility (10 to 15 $\times$ 10^6/mL and 20–40% motility) should begin with IUI alone or in combination with treatment of the female partner with clomiphene or gonadotropins, but it may require IVF with or without intracytoplasmic sperm injection (ICSI). For men with a severe defect (sperm count of <10 $\times$ 10^6/mL, 10% motility), IVF with ICSI or donor sperm should be used. If ICSI is performed because of azoospermia due to congenital bilateral absence of the vas deferens, genetic testing and counseling should be provided because of the risk of cystic fibrosis.

ASSISTED REPRODUCTIVE TECHNOLOGIES The development of assisted reproductive technologies (ARTs) has dramatically altered the treatment of male and female infertility. IVF is indicated for patients with many causes of infertility that have not been successfully managed with more conservative approaches. IVF or ICSI is often the treatment of choice in couples with a significant male factor or tubal disease, whereas IVF using donor oocytes is used in patients with premature ovarian failure and in women of advanced reproductive age. Success rates depend on the age of the woman and the cause of the infertility and are generally 18–24% per cycle when initiated in women <40. In women >40, there is a marked decrease in both the number of oocytes retrieved and their ability to be fertilized. Though often effective, IVF is expensive and requires careful monitoring of ovulation induction and invasive techniques including the aspiration of multiple follicles. IVF is associated with a significant risk of multiple gestation (31% twins, 6% triplets, and 0.2% higher-order multiples).

CONTRACEPTION

Though various forms of contraception are widely available, ~30% of births in the United States are the result of unintended pregnancy. Teenage pregnancies continue to represent a serious public health problem in the United States, with >1 million unintended pregnancies each year—a significantly greater incidence than in other industrialized nations.

Contraceptive methods are widely used (**Table 10-5**). Only 15% of couples report having unprotected sexual intercourse in the past 3 months. A reversible form of contraception is used by >50% of couples, while sterilization (in either the male or female) has been employed as a permanent form of contraception by over a third of couples. Pregnancy termination is relatively safe when directed by health care professionals but is rarely the option of choice.

No single contraceptive method is ideal, although all are safer than carrying a pregnancy to term. The effectiveness of a given method of contraception depends not only on the efficacy of the method itself. Discrepancies between theoretical and actual effectiveness emphasize the importance of patient education and compliance when considering various forms of contraception (Table 10-5). Knowledge of the advantages and disadvantages of each contraceptive is essential for counseling an individual about the methods that are safest and most consistent with his or her lifestyle. The World Health Organization (WHO) has extensive family planning resources for the physician and patient that can be accessed online.

BARRIER METHODS

Barrier contraceptives (such as condoms, diaphragms, and cervical caps) and spermicides are easily available, are reversible, and have fewer side effects than hormonal methods. However, their effectiveness is highly dependent on adherence and proper use (Table 10-5). A major advantage of barrier contraceptives is the protection provided against sexually transmitted infections (STIs). Consistent use is associated with a decreased risk of HIV, gonorrhea, nongonococcal urethritis, and genital herpes, probably due in part to the concomitant use of spermicides. Natural membrane condoms may be less effective than latex condoms, and petroleum-based lubricants can

TABLE 10-5

EFFECTIVENESS OF DIFFERENT FORMS OF CONTRACEPTION

METHOD OF CONTRACEPTION	THEORETICAL[a] EFFECTIVENESS, %	ACTUAL[a] EFFECTIVENESS, %	PERCENT CONTINUING USE AT 1 YEAR[b]	CONTRACEPTIVE METHODS USED BY U.S. WOMEN[c]
Barrier methods				
Condoms	98	88	63	20
Diaphragm	94	82	58	2
Cervical cap	94	82	50	<1
Spermicides	97	79	43	1
Sterilization				
Male	99.9	99.9	100	11
Female	99.8	99.6	100	28
Intrauterine device				1
Copper T380	99	97	78	
Progestasert	98	97	81	
Mirena	99.9	99.8		
Oral contraceptive pill			72	27
Combination	99.9	97		
Progestin only	99.5	97		
Long-acting progestins				
Depo-Provera	99.7	99.7	70	<1

[a]Adapted from J Trussel et al: Obstet Gynecol 76:558, 1990.
[b]Adapted from Contraceptive Technology Update. Contraceptive Technology, Feb. 1996, Vol 17, No 1, pp 13–24.
[c]Adapted from LJ Piccinino and WD Mosher: Fam Plan Perspective 30:4, 1998.

degrade condoms and decrease their efficacy for preventing HIV infection. A highly effective female condom, which also provides protection against STIs, was approved in 1994 but has not achieved widespread use.

STERILIZATION

Sterilization is the method of birth control most frequently chosen by fertile men and multiparous women >30 (Table 10-5). Sterilization refers to a procedure that prevents fertilization by surgical interruption of the fallopian tubes in women or the vas deferens in men. Although tubal ligation and vasectomy are potentially reversible, these procedures should be considered permanent and should not be undertaken without patient counseling.

Several methods of *tubal ligation* have been developed, all of which are highly effective with a 10-year cumulative pregnancy rate of 1.85 per 100 women. However, when pregnancy does occur, the risk of ectopic pregnancy may be as high as 30%. The success rate of tubal reanastomosis depends on the method used, but even after successful reversal, the risk of ectopic pregnancy remains high. In addition to prevention of pregnancy, tubal ligation reduces the risk of ovarian cancer, possibly by limiting the upward migration of potential carcinogens.

Vasectomy is a highly effective outpatient surgical procedure that has little risk. The development of azoospermia may be delayed for 2–6 months, and other forms of contraception must be used until two sperm-free ejaculations provide proof of sterility. Reanastomosis may restore fertility in 30–50% of men, but the success rate declines with time after vasectomy and may be influenced by factors such as the development of antisperm antibodies.

INTRAUTERINE DEVICES

IUDs inhibit pregnancy primarily through a spermicidal effect caused by a sterile inflammatory reaction produced by the presence of a foreign body in the uterine cavity (copper IUDs) or by the release of progestins (Progestasert, Mirena). IUDs provide a high level of efficacy in the absence of systemic metabolic effects, and ongoing motivation is not required to ensure efficacy once the device has been placed. However, only 1% of women in the United States use this method compared to a utilization rate of 15–30% in much of Europe and Canada, despite evidence that the newer devices are not associated with increased rates of pelvic infection and infertility, as occurred with earlier devices. An IUD should not be used in women at high risk for development of STI or in women at high risk for bacterial endocarditis. The IUD may not be effective in women with uterine leiomyomas because they alter the size or shape of the uterine cavity. IUD use is associated with increased menstrual blood flow, although this is less pronounced with the progesterone-releasing IUD than the copper-containing device.

HORMONAL METHODS

Oral Contraceptive Pills

Because of their ease of use and efficacy, oral contraceptive pills are the most widely used form of hormonal contraception. They act by suppressing ovulation, changing cervical mucus, and altering the endometrium. The current formulations are made from synthetic estrogens and progestins. The estrogen component of the pill consists of ethinyl estradiol or mestranol, which is metabolized to ethinyl estradiol. Multiple synthetic progestins are used. Norethindrone and its derivatives are used in many formulations. Low-dose norgestimate and the more recently developed progestins (desogestrel, gestodene, drospirenone) have a less androgenic profile; levonorgestrel appears to be the most androgenic of the progestins and should be avoided in patients with hyperandrogenic symptoms. The three major formulations of oral contraceptives are (1) fixed-dose estrogen-progestin combination, (2) phasic estrogen-progestin combination, and (3) progestin only. Each of these formulations is administered daily for 3 weeks followed by a week of no medication during which menstrual bleeding generally occurs. Two extended oral contraceptives have recently been approved for use in the United States: Seasonalle is a 3-month preparation with 84 days of active drug and 7 days of placebo; Lybrel is a continuous preparation containing 90 μg of levonorgestrel and 20 μg of ethinyl estradiol. Current doses of ethinyl estradiol range from 20–50 μg. However, indications for the 50-μg dose are rare, and the majority of formulations contain 35 μg of ethinyl estradiol. The reduced estrogen and progesterone content in the second- and third-generation pills has decreased both side effects and risks associated with oral contraceptive use (Table 10-6). At the currently used doses, patients must be cautioned not to miss pills due to the potential for ovulation. Side effects, including breakthrough bleeding, amenorrhea, breast tenderness, and weight gain, are often responsive to a change in formulation.

The microdose progestin-only minipill is less effective as a contraceptive, having a pregnancy rate of 2–7 per 100 woman-years. However, it may be appropriate for women with cardiovascular disease or for women who cannot tolerate synthetic estrogens.

TABLE 10-6

ORAL CONTRACEPTIVES: CONTRAINDICATIONS AND DISEASE RISK

Contraindications
- Absolute
  - Previous thromboembolic event or stroke
  - History of an estrogen-dependent tumor
  - Active liver disease
  - Pregnancy
  - Undiagnosed abnormal uterine bleeding
  - Hypertriglyceridemia
  - Women >35 who smoke heavily (>15 cigarettes per day)
- Relative
  - Hypertension
  - Women receiving anticonvulsant drug therapy

Disease risks
- Increased
  - Coronary heart disease—increased only in smokers >35; no relation to progestin type
  - Hypertension—relative risk 1.8 (current users) and 1.2 (previous users)
  - Venous thrombosis—relative risk ~4; markedly increased with factor V Leiden or prothrombin-gene mutations
  - Stroke—increased only in combination with hypertension; unclear relation to migraine headache
  - Cerebral vein thrombosis—relative risk ~13–15; synergistic with prothrombin-gene mutation
  - Cervical cancer—relative risk 2–4
- Decreased
  - Ovarian cancer—50% reduction in risk
  - Endometrial cancer—40% reduction in risk

New Methods

A *weekly contraceptive patch* (Ortho Evra) is available and has similar efficacy to oral contraceptives but may be associated with less breakthrough bleeding. Approximately 2% of patches fail to adhere, and a similar percentage of women have skin reactions. Efficacy is lower in women >90 kg. The amount of estrogen delivered may be comparable to that of a 40-μg ethinyl estradiol oral contraceptive, raising the possibility of increased risk of venous thromboembolism, which must be balanced against potential benefits for women not able to successfully use other methods. A *monthly contraceptive estrogen/progestin injection* (Lunelle) is highly effective, with a first-year failure rate of <0.2%, but it may be less effective in obese women. Its use is associated with bleeding irregularities that diminish over time. Fertility returns rapidly after discontinuation. A *monthly vaginal ring* (NuvaRing) that is intended to be left in place during intercourse is also available for contraceptive use. It is highly effective, with a 12-month failure rate of 0.7%. Ovulation returns within the first recovery cycle after discontinuation.

Long-Term Contraceptives

Long-term progestin administration in the form of Depo-Provera acts primarily by inhibiting ovulation and causing changes in the endometrium and cervical mucus that result in decreased implantation and sperm transport. Depo-Provera requires an IM injection and is effective for 3 months, but return of fertility after discontinuation may be delayed for up to 12–18 months. Although highly effective, Norplant is no longer being manufactured.

Amenorrhea, irregular bleeding, and weight gain are the most common adverse effects associated with both injectable forms of contraception. A major advantage of the injectable progestin-based contraceptives is the apparent lack of increased arterial and venous thromboembolic events, but increased gallbladder disease and decreased bone density may result.

POSTCOITAL CONTRACEPTION

Postcoital contraceptive methods prevent implantation or cause regression of the corpus luteum and are highly efficacious if used appropriately. Unprotected intercourse without regard to the time of the month carries an 8% incidence of pregnancy, an incidence that can be reduced to 2% by the use of emergency contraceptives within 72 h of unprotected intercourse. A notice published in 1997 by the U.S. Food and Drug Administration indicated that certain oral contraceptive pills could be used within 72 h of unprotected intercourse [Ovral (2 tablets, 12 h apart) and Lo/Ovral (4 tablets, 12 h apart)]. Preven (50 mg ethinyl estradiol and 0.25 mg levonorgestrel) and Plan B (0.75 mg Levonorgestrel) are now approved for postcoital contraception. Side effects are common with these high doses of hormones and include nausea, vomiting, and breast soreness. Recent studies suggest that 600 mg mifepristone (RU486), a progesterone receptor antagonist, may be equally as effective as or more effective than hormonal regimens, with fewer side effects. Mifepristone is now available in the United States as Mifeprex, to be used with or without misoprostol (synthetic prostaglandin E_1, an off-label indication for this use of misoprostol).

FURTHER READINGS

Boivin J et al: International estimates of infertility prevalence and treatment-seeking: Potential need and demand for infertility medical care. Hum Reprod 22:1506, 2007

Bulun SE: Endometriosis. N Engl J Med 360:268, 2009

Fisher WA, Black A: Contraception in Canada: A review of method choices, characteristics, adherence and approaches to counseling. CMAJ 176:953, 2007

Kaunitz AM: Clinical practice. Hormonal contraception in women of older reproductive age. N Engl J Med 358:1262, 2008

Knight PG, Glister C: TGF-β superfamily members and ovarian follicle development. Reproduction 132:191, 2006

Olive DL: Gonadotropin-releasing hormone agonists for endometriosis. N Engl J Med 359:1136, 2008

Palomba S et al: Clomiphene citrate, metformin or both as first-step approach in treating anovulatory infertility in patients with polycystic ovary syndrome (PCOS): A systematic review of head-to-head randomized controlled studies and meta-analysis. Clin Endocrinol (Oxf) 70:311, 2009

Practice Committee of the American Society of Reproductive Medicine: Hormonal contraception: Recent advances and controversies. Fertil Steril 86:S229, 2006

Roy A, Matzuk MM: Deconstructing mammalian reproduction: Using knockouts to define fertility pathways. Reproduction 131:207, 2006

Seminara SB: Mechanisms of disease: The first kiss—a crucial role for kisspeptin-1 and its receptor, G-protein-coupled receptor 54, in puberty and reproduction. Nat Clin Pract Endocrinol Metab 2:328, 2006

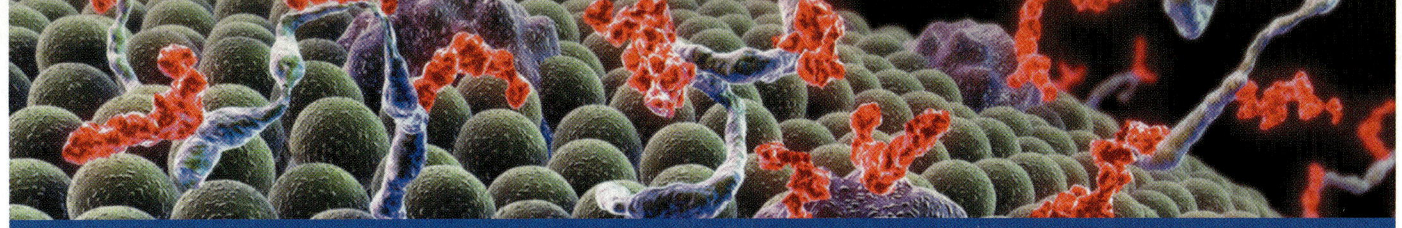

CHAPTER 11

MENSTRUAL DISORDERS AND PELVIC PAIN

Janet E. Hall

Menstrual dysfunction can signal an underlying abnormality that may have long-term health consequences. Although frequent or prolonged bleeding usually prompts a woman to seek medical attention, infrequent or absent bleeding may seem less troubling, and the patient may not bring it to the attention of the physician. Thus, a focused menstrual history is a critical part of every female patient encounter. Pelvic pain is a common complaint that may relate to an abnormality of the reproductive organs but may also be of gastrointestinal, urinary tract, or musculoskeletal origin. Depending on its cause, pelvic pain may require urgent surgical attention.

MENSTRUAL DISORDERS

DEFINITION AND PREVALENCE

Amenorrhea refers to the absence of menstrual periods. Amenorrhea is classified as *primary* if menstrual bleeding has never occurred in the absence of hormonal treatment or *secondary* if menstrual periods are absent for 3–6 months. *Oligoamenorrhea* is defined as a cycle length >35 days or <10 menses per year. Both the frequency and amount of vaginal bleeding are irregular in oligoamenorrhea. It is often associated with anovulation, which can also occur with intermenstrual intervals of <24 days or vaginal bleeding for >7 days. Frequent or heavy irregular bleeding is termed *dysfunctional uterine bleeding* if anatomic uterine lesions or a bleeding diathesis have been excluded.

Primary Amenorrhea

This is a rare disorder occurring in <1% of the female population. However, between 3 and 5% of women experience at least 3 months of secondary amenorrhea in a given year. There is no evidence that race or ethnicity influence the prevalence of amenorrhea. However, because of the importance of adequate nutrition for normal reproductive function, both the age at menarche and the prevalence of secondary amenorrhea vary significantly in different parts of the world.

The absence of menses by age 16 has been used traditionally to define primary amenorrhea. However, other factors such as growth, secondary sexual characteristics, the presence of cyclic pelvic pain, and the secular trend to an earlier age of menarche, particularly in African-American girls, also influence the age at which primary amenorrhea should be investigated. Thus, an evaluation for amenorrhea should be initiated by age 15 or 16 in the presence of normal growth and secondary sexual characteristics; by age 13 in the absence of secondary sexual characteristics or if height is less than the third percentile; by age 12 or 13 in the presence of breast development and cyclic pelvic pain; or within 2 years of breast development if menarche has not occurred.

Secondary Amenorrhea or Oligoamenorrhea

Anovulation and irregular cycles are relatively common for 2–4 years after menarche and for 1–2 years before the final menstrual period. In the intervening years, menstrual cycle length is ~28 days, with an intermenstrual interval normally ranging between 25 and 35 days. Cycle-to-cycle variability in an individual woman who is consistently ovulating is generally ± 2 days. Pregnancy is the most common cause of amenorrhea and should be excluded early in any evaluation of menstrual irregularity. However, many women will occasionally miss a single period. Three or more months of secondary amenorrhea should prompt an evaluation, as should a history of intermenstrual intervals of >35 or <21 days, or bleeding that persists for >7 days.

DIAGNOSIS

Evaluation of menstrual dysfunction depends on understanding the interrelationships between the four critical components of the reproductive tract: (1) the hypothalamus, (2) the pituitary, (3) the ovaries, and (4) the uterus and outflow tract (**Fig. 11-1**; Chap. 10). This system is maintained by complex negative and positive feedback loops involving the ovarian steroids (estradiol and progesterone) and peptides (inhibin B and inhibin A) and the hypothalamic [gonadotropin-releasing hormone (GnRH)] and pituitary [follicle-stimulating hormone (FSH) and luteinizing hormone (LH)] components of this system (Fig. 11-1).

Disorders of menstrual function can be thought of in two main categories: disorders of the uterus and outflow tract and disorders of ovulation. Many of the conditions that cause primary amenorrhea are congenital but go unrecognized until the time of normal puberty (e.g., genetic, chromosomal, and anatomic abnormalities). All causes of secondary amenorrhea can also cause primary amenorrhea.

Disorders of the Uterus or Outflow Tract

Abnormalities of the uterus and outflow tract typically present as primary amenorrhea. In patients with normal pubertal development and a blind vagina, the differential diagnosis includes *obstruction* by a transverse vaginal septum or imperforate hymen; *müllerian agenesis* (Mayer-Rokitansky-Kuster-Hauser syndrome), which has been associated with mutations in the *WNT4* gene; and *androgen insensitivity syndrome* (AIS), which is an X-linked recessive disorder that accounts for ~10% of all cases of primary amenorrhea (Chap. 8). Patients with AIS have a 46,XY karyotype, but because of the lack of androgen receptor responsiveness, they have severe underandrogenization and female external genitalia. The absence of pubic and axillary hair distinguishes them clinically from patients with müllerian agenesis. *Asherman syndrome* presents as

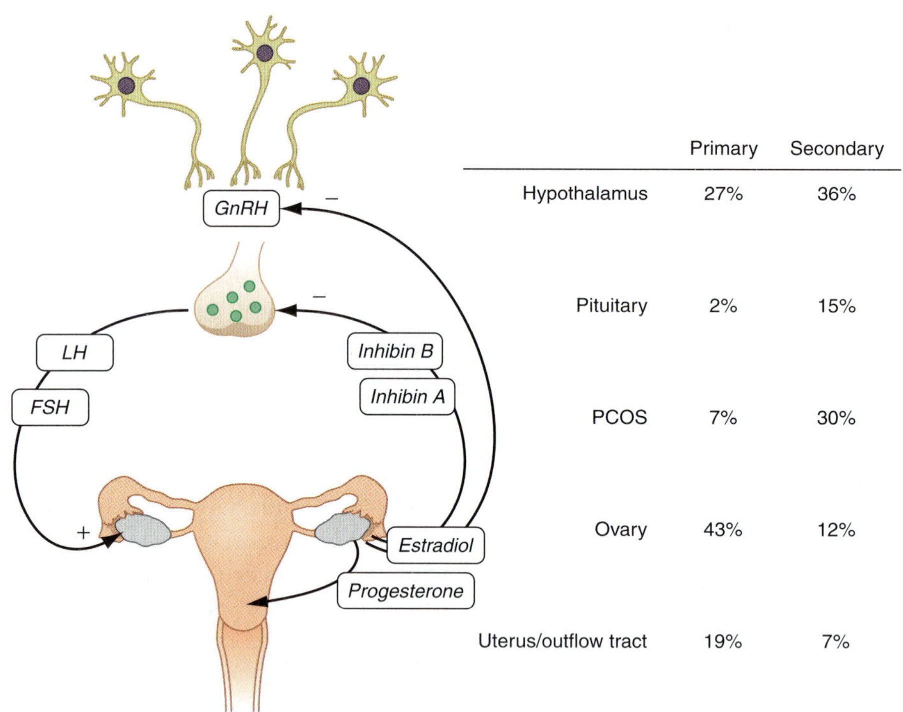

	Primary	Secondary
Hypothalamus	27%	36%
Pituitary	2%	15%
PCOS	7%	30%
Ovary	43%	12%
Uterus/outflow tract	19%	7%

FIGURE 11-1

Role of the hypothalamic-pituitary-gonadal axis in the etiology of amenorrhea. Gonadotropin-releasing hormone (GnRH) secretion from the hypothalamus stimulates follicle-stimulating hormone (FSH) and luteinizing hormone (LH) secretion from the pituitary to induce ovarian folliculogenesis and steroidogenesis. Ovarian secretion of estradiol and progesterone controls the shedding of the endometrium, resulting in menses, and, in combination with the inhibins, provides feedback regulation of the hypothalamus and pituitary to control secretion of FSH and LH. The prevalence of amenorrhea resulting from abnormalities at each level of the reproductive system (hypothalamus, pituitary, ovary, uterus, and outflow tract) varies depending on whether amenorrhea is primary or secondary. PCOS, polycystic ovarian syndrome.

secondary amenorrhea or hypomenorrhea and results from partial or complete obliteration of the uterine cavity by adhesions that prevent normal growth and shedding of the endometrium. Curettage performed for pregnancy complications accounts for >90% of cases; genital tuberculosis is an important cause in endemic regions.

℞ Treatment: DISORDERS OF UTERUS OR OUTFLOW TRACT

Obstruction of the outflow tract requires surgical correction. The risk of endometriosis is increased with this condition, perhaps because of retrograde menstrual flow. *Müllerian agenesis* may also require surgical intervention, although vaginal dilatation is adequate in some patients. Because ovarian function is normal, assisted reproductive techniques can be used with a surrogate carrier. *Androgen resistance syndrome* requires gonadectomy because there is risk of gonadoblastoma in the dysgenetic gonads. Whether this should be performed in early childhood or after completion of breast development is controversial. Estrogen replacement is indicated after gonadectomy, and vaginal dilatation may be required to allow sexual intercourse.

Disorders of Ovulation

Once uterus and outflow tract abnormalities have been excluded, all other causes of amenorrhea involve disorders of ovulation. The differential diagnosis is based on the results of initial tests including a pregnancy test, gonadotropins, and assessment of hyperandrogenism (Fig. 11-2).

Hypogonadotropic Hypogonadism

Low estrogen levels in combination with normal or low levels of LH and FSH are seen with anatomic, genetic, or functional abnormalities that interfere with hypothalamic GnRH secretion or normal pituitary responsiveness to GnRH. Although relatively uncommon, tumors and infiltrative diseases should be considered in the differential diagnosis of hypogonadotropic hypogonadism (Chap. 2). These disorders may present with primary or secondary amenorrhea. They may occur in association with other features suggestive of hypothalamic or pituitary dysfunction such as short stature, diabetes insipidus, galactorrhea, or headache. Hypogonadotropic hypogonadism may also be seen following cranial irradiation. In the postpartum period, it may be due to pituitary necrosis (Sheehan syndrome) or lymphocytic

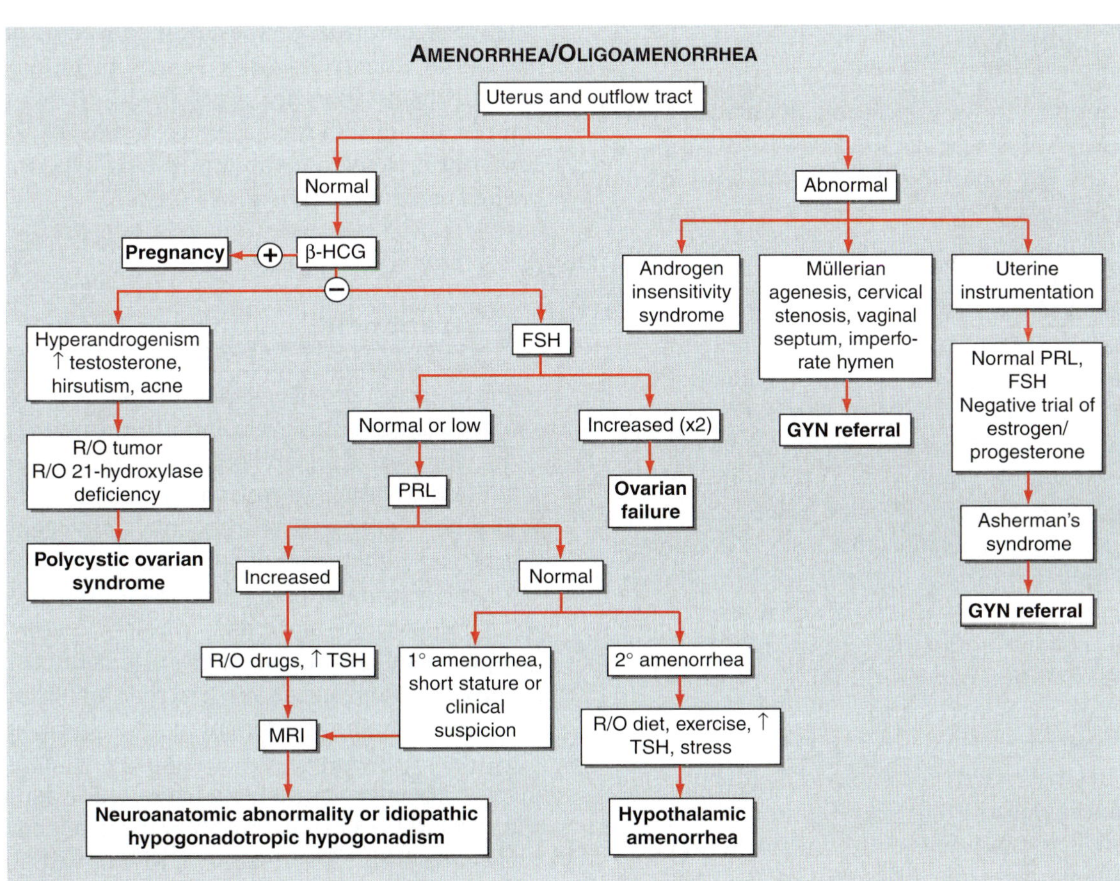

FIGURE 11-2

Algorithm for evaluation of amenorrhea. β-hCG, human chorionic gonadotropin; PRL, prolactin; FSH, follicle-stimulating hormone; TSH, thyroid-stimulating hormone.

hypophysitis. Because reproductive dysfunction is commonly associated with hyperprolactinemia, either from neuroanatomic lesions or medications, prolactin should be measured in all patients with hypogonadotropic hypogonadism (Chap. 2).

Isolated hypogonadotropic hypogonadism (IHH) is more common in men than women and is often associated with anosmia. IHH generally presents with primary amenorrhea. A number of genetic causes of IHH have been identified (Chaps. 8 and 10).

Functional hypothalamic amenorrhea (HA) is caused by a mismatch between energy expenditure and energy intake. Leptin secretion may play a key role in transducing the signals from the periphery to the hypothalamus in HA. The hypothalamic-pituitary-adrenal axis may also play a role. The diagnosis of HA can generally be made on the basis of a careful history, physical examination, and the demonstration of low levels of gonadotropins and normal prolactin levels. Eating disorders and chronic disease must be specifically excluded. An atypical history, headache, signs of other hypothalamic dysfunction, or hyperprolactinemia, even if mild, necessitates cranial imaging with CT or MRI to exclude a neuroanatomic cause.

Hypergonadotropic Hypogonadism

Ovarian failure is considered premature when it occurs in women younger than age 40. Ovarian failure is associated with the loss of negative-feedback restraint on the hypothalamus and pituitary, resulting in increased FSH and LH levels. FSH is a better marker of ovarian failure as its levels are less variable than LH. As with natural menopause, premature ovarian failure (POF) may wax and wane, and serial measurements may be necessary to establish the diagnosis.

Once the diagnosis of POF has been established, further evaluation is indicated because of other health problems that may be associated with POF. For example, POF is seen in association with a variety of chromosomal abnormalities including Turner syndrome, autoimmune polyglandular failure syndromes, radio- and chemotherapy, and galactosemia. In the majority of cases, however, a cause is not determined. The recognition that early ovarian failure occurs in premutation carriers of the fragile X syndrome is important because of increased risk of severe mental retardation in male children with *FMR1* mutations.

Hypergonadotropic hypogonadism occurs rarely in other disorders, such as mutations in the FSH or LH receptors. Aromatase deficiency and 17α-hydroxylase deficiency are associated with elevated gonadotropins with hyperandrogenism and hypertension, respectively. Gonadotropin-secreting tumors in women of reproductive age generally present with high, rather than low, estrogen levels and cause ovarian hyperstimulation or dysfunctional bleeding.

℞ Treatment: AMENORRHEA CAUSED BY OVULATORY DISORDERS

Amenorrhea is almost always associated with chronically low levels of estrogen, whether it is caused by hypogonadotropic hypogonadism or ovarian failure. Development of secondary sexual characteristics requires gradual titration of estradiol replacement with eventual addition of a progestin. Symptoms of hypoestrogenism can be treated with hormone replacement therapy or oral contraceptive pills. Patients with hypogonadotropic hypogonadism who are interested in fertility require treatment with pulsatile GnRH or exogenous FSH and LH, whereas patients with ovarian failure can consider oocyte donation, which has a high chance of success in this population.

Polycystic Ovarian Syndrome (PCOS)

This is diagnosed based on the presence of clinical or biochemical evidence of hyperandrogenism in association with amenorrhea or oligomenorrhea. Symptoms generally begin shortly after menarche and are slowly progressive. Lean patients with PCOS generally have high LH levels in the presence of normal to low levels of FSH and estradiol. The LH/FSH abnormality is less pronounced in obese patients in whom insulin resistance is a more prominent feature. Most patients also have a polycystic ovarian morphology on ultrasound, although there is controversy as to whether this morphology in combination with hyperandrogenism is sufficient for the diagnosis of PCOS.

℞ Treatment: POLYCYSTIC OVARIAN SYNDROME

The major abnormality in patients with PCOS is the failure of regular, predictable ovulation. Thus, these patients are at risk for the development of dysfunctional bleeding and endometrial hyperplasia associated with unopposed estrogen exposure. Endometrial protection can be achieved with the use of oral contraceptives or progestins (medroxyprogesterone acetate, 5–10 mg, or Prometrium, 200 mg daily for 10–14 days of each month). Oral contraceptives are also useful for management of hyperandrogenic symptoms, as is spironolactone, which functions as a weak androgen receptor antagonist. Management of the associated metabolic syndrome may be appropriate for some patients. For patients interested in fertility, weight control is a critical first step. Clomiphene citrate is highly effective as first-line treatment, with or without the addition of metformin. Exogenous gonadotropins can be used by experienced practitioners.

PELVIC PAIN

The mechanisms causing pelvic pain are similar to those causing abdominal pain and include inflammation of the parietal peritoneum, obstruction of hollow viscera, vascular disturbances, and pain originating in the abdominal wall. Pelvic pain may reflect pelvic disease per se but may also reflect extrapelvic disorders that refer pain to the pelvis. In up to 60% of cases, pelvic pain can be attributed to gastrointestinal problems including appendicitis, cholecystitis, infections, intestinal obstruction, diverticulitis, or inflammatory bowel disease. Urinary tract and musculoskeletal disorders are also common causes of pelvic pain.

Approach to the Patient: PELVIC PAIN

A thorough history including the type, location, radiation, and status with respect to increasing or decreasing severity can help to identify the cause of acute pelvic pain. Specific associations with vaginal bleeding, sexual activity, defecation, urination, movement, or eating should be specifically sought. A careful menstrual history is essential to assess the possibility of pregnancy. Determination of whether the pain is acute versus chronic and cyclic versus noncyclic will direct further investigation (Table 11-1). However, disorders that cause cyclic pain may occasionally cause noncyclic pain, and the converse is also true.

TABLE 11-1

CAUSES OF PELVIC PAIN

	ACUTE	CHRONIC
Cyclic pelvic pain		Premenstrual symptoms Mittelschmerz Dysmenorrhea Endometriosis
Noncyclic pelvic pain	Pelvic inflammatory disease Ruptured or hemorrhagic ovarian cyst or ovarian torsion Ectopic pregnancy Endometritis Acute growth or degeneration of uterine myoma	Pelvic congestion syndrome Adhesions and retroversion of the uterus Pelvic malignancy Vulvodynia History of sexual abuse

ACUTE PELVIC PAIN

Pelvic inflammatory disease most commonly presents with bilateral lower abdominal pain. It is generally of recent onset and is exacerbated by intercourse or jarring movements. Fever is present in about half of patients; abnormal uterine bleeding occurs in about one-third. New vaginal discharge, urethritis, and chills may be present but are less specific signs. *Adnexal pathology* can present acutely and may be due to rupture, bleeding or torsion of cysts, or, much less commonly, neoplasms of the ovary, fallopian tubes, or paraovarian areas. Fever may be present with ovarian torsion. *Ectopic pregnancy* is associated with right- or left-sided lower abdominal pain, vaginal bleeding, and menstrual cycle abnormalities, with clinical signs generally appearing 6–8 weeks after the last normal menstrual period. Orthostatic signs and fever may be present. Risk factors include the presence of known tubal disease, previous ectopic pregnancies, or a history of infertility, diethylstilbestrol (DES) exposure of the mother in utero, or pelvic infections. *Uterine pathology* includes endometritis and, less frequently, degenerating leiomyomas (fibroids). Endometritis is often associated with vaginal bleeding and systemic signs of infection. It occurs in the setting of sexually transmitted infections, uterine instrumentation, or postpartum infection.

A sensitive pregnancy test, complete blood count with differential, urinalysis, tests for chlamydial and gonococcal infections, and abdominal ultrasound aid in making the diagnosis and directing further management.

℞ Treatment: ACUTE PELVIC PAIN

Treatment of acute pelvic pain depends on the suspected etiology but may require surgical or gynecologic intervention. Conservative management is an important consideration for ovarian cysts, if torsion is not suspected, to avoid unnecessary pelvic surgery and the subsequent risk of infertility due to adhesions. The majority of unruptured ectopic pregnancies are now treated with methotrexate, which is effective in 84–96% of cases. However, surgical treatment may be required.

CHRONIC PELVIC PAIN

Some women experience discomfort at the time of ovulation (*mittelschmerz*). Pain can be quite intense but is generally of short duration. The mechanism is thought to involve rapid expansion of the dominant follicle, although it may also be caused by peritoneal irritation by follicular fluid released at the time of ovulation. Many women experience premenstrual symptoms such as breast discomfort, food cravings, and abdominal bloating or discomfort. These moliminal symptoms are a good predictor of ovulation, although their absence is less helpful.

Dysmenorrhea refers to the crampy lower abdominal discomfort that begins with the onset of menstrual bleeding and gradually decreases over the next 12–72 h. It may be associated with nausea, diarrhea, fatigue, and headache and occurs in 60–93% of adolescents, beginning with the establishment of regular ovulatory cycles. Its prevalence decreases after pregnancy and with the use of oral contraceptives.

Primary dysmenorrhea results from increased stores of prostaglandin precursors, which are generated by sequential stimulation of the uterus by estrogen and progesterone. During menstruation, these precursors are converted to prostaglandins, which cause intense uterine contractions, decreased blood flow, and increased peripheral nerve hypersensitivity, resulting in pain.

Secondary dysmenorrhea is caused by underlying pelvic pathology. *Endometriosis* results from the presence of endometrial glands and stroma outside of the uterus. These deposits of ectopic endometrium respond to hormonal stimulation and cause dysmenorrhea, which generally precedes menstruation by several days. Endometriosis may also be associated with painful intercourse, painful bowel movements, and tender nodules in the uterosacral ligament. Fibrosis and adhesions can produce lateral displacement of the cervix. The CA125 level may be increased, but it has low negative predictive value. Definitive diagnosis requires laparoscopy. Symptomatology does not always predict the extent of endometriosis. Other secondary causes of dysmenorrhea include adenomyosis, a condition caused by the presence of ectopic endometrial glands and stroma within the myometrium. Cervical stenosis may result from trauma, infection, or surgery.

℞ Treatment: DYSMENORRHEA

Local application of heat; use of vitamins B_1, B_6, and E and magnesium; acupuncture; yoga; and exercise are of some benefit for the treatment of dysmenorrhea. However, nonsteroidal anti-inflammatory drugs (NSAIDs) are the most effective treatment and provide >80% sustained response rates. Ibuprofen, naproxen, ketoprofen, mefenamic acid, and nimesulide are all superior to placebo. Treatment should be started a day before expected menses and is generally continued for 2–3 days. Oral contraceptives also reduce symptoms of dysmenorrhea. Failure of response to NSAIDs and oral contraceptives is suggestive of a pelvic disorder, such as endometriosis, and diagnostic laparoscopy should be considered to guide further treatment.

FURTHER READINGS

Dawood MY: Primary dysmenorrhea: Advances in pathogenesis and management. Obstet Gynecol 108:428, 2006

Dunaif A: Drug insight: Insulin-sensitizing drugs in the treatment of polycystic ovary syndrome—A reappraisal. Nat Clin Pract Endocrinol Metab 4:272, 2008

Genazzani AD et al: Diagnostic and therapeutic approach to hypothalamic amenorrhea. Ann NY Acad Sci 1092:103, 2006

Hall JE: Neuroendocrine control of the menstrual cycle, in *Yen and Jaffe's Reproductive Endocrinology*, 5th ed. JF Strauss, RL Barbieri (eds). Philadelphia, Elsevier, 2004, pp 195–211

Latthe P et al: Factors predisposing women to chronic pelvic pain: Systematic review. BMJ 332(7544):749, 2006

Misra M: What is the best strategy to combat low bone mineral density in functional hypothalamic amenorrhea? Nat Clin Pract Endocrinol Metab 4:542, 2008

Murray A: Premature ovarian failure and the FMR1 gene. Semin Reprod Med 18:59, 2000

Palomba S et al: Clomiphene citrate, metformin or both as first-step approach in treating anovulatory infertility in patients with polycystic ovary syndrome (PCOS): A systematic review of head-to-head randomized controlled studies and meta-analysis. Clin Endocrinol (Oxf) 70:311, 2009

Warren MP, Fried JL: Hypothalamic amenorrhea. The effects of environmental stresses on the reproductive system: A central effect of the central nervous system. Endocrinol Metab Clin North Am 30:611, 2001

Wittenberger MD et al: The FMR1 premutation and reproduction. Fertil Steril 87:456, 2007

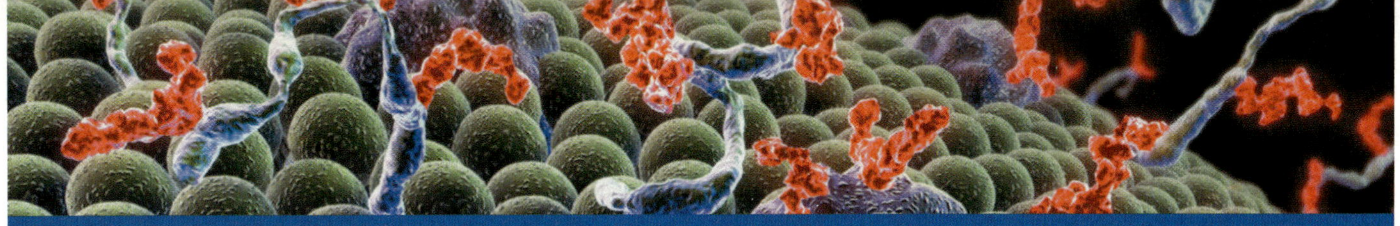

CHAPTER 12

THE MENOPAUSE TRANSITION AND POSTMENOPAUSAL HORMONE THERAPY

JoAnn E. Manson ■ Shari S. Bassuk

Menopause is the permanent cessation of menstruation due to loss of ovarian follicular function. It is diagnosed retrospectively after 12 months of amenorrhea. The average age at menopause is 51 years among U.S. women. *Perimenopause* refers to the time period preceding menopause, when fertility wanes and menstrual cycle irregularity increases, until the first year after cessation of menses. The onset of perimenopause precedes the final menses by 2–8 years, with a mean duration of 4 years. Smoking accelerates the menopausal transition by 2 years.

Although the peri- and postmenopausal transitions share many symptoms, the physiology and clinical management differ. Low-dose oral contraceptives have become a therapeutic mainstay in perimenopause, whereas postmenopausal hormone therapy (HT) has been a common method of symptom alleviation after menstruation ceases.

PERIMENOPAUSE

PHYSIOLOGY

Ovarian mass and fertility decline sharply after age 35 and even more precipitously during perimenopause; depletion of primary follicles, a process that begins before birth, occurs steadily until menopause (Chap. 10). In perimenopause, intermenstrual intervals shorten significantly (typically by 3 days) due to an accelerated follicular phase. Follicle-stimulating hormone (FSH) levels rise, due to altered folliculogenesis and reduced inhibin secretion. In contrast to the consistently high FSH and low estradiol levels seen in menopause, perimenopause is characterized by "irregularly irregular" hormone levels. The propensity for anovulatory cycles can produce a hyperestrogenic, hypoprogestagenic environment that may account for the increased incidence of endometrial hyperplasia or carcinoma, uterine polyps, and leiomyoma observed among women of perimenopausal age. Mean serum levels of selected ovarian and pituitary hormones during the menopausal transition are shown in **Fig. 12-1**. With transition into menopause, estradiol levels fall markedly, whereas estrone levels are relatively preserved, reflecting peripheral aromatization of adrenal and ovarian androgens. FSH levels increase more than those of luteinizing hormone (LH), presumably because of the loss of inhibin, as well as estrogen feedback.

DIAGNOSTIC TESTS

Because of their extreme intraindividual variability, FSH and estradiol levels are imperfect diagnostic indicators of perimenopause in menstruating women. However, a low FSH in the early follicular phase (days 2–5) of the menstrual cycle is inconsistent with a diagnosis of perimenopause.

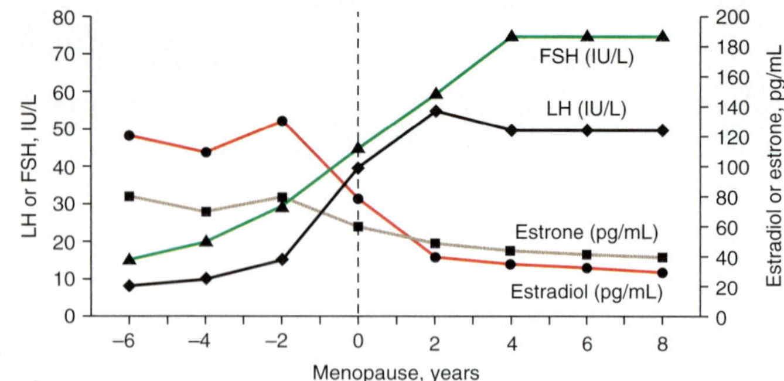

FIGURE 12-1

Mean serum levels of ovarian and pituitary hormones during the menopausal transition. FSH, follicle-stimulating hormone; LH, luteinizing hormone. *(From JL Shifren, I Schiff: The aging ovary. J Womens Health Gend Based Med 9:S-3, 2000, with permission.)*

FSH measurement can also aid in assessing fertility; levels of <20 mIU/mL, 20 to <30 mIU/mL, and ≥30 mIU/mL measured on day 3 of the cycle indicate a good, fair, and poor likelihood of achieving pregnancy, respectively.

SYMPTOMS

Determining whether symptoms that develop in midlife are due to ovarian senescence or to other age-related changes is difficult. There is strong evidence that the menopausal transition can cause hot flashes, night sweats, irregular bleeding, and vaginal dryness, and moderate evidence that it can cause sleep disturbances in some women. There is inconclusive or insufficient evidence that ovarian aging is a major cause of mood swings, depression, impaired memory or concentration, somatic symptoms, urinary incontinence, or sexual dysfunction. In one U.S. study, nearly 60% of women reported hot flashes in the 2 years before their final menses. Symptom intensity, duration, frequency, and effects on quality of life are highly variable.

℞ Treatment: PERIMENOPAUSE

For women with irregular or heavy menses or hormonally related symptoms that impair quality of life, low-dose combined oral contraceptives are a staple of therapy. Static doses of estrogen and progestin (e.g., 20 μg of ethinyl estradiol and 1 mg of norethindrone acetate daily for 21 days each month) can eliminate vasomotor symptoms and restore regular cyclicity. Oral contraceptives provide other benefits, including protection against ovarian and endometrial cancers and increased bone density, although it is not clear whether use during perimenopause decreases fracture risk later in life. Moreover, the contraceptive benefit is important, given that the unintentional pregnancy rate among women in their forties rivals that of adolescents. Contraindications to oral contraceptive use include cigarette smoking, liver disease, a history of thromboembolism or cardiovascular disease, breast cancer, or unexplained vaginal bleeding. Progestin-only formulations (e.g., 0.35 mg norethindrone daily) or medroxyprogesterone (Depo-Provera) injections (e.g., 150 mg IM every 3 months) may provide an alternative for the treatment of perimenopausal menorrhagia in women who smoke or have cardiovascular risk factors. Although progestins neither regularize cycles nor reduce the number of bleeding days, they reduce the volume of menstrual flow.

Nonhormonal strategies to reduce menstrual flow include use of nonsteroidal anti-inflammatory agents such as mefenamic acid (initial dose of 500 mg at start of menses, then 250 mg qid for 2–3 days) or, when medical approaches fail, endometrial ablation. It should be noted that menorrhagia requires an evaluation to rule out uterine disorders. Transvaginal ultrasound with saline enhancement is useful for detecting leiomyomata or polyps, and endometrial aspiration can identify hyperplastic changes.

TRANSITION TO MENOPAUSE For sexually active women using contraceptive hormones to alleviate perimenopausal symptoms, the question of when and if to switch to HT must be individualized. Doses of estrogen and progestogen (either synthetic progestins or natural forms of progesterone) in HT are lower than those in oral contraceptives and have not been documented to prevent pregnancy. Although a 1-year absence of spontaneous menses reliably indicates ovulation cessation, it is not possible to assess the natural menstrual pattern while a woman is taking an oral contraceptive. Women willing to switch to a barrier method of contraception should do so; if menses occur spontaneously, oral contraceptive use can be resumed. The average age of final menses among relatives can serve as a guide for when to initiate this process, which can be repeated yearly until menopause has occurred.

MENOPAUSE AND POSTMENOPAUSAL HORMONE THERAPY

One of the most complex health care decisions facing women is whether to use postmenopausal HT. Once prescribed primarily to relieve vasomotor symptoms, HT has been promoted as a strategy to forestall various disorders that accelerate after menopause, including osteoporosis and cardiovascular disease. In 2000, nearly 40% of postmenopausal women age 50–74 in the United States had used HT. This widespread use occurred despite the paucity of conclusive data, until recently, on the health consequences of such therapy. Although many women rely on their health care providers for a definitive answer to the question of whether to use postmenopausal hormones, balancing the benefits and risks for an individual patient is challenging.

Although observational studies suggest that HT prevents cardiovascular and other chronic diseases, the apparent benefits may result at least in part from differences between women who opt to take postmenopausal hormones and women who do not. Those choosing HT tend to be healthier, have greater access to medical care, be more compliant with prescribed treatments, and maintain a more health-promoting lifestyle. Randomized trials, which eliminate these confounding factors, have not consistently confirmed the benefits found in observational studies. Indeed, the largest HT trial to date, the Women's Health Initiative (WHI), which examined more than 27,000 postmenopausal women age 50–79 (mean age, 63) for an average of 5–7 years, was stopped early because of an overall unfavorable risk-versus-benefit ratio in the estrogen-progestin arm and an excess risk of stroke that was not offset by a reduced risk of coronary heart disease (CHD) in the estrogen-only arm.

The following summary offers a decision-making guide based on a synthesis of currently available evidence. Prevention of cardiovascular disease is eliminated from the equation due to lack of evidence for such benefits in recent randomized clinical trials.

BENEFITS AND RISKS OF POSTMENOPAUSAL HORMONE THERAPY

(**Table 12-1**)

Definite Benefits

Symptoms of Menopause

Compelling evidence, including data from randomized clinical trials, indicates that estrogen therapy is highly effective for controlling vasomotor and genitourinary symptoms. Alternative approaches, including the use of antidepressants (such as venlafaxine, 75–150 mg/d), gabapentin (300–900 mg/d), clonidine (0.1–0.2 mg/d), or vitamin E (400–800 IU/d), or the consumption of soy-based products or other phytoestrogens, may also alleviate vasomotor symptoms, although they are less effective than HT. For genitourinary symptoms, the efficacy of vaginal estrogen is similar to that of oral or transdermal estrogen.

Osteoporosis

(See also Chap. 28)

Bone Density

By reducing bone turnover and resorption rates, estrogen slows the aging-related bone loss experienced by most postmenopausal women. More than 50 randomized trials have demonstrated that postmenopausal estrogen therapy, with or without a progestogen, rapidly increases bone mineral density at the spine by 4–6% and at the hip by 2–3%, and maintains those increases during treatment.

Fractures

Data from observational studies indicate a 50–80% lower risk of vertebral fracture and a 25–30% lower risk of hip, wrist, and other peripheral fractures among current estrogen users; addition of a progestogen does not appear to modify this benefit. Discontinuation of estrogen therapy leads to a diminution of protection. In the WHI, 5–7 years of either combined estrogen-progestin or estrogen-only therapy was associated with a 30–40% reduction in hip fracture and 20–30% fewer total fractures among a population unselected for osteoporosis. Bisphosphonates (such as alendronate, 10 mg/d or 70 mg once per week; risedronate, 5 mg/d or 35 mg once per week; or ibandronate, 2.5 mg/d or 150 mg once per month or 3 mg every 3 months IV) and raloxifene (60 mg/d), a selective estrogen receptor modulator (SERM), have been shown in randomized trials to increase bone mass density and decrease fracture rates. A recently available option for treatment of osteoporosis is parathyroid hormone (teriparatide, 20 μg/d SC). These agents, unlike estrogen, do not appear to have adverse effects on the endometrium or breast. Increased physical activity and adequate calcium (1000–1500 mg/d through diet or supplements in two to three divided doses) and vitamin D (400–800 IU/d) intakes may also reduce the risk of osteoporosis-related fractures.

Definite Risks

Endometrial Cancer (*with Estrogen Alone*)

A combined analysis of 30 observational studies found a tripling of endometrial cancer risk among short-term (1–5 years) users of unopposed estrogen and a nearly tenfold increased risk among users for 10 or more years. These findings are supported by results from the randomized Postmenopausal Estrogen/Progestin Interventions (PEPI) trial, in which 24% of women assigned to unopposed estrogen for 3 years developed atypical endometrial hyperplasia, a premalignant lesion, compared with only 1% of women assigned to placebo. Use of a progestogen, which opposes the effects of estrogen on the endometrium, eliminates these risks.

Venous Thromboembolism

A meta-analysis of 12 studies—8 case-control, 1 cohort, and 3 randomized trials—found that current estrogen use was associated with a doubling of venous thromboembolism risk in postmenopausal women. Relative risks of thromboembolic events were even greater (2.7–5.1) in the three trials included in the meta-analysis. Results from the WHI indicate a twofold increase in risk of venous and pulmonary thromboembolism associated

TABLE 12-1

BENEFITS AND RISKS OF POSTMENOPAUSAL HORMONE THERAPY (HT) IN PRIMARY PREVENTION SETTINGS[a]

		BENEFIT OR RISK		
		RELATIVE		ABSOLUTE
OUTCOME	EFFECT	OBSERVATIONAL STUDIES	WHI,[b] EXCEPT WHERE NOTED	WHI,[b] EXCEPT WHERE NOTED
Definite Benefits				
Symptoms of menopause	Definite improvement	↓ 70–80% decreased risk	↓ 65–90% decreased risk[c]	
Osteoporosis	Definite increase in bone mineral density and decrease in fracture risk	↓ 20–50% decreased risk for fracture	E+P: ↓ 33% decreased risk for hip fracture E: ↓ 39% decreased risk for hip fracture	E+P: 50 fewer hip fractures (110 vs 160) per 100,000 woman-years E: 60 fewer hip fractures (110 vs 170) per 100,000 woman-years
Definite Risks				
Endometrial cancer	Definite increase in risk with estrogen alone; no increase in risk with estrogen-progestin	E+P: No increase in risk E: ↑ >300% increased risk (1–5 years); >600% increased risk (≥5 years)	E+P: No increase in risk E: Not applicable	E+P: No difference in risk E: 46 excess cases per 100,000 woman-years with unopposed estrogen (observational studies)[d]
Venous thrombo-embolism	Definite increase in risk	↑ 110% increased risk	E+P: ↑ 106% increased risk E: ↑ 32% increased risk	E+P: 180 excess cases (350 vs 170) per 100,000 woman-years E: 80 excess cases (300 vs 220) per 100,000 woman-years
Breast cancer	Increase in risk with long-term use (≥5 years) of estrogen-progestin	E+P: ↑ 63% increased risk (≥5 years) E: ↑ 20% increased risk (≥5 years)	E+P: ↑ 24% increased risk E: No increase in risk	10–30 excess cases per 10,000 women using HT for 5 years; 30–90 excess cases per 10,000 women after 10 years' use; 50–200 excess cases per 10,000 women after 15 years' use (estimate derived from observational data and WHI E+P findings)
Gallbladder disease	Definite increase in risk	↑ 110% increased risk	E+P: ↑ 67% increased risk E: ↑ 93% increased risk	E+P: 180 excess cases (460 vs 280) per 100,000 woman-years E: 310 excess cases (650 vs 340) per 100,000 woman-years
Probable or Uncertain Risks and Benefits				
Coronary heart disease	Probable increase in risk among older women and women many years past menopause; possible decrease in risk or no effect in younger or recently menopausal women	E+P: ↓ 36% decreased risk E: ↓ 45% decreased risk	E+P: ↑ 24% increased risk E: No increase or decrease in risk	E+P: 60 excess cases (390 vs 330) per 100,000 woman-years E: No difference in risk
Stroke	Probable increase in risk	↑ 12% increased risk	E+P: ↑ 31% increased risk E: ↑ 39% increased risk	E+P: 70 excess cases (310 vs 240) per 100,000 woman-years E: 120 excess cases (440 vs 320) per 100,000 woman-years

TABLE 12-1 (CONTINUED)

BENEFITS AND RISKS OF POSTMENOPAUSAL HORMONE THERAPY (HT) IN PRIMARY PREVENTION SETTINGS[a]

		BENEFIT OR RISK		
		RELATIVE		ABSOLUTE
OUTCOME	EFFECT	OBSERVATIONAL STUDIES	WHI,[b] EXCEPT WHERE NOTED	WHI,[b] EXCEPT WHERE NOTED
Ovarian cancer	Probable increase in risk with long-term use (≥5 years)	E+P: No effect (<4 years' use)	E+P: ↑ 58% increased risk[e]	E+P: 10 excess cases (40 vs 30) per 100,000 woman-years[e]
		E: ↑ 80% increased risk (≥10 years)	E: Not yet available	
Colorectal cancer	Probable decrease in risk with estrogen-progestin	↓ 34% decreased risk	E+P: ↓ 37% decreased risk	E+P: 70 fewer cases (90 vs 160) per 100,000 woman-years
			E: No increase or decrease in risk	E: No difference in risk
Diabetes mellitus	Probable decrease in risk	↓ 20% decreased risk	E+P: ↓ 21% decreased risk	E+P: 150 fewer cases (610 vs 760) per 100,000 woman-years
			E: ↓ 12% decreased risk[e]	E: 140 fewer cases (1160 vs 1300) per 100,000 woman-years[e]
Cognitive dysfunction	Unproven decrease in risk (inconsistent data from observational studies and randomized trials)	↓ 34% decreased risk	↑ 76% increased risk for dementia at age ≥65	120–230 excess cases of dementia per 100,000 woman-years

[a]E, estrogen alone; E+P, estrogen plus progestin. Most studies have assessed conjugated equine estrogen alone or in combination with medroxyprogesterone acetate.

[b]WHI, Women's Health Initiative. The estrogen-plus-progestin arm of the WHI assessed 5.6 years of conjugated equine estrogen (0.625 mg/d) plus medroxyprogesterone acetate (2.5 mg/d) versus placebo. The estrogen-alone arm of the WHI assessed 7.1 years of conjugated equine estrogen (0.625 mg/d) versus placebo.

[c]Data are from other randomized trials. The WHI was not designed to assess effect of HT on menopausal symptoms.

[d]JE Manson, KA Martin: N Engl J Med 345:34, 2001.

[e]Not statistically significant.

with estrogen-progestin and a one-third increase in this risk with estrogen-only therapy.

Breast Cancer (with Estrogen-Progestin)

An increased risk of breast cancer has been found among current or recent estrogen users in observational studies; this risk is directly related to duration of use. In a meta-analysis of 51 case-control and cohort studies, short-term use (<5 years) of postmenopausal HT did not appreciably elevate breast cancer incidence, whereas long-term use (≥5 years) was associated with a 35% increase in risk. In contrast to findings for endometrial cancer, combined estrogen-progestin regimens appear to increase breast cancer risk more than estrogen alone. Data from randomized trials also indicate that estrogen-progestin raises breast cancer risk. In the WHI, women assigned to receive combination hormones for an average of 5.6 years were 24% more likely to develop breast cancer than women assigned to placebo, but 7.1 years of estrogen-only therapy did not increase risk. Indeed, the WHI showed a trend toward a reduction in breast cancer risk with estrogen alone, although it is unclear whether this finding would pertain to formulations of estrogen other than conjugated equine estrogens or to treatment durations longer than 7 years. In the Heart and Estrogen/progestin Replacement Study (HERS), 4 years of combination therapy was associated with a 27% increase in breast cancer risk. Although the latter finding was not statistically significant, the totality of evidence strongly implicates estrogen-progestin therapy in breast carcinogenesis.

Gallbladder Disease

Large observational studies report a two- to threefold increased risk of gallstones or cholecystectomy among postmenopausal women taking oral estrogen. In the WHI, women randomized to estrogen-progestin or estrogen alone had a 67% and 93% greater risk, respectively, of undergoing cholecystectomy than those assigned to placebo. Increased risks were also observed in the HERS. Transdermal HT may not increase the risk of gallbladder disease, but further research is needed.

Probable or Uncertain Risks and Benefits

Coronary Heart Disease/Stroke

Until recently, HT had been enthusiastically recommended as a possible cardioprotective agent. In the past three decades, multiple observational studies suggested, in the aggregate, that estrogen use leads to a 35–50% reduction in CHD incidence among postmenopausal women. The biologic plausibility of such an association is supported by data from randomized trials demonstrating that exogenous estrogen lowers plasma low-density lipoprotein (LDL) cholesterol and raises high-density lipoprotein (HDL) cholesterol levels by 10–15%. Administration of estrogen also favorably affects lipoprotein(a) levels, LDL oxidation, endothelial vascular function, fibrinogen, and plasminogen activator inhibitor-1. However, estrogen therapy also has unfavorable effects on other biomarkers of cardiovascular risk: it boosts triglyceride levels; promotes coagulation via factor VII, prothrombin fragments 1 and 2, and fibrinopeptide A elevations; and raises levels of the inflammatory marker C-reactive protein.

Randomized trials of estrogen or combined estrogen-progestin in women with preexisting cardiovascular disease have not confirmed the benefits reported in observational studies. In the HERS, a secondary prevention trial designed to test the efficacy and safety of estrogen-progestin therapy on clinical cardiovascular outcomes, the 4-year incidence of coronary mortality and nonfatal myocardial infarction was similar in the active treatment and placebo groups, and a 50% increase in risk of coronary events was noted during the first year of the study among participants assigned to the active treatment group. Although it is possible that progestin may mitigate estrogen's benefits, the Estrogen Replacement and Atherosclerosis (ERA) trial indicated that angiographically determined progression of coronary atherosclerosis was unaffected by either opposed or unopposed estrogen treatment. Moreover, the Papworth Hormone Replacement Therapy Atherosclerosis Study, a trial of transdermal estradiol with and without norethindrone; the Women's Estrogen for Stroke Trial (WEST), a trial of oral 17β-estradiol; and the EStrogen in the Prevention of ReInfarction Trial (ESPRIT), a trial of oral estradiol valerate, found no cardiovascular benefits of the regimens studied. Thus, in clinical trials, HT has not proved effective for the secondary prevention of cardiovascular disease in postmenopausal women.

Primary prevention trials also suggest an early increase in cardiovascular risk and absence of cardioprotection with postmenopausal HT. Results from the WHI suggest a deleterious cardiovascular effect of HT. Women assigned to 5.6 years of estrogen-progestin therapy were 24% more likely to develop CHD and 31% more likely to suffer a stroke than those assigned to placebo. In the estrogen-only arm of the WHI, a similar increase in stroke and no effect on CHD were observed.

However, a closer look at available data suggests that timing of initiation of HT may critically influence the association between such therapy and CHD. Estrogen may slow early stages of atherosclerosis but have adverse effects on advanced atherosclerotic lesions. It has been hypothesized that the prothrombotic and proinflammatory effects of estrogen manifest themselves predominantly among women with subclinical lesions who initiate HT well after the menopausal transition, whereas women with less arterial damage who start HT early in menopause may derive cardiovascular benefit because they have not yet developed advanced lesions. Nonhuman primate data support this concept. Conjugated estrogens had no effect on the extent of coronary artery plaque in cynomolgus monkeys assigned to estrogen alone or combined with progestin starting 2 years (approximately 6 human years) after oophorectomy and well after the establishment of atherosclerosis. However, administration of exogenous hormones immediately after oophorectomy, during the early stages of atherosclerosis, reduced the extent of plaque by 70%.

Lending further credence to this hypothesis are results of subgroup analyses of observational and clinical trial data. For example, although there was no association between estrogen-only therapy and CHD in the WHI study cohort as a whole, such therapy was associated with a CHD risk reduction of 37% among participants age 50–59. By contrast, a risk reduction of only 8% was observed among those age 60–69, and a risk increase of 11% was found among those age 70–79. Due to the relatively small number of cases of myocardial infarction or coronary death (the primary definition of CHD in the WHI), especially in the younger women, these intra- and inter-age group differences were not statistically significant. However, when the definition of CHD was widened to include coronary bypass surgery or percutaneous coronary interventions, estrogen-only therapy was associated with a significant 45% reduction in CHD among women in the youngest age group. Moreover, estrogen was associated with lower levels of coronary artery calcified plaque.

Although age did not have a similar effect in the estrogen-progestin arm of the WHI, CHD risks steadily increased with years since menopause. Estrogen-progestin was associated with an 11% risk reduction for women less than 10 years beyond menopause but was associated with a 22% increase in risk for women 10–19 years from menopause, and a 71% increase in risk for women 20 years or more from menopause (only the latter was statistically significant). In the large observational Nurses' Health Study, women who chose to start HT within 4 years of menopause experienced a lower risk of CHD than did nonusers, whereas those who began therapy 10 or more years after menopause appeared to receive little coronary benefit. Because observational studies include a high proportion of women who begin HT within 3–4 years of menopause and clinical trials include a high proportion of women 12 or more years past menopause, these findings help to reconcile some of the apparent discrepancies between the two types of studies.

Whether age at initiation of HT influences stroke risk is not well understood. Further research is needed on age, time since menopause, and other clinical characteristics as well as on biomarkers that predict increases or decreases in cardiovascular risk associated with exogenous HT. Furthermore, it remains uncertain whether different doses, formulations, or routes of administration of HT will produce different cardiovascular effects.

Colorectal Cancer

Observational studies have suggested that HT reduces risks of colon and rectal cancer, although the estimated magnitudes of the relative benefits ranged from 8 to 34% in various meta-analyses. In the WHI, the sole trial to examine the issue, estrogen-progestin was associated with a significant 44% reduction in colorectal cancer over a 5.6-year period, although no benefit was seen with 7 years of estrogen-only therapy.

Cognitive Decline and Dementia

A meta-analysis of 10 case-control and 2 cohort studies suggested that postmenopausal HT is associated with a 34% decreased risk of dementia. Subsequent randomized trials, including the WHI, however, have failed to demonstrate any benefit of estrogen or estrogen-progestin therapy on the progression of mild to moderate Alzheimer's disease and/or have indicated a potential adverse effect of HT on the incidence of dementia, at least in women age 65 and older. Determining whether timing of initiation of HT influences cognitive outcomes will require further study.

Ovarian Cancer and Other Disorders

On the basis of limited observational and randomized data, it has been hypothesized that HT increases the risk of ovarian cancer and reduces the risk of type 2 diabetes mellitus. Results from the WHI support these hypotheses.

Approach to the Patient: POSTMENOPAUSAL HORMONE THERAPY

The rational use of postmenopausal HT requires balancing the potential benefits and risks. Figure 12-2 provides one approach to decision-making. The clinician should first determine whether the patient has moderate to severe menopausal symptoms, the only indication for initiating systemic HT (urogenital symptoms in the absence of vasomotor symptoms may be treated with vaginal estrogen). The benefits and risks of such therapy should then be reviewed with the patient, giving more emphasis to absolute than to relative measures of effect, and pointing out uncertainties in clinical knowledge where relevant. (Because chronic disease rates generally increase with age, absolute risks tend to be greater in older women, even when relative risks remain similar.) Potential side effects—especially vaginal bleeding that may result from use of combined estrogen-progestogen formulations recommended for women with an intact uterus—should be noted. The patient's own preference regarding therapy should be elicited and factored into the decision. Contraindications to HT should be assessed routinely and include unexplained vaginal bleeding; active liver disease; venous thromboembolism; history of endometrial cancer (except stage 1 without deep invasion) or breast cancer; and history of CHD, stroke, transient ischemic attack, or diabetes. Relative contraindications include hypertriglyceridemia (>400 mg/dL) and active gallbladder disease; in such cases, transdermal estrogen may be an option. Primary prevention of heart disease should not be viewed as an expected benefit of HT, and an increase in stroke and a small early increase in coronary artery disease risk should be considered. Nevertheless, such therapy may be appropriate if the noncoronary benefits of treatment clearly outweigh risks. A woman who suffers an acute coronary event or stroke while on HT should stop therapy immediately.

Short-term use (<5 years) of HT is appropriate for relief of menopausal symptoms among women without contraindications to such use. However, such therapy should be avoided among women with an elevated baseline risk of future cardiovascular events. Women who have contraindications, or are opposed to HT, may derive benefit from the use of certain antidepressants (including venlafaxine, fluoxetine, or paroxetine), gabapentin, clonidine, soy, or black cohosh, and, for genitourinary symptoms, intravaginal estrogen creams or devices.

Long-term use (≥5 years) of HT, especially estrogen-progestogen, is more problematic because a heightened risk of breast cancer must be factored into the decision. Reasonable candidates for such use include a small percentage of postmenopausal women and comprise those who have persistent severe vasomotor symptoms along with an increased risk of osteoporosis (e.g., those with osteopenia, a personal or family history of nontraumatic fracture, or a weight below 125 lb), who also have no personal or family history of breast cancer in a first-degree relative or other contraindications, and who have a strong personal preference for therapy. Poor candidates are women with elevated cardiovascular risk, those at increased risk of breast cancer (e.g., women who have a first-degree relative with breast cancer, susceptibility genes such as *BRCA1* or *BRCA2*, or a personal history of

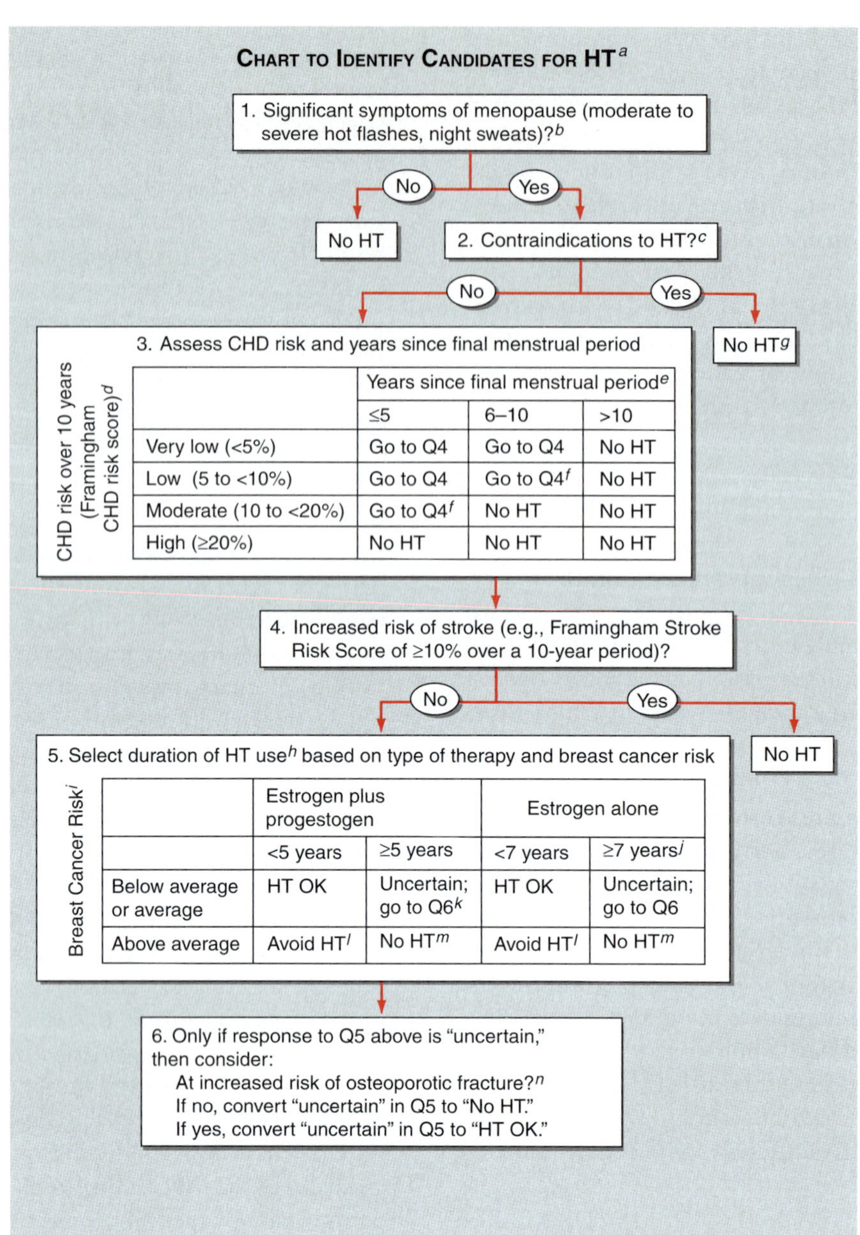

FIGURE 12-2

Flowchart for identifying appropriate candidates for postmenopausal hormone therapy (HT). CHD, coronary heart disease.

[a]Reassess each step at least once every 6–12 months (assuming patient's continued preference for HT).

[b]Women who have vaginal dryness without moderate to severe vasomotor symptoms may be candidates for vaginal estrogen.

[c]Traditional contraindications: unexplained vaginal bleeding; active liver disease; history of venous thromboembolism due to pregnancy, oral contraceptive use, or unknown etiology; blood clotting disorder; history of breast or endometrial cancer; history of CHD, stroke, transient ischemic attack, or diabetes. For other contraindications, including high triglycerides (>400 mg/dL); active gallbladder disease; and history of venous thromboembolism due to past immobility, surgery, or bone fracture, oral HT should be avoided but transdermal HT may be an option (see *f*).

[d]Ten-year risk of CHD, based on Framingham Coronary Heart Disease Risk Score (Expert Panel on Detection, Evaluation, and Treatment of High Blood Cholesterol in Adults: JAMA 285:2486, 2001), as modified by JE Manson, with SS Bassuk: *Hot Flashes, Hormones & Your Health*. New York, McGraw-Hill, 2007.

[e]Women >10 years past menopause are not good candidates for starting (first use of) HT.

[f]Avoid oral HT. Transdermal HT may be an option because it has a less adverse effect on clotting factors, triglyceride levels, and inflammation factors than oral HT.

[g]Consider selective serotonin or serotonin-norepinephrine reuptake inhibitor, gabapentin, clonidine, soy, or alternative.

[h]HT should be continued only if moderate to severe menopausal symptoms persist. The recommended cutpoints for duration are based on results of the Women's Health Initiative estrogen-progestin and estrogen-alone trials, which lasted 5.6 and 7.1 years, respectively. For longer durations of HT use, balance of benefits and risks is not known.

FIGURE 12-2 (*CONTINUED*)

[i]Above-average risk of breast cancer: one or more first-degree relatives with breast cancer; susceptibility genes such as *BRCA1* or *BRCA2*; or a personal history of breast biopsy demonstrating atypia.

[j]Women with premature surgical menopause may take HT until average age at menopause (age 51 in the United States) and then follow flowchart for subsequent decision-making.

[k]If progestogen is taken daily, avoid extending duration. If progestogen is cyclical or infrequent, avoid extending duration more than 1–2 years.

[l]If menopausal symptoms are severe, estrogen plus progestin can be taken for 2–3 years maximum and estrogen alone for 4–5 years maximum.

[m]If at high risk of osteoporotic fracture (see Q6), consider bisphosphonate, raloxifene, or alternative.

[n]Increased risk of osteoporotic fracture: documented osteopenia, personal or family history of nontraumatic fracture, current smoking, or weight <125 lb.

Source: Adapted from JE Manson, with SS Bassuk: *Hot Flashes, Hormones & Your Health*. New York, McGraw-Hill, 2007.

cellular atypia detected by breast biopsy), and those at low risk of osteoporosis. Even in reasonable candidates, strategies to minimize dose and duration of use should be employed. For example, women using HT to relieve intense vasomotor symptoms in early postmenopause should consider discontinuing therapy before 5 years, resuming it only if such symptoms persist. Because of the role of progestogens in increasing breast cancer risk, regimens that employ cyclic rather than continuous progestogen exposure should be considered if treatment is extended. For prevention of osteoporosis, alternative therapies such as bisphosphonates or SERMs should be considered. Research on androgen-containing preparations has been limited, particularly in terms of long-term safety. Additional research on the effects of these agents on cardiovascular disease, glucose tolerance, and breast cancer will be of particular interest.

In addition to HT, control of symptoms and prevention of chronic disease can be accomplished by lifestyle choices, including smoking abstention, adequate physical activity, and a healthy diet. An expanding array of pharmacologic options—e.g., bisphosphonates, SERMs, and other agents for osteoporosis, and cholesterol-lowering or antihypertensive agents for cardiovascular disease—should also reduce the widespread reliance on hormone use. However, short-term HT may still benefit some women.

FURTHER READINGS

Advisory panel of the North American Menopause Society: Estrogen and progestin use in peri- and postmenopausal women: March 2007 Position Statement of the North American Menopause Society. Menopause 14:168, 2007

American College of Obstetricians and Gynecologists Task Force on Hormone Therapy: Hormone therapy. Obstet Gynecol 104:S1, 2004

Manson JE et al: Estrogen plus progestin and the risk of coronary heart disease. N Engl J Med 349:523, 2003

——— et al: Estrogen therapy and coronary-artery calcification. N Engl J Med 356:2591, 2007

Manson JE, with Bassuk SS: *Hot Flashes, Hormones & Your Health*. New York: McGraw-Hill, 2007

Nachtigall L: Does combined hormone replacement therapy improve the health-related quality of life of postmenopausal women? Nat Clin Pract Endocrinol Metab 5:136, 2009

Nelson HD: Menopause. Lancet 371:760, 2008

Roberts H: Managing the menopause. BMJ 334(7596):736, 2007

Rossouw JE et al: Postmenopausal hormone therapy and risk of cardiovascular disease by age and years since menopause. JAMA 297:1465, 2007

Warren MP: Historical perspectives in postmenopausal hormone therapy: Defining the right dose and duration. Mayo Clin Proc 82(2):219, 2007

Writing Group for the Women's Health Initiative Investigators: Risks and benefits of estrogen plus progestin in healthy postmenopausal women. Principal results from the Women's Health Initiative randomized controlled trial. JAMA 288:321, 2002

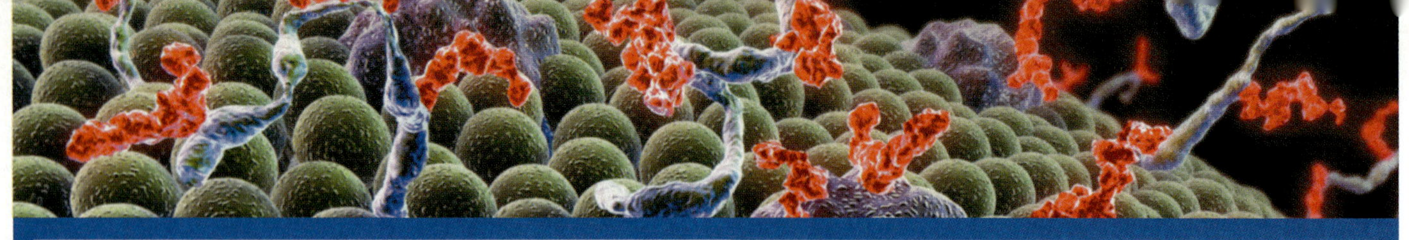

CHAPTER 13

HIRSUTISM AND VIRILIZATION

David A. Ehrmann

Hirsutism, defined as excessive male-pattern hair growth, affects approximately 10% of women. It usually represents a variation of normal hair growth, but rarely, it is a harbinger of a serious underlying condition. Hirsutism is often idiopathic but may be caused by conditions associated with androgen excess, such as polycystic ovarian syndrome (PCOS) or congenital adrenal hyperplasia (CAH) (**Table 13-1**). Cutaneous manifestations commonly associated with hirsutism include acne and male-pattern balding (androgenic alopecia). *Virilization* refers to a condition in which androgen levels are sufficiently high to cause additional signs and symptoms such as deepening of the voice, breast atrophy, increased muscle bulk, clitoromegaly, and increased libido; virilization is an ominous sign that suggests the possibility of an ovarian or adrenal neoplasm.

HAIR FOLLICLE GROWTH AND DIFFERENTIATION

Hair can be categorized as either *vellus* (fine, soft, and not pigmented) or *terminal* (long, coarse, and pigmented). The number of hair follicles does not change over an individual's lifetime, but the follicle size and type of hair can change in response to numerous factors, particularly androgens. Androgens are necessary for terminal hair and sebaceous gland development and mediate differentiation of pilosebaceous units (PSUs) into either a terminal hair follicle or a sebaceous gland. In the former case, androgens transform the vellus hair into a terminal hair; in the latter, the sebaceous component proliferates and the hair remains vellus.

There are three phases in the cycle of hair growth: (1) *anagen* (growth phase), (2) *catagen* (involution phase), and (3) *telogen* (rest phase). Depending on the body site, hormonal regulation may play an important role in the hair growth cycle. For example, the eyebrows, eyelashes, and vellus hairs are androgen-insensitive, whereas the axillary and pubic areas are sensitive to low levels of androgens. Hair growth on the face, chest, upper abdomen, and back requires greater levels of androgens and is therefore more characteristic of the pattern typically seen in men. Androgen excess in women leads to increased hair growth in most androgen-sensitive sites except in the scalp region, where hair loss occurs because androgens cause scalp hairs to spend less time in the anagen phase.

Although androgen excess underlies most cases of hirsutism, there is only a modest correlation between androgen levels and the quantity of hair growth. This is due to the fact that hair growth from the follicle also depends on local growth factors, and there is variability in end organ sensitivity. Genetic factors and ethnic background also influence hair growth. In general, dark-haired individuals tend to be more hirsute than blonde or fair individuals. Asians and Native Americans have relatively sparse hair in regions sensitive to high androgen levels, whereas people of Mediterranean descent are more hirsute.

CLINICAL ASSESSMENT

Historic elements relevant to the assessment of hirsutism include the age of onset and rate of progression of hair growth and associated symptoms or signs (e.g., acne).

TABLE 13-1

CAUSES OF HIRSUTISM
Gonadal hyperandrogenism
Ovarian hyperandrogenism
Polycystic ovary syndrome/functional ovarian hyperandrogenism
Ovarian steroidogenic blocks
Syndromes of extreme insulin resistance
Ovarian neoplasms
Adrenal hyperandrogenism
Premature adrenarche
Functional adrenal hyperandrogenism
Congenital adrenal hyperplasia (nonclassic and classic)
Abnormal cortisol action/metabolism
Adrenal neoplasms
Other endocrine disorders
Cushing's syndrome
Hyperprolactinemia
Acromegaly
Peripheral androgen overproduction
Obesity
Idiopathic
Pregnancy-related hyperandrogenism
Hyperreactio luteinalis
Thecoma of pregnancy
Drugs
Androgens
Oral contraceptives containing androgenic progestins
Minoxidil
Phenytoin
Diazoxide
Cyclosporine
True hermaphroditism

Depending on the cause, excess hair growth is typically first noted during the second and third decades. The growth is usually slow but progressive. Sudden development and rapid progression of hirsutism suggest the possibility of an androgen-secreting neoplasm, in which case virilization also may be present.

The age of onset of menstrual cycles (menarche) and the pattern of the menstrual cycle should be ascertained; irregular cycles from the time of menarche onward are more likely to result from ovarian rather than adrenal androgen excess. Associated symptoms such as galactorrhea should prompt evaluation for hyperprolactinemia (Chap. 2) and possibly hypothyroidism (Chap. 4). Hypertension, striae, easy bruising, centripetal weight gain, and weakness suggest hypercortisolism (Cushing's syndrome; Chap. 5). Rarely, patients with growth hormone excess (i.e., acromegaly) will present with hirsutism. Use of medications such as phenytoin, minoxidil, or cyclosporine may be associated with androgen-independent excess hair growth (i.e., hypertrichosis). A family history of infertility and/or hirsutism may indicate disorders such as nonclassic CAH (Chap. 5).

Physical examination should include measurement of height and weight and calculation of body mass index (BMI). A BMI >25 kg/m^2 is indicative of excess weight for height, and values >30 kg/m^2 are often seen in association with hirsutism. Notation should be made of blood pressure, as adrenal causes may be associated with hypertension. Cutaneous signs sometimes associated with androgen excess and insulin resistance include acanthosis nigricans and skin tags.

An objective clinical assessment of hair distribution and quantity is central to the evaluation in any woman presenting with hirsutism. This assessment permits the distinction between hirsutism and hypertrichosis and provides a baseline reference point to gauge the response to treatment. A simple and commonly used method to grade hair growth is the modified scale of Ferriman and Gallwey (**Fig. 13-1**), where each of nine androgen-sensitive sites is graded from 0 to 4. Approximately 95% of Caucasian women have a score below 8 on this scale; thus, it is normal for most women to have some hair growth in androgen-sensitive sites. Scores above 8 suggest excess androgen-mediated hair growth, a finding that should be assessed further by hormonal evaluation (see below). In racial/ethnic groups that are less likely to manifest hirsutism (e.g., Asian women), additional cutaneous evidence of androgen excess should be sought, including pustular acne or thinning hair.

HORMONAL EVALUATION

Androgens are secreted by the ovaries and adrenal glands in response to their respective tropic hormones, luteinizing hormone (LH) and adrenocorticotropic hormone (ACTH). The principal circulating steroids involved in the etiology of hirsutism are testosterone, androstenedione, and dehydroepiandrosterone (DHEA) and its sulfated form (DHEAS). The ovaries and adrenal glands normally contribute about equally to testosterone production. Approximately half of the total testosterone originates from direct glandular secretion, and the remainder is derived from the peripheral conversion of androstenedione and DHEA (Chap. 8).

Although it is the most important circulating androgen, testosterone is, in effect, the penultimate androgen in mediating hirsutism; it is converted to the more potent dihydrotestosterone (DHT) by the enzyme 5α-reductase, which is located in the PSU. DHT has a higher affinity for, and slower dissociation from, the androgen receptor. The local production of DHT allows it to serve as the primary mediator of androgen action at the level of the pilosebaceous unit. There are two isoenzymes of 5α-reductase: type 2 is found in the prostate gland and in hair follicles, whereas type 1 is found primarily in sebaceous glands.

One approach to testing for hyperandrogenemia is depicted in **Fig. 13-2**. In addition to measuring blood levels of testosterone and DHEAS, it is also important to

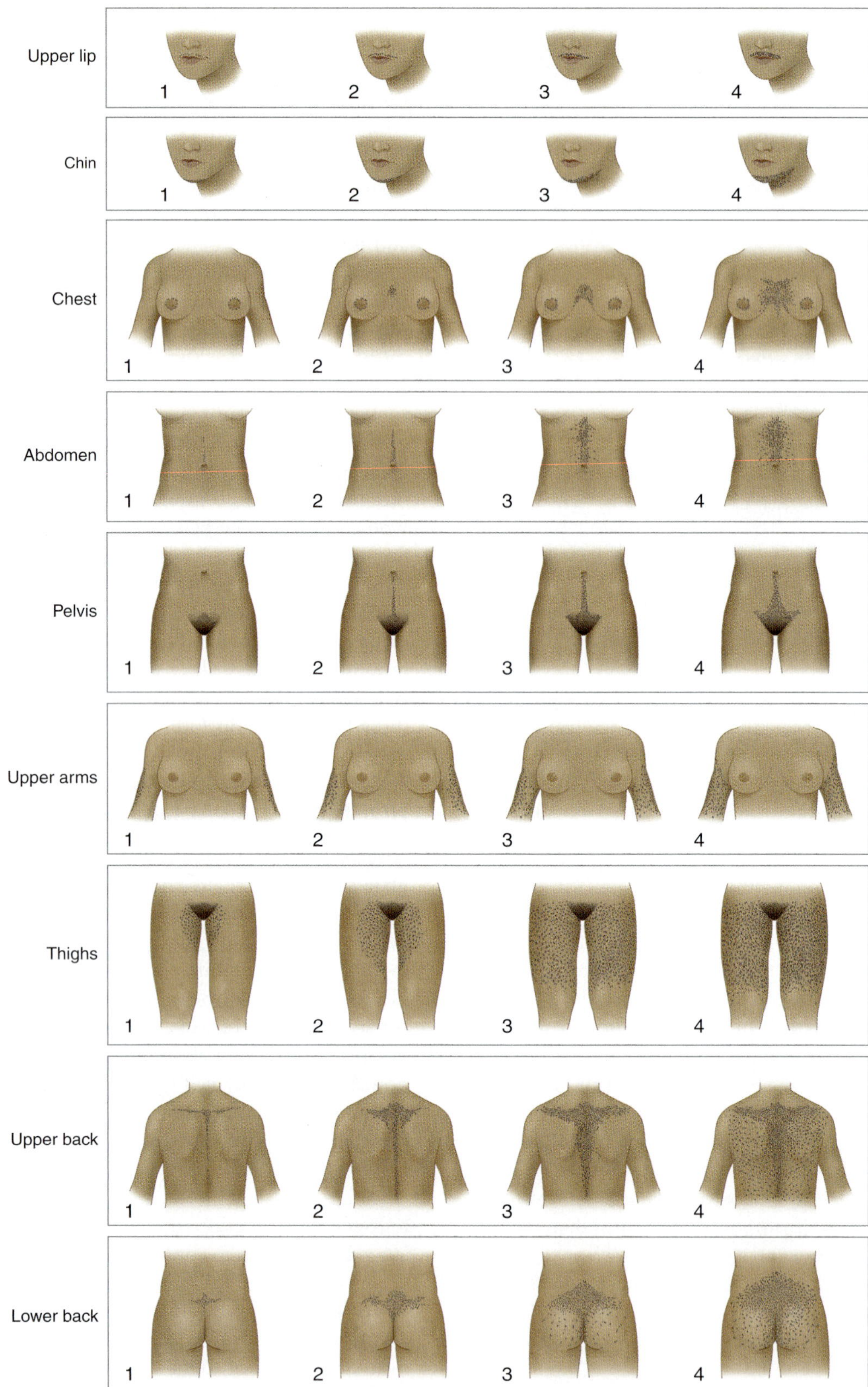

FIGURE 13-1

Hirsutism scoring scale of Ferriman and Gallwey. The nine body areas possessing androgen-sensitive areas are graded from 0 (no terminal hair) to 4 (frankly virile) to obtain a total score. A normal hirsutism score is less than 8. [*Modified from DA Ehrmann et al: Hyperandrogenism, hirsutism, and polycystic ovary syndrome, in LJ DeGroot and JL Jameson (eds), Endocrinology, 5th ed. Philadelphia, Saunders, 2006; with permission.*]

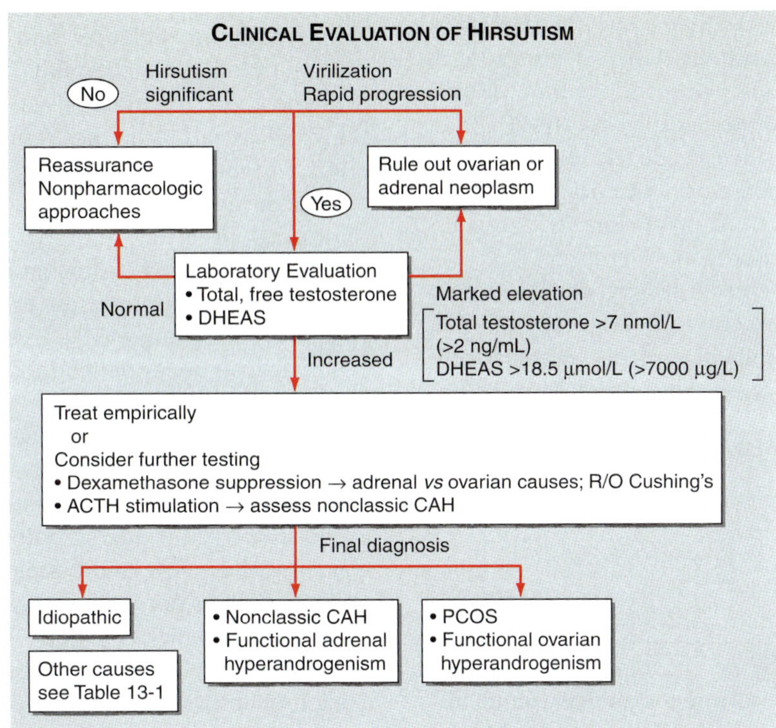

FIGURE 13-2

Algorithm for the evaluation and differential diagnosis of hirsutism. ACTH, adrenocorticotropic hormone; CAH, congenital adrenal hyperplasia; DHEAS, sulfated form of dehydroepiandrosterone; PCOS, polycystic ovarian syndrome.

measure the level of free (or unbound) testosterone. The fraction of testosterone that is not bound to its carrier protein, sex hormone–binding globulin (SHBG), is biologically available for conversion to DHT and for binding to androgen receptors. Hyperinsulinemia and/or androgen excess decrease hepatic production of SHBG, resulting in levels of total testosterone within the high-normal range, whereas the unbound hormone is more substantially elevated. Although there is a decline in ovarian testosterone production after menopause, ovarian estrogen production decreases to an even greater extent, and the concentration of SHBG is reduced. Consequently, there is an increase in the relative proportion of unbound testosterone, and it may exacerbate hirsutism after menopause.

A baseline plasma total testosterone level >12 nmol/L (>3.5 ng/mL) usually indicates a virilizing tumor, whereas a level >7 nmol/L (>2 ng/mL) is suggestive. A basal DHEAS level >18.5 μmol/L (>7000 μg/L) suggests an adrenal tumor. Although DHEAS has been proposed as a "marker" of predominant adrenal androgen excess, it is not unusual to find modest elevations in DHEAS among women with PCOS. CT or MRI should be used to localize an adrenal mass, and ultrasound will usually suffice to identify an ovarian mass if clinical evaluation and hormonal levels suggest these possibilities.

PCOS is the most common cause of ovarian androgen excess (Chap. 10). However, the increased ratio of LH to follicle-stimulating hormone that is characteristic of carefully studied patients with PCOS is not seen in up to half of these women due to the pulsatility of gonadotropins. If performed, ultrasound shows enlarged ovaries and increased stroma in many women with PCOS. However, polycystic ovaries may also be found in women without clinical or laboratory features of PCOS. Therefore, polycystic ovaries are a relatively insensitive and nonspecific finding for the diagnosis of ovarian hyperandrogenism. Although not usually necessary, gonadotropin-releasing hormone agonist testing can be used to make a specific diagnosis of ovarian hyperandrogenism. A peak 17-hydroxyprogesterone level ≥7.8 nmol/L (≥2.6 μg/L), after the administration of 100 μg nafarelin (or 10 μg/kg leuprolide) SC, is virtually diagnostic of ovarian hyperandrogenism.

Because adrenal androgens are readily suppressed by low doses of glucocorticoids, the dexamethasone androgen suppression test may broadly distinguish ovarian from adrenal androgen overproduction. A blood sample is obtained before and after administering dexamethasone (0.5 mg PO every 6 h for 4 days). An adrenal source is suggested by suppression of unbound testosterone into the normal range; incomplete suppression suggests ovarian androgen excess. An overnight 1-mg dexamethasone suppression test, with measurement of 8:00 A.M. serum cortisol, is useful when there is clinical suspicion of Cushing's syndrome (Chap. 5).

Nonclassic CAH is most commonly due to 21-hydroxylase deficiency but can also be caused by autosomal recessive defects in other steroidogenic enzymes necessary for adrenal corticosteroid synthesis (Chap. 5). Because of the enzyme defect, the adrenal gland cannot secrete glucocorticoids efficiently (especially cortisol). This results in diminished negative feedback inhibition of ACTH, leading to compensatory adrenal hyperplasia and the accumulation of steroid precursors that are subsequently converted to androgen. Deficiency of 21-hydroxylase can be reliably excluded by determining a morning 17-hydroxyprogesterone level <6 nmol/L (<2 μg/L) (drawn in the follicular phase). Alternatively, 21-hydroxylase deficiency can be diagnosed by measurement of 17-hydroxyprogesterone 1 h after administration of 250 μg of synthetic ACTH (cosyntropin) IV.

℞ Treatment: HIRSUTISM

Treatment of hirsutism may be accomplished pharmacologically or by mechanical means of hair removal. Nonpharmacologic treatments should be considered in all patients, either as the only treatment or as an adjunct to drug therapy.

Nonpharmacologic treatments include (1) bleaching; (2) depilatory (removal from the skin surface) such as shaving and chemical treatments; or (3) epilatory (removal of the hair including the root) such as plucking, waxing, electrolysis, and laser therapy. Despite perceptions to the contrary, shaving does not increase the rate or density of hair growth. Chemical depilatory treatments may be useful for mild hirsutism that affects only limited skin areas, though they can cause skin irritation. Wax treatment removes hair temporarily but is uncomfortable. Electrolysis is effective for more permanent hair removal, particularly in the hands of a skilled electrologist. Laser phototherapy appears to be efficacious for hair removal. It delays hair regrowth and causes permanent hair removal in most patients. The long-term effects and complications associated with laser treatment are still being evaluated.

Pharmacologic therapy is directed at interrupting one or more of the steps in the pathway of androgen synthesis and action: (1) suppression of adrenal and/or ovarian androgen production; (2) enhancement of androgen-binding to plasma-binding proteins, particularly SHBG; (3) impairment of the peripheral conversion of androgen precursors to active androgen; and (4) inhibition of androgen action at the target tissue level. Attenuation of hair growth is typically not evident until 4–6 months after initiation of medical treatment and, in most cases, leads to only a modest reduction in hair growth.

Combination estrogen-progestin therapy, in the form of an oral contraceptive, is usually the first-line endocrine treatment for hirsutism and acne, after cosmetic and dermatologic management. The estrogenic component of most oral contraceptives currently in use is either ethinyl estradiol or mestranol. The suppression of LH leads to reduced production of ovarian androgens. The reduced androgen levels also result in a dose-related increase in SHBG, thereby lowering the fraction of unbound plasma testosterone. Combination therapy has also been demonstrated to decrease DHEAS, perhaps by reducing ACTH levels. Estrogens also have a direct, dose-dependent suppressive effect on sebaceous cell function.

The choice of a specific oral contraceptive should be predicated on the progestational component, as progestins vary in their suppressive effect on SHBG levels and in their androgenic potential. Ethynodiol diacetate has relatively low androgenic potential, whereas progestins such as norgestrel and levonorgestrel are particularly androgenic, as judged from their attenuation of the estrogen-induced increase in SHBG. Norgestimate exemplifies the newer generation of progestins that are virtually nonandrogenic. Drospirenone, an analogue of spironolactone that has both antimineralocorticoid and antiandrogenic activities, has been approved for use as a progestational agent in combination with ethinyl estradiol. Its properties suggest that it should be the preferred choice for the treatment of hirsutism.

Oral contraceptives are contraindicated in women with a history of thromboembolic disease or in women with increased risk of breast or other estrogen-dependent cancers (Chap. 12). There is a relative contraindication to the use of oral contraceptives in smokers or in those with hypertension or a history of migraine headaches. In most trials, estrogen-progestin therapy alone improves the extent of acne by a maximum of 50–70%. The effect on hair growth may not be evident for 6 months, and the maximum effect may require 9–12 months owing to the length of the hair growth cycle. Improvements in hirsutism are typically in the range of 20%, but there may be an arrest of further progression of hair growth.

Adrenal androgens are more sensitive than cortisol to the suppressive effects of glucocorticoids. Therefore, glucocorticoids are the mainstay of treatment in patients with CAH. Although glucocorticoids have been reported to restore ovulatory function in some women with PCOS, this effect is highly variable. Because of side effects from excessive glucocorticoids, low doses should be used. Dexamethasone (0.2–0.5 mg) or prednisone (5–10 mg) should be taken at bedtime to achieve maximal suppression by inhibiting the nocturnal surge of ACTH.

Cyproterone acetate is the prototypic antiandrogen. It acts mainly by competitive inhibition of the binding of testosterone and DHT to the androgen receptor. In addition, it may enhance the metabolic clearance of testosterone by inducing hepatic enzymes. Although not available for use in the United States, cyproterone acetate is widely used in Canada, Mexico, and Europe. Cyproterone (50–100 mg) is given on days 1–15 and ethinyl estradiol (50 μg) is given on days 5–26 of the menstrual cycle. Side effects include irregular uterine bleeding, nausea, headache, fatigue, weight gain, and decreased libido.

Spironolactone, usually used as a mineralocorticoid antagonist, is also a weak antiandrogen. It is almost as effective as cyproterone acetate when used at high enough doses (100–200 mg daily). Patients should be monitored intermittently for hyperkalemia or hypotension, though these side effects are uncommon. Pregnancy should be avoided because of the risk of feminization of a male fetus. Spironolactone can also cause menstrual irregularity. It is often used in combination with an oral contraceptive, which suppresses ovarian androgen production and helps prevent pregnancy.

Flutamide is a potent nonsteroidal antiandrogen that is effective in treating hirsutism, but concerns about the induction of hepatocellular dysfunction have limited its use. Finasteride is a competitive inhibitor of 5α-reductase type 2. Beneficial effects on hirsutism have been reported, but the predominance of 5α-reductase type 1 in the PSU appears to account for its limited efficacy. Finasteride would also be expected to impair sexual differentiation in a male fetus, and it should not be used in women who may become pregnant.

Eflornithine cream (Vaniqa) has been approved as a novel treatment for unwanted facial hair in women, but long-term efficacy remains to be established. It can cause skin irritation under exaggerated conditions of use. Ultimately, the choice of any specific agent(s) must be tailored to the unique needs of the patient being treated. As noted previously, pharmacologic treatments for hirsutism should be used in conjunction with nonpharmacologic approaches. It is also helpful to review the pattern of female hair distribution in the normal population to dispel unrealistic expectations.

FURTHER READINGS

Carmina E: Antiandrogens for the treatment of hirsutism. Expert Opin Investig Drugs 11:357, 2002

Cosma M et al: Clinical review: Insulin sensitizers for the treatment of hirsutism: A systematic review and metaanalyses of randomized controlled trials. J Clin Endocrinol Metab 93:1135, 2008

Ehrmann DA: Polycystic ovary syndrome. N Engl J Med 352:1223, 2005

Hordinsky M et al: Hair loss and hirsutism in the elderly. Clin Geriatr Med 18:121, 2002

Martin KA et al: Evaluation and treatment of hirsutism in premenopausal women: An Endocrine Society clinical practice guideline. J Clin Endocrinol Metab 93:1105, 2008

Rosenfield RL: Clinical practice. Hirsutism. N Engl J Med 353:2578, 2005

Swiglo BA et al: Clinical review: Antiandrogens for the treatment of hirsutism: A systematic review and metaanalyses of randomized controlled trials. J Clin Endocrinol Metab 93:1153, 2008

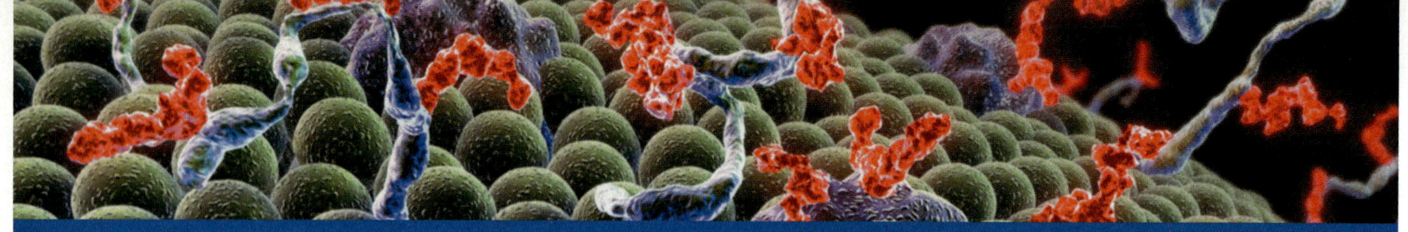

CHAPTER 14

GYNECOLOGIC MALIGNANCIES

Robert C. Young

OVARIAN CANCER

INCIDENCE AND EPIDEMIOLOGY

Ovarian cancer can develop from three distinctive cell types (germ cells, stromal cells, and epithelial cells), and each of these presents with distinctive features and outcomes and requires widely different management approaches. Epithelial ovarian cancer is the most common of the three and the leading cause of death from gynecologic cancer in the United States. In 2007, 22,430 new cases were diagnosed, and 15,280 women died from ovarian cancer. Epithelial ovarian cancer accounts for 5% of all cancer deaths in women in the United States; more women die of this disease than from cervical and endometrial cancer combined.

The age-specific incidence of the common epithelial type of ovarian cancer increases progressively and peaks in the eighth decade. Epithelial tumors, unlike germ cell and stromal tumors, are uncommon before the age of 40. Epidemiologic studies suggest higher incidences in women with a family history; in those who have been exposed to asbestos or talc; in industrialized nations; and in women with disordered ovarian function, including infertility, nulliparity, and frequent miscarriages. The use of ovulation-inducing drugs such as clomiphene has been implicated, but the studies have produced mixed results. Reduction in ovarian cancer risk is associated with pregnancy (each pregnancy reduces the ovarian cancer risk by about 10%), breast-feeding, and tubal ligation. Oral contraceptives reduce the risk of ovarian cancer in patients with a family history of cancer and in the general population. Many of these risk-reduction factors support the "incessant ovulation" hypothesis for ovarian cancer etiology, which implies that an aberrant repair process of the surface epithelium is central to ovarian cancer development. Estrogen replacement after menopause does not appear to increase the risk of ovarian cancer, although its use has declined substantially since the hormone replacement therapy (HRT) trials demonstrated an increased cardiovascular risk.

Familial cases account for about 10% of all ovarian cancer. Compared to a lifetime risk of 1.6% in the general population, women with one affected first-degree relative have a 5% risk. In families with two or more affected first-degree relatives, the risk may exceed 50%. Two types of autosomal dominant familial cancers have been identified: (1) breast/ovarian cancer syndrome and (2) the Lynch type II cancer family syndrome with nonpolyposis colorectal cancer, endometrial cancer, and ovarian cancer.

ETIOLOGY AND GENETICS

In women with hereditary breast/ovarian cancer, two susceptibility loci have been identified: *BRCA1*, located on chromosome 17q12-21, and *BRCA2*, on 13q12-13. Both are tumor-suppressor genes that produce nuclear proteins that interact with RAD 51, which affects genomic integrity. Both genes are large, and numerous mutations have been described; most are frameshift or nonsense mutations, and 86% produce truncated protein products. The implications of the many other mutations, including many missense mutations, are not known. The cumulative risk of ovarian cancer with critical mutations of *BRCA1* or *-2* is 25%. Mutated genes can be inherited from either parent, so a complete family history is required. Men in such families have an increased risk of prostate cancer.

The Lynch type II syndrome is associated with an increased risk of ovarian cancer. Affected women often present at a younger age (<50 years). The predisposition results from germline mutations of mismatch repair genes (*MSH2*, *MLH1*, *MLH6*, *PMS1*, and *PMS2*). Because the risk of both endometrial and ovarian cancer is high, intensified screening and prophylactic surgery are often considered.

CLINICAL PRESENTATION AND DIFFERENTIAL DIAGNOSIS

Seventy percent of patients with ovarian cancer are first diagnosed when the disease has already spread beyond the true pelvis. The occurrence of abdominal pain, bloating, and urinary symptoms usually indicates advanced disease. Localized ovarian cancer is generally asymptomatic. However, progressive enlargement of a localized ovarian tumor can produce urinary frequency or constipation. Rarely, torsion of an ovarian mass causes acute abdominal pain or a surgical abdomen. In contrast to cervical or endometrial cancer, vaginal bleeding or discharge is rarely seen with early ovarian cancer. The diagnosis of early disease usually occurs with palpation of an asymptomatic adnexal mass during routine pelvic examination or as an incidental finding at surgery. However, most ovarian enlargements discovered on physical examination, especially in premenopausal women, are benign functional cysts that characteristically resolve over one to three menstrual cycles. Adnexal masses in premenarchal or postmenopausal women are more likely to be pathologic. A solid, irregular, fixed pelvic mass is usually ovarian cancer. Ultrasound studies usually show complex cysts with solid elements. Other causes of adnexal masses include pedunculated uterine fibroids, endometriosis, benign ovarian neoplasms, and inflammatory lesions of the bowel.

Evaluation of patients with suspected ovarian cancer should include measurement of CA-125. Between 80 and 85% of patients with epithelial ovarian cancer have levels of CA-125 ≥35 U/mL. Other malignant tumors can also elevate CA-125 levels, including cancers of the endometrium, cervix, fallopian tubes, pancreas, breast, lung, and colon. Certain nonmalignant conditions that can produce moderate elevations of CA-125 levels include pregnancy, endometriosis, pelvic inflammatory disease, and uterine fibroids. About 1% of normal females have serum CA-125 levels >35 U/mL. However, in postmenopausal women with an asymptomatic pelvic mass and CA-125 levels ≥65 U/mL, the test has a sensitivity of 97% and a specificity of 78%.

SCREENING

In contrast to patients who present with advanced disease, patients with early ovarian cancers (stages I and II) are commonly curable with conventional therapy. Thus, effective screening procedures would improve the cure rate in this disease. Although pelvic examination and CA-125 can occasionally detect early disease, these are relatively insensitive screening procedures. Transvaginal sonography is often used, but significant false-positive results are noted, particularly in premenopausal women. Doppler flow imaging coupled with transvaginal ultrasound may improve accuracy and reduce the high rate of false positives.

CA-125 has significant limitations as a screening test. Half of women with stages I and II ovarian cancer have normal CA-125 levels. Attempts have been made to improve the sensitivity and specificity by combinations of procedures, commonly transvaginal ultrasound and CA-125. In a screening study of 22,000 women, 42 had a positive screen and 11 had ovarian cancer (7 with advanced disease). In addition, eight women with a negative screen developed ovarian cancer. Thus, the false-positive rate would lead to a large number of unnecessary (i.e., negative) laparotomies if each positive screen resulted in a surgical exploration. In the United Kingdom, a large collaborative screening trial is underway to prospectively compare various screening techniques with controls. Until the results of such trials are available, the National Institutes of Health Consensus Conference recommended against screening for ovarian cancer among the general population without known risk factors for the disease. Although no evidence shows that screening saves lives, many physicians use annual pelvic examinations, transvaginal ultrasound, and CA-125 to screen women with a family history of ovarian cancer, Lynch type II, or breast/ovarian cancer syndrome.

Proteomic technologies have been used to identify patterns of proteins associated with early disease. Preliminary studies identified all 50 stage I patients with a sensitivity of 100%, a specificity of 95%, and a positive predictive value of 94%. However, difficulty in consistency of replicate samples, variability of results from different spectroscopy equipment, and the tendency of the artificial intelligence algorithms to overfit the data have limited its utility. Most proteins identified to date have been acute phase reactants, and extensive fractionation is necessary to identify unique cancer-specific proteins.

PATHOLOGY

Common epithelial tumors comprise most (85%) of the ovarian neoplasms. These may be benign (50%), malignant (33%), or tumors of low malignant potential (16%) (i.e., tumors of borderline malignancy). Epithelial tumors of low malignant potential have the cytologic features of malignancy but do not invade the ovarian stroma. More than 75% of borderline malignancies present in early stage and generally occur in the fourth or fifth decade of life. They usually have 10-year survival of 80–90%.

There are five major subtypes of common epithelial tumors: serous (50%), mucinous (25%), endometrioid (15%), clear cell (5%), and Brenner tumors (1%), the latter derived from the urothelium. Benign common epithelial tumors are almost always serous or mucinous and develop in women ages 20–60. They are frequently large (20–30 cm), bilateral, and cystic. Malignant epithelial tumors are usually seen in women over 40.

Although most ovarian tumors are epithelial, two other ovarian tumor types, stromal and germ cell tumors, are distinct in their cell of origin, have different clinical presentations and natural histories, and require different management.

Metastasis to the ovary can occur from breast, colon, gastric, and pancreatic cancers. The Krukenberg tumor was classically described as bilateral ovarian masses from metastatic mucin-secreting gastrointestinal cancers.

STAGING AND PROGNOSTIC FACTORS

Laparotomy is the primary procedure used to establish the diagnosis and provide accurate staging. Less invasive studies may help define the extent of spread, including chest x-rays, abdominal CT or MRI scans, and abdominal and pelvic sonography. Symptoms of bladder or renal dysfunction are evaluated by cystoscopy or IV pyelography.

A careful staging laparotomy with a total abdominal hysterectomy and bilateral salpingo-oophorectomy will establish the stage and extent of disease and allow for the cytoreduction of tumor masses in patients with advanced disease. Proper laparotomy requires a vertical incision of sufficient length to ensure adequate examination of the abdominal contents. The presence, amount, and cytology of any ascitic fluid should be noted. The primary tumor should be evaluated for rupture, excrescences, or dense adherence. Careful visual and manual inspection of the diaphragm and peritoneal surfaces is required. A partial omentectomy should be performed and the paracolic gutters inspected. Pelvic lymph nodes as well as para-aortic nodes in the region of the renal hilus should be biopsied. Since this surgical procedure defines stage, establishes prognosis, and determines the necessity for subsequent therapy, it should be performed by a surgeon with special expertise in ovarian cancer staging. Studies have shown that patients operated on by gynecologic oncologists were properly staged 97% of the time, compared to 52 and 35% of cases staged by obstetricians/gynecologists and general surgeons, respectively. After staging, ~23% of women have stage I disease (cancer confined to the ovary or ovaries), 13% have stage II (disease confined to the true pelvis), 47% have stage III (disease spread into but confined to the abdomen), and 16% have stage IV disease (spread outside the pelvis and abdomen). The 5-year survival correlates with stage of disease: stage I, 90–95%; stage II, 70–80%; stage III, 25–50%; and stage IV, 1–5% (**Table 14-1**).

Prognosis in ovarian cancer is dependent not only on stage but also on the extent of residual disease and histologic grade. Patients presenting with advanced disease but left without significant residual disease after surgery have a median survival of 39 months, compared to 17 months for those with suboptimal tumor resection.

If initial surgery does not produce minimal residual disease, a second cytoreductive surgery has been used after the first three cycles of chemotherapy; in one trial it was associated with a 6-month improvement in median duration of survival. Another randomized trial where more aggressive debulking surgery was initially carried out was unable to confirm this benefit.

Prognosis of epithelial tumors is also highly influenced by histologic grade but less so by histologic type. Although grading systems differ among pathologists, all grading systems show a better prognosis for well- or moderately differentiated tumors than for poorly differentiated histologies. Estimated 5-year survivals for patients by tumor grade are well-differentiated, 88%; moderately differentiated, 58%; poorly differentiated, 27%.

The prognostic significance of pre- and postoperative CA-125 levels is uncertain. CA-125 levels generally reflect volume of disease, and high levels usually indicate unresectability and a poorer survival. Postoperative levels, if elevated, usually indicate residual disease. The rate of decline of CA-125 levels during initial therapy or the absolute level after one to three cycles of chemotherapy correlates with prognosis but is not sufficiently accurate to guide individual treatment decisions. Even when the CA-125 level falls to normal after surgery or chemotherapy, "second-look" laparotomy identifies residual disease in 60% of women.

TABLE 14-1

STAGING AND SURVIVAL IN GYNECOLOGIC MALIGNANCIES

STAGE	OVARIAN	5-YEAR SURVIVAL, %	ENDOMETRIAL	5-YEAR SURVIVAL, %	CERVIX	5-YEAR SURVIVAL, %
0	—		—		Carcinoma in situ	100
I	Confined to ovary	90	Confined to corpus	89	Confined to uterus	85
II	Confined to pelvis	70	Involves corpus and cervix	73	Invades beyond uterus but not to pelvic wall	65
III	Intraabdominal spread	25–500	Extends outside the uterus but not outside the true pelvis	52	Extends to pelvic wall and/or lower third of vagina, or hydronephrosis	35
IV	Spread outside abdomen	1–5	Extends outside the true pelvis or involves the bladder or rectum	17	Invades mucosa of bladder or rectum or extends beyond the true pelvis	7

Genetic and biologic factors may influence prognosis. Increased tumor levels of p53 are associated with a poorer prognosis in advanced disease. Epidermal growth factor receptors in ovarian cancer are associated with a decrease in disease-free survival, but the increased expression of HER-2/neu has given conflicting prognostic results. HER-2/neu is overexpressed in 20% of ovarian cancers, and responses have been seen to trastuzumab in this subset of patients.

℞ Treatment: OVARIAN CANCER

The selection of therapy for patients with epithelial ovarian cancer depends on the stage, extent of residual tumor, and histologic grade. In general, patients are considered in three separate treatment groups: (1) those with early (stages I and II) ovarian cancer and microscopic or no residual disease, (2) patients with advanced (stage III) disease but minimal residual tumor (<1 cm) after initial surgery, and (3) patients with bulky residual tumor and advanced (stage III or IV) disease.

Patients with stage I disease, no residual tumor, and well or moderately differentiated tumors need no adjuvant therapy after definitive surgery, and 5-year survival exceeds 95%. For all other patients with early disease and those stage I patients with poor prognosis histologic grade, adjuvant platinum-based therapy is warranted. Large prospective randomized trials have demonstrated that adjuvant therapy improves disease-free and overall survival by 8% (82% vs. 74%, $p = .008$).

For patients with advanced (stage III) disease but with limited or no residual disease after definitive cytoreductive surgery (about half of all stage III patients), the primary therapy is platinum-based combination chemotherapy. Approximately 70% of women respond to initial combination chemotherapy, and 40–50% have a complete regression of disease. Unfortunately, only about half of these patients are free of disease if surgically restaged. Although a variety of combinations are active, a randomized prospective trial of paclitaxel and cisplatin compared to paclitaxel and carboplatin in patients with optimally resected advanced disease demonstrated equivalent disease-free and overall survivals but with significantly reduced toxicity with the carboplatin combination. This regimen of paclitaxel, 175 mg/m^2 by 3-h infusion, and carboplatin, dosed to an AUC (area under the curve) of 7.5, is the preferred treatment choice for patients with previously untreated advanced-stage disease.

Three randomized trials using intraperitoneal (IP) chemotherapy have demonstrated improved disease-free and overall survival compared to the IV administration of the same drugs. However, the increased toxicity (neuropathy, nephropathy, and catheter complications) is significant, and only about 40% of patients were able to receive full courses of therapy. Furthermore, the optimal dose and schedule of IP therapy has not been established, nor have any of the IP regimens been prospectively compared to the standard IV carboplatin-paclitaxel regimen. The ultimate role of IP therapy in the treatment of advanced ovarian cancer is unresolved.

Patients with advanced disease (stages III and IV) and bulky residual tumor are generally treated with IV paclitaxel-platinum combination, and while the overall prognosis is poorer, 5-year survival may reach 15–20%.

Historically, patients who had an excellent initial response to chemotherapy and no clinical evidence of disease had a second-look laparotomy. The second-look surgical procedure itself does not prolong overall survival, and outside of clinical trials its routine use is no longer recommended. Maintenance therapy may extend progression-free survival but has not improved overall survival.

Patients with advanced disease whose disease recurs after initial treatment are usually not curable but may benefit significantly from limited surgery to relieve intestinal obstruction, localized radiation therapy to relieve pressure or pain from mass lesions or metastasis, or palliative chemotherapy. The selection of chemotherapy for palliation depends on the initial regimen and evidence of drug resistance. Patients who had a complete regression of disease lasting ≥6 months often respond to reinduction with the same agents; patients relapsing within the first 6 months of initial therapy rarely do. Progestational agents, tamoxifen, or aromatase inhibitors produce responses in 5–15% of patients and have minimal side effects. Agents with >15% response rates in patients relapsing after initial combination chemotherapy include gemcitabine, topotecan, liposomal doxorubicin, and bevacizumab.

Bevacizumab is a monoclonal antibody that targets the vascular endothelial growth factor. Initial trials produced a 17% overall response rate in heavily pretreated patients. However, hypertension, thrombosis, and bowel perforations have been reported in some trials.

Patients with tumors of low malignant potential, even with advanced-stage disease, have longer survivals (80–90%) when managed with surgery alone. Radiation and chemotherapy do not improve outcome.

OVARIAN GERM CELL TUMORS

Fewer than 5% of all ovarian tumors are germ cell in origin. They include teratoma, dysgerminoma, endodermal sinus tumor, and embryonal carcinoma. Germ cell tumors of the ovary generally occur in younger women (75% of ovarian malignancies in women <30), display an unusually aggressive natural history, and are commonly cured with less extensive nonsterilizing surgery and chemotherapy. Women cured of these malignancies are able to conceive and have normal children.

These neoplasms can be divided into three major groups: (1) benign tumors (usually dermoid cysts); (2) malignant tumors that arise from dermoid cysts; and (3) primitive malignant germ cell tumors, including dysgerminoma, yolk sac tumors, immature teratomas, embryonal carcinomas, and choriocarcinoma.

Dermoid cysts are teratomatous cysts usually lined by epidermis and skin appendages. They often contain hair, and calcified bone or teeth can sometimes be seen on conventional pelvic x-ray. They are almost always curable by surgical resection. Approximately 1% of these tumors have malignant elements, usually squamous cell carcinoma.

Malignant germ cell tumors are usually large (median, 16 cm). Bilateral disease is rare except in dysgerminoma (10–15% bilaterality). Abdominal or pelvic pain in young women is the usual presenting symptom. Serum human chorionic gonadotropin (β-hCG) and α-fetoprotein levels are useful in the diagnosis and management of these patients. Before the advent of chemotherapy, extensive surgery was routine, but it has now been replaced by careful evaluation of extent of spread, followed by resection of bulky disease and preservation of one ovary, the uterus, and the cervix, if feasible. This allows many affected women to preserve fertility. After surgical staging, 60–75% of women have stage I disease and 25–30% have stage III disease. Stages II and IV are infrequent.

Most of the malignant germ cell tumors are managed with chemotherapy after surgery. Regimens similar to those used in testicular cancer, such as BEP (bleomycin, etoposide, and cisplatin), with three or four courses given at 21-day intervals, have produced 95% long-term survival in patients with disease stages I–III. This regimen is the treatment of choice for all malignant germ cell tumors except grade I, stage I immature teratoma, where surgery alone is adequate, and perhaps early-stage dysgerminoma, where surgery and radiation therapy are used.

Dysgerminoma is the ovarian counterpart of testicular seminoma. The tumor is very sensitive to radiation therapy. The 5-year disease-free survival is 100% in early-stage patients and 61% in stage III disease. Unfortunately, the use of radiation therapy makes many patients infertile. BEP chemotherapy is equally or more effective and does not cause infertility. In incompletely resected patients with dysgerminoma treated with BEP, the 2-year disease-free survival is 95% and infertility is not observed. Combination chemotherapy (BEP) has replaced postoperative radiation therapy as the treatment of choice in women with ovarian dysgerminoma.

OVARIAN STROMAL TUMORS

Stromal tumors make up <10% of ovarian tumors. They are named for the stromal tissue involved: granulosa, theca, Sertoli, Leydig, and collagen-producing stromal cells. The granulosa and theca cell stromal cell tumors occur most frequently in the first three decades of life. Granulosa cell tumors frequently produce estrogen and cause menstrual abnormalities, bleeding, and precocious puberty. Endometrial carcinoma can be seen in 5% of these women, perhaps related to the persistent hyperestrogenism. Sertoli and Leydig cell tumors, when functional, produce androgens with resultant virilization or hirsutism. Some 75% of these stromal cell tumors present in stage I and can be cured with total abdominal hysterectomy and bilateral salpingo-oophorectomy. Stromal tumors generally grow slowly, and recurrences can occur 5–10 years after initial surgery; serum markers such as estradiol, inhibin, and müllerian inhibitory substance may be useful in monitoring patients. Neither radiation therapy nor chemotherapy has been documented to be consistently effective, and surgical management remains the primary treatment.

Ovarian stromal and germ cell tumors are sometimes components of complex genetic syndromes. Peutz-Jeghers syndrome (mucocutaneous pigmentation and intestinal polyps) is associated with ovarian sex cord stromal tumors and Sertoli cell tumors in men. Patients with gonadal dysgenesis (46,XY genotype or mosaic for Y-containing cell lines) develop gonadoblastomas, and women with nevoid basal cell carcinomas have an increased risk of ovarian fibromas.

CARCINOMA OF THE FALLOPIAN TUBE

The fallopian tube is a very rare site of cancer in the female genital tract, although its epithelial surface far exceeds that of the ovary, where epithelial cancer is 20 times more common. Approximately 300 new cases occur yearly; 90% are papillary serous adenocarcinomas, with the remainder being mixed mesodermal, endometrioid, and transitional cell tumors. *BRCA1* and *-2* mutations are found in 16% of cases. The gross and microscopic characteristics and the spread of tumor are similar to those of ovarian cancer but can be distinguished if the tumor arises from the endosalpinx, where the tubal epithelium shows a transition between benign and malignant, and the ovaries and endometrium are normal or minimally involved. The differential diagnosis includes primary or metastatic ovarian cancer, chronic salpingitis, tuberculous salpingitis, salpingitis isthmica nodosa, and cautery artifact.

Unlike patients with ovarian cancer, patients often present with early symptoms, usually postmenopausal vaginal bleeding, pain, and leukorrhea. Surgical staging is similar to that used for ovarian cancer, and prognosis is related to stage and extent of residual disease. Patients with stages I and II disease are generally treated with surgery alone or with surgery and pelvic radiation therapy, although radiation therapy does not clearly improve 5-year survival (5-year survival, stage I: 74% vs. 75%; stage II: 43% vs. 48%). Patients with stages III and IV disease are treated with the same chemotherapy regimens used in advanced ovarian cancer; 5-year survival is similar (stage III, 20%; stage IV, 5%).

UTERINE CANCER

INCIDENCE AND EPIDEMIOLOGY

Carcinoma of the endometrium is the most common female pelvic malignancy. Approximately 39,080 new cases are diagnosed yearly, although in most (75%), tumor is confined to the uterine corpus at diagnosis, and therefore most can be cured. The 7400 deaths yearly make uterine cancer only the eighth leading cause of cancer death in females. It is primarily a disease of postmenopausal women, although 25% of cases occur in women ages <50 and 5% ages <40. The disease is common in Eastern Europe and the United States and uncommon in Asia.

Proliferation of the endometrium is under the control of estrogen, and prolonged exposure to unopposed estrogen from either endogenous or exogenous sources plays a central etiologic role. Risk factors for endometrial cancer include obesity, low fertility index, early menarche, late menopause, and chronic anovulation. Granulosa cell tumors of the ovary that secrete estrogen may present with synchronous endometrial cancers. Chronic unopposed estrogen replacement increases the risk, and women taking tamoxifen for breast cancer treatment or prevention have a twofold increased risk.

The Lynch syndrome occurs in families with an autosomal dominant mutation of mismatch repair genes *MLH1*, *MSH2*, *MSH6*, and *PMS2*, which predispose to nonpolyposis colon cancer as well as endometrial and ovarian cancer. The estimated lifetime risk for endometrial cancer is 40–60%, with a mean age around 50 years. Unlike colorectal cancer, endometrial cancer risk is not lower in *MSH6* mutation carriers. Most women present with stage I disease, and the survival rate is generally good (5-year survival 88%). No unique endometrial screening strategies have been established for Lynch family gene carriers.

CLINICAL PRESENTATION

Endometrial carcinoma occurs most often in the sixth and seventh decades of life. Symptoms often include abnormal vaginal discharge (90%), abnormal postmenopausal bleeding (80%), and leukorrhea (10%). The risk of endometrial cancer associated with postmenopausal bleeding increases with advancing age (9% at age 50 vs. 60% at age 80). Evaluation of such patients should include a history and physical with pelvic examination followed by an endometrial biopsy or a fractional dilation and curettage. Outpatient procedures such as endometrial biopsy or aspiration curettage can be used but are definitive only when positive.

PATHOLOGY

Between 75 and 80% of all endometrial carcinomas are adenocarcinomas, and the prognosis depends on stage, histologic grade, and extent of myometrial invasion. Grade I tumors are highly differentiated adenocarcinomas, grade II tumors contain some solid areas, and grade III tumors are largely solid or undifferentiated. Adenocarcinoma with squamous differentiation is seen in 10% of patients; the most differentiated form is known as *adenoacanthoma*, and the poorly differentiated form is called *adenosquamous carcinoma*. Other less common pathologies include mucinous carcinoma (5%) and papillary serous carcinoma (<10%). This latter type has a natural history similar to ovarian carcinoma and should be managed in the same way. Rarer histologies include secretory (2%), ciliated, clear cell, and undifferentiated carcinomas.

STAGING

The staging of endometrial cancer requires surgery to establish the extent of disease and the depth of myometrial invasion. A total abdominal hysterectomy and bilateral salpingo-oophorectomy should be performed and peritoneal fluid sampled. Frozen sections of the uterine specimen are used to determine the histology and grade and depth of invasion. If indicated, pelvic and para-aortic lymphadenectomy is performed. After evaluation and staging, ~75% of patients are stage I, 13% are stage II, 9% are stage III, and 3% are stage IV. Five-year survival declines with advancing stage: stage I, 89%; stage II, 73%; stage III, 52%; and stage IV, 17% (Table 14-1).

℞ Treatment: UTERINE CANCER

Patients with uncomplicated stage I endometrial carcinoma are effectively managed with total abdominal hysterectomy and bilateral salpingo-oophorectomy. Pre- or postoperative irradiation has been used, and although vaginal cuff recurrence is reduced, survival is not altered. In women with poor histologic grade, deep myometrial invasion, or extensive involvement of the lower uterine segment or cervix, intracavitary or external beam irradiation is warranted.

About 15% of women have endometrial carcinoma with extension to the cervix only (stage II), and management depends on the extent of cervical invasion. Superficial cervical invasion can be managed like stage I disease, but extensive cervical invasion requires radical hysterectomy or preoperative radiotherapy followed by extrafascial hysterectomy. Once disease is outside the uterus but still confined to the true pelvis (stage III), management generally includes surgery and irradiation. Patients who have involvement only of the ovary or fallopian tubes generally do well with such therapy (5-year survival of 80%). Other stage III patients with disease extending beyond the adnexa or those with serous carcinomas of the endometrium have a significantly poorer prognosis (5-year survival of 15%). Patients with positive para-aortic nodes (stage IIIC) or those with upper abdominal involvement (stage IV) have shown improved survival with platinum-based chemotherapy compared to whole-abdominal irradiation alone.

Patients with stage IV disease (outside the abdomen or invading the bladder or rectum) are treated palliatively with irradiation, surgery, and platinum-based chemotherapy. Progestational agents produce responses in ~10–20% of patients. Well-differentiated tumors respond most frequently, and response can be correlated with the level of progesterone receptor expression in the tumor. The commonly used progestational agents hydroxyprogesterone (Delalutin), megestrol (Megace), and deoxyprogesterone (Provera) all produce similar response rates, and the antiestrogen tamoxifen (Nolvadex) produces responses in 10–25% of patients in a salvage setting.

Chemotherapy is not very successful in advanced endometrial carcinoma. The most active single agents with consistent response rates of ≥20% include cisplatin, carboplatin, doxorubicin, epirubicin, and paclitaxel. Combinations of drugs with or without progestational agents have generally produced response rates similar to single agents.

CERVIX CANCER

INCIDENCE AND EPIDEMIOLOGY

Carcinoma of the cervix was once the most common cause of cancer death in women, but over the past 40 years, the mortality rate has decreased by 50% due to widespread screening with the Pap smear. In 2007, ~11,150 new cases of invasive cervix cancer occurred, and >50,000 cases of carcinoma in situ were detected. There were 3670 deaths from the disease, and of those patients, ~85% had never had a Pap smear. Worldwide, cervical cancer is the third commonest cancer diagnosed, and it remains the major gynecologic cancer in underdeveloped countries. It is more common in lower socioeconomic groups, in women with early initial sexual activity and/or multiple sexual partners, and in smokers.

ETIOLOGY AND GENETICS

Venereal transmission of human papilloma virus (HPV) has an important etiologic role. Over 66 types of HPVs have been isolated, and many are associated with genital warts. Those types commonly associated with cervical carcinoma are 16, 18, 31, 33, 52, and 58, but 70% of cases are caused by HPV-16 and -18. These, along with many other types, are also associated with cervical intraepithelial neoplasia (CIN). The protein product of HPV-16, the E7 protein, binds and inactivates the tumor-suppressor gene Rb, and the E6 protein of HPV-18 has sequence homology to the SV40 large T antigen and the capacity to bind and inactivate the tumor-suppressor gene p53. E6 and E7 are both necessary and sufficient to cause cell transformation in vitro. These binding and inactivation events may explain the carcinogenic effects of the viruses.

SCREENING AND PREVENTION

Vaccination against pathologic HPV appears to be an effective cervix cancer prevention strategy. Vaccines are made with inactivated virus-like particles that are noninfectious but highly immunogenic. The administration of a quadrivalent HPV vaccine against types 16, 18, 6, and 11 in a double-blind study of 2392 women completely prevented infection with the virus, and no cases of HPV-16–related CIN were seen in vaccinated women. This quadrivalent vaccine has been approved for use by the U.S. Food and Drug Administration (FDA) for patients 9–26 years old and must be administered before HPV exposure to be effective. A second study with a bivalent vaccine (types 16 and 18) is underway. Both vaccines appear highly effective in preventing their particular HPV infections, and protection has persisted for at least 4.5 years after three injections over a 6-month period. Since not all oncogenic HPVs are targeted, patients will need to continue Pap smear surveillance.

Uncomplicated HPV infection in the lower genital tract can progress to CIN. This lesion precedes invasive cervical carcinoma and is classified as low-grade squamous intraepithelial lesion (SIL), high-grade SIL, and carcinoma in situ. Carcinoma in situ demonstrates cytologic evidence of neoplasia without invasion through the basement membrane and can persist unchanged for 10–20 years, but most of these eventually progress to invasive carcinoma.

The Pap smear is 90–95% accurate in detecting early lesions such as CIN but is less sensitive in detecting cancer when frankly invasive cancer or fungating masses are present. Inflammation, necrosis, and hemorrhage may produce false-positive smears, and colposcopic-directed biopsy is required when any lesion is visible on the cervix, regardless of Pap smear findings. The American Cancer Society recommends that women after onset of sexual activity, or age >20, have two consecutive yearly smears. If negative, smears should be repeated every 3 years until age 65. The Pap smear can be reported as normal (includes benign, reactive, or reparative changes); atypical squamous cells of undetermined significance (ASCUS) or cannot exclude high-grade SIL (ASC-H); low- or high-grade CIN; or frankly malignant. Women with ASCUS, ASC-H, or low-grade CIN should have repeat smears in 3–6 months and be tested for HPV. Women with high-grade CIN or frankly malignant Pap smears should have colposcopic-directed cervical biopsy. Colposcopy is a technique using a binocular microscope and 3% acetic acid applied to the cervix in which abnormal areas appear white and can be biopsied directly. Cone biopsy is still required when endocervical tumor is suspected, colposcopy is inadequate, the biopsy shows microinvasive carcinoma, or a discrepancy is noted between the Pap smear and the colposcopic findings. Cone biopsy alone is therapeutic for CIN in many patients, although a less radical electrocautery excision may be sufficient.

Approximately 70% of invasive cervix cancers are squamous cell tumors, 20–25% are adenocarcinomas, and 2–5% are adenosquamous with epithelial and glandular structures.

CLINICAL PRESENTATION AND STAGING

Patients with cervix cancer generally are asymptomatic, and the disease is detected on routine pelvic examination. Others present with abnormal bleeding or postcoital spotting that may increase to intermenstrual or prominent menstrual bleeding. Yellowish vaginal discharge, lumbosacral back pain, lower extremity edema, and urinary symptoms may be present.

The staging of cervical carcinoma is clinical and generally completed with a pelvic examination under anesthesia with cystoscopy and proctoscopy. Chest x-rays, IV pyelograms, and CT are generally required, and MRI may be used to assess extracervical extension. Stage 0 is carcinoma in situ, stage I is disease confined to the cervix, stage II disease invades beyond the cervix but not to the pelvic wall or lower third of the vagina, stage III disease extends to the pelvic wall or lower third of the vagina or causes hydronephrosis, and stage IV is present when the tumor invades the mucosa of bladder or rectum or extends beyond the true pelvis (Fig. 14-1). Five-year survivals by stage are stage I, 85%; stage II, 65%; stage III, 35%; and stage IV, 7% (Table 14-1).

Rx Treatment: CERVIX CANCER

Carcinoma in situ (stage 0) can be managed successfully by cone biopsy or by abdominal hysterectomy. For stage I disease, results appear equivalent for either radical hysterectomy or radiation therapy. Patients with disease stages II–IV are primarily managed with external beam irradiation and intracavitary treatment or combined modality therapy. Retroperitoneal lymphadenectomy has no proven therapeutic role. Pelvic exenterations have become increasingly rare due to improved radiation control. However, they are sometimes performed for centrally recurrent or persistent disease.

In women with locally advanced disease (stages IIB–IVA), platinum-based chemotherapy given concomitantly with radiation therapy improves survival compared to radiation therapy alone. Cisplatin, 75 mg/m^2 over 4 h, followed by 5-fluorouracil (5-FU), 4 g given by 96-h infusion on days 1–5 of radiation therapy, is a common regimen. Two additional cycles of chemotherapy are given at

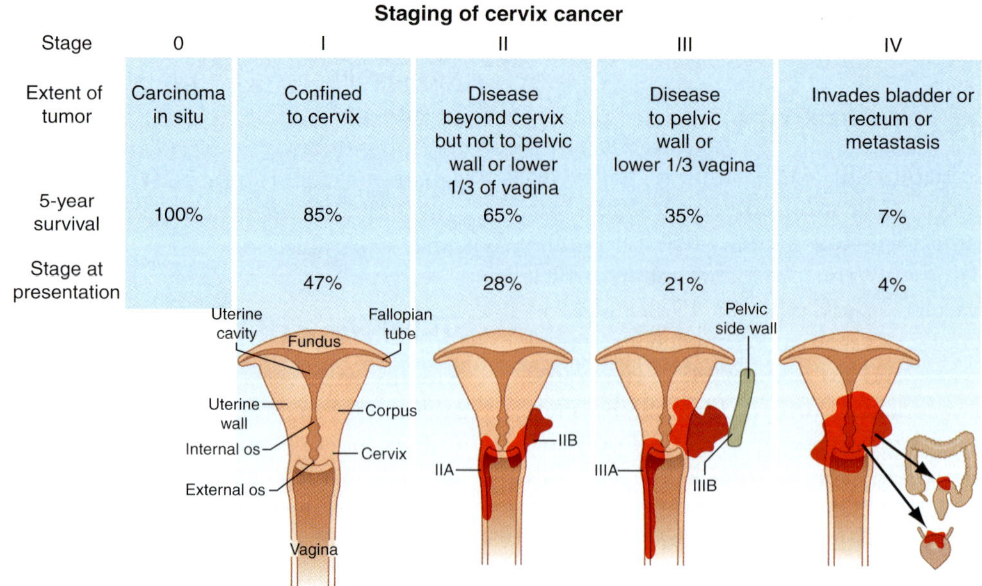

FIGURE 14-1

Anatomic display of the stages of cervix cancer defined by location, extent of tumor, frequency of presentation, and 5-year survival.

3-week intervals. Three randomized trials of platinum-based chemotherapy reduced the risk of recurrence by 30–50% across a wide spectrum of stages and presentations and were found to improve the survival rate in bulky stage I as well as locally advanced (stages IIB–IV) cervical cancer.

Chemotherapy has some palliative benefit in patients with unresectable advanced disease or recurrent disease. Active agents with ≥20% response rates include cisplatin, paclitaxel, vinorelbine, ifosfamide, and topotecan. The combination of topotecan and cisplatin has a modest survival advantage over cisplatin alone.

GESTATIONAL TROPHOBLASTIC NEOPLASIA

Gestational trophoblastic diseases are a group of related diseases that form a spectrum from benign hydatidiform mole to trophoblastic malignancy (placental-site trophoblastic tumor and choriocarcinoma). Malignant forms account for <1% of female gynecologic malignancies and can be cured with appropriate chemotherapy. Deaths from this disease have become rare in the United States.

EPIDEMIOLOGY

The incidence is about 1 per 1500 pregnancies in the United States and is nearly tenfold higher in Asia. Maternal age >45 years is a risk factor for hydatidiform mole as is a prior history of molar pregnancy. Choriocarcinoma occurs in ~1 in 25,000 pregnancies or 1 in 20,000 live births. Prior history of hydatidiform mole is a risk factor for choriocarcinoma. A woman with a previous molar pregnancy is 1000 times more likely to develop choriocarcinoma than a woman with a prior normal-term pregnancy.

PATHOLOGY AND ETIOLOGY

The trophoblastic neoplasms have been divided by morphology into complete or partial hydatidiform mole, invasive mole, placental-site trophoblastomas, and choriocarcinomas. Hydatidiform moles contain clusters of villi with hydropic changes, hyperplasia of the trophoblast, and the absence of fetal vessels. Invasive moles differ only by invasion into the uterine myometrium. Placental-site trophoblastic tumors are predominately made up of cytotrophoblast cells arising from the placental implantation site. Choriocarcinomas consist of anaplastic trophoblastic tissue with both cytotrophoblastic and syncytiotrophoblastic elements and no identifiable villi.

Complete moles result from uniparental disomy in which loss of the maternal genes (23 autosomes plus X) occurs by unknown mechanisms and is followed by duplication of the paternal haploid genome (23 autosomes plus X). Uncommonly (5%), moles result from dispermic fertilization of an empty egg, resulting in either 46,XY or 46,XX genotype. Partial moles result from dispermic fertilization of an egg with retention of the maternal haploid set of chromosomes, resulting in diandric triploidy.

CLINICAL PRESENTATION

Molar pregnancies are generally associated with first-trimester bleeding and excessive uterine size. About 45% of patients have ovarian theca lutein cysts present on ultrasound. The β-hCG levels are generally markedly elevated. Fetal parts and heart sounds are not present. The diagnosis is generally made by the passage of grapelike clusters from the uterus, but ultrasound demonstration of the hydropic mole can be diagnostic. Patients suspected of a molar pregnancy require a chest film, careful pelvic examinations, and weekly serial monitoring of β-hCG levels.

℞ Treatment: GESTATIONAL TROPHOBLASTIC NEOPLASIA

Patients with hydatidiform moles require suction curettage coupled with postevacuation monitoring of β-hCG levels. In most women (80%), the β-hCG titer progressively declines within 8–10 days of evacuation (serum half-life is 24–36 h). Patients should be monitored on a monthly basis and should not become pregnant for at least a year. Patients found to have invasive mole at curettage are generally treated with hysterectomy and chemotherapy. Approximately half of patients with choriocarcinoma develop the malignancy after a molar pregnancy, and the other half develop the malignancy after abortion, after ectopic pregnancy, or occasionally after a normal full-term pregnancy.

Chemotherapy is used for gestational trophoblastic neoplasia and often as chemoprophylaxis after molar evacuation to reduce postmolar tumors. It is also used in hydatidiform mole if β-hCG levels rise or plateau or if metastases develop. Patients with invasive mole or choriocarcinoma require chemotherapy. Several regimens are effective for low-risk patients, including methotrexate at 30 mg/m^2 IM on a weekly basis until β-hCG titers are normal. However, methotrexate (1 mg/kg) every other day for four doses, followed by leukovorin[D2] (0.1 mg/kg) IV 24 h after methotrexate, is associated with a cure rate of ≥90% and low toxicity. Intermittent courses are continued until the β-hCG titer becomes undetectable for 3 consecutive weeks, then patients are monitored monthly for a year.

Patients with high-risk tumors (high β-hCG levels, disease presenting ≥4 months after antecedent pregnancy, brain or liver metastasis, or failure of single-agent methotrexate) are initially treated with combination chemotherapy. EMA-CO (a cyclic non-cross-resistant combination of etoposide, methotrexate, and dactinomycin alternating with cyclophosphamide and vincristine); cisplatin, bleomycin, and vinblastine; and cisplatin, etoposide, and bleomycin are effective regimens. EMA-CO is now the regimen of choice for patients with high-risk disease because of excellent survival rates (>80%) and less toxicity. The use of etoposide carries a 1.5% lifetime risk of acute myeloid leukemia (sixteenfold relative risk) and other solid tumors. As a result, etoposide-containing regimens should be reserved for patients with high-risk features. Patients with brain or liver metastases are usually treated with local irradiation to metastatic sites in conjunction with chemotherapy. Long-term studies of patients cured of trophoblastic disease have not demonstrated an increased risk of maternal complications or fetal abnormalities with subsequent pregnancies.

FURTHER READINGS

Beral V et al: Ovarian cancer and oral contraceptives: Collaborative reanalysis of data from 45 epidemiological studies including 23,257 women with ovarian cancer and 87,303 controls. Lancet 371:303, 2008

Champion V et al: Quality of life in long-term survivors of ovarian germ cell tumors: A gynecologic oncology group study. Gynecol Oncol 105:687, 2007

Clarke-Pearson DL: Clinical practice. Screening for ovarian cancer. N Engl J Med 361:170, 2009

Koutsky LA: A controlled trial of a human papilloma virus type 16 vaccine. N Engl J Med 347:1645, 2002

Lindor NM et al: Recommendations for the care of individuals with an inherited predisposition to Lynch syndrome. JAMA 296:1507, 2006

Merritt WM et al: Dicer, Drosha, and outcomes in patients with ovarian cancer. N Engl J Med 359:2641, 2008

Modugno F: Ovarian Cancer and High Risk Women Symposium Presenters. Ovarian cancer and high-risk women: Implications for prevention, screening and early detection. Gynecol Oncol 91:15, 2003

Morch LS et al: Hormone therapy and ovarian cancer. JAMA 302:298, 2009

Ozols RF et al: Phase III study of cisplatin/paclitaxel compared with carboplatin/paclitaxel in patients with optimally resected stage III epithelial ovarian cancer. J Clin Oncol 21:3194, 2003

Randall ME et al: Randomized phase III trial of whole abdominal irradiation vs. doxorubicin and cisplatin chemotherapy in advanced endometrial carcinoma: A Gynecologic Oncology Group study. J Clin Oncol 24:36, 2006

Rose PG: Secondary surgical cytoreduction for advanced ovarian cancer. N Engl J Med 351:2489, 2004

Schiffman M et al: From India to the world—a better way to prevent cervical cancer. N Engl J Med 360:1453, 2009

Solomon D et al: The 2001 Bethesda System. JAMA 287:2114, 2002

Stehman FB et al: Innovations in the treatment of invasive cervical cancer. Cancer 98:2052, 2003

Trimbos JB: International Collaborative Neoplasm Trial I and Adjuvant Chemotherapy in Ovarian Neoplasm Trial: Two parallel randomized phase III trials of adjuvant chemotherapy in patients with early stage ovarian carcinoma. J Natl Cancer Inst 95:105, 2003

Wright JD, Mutch DG: Treatment of high-risk gestational trophoblastic tumors. Clin Obstet Gynecol 46:593, 2003

Young RC et al: Adjuvant therapy in stage I and stage II epithelial ovarian cancer. Results of two prospective trials. N Engl J Med 327:1021, 1990

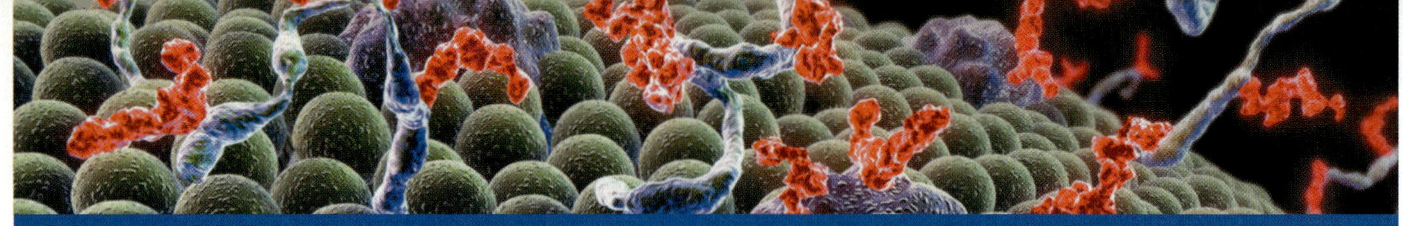

CHAPTER 15

SEXUAL DYSFUNCTION

Kevin T. McVary

Male sexual dysfunction affects 10–25% of middle-aged and elderly men. Female sexual dysfunction occurs with a similar frequency. Demographic changes, the popularity of newer treatments, and greater awareness of sexual dysfunction by patients and society have led to increased diagnosis and associated health care expenditures for the management of this common disorder. Because many patients are reluctant to initiate discussion of their sex lives, the physician should address this topic directly to elicit a history of sexual dysfunction.

MALE SEXUAL DYSFUNCTION

PHYSIOLOGY OF MALE SEXUAL RESPONSE

Normal male sexual function requires (1) an intact libido, (2) the ability to achieve and maintain penile erection, (3) ejaculation, and (4) detumescence. *Libido* refers to sexual desire and is influenced by a variety of visual, olfactory, tactile, auditory, imaginative, and hormonal stimuli. Sex steroids, particularly testosterone, act to increase libido. Libido can be diminished by hormonal or psychiatric disorders or by medications.

Penile tumescence leading to erection depends on the increased flow of blood into the lacunar network accompanied by the complete relaxation of the arteries and corporal smooth muscle. The microarchitecture of the corpora is composed of a mass of smooth muscle (trabecula), which contains a network of endothelial-lined vessels (lacunar spaces). Subsequent compression of the trabecular smooth muscle against the fibroelastic tunica albuginea causes a passive closure of the emissary veins and accumulation of blood in the corpora. In the presence of a full erection and a competent valve mechanism, the corpora become noncompressible cylinders from which blood does not escape.

The central nervous system (CNS) exerts an important influence by either stimulating or antagonizing spinal pathways that mediate erectile function and ejaculation. The erectile response is mediated by a combination of central (psychogenic) and peripheral (reflexogenic) innervation. Sensory nerves that originate from receptors in the penile skin and glans converge to form the dorsal nerve of the penis, which travels to the S2-S4 dorsal root ganglia via the pudendal nerve. Parasympathetic nerve fibers to the penis arise from neurons in the intermediolateral columns of S2-S4 sacral spinal segments. Sympathetic innervation originates from the T-11 to the L-2 spinal segments and descends through the hypogastric plexus.

Neural input to smooth-muscle tone is crucial to the initiation and maintenance of an erection. There is also an intricate interaction between the corporal smooth muscle cell and its overlying endothelial cell lining (**Fig. 15-1*A***). Nitric oxide, which induces vascular relaxation, promotes erection and is opposed by endothelin-1 (ET-1) and Rho kinase, which mediate vascular contraction. Nitric oxide is synthesized from L-arginine by nitric oxide

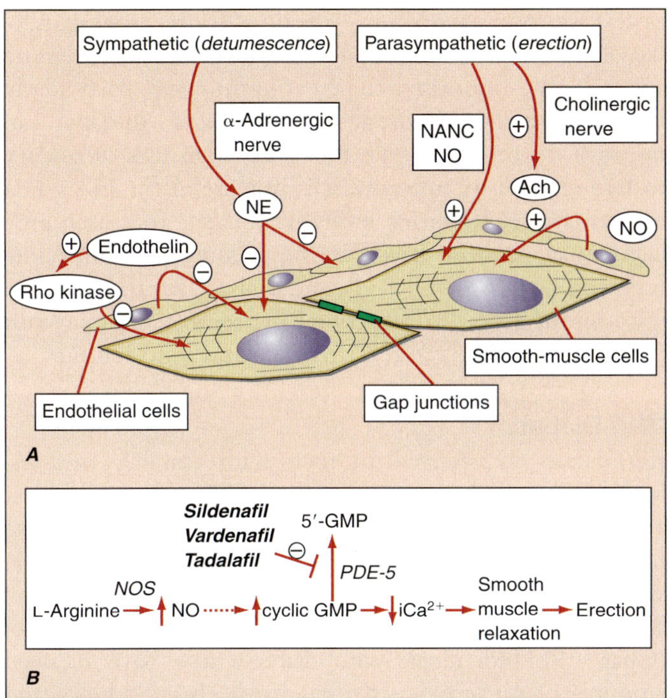

FIGURE 15-1

Pathways that control erection and detumescence. ***A.*** Erection is mediated by cholinergic parasympathetic pathways, and nonadrenergic, noncholinergic (NANC) pathways, which release nitric oxide (NO). Endothelial cells also release NO, which induces vascular smooth-muscle cell relaxation, allowing enhanced blood flow, and leading to erection. Detumescence is mediated by sympathetic pathways that release norepinephrine and stimulate α-adrenergic pathways, leading to contraction of vascular smooth-muscle cells. Endothelin, released from endothelial cells, also induces contraction. Rho kinase activation via endothelin activity (among others) also contributes to detumescence by alteration of calcium signaling. ***B.*** Biochemical pathways of NO synthesis and action. Sildenafil, vardenafil, and tadalafil enhance erectile function by inhibiting phosphodiesterase type 5 (PDE-5), thereby maintaining high levels of cyclic 3′,5′-guanosine monophosphate (cyclic GMP). NOS, nitric oxide synthase; iCa^{2+}, intracellular calcium.

synthase and is released from the nonadrenergic, noncholinergic (NANC) autonomic nerve supply to act postjunctionally on smooth-muscle cells. Nitric oxide increases the production of cyclic 3′,5′-guanosine monophosphate (cyclic GMP), which induces relaxation of the smooth muscle (Fig. 15-1*B*). Cyclic GMP is gradually broken down by phosphodiesterase type 5 (PDE-5). Inhibitors of PDE-5, such as the oral medications sildenafil, vardenafil, and tadalafil maintain erections by reducing the breakdown of cyclic GMP. However, if nitric oxide is not produced at some level, PDE-5 inhibitors are ineffective, as these drugs facilitate, but do not initiate, the initial enzyme cascade. In addition to nitric oxide, vasoactive prostaglandins (PGE_1, $PGF_2\alpha$) are synthesized within the cavernosal tissue and increase cyclic AMP levels, also leading to relaxation of cavernosal smooth-muscle cells.

Ejaculation is stimulated by the sympathetic nervous system, which results in contraction of the epididymis, vas deferens, seminal vesicles, and prostate, causing seminal fluid to enter the urethra. Seminal fluid emission is followed by rhythmic contractions of the bulbocavernosus and ischiocavernosus muscles, leading to ejaculation. *Premature ejaculation* is usually related to anxiety or a learned behavior and is amenable to behavioral therapy or treatment with medications such as selective serotonin reuptake inhibitors (SSRIs). *Retrograde ejaculation* results when the internal urethral sphincter does not close; it may occur in men with diabetes or after surgery involving the bladder neck.

Detumescence is mediated by norepinephrine from the sympathetic nerves, endothelin from the vascular surface, and smooth-muscle contraction induced by postsynaptic α-adrenergic receptors and activation of Rho kinase. These events increase venous outflow and restore the flaccid state. Venous leak can cause premature detumescence and is caused by insufficient relaxation of the corporal smooth muscle rather than a specific anatomic defect. *Priapism* refers to a persistent and painful erection and may be associated with sickle cell anemia, hypercoagulable states, spinal cord injury, or injection of vasodilator agents into the penis.

ERECTILE DYSFUNCTION

Epidemiology

Erectile dysfunction (ED) is not considered a normal part of the aging process. Nonetheless, it is associated with certain physiologic and psychological changes related to age. In the Massachusetts Male Aging Study (MMAS), a community-based survey of men between the ages of 40 and 70, 52% of responders reported some degree of ED. Complete ED occurred in 10% of respondents, moderate ED occurred in 25%, and minimal ED in 17%. The incidence of moderate or severe ED more than doubled between the ages of 40 and 70. In the National Health and Social Life Survey (NHSLS), which was a nationally representative sample of men and women ages 18–59, 10% of men reported being unable to maintain an erection (corresponding to the proportion of men in the MMAS reporting severe ED). Incidence was highest among men in the 50–59 age group (21%) and among men who were poor (14%), divorced (14%), and less educated (13%).

The incidence of ED is also higher among men with certain medical disorders such as diabetes mellitus, obesity, lower urinary tract symptoms secondary to benign prostatic hyperplasia (BPH), heart disease, hypertension, and decreased high-density lipoprotein (HDL) levels. Smoking is a significant risk factor in the development of ED. Medications used to treat diabetes or cardiovascular disease are additional risk factors. There is a higher incidence of ED among men who have undergone radiation or surgery for prostate cancer and in those with a lower spinal cord injury. Psychological causes of ED include depression, anger, or stress from unemployment or other causes.

Pathophysiology

ED may result from three basic mechanisms: (1) failure to initiate (psychogenic, endocrinologic, or neurogenic); (2) failure to fill (arteriogenic); or (3) failure to store adequate blood volume within the lacunar network (venoocclusive dysfunction). These categories are not mutually exclusive, and multiple factors contribute to ED in many patients. For example, diminished filling pressure can lead secondarily to venous leak. Psychogenic factors frequently coexist with other etiologic factors and should be considered in all cases. Diabetic, atherosclerotic, and drug-related causes account for >80% of cases of ED in older men.

Vasculogenic

The most frequent organic cause of ED is a disturbance of blood flow to and from the penis. Atherosclerotic or traumatic arterial disease can decrease flow to the lacunar spaces, resulting in decreased rigidity and an increased time to full erection. Excessive outflow through the veins, despite adequate inflow, may also contribute to ED. Structural alterations to the fibroelastic components of the corpora may cause a loss of compliance and an inability to compress the tunical veins. This condition may result from aging, increased cross-linking of collagen fibers induced by nonenzymatic glycosylation, hypoxia, or altered synthesis of collagen associated with hypercholesterolemia.

Neurogenic

Disorders that affect the sacral spinal cord or the autonomic fibers to the penis preclude nervous system relaxation of penile smooth muscle, thus leading to ED. In patients with spinal cord injury, the degree of ED depends on the completeness and level of the lesion. Patients with incomplete lesions or injuries to the upper part of the spinal cord are more likely to retain erectile capabilities than those with complete lesions or injuries to the lower part. Although 75% of patients with spinal cord injuries have some erectile capability, only 25% have erections sufficient for penetration. Other neurologic disorders commonly associated with ED include multiple sclerosis and peripheral neuropathy. The latter is often due to either diabetes or alcoholism. Pelvic surgery may cause ED through disruption of the autonomic nerve supply.

Endocrinologic

Androgens increase libido, but their exact role in erectile function remains unclear. Individuals with castrate levels of testosterone can achieve erections from visual or sexual stimuli. Nonetheless, normal levels of testosterone appear to be important for erectile function, particularly in older males. Androgen replacement therapy can improve depressed erectile function when it is secondary to hypogonadism; however, it is not useful for ED when endogenous testosterone levels are normal. Increased prolactin may decrease libido by suppressing gonadotropin-releasing hormone (GnRH), and it also leads to decreased testosterone levels. Treatment of hyperprolactinemia with dopamine agonists can restore libido and testosterone.

Diabetic

ED occurs in 35–75% of men with diabetes mellitus. Pathologic mechanisms are primarily related to diabetes-associated vascular and neurologic complications. Diabetic macrovascular complications are mainly related to age, whereas microvascular complications correlate with the duration of diabetes and the degree of glycemic control (Chap. 19). Individuals with diabetes also have reduced amounts of nitric oxide synthase in both endothelial and neural tissues.

Psychogenic

Two mechanisms contribute to the inhibition of erections in psychogenic ED. First, psychogenic stimuli to the sacral cord may inhibit reflexogenic responses, thereby blocking activation of vasodilator outflow to the penis. Second, excess sympathetic stimulation in an anxious man may increase penile smooth-muscle tone. The most common causes of psychogenic ED are performance anxiety, depression, relationship conflict, loss of attraction, sexual inhibition, conflicts over sexual preference, sexual abuse in childhood, and fear of pregnancy or sexually transmitted disease. Almost all patients with ED, even when it has a clear-cut organic basis, develop a psychogenic component as a reaction to ED.

Medication-Related

Medication-induced ED (Table 15-1) is estimated to occur in 25% of men seen in general medical outpatient clinics. Among the antihypertensive agents, the thiazide diuretics and beta blockers have been implicated most frequently. Calcium channel blockers and angiotensin-converting enzyme inhibitors are less frequently cited. These drugs may act directly at the corporal level (e.g., calcium channel blockers) or indirectly by reducing pelvic blood pressure, which is important in the development of penile rigidity. α-Adrenergic blockers are less likely to cause ED. Estrogens, GnRH agonists, H_2 antagonists, and spironolactone cause ED by suppressing gonadotropin production or by blocking androgen action. Antidepressant and antipsychotic agents—particularly neuroleptics, tricyclics, and SSRIs—are associated with erectile, ejaculatory, orgasmic, and sexual desire difficulties.

TABLE 15-1

DRUGS ASSOCIATED WITH ERECTILE DYSFUNCTION

CLASSIFICATION	DRUGS
Diuretics	Thiazides Spironolactone
Antihypertensives	Calcium channel blockers Methyldopa Clonidine Reserpine β Blockers Guanethidine
Cardiac/antihyperlipidemics	Digoxin Gemfibrozil Clofibrate
Antidepressants	Selective serotonin reuptake inhibitors Tricyclic antidepressants Lithium Monoamine oxidase inhibitors
Tranquilizers	Butyrophenones Phenothiazines
H_2 antagonists	Ranitidine Cimetidine
Hormones	Progesterone Estrogens Corticosteroids GnRH agonists 5α-Reductase inhibitors Cyproterone acetate
Cytotoxic agents	Cyclophosphamide Methotrexate Roferon-A
Anticholinergics	Disopyramide Anticonvulsants
Recreational	Ethanol Cocaine Marijuana

GnRH, gonadotropin-releasing hormone.

Although many medications can cause ED, patients frequently have concomitant risk factors that confound the clinical picture. If there is a strong association between the institution of a drug and the onset of ED, alternative medications should be considered. Otherwise, it is often practical to treat the ED without attempting multiple changes in medications, as it may be difficult to establish a causal role for the drug.

Approach to the Patient: ERECTILE DYSFUNCTION

A good physician-patient relationship helps to unravel the possible causes of ED, many of which require discussion of personal and sometimes embarrassing topics. For this reason, a primary care provider is often ideally suited to initiate the evaluation. A complete medical and sexual history should be taken in an effort to assess whether the cause of ED is organic, psychogenic, or multifactorial (Fig. 15-2). Initial questions should focus on the onset of symptoms, the presence and duration of partial erections, and the progression of ED. A history of nocturnal or early morning erections is useful for distinguishing physiologic from psychogenic ED. Nocturnal erections occur during rapid eye movement (REM) sleep and require intact neurologic and circulatory systems. Organic causes of ED are generally characterized by a gradual and persistent change in rigidity or the inability to sustain nocturnal, coital, or self-stimulated erections. The patient should be questioned about the presence of penile curvature or pain with coitus. It is also important to address libido, as decreased sexual drive and ED are sometimes the earliest signs of endocrine abnormalities (e.g., increased prolactin, decreased testosterone levels). It is useful to ask whether the problem is confined to coitus with one or other partners; ED arises not uncommonly in association with new or extramarital sexual relationships. Situational ED, as opposed to consistent ED, suggests psychogenic causes. Ejaculation is much less commonly affected than erection, but questions should be asked about whether ejaculation is normal, premature, delayed, or absent. Relevant risk factors should be identified, such as diabetes mellitus, coronary artery disease (CAD), or neurologic disorders. The patient's surgical history should be explored with

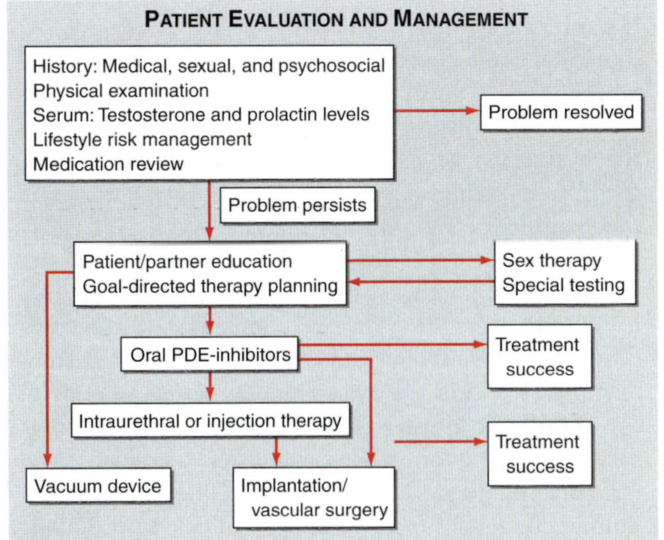

FIGURE 15-2

Algorithm for the evaluation and management of patients with ED.

an emphasis on bowel, bladder, prostate, or vascular procedures. A complete drug history is also important. Social changes that may precipitate ED are also crucial to the evaluation, including health worries, spousal death, divorce, relationship difficulties, and financial concerns.

Because ED commonly involves a host of endothelial cell risk factors, men with ED report higher rates of overt and silent myocardial infarction. As such, ED in an otherwise asymptomatic male warrants consideration of other vascular disorders including CAD.

The physical examination is an essential element in the assessment of ED. Signs of hypertension as well as evidence of thyroid, hepatic, hematologic, cardiovascular, or renal diseases should be sought. An assessment should be made of the endocrine and vascular systems, the external genitalia, and the prostate gland. The penis should be carefully palpated along the corpora to detect fibrotic plaques. Reduced testicular size and loss of secondary sexual characteristics are suggestive of hypogonadism. Neurologic examination should include assessment of anal sphincter tone and the bulbocavernosus reflex, and testing for peripheral neuropathy.

Although hyperprolactinemia is uncommon, a serum prolactin level should be measured, as decreased libido and/or erectile dysfunction may be the presenting symptoms of a prolactinoma or other mass lesions of the sella (Chap. 2). The serum testosterone level should be measured and, if low, gonadotropins should be measured to determine whether hypogonadism is primary (testicular) or secondary (hypothalamic-pituitary) in origin (Chap. 8). If not performed recently, serum chemistries, complete blood count (CBC), and lipid profiles may be of value, as they can yield evidence of anemia, diabetes, hyperlipidemia, or other systemic diseases associated with ED. Determination of serum prostate-specific antigen (PSA) should be conducted according to recommended clinical guidelines.

Additional diagnostic testing is rarely necessary in the evaluation of ED. However, in selected patients, specialized testing may provide insight into pathologic mechanisms of ED and aid in the selection of treatment options. Optional specialized testing includes (1) studies of nocturnal penile tumescence and rigidity; (2) vascular testing (in-office injection of vasoactive substances, penile Doppler ultrasound, penile angiography, dynamic infusion cavernosography/cavernosometry); (3) neurologic testing (biothesiometry-graded vibratory perception; somatosensory evoked potentials); and (4) psychological diagnostic tests. The information potentially gained from these procedures must be balanced against their invasiveness and cost.

℞ Treatment: MALE SEXUAL DYSFUNCTION

PATIENT EDUCATION Patient and partner education is essential in the treatment of ED. In goal-directed therapy, education facilitates understanding of the disease, results of the tests, and selection of treatment. Discussion of treatment options helps to clarify how treatment is best offered and stratify first- and second-line therapies. Patients with high-risk lifestyle issues, such as smoking, alcohol abuse, or recreational drug use, should be counseled on the role these factors play in the development of ED.

ORAL AGENTS Sildenafil, tadalafil, and vardenafil are the only approved and effective oral agents for the treatment of ED. These three medications have markedly improved the management of ED because they are effective for the treatment of a broad range of causes, including psychogenic, diabetic, vasculogenic, postradical prostatectomy (nerve-sparing procedures), and spinal cord injury. They belong to a class of medications that are selective and potent inhibitors of PDE-5, the predominant phosphodiesterase isoform found in the penis. They are administered in graduated doses and enhance erections after sexual stimulation. The onset of action is approximately 60–120 min, depending on the medication used and other factors such as recent food intake. Reduced initial doses should be considered for patients who are elderly, taking concomitant alpha blockers, have renal insufficiency, or are taking medications that inhibit the CYP3A4 metabolic pathway in the liver (e.g., erythromycin, cimetidine, ketoconazole, and, possibly, itraconazole and mibefradil), as they may increase the serum concentration of the PDE-5 inhibitors or promote hypotension. Testosterone supplementation combined with a PDE-5 inhibitor may be beneficial in improving erectile function in hypogonadal men with erectile dysfunction who are unresponsive to PDE-5 inhibitors alone. These drugs do not affect ejaculation, orgasm, or sexual drive. Side effects associated with PDE-5 inhibitors include headaches (19%), facial flushing (9%), dyspepsia (6%), and nasal congestion (4%). Approximately 7% of men using sildenafil may experience transient altered color vision (blue halo effect), while 6% of men taking tadalafil may experience loin pain. PDE-5 inhibitors are contraindicated in men receiving nitrate therapy for cardiovascular disease, including agents delivered by oral, sublingual, transnasal, or topical routes. These agents can potentiate its hypotensive effect and may result in profound shock. Likewise, amyl/butyl nitrate "poppers" may have a fatal synergistic effect on blood pressure. PDE-5 inhibitors should also be avoided in patients with congestive heart failure and cardiomyopathy because of the risk of vascular collapse.

Because sexual activity leads to an increase in physiologic expenditure [5–6 metabolic equivalents (METS)], physicians have been advised to exercise caution in prescribing any drug for sexual activity to those with active coronary disease, heart failure, borderline hypotension, or hypovolemia, and to those on complex antihypertensive regimens.

Although the PDE-5 inhibitors share a common mechanism of action, there are a few differences among the three agents. Having been on the market the longest, sildenafil has the most robust data confirming its activity, safety, and tolerability. It has recently been released for use in pulmonary hypertension as well as ED. Tadalafil is unique in its longer half-life. All three drugs are effective for patients with ED of all ages, severities, and etiologies. While there are pharmacokinetic and pharmacodynamic differences among these agents, clinically relevant differences are not clear.

ANDROGEN THERAPY Testosterone replacement is used to treat both primary and secondary causes of hypogonadism (Chap. 8). Androgen supplementation in the setting of normal testosterone is rarely efficacious and is discouraged. Methods of androgen replacement include transdermal patches and gels, parenteral administration of long-acting testosterone esters (enanthate and cypionate), and oral preparations (17α-alkylated derivatives) (Chap. 8). Transdermal delivery of testosterone using patches or gels (50–100 mg/d) more closely mimics physiologic testosterone levels, but it is unclear whether this translates into improved sexual function. The administration of 200–300 mg IM every 2–3 weeks provides another option but is far from an ideal physiologic replacement. Oral androgen preparations have the potential for hepatotoxicity and should be avoided. Testosterone therapy is contraindicated in men with androgen-sensitive cancers (e.g., prostate) and may be inappropriate for men with bladder neck obstruction. It is generally advisable to measure PSA before giving androgen. Hepatic function should be tested before and during testosterone therapy.

VACUUM CONSTRICTION DEVICES Vacuum constriction devices (VCDs) are a well-established, noninvasive therapy. They are a reasonable treatment alternative for select patients who cannot take sildenafil or do not desire other interventions. VCDs draw venous blood into the penis and use a constriction ring to restrict venous return and maintain tumescence. Adverse events with VCDs include pain, numbness, bruising, and altered ejaculation. Additionally, many patients complain that the devices are cumbersome and that the induced erections have a nonphysiologic appearance and feel.

INTRAURETHRAL ALPROSTADIL If a patient fails to respond to oral agents, a reasonable next choice is intraurethral or self-injection of vasoactive substances. Intraurethral prostaglandin E_1 (alprostadil), in the form of a semisolid pellet (doses of 125–1000 μg), is delivered with an applicator. Approximately 65% of men receiving intraurethral alprostadil respond with an erection when tested in the office, but only 50% of those achieve successful coitus at home. Intraurethral insertion is associated with a markedly reduced incidence of priapism in comparison to intracavernosal injection.

INTRACAVERNOSAL SELF-INJECTION Injection of synthetic formulations of alprostadil is effective in 70–80% of patients with ED, but discontinuation rates are high because of the invasive nature of administration. Doses range between 1 and 40 μg. Injection therapy is contraindicated in men with a history of hypersensitivity to the drug and in men at risk for priapism (hypercoagulable states, sickle cell disease). Side effects include local adverse events, prolonged erections, pain, and fibrosis with chronic use. Various combinations of alprostadil, phentolamine, and/or papaverine are sometimes used.

SURGERY A less frequently used form of therapy for ED involves the surgical implantation of a semirigid or inflatable penile prosthesis. These surgical treatments are invasive, associated with potential complications, and generally reserved for treatment of refractory ED. Despite their high cost and invasiveness, penile prostheses are associated with high rates of patient and partner satisfaction.

SEX THERAPY A course of sex therapy may be useful for addressing specific interpersonal factors that may affect sexual functioning. Sex therapy generally consists of in-session discussion and at-home exercises specific to the person and the relationship. It is preferable if therapy includes both partners, provided the patient is involved in an ongoing relationship.

FEMALE SEXUAL DYSFUNCTION

Female sexual dysfunction (FSD) has traditionally included disorders of desire, arousal, pain, and muted orgasm. The associated risk factors for FSD are similar to those in males: cardiovascular disease, endocrine disorders, hypertension, neurologic disorders, and smoking (Table 15-2).

EPIDEMIOLOGY

Epidemiologic data are limited, but the available estimates suggest that as many as 43% of women complain

TABLE 15-2

RISK FACTORS FOR FEMALE SEXUAL DYSFUNCTION
Neurologic disease: stroke, spinal cord injury, Parkinsonism
Trauma, genital surgery, radiation
Endocrinopathies: diabetes, hyperprolactinemia
Liver and/or renal failure
Cardiovascular disease
Psychological factors and interpersonal relationship disorders: sexual abuse, life stressors
Medications
Antiandrogens: cimetidine, spironolactone
Antidepressants, alcohol, hypnotics, sedatives
Antiestrogens or GnRH antagonists
Antihistamines, sympathomimetic amines
Antihypertensives: diuretics, calcium channel blockers
Alkylating agents
Anticholinergics

GnRH, gonadotropin-releasing hormone.

of at least one sexual problem. Despite the recent interest in organic causes of FSD, desire and arousal phase disorders (including lubrication complaints) remain the most common presenting problems when surveyed in a community-based population.

PHYSIOLOGY OF THE FEMALE SEXUAL RESPONSE

The female sexual response requires the presence of estrogens. A role for androgens is also likely but less well established. In the CNS, estrogens and androgens work synergistically to enhance sexual arousal and response. A number of studies report enhanced libido in women during preovulatory phases of the menstrual cycle, suggesting that hormones involved in the ovulatory surge (e.g., estrogens) increase desire.

Sexual motivation is heavily influenced by context, including the environment and partner factors. Once sufficient sexual desire is reached, sexual arousal is mediated by the central and autonomic nervous systems. Cerebral sympathetic outflow is thought to increase desire, while peripheral parasympathetic activity results in clitoral vasocongestion and vaginal secretion (lubrication).

The neurotransmitters for clitoral corporal engorgement are similar to those in the male, with a prominent role for neural, smooth muscle, and endothelial released nitric oxide (NO). A fine network of vaginal nerves and arterioles promote a vaginal transudate. The major transmitters of this complex vaginal response are not certain, but roles for NO and vasoactive intestinal polypeptide (VIP) are suspected. Investigators studying the normal female sexual response have challenged the long-held construct of a linear and unmitigated relationship between initial desire, arousal, vasocongestion, lubrication, and eventual orgasm. Caregivers should consider a paradigm of a positive emotional and physical outcome with one, many, or no orgasmic peak and release.

Although there are the obvious anatomic differences as well as variation in the density of vascular and neural beds in males and females, the primary effectors of sexual response are strikingly similar. Intact sensation is important for arousal. Thus, reduced levels of sexual functioning are more common in women with peripheral neuropathies (e.g., diabetes). Vaginal lubrication is a transudate of serum that results from the increased pelvic blood flow associated with arousal. Vascular insufficiency from a variety of causes may compromise adequate lubrication and result in dyspareunia. Cavernosal and arteriole smooth-muscle relaxation occurs via increased nitric oxide synthase (NOS) activity and produces engorgement in the clitoris and surrounding vestibule. Orgasm requires an intact sympathetic outflow tract; hence, orgasmic disorders are common in female patients with spinal cord injuries.

Approach to the Patient: FEMALE SEXUAL DYSFUNCTION

Many women do not volunteer information concerning their sexual response. Open-ended questions in a supportive atmosphere are helpful for initiating a discussion of sexual fitness in women who are reluctant to discuss such issues. Once a complaint has been voiced, a comprehensive evaluation should be performed, including a medical history, psychosocial history, physical examination, and limited laboratory testing.

The history should include the usual medical, surgical, obstetric, psychological, gynecologic, sexual, and social information. Past experiences, intimacy, knowledge, and partner availability should also be ascertained. Medical disorders that may impact sexual health should be delineated. These include diabetes, cardiovascular disease, gynecologic conditions, obstetric history, depression, anxiety disorders, and neurologic disease. Medications should be reviewed as they may impact arousal, libido, and orgasm. The need for counseling and life stresses should be identified. The physical examination should assess the genitalia, including clitoris. Pelvic floor examination may identify prolapse or other disorders. Laboratory studies are needed, especially if menopausal status is uncertain. Estradiol, follicle-stimulating hormone (FSH), and luteinizing hormone (LH) are usually obtained, and dehydroepiandrosterone (DHEA) should be considered as it reflects adrenal androgen secretion. A complete blood count, liver function assessment, and lipid studies may be useful, if not otherwise obtained. Complicated diagnostic evaluation, such as clitoral Doppler ultrasonography and biothesiometry, require expensive equipment and are of uncertain utility. It is important for the patient to identify which symptoms are most distressing.

The evaluation of FSD previously occurred mainly in a psychosocial context. However, inconsistencies between diagnostic categories based on only psychosocial considerations, and the emerging recognition of organic etiologies, have led to a new classification of FSD. This diagnostic scheme is based on four components that are not mutually exclusive: (1) *Hypoactive sexual desire*—the persistent or recurrent lack of sexual thoughts and/or receptivity to sexual activity, which causes personal distress. Hypoactive sexual desire may result from endocrine failure or may be associated with psychological or emotional disorders; (2) *Sexual arousal disorder*—the persistent or recurrent inability to attain or maintain sexual excitement, which causes personal distress; (3) *Orgasmic disorder*—the persistent or recurrent loss of orgasmic potential after sufficient sexual stimulation and arousal, which causes personal distress; (4) *Sexual pain disorder*—persistent or recurrent genital pain associated with noncoital sexual stimulation, which causes personal distress. This newer classification emphasizes "personal distress" as a requirement for dysfunction and provides clinicians with an organized framework for evaluation prior to or in conjunction with more traditional counseling methods.

℞ Treatment: FEMALE SEXUAL DYSFUNCTION

GENERAL An open discussion with the patient is important as couples may need to be educated about normal anatomy and physiologic responses, including role of orgasm in sexual encounters. Physiologic changes associated with aging and/or disease should be explained. Couples may need to be reminded that clitoral stimulation rather than coital intromission may be more beneficial.

Behavioral modification and nonpharmacologic therapies should be a first step. Patient and partner counseling may improve communication and relationship strains. Lifestyle changes involving known risk factors can be an important part of the treatment process. Emphasis on maximizing physical health and avoiding lifestyles (e.g., smoking, alcohol abuse) and medications likely to produce FSD is important (Table 15-2). The use of topical lubricants may address complaints of dyspareunia and dryness. Contributing medications, such as antidepressants, may need to be altered, including the use of medications with less impact on sexual function, dose reduction, medication switching, or drug holidays.

HORMONAL THERAPY In postmenopausal women, estrogen replacement therapy may be helpful in treating vaginal atrophy, decreasing coital pain, and improving clitoral sensitivity (Chap. 12). Estrogen replacement in the form of local cream is the preferred method, as it avoids systemic side effects. Androgen levels in women decline substantially before menopause. However, low levels of testosterone or DHEA are not effective predictors of a positive therapeutic outcome with androgen therapy. The widespread use of exogenous androgens is not supported by the literature except in select circumstances (premature ovarian failure or menopausal states) and in secondary arousal disorders.

ORAL AGENTS The efficacy of PDE-5 inhibitors in FDS has been a marked disappointment given the proposed role of nitric oxide–dependent physiology in the normal female sexual response. The use of PDE-5 inhibitors for FSD should be discouraged pending proof that it is effective.

CLITORAL VACUUM DEVICE In patients with arousal and orgasmic difficulties, the option of using a clitoral vacuum device may be explored. This handheld battery-operated device has a small soft plastic cup that applies a vacuum over the stimulated clitoris. This causes increased cavernosal blood flow, engorgement, and vaginal lubrication.

FURTHER READINGS

Araujo AB et al: Changes in sexual function in middle-aged and older men: Longitudinal data from the Massachusetts male aging study. J Am Geriatr Soc 52:1502, 2004

Basson R: Recent advances in women's sexual function and dysfunction. Menopause 11:714, 2004

Bhasin S et al: Sexual dysfunction in men and women with endocrine disorders. Lancet 369(9561):597, 2007

Burnett AL: Erectile dysfunction. J Urol 175:S25, 2006

Davis SR et al: Endocrine aspects of female sexual dysfunction. J Sex Med 1:82, 2004

Doggrell SA: Comparison of clinical trials with sildenafil, vardenafil, and tadalafil in erectile dysfunction. Expert Opin Pharmacother 6:75, 2005

Enzlin P et al: Sexual dysfunction in women with type 1 diabetes: Long-term findings from the DCCT/EDIC study cohort. Diabetes Care 32:780, 2009

Nurnberg HG et al: Sildenafil treatment of women with antidepressant-associated sexual dysfunction: A randomized controlled trial. JAMA 300:395, 2008

Pauls RN et al: Female sexual dysfunction: Principles of diagnosis and therapy. Obstet Gynecol Surv 60:196, 2005

Rees PM et al: Sexual function in men and women with neurological disorders. Lancet 369(9560):512, 2007

SECTION III

DIABETES MELLITUS, OBESITY, LIPOPROTEIN METABOLISM

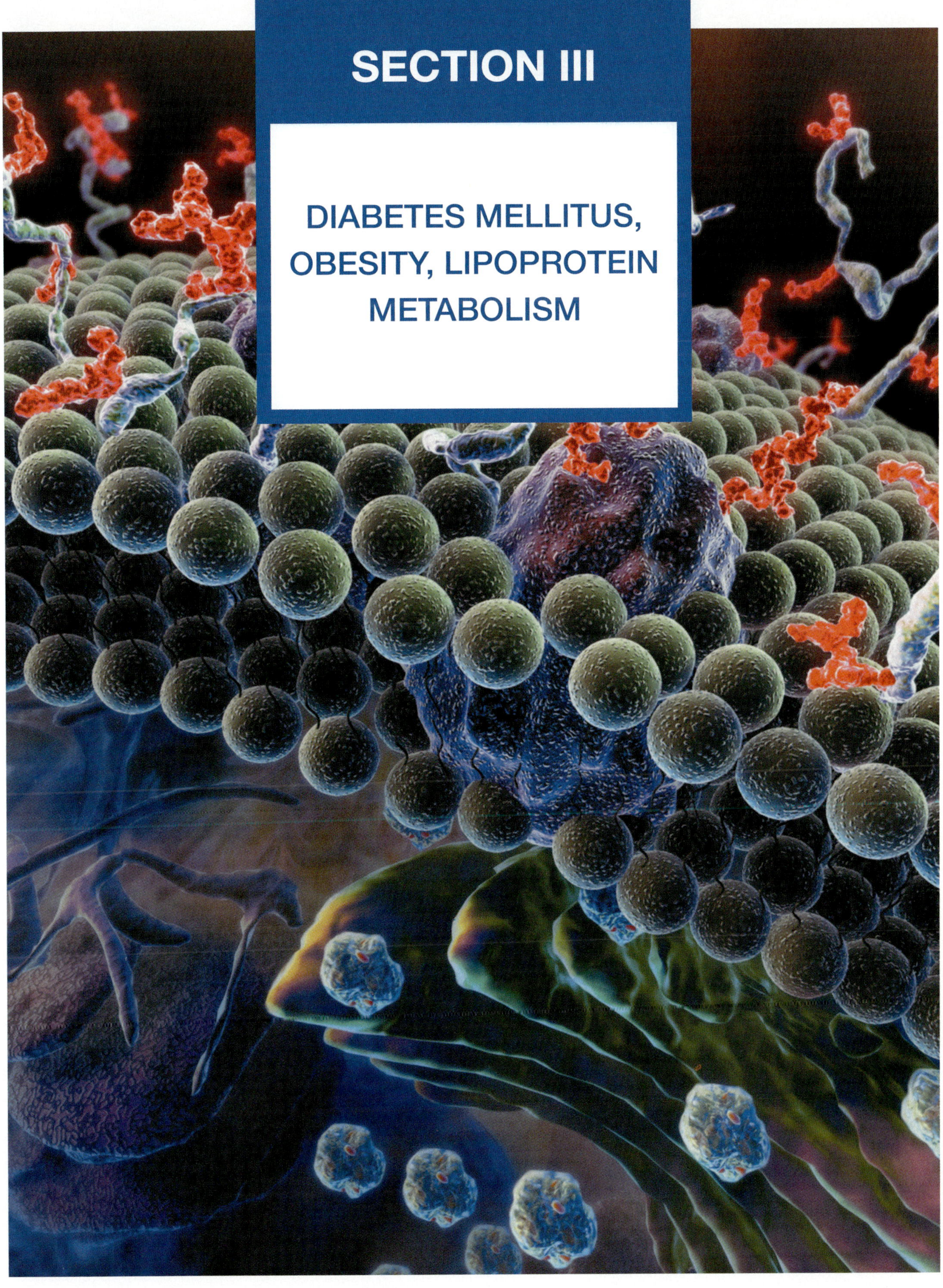

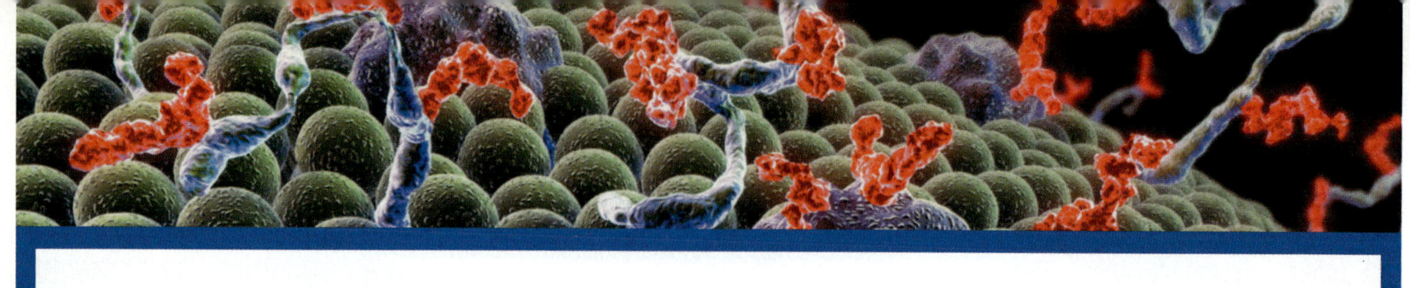

CHAPTER 16

BIOLOGY OF OBESITY

Jeffrey S. Flier ■ Eleftheria Maratos-Flier

In a world where food supplies are intermittent, the ability to store energy in excess of what is required for immediate use is essential for survival. Fat cells, residing within widely distributed adipose tissue depots, are adapted to store excess energy efficiently as triglyceride and, when needed, to release stored energy as free fatty acids for use at other sites. This physiologic system, orchestrated through endocrine and neural pathways, permits humans to survive starvation for as long as several months. However, in the presence of nutritional abundance and a sedentary lifestyle, and influenced importantly by genetic endowment, this system increases adipose energy stores and produces adverse health consequences.

DEFINITION AND MEASUREMENT

Obesity is a state of excess adipose tissue mass. Although often viewed as equivalent to increased body weight, this need not be the case—lean but very muscular individuals may be overweight by numerical standards without having increased adiposity. Body weights are distributed continuously in populations, so that choice of a medically meaningful distinction between lean and obese is somewhat arbitrary. Obesity is therefore more effectively defined by assessing its linkage to morbidity or mortality.

Although not a direct measure of adiposity, the most widely used method to gauge obesity is the *body mass index* (BMI), which is equal to weight/height^2 (in kg/m^2) (**Fig. 16-1**). Other approaches to quantifying obesity include anthropometry (skinfold thickness), densitometry (underwater weighing), CT or MRI, and electrical impedance. Using data from the Metropolitan Life Tables, BMIs for the midpoint of all heights and frames among both men and women range from 19–26 kg/m^2; at a similar BMI, women have more body fat than men. Based on data of substantial morbidity, a BMI of 30 is most commonly used as a threshold for obesity in both men and women. Large-scale epidemiologic studies suggest that all-cause, metabolic, cancer, and cardiovascular morbidity begin to rise (albeit at a slow rate) when BMIs are ≥25, suggesting that the cut-off for obesity should be lowered. Most authorities use the term *overweight* (rather than obese) to describe individuals with BMIs between 25 and 30. A BMI between 25 and 30 should be viewed as medically significant and worthy of therapeutic intervention, especially in the presence of risk factors that are influenced by adiposity, such as hypertension and glucose intolerance.

The distribution of adipose tissue in different anatomic depots also has substantial implications for morbidity. Specifically, intraabdominal and abdominal subcutaneous fat have more significance than subcutaneous fat present in the buttocks and lower extremities. This distinction is most easily made clinically by determining the waist-to-hip ratio, with a ratio >0.9 in women and >1.0 in men being abnormal. Many of the most important complications of obesity, such as insulin resistance, diabetes, hypertension, hyperlipidemia, and hyperandrogenism in women, are linked more strongly to intraabdominal and/or upper body fat than to overall adiposity (Chap. 18). The mechanism underlying this association

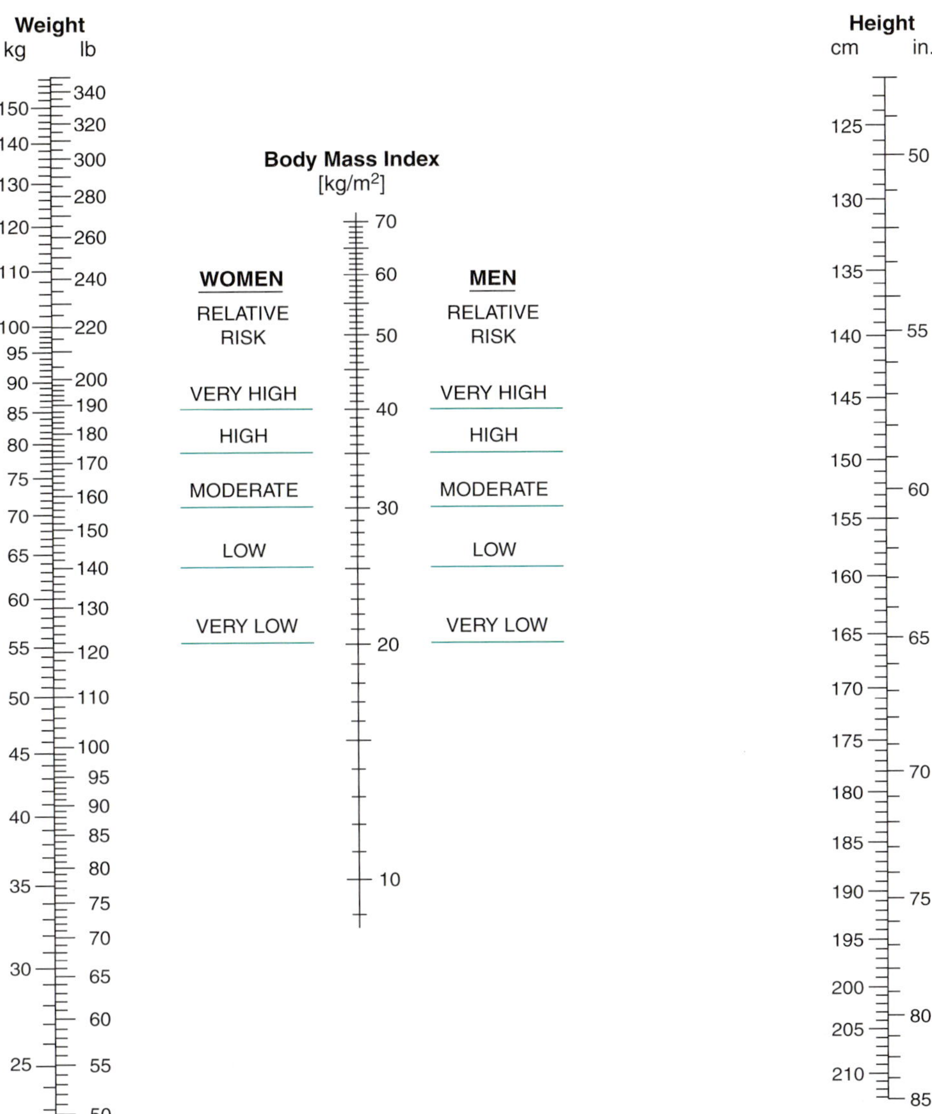

FIGURE 16-1

Nomogram for determining body mass index. To use this nomogram, place a ruler or other straight edge between the body weight (without clothes) in kilograms or pounds located on the left-hand line and the height (without shoes) in centimeters or inches located on the right-hand line. The body mass index is read from the middle of the scale and is in metric units. (*Copyright 1979, George A. Bray, M.D.; used with permission.*)

is unknown but may relate to the fact that intraabdominal adipocytes are more lipolytically active than those from other depots. Release of free fatty acids into the portal circulation has adverse metabolic actions, especially on the liver. Whether adipokines and cytokines secreted by visceral adipocytes play an additional role in systemic complications of obesity is an area of active investigation.

PREVALENCE

Data from the National Health and Nutrition Examination Surveys (NHANES) show that the percent of the American adult population with obesity (BMI >30) has increased from 14.5% (between 1976 and 1980) to 30.5% (between 1999 and 2000). As many as 64% of U.S. adults ≥20 years of age were overweight (defined as BMI >25) between the years of 1999 and 2000. Extreme obesity (BMI ≥40) has also increased and affects 4.7% of the population. The increasing prevalence of medically significant obesity raises great concern. Obesity is more common among women and in the poor; the prevalence in children is also rising at a worrisome rate.

PHYSIOLOGIC REGULATION OF ENERGY BALANCE

Substantial evidence suggests that body weight is regulated by both endocrine and neural components that ultimately influence the effector arms of energy intake and expenditure. This complex regulatory system is necessary because even small imbalances between energy intake and expenditure will ultimately have large effects on body weight. For example, a 0.3% positive imbalance over 30 years would result in a 9-kg (20-lb) weight gain. This exquisite regulation of energy balance cannot be monitored easily by calorie-counting in relation to physical activity. Rather, body weight regulation or dysregulation depends on a complex interplay of hormonal and neural signals. Alterations in stable weight by forced overfeeding or food deprivation induce physiologic changes that resist these perturbations: with weight loss, appetite increases and energy expenditure falls; with overfeeding, appetite falls and energy expenditure increases. This latter compensatory mechanism frequently fails, however, permitting obesity to develop when food is abundant and physical activity is limited. A major regulator of these adaptive responses is the adipocyte-derived hormone leptin, which acts through brain circuits (predominantly in the hypothalamus) to influence appetite, energy expenditure, and neuroendocrine function.

Appetite is influenced by many factors that are integrated by the brain, most importantly within the hypothalamus (**Fig. 16-2**). Signals that impinge on the hypothalamic center include neural afferents, hormones, and metabolites. Vagal inputs are particularly important, bringing information from viscera, such as gut distention. Hormonal signals include leptin, insulin, cortisol, and gut peptides. Among the latter are ghrelin, which is made in the stomach and stimulates feeding, and peptide YY (PYY) and cholecystokinin, which are made in the small intestine and signal to the brain through direct action on hypothalamic control centers and/or via the vagus nerve. Metabolites, including glucose, can influence appetite, as seen by the effect of hypoglycemia to induce hunger; however, glucose is not normally a major regulator of appetite. These diverse hormonal, metabolic, and neural signals act by influencing the expression and release of various hypothalamic peptides [e.g., neuropeptide Y (NPY), Agouti-related peptide (AgRP), α-melanocyte-stimulating hormone (α-MSH), and melanin-concentrating hormone (MCH)] that are integrated with serotonergic, catecholaminergic, endocannabinoid, and opioid signaling pathways. Psychological and cultural factors also play a role in the final expression of appetite. Apart from rare genetic syndromes involving leptin, its receptor, and the melanocortin system, specific defects in this complex appetite control network that influence common cases of obesity are not well defined.

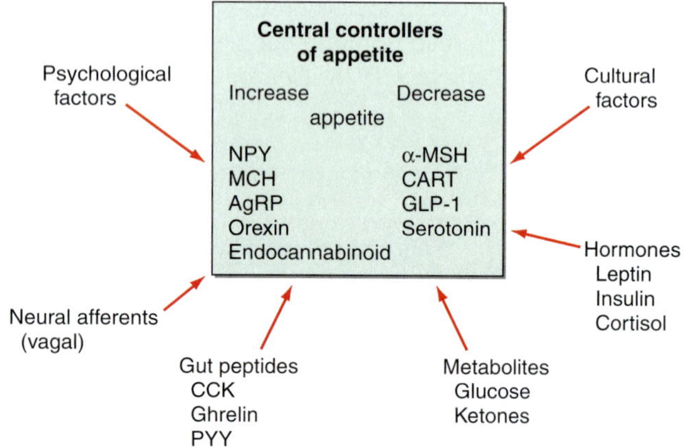

FIGURE 16-2

The factors that regulate appetite through effects on central neural circuits. Some factors that increase or decrease appetite are listed. NPY, neuropeptide Y; MCH, melanin-concentrating hormone; AgRP, Agouti-related peptide; MSH, melanocyte-stimulating hormone; CART, cocaine- and amphetamine-related transcript; GLP-1, glucagon-related peptide-1; CCK, cholecystokinin.

Energy expenditure includes the following components: (1) resting or basal metabolic rate; (2) the energy cost of metabolizing and storing food; (3) the thermic effect of exercise; and (4) adaptive thermogenesis, which varies in response to chronic caloric intake (rising with increased intake). Basal metabolic rate accounts for ~70% of daily energy expenditure, whereas active physical activity contributes 5–10%. Thus, a significant component of daily energy consumption is fixed.

Genetic models in mice indicate that mutations in certain genes (e.g., targeted deletion of the insulin receptor in adipose tissue) protect against obesity, apparently by increasing energy expenditure. Adaptive thermogenesis occurs in *brown adipose tissue* (BAT), which plays an important role in energy metabolism in many mammals. In contrast to white adipose tissue, which is used to store energy in the form of lipids, BAT expends stored energy as heat. A mitochondrial *uncoupling protein* (UCP-1) in BAT dissipates the hydrogen ion gradient in the oxidative respiration chain and releases energy as heat. The metabolic activity of BAT is increased by a central action of leptin, acting through the sympathetic nervous system, which heavily innervates this tissue. In rodents, BAT deficiency causes obesity and diabetes; stimulation of BAT with a specific adrenergic agonist (β_3 agonist) protects against diabetes and obesity. Although BAT exists in humans (especially neonates), its physiologic role is not yet established. Homologues of UCP-1 (UCP-2 and -3) may mediate uncoupled mitochondrial respiration in other tissues.

THE ADIPOCYTE AND ADIPOSE TISSUE

Adipose tissue is composed of the lipid-storing adipose cell and a stromal/vascular compartment in which cells including preadipocytes and macrophages reside. Adipose mass increases by enlargement of adipose cells through lipid deposition, as well as by an increase in the number of adipocytes. Obese adipose tissue is also characterized by increased numbers of infiltrating macrophages. The process by which adipose cells are derived from a mesenchymal preadipocyte involves an orchestrated series of differentiation steps mediated by a cascade of specific

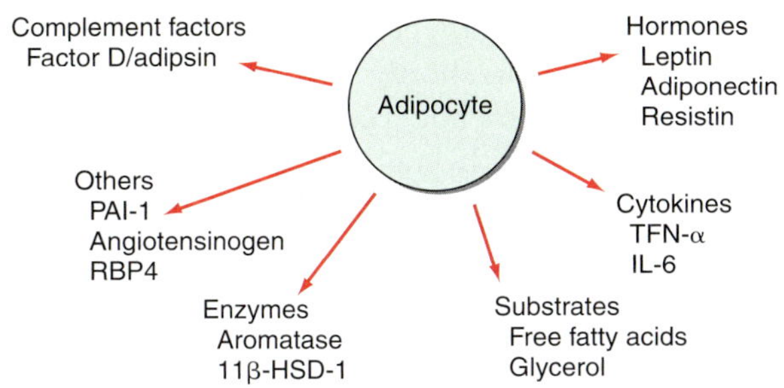

FIGURE 16-3

Factors released by the adipocyte that can affect peripheral tissues. PAI, plasminogen activator inhibitor; TNF, tumor necrosis factor; RBP4, retinal binding protein 4.

transcription factors. One of the key transcription factors is *peroxisome proliferator-activated receptor* γ (PPARγ), a nuclear receptor that binds the thiazolidinedione class of insulin-sensitizing drugs used in the treatment of type 2 diabetes (Chap. 19).

Although the adipocyte has generally been regarded as a storage depot for fat, it is also an endocrine cell that releases numerous molecules in a regulated fashion (Fig. 16-3). These include the energy balance–regulating hormone leptin, cytokines such as tumor necrosis factor (TNF) α and interleukin (IL) 6, complement factors such as factor D (also known as *adipsin*), prothrombotic agents such as plasminogen activator inhibitor I, and a component of the blood pressure–regulating system, angiotensinogen. Adiponectin, an abundant adipose-derived protein whose levels are reduced in obesity, enhances insulin sensitivity and lipid oxidation and it has vascular protective effects, whereas resistin and RBP4, whose levels are increased in obesity, may induce insulin resistance. These factors, and others not yet identified, play a role in the physiology of lipid homeostasis, insulin sensitivity, blood pressure control, coagulation, and vascular health, and are likely to contribute to obesity-related pathologies.

ETIOLOGY OF OBESITY

Though the molecular pathways regulating energy balance are beginning to be illuminated, the causes of obesity remain elusive. In part, this reflects the fact that obesity is a heterogeneous group of disorders. At one level, the pathophysiology of obesity seems simple: a chronic excess of nutrient intake relative to the level of energy expenditure. However, due to the complexity of the neuroendocrine and metabolic systems that regulate energy intake, storage, and expenditure, it has been difficult to quantitate all the relevant parameters (e.g., food intake and energy expenditure) over time in human subjects.

Role of Genes versus Environment

Obesity is commonly seen in families, and the heritability of body weight is similar to that for height. Inheritance is usually not Mendelian, however, and it is difficult to distinguish the role of genes and environmental factors. Adoptees more closely resemble their biologic than adoptive parents with respect to obesity, providing strong support for genetic influences. Likewise, identical twins have very similar BMIs whether reared together or apart, and their BMIs are much more strongly correlated than those of dizygotic twins. These genetic effects appear to relate to both energy intake and expenditure.

Whatever the role of genes, it is clear that the environment plays a key role in obesity, as evidenced by the fact that famine prevents obesity in even the most obesity-prone individual. In addition, the recent increase in the prevalence of obesity in the United States is far too rapid to be due to changes in the gene pool. Undoubtedly, genes influence the susceptibility to obesity in response to specific diets and availability of nutrition. Cultural factors are also important—these relate to both availability and composition of the diet and to changes in the level of physical activity. In industrial societies, obesity is more common among poor women, whereas in underdeveloped countries, wealthier women are more often obese. In children, obesity correlates to some degree with time spent watching television. Although the role of diet composition in obesity continues to generate controversy, it appears that high-fat diets may promote obesity, especially when combined with diets rich in simple (as opposed to complex) carbohydrates.

Additional environmental factors may contribute to the increasing obesity prevalence. Both epidemiologic correlations and experimental data suggest that sleep deprivation leads to increased obesity. Less well supported in humans are potential changes in gut flora with capacity to alter energy balance and a possible role for obesogenic viral infections.

Specific Genetic Syndromes

For many years obesity in rodents has been known to be caused by a number of distinct mutations distributed through the genome. Most of these single-gene mutations cause both hyperphagia and diminished energy expenditure, suggesting a physiologic link between these two parameters of energy homeostasis. Identification of the *ob* gene mutation in genetically obese (ob/ob) mice represented a major breakthrough in the field. The ob/ob mouse develops severe obesity, insulin resistance, and hyperphagia, as well as efficient metabolism (e.g., it gets fat even when ingesting the same number of calories as lean litter mates). The product of the *ob* gene is the peptide leptin, a name derived from the Greek root *leptos*, meaning "thin." Leptin is secreted by adipose cells and acts primarily through the hypothalamus. Its level of production provides an index of adipose energy stores (Fig. 16-4). High leptin levels decrease food intake and increase energy expenditure. Another mouse mutant, db/db, which is resistant to leptin, has a mutation in the leptin receptor and develops a

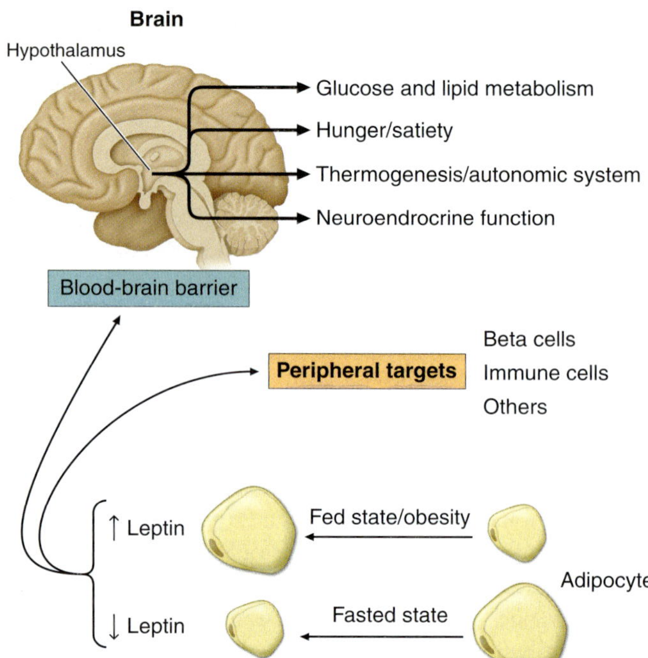

FIGURE 16-4

The physiologic system regulated by leptin. Rising or falling leptin levels act through the hypothalamus to influence appetite, energy expenditure, and neuroendocrine function and through peripheral sites to influence systems such as the immune system.

similar syndrome. The *OB* gene is present in humans and expressed in fat. Several families with morbid, early-onset obesity caused by inactivating mutations in either leptin or the leptin receptor have been described, thus demonstrating the biologic relevance of leptin in humans. The obesity in these individuals begins shortly after birth, is severe, and is accompanied by neuroendocrine abnormalities. The most prominent of these is hypogonadotropic hypogonadism, which is reversed by leptin replacement. Central hypothyroidism and growth retardation are seen in the mouse model, but their occurrence in leptin-deficient humans is less clear. To date, there is no evidence to suggest that mutations or polymorphisms in the leptin or leptin receptor genes play a prominent role in common forms of obesity.

Mutations in several other genes cause severe obesity in humans (Table 16–1); each of these syndromes is rare. Mutations in the gene encoding proopiomelanocortin (POMC) cause severe obesity through failure to synthesize α-MSH, a key neuropeptide that inhibits appetite in the hypothalamus. The absence of POMC also causes secondary adrenal insufficiency due to absence of adrenocorticotropic hormone (ACTH), as well as pale skin and red hair due to absence of α-MSH. Proenzyme convertase 1 (PC-1) mutations are thought to cause obesity by preventing synthesis of α-MSH from its precursor peptide, POMC. α-MSH binds to the type 4 melanocortin receptor (MC4R), a key hypothalamic receptor that inhibits eating. Heterozygous loss-of-function mutations of this receptor account for as much as 5% of severe obesity. These five genetic defects define a pathway through which leptin (by stimulating POMC and increasing α-MSH) restricts food intake and limits weight (Fig. 16–5).

In addition to these human obesity genes, studies in rodents reveal several other molecular candidates for hypothalamic mediators of human obesity or leanness. The *tub* gene encodes a hypothalamic peptide of unknown function;

TABLE 16-1

SOME OBESITY GENES IN HUMANS AND MICE

GENE	GENE PRODUCT	MECHANISM OF OBESITY	IN HUMAN	IN RODENT
Lep (*ob*)	Leptin, a fat-derived hormone	Mutation prevents leptin from delivering satiety signal; brain perceives starvation	Yes	Yes
LepR (*db*)	Leptin receptor	Same as above	Yes	Yes
POMC	Proopiomelanocortin, a precursor of several hormones and neuropeptides	Mutation prevents synthesis of melanocyte-stimulating hormone (MSH), a satiety signal	Yes	Yes
MC4R	Type 4 receptor for MSH	Mutation prevents reception of satiety signal from MSH	Yes	Yes
AgRP	Agouti-related peptide, a neuropeptide expressed in the hypothalamus	Overexpression inhibits signal through MC4R	No	Yes
PC-1	Prohormone convertase 1, a processing enzyme	Mutation prevents synthesis of neuropeptide, probably MSH	Yes	No
Fat	Carboxypeptidase E, a processing enzyme	Same as above	No	Yes
Tub	Tub, a hypothalamic protein of unknown function	Hypothalamic dysfunction	No	Yes
TrkB	TrkB, a neurotrophin receptor	Hyperphagia due to uncharacterized hypothalamic defect	Yes	Yes

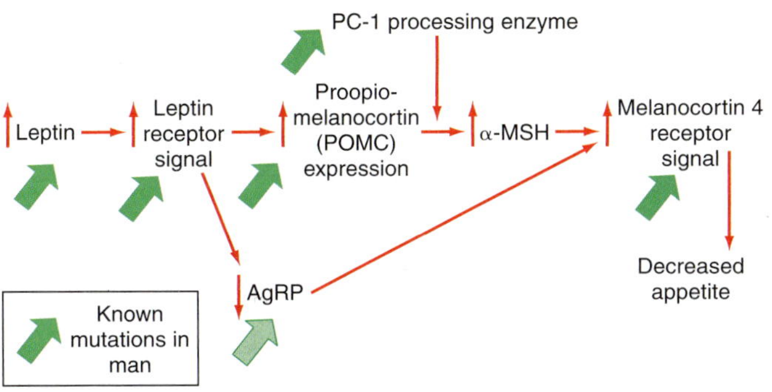

FIGURE 16-5

A central pathway through which leptin acts to regulate appetite and body weight. Leptin signals through proopiomelanocortin (POMC) neurons in the hypothalamus to induce increased production of α-melanocyte-stimulating hormone (α-MSH), requiring the processing enzyme PC-1 (proenzyme convertase 1). α-MSH acts as an agonist on melanocortin-4 receptors to inhibit appetite, and the neuropeptide AgRp (Agouti-related peptide) acts as an antagonist of this receptor. Mutations that cause obesity in humans are indicated by the solid green arrows.

mutation of this gene causes late-onset obesity. The *fat* gene encodes carboxypeptidase E, a peptide-processing enzyme; mutation of this gene is thought to cause obesity by disrupting production of one or more neuropeptides. AgRP is coexpressed with NPY in arcuate nucleus neurons. AgRP antagonizes α-MSH action at MC4 receptors, and its overexpression induces obesity. In contrast, a mouse deficient in the peptide MCH, whose administration causes feeding, is lean.

A number of complex human syndromes with defined inheritance are associated with obesity (Table 16-2). Although specific genes are undefined at present, their identification will likely enhance our understanding of more common forms of human obesity. In Prader-Willi syndrome, obesity coexists with short stature, mental retardation, hypogonadotropic hypogonadism, hypotonia, small hands and feet, fish-shaped mouth, and hyperphagia. Most patients have a chromosome 15 deletion, and reduced expression of the signaling protein necdin may be an important cause of defective hypothalamic neural development in this disorder. Bardet-Biedl syndrome (BBS) is a genetically heterogeneous disorder characterized by obesity, mental

TABLE 16-2

A COMPARISON OF SYNDROMES OF OBESITY—HYPOGONADISM AND MENTAL RETARDATION

	SYNDROME				
FEATURE	PRADER-WILLI	LAURENCE-MOON-BIEDL	AHLSTROM	COHEN	CARPENTER
Inheritance	Sporadic; two-thirds have defect	Autosomal recessive	Autosomal recessive	Probably autosomal recessive	Autosomal recessive
Stature	Short	Normal; infrequently short	Normal; infrequently short	Short or tall	Normal
Obesity	Generalized Moderate to severe Onset 1–3 years	Generalized Early onset, 1–2 years	Truncal Early onset, 2–5 years	Truncal Mid-childhood, age 5	Truncal, gluteal
Craniofacies	Narrow bifrontal diameter Almond-shaped eyes Strabismus V-shaped mouth High-arched palate	Not distinctive	Not distinctive	High nasal bridge Arched palate Open mouth Short philtrum	Acrocephaly Flat nasal bridge High-arched palate
Limbs	Small hands and feet Hypotonia	Polydactyly	No abnormalities	Hypotonia Narrow hands and feet	Polydactyly Syndactyly Genu valgum
Reproductive status	1°Hypogonadism	1°Hypogonadism	Hypogonadism in males but not in females	Normal gonadal function or hypogonadotrophic hypogonadism	2°Hypogonadism
Other features	Enamel hypoplasia Hyperphagia Temper tantrums Nasal speech			Dysplastic ears Delayed puberty	
Mental retardation	Mild to moderate		Normal intelligence	Mild	Slight

retardation, retinitis pigmentosa, renal and cardiac malformations, polydactyly, and hypogonadotropic hypogonadism. At least eight genetic loci have been identified, and BBS may involve defects in ciliary function.

Other Specific Syndromes Associated with Obesity

Cushing's Syndrome

Although obese patients commonly have central obesity, hypertension, and glucose intolerance, they lack other specific stigmata of Cushing's syndrome (Chap. 5). Nonetheless, a potential diagnosis of Cushing's syndrome is often entertained. Cortisol production and urinary metabolites (17OH steroids) may be increased in simple obesity. Unlike in Cushing's syndrome, however, cortisol levels in blood and urine in the basal state and in response to corticotropin-releasing hormone (CRH) or ACTH are normal; the overnight 1-mg dexamethasone suppression test is normal in 90%, with the remainder being normal on a standard 2-day low-dose dexamethasone suppression test. Obesity may be associated with excessive local reactivation of cortisol in fat by 11β-hydroxysteroid dehydrogenase 1, an enzyme that converts inactive cortisone to cortisol.

Hypothyroidism

The possibility of hypothyroidism should be considered, but it is an uncommon cause of obesity; hypothyroidism is easily ruled out by measuring thyroid-stimulating hormone (TSH). Much of the weight gain that occurs in hypothyroidism is due to myxedema (Chap. 4).

Insulinoma

Patients with insulinoma often gain weight as a result of overeating to avoid hypoglycemic symptoms (Chap. 20). The increased substrate plus high insulin levels promote energy storage in fat. This can be marked in some individuals but is modest in most.

Craniopharyngioma and Other Disorders Involving the Hypothalamus

Whether through tumors, trauma, or inflammation, hypothalamic dysfunction of systems controlling satiety, hunger, and energy expenditure can cause varying degrees of obesity (Chap. 2). It is uncommon to identify a discrete anatomic basis for these disorders. Subtle hypothalamic dysfunction is probably a more common cause of obesity that can be documented using currently available imaging techniques. Growth hormone (GH), which exerts lipolytic activity, is diminished in obesity and is increased with weight loss. Despite low GH levels, insulin-like growth factor (IGF) I (somatomedin) production is normal, suggesting that GH suppression is a compensatory response to increased nutritional supply.

Pathogenesis of Common Obesity

Obesity can result from increased energy intake, decreased energy expenditure, or a combination of the two. Thus, identifying the etiology of obesity should involve measurements of both parameters. However, it is nearly impossible to perform direct and accurate measurements of energy intake in free-living individuals, and the obese, in particular, often underreport intake. Measurements of chronic energy expenditure have only recently become available using doubly labeled water or metabolic chamber rooms. In subjects at stable weight and body composition, energy intake equals expenditure. Consequently, these techniques allow assessment of energy intake in free-living individuals. The level of energy expenditure differs in established obesity, during periods of weight gain or loss, and in the pre- or postobese state. Studies that fail to take note of this phenomenon are not easily interpreted.

There is continued interest in the concept of a body weight "set point." This idea is supported by physiologic mechanisms centered around a sensing system in adipose tissue that reflects fat stores and a receptor, or "adipostat," that is in the hypothalamic centers. When fat stores are depleted, the adipostat signal is low, and the hypothalamus responds by stimulating hunger and decreasing energy expenditure to conserve energy. Conversely, when fat stores are abundant, the signal is increased, and the hypothalamus responds by decreasing hunger and increasing energy expenditure. The recent discovery of the *ob* gene, and its product leptin, and the *db* gene, whose product is the leptin receptor, provides important elements of a molecular basis for this physiologic concept.

What Is the Status of Food Intake in Obesity? (Do the Obese Eat More Than the Lean?)

This question has stimulated much debate, due in part to the methodologic difficulties inherent in determining food intake. Many obese individuals believe that they eat small quantities of food, and this claim has often been supported by the results of food intake questionnaires. However, it is now established that average energy expenditure increases as individuals get more obese, due primarily to the fact that metabolically active lean tissue mass increases with obesity. Given the laws of thermodynamics, the obese person must therefore eat more than the average lean person to maintain their increased weight. It may be the case, however, that a subset of individuals who are predisposed to obesity have the capacity to become obese initially without an absolute increase in caloric consumption.

What Is the State of Energy Expenditure in Obesity?

The average total daily energy expenditure is higher in obese than lean individuals when measured at stable weight. However, energy expenditure falls as weight is lost, due in part to loss of lean body mass and to decreased sympathetic nerve activity. When reduced to near-normal weight and maintained there for a while, (some) obese individuals have lower energy expenditure than (some) lean individuals. There is also a tendency for those who will develop obesity as infants or children to have lower resting energy expenditure rates than those who remain lean.

The physiologic basis for variable rates of energy expenditure (at a given body weight and level of energy intake) is essentially unknown. A mutation in the human β_3-adrenergic receptor may be associated with increased risk of obesity and/or insulin resistance in certain (but not all) populations. Homologues of the BAT uncoupling protein, named UCP-2 and UCP-3, have been identified in both rodents and humans. UCP-2 is expressed widely, whereas UCP-3 is primarily expressed in skeletal muscle. These proteins may play a role in disordered energy balance.

One newly described component of thermogenesis, called *nonexercise activity thermogenesis* (NEAT), has been linked to obesity. It is the thermogenesis that accompanies physical activities other than volitional exercise, such as the activities of daily living, fidgeting, spontaneous muscle contraction, and maintaining posture. NEAT accounts for about two-thirds of the increased daily energy expenditure induced by overfeeding. The wide variation in fat storage seen in overfed individuals is predicted by the degree to which NEAT is induced. The molecular basis for NEAT and its regulation is unknown.

Leptin in Typical Obesity

The vast majority of obese persons have increased leptin levels but do not have mutations of either leptin or its receptor. They appear, therefore, to have a form of functional "leptin resistance." Data suggesting that some individuals produce less leptin per unit fat mass than others or have a form of relative leptin deficiency that predisposes to obesity are at present contradictory and unsettled. The mechanism for leptin resistance, and whether it can be overcome by raising leptin levels, is not yet established. Some data suggest that leptin may not effectively cross the blood-brain barrier as levels rise. It is also apparent from animal studies that leptin signaling inhibitors, such as SOCS3 and PTP1b, are involved in the leptin-resistant state.

PATHOLOGIC CONSEQUENCES OF OBESITY

(See also Chap. 17) Obesity has major adverse effects on health. Obesity is associated with an increase in mortality, with a 50–100% increased risk of death from all causes compared to normal-weight individuals, mostly due to cardiovascular causes. Obesity and overweight together are the second leading cause of preventable death in the United States, accounting for 300,000 deaths per year. Mortality rates rise as obesity increases, particularly when obesity is associated with increased intraabdominal fat. Life expectancy of a moderately obese individual could be shortened by 2–5 years, and a 20- to 30-year-old male with a BMI >45 may lose 13 years of life. It is also apparent that the degree to which obesity affects particular organ systems is influenced by susceptibility genes that vary in the population.

Insulin Resistance and Type 2 Diabetes Mellitus

Hyperinsulinemia and insulin resistance are pervasive features of obesity, increasing with weight gain and diminishing with weight loss (Chap. 18). Insulin resistance is more strongly linked to intraabdominal fat than to fat in other depots. The molecular link between obesity and insulin resistance in tissues such as fat, muscle, and liver has been sought for many years. Major factors under investigation include (1) insulin itself, by inducing receptor downregulation; (2) free fatty acids, known to be increased and capable of impairing insulin action; (3) intracellular lipid accumulation; and (4) various circulating peptides produced by adipocytes, including the cytokines TNF-α and IL-6, RBP4, and the "adipokines" adiponectin and resistin, which are produced by adipocytes, have altered expression in obese adipocytes, and are capable of modifying insulin action. Despite nearly universal insulin resistance, most obese individuals do not develop diabetes, suggesting that the onset of diabetes requires an interaction between obesity-induced insulin resistance and other factors that predispose to diabetes, such as impaired insulin secretion (Chap. 19). Obesity, however, is a major risk factor for diabetes, and as many as 80% of patients with type 2 diabetes mellitus are obese. Weight loss and exercise, even of modest degree, are associated with increased insulin sensitivity and often improve glucose control in diabetes.

Reproductive Disorders

Disorders that affect the reproductive axis are associated with obesity in both men and women. Male hypogonadism is associated with increased adipose tissue, often distributed in a pattern more typical of females. In men >160% ideal body weight, plasma testosterone and sex hormone–binding globulin (SHBG) are often reduced, and estrogen levels (derived from conversion of adrenal androgens in adipose tissue) are increased (Chap. 8). Gynecomastia may be seen. However, masculinization, libido, potency, and spermatogenesis are preserved in most of these individuals. Free testosterone may be decreased in morbidly obese men whose weight is >200% ideal body weight.

Obesity has long been associated with menstrual abnormalities in women, particularly in women with upper body obesity (Chap. 10). Common findings are increased androgen production, decreased SHBG, and increased peripheral conversion of androgen to estrogen. Most obese women with oligomenorrhea have the polycystic ovarian syndrome (PCOS), with its associated anovulation and ovarian hyperandrogenism; 40% of women with PCOS are obese. Most nonobese women with PCOS are also insulin-resistant, suggesting that insulin resistance, hyperinsulinemia, or the combination of the two are causative or contribute to the ovarian pathophysiology in PCOS in both obese and lean individuals. In obese women with PCOS, weight loss or treatment with insulin-sensitizing drugs often restores normal menses. The increased conversion of androstenedione to estrogen, which occurs to a greater degree in women with lower body obesity, may contribute to the increased incidence of uterine cancer in postmenopausal women with obesity.

Cardiovascular Disease

The Framingham Study revealed that obesity was an independent risk factor for the 26-year incidence of cardiovascular disease in men and women [including coronary disease, stroke, and congestive heart failure (CHF)]. The waist/hip ratio may be the best predictor of these risks. When the additional effects of hypertension and glucose intolerance associated with obesity are included, the adverse impact of obesity is even more evident. The effect of obesity on cardiovascular mortality in women may be seen at BMIs as low as 25. Obesity, especially abdominal obesity, is associated with an atherogenic lipid profile; with increased low-density lipoprotein (LDL) cholesterol, very low density lipoprotein, and triglyceride; and with decreased high-density lipoprotein cholesterol and decreased levels of the vascular protective adipokine adiponectin (Chap. 21). Obesity is also associated with hypertension. Measurement of blood pressure in the obese requires use of a larger cuff size to avoid artifactual increases. Obesity-induced hypertension is associated with increased peripheral resistance and cardiac output, increased sympathetic nervous system tone, increased salt sensitivity, and insulin-mediated salt retention; it is often responsive to modest weight loss.

Pulmonary Disease

Obesity may be associated with a number of pulmonary abnormalities. These include reduced chest wall compliance, increased work of breathing, increased minute ventilation due to increased metabolic rate, and decreased functional residual capacity and expiratory reserve volume. Severe obesity may be associated with obstructive sleep apnea and the "obesity hypoventilation syndrome" with attenuated hypoxic and hypercapnic ventilatory responses. Sleep apnea can be obstructive (most common), central, or mixed and is associated with hypertension. Weight loss (10–20 kg) can bring substantial improvement, as can major weight loss following gastric bypass or restrictive surgery. Continuous positive airway pressure has been used with some success.

Gallstones

Obesity is associated with enhanced biliary secretion of cholesterol, supersaturation of bile, and a higher incidence of gallstones, particularly cholesterol gallstones. A person 50% above ideal body weight has about a sixfold increased incidence of symptomatic gallstones. Paradoxically, fasting increases supersaturation of bile by decreasing the phospholipid component. Fasting-induced cholecystitis is a complication of extreme diets.

Cancer

Obesity in males is associated with higher mortality from cancer, including cancer of the esophagus, colon, rectum, pancreas, liver, and prostate; obesity in females is associated with higher mortality from cancer of the gallbladder, bile ducts, breasts, endometrium, cervix, and ovaries. Some of the latter may be due to increased rates of conversion of androstenedione to estrone in adipose tissue of obese individuals. It was recently estimated that obesity accounts for 14% of cancer deaths in men and 20% in women in the United States.

Bone, Joint, and Cutaneous Disease

Obesity is associated with an increased risk of osteoarthritis, no doubt partly due to the trauma of added weight bearing and joint malalignment. The prevalence of gout may also be increased. Among the skin problems associated with obesity is acanthosis nigricans, manifested by darkening and thickening of the skin folds on the neck, elbows, and dorsal interphalangeal spaces. Acanthosis reflects the severity of underlying insulin resistance and diminishes with weight loss. Friability of skin may be increased, especially in skinfolds, enhancing the risk of fungal and yeast infections. Finally, venous stasis is increased in the obese.

FURTHER READINGS

Cecil JE et al: An obesity-associated FTO gene variant and increased energy intake in children. N Engl J Med 359:2558, 2008

Farooqi IS, O'Rahilly S: Genetics of obesity. Philos Trans R Soc Lond B Biol Sci 361:1095, 2006

Flier JS: Obesity wars: Molecular progress confronts an expanding epidemic. Cell 116:337, 2004

Morton GJ et al: Central nervous system control of food intake and body weight. Nature 443:289, 2006

Murphy KG et al: Gut peptides in the regulation of food intake and energy homeostasis. Endocr Rev 27:719, 2006

Ogden CL et al: The epidemiology of obesity. Gastroenterology 132(6):2087, 2007

Ogden CL et al: Prevalence of overweight and obesity in the United States, 1999–2004. JAMA 295:1549, 2006

Zobel DP et al: Variants near MC4R are associated with obesity and influence obesity-related quantitative traits in a population of middle-aged people: Studies of 14,940 Danes. Diabetes 58:757, 2009

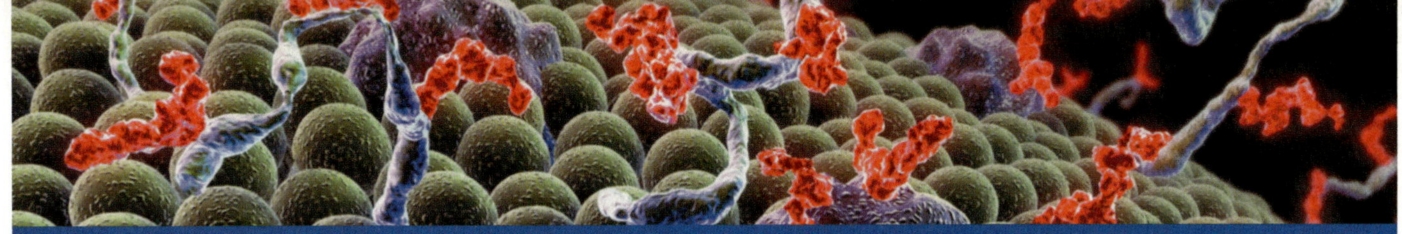

CHAPTER 17

EVALUATION AND MANAGEMENT OF OBESITY

Robert F. Kushner

Over 66% of U.S. adults are currently categorized as overweight or obese, and the prevalence of obesity is increasing rapidly throughout most of the industrialized world. Based on statistics from the World Health Organization, overweight and obesity may soon replace more traditional public health concerns such as undernutrition and infectious diseases as the most significant contributors to ill health. Children and adolescents are also becoming more obese, indicating that the current trends will accelerate over time. Obesity is associated with an increased risk of multiple health problems, including hypertension, type 2 diabetes, dyslipidemia, degenerative joint disease, and some malignancies. Thus, it is important for physicians to routinely identify, evaluate, and treat patients for obesity and associated comorbid conditions.

EVALUATION

The U.S. Preventive Services Task Force recommends that physicians screen all adult patients for obesity and offer intensive counseling and behavioral interventions to promote sustained weight loss. This recommendation is consistent with previously released guidelines from the National Heart, Lung, and Blood Institute (NHLBI) and a number of medical societies. The five main steps in the evaluation of obesity are described below and include (1) focused obesity-related history, (2) physical examination to determine the degree and type of obesity, (3) comorbid conditions, (4) fitness level, and (5) the patient's readiness to adopt lifestyle changes.

The Obesity-Focused History

Information from the history should address the following six questions:

- What factors contribute to the patient's obesity?
- How is the obesity affecting the patient's health?
- What is the patient's level of risk from obesity?
- What are the patient's goals and expectations?
- Is the patient motivated to begin a weight management program?
- What kind of help does the patient need?

Although the vast majority of obesity can be attributed to behavioral features that affect diet and physical activity patterns, the history may suggest secondary causes that merit further evaluation. Disorders to consider include polycystic ovarian syndrome, hypothyroidism, Cushing's syndrome, and hypothalamic disease. Drug-induced weight gain should also be considered. Common causes include antidiabetes agents (insulin, sulfonylureas, thiazolidinediones), steroid hormones, psychotropic agents, mood stabilizers (lithium), antidepressants (tricyclics, monoamine oxidase inhibitors, paroxetine, mirtazapine), and antiepileptic drugs (valproate, gabapentin, carbamazepine). Other medications such as nonsteroidal anti-inflammatory drugs and calcium channel blockers may cause peripheral edema, but they do not increase body fat.

The patient's current diet and physical activity patterns may reveal factors that contribute to the development of obesity in addition to identifying behaviors to target for treatment. This type of historical information is best obtained by using a questionnaire in combination with an interview.

BMI and Waist Circumference

Three key anthropometric measurements are important to evaluate the degree of obesity—weight, height, and waist circumference. The body mass index (BMI), calculated

TABLE 17-1

BODY MASS INDEX (BMI) TABLE

HEIGHT, INCHES — BODY WEIGHT, POUNDS

BMI	19	20	21	22	23	24	25	26	27	28	29	30	31	32	33	34	35
58	91	96	100	105	110	115	119	124	129	134	138	143	148	153	158	162	167
59	94	99	104	109	114	119	124	128	133	138	143	148	153	158	163	168	173
60	97	102	107	112	118	123	128	133	138	143	148	153	158	163	168	174	179
61	100	106	111	116	122	127	132	137	143	148	153	158	164	169	174	180	185
62	104	109	115	120	126	131	136	142	147	153	158	164	169	175	180	186	191
63	107	113	118	124	130	135	141	146	152	158	163	169	175	180	186	191	197
64	110	116	122	128	134	140	145	151	157	163	169	174	180	186	192	197	204
65	114	120	126	132	138	144	150	156	162	168	174	180	186	192	198	204	210
66	118	124	130	136	142	148	155	161	167	173	179	186	192	198	204	210	216
67	121	127	134	140	146	153	159	166	172	178	185	191	198	204	211	217	223
68	125	131	138	144	151	158	164	171	177	184	190	197	203	210	216	223	230
69	128	135	142	149	155	162	169	176	182	189	196	203	209	216	223	230	236
70	132	139	146	153	160	167	174	181	188	195	202	209	216	222	229	236	243
71	136	143	150	157	165	172	179	186	193	200	208	215	222	229	236	243	250
72	140	147	154	162	169	177	184	191	199	206	213	221	228	235	242	250	258
73	144	151	159	166	174	182	189	197	204	212	219	227	235	242	250	257	265
74	148	155	163	171	179	186	194	202	210	218	225	233	241	249	256	264	272
75	152	160	168	176	184	192	200	208	216	224	232	240	248	256	264	272	279
76	156	164	172	180	189	197	205	213	221	230	238	246	254	263	271	279	287

BMI	36	37	38	39	40	41	42	43	44	45	46	47	48	49	50	51	52	53	54
58	172	177	181	186	191	196	201	205	210	215	220	224	229	234	239	244	248	253	258
59	178	183	188	193	198	203	208	212	217	222	227	232	237	242	247	252	257	262	267
60	184	189	194	199	204	209	215	220	225	230	235	240	245	250	255	261	266	271	276
61	190	195	201	206	211	217	222	227	232	238	243	248	254	259	264	269	275	280	285
62	196	202	207	213	218	224	229	235	240	246	251	256	262	267	273	278	284	289	295
63	203	208	214	220	225	231	237	242	248	254	259	265	270	278	282	287	293	299	304
64	209	215	221	227	232	238	244	250	256	262	267	273	279	285	291	296	302	308	314
65	216	222	228	234	240	246	252	258	264	270	276	282	288	294	300	306	312	318	324
66	223	229	235	241	247	253	260	266	272	278	284	291	297	303	309	315	322	328	334
67	230	236	242	249	255	261	268	274	280	287	293	299	306	312	319	325	331	338	344
68	236	243	249	256	262	269	276	282	289	295	302	308	315	322	328	335	341	348	354
69	243	250	257	263	270	277	284	291	297	304	311	318	324	331	338	345	351	358	365
70	250	257	264	271	278	285	292	299	306	313	320	327	334	341	348	355	362	369	376
71	257	265	272	279	286	293	301	308	315	322	329	338	343	351	358	365	372	379	386
72	265	272	279	287	294	302	309	316	324	331	338	346	353	361	368	375	383	390	397
73	272	280	288	295	302	310	318	325	333	340	348	355	363	371	378	386	393	401	408
74	280	287	295	303	311	319	326	334	342	350	358	365	373	381	389	396	404	412	420
75	287	295	303	311	319	327	335	343	351	359	367	375	383	391	399	407	415	423	431
76	295	304	312	320	328	336	344	353	361	369	377	385	394	402	410	418	426	435	443

as weight (kg)/height (m)^2, or as weight (lb)/height (inches)^2 × 703, is used to classify weight status and risk of disease (Tables 17-1 and 17-2). BMI is used since it provides an estimate of body fat and is related to risk of disease. Lower BMI thresholds for overweight and obesity have been proposed for the Asia-Pacific region since this population appears to be at risk at lower body weights for glucose and lipid abnormalities.

Excess abdominal fat, assessed by measurement of waist circumference or waist-to-hip ratio, is independently associated with higher risk for diabetes mellitus and cardiovascular disease. Measurement of the waist circumference is a surrogate for visceral adipose tissue and should be performed in the horizontal plane above the iliac crest. Cut points that define higher risk for men and women based on ethnicity have been proposed by the International Diabetes Federation (Table 17-3).

Physical Fitness

Several prospective studies have demonstrated that physical fitness, reported by questionnaire or measured by a

TABLE 17-2

CLASSIFICATION OF WEIGHT STATUS AND RISK OF DISEASE

	BMI (kg/m^2)	OBESITY CLASS	RISK OF DISEASE
Underweight	<18.5		
Healthy weight	18.5–24.9		
Overweight	25.0–29.9		Increased
Obesity	30.0–34.9	I	High
Obesity	35.0–39.9	II	Very high
Extreme obesity	≥40	III	Extremely high

Source: Adapted from National Institutes of Health, National Heart, Lung, and Blood Institute: *Clinical Guidelines on the Identification, Evaluation, and Treatment of Overweight and Obesity in Adults*. U.S. Department of Health and Human Services, Public Health Service, 1998.

maximal treadmill exercise test, is an important predictor of all-cause mortality independent of BMI and body composition. These observations highlight the importance of taking an exercise history during examination as well as emphasizing physical activity as a treatment approach.

Obesity-Associated Comorbid Conditions

The evaluation of comorbid conditions should be based on presentation of symptoms, risk factors, and index of suspicion. All patients should have a fasting lipid panel [total, low-density lipoprotein (LDL), and high-density lipoprotein (HDL) cholesterol and triglyceride levels] and blood glucose measured at presentation along with blood pressure determination. Symptoms and diseases that are directly or indirectly related to obesity are listed in Table 17-4. Although individuals vary, the number and severity of organ-specific comorbid conditions usually rise with increasing levels of obesity. Patients at very high absolute risk include the following: established coronary heart disease; presence of other atherosclerotic diseases such as peripheral arterial disease, abdominal aortic aneurysm, and symptomatic carotid artery disease; type 2 diabetes; and sleep apnea.

TABLE 17-3

ETHNIC-SPECIFIC VALUES FOR WAIST CIRCUMFERENCE

ETHNIC GROUP	WAIST CIRCUMFERENCE
Europeans	
Men	>94 cm (37 in.)
Women	>80 cm (31.5 in.)
South Asians and Chinese	
Men	>90 cm (35 in.)
Women	>80 cm (31.5 in.)
Japanese	
Men	>85 cm (33.5 in.)
Women	>90 cm (35 in.)
Ethnic south and central Americans	Use south Asian recommendations until more specific data are available.
Sub-Saharan Africans	Use European data until more specific data are available.
Eastern Mediterranean and Middle East (Arab) populations	Use European data until more specific data are available.

Source: From KGMM Alberti et al for the IDF Epidemiology Task Force Consensus Group: The metabolic syndrome—a new worldwide definition. Lancet 366:1059, 2005.

TABLE 17-4

OBESITY-RELATED ORGAN SYSTEMS REVIEW

Cardiovascular	**Respiratory**
Hypertension	Dyspnea
Congestive heart failure	Obstructive sleep apnea
Cor pulmonale	Hypoventilation syndrome
Varicose veins	Pickwickian syndrome
Pulmonary embolism	Asthma
Coronary artery disease	**Gastrointestinal**
Endocrine	Gastroesophageal reflux disease
Metabolic syndrome	Nonalcoholic fatty liver disease
Type 2 diabetes	Cholelithiasis
Dyslipidemia	Hernias
Polycystic ovarian syndrome	Colon cancer
Musculoskeletal	**Genitourinary**
Hyperuricemia and gout	Urinary stress incontinence
Immobility	Obesity-related glomerulopathy
Osteoarthritis (knees and hips)	Hypogonadism (male)
Low back pain	Breast and uterine cancer
Carpal tunnel syndrome	Pregnancy complications
Psychological	**Neurologic**
Depression/low self-esteem	Stroke
Body image disturbance	Idiopathic intracranial hypertension
Social stigmatization	Meralgia paresthetica
Integument	Dementia
Striae distensae	
Stasis pigmentation of legs	
Lymphedema	
Cellulitis	
Intertrigo, carbuncles	
Acanthosis nigricans	
Acrochordon (skin tags)	
Hidradenitis suppurativa	

Assessing the Patient's Readiness to Change

An attempt to initiate lifestyle changes when the patient is not ready usually leads to frustration and may hamper future weight-loss efforts. Assessment includes patient motivation and support, stressful life events, psychiatric status, time availability and constraints, and appropriateness of goals and expectations. Readiness can be viewed as the balance of two opposing forces: (1) motivation, or the patient's desire to change, and (2) resistance, or the patient's resistance to change.

A helpful method to begin a readiness assessment is to "anchor" the patient's interest and confidence to change on a numerical scale. Using this technique, the patient is asked to rate his or her level of interest and confidence on a scale from 0 to 10, with 0 being not so important (or confident) and 10 being very important (or confident) to lose weight at this time. This exercise helps to establish readiness to change and also serves as a basis for further dialogue.

℞ Treatment: OBESITY

THE GOAL OF THERAPY The primary goal of treatment is to improve obesity-related comorbid conditions and reduce the risk of developing future comorbidities. Information obtained from the history, physical examination, and diagnostic tests is used to determine risk and develop a treatment plan (Fig. 17-1). The decision

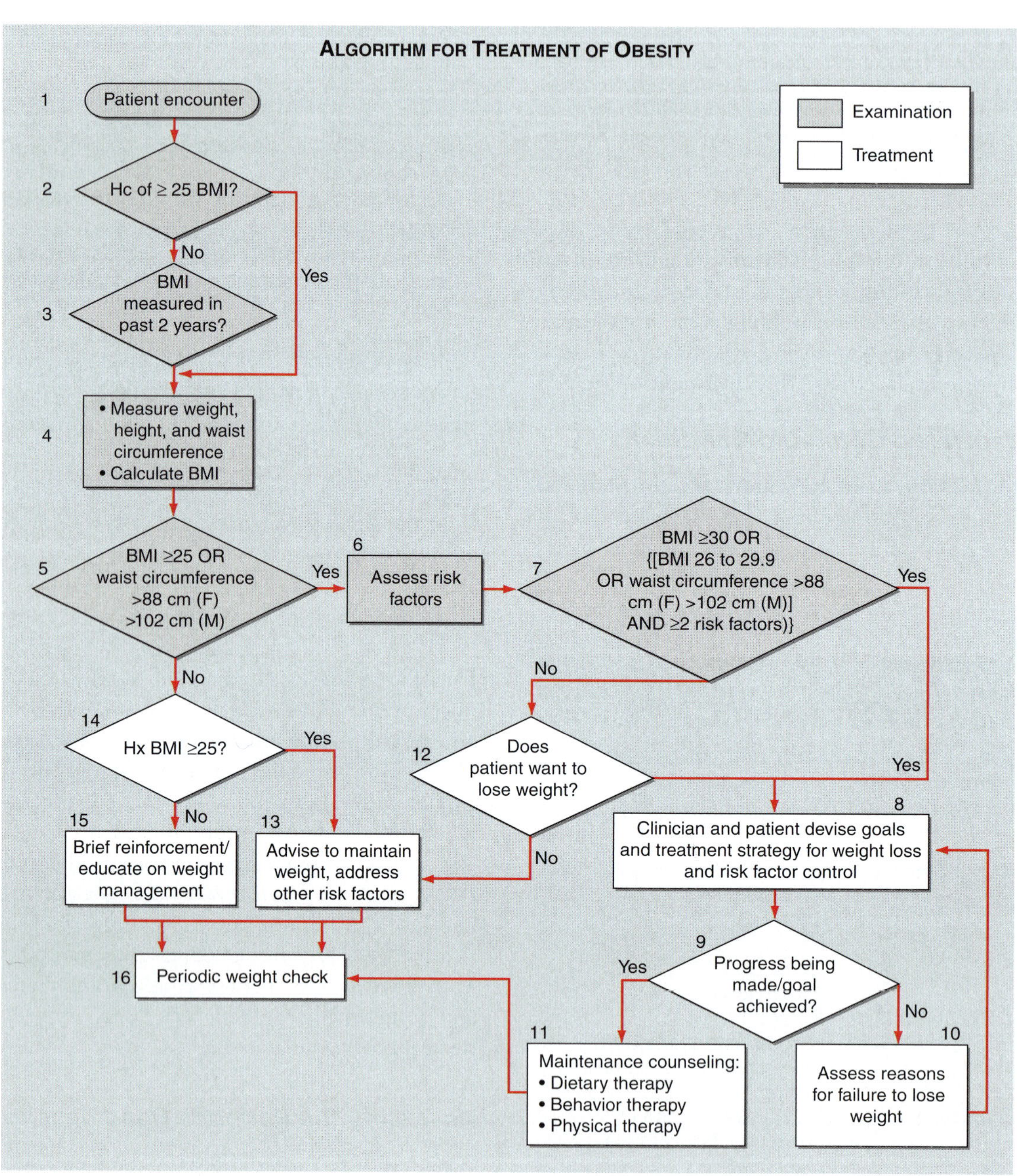

FIGURE 17-1

Treatment algorithm. This algorithm applies only to the assessment for overweight and obesity and subsequent decisions on that assessment. It does not reflect any initial overall assessment for other conditions that the physician may wish to perform. Ht, height; Hx, history; Wt, weight. (*From National, Heart, Lung, and Blood Institute: Clinical Guidelines on the Identification, Evaluation, and Treatment of Overweight and Obesity in Adults: The Evidence Report. Washington, DC, US Department of Health and Human Services, 1998.*)

of how aggressively to treat the patient, and which modalities to use, is determined by the patient's risk status, expectations, and available resources. Therapy for obesity always begins with lifestyle management and may include pharmacotherapy or surgery, depending on BMI risk category (**Table 17-5**). Setting an initial weight-loss goal of 10% over 6 months is a realistic target.

LIFESTYLE MANAGEMENT Obesity care involves attention to three essential elements of lifestyle: dietary habits, physical activity, and behavior modification. Because obesity is fundamentally a disease of energy imbalance, all patients must learn how and when energy is consumed (diet), how and when energy is expended (physical activity), and how to incorporate this information into their daily life (behavior therapy). Lifestyle management has been shown to result in a modest (typically 3–5 kg) weight loss compared to no treatment or usual care.

Diet Therapy The primary focus of diet therapy is to reduce overall calorie consumption. The NHLBI guidelines recommend initiating treatment with a calorie deficit of 500–1000 kcal/d compared to the patient's habitual diet. This reduction is consistent with a goal of losing approximately 1–2 lb per week. This calorie deficit can be accomplished by suggesting substitutions or alternatives to the diet. Examples include choosing smaller portion sizes, eating more fruits and vegetables, consuming more whole-grain cereals, selecting leaner cuts of meat and skimmed dairy products, reducing fried foods and other added fats and oils, and drinking water instead of caloric beverages. It is important that the dietary counseling remains patient-centered and that the goals are practical, realistic, and achievable.

The macronutrient composition of the diet will vary depending on the patient's preference and medical condition. The 2005 U.S. Department of Agriculture Dietary Guidelines for Americans, which focus on health promotion and risk reduction, can be applied to treatment of the overweight or obese patient. The recommendations include maintaining a diet rich in whole grains, fruits, vegetables, and dietary fiber; consuming two servings (8 oz) of fish high in omega-3 fatty acids per week; decreasing sodium to <2300 mg/d; consuming 3 cups of milk (or equivalent low-fat or fat-free dairy products) per day; limiting cholesterol to <300 mg/d; and keeping total fat between 20 and 35% of daily calories and saturated fats to <10% of daily calories. Application of these guidelines to specific calorie goals can be found on the website *www.mypyramid.gov*. The revised Dietary Reference Intakes for Macronutrients released by the Institute of Medicine recommends 45–65% of calories from carbohydrates, 20–35% from fat, and 10–35% from protein. The guidelines also recommend daily fiber intake of 38 g (men) and 25 g (women) for persons over 50 years of age and 30 g (men) and 21 g (women) for those under 50.

Since portion control is one of the most difficult strategies for patients to manage, the use of pre-prepared products, such as meal replacements, is a simple and convenient suggestion. Examples include frozen entrees, canned beverages, and bars. Use of meal replacements in the diet has been shown to result in a 7–8% weight loss.

A current area of controversy is the use of low-carbohydrate, high-protein diets for weight loss. These diets are based on the concept that carbohydrates are the primary cause of obesity and lead to insulin resistance. Most low-carbohydrate diets (e.g., South Beach, Zone, and Sugar Busters!) recommend a carbohydrate level of approximately 40–46% of energy. The Atkins diet contains 5–15% carbohydrate, depending on the phase of the diet. Several randomized, controlled trials of these low-carbohydrate diets have demonstrated greater weight loss at 6 months with improvement in coronary heart disease risk factors, including an increase in HDL cholesterol and a decrease in triglyceride levels. Weight loss between groups did not remain statistically significant at 1 year; however, low-carbohydrate diets appear to be at least as effective as low-fat diets in inducing weight loss for up to 1 year.

Another dietary approach to consider is the concept of energy density, which refers to the number of calories (energy) a food contains per unit of weight. People tend to ingest a constant volume of food, regardless of caloric or macronutrient content. Adding water or fiber to a food decreases its energy density by increasing weight without affecting caloric content. Examples of foods with

TABLE 17-5

A GUIDE TO SELECTING TREATMENT

	BMI CATEGORY				
TREATMENT	**25–26.9**	**27–29.9**	**30–35**	**35–39.9**	**≥40**
Diet, exercise, behavior therapy	With comorbidities	With comorbidities	+	+	+
Pharmacotherapy		With comorbidities	+	+	+
Surgery				With comorbidities	+

Source: From National Heart, Lung, and Blood Institute, North American Association for the Study of Obesity (2000).

low-energy density include soups, fruits, vegetables, oatmeal, and lean meats. Dry foods and high-fat foods such as pretzels, cheese, egg yolks, potato chips, and red meat have a high-energy density. Diets containing low-energy dense foods have been shown to control hunger and result in decreased caloric intake and weight loss.

Occasionally, very-low-calorie diets (VLCDs) are prescribed as a form of aggressive dietary therapy. The primary purpose of a VLCD is to promote a rapid and significant (13–23 kg) short-term weight loss over a 3–6-month period. These propriety formulas typically supply ≤800 kcal, 50–80 g protein, and 100% of the recommended daily intake for vitamins and minerals. According to a review by the National Task Force on the Prevention and Treatment of Obesity, indications for initiating a VLCD include well-motivated individuals who are moderately to severely obese (BMI >30), have failed at more conservative approaches to weight loss, and have a medical condition that would be immediately improved with rapid weight loss. These conditions include poorly controlled type 2 diabetes, hypertriglyceridemia, obstructive sleep apnea, and symptomatic peripheral edema. The risk for gallstone formation increases exponentially at rates of weight loss >1.5 kg/week (3.3 lb/week). Prophylaxis against gallstone formation with ursodeoxycholic acid, 600 mg/d, is effective in reducing this risk. Because of the need for close metabolic monitoring, these diets are usually prescribed by physicians specializing in obesity care.

Physical Activity Therapy Although exercise alone is only moderately effective for weight loss, the combination of dietary modification and exercise is the most effective behavioral approach for the treatment of obesity. The most important role of exercise appears to be in the maintenance of the weight loss. Currently, the *minimum* public health recommendation for physical activity is 30 min of moderate-intensity physical activity on most, and preferably all, days of the week. Focusing on simple ways to add physical activity into the normal daily routine through leisure activities, travel, and domestic work should be suggested. Examples include walking, using the stairs, doing home and yard work, and engaging in sport activities. Asking the patient to wear a pedometer to monitor total accumulation of steps as part of the activities of daily living is a useful strategy. Step counts are highly correlated with activity level. Studies have demonstrated that lifestyle activities are as effective as structured exercise programs for improving cardiorespiratory fitness and weight loss. The 2005 Dietary Guidelines for Americans summarizes compelling evidence that at least 60–90 min of daily moderate-intensity physical activity (420–630 min per week) is needed to sustain weight loss (*http://www.health.gov/dietaryguidelines/dga2005/*). The American College of Sports Medicine recommends that overweight and obese individuals progressively increase to a minimum of 150 min of moderate-intensity physical activity per week as a first goal. However, for long-term weight loss, a higher level of exercise (e.g., 200–300 min or ≥2000 kcal per week) is needed. These recommendations are daunting to most patients and need to be implemented gradually. Consultation with an exercise physiologist or personal trainer may be helpful.

Behavioral Therapy Cognitive behavioral therapy is used to help change and reinforce new dietary and physical activity behaviors. Strategies include self-monitoring techniques (e.g., journaling, weighing, and measuring food and activity), stress management, stimulus control (e.g., using smaller plates, not eating in front of the television or in the car), social support, problem solving, and cognitive restructuring to help patients develop more positive and realistic thoughts about themselves. When recommending any behavioral lifestyle change, have the patient identify what, when, where, and how the behavioral change will be performed. The patient should keep a record of the anticipated behavioral change so that progress can be reviewed at the next office visit. Because these techniques are time-consuming to implement, they are often provided by ancillary office staff such as a nurse clinician or registered dietitian.

PHARMACOTHERAPY Adjuvant pharmacologic treatments should be considered for patients with a BMI >30 kg/m^2 or with a BMI >27 kg/m^2 who also have concomitant obesity-related diseases and for whom dietary and physical activity therapy has not been successful. When prescribing an antiobesity medication, patients should be actively engaged in a lifestyle program that provides the strategies and skills needed to effectively use the drug since this support increases total weight loss.

There are several potential targets of pharmacologic therapy for obesity. The most thoroughly explored treatment is suppression of appetite via centrally active medications that alter monoamine neurotransmitters. A second strategy is to reduce the absorption of selective macronutrients from the gastrointestinal (GI) tract, such as fat. These two mechanisms form the basis for all currently prescribed antiobesity agents. A third target, selective blocking of the endocannabinoid system, has recently been identified.

Centrally Acting Anorexiant Medications Appetite-suppressing drugs, or anorexiants, affect satiety—the absence of hunger after eating—and hunger—a biologic sensation that initiates eating. By increasing satiety and decreasing hunger, these agents help patients reduce caloric intake without a sense of deprivation. The target site for the actions of anorexiants is the ventromedial and lateral hypothalamic regions in the central nervous system (Chap. 16). Their biologic effect on appetite regulation is produced by augmenting the neurotransmission of three monoamines: norepinephrine, serotonin [5-hydroxytryptamine (5-HT)], and, to a lesser degree, dopamine. The classic sympathomimetic adrenergic agents (benzphetamine, phendimetrazine, diethylpropion, mazindol, and phentermine) function by stimulating norepinephrine release or by blocking its reuptake. In contrast, sibutramine (Meridia) functions as a serotonin and norepinephrine reuptake inhibitor. Unlike other previously used anorexiants, sibutramine is not pharmacologically related to amphetamine and has no addictive potential.

Sibutramine is the only anorexiant that is currently approved by the U.S. Food and Drug Administration (FDA) for long-term use. It produces an average loss of about 5–9% of initial body weight at 12 months. Sibutramine has been demonstrated to maintain weight loss for up to 2 years. The most commonly reported adverse events of sibutramine are headache, dry mouth, insomnia, and constipation. These are generally mild and well tolerated. The principal concern is a dose-related increase in blood pressure and heart rate that may require discontinuation of the medication. A dose of 10–15 mg/d causes an average increase in systolic and diastolic blood pressure of 2–4 mmHg and an increase in heart rate of 4–6 beats/min. For this reason, all patients should be monitored closely and evaluated within 1 month after initiating therapy. The risk of adverse effects on blood pressure are no greater in patients with controlled hypertension than in those who do not have hypertension, and the drug does not appear to cause cardiac valve dysfunction. Contraindications to sibutramine use include uncontrolled hypertension, congestive heart failure, symptomatic coronary heart disease, arrhythmias, or history of stroke. Similar to other antiobesity medications, weight reduction is enhanced when the drug is used along with behavioral therapy, and body weight increases when the medication is discontinued.

Peripherally Acting Medications Orlistat (Xenical) is a synthetic hydrogenated derivative of a naturally occurring lipase inhibitor, lipostatin, produced by the mold *Streptomyces toxytricini*. Orlistat is a potent, slowly reversible inhibitor of pancreatic, gastric, and carboxyl ester lipases and phospholipase A_2, which are required for the hydrolysis of dietary fat into fatty acids and monoacylglycerols. The drug acts in the lumen of the stomach and small intestine by forming a covalent bond with the active site of these lipases. Taken at a therapeutic dose of 120 mg tid, orlistat blocks the digestion and absorption of about 30% of dietary fat. After discontinuation of the drug, fecal fat usually returns to normal concentrations within 48–72 h.

Multiple randomized, 1–2-year double-blind, placebo-controlled studies have shown that after 1 year, orlistat produces a weight loss of about 9–10%, compared with a 4–6% weight loss in the placebo-treated groups. Because orlistat is minimally (<1%) absorbed from the GI tract, it has no systemic side effects. Tolerability to the drug is related to the malabsorption of dietary fat and subsequent passage of fat in the feces. GI tract adverse effects are reported in at least 10% of orlistat-treated patients. These include flatus with discharge, fecal urgency, fatty/oily stool, and increased defecation. These side effects are generally experienced early, diminish as patients control their dietary fat intake, and infrequently cause patients to withdraw from clinical trials. Psyllium mucilloid is helpful in controlling the orlistat-induced GI side effects when taken concomitantly with the medication. Serum concentrations of the fat-soluble vitamins D and E and β-carotene may be reduced, and vitamin supplements are recommended to prevent potential deficiencies. Orlistat was approved for over-the-counter use in 2007.

The Endocannabinoid System Cannabinoid receptors and their endogenous ligands have been implicated in a variety of physiologic functions, including feeding, modulation of pain, emotional behavior, and peripheral lipid metabolism. Cannabis and its main ingredient, Δ^9-tetrahydrocannabinol (THC), is an exogenous cannabinoid compound. Two endocannabinoids have been identified, anandamide and 2-arachidonyl glyceride. Two cannabinoid receptors have been identified: CB_1 (abundant in the brain) and CB_2 (present in immune cells). The brain endocannabinoid system is thought to control food intake through reinforcing motivation to find and consume foods with high incentive value and to regulate actions of other mediators of appetite. The first selective cannabinoid CB_1 receptor antagonist, rimonabant, was discovered in 1994. The medication antagonizes the orexigenic effect of THC and suppresses appetite when given alone in animal models. Several large prospective, randomized controlled trials have demonstrated the effectiveness of rimonabant as a weight-loss agent. Taken as a 20-mg dose, subjects lost an average of 6.5 kg (14.32 lb) compared to 1.5 kg (3.3 lb) for placebo at 1 year. Concomitant improvements were seen in waist circumference and cardiovascular risk factors. The most common reported side effects include depression, anxiety, and nausea. FDA approval of rimonabant is still pending.

SURGERY Bariatric surgery can be considered for patients with severe obesity (BMI ≥40 kg/m^2) or those with moderate obesity (BMI ≥35 kg/m^2) associated with a serious medical condition. Surgical weight loss functions by reducing caloric intake and, depending on the procedure, macronutrient absorption.

Weight-loss surgeries fall into one of two categories: restrictive and restrictive-malabsorptive (Fig. 17-2). Restrictive surgeries limit the amount of food the stomach can hold and slow the rate of gastric emptying. The vertical banded gastroplasty (VBG) is the prototype of this category but is currently performed on a very limited basis due to lack of effectiveness in long-term trials. Laparoscopic adjustable silicone gastric banding (LASGB)

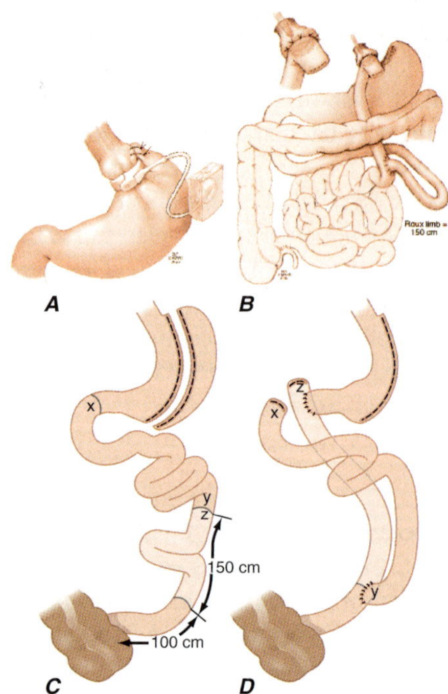

FIGURE 17-2

Bariatric surgical procedures. Examples of operative interventions used for surgical manipulation of the gastrointestinal tract. ***A.*** Laparoscopic gastric band (LAGB). ***B.*** The Roux-en-Y gastric bypass. ***C.*** Biliopancreatic diversion with duodenal switch. ***D.*** Biliopancreatic diversion. (*From ML Kendrick, GF Dakin. Surgical approaches to obesity. Mayo Clin Proc 815:518, 2006; with permission.*)

has replaced the VBG as the most commonly performed restrictive operation. The first banding device, the lap-band, was approved for use in the United States in 2001. In contrast to previous devices, the diameter of this band is adjustable by way of its connection to a reservoir that is implanted under the skin. Injection or removal of saline into the reservoir tightens or loosens the band's internal diameter, thus changing the size of the gastric opening.

The three restrictive-malabsorptive bypass procedures combine the elements of gastric restriction and selective malabsorption. These procedures include Roux-en-Y gastric bypass (RYGB), biliopancreatic diversion (BPD), and biliopancreatic diversion with duodenal switch (BPDDS) (Fig. 17-2). RYGB is the most commonly performed and accepted bypass procedure. It may be performed with an open incision or laparoscopically.

Although no recent randomized controlled trials compare weight loss after surgical and nonsurgical interventions, data from meta-analyses and large databases, primarily obtained from observational studies, suggest that bariatric surgery is the most effective weight-loss therapy for those with clinically severe obesity. These procedures generally produce a 30–35% average total body weight loss that is maintained in nearly 60% of patients at 5 years. In general, mean weight loss is greater after the combined restrictive-malabsorptive procedures compared to the restrictive procedures. An abundance of data supports the positive impact of bariatric surgery on obesity-related morbid conditions, including diabetes mellitus, hypertension, obstructive sleep apnea, dyslipidemia, and nonalcoholic fatty liver disease.

Surgical mortality from bariatric surgery is generally <1% but varies with the procedure, patient's age and comorbid conditions, and experience of the surgical team. The most common surgical complications include stomal stenosis or marginal ulcers (occurring in 5–15% of patients) that present as prolonged nausea and vomiting after eating or inability to advance the diet to solid foods. These complications are typically treated by endoscopic balloon dilatation and acid suppression therapy, respectively. For patients who undergo LASGB, there are no intestinal absorptive abnormalities other than mechanical reduction in gastric size and outflow. Therefore, selective deficiencies occur uncommonly unless eating habits become unbalanced. In contrast, the restrictive-malabsorptive procedures increase risk for micronutrient deficiencies of vitamin B_{12}, iron, folate, calcium, and vitamin D. Patients with restrictive-malabsorptive procedures require lifelong supplementation with these micronutrients.

FURTHER READINGS

Bray GA, Greenway FL: Pharmacologic treatment of the overweight patient. Pharmacol Rev 59:151, 2007

Bray GA, Ryan DH: Drug treatment of the overweight patient. Gastroenterology 132(6):2239, 2007

Buchwald H et al: Bariatric surgery: A systematic review and meta-analysis. JAMA 292:1724, 2004

DeMaria EJ: Bariatric surgery for morbid obesity. N Engl J Med 356:2176, 2007

Eckel RH: Clinical practice. Nonsurgical management of obesity in adults. N Engl J Med 358:1941, 2008

Haslam DW, James WPT: Obesity. Lancet 366:1197, 2005

Katan MB: Weight-loss diets for the prevention and treatment of obesity. N Engl J Med 360:923, 2009

Kramer H et al: Obesity management in adults with CKD. Am J Kidney Dis 53:151, 2009

Kushner RF: Roadmaps for clinical practice: Case studies in disease prevention and health promotion—assessment and management of adult obesity: A primer for physicians. Chicago, American Medical Association, 2003. (Available online at *www.ama-assn.org/ama/pub/category/10931.html*)

National Heart, Lung, and Blood Institute, North American Association for the Study of Obesity: Practical guide: Identification, evaluation, and treatment of overweight and obesity in adults. Bethesda, MD, National Institutes of Health pub number 00-4084, Oct. 2000. Available online: *http://www.nhlbi.nih.gov/guidelines/obesity/practgde.htm*

Polonsky KS et al: Gastric banding to treat obesity: Band-aid or breakthrough? Nat Clin Pract Endocrinol Metab 4:421, 2008

Wadden TA et al: Lifestyle modification for the management of obesity. Gastroenterology 132(6):2226, 2007

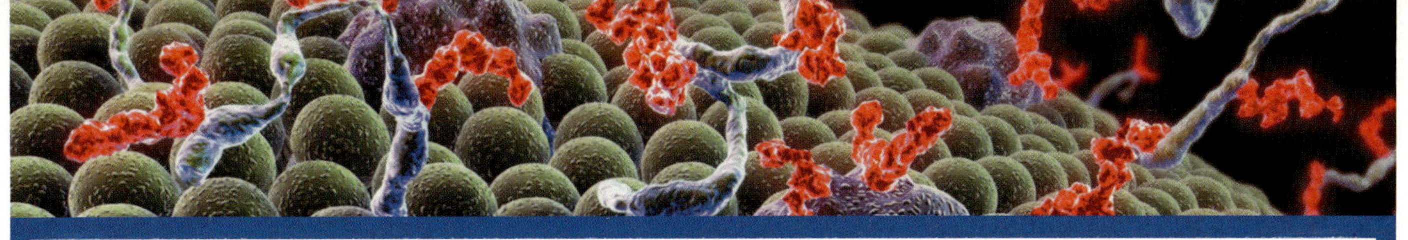

CHAPTER 18

THE METABOLIC SYNDROME

Robert H. Eckel

The metabolic syndrome (syndrome X, insulin resistance syndrome) consists of a constellation of metabolic abnormalities that confer increased risk of cardiovascular disease (CVD) and diabetes mellitus (DM). The criteria for the metabolic syndrome have evolved since the original definition by the World Health Organization in 1998, reflecting growing clinical evidence and analysis by a variety of consensus conferences and professional organizations. The major features of the metabolic syndrome include central obesity, hypertriglyceridemia, low high-density lipoprotein (HDL) cholesterol, hyperglycemia, and hypertension (Table 18-1).

EPIDEMIOLOGY

Prevalence of the metabolic syndrome varies across the globe, in part reflecting the age and ethnicity of the populations studied and the diagnostic criteria applied. In general, the prevalence of metabolic syndrome increases with age. The highest recorded prevalence worldwide is in Native Americans, with nearly 60% of women ages 45–49 and 45% of men ages 45–49 meeting National Cholesterol Education Program, Adult Treatment Panel III (NCEP:ATPIII) criteria. In the United States, metabolic syndrome is less common in African-American men but more common in Mexican-American women. Based on data from the National Health and Nutrition Examination Survey (NHANES) III, the age-adjusted prevalence of the metabolic syndrome in the United States is 34% for men and 35% for women. In France, a 30–64-year-old cohort shows a <10% prevalence for each gender, although 17.5% are affected in the 60–64 age range. Greater industrialization worldwide is associated with rising rates of obesity, which is anticipated to dramatically increase prevalence of the metabolic syndrome, especially as the population ages. Moreover, the rising prevalence and severity of obesity in children is initiating features of the metabolic syndrome in a younger population.

The frequency distribution of the five components of the syndrome for the U.S. population (NHANES III) is summarized in Fig. 18-1. Increases in waist circumference predominate in women, whereas fasting triglycerides >150 mg/dL and hypertension are more likely in men.

RISK FACTORS

Overweight/Obesity

Although the first description of the metabolic syndrome occurred in the early twentieth century, the worldwide overweight/obesity epidemic has been the driving force for more recent recognition of the syndrome. Central adiposity is a key feature of the syndrome, reflecting the fact that the syndrome's prevalence is driven by the strong relationship between waist circumference and increasing adiposity. However, despite the importance of obesity, patients who are normal weight may also be insulin-resistant and have the syndrome.

TABLE 18-1

NCEP:ATPIII 2001 AND IDF CRITERIA FOR THE METABOLIC SYNDROME

NCEP:ATPIII 2001	IDF CRITERIA FOR CENTRAL ADIPOSITY[a]		
Three or more of the following:	**Waist Circumference**		
	Men	**Women**	**Ethnicity**
Central obesity: Waist circumference >102 cm (M), >88 cm (F)	≥94 cm	≥80 cm	Europid, Sub-Saharan African, Eastern and Middle Eastern
Hypertriglyceridemia: Triglycerides 150 mg/dL or specific medication	≥90 cm	≥80 cm	South Asian, Chinese, and ethnic South and Central American
Low HDL cholesterol: <40 mg/dL and <50 mg/dL, respectively, or specific medication	≥85 cm	≥90 cm	Japanese
Hypertension: Blood pressure ≥130 mmHg systolic or ≥85 mmHg diastolic or specific medication	**Two or more of the following:** Fasting triglycerides >150 mg/dL or specific medication HDL cholesterol <40 mg/dL and <50 mg/dL for men and women, respectively, or specific medication		
Fasting plasma glucose ≥100 mg/dL or specific medication or previously diagnosed type 2 diabetes	Blood pressure >130 mmHg systolic or >85 mmHg diastolic or previous diagnosis or specific medication Fasting plasma glucose ≥100 mg/dL or previously diagnosed type 2 diabetes		

[a]In this analysis, the following thresholds for waist circumference were used: White men, ≥94 cm; African-American men, ≥94 cm; Mexican-American men, ≥90 cm; white women, ≥80 cm; African-American women, ≥80 cm; Mexican-American women, ≥80 cm. For participants whose designation was "other race—including multiracial," thresholds that were once based on Europid cut points (≥94 cm for men and ≥80 cm for women) and once based on South Asian cut points (≥90 cm for men and ≥80 cm for women) were used. For participants who were considered "other Hispanic," the IDF thresholds for ethnic South and Central Americans were used.

Note: NCEP:ATPIII, National Cholesterol Education Program, Adult Treatment Panel III; IDF, International Diabetes Foundation; HDL, high-density lipoprotein.

Sedentary Lifestyle

Physical inactivity is a predictor of CVD events and related mortality. Many components of the metabolic syndrome are associated with a sedentary lifestyle, including increased adipose tissue (predominantly central); reduced HDL cholesterol; and a trend toward increased triglycerides, blood pressure, and glucose in the genetically susceptible. Compared with individuals who watched television or videos or used their computer <1 h daily, those who carried out these behaviors for >4 h daily have a twofold increased risk of the metabolic syndrome.

Population (%)
5.0
4.5
4.0
3.5
3.0
2.5
2.0
1.5
1.0
.5
0
Waist circ
TG150
↓ HDL chol
↑ BP
Glucose
Men
Women

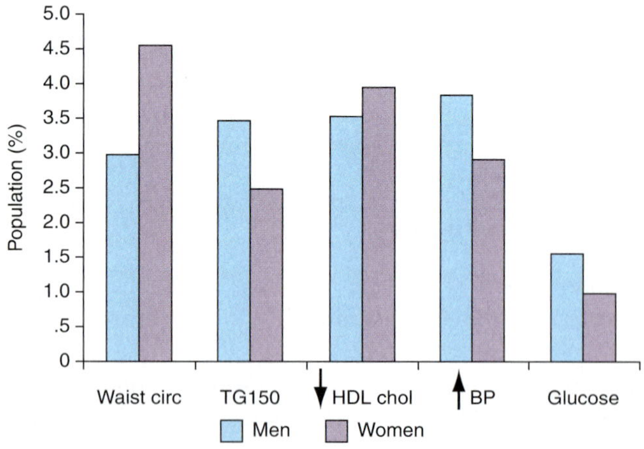

FIGURE 18-1

Prevalence of the metabolic syndrome components, from NHANES III. NHANES, National Health and Nutrition Examination Survey; TG, triglyceride; HDL, high-density lipoprotein; BP, blood pressure. (*From ES Ford et al: JAMA 287:356, 2002; with permission.*)

Aging

The metabolic syndrome affects 44% of the U.S. population older than age 50. A greater percentage of women older than age 50 have the syndrome than men. The age dependency of the syndrome's prevalence is seen in most populations around the world.

Diabetes Mellitus

DM is included in both the NCEP and International Diabetes Foundation (IDF) definitions of the metabolic syndrome. It is estimated that the large majority (~75%) of patients with type 2 diabetes or impaired glucose tolerance (IGT) have the metabolic syndrome. The presence of the metabolic syndrome in these populations relates to a higher prevalence of CVD compared to patients with type 2 diabetes or IGT without the syndrome.

Coronary Heart Disease

The approximate prevalence of the metabolic syndrome in patients with coronary heart disease (CHD) is 50%, with a prevalence of 37% in patients with premature coronary artery disease (age ≤45), particularly in women. With appropriate cardiac rehabilitation and changes in lifestyle (e.g., nutrition, physical activity, weight reduction, and, in some cases, pharmacologic agents), the prevalence of the syndrome can be reduced.

Lipodystrophy

Lipodystrophic disorders in general are associated with the metabolic syndrome. Both genetic (e.g., Berardinelli-Seip congenital lipodystrophy, Dunnigan familial partial lipodystrophy) and acquired (e.g., HIV-related lipodystrophy in patients treated with highly active antiretroviral therapy) forms of lipodystrophy may give rise to severe insulin resistance and many of the metabolic syndrome's components.

ETIOLOGY

Insulin Resistance

The most accepted and unifying hypothesis to describe the pathophysiology of the metabolic syndrome is insulin resistance, caused by an incompletely understood defect in insulin action (Chap. 19). The onset of insulin resistance is heralded by postprandial hyperinsulinemia, followed by fasting hyperinsulinemia and, ultimately, hyperglycemia.

An early major contributor to the development of insulin resistance is an overabundance of circulating fatty acids (Fig. 18-2). Plasma albumin-bound free fatty acids (FFAs) are derived predominantly from adipose tissue triglyceride stores released by hormone-sensitive lipase. Fatty acids are also derived through the lipolysis of triglyceride-rich lipoproteins in tissues by lipoprotein lipase (LPL). Insulin mediates both antilipolysis and the stimulation of LPL in adipose tissue. Of note, the inhibition of lipolysis in adipose tissue is the most sensitive pathway of insulin action. Thus, when insulin resistance develops, increased lipolysis produces more fatty acids, which further decrease the antilipolytic effect of insulin. Excessive fatty acids enhance substrate availability and create insulin resistance

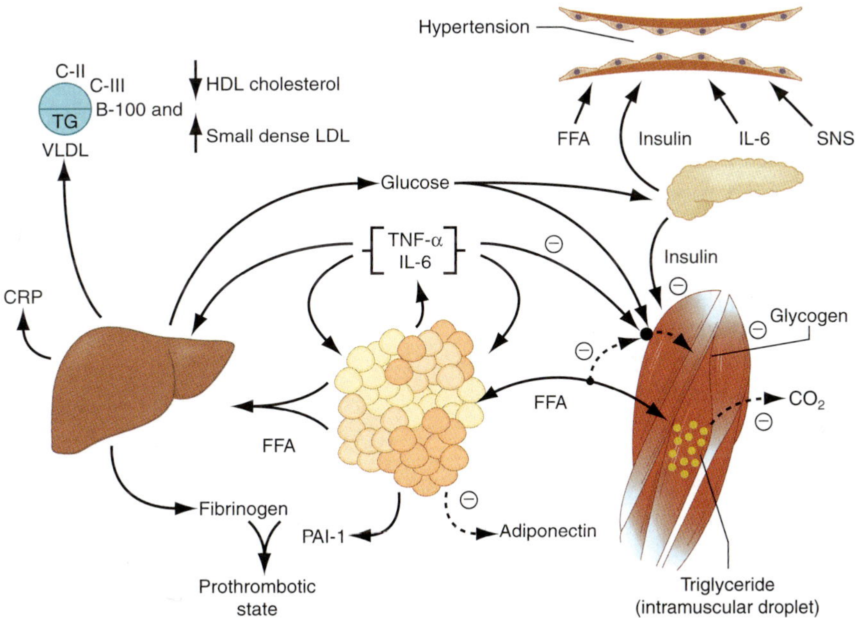

FIGURE 18-2

Pathophysiology of the metabolic syndrome. Free fatty acids (FFAs) are released in abundance from an expanded adipose tissue mass. In the liver, FFAs result in an increased production of glucose and triglycerides and secretion of very low density lipoproteins (VLDLs). Associated lipid/lipoprotein abnormalities include reductions in high-density lipoprotein (HDL) cholesterol and an increased density of low-density lipoproteins (LDLs). FFAs also reduce insulin sensitivity in muscle by inhibiting insulin-mediated glucose uptake. Associated defects include a reduction in glucose partitioning to glycogen and increased lipid accumulation in triglyceride (TG). Increases in circulating glucose, and to some extent FFA, increase pancreatic insulin secretion, resulting in hyperinsulinemia. Hyperinsulinemia may result in enhanced sodium reabsorption and increased sympathetic nervous system (SNS) activity and contribute to the hypertension, as might increased levels of circulating FFAs. The proinflammatory state is superimposed and contributory to the insulin resistance produced by excessive FFAs. The enhanced secretion of interleukin 6 (IL-6) and tumor necrosis factor α (TNF-α) produced by adipocytes and monocyte-derived macrophages results in more insulin resistance and lipolysis of adipose tissue triglyceride stores to circulating FFAs. IL-6 and other cytokines also enhance hepatic glucose production, VLDL production by the liver, and insulin resistance in muscle. Cytokines and FFAs also increase the hepatic production of fibrinogen and adipocyte production of plasminogen activator inhibitor 1 (PAI-1), resulting in a prothrombotic state. Higher levels of circulating cytokines also stimulate the hepatic production of C-reactive protein (CRP). Reduced production of the anti-inflammatory and insulin-sensitizing cytokine adiponectin are also associated with the metabolic syndrome. (*Reprinted from Eckel et al., with permission from Elsevier.*)

by modifying downstream signaling. Fatty acids impair insulin-mediated glucose uptake and accumulate as triglycerides in both skeletal and cardiac muscle, whereas increased glucose production and triglyceride accumulation are seen in liver.

The oxidative stress hypothesis provides unifying theory for aging and the predisposition to the metabolic syndrome. In studies carried out in insulin-resistant subjects with obesity or type 2 diabetes, in the offspring of patients with type 2 diabetes, and in the elderly, a defect has been identified in mitochondrial oxidative phosphorylation, leading to the accumulation of triglycerides and related lipid molecules in muscle. The accumulation of lipids in muscle is associated with insulin resistance.

Increased Waist Circumference

Waist circumference is an important component of the most recent and frequently applied diagnostic criteria for the metabolic syndrome. However, measuring waist circumference does not reliably distinguish between a large waist due to increases in subcutaneous adipose tissue versus visceral fat; this distinction requires CT or MRI. With increases in visceral adipose tissue, adipose tissue–derived FFAs are directed to the liver. On the other hand, increases in abdominal subcutaneous fat release lipolysis products into the systemic circulation and avoid more direct effects on hepatic metabolism. Relative increases in visceral versus subcutaneous adipose tissue with increasing waist circumference in Asians and Asian Indians may explain the greater prevalence of the syndrome in these populations compared to African-American men in whom subcutaneous fat predominates. It is also possible that visceral fat is a marker for, but not the source of, excess postprandial FFAs in obesity.

Dyslipidemia

(See also Chap. 21) In general, FFA flux to the liver is associated with increased production of apoB-containing, triglyceride-rich very low density lipoproteins (VLDLs). The effect of insulin on this process is complex, but *hypertriglyceridemia* is an excellent marker of the insulin-resistant condition.

The other major lipoprotein disturbance in the metabolic syndrome is a *reduction in HDL cholesterol.* This reduction is a consequence of changes in HDL composition and metabolism. In the presence of hypertriglyceridemia, a decrease in the cholesterol content of HDL is a consequence of reduced cholesteryl ester content of the lipoprotein core in combination with cholesteryl ester transfer protein–mediated alterations in triglyceride making the particle small and dense. This change in lipoprotein composition also results in an increased clearance of HDL from the circulation. The relationships of these changes in HDL to insulin resistance are likely indirect, occurring in concert with the changes in triglyceride-rich lipoprotein metabolism.

In addition to HDL, low-density lipoproteins (LDLs) are also modified in composition. With fasting serum triglycerides >2.0 mM (~180 mg/dL), there is almost always a predominance of small dense LDLs. Small dense LDLs are thought to be more atherogenic. They may be toxic to the endothelium, and they are able to transit through the endothelial basement membrane and adhere to glycosaminoglycans. They also have increased susceptibility to oxidation and are selectively bound to scavenger receptors on monocyte-derived macrophages. Subjects with increased small dense LDL particles and hypertriglyceridemia also have increased cholesterol content of both VLDL1 and VLDL2 subfractions. This relatively cholesterol-rich VLDL particle may also contribute to the atherogenic risk in patients with metabolic syndrome.

Glucose Intolerance

(See also Chap. 19) The defects in insulin action lead to impaired suppression of glucose production by the liver and kidney and reduced glucose uptake and metabolism in insulin-sensitive tissues, i.e., muscle and adipose tissue. The relationship between impaired fasting glucose (IFG) or IGT and insulin resistance is well supported by human, nonhuman primate, and rodent studies. To compensate for defects in insulin action, insulin secretion and/or clearance must be modified to sustain euglycemia. Ultimately, this compensatory mechanism fails, usually because of defects in insulin secretion, resulting in progress from IFG and/or IGT to DM.

Hypertension

The relationship between insulin resistance and hypertension is well established. Paradoxically, under normal physiologic conditions, insulin is a vasodilator with secondary effects on sodium reabsorption in the kidney. However, in the setting of insulin resistance, the vasodilatory effect of insulin is lost, but the renal effect on sodium reabsorption is preserved. Sodium reabsorption is increased in Caucasians with the metabolic syndrome but not in Africans or Asians. Insulin also increases the activity of the sympathetic nervous system, an effect that may also be preserved in the setting of the insulin resistance. Finally, insulin resistance is characterized by pathway-specific impairment in phosphatidylinositol 3-kinase signaling. In the endothelium, this may cause an imbalance between the production of nitric oxide and secretion of endothelin-1, leading to decreased blood flow. Although these mechanisms are provocative, when insulin action is assessed by levels of fasting insulin or by the Homeostasis Model Assessment (HOMA), insulin resistance contributes only modestly to the increased prevalence of hypertension in the metabolic syndrome.

Proinflammatory Cytokines

The increases in proinflammatory cytokines, including interleukin (IL)-1, IL-6, IL-18, resistin, tumor necrosis factor (TNF) α, and C-reactive protein (CRP), reflect overproduction by the expanded adipose tissue mass (Fig. 18-2). Adipose tissue–derived macrophages may be the primary source of proinflammatory cytokines locally and in the systemic circulation. It remains unclear, however, how much of the insulin resistance is caused by the paracrine versus endocrine effects of these cytokines.

Adiponectin

Adiponectin is an anti-inflammatory cytokine produced exclusively by adipocytes. Adiponectin enhances insulin sensitivity and inhibits many steps in the inflammatory process. In the liver, adiponectin inhibits the expression of gluconeogenic enzymes and the rate of glucose production. In muscle, adiponectin increases glucose transport and enhances fatty acid oxidation, partially due to activation of AMP kinase. Adiponectin is reduced in the metabolic syndrome. The relative contribution of adiponectin deficiency versus overabundance of the proinflammatory cytokines remains unclear.

CLINICAL FEATURES

Symptoms and Signs

The metabolic syndrome is typically unassociated with symptoms. On physical examination, waist circumference may be expanded and blood pressure elevated. The presence of one or either of these signs should alert the clinician to search for other biochemical abnormalities that may be associated with the metabolic syndrome. Less frequently, lipoatrophy or acanthosis nigricans is found on exam. Because these physical findings are typically associated with severe insulin resistance, other components of the metabolic syndrome should be expected.

Associated Diseases

Cardiovascular Disease

The relative risk for new-onset CVD in patients with the metabolic syndrome, in the absence of diabetes, averages between 1.5- and threefold. In an 8-year follow-up of middle-aged men and women in the Framingham Offspring Study (FOS), the population-attributable risk for patients with the metabolic syndrome to develop CVD was 34% in men and 16% in women. In the same study, both the metabolic syndrome and diabetes predicted ischemic stroke with greater risk for patients with the metabolic syndrome than for diabetes alone (19% vs 7%), particularly in women (27% vs 5%). Patients with metabolic syndrome are also at increased risk for peripheral vascular disease.

Type 2 Diabetes

Overall, the risk for type 2 diabetes in patients with the metabolic syndrome is increased three- to fivefold. In the FOS's 8-year follow-up of middle-aged men and women, the population-attributable risk for developing type 2 diabetes was 62% in men and 47% in women.

Other Associated Conditions

In addition to the features specifically associated with metabolic syndrome, insulin resistance is accompanied by other metabolic alterations. These included increases in apoB and C III, uric acid, prothrombotic factors (fibrinogen, plasminogen activator inhibitor 1), serum viscosity, asymmetric dimethylarginine, homocysteine, white blood cell count, proinflammatory cytokines, CRP, microalbuminuria, nonalcoholic fatty liver disease (NAFLD) and/or nonalcoholic steatohepatitis (NASH), polycystic ovarian disease (PCOS), and obstructive sleep apnea (OSA).

Nonalcoholic Fatty Liver Disease

Fatty liver is relatively common. However, in NASH, both triglyceride accumulation and inflammation coexist. NASH is now present in 2–3% of the population in the United States and other Western countries. As the prevalence of overweight/obesity and the metabolic syndrome increases, NASH may become one of the more frequent causes of end-stage liver disease and hepatocellular carcinoma.

Hyperuricemia

Hyperuricemia reflects defects in insulin action on the renal tubular reabsorption of uric acid, whereas the increase in asymmetric dimethylarginine, an endogenous inhibitor of nitric oxide synthase, relates to endothelial dysfunction. Microalbuminuria may also be caused by altered endothelial pathophysiology in the insulin-resistant state.

Polycystic Ovary Syndrome

(See also Chap. 10) PCOS is highly associated with the metabolic syndrome, with a prevalence between 40 and 50%. Women with PCOS are two to four times more likely to have the metabolic syndrome compared to women without PCOS.

Obstructive Sleep Apnea

OSA is commonly associated with obesity, hypertension, increased circulating cytokines, IGT, and insulin resistance. With these associations, it is not surprising that the metabolic syndrome is frequently present. Moreover, when biomarkers of insulin resistance are compared between patients with OSA and weight-matched controls, insulin resistance is more severe in patients with OSA. Continuous positive airway pressure (CPAP) treatment in OSA patients improves insulin sensitivity.

DIAGNOSIS

The diagnosis of the metabolic syndrome relies on satisfying the criteria listed in Table 18-1 using tools at the bedside and in the laboratory. Because the NCEP:ATPIII and IDF criteria are similar, either can be used. The medical history should include evaluation of symptoms for OSA in all patients and PCOS in premenopausal women. Family history will help determine risk for CVD and DM. Blood pressure and waist circumference measurements provide information necessary for the diagnosis.

Laboratory Tests

Fasting lipids and glucose are needed to determine if the metabolic syndrome is present. The measurement of additional biomarkers associated with insulin resistance must be individualized. Such tests might include apoB, high-sensitivity CRP, fibrinogen, uric acid, urinary microalbumin, and liver function tests. A sleep study should be performed if symptoms of OSA are present. If PCOS is suspected based on clinical features and anovulation, testosterone, luteinizing hormone, and follicle-stimulating hormone should be measured.

℞ Treatment: THE METABOLIC SYNDROME

LIFESTYLE (See also Chap. 17) Obesity is the driving force behind the metabolic syndrome. Thus, weight reduction is the primary approach to the disorder. With weight reduction, the improvement in insulin sensitivity is often accompanied by favorable modifications in many components of the metabolic syndrome. In general, recommendations for weight loss include a combination of caloric restriction, increased physical activity, and behavior modification. For weight reduction, caloric restriction is the most important component, whereas increases in physical activity are important for maintenance of weight loss. Some, but not all, evidence suggests that the addition of exercise to caloric restriction may promote relatively greater weight loss from the visceral depot. The tendency for weight regain after successful weight reduction underscores the need for long-lasting behavioral changes.

Diet Before prescribing a weight-loss diet, it is important to emphasize that it takes a long time for a patient to achieve an expanded fat mass; thus, the correction need not occur quickly. On the basis of ~3500 kcal = 1 lb of fat, ~500 kcal restriction daily equates to a weight reduction of 1 lb per week. Diets restricted in carbohydrate typically provide a rapid initial weight loss. However, after 1 year, the amount of weight reduction is usually unchanged. Thus, adherence to the diet is more important than which diet is chosen. Moreover, there is concern about diets enriched in saturated fat, particularly for patients at risk for CVD. Therefore, a high quality of the diet—i.e., enriched in fruits, vegetables, whole grains, lean poultry, and fish—should be encouraged to provide the maximum overall health benefit.

Physical Activity Before a physical activity recommendation is provided to patients with the metabolic syndrome, it is important to ensure that this increased activity does not incur risk. Some high-risk patients should undergo formal cardiovascular evaluation before initiating an exercise program. For the inactive participant, gradual increases in physical activity should be encouraged to enhance adherence and to avoid injury. Although increases in physical activity can lead to modest weight reduction, 60–90 min of daily activity is required to achieve this goal. Even if an overweight or obese adult is unable to achieve this level of activity, they still derive a significant health benefit from at least 30 min of moderate intensity daily activity. The caloric value of 30 min of a variety of activities can be found at *http://www.americanheart.org/presenter.jhtml?identifier=3040364*. Of note, a variety of routine activities—such as gardening, walking, and housecleaning—require moderate caloric expenditure. Thus, physical activity need not be defined solely in terms of formal exercise such as jogging, swimming, or tennis.

Obesity (See also Chap. 17) In some patients with the metabolic syndrome, treatment options need to extend beyond lifestyle intervention. Weight-loss drugs come in two major classes: appetite suppressants and absorption inhibitors. Appetite suppressants approved by the U.S. Food and Drug Administration include phentermine (for short-term use only, 3 months) and sibutramine. Orlistat inhibits fat absorption by ~30% and is moderately effective compared to placebo (~5% weight loss). Orlistat has been shown to reduce the incidence of type 2 diabetes, an effect that was especially evident in patients with baseline IGT.

Bariatric surgery is an option for patients with the metabolic syndrome who have a body mass index (BMI) of >40 kg/m^2 or >35 kg/m^2 with comorbidities. Gastric bypass results in a dramatic weight reduction and improvement in the features of metabolic syndrome. At present, however, a survival benefit has yet to be realized.

LDL CHOLESTEROL (See also Chap. 21) The rationale for the NCEP:ATP III panel to develop criteria for the metabolic syndrome was to go beyond LDL cholesterol in identifying and reducing risk for CVD. The working assumption by the panel was that LDL cholesterol goals had already been achieved, and increasing evidence supports a linear reduction in CVD events with progressive lowering of LDL cholesterol. For patients with the metabolic syndrome and diabetes, LDL cholesterol should be reduced to <100 mg/dL and perhaps further in patients with a history of CVD events. For patients with the metabolic syndrome without diabetes, the Framingham risk score may predict a 10-year CVD risk that exceeds 20%. In these subjects, LDL cholesterol should also be reduced to <100 mg/dL. With a 10-year risk of <20%, however, the targeted LDL cholesterol goal is <130 mg/dL.

Diets restricted in saturated fats (<7% of calories), trans fat (as few as possible), and cholesterol (<200 mg daily) should be applied aggressively. If LDL cholesterol remains above goal, then pharmacologic intervention is needed. Statins (HMG-CoA reductase inhibitors), which produce a 20–60% lowering of LDL cholesterol, are generally the first choice for medication intervention. Of note, for each doubling of the statin dose, there is only ~6% additional lowering of LDL cholesterol. Side effects are rare and include an increase in hepatic transaminases and/or myopathy. The cholesterol absorption inhibitor ezetimibe is well tolerated and should be the second choice. Ezetimibe typically reduces LDL cholesterol by 15–20%. The bile acid sequestrants cholestyramine and colestipol are more effective than ezetimibe but must be used with caution in patients with the metabolic syndrome because they often increase triglycerides. In general, bile sequestrants should not be administered when fasting triglycerides are >200 mg/dL. Side effects include gastrointestinal symptoms (palatability, bloating, belching, constipation, anal irritation). Nicotinic acid has modest LDL cholesterol–lowering capabilities (<20%). Fibrates are best employed to lower LDL cholesterol when both LDL cholesterol and nontriglycerides are elevated. Fenofibrate may be more effective than gemfibrozil in this group.

TRIGLYCERIDES The NCEP:ATPIII has focused on non-HDL cholesterol rather than triglycerides. However, a fasting triglyceride value of <150 mg/dL is recommended. In general, the response of fasting triglycerides relates to the amount of weight reduction achieved. A weight reduction of >10% is necessary to lower fasting triglycerides.

A fibrate (gemfibrozil or fenofibrate) is the drug of choice to lower fasting triglycerides and typically achieves a 35–50% reduction. Concomitant administration with drugs metabolized by the 3A4 cytochrome P450 system (including some statins) greatly increases the risk of myopathy. In these cases, fenofibrate may be preferable to gemfibrozil. In the Veterans Affairs HDL Intervention Trial (VA-HIT), gemfibrozil was administered to men with known CHD and levels of HDL cholesterol <40 mg/dL. A coronary disease event and mortality benefit was experienced predominantly in men with hyperinsulinemia and/or diabetes, many of whom retrospectively had the metabolic syndrome. Of note, the amount of triglyceride lowering in the VA-HIT did not predict benefit. Although levels of LDL cholesterol did not change, a decrease in LDL particle number related to benefit. Although several additional clinical trials have been performed, these have not shown clear evidence that fibrates reduce CVD risk as a consequence of triglyceride lowering.

Other drugs that lower triglycerides include statins, nicotinic acid, and high doses of omega-3 fatty acids. When choosing a statin for this purpose, the dose must be high for the "less potent" statins (lovastatin, pravastatin, fluvastatin) or intermediate for the "more potent" statins (simvastatin, atorvastatin, rosuvastatin). The effect of nicotinic acid on fasting triglycerides is dose-related and less than fibrates (~20–40%). In patients with the metabolic syndrome and diabetes, nicotinic acid may increase fasting glucose. Omega-3 fatty acid preparations that include high doses of docosahexaenoic acid and eicosapentaenoic acid (~3.0–4.5 g daily) lower fasting triglycerides by ~40%. No interactions with fibrates or statins occur, and the main side effect is eructation with a fishy taste. This can be partially blocked by ingesting the nutraceutical after freezing. Clinical trials of nicotinic acid or high-dose omega-3 fatty acids in patients with the metabolic syndrome have not been reported.

HDL CHOLESTEROL Beyond weight reduction, there are very few lipid-modifying compounds that increase HDL cholesterol. Statins, fibrates, and bile acid sequestrants have modest effects (5–10%), and there is no effect on HDL cholesterol with ezetimibe or omega-3 fatty acids. Nicotinic acid is the only currently available drug with predictable HDL cholesterol–raising properties. The response is dose-related and can increase HDL cholesterol ~30% above baseline. There is little evidence at present that raising HDL has a benefit on CVD events independent of lowering LDL cholesterol, particularly in patients with the metabolic syndrome.

BLOOD PRESSURE The direct relationship between blood pressure and all-cause mortality has been well established, including patients with hypertension (>140/90) versus prehypertension (>120/80 but <140/90) versus individuals with normal blood pressure (<120/80). In patients with the metabolic syndrome without diabetes, the best choice for the first antihypertensive should usually be an angiotensin-converting enzyme (ACE) inhibitor or an angiotensin II receptor blocker, as these two classes of drugs appear to reduce the incidence of new-onset type 2 diabetes. In all patients with hypertension, a sodium-restricted diet enriched in fruits and vegetables and low-fat dairy products should be advocated. Home monitoring of blood pressure may assist in maintaining good blood pressure control.

IMPAIRED FASTING GLUCOSE (See also Chap. 19) In patients with the metabolic syndrome and type 2 diabetes, aggressive glycemic control may favorably modify fasting triglycerides and/or HDL cholesterol. In those patients with IFG without a diagnosis of diabetes, a lifestyle intervention that includes weight reduction, dietary fat restriction, and increased physical activity has been shown to reduce the incidence of type 2 diabetes. Metformin has also been shown to reduce the incidence of diabetes, although the effect was less than that seen with lifestyle intervention.

INSULIN RESISTANCE (See also Chap. 19) Several drug classes [biguanides, thiazolidinediones (TZDs)] increase insulin sensitivity. If insulin resistance is the primary pathophysiologic mechanism for the metabolic syndrome, then representative drugs in these classes should reduce its prevalence. Both metformin and TZDs enhance insulin action in the liver and suppress endogenous glucose production. TZDs, but not metformin, also improve insulin-mediated glucose uptake in muscle and adipose tissue. Benefits of both drugs have also been seen in patients with NAFLD and PCOS, and they have been shown to reduce markers of inflammation and small dense LDL. In general, the beneficial effects of TZDs appear superior to those of metformin.

FURTHER READINGS

Alberti KG et al: The IDF Epidemiology Task Force Consensus Group. The metabolic syndrome—A new worldwide definition. Lancet 366:1059, 2005

Cornier MA et al: The metabolic syndrome. Endocr Rev 29:777, 2008

Eckel RH et al: The metabolic syndrome. Lancet 365:1415, 2005

Expert Panel on Detection, Evaluation, and Treatment of High Blood Cholesterol in Adults: Executive summary of the third report of the National Cholesterol Education Program (NCEP) expert panel on detection, evaluation, and treatment of high blood cholesterol in adults (Adult Treatment Panel III). JAMA 285:2486, 2001

Ford ES: Prevalence of the metabolic syndrome defined by the International Diabetes Federation among adults in the U.S. Diabetes Care 28:2745, 2005

Grundy SM et al: Diagnosis and management of the metabolic syndrome. An American Heart Association/National Heart, Lung, and Blood Institute Scientific statement. Circulation 112:2735, 2005

Kahn R et al: The metabolic syndrome: Time for a critical appraisal. Joint statement from the American Diabetes Association and the European Association for the Study of Diabetes. Diabetes Care 28:2289, 2005

Saleem U et al: Plasma carboxy-terminal provasopressin (copeptin): A novel marker of insulin resistance and metabolic syndrome. J Clin Endocrinol Metab 94:2558, 2009

Stewart PM et al: Selective inhibitors of 11beta-hydroxysteroid dehydrogenase type 1 for patients with metabolic syndrome: Is the target liver, fat, or both? Diabetes 58:14, 2009

Zimmet P et al: The metabolic syndrome: Progress towards one definition for an epidemic of our time. Nat Clin Pract Endocrinol Metab 4:239, 2008

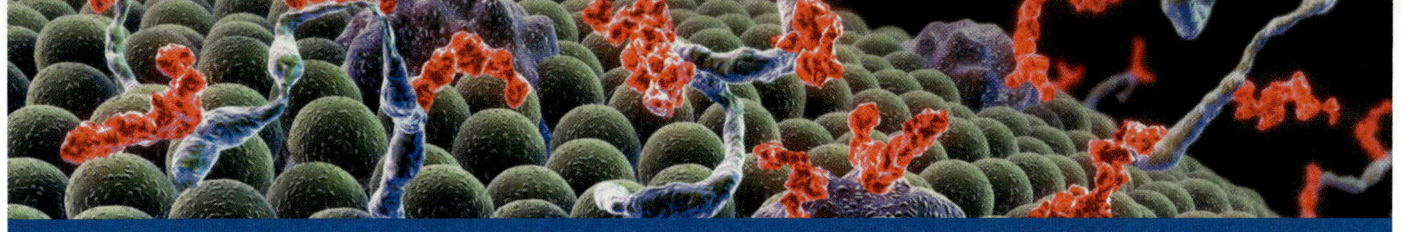

CHAPTER 19

DIABETES MELLITUS

Alvin C. Powers

Diabetes mellitus (DM) refers to a group of common metabolic disorders that share the phenotype of hyperglycemia. Several distinct types of DM exist and are caused by a complex interaction of genetics and environmental factors. Depending on the etiology of the DM, factors contributing to hyperglycemia include reduced insulin secretion, decreased glucose utilization, and increased glucose production. The metabolic dysregulation associated with DM causes secondary pathophysiologic changes in multiple organ systems that impose a tremendous burden on the individual with diabetes and on the health care system. In the United States, DM is the leading cause of end-stage renal disease (ESRD), nontraumatic lower extremity amputations, and adult blindness. It also predisposes to cardiovascular diseases. With an increasing incidence worldwide, DM will be a leading cause of morbidity and mortality for the foreseeable future.

CLASSIFICATION

DM is classified on the basis of the pathogenic process that leads to hyperglycemia, as opposed to earlier criteria such as age of onset or type of therapy (**Fig. 19-1**). The two broad categories of DM are designated type 1 and type 2 (**Table 19-1**). Both types of diabetes are preceded by a phase of abnormal glucose homeostasis as the pathogenic process progresses. Type 1 diabetes is the result of complete or near-total insulin deficiency. Type 2 DM is a heterogeneous group of disorders characterized by variable degrees of insulin resistance, impaired insulin secretion, and increased glucose production. Distinct genetic and metabolic defects in insulin action and/or secretion give rise to the common phenotype of hyperglycemia in type 2 DM and have important potential therapeutic implications now that pharmacologic agents are available to target specific

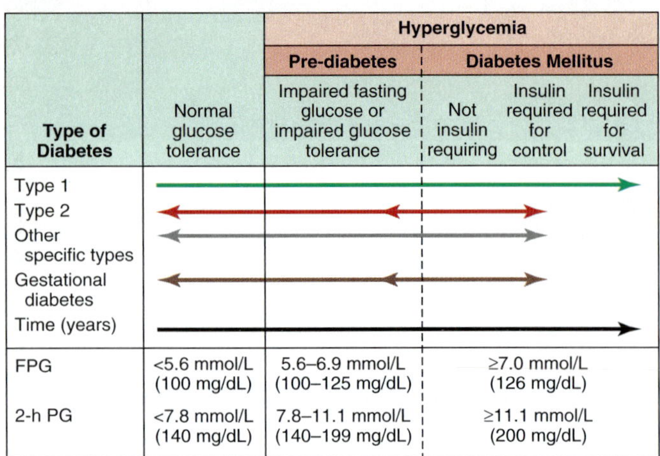

FIGURE 19-1

Spectrum of glucose homeostasis and diabetes mellitus (DM). The spectrum from normal glucose tolerance to diabetes in type 1 DM, type 2 DM, other specific types of diabetes, and gestational DM is shown from left to right. In most types of DM, the individual traverses from normal glucose tolerance to impaired glucose tolerance to overt diabetes. Arrows indicate that changes in glucose tolerance may be bi-directional in some types of diabetes. For example, individuals with type 2 DM may return to the impaired glucose tolerance category with weight loss; in gestational DM, diabetes may revert to impaired glucose tolerance or even normal glucose tolerance after delivery. The fasting plasma glucose (FPG) and 2-h plasma glucose (PG), after a glucose challenge for the different categories of glucose tolerance, are shown at the lower part of the figure. These values do not apply to the diagnosis of gestational DM. Some types of DM may or may not require insulin for survival, hence the dotted line. (Conventional units are used in the figure.) (*Adapted from the American Diabetes Association, 2007.*)

metabolic derangements. Type 2 DM is preceded by a period of abnormal glucose homeostasis classified as impaired fasting glucose (IFG) or impaired glucose tolerance (IGT).

Two features of the current classification of DM diverge from previous classifications. First, the terms *insulin-dependent diabetes mellitus* (IDDM) and *non-insulin-dependent diabetes mellitus* (NIDDM) are obsolete. Since many individuals with type 2 DM eventually require insulin treatment for control of glycemia, the use of the term NIDDM generated considerable confusion. A second difference is that age is not a criterion in the classification system. Although type 1 DM most commonly develops before the age of 30, an autoimmune beta cell destructive process can develop at any age. It is estimated that between 5 and 10% of individuals who develop DM after age 30 have type 1 DM. Likewise, type 2 DM more typically develops with increasing age but is now being diagnosed more frequently in children and young adults, particularly in obese adolescents.

TABLE 19-1

ETIOLOGIC CLASSIFICATION OF DIABETES MELLITUS

I. Type 1 diabetes (β-cell destruction, usually leading to absolute insulin deficiency)
   A. Immune-mediated
   B. Idiopathic
II. Type 2 diabetes (may range from predominantly insulin resistance with relative insulin deficiency to a predominantly insulin secretory defect with insulin resistance)
III. Other specific types of diabetes
   A. Genetic defects of β-cell function characterized by mutations in:
      1. Hepatocyte nuclear transcription factor (HNF) 4α (MODY 1)
      2. Glucokinase (MODY 2)
      3. HNF-1α (MODY 3)
      4. Insulin promoter factor-1 (IPF-1; MODY 4)
      5. HNF-1β (MODY 5)
      6. NeuroD1 (MODY 6)
      7. Mitochondrial DNA
      8. Subunits of ATP-sensitive potassium channel
      9. Proinsulin or insulin conversion
   B. Genetic defects in insulin action
      1. Type A insulin resistance
      2. Leprechaunism
      3. Rabson-Mendenhall syndrome
      4. Lipodystrophy syndromes
   C. Diseases of the exocrine pancreas—pancreatitis, pancreatectomy, neoplasia, cystic fibrosis, hemochromatosis, fibrocalculous pancreatopathy, mutations in carboxyl ester lipase
   D. Endocrinopathies—acromegaly, Cushing's syndrome, glucagonoma, pheochromocytoma, hyperthyroidism, somatostatinoma, aldosteronoma
   E. Drug- or chemical-induced—Vacor, pentamidine, nicotinic acid, glucocorticoids, thyroid hormone, diazoxide, β-adrenergic agonists, thiazides, phenytoin, α-interferon, protease inhibitors, clozapine
   F. Infections—congenital rubella, cytomegalovirus, coxsackie
   G. Uncommon forms of immune-mediated diabetes—"stiff-person" syndrome, anti-insulin receptor antibodies

Note: MODY, maturity-onset diabetes of the young.
Source: Adapted from American Diabetes Association, 2007.

OTHER TYPES OF DM

Other etiologies for DM include specific genetic defects in insulin secretion or action, metabolic abnormalities that impair insulin secretion, mitochondrial abnormalities, and a host of conditions that impair glucose tolerance (Table 19-1). *Maturity-onset diabetes of the young* (MODY) is a subtype of DM characterized by autosomal dominant inheritance, early onset of hyperglycemia (usually <25 years), and impairment in insulin secretion. Mutations in the insulin receptor cause a group of rare disorders characterized by severe insulin resistance.

DM can result from pancreatic exocrine disease when the majority of pancreatic islets are destroyed. Hormones that antagonize insulin action can also lead to DM. Thus, DM is often a feature of endocrinopathies such as acromegaly and Cushing's disease. Viral infections have been implicated in pancreatic islet destruction but are an extremely rare cause of DM. A form of acute onset of type 1 diabetes, termed *fulminant diabetes*, has been noted in Japan and may be related to viral infection of islets.

GESTATIONAL DIABETES MELLITUS

Glucose intolerance may develop during pregnancy. Insulin resistance is related to the metabolic changes of late pregnancy, and the increased insulin requirements may lead to IGT. Gestational diabetes mellitus (GDM) occurs in ~4% of pregnancies in the United States; most women revert to normal glucose tolerance post-partum but have a substantial risk (30–60%) of developing DM later in life.

EPIDEMIOLOGY

The worldwide prevalence of DM has risen dramatically over the past two decades, from an estimated 30 million cases in 1985 to 177 million in 2000. Based on current trends, >360 million individuals will have diabetes by the year 2030 (**Fig. 19-2**). Although the prevalence of both type 1 and type 2 DM is increasing worldwide, the prevalence of type 2 DM is rising much more rapidly because of increasing obesity and reduced activity levels as countries become more industrialized. This is true in most countries, and 6 of the top 10 countries with the highest rates are in Asia. In the United States, the Centers for Disease Control and Prevention (CDC) estimated that 20.8 million persons, or 7% of the population, had diabetes in 2005 (~30% of individuals with diabetes were undiagnosed). Approximately 1.5 million individuals (>20 years) were newly diagnosed with diabetes in 2005. DM increases with aging. In 2005, the prevalence of DM in the United Sates was estimated to be 0.22% in those <20 years and 9.6% in those >20 years. In individuals >60 years, the prevalence of DM was 20.9%. The prevalence is similar in men and women throughout most age ranges (10.5% and 8.8% in individuals >20 years) but is slightly greater in men >60 years. Worldwide estimates project that in 2030 the greatest number of individuals with diabetes will be 45–64 years of age.

There is considerable geographic variation in the incidence of both type 1 and type 2 DM. Scandinavia has the highest incidence of type 1 DM (e.g., in Finland, the incidence is 35/100,000 per year). The Pacific Rim has a much lower rate (in Japan and China, the incidence is 1–3/100,000 per year) of type 1 DM; Northern Europe and the United States have an intermediate rate (8–17/100,000 per year). Much of the increased risk of type 1 DM is believed to reflect the frequency of high-risk HLA alleles among ethnic groups in different geographic locations. The prevalence of type 2 DM and its harbinger, IGT, is highest in certain Pacific islands, intermediate in countries such as India and the United States, and relatively low in Russia. This variability is likely due to

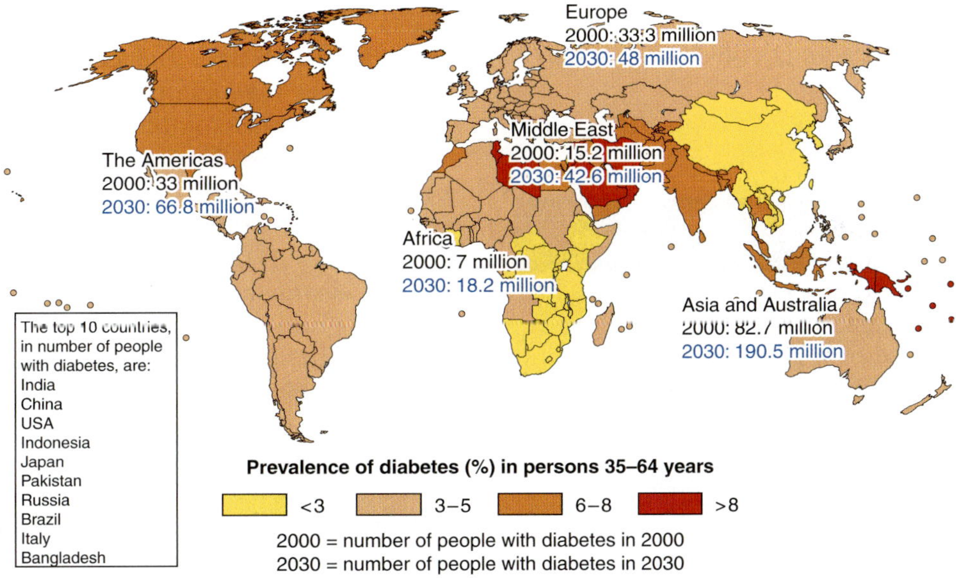

FIGURE 19-2

Worldwide prevalence of diabetes mellitus. The prevalence of diabetes in 2000 and the projected prevalence in 2030 are shown by geographical region. (*Used with permission from Diabetes Action Now: An Initiative of the World Health Organization and the International Diabetes Federation, 2004, as adapted from S Wild et al: Diabetes Care 27:1047, 2004.*)

genetic, behavioral, and environmental factors. DM prevalence also varies among different ethnic populations within a given country. In 2005, the CDC estimated that the prevalence of DM in the United States (age >20 years) was 13.3% in African Americans, 9.5% in Latinos, 15.1% in Native Americans (American Indians and Alaska natives), and 8.7% in non-Hispanic whites. Individuals belonging to Asian-American or Pacific-Islander ethnic groups in Hawaii are twice as likely to have diabetes compared to non-Hispanic whites. The onset of type 2 DM occurs, on average, at an earlier age in ethnic groups other than non-Hispanic whites.

Diabetes is a major cause of mortality, but several studies indicate that diabetes is likely underreported as a cause of death. In the United States, diabetes was listed as the sixth leading cause of death in 2002; a recent estimate suggested that diabetes was the fifth leading cause of death worldwide and was responsible for almost 3 million deaths annually (1.7–5.2% of deaths worldwide).

DIAGNOSIS

The National Diabetes Data Group and World Health Organization have issued diagnostic criteria for DM (Table 19-2) based on the following premises: (1) the spectrum of fasting plasma glucose (FPG) and the response to an oral glucose load (OGTT—oral glucose tolerance test) varies among normal individuals, and (2) DM is defined as the level of glycemia at which diabetes-specific complications occur rather than on deviations from a population-based mean. For example, the prevalence of retinopathy in Native Americans (Pima Indian population) begins to increase at a FPG >6.4 mmol/L (116 mg/dL) (Fig. 19-3).

Glucose tolerance is classified into three categories based on the FPG (Fig. 19-1): (1) FPG <5.6 mmol/L

TABLE 19-2

CRITERIA FOR THE DIAGNOSIS OF DIABETES MELLITUS

- Symptoms of diabetes plus random blood glucose concentration ≥11.1 mmol/L (200 mg/dL)[a] *or*
- Fasting plasma glucose ≥7.0 mmol/L (126 mg/dL)[b] *or*
- Two-hour plasma glucose ≥11.1 mmol/L (200 mg/dL) during an oral glucose tolerance test[c]

[a]Random is defined as without regard to time since the last meal.
[b]Fasting is defined as no caloric intake for at least 8 h.
[c]The test should be performed using a glucose load containing the equivalent of 75 g anhydrous glucose dissolved in water; not recommended for routine clinical use.
Note: In the absence of unequivocal hyperglycemia and acute metabolic decompensation, these criteria should be confirmed by repeat testing on a different day.
Source: Adapted from American Diabetes Association, 2007.

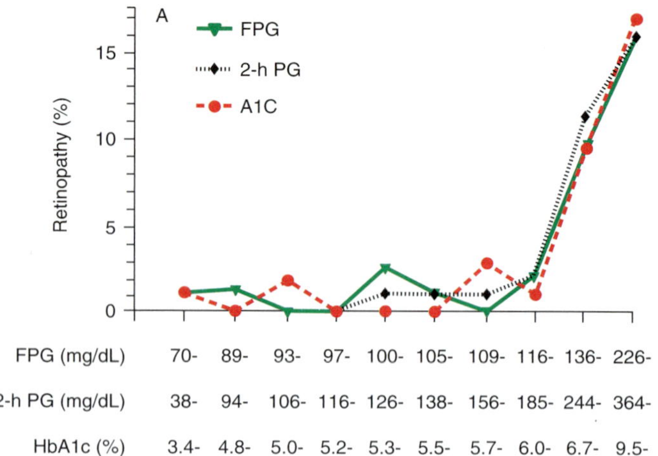

FIGURE 19-3

Relationship of diabetes-specific complication and glucose tolerance. This figure shows the incidence of retinopathy in Pima Indians as a function of the fasting plasma glucose (FPG), the 2-h plasma glucose after a 75-g oral glucose challenge (2-h PG), or glycated hemoglobin (A1C). Note that the incidence of retinopathy greatly increases at a fasting plasma glucose >116 mg/dL, or a 2-h plasma glucose of 185 mg/dL, or a A1C >6.0%. (Blood glucose values are shown in mg/dL; to convert to mmol/L, divide value by 18.) [*Copyright 2002, American Diabetes Association. From Diabetes Care 25(Suppl 1): S5–S20, 2002.*]

(100 mg/dL) is considered normal; (2) FPG = 5.6–6.9 mmol/L (100–125 mg/dL) is defined as IFG; and (3) FPG ≥7.0 mmol/L (126 mg/dL) warrants the diagnosis of DM. Based on the OGTT, IGT is defined as plasma glucose levels between 7.8 and 11.1 mmol/L (140 and 199 mg/dL) and diabetes is defined as a glucose >11.1 mmol/L (200 mg/dL) 2 h after a 75-g oral glucose load (Table 19-2). Some individuals have both IFG and IGT. Individuals with IFG and/or IGT, recently designated *pre-diabetes* by the American Diabetes Association (ADA), are at substantial risk for developing type 2 DM (25–40% risk over the next 5 years) and have an increased risk of cardiovascular disease.

The current criteria for the diagnosis of DM emphasize that the FPG is the most reliable and convenient test for identifying DM in asymptomatic individuals. A random plasma glucose concentration ≥11.1 mmol/L (200 mg/dL) accompanied by classic symptoms of DM (polyuria, polydipsia, weight loss) is sufficient for the diagnosis of DM (Table 19-2). Oral glucose tolerance testing, although still a valid means for diagnosing DM, is not recommended as part of routine care.

Some investigators have advocated the hemoglobin A1C (A1C) as a diagnostic test for DM. Though there is a strong correlation between elevations in the plasma glucose and the A1C, the relationship between the FPG and the A1C in individuals with normal glucose tolerance or mild glucose intolerance is less clear, and thus the use of the A1C is not currently recommended to diagnose diabetes.

The diagnosis of DM has profound implications for an individual from both a medical and financial standpoint. Thus, these diagnostic criteria must be satisfied before assigning the diagnosis of DM. Abnormalities on screening tests for diabetes should be repeated before making a definitive diagnosis of DM, unless acute metabolic derangements or a markedly elevated plasma glucose is present (Table 19-2). The revised criteria also allow for the diagnosis of DM to be withdrawn in situations where the FPG reverts to normal.

SCREENING

Widespread use of the FPG as a screening test for type 2 DM is recommended because (1) a large number of individuals who meet the current criteria for DM are asymptomatic and unaware that they have the disorder, (2) epidemiologic studies suggest that type 2 DM may be present for up to a decade before diagnosis, (3) as many as 50% of individuals with type 2 DM have one or more diabetes-specific complications at the time of their diagnosis, and (4) treatment of type 2 DM may favorably alter the natural history of DM. The ADA recommends screening all individuals >45 years every 3 years and screening individuals at an earlier age if they are overweight [body mass index (BMI) >25 kg/m^2] and have one additional risk factor for diabetes (**Table 19-3**). In contrast to type 2 DM, a long asymptomatic period of hyperglycemia is rare prior to the diagnosis of type 1 DM. A number of immunologic markers for type 1 DM are becoming available, but their routine use is discouraged pending the identification of clinically beneficial interventions for individuals at high risk for developing type 1 DM.

TABLE 19-3

RISK FACTORS FOR TYPE 2 DIABETES MELLITUS
Family history of diabetes (i.e., parent or sibling with type 2 diabetes)
Obesity (BMI ≥25 kg/m^2)
Habitual physical inactivity
Race/ethnicity (e.g., African American, Latino, Native American, Asian American, Pacific Islander)
Previously identified IFG or IGT
History of GDM or delivery of baby >4 kg (>9 lb)
Hypertension (blood pressure ≥140/90 mmHg)
HDL cholesterol level <35 mg/dL (0.90 mmol/L) and/or a triglyceride level >250 mg/dL (2.82 mmol/L)
Polycystic ovary syndrome or acanthosis nigricans
History of vascular disease

Note: BMI, body mass index; IFG, impaired fasting glucose; IGT, impaired glucose tolerance; GDM, gestational diabetes mellitus; HDL, high-density lipoprotein.
Source: Adapted from American Diabetes Association, 2007.

INSULIN BIOSYNTHESIS, SECRETION, AND ACTION

BIOSYNTHESIS

Insulin is produced in the beta cells of the pancreatic islets. It is initially synthesized as a single-chain 86-amino-acid precursor polypeptide, preproinsulin. Subsequent proteolytic processing removes the amino-terminal signal peptide, giving rise to proinsulin. Proinsulin is structurally related to insulin-like growth factors I and II, which bind weakly to the insulin receptor. Cleavage of an internal 31-residue fragment from proinsulin generates the C peptide and the A (21 amino acids) and B (30 amino acids) chains of insulin, which are connected by disulfide bonds. The mature insulin molecule and C peptide are stored together and cosecreted from secretory granules in the beta cells. Because the C peptide is cleared more slowly than insulin, it is a useful marker of insulin secretion and allows discrimination of endogenous and exogenous sources of insulin in the evaluation of hypoglycemia (Chaps. 20 and 22). Pancreatic beta cells cosecrete islet amyloid polypeptide (IAPP) or amylin, a 37-amino-acid peptide, along with insulin. The role of IAPP in normal physiology is unclear, but it is the major component of the amyloid fibrils found in the islets of patients with type 2 diabetes, and an analogue is sometimes used in treating both type 1 and type 2 DM. Human insulin is now produced by recombinant DNA technology; structural alterations at one or more residues are useful for modifying its physical and pharmacologic characteristics.

SECRETION

Glucose is the key regulator of insulin secretion by the pancreatic beta cell, although amino acids, ketones, various nutrients, gastrointestinal peptides, and neurotransmitters also influence insulin secretion. Glucose levels >3.9 mmol/L (70 mg/dL) stimulate insulin synthesis, primarily by enhancing protein translation and processing. Glucose stimulation of insulin secretion begins with its transport into the beta cell by the GLUT2 glucose transporter (**Fig. 19-4**). Glucose phosphorylation by glucokinase is the rate-limiting step that controls glucose-regulated insulin secretion. Further metabolism of glucose-6-phosphate via glycolysis generates ATP, which inhibits the activity of an ATP-sensitive K^+ channel. This channel consists of two separate proteins: one is the binding site for certain oral hypoglycemics (e.g., sulfonylureas, meglitinides); the other is an inwardly rectifying K^+ channel protein (Kir6.2). Inhibition of this K^+ channel induces beta cell membrane depolarization, which opens voltage-dependent calcium channels (leading to an influx of calcium) and stimulates insulin secretion. Insulin secretory profiles reveal a pulsatile pattern of hormone release, with small secretory bursts occurring about every 10 min, superimposed

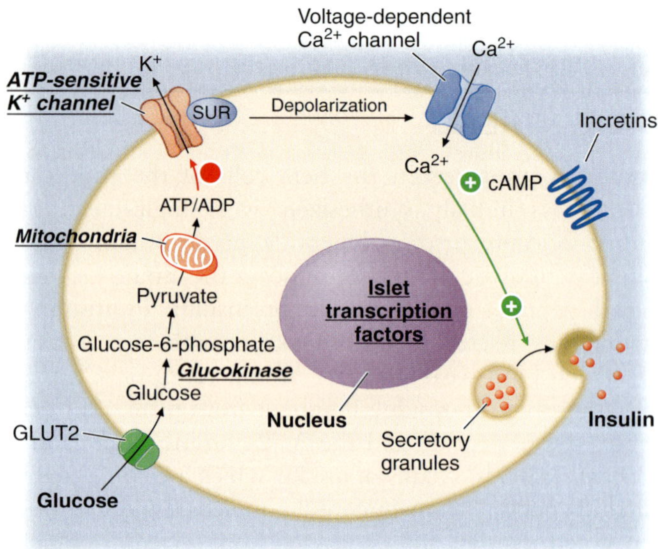

FIGURE 19-4

Diabetes and abnormalities in glucose-stimulated insulin secretion. Glucose and other nutrients regulate insulin secretion by the pancreatic beta cell. Glucose is transported by the GLUT2 glucose transporter; subsequent glucose metabolism by the beta cell alters ion channel activity, leading to insulin secretion. The SUR receptor is the binding site for drugs that act as insulin secretagogues. Mutations in the events or proteins underlined are a cause of maturity-onset diabetes of the young (MODY) or other forms of diabetes. SUR, sulfonylurea receptor; ATP, adenosine triphosphate; ADP, adenosine diphosphate, cAMP, cyclic adenosine monophosphate. [*Adapted from WL Lowe, in JL Jameson (ed): Principles of Molecular Medicine. Totowa, NJ, Humana, 1998.*]

on greater-amplitude oscillations of about 80–150 min. Incretins are released from neuroendocrine cells of the gastrointestinal tract following food ingestion and amplify glucose-stimulated insulin secretion and suppress glucagon secretion. Glucagon-like peptide 1 (GLP-1), the most potent incretin, is released from L cells in the small intestine and stimulates insulin secretion only when the blood glucose is above the fasting level. Incretin analogues, such as exena-tide, are being used to enhance endogenous insulin secretion.

ACTION

Once insulin is secreted into the portal venous system, ~50% is degraded by the liver. Unextracted insulin enters the systemic circulation where it binds to receptors in target sites. Insulin binding to its receptor stimulates intrinsic tyrosine kinase activity, leading to receptor autophosphorylation and the recruitment of intracellular signaling molecules, such as insulin receptor substrates (IRSs) (Fig. 19-5). IRSs and other adaptor proteins initiate a complex cascade of phosphorylation and dephosphorylation reactions, resulting in the widespread metabolic and mitogenic effects of insulin. As an example, activation of the phosphatidylinositol-3′-kinase (PI-3-kinase) pathway stimulates translocation of glucose transporters (e.g., GLUT4) to the cell surface, an event that is crucial for glucose uptake by skeletal muscle and fat. Activation of other insulin receptor signaling pathways induces glycogen synthesis, protein synthesis, lipogenesis, and regulation of various genes in insulin-responsive cells.

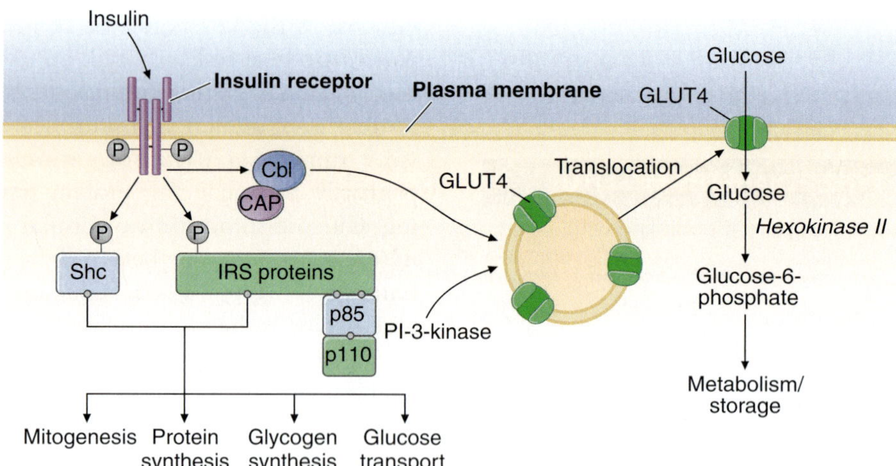

FIGURE 19-5

Insulin signal transduction pathway in skeletal muscle. The insulin receptor has intrinsic tyrosine kinase activity and interacts with insulin receptor substrate (IRS and Shc) proteins. A number of "docking" proteins bind to these cellular proteins and initiate the metabolic actions of insulin [GrB-2, SOS, SHP-2, p65, p110, and phosphatidylinositol-3′-kinase (PI-3-kinase)]. Insulin increases glucose transport through PI-3-kinase and the Cbl pathway, which promotes the translocation of intracellular vesicles containing GLUT4 glucose transporter to the plasma membrane. [*Adapted from WL Lowe, in Principles of Molecular Medicine, JL Jameson (ed). Totowa, NJ, Humana, 1998; A Virkamaki et al: J Clin Invest 103:931, 1999. For additional details see AR Saltiel, CR Kahn: Nature 414:799, 2001.*]

Glucose homeostasis reflects a balance between hepatic glucose production and peripheral glucose uptake and utilization. Insulin is the most important regulator of this metabolic equilibrium, but neural input, metabolic signals, and other hormones (e.g., glucagon) result in integrated control of glucose supply and utilization (Chap. 20; see Fig. 20-1). In the fasting state, low insulin levels increase glucose production by promoting hepatic gluconeogenesis and glycogenolysis and reduce glucose uptake in insulin-sensitive tissues (skeletal muscle and fat), thereby promoting mobilization of stored precursors such as amino acids and free fatty acids (lipolysis). Glucagon, secreted by pancreatic alpha cells when blood glucose or insulin levels are low, stimulates glycogenolysis and gluconeogenesis by the liver and renal medulla. Postprandially, the glucose load elicits a rise in insulin and fall in glucagon, leading to a reversal of these processes. Insulin, an anabolic hormone, promotes the storage of carbohydrate and fat and protein synthesis. The major portion of postprandial glucose is utilized by skeletal muscle, an effect of insulin-stimulated glucose uptake. Other tissues, most notably the brain, utilize glucose in an insulin-independent fashion.

PATHOGENESIS

TYPE 1 DM

Type 1 DM is the result of interactions of genetic, environmental, and immunologic factors that ultimately lead to the destruction of the pancreatic beta cells and insulin deficiency. Type 1 DM results from autoimmune beta cell destruction and most, but not all, individuals have evidence of islet-directed autoimmunity. Some individuals who have the clinical phenotype of type 1 DM lack immunologic markers indicative of an autoimmune process involving the beta cells. These individuals are thought to develop insulin deficiency by unknown, nonimmune mechanisms and are ketosis prone; many are African American or Asian in heritage. The temporal development of type 1 DM is shown schematically as a function of beta cell mass in Fig. 19-6. Individuals with a genetic susceptibility have normal beta cell mass at birth but begin to lose beta cells secondary to autoimmune destruction that occurs over months to years. This autoimmune process is thought to be triggered by an infectious or environmental stimulus and to be sustained by a beta cell–specific molecule. In the majority, immunologic markers appear after the triggering event but before diabetes becomes clinically overt. Beta cell mass then begins to decline, and insulin secretion becomes progressively impaired, although normal glucose tolerance is maintained. The rate of decline in beta cell mass varies widely among individuals, with some patients progressing rapidly to clinical diabetes and others evolving more slowly. Features of diabetes do not become evident until a majority of beta cells are destroyed (~80%). At this point, residual functional

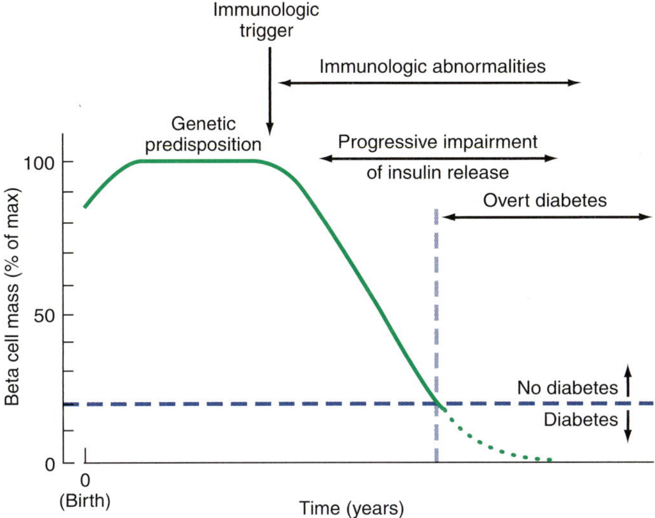

FIGURE 19-6

Temporal model for development of type 1 diabetes. Individuals with a genetic predisposition are exposed to an immunologic trigger that initiates an autoimmune process, resulting in a gradual decline in beta cell mass. The downward slope of the beta cell mass varies among individuals and may not be continuous. This progressive impairment in insulin release results in diabetes when ~80% of the beta cell mass is destroyed. A "honeymoon" phase may be seen in the first 1 or 2 years after the onset of diabetes and is associated with reduced insulin requirements. [*Adapted from Medical Management of Type 1 Diabetes, 3d ed, JS Skyler (ed). American Diabetes Association, Alexandria, VA, 1998.*]

beta cells still exist but are insufficient in number to maintain glucose tolerance. The events that trigger the transition from glucose intolerance to frank diabetes are often associated with increased insulin requirements, as might occur during infections or puberty. After the initial clinical presentation of type 1 DM, a "honeymoon" phase may ensue during which time glycemic control is achieved with modest doses of insulin or, rarely, insulin is not needed. However, this fleeting phase of endogenous insulin production from residual beta cells disappears as the autoimmune process destroys the remaining beta cells, and the individual becomes completely insulin deficient.

GENETIC CONSIDERATIONS

Susceptibility to type 1 DM involves multiple genes. The concordance of type 1 DM in identical twins ranges between 30 and 70%, indicating that additional modifying factors are likely involved in determining whether diabetes develops. The major susceptibility gene for type 1 DM is located in the HLA region on chromosome 6. Polymorphisms in the HLA complex account for 40–50% of the genetic risk of developing type 1 DM. This region contains genes that encode the class II MHC molecules, which present antigen to helper

T cells and thus are involved in initiating the immune response. The ability of class II MHC molecules to present antigen is dependent on the amino acid composition of their antigen-binding sites. Amino acid substitutions may influence the specificity of the immune response by altering the binding affinity of different antigens for class II molecules.

Most individuals with type 1 DM have the HLA DR3 and/or DR4 haplotype. Refinements in genotyping of HLA loci have shown that the haplotypes DQA1*0301, DQB1*0302, and DQB1*0201 are most strongly associated with type 1 DM. These haplotypes are present in 40% of children with type 1 DM as compared to 2% of the normal U.S. population. However, most individuals with predisposing haplotypes do not develop diabetes.

In addition to MHC class II associations, at least 10 different genetic loci contribute susceptibility to type 1 DM (loci recently identified include polymorphisms in the promoter region of the insulin gene, the CTLA-4 gene, interleukin-2 receptor, *IFIH1*, and PTPN22). Genes that confer protection against the development of the disease also exist. The haplotype DQA1*0102, DQB1*0602 is extremely rare in individuals with type 1 DM (<1%) and appears to provide protection from type 1 DM.

Although the risk of developing type 1 DM is increased tenfold in relatives of individuals with the disease, the risk is relatively low: 3–4% if the parent has type 1 diabetes and 5–15% in a sibling (depending on which HLA haplotypes are shared). Hence, most individuals with type 1 DM do not have a first-degree relative with this disorder.

Pathophysiology

Although other islet cell types [alpha cells (glucagon-producing), delta cells (somatostatin-producing), or PP cells (pancreatic polypeptide-producing)] are functionally and embryologically similar to beta cells and express most of the same proteins as beta cells, they are inexplicably spared from the autoimmune process. Pathologically, the pancreatic islets are infiltrated with lymphocytes (in a process termed *insulitis*). After all beta cells are destroyed, the inflammatory process abates, the islets become atrophic, and most immunologic markers disappear. Studies of the autoimmune process in humans and in animal models of type 1 DM (NOD mouse and BB rat) have identified the following abnormalities in the humoral and cellular arms of the immune system: (1) islet cell autoantibodies; (2) activated lymphocytes in the islets, peripancreatic lymph nodes, and systemic circulation; (3) T lymphocytes that proliferate when stimulated with islet proteins; and (4) release of cytokines within the insulitis. Beta cells seem to be particularly susceptible to the toxic effect of some cytokines [tumor necrosis factor α (TNF-α), interferon γ, and interleukin 1 (IL-1)]. The precise mechanisms of beta cell death are not known but may involve formation of nitric oxide metabolites, apoptosis, and direct CD8+ T cell cytotoxicity. The islet destruction is mediated by T lymphocytes rather than islet autoantibodies, as these antibodies do not generally react with the cell surface of islet cells and are not capable of transferring DM to animals. Suppression of the autoimmune process (cyclosporine, T lymphocyte antibodies) at the time of diagnosis of diabetes slows the decline in beta cell destruction, but the safety of such interventions is unknown.

Pancreatic islet molecules targeted by the autoimmune process include insulin, glutamic acid decarboxylase (GAD, the biosynthetic enzyme for the neurotransmitter GABA), ICA-512/IA-2 (homology with tyrosine phosphatases), and phogrin (insulin secretory granule protein). With the exception of insulin, none of the autoantigens are beta cell specific, which raises the question of how the beta cells are selectively destroyed. Current theories favor initiation of an autoimmune process directed at one beta cell molecule, which then spreads to other islet molecules as the immune process destroys beta cells and creates a series of secondary autoantigens. The beta cells of individuals who develop type 1 DM do not differ from beta cells of normal individuals, since islets transplanted from a genetically identical twin are destroyed by a recurrence of the autoimmune process of type 1 DM.

Immunologic Markers

Islet cell autoantibodies (ICAs) are a composite of several different antibodies directed at pancreatic islet molecules such as GAD, insulin, and IA-2/ICA-512 and serve as a marker of the autoimmune process of type 1 DM. Assays for autoantibodies to GAD-65 are commercially available. Testing for ICAs can be useful in classifying the type of DM as type 1 and in identifying nondiabetic individuals at risk for developing type 1 DM. ICAs are present in the majority of individuals (>75%) diagnosed with new-onset type 1 DM, in a significant minority of individuals with newly diagnosed type 2 DM (5–10%), and occasionally in individuals with GDM (<5%). ICAs are present in 3–4% of first-degree relatives of individuals with type 1 DM. In combination with impaired insulin secretion after IV glucose tolerance testing, they predict a >50% risk of developing type 1 DM within 5 years. Without this impairment in insulin secretion, the presence of ICAs predicts a 5-year risk of <25%. Based on these data, the risk of a first-degree relative developing type 1 DM is relatively low. At present, the measurement of ICAs in nondiabetic individuals is a research tool because no treatments have been approved to prevent the occurrence or progression to type 1 DM.

Environmental Factors

Numerous environmental events have been proposed to trigger the autoimmune process in genetically susceptible individuals; however, none have been conclusively linked to diabetes. Identification of an environmental trigger has been difficult because the event may precede the onset of DM by several years (Fig. 19-6). Putative environmental triggers include viruses (coxsackie and rubella most prominently), bovine milk proteins, and nitrosourea compounds.

Prevention of Type 1 DM

A number of interventions have successfully delayed or prevented diabetes in animal models. Some interventions have targeted the immune system directly (immunosuppression, selective T cell subset deletion, induction of immunologic tolerance to islet proteins), whereas others have prevented islet cell death by blocking cytotoxic cytokines or increasing islet resistance to the destructive process. Though results in animal models are promising, these interventions have not been successful in preventing type 1 DM in humans. The Diabetes Prevention Trial—type 1 concluded that administering insulin (IV or PO) to individuals at high risk for developing type 1 DM did not prevent type 1 DM.

In patients with new-onset type 1 diabetes, treatment with anti-CD3 monoclonal antibodies has recently been shown to slow the decline in C-peptide levels.

TYPE 2 DM

Insulin resistance and abnormal insulin secretion are central to the development of type 2 DM. Although the primary defect is controversial, most studies support the view that insulin resistance precedes an insulin secretory defect but that diabetes develops only when insulin secretion becomes inadequate.

GENETIC CONSIDERATIONS

Type 2 DM has a strong genetic component. The concordance of type 2 DM in identical twins is between 70 and 90%. Individuals with a parent with type 2 DM have an increased risk of diabetes; if both parents have type 2 DM, the risk approaches 40%. Insulin resistance, as demonstrated by reduced glucose utilization in skeletal muscle, is present in many nondiabetic, first-degree relatives of individuals with type 2 DM. The disease is polygenic and multifactorial since in addition to genetic susceptibility, environmental factors (such as obesity, nutrition, and physical activity) modulate the phenotype. The genes that predispose to type 2 DM are incompletely identified, but recent genome-wide association studies have identified several genes that convey a relatively small risk for type 2 DM (relative risk of 1.1–1.5). Most prominent is a variant of the transcription factor 7–like 2 gene that has been associated with type 2 diabetes in several populations and with impaired glucose tolerance in one population at high risk for diabetes. Genetic polymorphisms associated with type 2 diabetes have also been found in the genes encoding the peroxisome proliferator-activated receptor-γ, inward rectifying potassium channel expressed in beta cells, zinc transporter expressed in beta cells, IRS, and calpain 10. The mechanisms by which these genetic alterations increase the susceptibility to type 2 diabetes are not clear, but several are predicted to alter insulin secretion. Investigation using genome-wide scanning for polymorphisms associated with type 2 DM is ongoing.

Pathophysiology

Type 2 DM is characterized by impaired insulin secretion, insulin resistance, excessive hepatic glucose production, and abnormal fat metabolism. Obesity, particularly visceral or central (as evidenced by the hip/waist ratio), is very common in type 2 DM. In the early stages of the disorder, glucose tolerance remains near-normal, despite insulin resistance, because the pancreatic beta cells compensate by increasing insulin output (**Fig. 19-7**). As insulin resistance and compensatory hyperinsulinemia progress, the pancreatic islets in certain individuals are unable to sustain the hyperinsulinemic state. IGT, characterized by elevations in postprandial glucose, then develops. A further decline in insulin secretion and an increase in hepatic glucose production lead to overt diabetes with fasting hyperglycemia. Ultimately, beta cell failure may ensue.

Metabolic Abnormalities

Abnormal Muscle and Fat Metabolism

Insulin resistance, the decreased ability of insulin to act effectively on target tissues (especially muscle, liver, and fat),

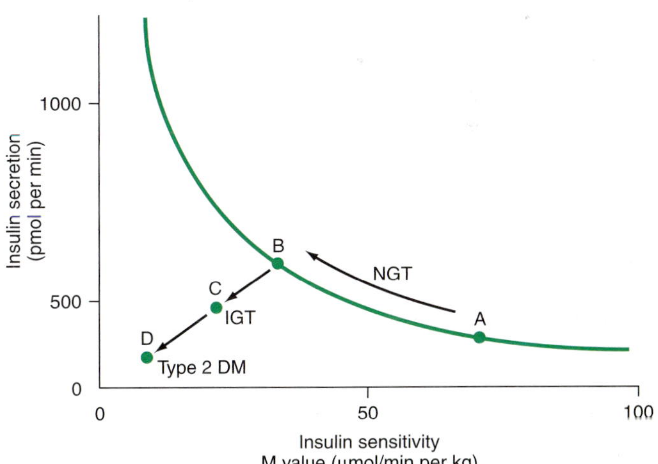

FIGURE 19-7

Metabolic changes during the development of type 2 diabetes mellitus (DM). Insulin secretion and insulin sensitivity are related, and as an individual becomes more insulin-resistant (by moving from point A to point B), insulin secretion increases. A failure to compensate by increasing the insulin secretion results initially in impaired glucose tolerance (IGT; point C) and ultimately in type 2 DM (point D). *(Adapted from SE Kahn: J Clin Endocrinol Metab 86:4047, 2001; RN Bergman, M Ader: Trends Endocrinol Metab 11:351, 2000.)*

is a prominent feature of type 2 DM and results from a combination of genetic susceptibility and obesity. Insulin resistance is relative, however, since supernormal levels of circulating insulin will normalize the plasma glucose. Insulin dose-response curves exhibit a rightward shift, indicating reduced sensitivity, and a reduced maximal response, indicating an overall decrease in maximum glucose utilization (30–60% lower than in normal individuals). Insulin resistance impairs glucose utilization by insulin-sensitive tissues and increases hepatic glucose output; both effects contribute to the hyperglycemia. Increased hepatic glucose output predominantly accounts for increased FPG levels, whereas decreased peripheral glucose usage results in postprandial hyperglycemia. In skeletal muscle, there is a greater impairment in nonoxidative glucose usage (glycogen formation) than in oxidative glucose metabolism through glycolysis. Glucose metabolism in insulin-independent tissues is not altered in type 2 DM.

The precise molecular mechanism leading to insulin resistance in type 2 DM has not been elucidated. Insulin receptor levels and tyrosine kinase activity in skeletal muscle are reduced, but these alterations are most likely secondary to hyperinsulinemia and are not a primary defect. Therefore, "postreceptor" defects in insulin-regulated phosphorylation/dephosphorylation may play the predominant role in insulin resistance (Fig. 19-5). For example, a PI-3-kinase signaling defect may reduce translocation of GLUT4 to the plasma membrane. Other abnormalities include the accumulation of lipid within skeletal myocytes, which may impair mitochondrial oxidative phosphorylation and reduce insulin-stimulated mitochondrial ATP production. Impaired fatty acid oxidation and lipid accumulation within skeletal myocytes may generate reactive oxygen species such as lipid peroxides. Of note, not all insulin signal transduction pathways are resistant to the effects of insulin (e.g., those controlling cell growth and differentiation using the mitogenic-activated protein kinase pathway). Consequently, hyperinsulinemia may increase the insulin action through these pathways, potentially accelerating diabetes-related conditions such as atherosclerosis.

The obesity accompanying type 2 DM, particularly in a central or visceral location, is thought to be part of the pathogenic process. The increased adipocyte mass leads to increased levels of circulating free fatty acids and other fat cell products (Chap. 16). For example, adipocytes secrete a number of biologic products (nonesterified free fatty acids, retinol-binding protein 4, leptin, TNF-α, resistin, and adiponectin). In addition to regulating body weight, appetite, and energy expenditure, adipokines also modulate insulin sensitivity. The increased production of free fatty acids and some adipokines may cause insulin resistance in skeletal muscle and liver. For example, free fatty acids impair glucose utilization in skeletal muscle, promote glucose production by the liver, and impair beta cell function. In contrast, the production by adipocytes of adiponectin, an insulin-sensitizing peptide, is reduced in obesity, and this may contribute to hepatic insulin resistance. Adipocyte products and adipokines also produce an inflammatory state and may explain why markers of inflammation such as IL-6 and C-reactive protein are often elevated in type 2 DM. Inhibition of inflammatory signaling pathways such as the nuclear factor κB (NFκB) pathway appears to reduce insulin resistance and improve hyperglycemia in animal models.

Impaired Insulin Secretion

Insulin secretion and sensitivity are interrelated (Fig. 19-7). In type 2 DM, insulin secretion initially increases in response to insulin resistance to maintain normal glucose tolerance. Initially, the insulin secretory defect is mild and selectively involves glucose-stimulated insulin secretion. The response to other nonglucose secretagogues, such as arginine, is preserved. Eventually, the insulin secretory defect progresses to a state of grossly inadequate insulin secretion.

The reason for the decline in insulin secretory capacity in type 2 DM is unclear. The assumption is that a second genetic defect—superimposed on insulin resistance—leads to beta cell failure. Islet amyloid polypeptide or amylin is cosecreted by the beta cell and forms the amyloid fibrillar deposit found in the islets of individuals with longstanding type 2 DM. Whether such islet amyloid deposits are a primary or secondary event is not known. The metabolic environment of diabetes may also negatively impact islet function. For example, chronic hyperglycemia paradoxically impairs islet function ("glucose toxicity") and leads to a worsening of hyperglycemia. Improvement in glycemic control is often associated with improved islet function. In addition, elevation of free fatty acid levels ("lipotoxicity") and dietary fat may also worsen islet function. Beta cell mass is decreased in individuals with longstanding type 2 diabetes.

Increased Hepatic Glucose and Lipid Production

In type 2 DM, insulin resistance in the liver reflects the failure of hyperinsulinemia to suppress gluconeogenesis, which results in fasting hyperglycemia and decreased glycogen storage by the liver in the postprandial state. Increased hepatic glucose production occurs early in the course of diabetes, though likely after the onset of insulin secretory abnormalities and insulin resistance in skeletal muscle. As a result of insulin resistance in adipose tissue and obesity, free fatty acid (FFA) flux from adipocytes is increased, leading to increased lipid [very low density lipoprotein (VLDL) and triglyceride] synthesis in hepatocytes. This lipid storage or steatosis in the liver may lead to nonalcoholic fatty liver disease and abnormal liver function tests. This is also responsible for the dyslipidemia found in type 2 DM [elevated triglycerides, reduced high-density lipoprotein (HDL), and increased small dense low-density lipoprotein (LDL) particles].

Insulin Resistance Syndromes

The insulin resistance condition is composed of a spectrum of disorders, with hyperglycemia representing one of the most readily diagnosed features. The *metabolic syndrome*, the *insulin resistance syndrome*, and *syndrome X* are terms used to describe a constellation of metabolic derangements that includes insulin resistance, hypertension, dyslipidemia (low HDL and elevated triglycerides), central or visceral obesity, type 2 diabetes or IGT/IFG, and accelerated cardiovascular disease. This syndrome is discussed in Chap. 18.

A number of relatively rare forms of severe insulin resistance include features of type 2 DM or IGT (Table 19-1). Acanthosis nigricans and signs of hyperandrogenism (hirsutism, acne, and oligomenorrhea in women) are also common physical features. Two distinct syndromes of severe insulin resistance have been described in adults: (1) type A, which affects young women and is characterized by severe hyperinsulinemia, obesity, and features of hyperandrogenism, and (2) type B, which affects middle-aged women and is characterized by severe hyperinsulinemia, features of hyperandrogenism, and autoimmune disorders. Individuals with the type A insulin resistance syndrome have an undefined defect in the insulin-signaling pathway; individuals with the type B insulin resistance syndrome have autoantibodies directed at the insulin receptor. These receptor autoantibodies may block insulin binding or may stimulate the insulin receptor, leading to intermittent hypoglycemia.

Polycystic ovary syndrome (PCOS) is a common disorder that affects premenopausal women and is characterized by chronic anovulation and hyperandrogenism (Chap. 10). Insulin resistance is seen in a significant subset of women with PCOS, and the disorder substantially increases the risk for type 2 DM, independent of the effects of obesity.

Prevention

Type 2 DM is preceded by a period of IGT, and a number of lifestyle modifications and pharmacologic agents prevent or delay the onset of DM. The Diabetes Prevention Program (DPP) demonstrated that intensive changes in lifestyle (diet and exercise for 30 min/d five times per week) in individuals with IGT prevented or delayed the development of type 2 DM by 58% compared to placebo. This effect was seen in individuals regardless of age, sex, or ethnic group. In the same study, metformin prevented or delayed diabetes by 31% compared to placebo. The lifestyle intervention group lost 5–7% of their body weight during the 3 years of the study. Studies in Finnish and Chinese populations noted similar efficacy of diet and exercise in preventing or delaying type 2 DM; acarbose, metformin, thiazolidinediones, and orlistat prevent or delay type 2 DM but are not approved for this purpose. When administered to nondiabetic individuals for other reasons (cardiac, cholesterol lowering, etc.), pravastatin reduced the number of new cases of diabetes. Individuals with a strong family history of type 2 DM and individuals with IFG or IGT should be strongly encouraged to maintain a normal BMI and engage in regular physical activity. Pharmacologic therapy for individuals with prediabetes is currently controversial because its cost-effectiveness and safety profile are not known. A recent ADA consensus panel concluded that metformin, but not other medications, could be considered in individuals with both IFG and IGT who are at very high risk for progression to diabetes (age <60 years, BMI ≥35 kg/m^2, family history of diabetes in first-degree relative, elevated triglycerides, reduced HDL, hypertension, or A1C >6.0%).

GENETICALLY DEFINED, MONOGENIC FORMS OF DIABETES MELLITUS

Several monogenic forms of DM have been identified. Six different variants of MODY, caused by mutations in genes encoding islet-enriched transcription factors or glucokinase (Fig. 19-4), are transmitted as autosomal dominant disorders. MODY 1, MODY 3, and MODY 5 are caused by mutations in the hepatocyte nuclear transcription factor (HNF) 4α, HNF-1α, and HNF-1β, respectively. As their names imply, these transcription factors are expressed in the liver but also in other tissues, including the pancreatic islets and kidney. These factors most likely affect islet development or the expression of genes important in glucose-stimulated insulin secretion or the maintenance of beta cell mass. For example, individuals with an HNF-1α mutation have a progressive decline in glycemic control but respond to sulfonylureas. In fact, some of these patients were initially thought to have type 1 DM but were later shown to respond to a sulfonylurea when insulin was discontinued. Individuals with a HNF-1β mutation have progressive impairment of insulin secretion and hepatic insulin resistance and require insulin treatment (minimal response to sulfonylureas). These individuals often have other abnormalities such as renal cysts, mild pancreatic exocrine insufficiency, and abnormal liver function tests. Individuals with MODY 2, the result of mutations in the glucokinase gene, have mild-to-moderate, stable hyperglycemia that does not respond to oral hypoglycemic agents. Glucokinase catalyzes the formation of glucose-6-phosphate from glucose, a reaction that is important for glucose sensing by the beta cells and for glucose utilization by the liver. As a result of glucokinase mutations, higher glucose levels are required to elicit insulin secretory responses, thus altering the set point for insulin secretion. MODY 4 is a rare variant caused by mutations in the insulin promoter factor (IPF) 1, which is a transcription factor that regulates pancreatic development and insulin gene transcription. Homozygous inactivating mutations cause pancreatic agenesis, whereas heterozygous mutations result in DM. Studies of populations with type 2 DM suggest that mutations in MODY-associated genes are rare (<5%) causes of type 2 DM.

Transient or permanent neonatal diabetes (onset <6 months of age) may be caused by several genetic mutations and requires treatment with insulin. Mutations in subunits of the ATP-sensitive potassium channel subunits (Kir6.2 and ABCC8) (Fig. 19-4) are the major causes of permanent neonatal diabetes. Although these activating mutations impair glucose-stimulated insulin secretion, these individuals may respond to sulfonylureas and improve their glycemic control and can be treated with these agents. Homozygous glucokinase mutations cause a severe form of neonatal diabetes.

ACUTE COMPLICATIONS OF DM

Diabetic ketoacidosis (DKA) and hyperglycemic hyperosmolar state (HHS) are acute complications of diabetes. DKA was formerly considered a hallmark of type 1 DM, but it also occurs in individuals who lack immunologic features of type 1 DM and who can subsequently be treated with oral glucose-lowering agents (these obese individuals with type 2 DM are often of Hispanic or African-American descent). HHS is primarily seen in individuals with type 2 DM. Both disorders are associated with absolute or relative insulin deficiency, volume depletion, and acid-base abnormalities. DKA and HHS exist along a continuum of hyperglycemia, with or without ketosis. The metabolic similarities and differences in DKA and HHS are highlighted in Table 19-4. Both disorders are associated with potentially serious complications if not promptly diagnosed and treated.

TABLE 19-4

LABORATORY VALUES IN DIABETIC KETOACIDOSIS (DKA) AND HYPERGLYCEMIC HYPEROSMOLAR STATE (HHS) (REPRESENTATIVE RANGES AT PRESENTATION)

	DKA	HHS
Glucose,[a] mmol/L (mg/dL)	13.9–33.3 (250–600)	33.3–66.6 (600–1200)
Sodium, meq/L	125–135	135–145
Potassium[a]	Normal to ↑	Normal
Magnesium[a]	Normal[b]	Normal
Chloride[a]	Normal	Normal
Phosphate[a]	↓	Normal
Creatinine	Slightly ↑	Moderately ↑
Osmolality (mOsm/mL)	300–320	330–380
Plasma ketones[a]	++++	+/–
Serum bicarbonate,[a] meq/L	<15 meq/L	Normal to slightly ↓
Arterial pH	6.8–7.3	>7.3
Arterial P_{CO_2},[a] mmHg	20–30	Normal
Anion gap[a] [Na – (Cl + HCO_3)]	↑	Normal to slightly ↑

[a]Large changes occur during treatment of DKA.

[b]Although plasma levels may be normal or high at presentation, total-body stores are usually depleted.

DIABETIC KETOACIDOSIS

Clinical Features

The symptoms and physical signs of DKA are listed in Table 19-5 and usually develop over 24 h. DKA may be the initial symptom complex that leads to a diagnosis of type 1 DM, but more frequently it occurs in individuals with established diabetes. Nausea and vomiting are often prominent, and their presence in an individual with diabetes warrants laboratory evaluation for DKA. Abdominal pain may be severe and can resemble acute pancreatitis or ruptured viscus. Hyperglycemia leads to glucosuria, volume depletion, and tachycardia. Hypotension can occur because of volume depletion in combination with peripheral vasodilatation. Kussmaul respirations and a fruity odor on the patient's breath (secondary to metabolic acidosis and increased acetone) are classic signs of the disorder. Lethargy and central nervous system depression may evolve into coma with severe DKA but should also prompt evaluation for other reasons for altered mental status (infection, hypoxia, etc.). Cerebral edema, an extremely serious complication of DKA, is seen most frequently in children. Signs of infection, which may precipitate DKA, should be sought on physical examination, even in the absence of fever. Tissue ischemia (heart, brain) can also be a precipitating factor.

Pathophysiology

DKA results from relative or absolute insulin deficiency combined with counterregulatory hormone excess (glucagon, catecholamines, cortisol, and growth hormone). Both insulin deficiency and glucagon excess, in particular,

TABLE 19-5

MANIFESTATIONS OF DIABETIC KETOACIDOSIS

Symptoms	Physical findings
Nausea/vomiting	Tachycardia
Thirst/polyuria	Dehydration/hypotension
Abdominal pain	Tachypnea/Kussmaul respirations/respiratory distress
Shortness of breath	Abdominal tenderness (may resemble acute pancreatitis or surgical abdomen)
Precipitating events	Lethargy/obtundation/cerebral edema/possibly coma
Inadequate insulin administration	
Infection (pneumonia/UTI/gastroenteritis/sepsis)	
Infarction (cerebral, coronary, mesenteric, peripheral)	
Drugs (cocaine)	
Pregnancy	

Note: UTI, urinary tract infection.

are necessary for DKA to develop. The decreased ratio of insulin to glucagon promotes gluconeogenesis, glycogenolysis, and ketone body formation in the liver, as well as increases in substrate delivery from fat and muscle (free fatty acids, amino acids) to the liver.

The combination of insulin deficiency and hyperglycemia reduces the hepatic level of fructose-2,6-biphosphate, which alters the activity of phosphofructokinase and fructose-1,6-bisphosphatase. Glucagon excess decreases the activity of pyruvate kinase, whereas insulin deficiency increases the activity of phosphoenolpyruvate carboxykinase. These changes shift the handling of pyruvate toward glucose synthesis and away from glycolysis. The increased levels of glucagon and catecholamines in the face of low insulin levels promote glycogenolysis. Insulin deficiency also reduces levels of the GLUT4 glucose transporter, which impairs glucose uptake into skeletal muscle and fat and reduces intracellular glucose metabolism (Fig. 19-5).

Ketosis results from a marked increase in free fatty acid release from adipocytes, with a resulting shift toward ketone body synthesis in the liver. Reduced insulin levels, in combination with elevations in catecholamines and growth hormone, increase lipolysis and the release of free fatty acids. Normally, these free fatty acids are converted to triglycerides or VLDL in the liver. However, in DKA, hyperglucagonemia alters hepatic metabolism to favor ketone body formation, through activation of the enzyme carnitine palmitoyltransferase I. This enzyme is crucial for regulating fatty acid transport into the mitochondria, where β-oxidation and conversion to ketone bodies occur. At physiologic pH, ketone bodies exist as ketoacids, which are neutralized by bicarbonate. As bicarbonate stores are depleted, metabolic acidosis ensues. Increased lactic acid production also contributes to the acidosis. The increased free fatty acids increase triglyceride and VLDL production. VLDL clearance is also reduced because the activity of insulin-sensitive lipoprotein lipase in muscle and fat is decreased. Hypertriglyceridemia may be severe enough to cause pancreatitis.

DKA is initiated by inadequate levels of plasma insulin (Table 19-5). Most commonly, DKA is precipitated by increased insulin requirements, as might occur during a concurrent illness. Failure to augment insulin therapy often compounds the problem. Occasionally, complete omission of insulin by the patient or health care team (in a hospitalized patient with type 1 DM) precipitates DKA. Patients using insulin infusion devices with short-acting insulin are at increased risk of DKA, since even a brief interruption in insulin delivery (e.g., mechanical malfunction) quickly leads to insulin deficiency.

Laboratory Abnormalities and Diagnosis

The timely diagnosis of DKA is crucial and allows for prompt initiation of therapy. DKA is characterized by hyperglycemia, ketosis, and metabolic acidosis (increased anion gap) along with a number of secondary metabolic derangements (Table 19-4). Occasionally, the serum glucose is only minimally elevated. Serum bicarbonate is frequently <10 mmol/L, and arterial pH ranges between 6.8 and 7.3, depending on the severity of the acidosis. Despite a total-body potassium deficit, the serum potassium at presentation may be mildly elevated, secondary to the acidosis. Total-body stores of sodium, chloride, phosphorous, and magnesium are also reduced in DKA but are not accurately reflected by their levels in the serum because of dehydration and hyperglycemia. Elevated blood urea nitrogen (BUN) and serum creatinine levels reflect intravascular volume depletion. Interference from acetoacetate may falsely elevate the serum creatinine measurement. Leukocytosis, hypertriglyceridemia, and hyperlipoproteinemia are commonly found as well. Hyperamylasemia may suggest a diagnosis of pancreatitis, especially when accompanied by abdominal pain. However, in DKA the amylase is usually of salivary origin and thus is not diagnostic of pancreatitis. Serum lipase should be obtained if pancreatitis is suspected.

The measured serum sodium is reduced as a consequence of the hyperglycemia [1.6-mmol/L (1.6 meq) reduction in serum sodium for each 5.6-mmol/L (100 mg/dL) rise in the serum glucose]. A normal serum sodium in the setting of DKA indicates a more profound water deficit. In "conventional" units, the calculated serum osmolality [2 × (serum sodium + serum potassium) + plasma glucose (mg/dL)/18 + BUN/2.8] is mildly to moderately elevated, though to a lesser degree than that found in HHS.

In DKA, the ketone body, β-hydroxybutyrate, is synthesized at a threefold greater rate than acetoacetate; however, acetoacetate is preferentially detected by a commonly used ketosis detection reagent (nitroprusside). Serum ketones are present at significant levels (usually positive at serum dilution of ≥1:8). The nitroprusside tablet, or stick, is often used to detect urine ketones; certain medications such as captopril or penicillamine may cause false-positive reactions. Serum or plasma assays for β-hydroxybutyrate more accurately reflect the true ketone body level.

The metabolic derangements of DKA exist along a spectrum, beginning with mild acidosis with moderate hyperglycemia evolving into more severe findings. The degree of acidosis and hyperglycemia do not necessarily correlate closely since a variety of factors determine the level of hyperglycemia (oral intake, urinary glucose loss). Ketonemia is a consistent finding in DKA and distinguishes it from simple hyperglycemia. The differential diagnosis of DKA includes starvation ketosis, alcoholic ketoacidosis (bicarbonate usually >15 meq/L), and other increased anion gap acidosis.

℞ Treatment: DIABETIC KETOACIDOSIS

The management of DKA is outlined in Table 19-6. After initiating IV fluid replacement and insulin therapy, the agent or event that precipitated the episode of DKA should be sought and aggressively treated. If the patient is vomiting or has altered mental status, a nasogastric tube should be inserted to prevent aspiration of gastric contents. Central to successful treatment of DKA is careful monitoring and frequent reassessment to ensure that the patient and the metabolic derangements are improving. A comprehensive flow sheet should record chronologic changes in vital signs, fluid intake and output, and laboratory values as a function of insulin administered.

After the initial bolus of normal saline, replacement of the sodium and free-water deficit is carried out over the next 24 h (fluid deficit is often 3–5 L). When hemodynamic stability and adequate urine output are achieved, IV fluids should be switched to 0.45% saline at a rate of 200–300 mL/h, depending on the calculated volume deficit. The change to 0.45% saline helps to reduce the trend toward hyperchloremia later in the course of DKA. Alternatively, initial use of lactated Ringer's IV solution may reduce the hyperchloremia that commonly occurs with normal saline.

A bolus of IV (0.1 units/kg) or IM (0.3 units/kg) short-acting insulin should be administered immediately (Table 19-6), and subsequent treatment should provide continuous and adequate levels of circulating insulin. IV administration is preferred (0.1 units/kg per h), because it ensures rapid distribution and allows adjustment of the infusion rate as the patient responds to therapy. In mild episodes of DKA, short-acting insulin analogues can be used subcutaneously. IV regular insulin should be continued until the acidosis resolves and the patient is metabolically stable. As the acidosis and insulin resistance associated with DKA resolve, the insulin infusion rate can be decreased (to 0.05–0.1 units/kg per h). Intermediate or long-acting insulin, in combination with SC short-acting insulin, should be administered as soon as the patient resumes eating, as this facilitates transition to an outpatient insulin regimen and reduces length of hospital stay. It is crucial to continue the insulin infusion until adequate insulin levels are achieved by the SC route. Even relatively brief periods of inadequate insulin administration in this transition phase may result in DKA relapse.

Hyperglycemia usually improves at a rate of 4.2–5.6 mmol/L (75–100 mg/dL) per h as a result of insulin-mediated glucose disposal, reduced hepatic glucose release, and rehydration. The latter reduces catecholamines, increases urinary glucose loss, and expands the intravascular volume. The decline in the plasma glucose within the first 1–2 h may be more rapid and is mostly related to volume expansion. When the plasma glucose reaches 13.9 mmol/L (250 mg/dL), glucose should be added to the 0.45% saline infusion to maintain the plasma glucose in the 11.1–13.9 mmol/L (200–250 mg/dL) range, and the insulin infusion should be continued. Ketoacidosis begins to resolve as insulin reduces lipolysis, increases peripheral ketone body use, suppresses hepatic ketone body formation, and promotes bicarbonate regeneration. However, the acidosis and ketosis resolve more slowly than hyperglycemia. As ketoacidosis improves, β-hydroxybutyrate is converted

TABLE 19-6

MANAGEMENT OF DIABETIC KETOACIDOSIS

1. Confirm diagnosis (↑ plasma glucose, positive serum ketones, metabolic acidosis).
2. Admit to hospital; intensive-care setting may be necessary for frequent monitoring or if pH <7.00 or unconscious.
3. Assess:
   Serum electrolytes (K^+, Na^+, Mg^{2+}, Cl^-, bicarbonate, phosphate)
   Acid-base status—pH, HCO_3^-, P_{CO_2}, β-hydroxybutyrate
   Renal function (creatinine, urine output)
4. Replace fluids: 2–3 L of 0.9% saline over first 1–3 h (10–15 mL/kg per h); subsequently, 0.45% saline at 150–300 mL/h; change to 5% glucose and 0.45% saline at 100–200 mL/h when plasma glucose reaches 250 mg/dL (14 mmol/L).
5. Administer short-acting insulin: IV (0.1 units/kg) or IM (0.3 units/kg), then 0.1 units/kg per h by continuous IV infusion; increase two- to threefold if no response by 2–4 h. If initial serum potassium is <3.3 mmol/L (3.3 meq/L), do not administer insulin until the potassium is corrected to >3.3 mmol/L (3.3.meq/L).
6. Assess patient: What precipitated the episode (noncompliance, infection, trauma, infarction, cocaine)? Initiate appropriate workup for precipitating event (cultures, CXR, ECG).
7. Measure capillary glucose every 1–2 h; measure electrolytes (especially K^+, bicarbonate, phosphate) and anion gap every 4 h for first 24 h.
8. Monitor blood pressure, pulse, respirations, mental status, fluid intake and output every 1–4 h.
9. Replace K^+: 10 meq/h when plasma K^+ is <5.5 meq/L, ECG normal, urine flow and normal creatinine documented; administer 40–80 meq/h when plasma K^+ is <3.5 meq/L or if bicarbonate is given.
10. Continue above until patient is stable, glucose goal is 150–250 mg/dL, and acidosis is resolved. Insulin infusion may be decreased to 0.05–0.1 units/kg per h.
11. Administer intermediate or long-acting insulin as soon as patient is eating. Allow for overlap in insulin infusion and SC insulin injection.

Note: CXR, chest x-ray; ECG, electrocardiogram.
Source: Adapted from M Sperling, in *Therapy for Diabetes Mellitus and Related Disorders*, American Diabetes Association, Alexandria, VA, 1998; and AE Kitabchi et al: *Diabetes Care* 29:2739, 2006.

to acetoacetate. Ketone body levels may appear to increase if measured by laboratory assays that use the nitroprusside reaction, which only detects acetoacetate and acetone. The improvement in acidosis and anion gap, a result of bicarbonate regeneration and decline in ketone bodies, is reflected by a rise in the serum bicarbonate level and the arterial pH. Depending on the rise of serum chloride, the anion gap (but not bicarbonate) will normalize. A hyperchloremic acidosis [serum bicarbonate of 15–18 mmol/L (15–18 meq/L)] often follows successful treatment and gradually resolves as the kidneys regenerate bicarbonate and excrete chloride.

Potassium stores are depleted in DKA [estimated deficit 3–5 mmol/kg (3–5 meq/kg)]. During treatment with insulin and fluids, various factors contribute to the development of hypokalemia. These include insulin-mediated potassium transport into cells, resolution of the acidosis (which also promotes potassium entry into cells), and urinary loss of potassium salts of organic acids. Thus, potassium repletion should commence as soon as adequate urine output and a normal serum potassium are documented. If the initial serum potassium level is elevated, then potassium repletion should be delayed until the potassium falls into the normal range. Inclusion of 20–40 meq of potassium in each liter of IV fluid is reasonable, but additional potassium supplements may also be required. To reduce the amount of chloride administered, potassium phosphate or acetate can be substituted for the chloride salt. The goal is to maintain the serum potassium >3.5 mmol/L (3.5 meq/L). If the initial serum potassium is <3.3 mmol/L (3.3 meq/L), do not administer insulin until the potassium is supplemented to >3.3 mmol/L (3.3 meq/L).

Despite a bicarbonate deficit, bicarbonate replacement is not usually necessary. In fact, theoretical arguments suggest that bicarbonate administration and rapid reversal of acidosis may impair cardiac function, reduce tissue oxygenation, and promote hypokalemia. The results of most clinical trials do not support the routine use of bicarbonate replacement, and one study in children found that bicarbonate use was associated with an increased risk of cerebral edema. However, in the presence of severe acidosis (arterial pH <7.0 after initial hydration), the ADA advises bicarbonate [50 mmol/L (meq/L) of sodium bicarbonate in 200 mL of sterile water with 10 meq/L KCl over 1 h if pH = 6.9–7.0; or 100 mmol/L (meq/L) of sodium bicarbonate in 400 mL of sterile water with 20 meq/L KCl over 2 h if pH <6.9]. Repeat the dose of bicarbonate every 2 h until the arterial pH is >7.0. Hypophosphatemia may result from increased glucose usage, but randomized clinical trials have not demonstrated that phosphate replacement is beneficial in DKA. If the serum phosphate is <0.32 mmol/L (1.0 mg/dL), then phosphate supplement should be considered and the serum calcium monitored. Hypomagnesemia may develop during DKA therapy and may also require supplementation.

With appropriate therapy, the mortality of DKA is low (<5%) and is related more to the underlying or precipitating event, such as infection or myocardial infarction. The major nonmetabolic complication of DKA therapy is cerebral edema, which most often develops in children as DKA is resolving. The etiology of and optimal therapy for cerebral edema are not well established, but overreplacement of free water should be avoided. Venous thrombosis, upper gastrointestinal bleeding, and acute respiratory distress syndrome occasionally complicate DKA.

Following treatment, the physician and patient should review the sequence of events that led to DKA to prevent future recurrences. Foremost is patient education about the symptoms of DKA, its precipitating factors, and the management of diabetes during a concurrent illness. During illness or when oral intake is compromised, patients should (1) frequently measure the capillary blood glucose; (2) measure urinary ketones when the serum glucose is >16.5 mmol/L (300 mg/dL); (3) drink fluids to maintain hydration; (4) continue or increase insulin; and (5) seek medical attention if dehydration, persistent vomiting, or uncontrolled hyperglycemia develop. Using these strategies, early DKA can be prevented or detected and treated appropriately on an outpatient basis.

HYPERGLYCEMIC HYPEROSMOLAR STATE

Clinical Features

The prototypical patient with HHS is an elderly individual with type 2 DM, with a several-week history of polyuria, weight loss, and diminished oral intake that culminates in mental confusion, lethargy, or coma. The physical examination reflects profound dehydration and hyperosmolality and reveals hypotension, tachycardia, and altered mental status. Notably absent are symptoms of nausea, vomiting, and abdominal pain and the Kussmaul respirations characteristic of DKA. HHS is often precipitated by a serious, concurrent illness such as myocardial infarction or stroke. Sepsis, pneumonia, and other serious infections are frequent precipitants and should be sought. In addition, a debilitating condition (prior stroke or dementia) or social situation that compromises water intake usually contributes to the development of the disorder.

Pathophysiology

Relative insulin deficiency and inadequate fluid intake are the underlying causes of HHS. Insulin deficiency increases hepatic glucose production (through glycogenolysis and gluconeogenesis) and impairs glucose utilization in skeletal muscle (see discussion of DKA earlier in the chapter).

Hyperglycemia induces an osmotic diuresis that leads to intravascular volume depletion, which is exacerbated by inadequate fluid replacement. The absence of ketosis in HHS is not completely understood. Presumably, the insulin deficiency is only relative and less severe than in DKA. Lower levels of counterregulatory hormones and free fatty acids have been found in HHS than in DKA in some studies. It is also possible that the liver is less capable of ketone body synthesis or that the insulin/glucagon ratio does not favor ketogenesis.

Laboratory Abnormalities and Diagnosis

The laboratory features in HHS are summarized in Table 19-4. Most notable are the marked hyperglycemia [plasma glucose may be >55.5 mmol/L (1000 mg/dL)], hyperosmolality (>350 mosmol/L), and prerenal azotemia. The measured serum sodium may be normal or slightly low despite the marked hyperglycemia. The corrected serum sodium is usually increased [add 1.6 meq to measured sodium for each 5.6-mmol/L (100 mg/dL) rise in the serum glucose]. In contrast to DKA, acidosis and ketonemia are absent or mild. A small anion gap metabolic acidosis may be present secondary to increased lactic acid. Moderate ketonuria, if present, is secondary to starvation.

Rx Treatment: HYPERGLYCEMIC HYPEROSMOLAR STATE

Volume depletion and hyperglycemia are prominent features of both HHS and DKA. Consequently, therapy of these disorders shares several elements (Table 19-6). In both disorders, careful monitoring of the patient's fluid status, laboratory values, and insulin infusion rate is crucial. Underlying or precipitating problems should be aggressively sought and treated. In HHS, fluid losses and dehydration are usually more pronounced than in DKA due to the longer duration of the illness. The patient with HHS is usually older, more likely to have mental status changes, and more likely to have a life-threatening precipitating event with accompanying comorbidities. Even with proper treatment, HHS has a substantially higher mortality than DKA (up to 15% in some clinical series).

Fluid replacement should initially stabilize the hemodynamic status of the patient (1–3 L of 0.9% normal saline over the first 2–3 h). Because the fluid deficit in HHS is accumulated over a period of days to weeks, the rapidity of reversal of the hyperosmolar state must balance the need for free-water repletion with the risk that too rapid a reversal may worsen neurologic function. If the serum sodium is >150 mmol/L (150 meq/L), 0.45% saline should be used. After hemodynamic stability is achieved, the IV fluid administration is directed at reversing the free-water deficit using hypotonic fluids (0.45% saline initially then 5% dextrose in water, D_5W). The calculated free-water deficit (which averages 9–10 L) should be reversed over the next 1–2 days (infusion rates of 200–300 mL/h of hypotonic solution). Potassium repletion is usually necessary and should be dictated by repeated measurements of the serum potassium. In patients taking diuretics, the potassium deficit can be quite large and may be accompanied by magnesium deficiency. Hypophosphatemia may occur during therapy and can be improved by using KPO_4 and beginning nutrition.

As in DKA, rehydration and volume expansion lower the plasma glucose initially, but insulin is also required. A reasonable regimen for HHS begins with an IV insulin bolus of 0.1 units/kg followed by IV insulin at a constant infusion rate of 0.1 units/kg per h. If the serum glucose does not fall, increase the insulin infusion rate by twofold. As in DKA, glucose should be added to IV fluid when the plasma glucose falls to 13.9 mmol/L (250 mg/dL), and the insulin infusion rate should be decreased to 0.05–0.1 units/kg per h. The insulin infusion should be continued until the patient has resumed eating and can be transferred to a SC insulin regimen. The patient should be discharged from the hospital on insulin, though some patients can later switch to oral glucose-lowering agents.

CHRONIC COMPLICATIONS OF DM

The chronic complications of DM affect many organ systems and are responsible for the majority of morbidity and mortality associated with the disease. Chronic complications can be divided into vascular and nonvascular complications (**Table 19-7**). The vascular complications of DM are further subdivided into microvascular (retinopathy, neuropathy, nephropathy) and macrovascular complications [coronary artery disease (CAD), peripheral arterial disease (PAD), cerebrovascular disease]. Nonvascular complications include problems such as gastroparesis, infections, and skin changes. Longstanding diabetes may be associated with hearing loss. Whether type 2 DM in elderly individuals is associated with impaired mental function is not clear.

The risk of chronic complications increases as a function of the duration of hyperglycemia; they usually become apparent in the second decade of hyperglycemia. Since type 2 DM often has a long asymptomatic period of hyperglycemia, many individuals with type 2 DM have complications at the time of diagnosis.

The microvascular complications of both type 1 and type 2 DM result from chronic hyperglycemia. Large, randomized clinical trials of individuals with type 1 or type 2 DM have conclusively demonstrated that a reduction in

TABLE 19-7

CHRONIC COMPLICATIONS OF DIABETES MELLITUS

Microvascular
Eye disease
Retinopathy (nonproliferative/proliferative)
Macular edema
Neuropathy
Sensory and motor (mono- and polyneuropathy)
Autonomic
Nephropathy
Macrovascular
Coronary artery disease
Peripheral arterial disease
Cerebrovascular disease
Other
Gastrointestinal (gastroparesis, diarrhea)
Genitourinary (uropathy/sexual dysfunction)
Dermatologic
Infectious
Cataracts
Glaucoma
Periodontal disease

chronic hyperglycemia prevents or delays retinopathy, neuropathy, and nephropathy. Other incompletely defined factors may modulate the development of complications. For example, despite longstanding DM, some individuals never develop nephropathy or retinopathy. Many of these patients have glycemic control that is indistinguishable from those who develop microvascular complications, suggesting that there is a genetic susceptibility for developing particular complications.

Evidence implicating a causative role for chronic hyperglycemia in the development of macrovascular complications is less conclusive. However, coronary heart disease events and mortality are two to four times greater in patients with type 2 DM. These events correlate with fasting and postprandial plasma glucose levels as well as with the A1C. Other factors (dyslipidemia and hypertension) also play important roles in macrovascular complications.

MECHANISMS OF COMPLICATIONS

Although chronic hyperglycemia is an important etiologic factor leading to complications of DM, the mechanism(s) by which it leads to such diverse cellular and organ dysfunction is unknown. Four prominent theories, which are not mutually exclusive, have been proposed to explain how hyperglycemia might lead to the chronic complications of DM.

One theory is that increased intracellular glucose leads to the formation of advanced glycosylation end products (AGEs) via the nonenzymatic glycosylation of intra- and extracellular proteins. Nonenzymatic glycosylation results from the interaction of glucose with amino groups on proteins. AGEs have been shown to cross-link proteins (e.g., collagen, extracellular matrix proteins), accelerate atherosclerosis, promote glomerular dysfunction, reduce nitric oxide synthesis, induce endothelial dysfunction, and alter extracellular matrix composition and structure. The serum level of AGEs correlates with the level of glycemia, and these products accumulate as the glomerular filtration rate declines.

A second theory is based on the observation that hyperglycemia increases glucose metabolism via the sorbitol pathway. Intracellular glucose is predominantly metabolized by phosphorylation and subsequent glycolysis, but when increased, some glucose is converted to sorbitol by the enzyme aldose reductase. Increased sorbitol concentration alters redox potential, increases cellular osmolality, generates reactive oxygen species, and likely leads to other types of cellular dysfunction. However, testing of this theory in humans, using aldose reductase inhibitors, has not demonstrated significant beneficial effects on clinical endpoints of retinopathy, neuropathy, or nephropathy.

A third hypothesis proposes that hyperglycemia increases the formation of diacylglycerol leading to activation of protein kinase C (PKC). Among other actions, PKC alters the transcription of genes for fibronectin, type IV collagen, contractile proteins, and extracellular matrix proteins in endothelial cells and neurons. Inhibitors of PKC are being studied in clinical trials.

A fourth theory proposes that hyperglycemia increases the flux through the hexosamine pathway, which generates fructose-6-phosphate, a substrate for O-linked glycosylation and proteoglycan production. The hexosamine pathway may alter function by glycosylation of proteins such as endothelial nitric oxide synthase or by changes in gene expression of transforming growth factor β (TGF-β) or plasminogen activator inhibitor-1 (PAI-1).

Growth factors appear to play an important role in DM-related complications, and their production is increased by most of these proposed pathways. Vascular endothelial growth factor A (VEGF-A) is increased locally in diabetic proliferative retinopathy and decreases after laser photocoagulation. TGF-β is increased in diabetic nephropathy and stimulates basement membrane production of collagen and fibronectin by mesangial cells. Other growth factors, such as platelet-derived growth factor, epidermal growth factor, insulin-like growth factor 1, growth hormone, basic fibroblast growth factor, and even insulin, have been suggested to play a role in DM-related complications. A possible unifying mechanism is that hyperglycemia leads to increased production of reactive oxygen species or superoxide in the mitochondria; these compounds may activate all four of the pathways described above. Although hyperglycemia serves as the initial trigger for complications of diabetes, it is still unknown whether the same pathophysiologic processes are operative in all complications or whether some pathways predominate in certain organs.

GLYCEMIC CONTROL AND COMPLICATIONS

The Diabetes Control and Complications Trial (DCCT) provided definitive proof that reduction in chronic hyperglycemia can prevent many of the early complications of type 1 DM. This large multicenter clinical trial randomized over 1400 individuals with type 1 DM to either intensive or conventional diabetes management and prospectively evaluated the development of retinopathy, nephropathy, and neuropathy. Individuals in the intensive diabetes management group received multiple administrations of insulin each day along with extensive educational, psychological, and medical support. Individuals in the conventional diabetes management group received twice-daily insulin injections and quarterly nutritional, educational, and clinical evaluation. The goal in the former group was normoglycemia; the goal in the latter group was prevention of symptoms of diabetes. Individuals in the intensive diabetes management group achieved a substantially lower hemoglobin A1C (7.3%) than individuals in the conventional diabetes management group (9.1%).

The DCCT demonstrated that improvement of glycemic control reduced nonproliferative and proliferative retinopathy (47% reduction), microalbuminuria (39% reduction), clinical nephropathy (54% reduction), and neuropathy (60% reduction). Improved glycemic control also slowed the progression of early diabetic complications. There was a nonsignificant trend in reduction of macrovascular events during the trial (most individuals were young and had a low risk of cardiovascular disease). The results of the DCCT predicted that individuals in the intensive diabetes management group would gain 7.7 additional years of vision, 5.8 additional years free from ESRD, and 5.6 years free from lower extremity amputations. If all complications of DM were combined, individuals in the intensive diabetes management group would experience 15.3 more years of life without significant microvascular or neurologic complications of DM, compared to individuals who received standard therapy. This translates into an additional 5.1 years of life expectancy for individuals in the intensive diabetes management group. The benefit of the improved glycemic control during the DCCT persisted even after the study concluded and glycemic control worsened. For example, individuals in the intensive diabetes management group for a mean of 6.5 years had a 42–57% reduction in cardiovascular events [nonfatal myocardial infarction (MI), stroke, or death from a cardiovascular event] at a mean follow-up of 17 years, even though their subsequent glycemic control was the same as those in the conventional diabetes management group.

The benefits of an improvement in glycemic control occurred over the entire range of A1C values (Fig. 19-8), suggesting that at any A1C level, an improvement in glycemic control is beneficial. The goal of therapy is to achieve an A1C level as close to normal as possible, without subjecting the patient to excessive risk of hypoglycemia.

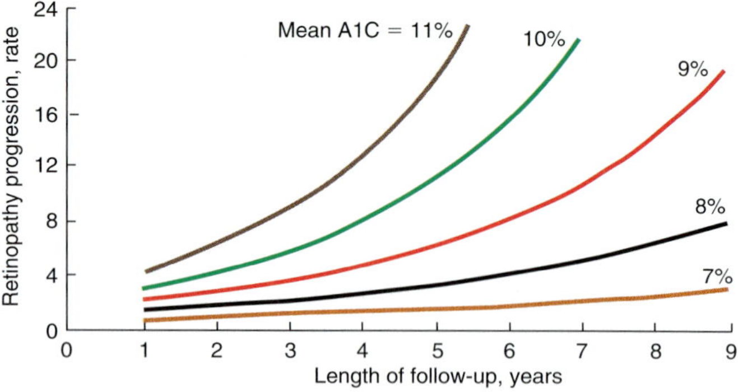

FIGURE 19-8

Relationship of glycemic control and diabetes duration to diabetic retinopathy. The progression of retinopathy in individuals in the Diabetes Control and Complications Trial is graphed as a function of the length of follow-up with different curves for different A1C values. (*Adapted from The Diabetes Control and Complications Trial Research Group: Diabetes 44:968, 1995.*)

The United Kingdom Prospective Diabetes Study (UKPDS) studied the course of >5000 individuals with type 2 DM for >10 years. This study utilized multiple treatment regimens and monitored the effect of intensive glycemic control and risk factor treatment on the development of diabetic complications. Newly diagnosed individuals with type 2 DM were randomized to (1) intensive management using various combinations of insulin, a sulfonylurea, or metformin or (2) conventional therapy using dietary modification and pharmacotherapy with the goal of symptom prevention. In addition, individuals were randomly assigned to different antihypertensive regimens. Individuals in the intensive treatment arm achieved an A1C of 7.0%, compared to a 7.9% A1C in the standard treatment group. The UKPDS demonstrated that each percentage point reduction in A1C was associated with a 35% reduction in microvascular complications. As in the DCCT, there was a continuous relationship between glycemic control and development of complications. Improved glycemic control did not conclusively reduce (nor worsen) cardiovascular mortality but was associated with improvement with lipoprotein risk profiles, such as reduced triglycerides and increased HDL.

One of the major findings of the UKPDS was that strict blood pressure control significantly reduced both macro- and microvascular complications. In fact, the beneficial effects of blood pressure control were greater than the beneficial effects of glycemic control. Lowering blood pressure to moderate goals (144/82 mmHg) reduced the risk of DM-related death, stroke, microvascular endpoints, retinopathy, and heart failure (risk reductions between 32 and 56%).

Similar reductions in the risks of retinopathy and nephropathy were also seen in a small trial of lean Japanese individuals with type 2 DM randomized to either intensive glycemic control or standard therapy with insulin (Kumamoto study). These results demonstrate the effectiveness of improved glycemic control in individuals of different ethnicity and, presumably, a different etiology of DM (i.e., phenotypically different from those in the DCCT and UKPDS).

The findings of the DCCT, UKPDS, and Kumamoto study support the idea that chronic hyperglycemia plays a causative role in the pathogenesis of diabetic microvascular complications. These landmark studies prove the value of metabolic control and emphasize the importance of (1) intensive glycemic control in all forms of DM and (2) early diagnosis and strict blood pressure control in type 2 DM.

OPHTHALMOLOGIC COMPLICATIONS OF DIABETES MELLITUS

DM is the leading cause of blindness between the ages of 20 and 74 in the United States. The gravity of this problem is highlighted by the finding that individuals with DM are 25 times more likely to become legally blind than individuals without DM. Blindness is primarily the result of progressive diabetic retinopathy and clinically significant macular edema. Diabetic retinopathy is classified into two stages: nonproliferative and proliferative. Nonproliferative diabetic retinopathy usually appears late in the first decade or early in the second decade of the disease and is marked by retinal vascular microaneurysms, blot hemorrhages, and cotton wool spots (Fig. 19-9). Mild nonproliferative retinopathy progresses to more extensive disease, characterized by changes in venous vessel caliber, intraretinal microvascular abnormalities, and more numerous microaneurysms and hemorrhages. The pathophysiologic mechanisms invoked in nonproliferative retinopathy include loss of retinal pericytes, increased retinal vascular permeability, alterations in retinal blood flow, and abnormal retinal microvasculature, all of which lead to retinal ischemia.

The appearance of neovascularization in response to retinal hypoxia is the hallmark of proliferative diabetic retinopathy (Fig. 19-9). These newly formed vessels appear near the optic nerve and/or macula and rupture easily, leading to vitreous hemorrhage, fibrosis, and ultimately retinal detachment. Not all individuals with nonproliferative retinopathy develop proliferative retinopathy, but the more severe the nonproliferative disease, the greater the chance of evolution to proliferative retinopathy within 5 years. This creates an important opportunity for early detection and treatment of diabetic retinopathy. Clinically significant macular edema can occur when only nonproliferative retinopathy is present. Fluorescein angiography is useful to detect macular edema, which is associated with a 25% chance of moderate visual loss over the next 3 years.

Duration of DM and degree of glycemic control are the best predictors of the development of retinopathy; hypertension is also a risk factor. Nonproliferative retinopathy is found in almost all individuals who have had DM for >20 years (25% incidence with 5 years, and 80% incidence with 15 years of type 1 DM). Although there is genetic susceptibility for retinopathy, it confers less influence than either the duration of DM or the degree of glycemic control.

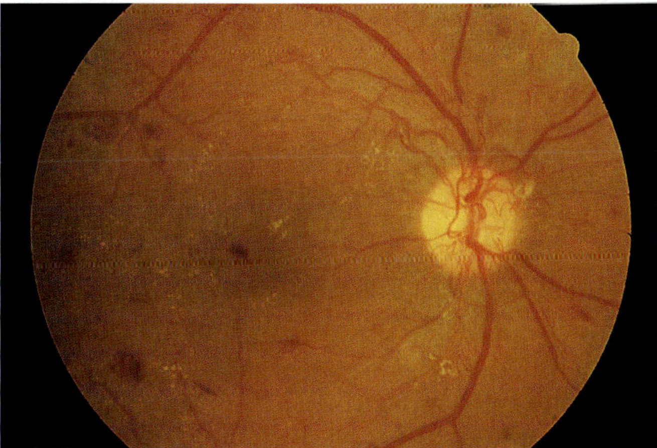

FIGURE 19-9
Diabetic retinopathy results in scattered hemorrhages, yellow exudates, and neovascularization. This patient has neovascular vessels proliferating from the optic disc, requiring urgent panretinal laser photocoagulation.

℞ Treatment: DIABETIC RETINOPATHY

The most effective therapy for diabetic retinopathy is prevention. Intensive glycemic and blood pressure control will delay the development or slow the progression of retinopathy in individuals with either type 1 or type 2 DM. Paradoxically, during the first 6–12 months of improved glycemic control, established diabetic retinopathy may transiently worsen. Fortunately, this progression is temporary, and in the long term, improved glycemic control is associated with less diabetic retinopathy. Individuals with known retinopathy are candidates for prophylactic photocoagulation when initiating intensive therapy. Once advanced retinopathy is present, improved glycemic control imparts less benefit, though adequate ophthalmologic care can prevent most blindness.

Regular, comprehensive eye examinations are essential for all individuals with DM. Most diabetic eye disease can be successfully treated if detected early. Routine, nondilated eye examinations by the primary care provider or diabetes specialist are inadequate to detect diabetic eye disease, which requires an ophthalmologist for optimal care of these disorders. Laser photocoagulation is very successful in preserving vision. Proliferative retinopathy is usually treated with panretinal laser photocoagulation, whereas macular edema is treated with focal laser photocoagulation. Although exercise has not been conclusively shown to worsen proliferative diabetic retinopathy, most ophthalmologists advise individuals with advanced diabetic eye disease to limit physical activities associated with repeated Valsalva maneuvers. Aspirin therapy (650 mg/d) does not appear to influence the natural history of diabetic retinopathy.

RENAL COMPLICATIONS OF DIABETES MELLITUS

Diabetic nephropathy is the leading cause of ESRD in the United States and a leading cause of DM-related morbidity and mortality. Both microalbuminuria and macroalbuminuria in individuals with DM are associated with increased risk of cardiovascular disease. Individuals with diabetic nephropathy commonly have diabetic retinopathy.

Like other microvascular complications, the pathogenesis of diabetic nephropathy is related to chronic hyperglycemia. The mechanisms by which chronic hyperglycemia leads to ESRD, though incompletely defined, involve the effects of soluble factors (growth factors, angiotensin II, endothelin, AGEs), hemodynamic alterations in the renal microcirculation (glomerular hyperfiltration or hyperperfusion, increased glomerular capillary pressure), and structural changes in the glomerulus (increased extracellular matrix, basement membrane thickening, mesangial expansion, fibrosis). Some of these effects may be mediated through angiotensin II receptors. Smoking accelerates the decline in renal function. Because only 20–40% of patients with diabetes develop diabetic nephropathy, additional susceptibility factors remain unidentified. One known risk factor is a family history of diabetic nephropathy.

The natural history of diabetic nephropathy is characterized by a fairly predictable sequence of events that was initially defined for individuals with type 1 DM but appears to be similar in type 2 DM (**Fig. 19-10**). Glomerular hyperperfusion and renal hypertrophy occur in the first years after the onset of DM and are associated with an increase of the glomerular filtration rate (GFR). During the first 5 years of DM, thickening of the glomerular basement membrane, glomerular hypertrophy, and mesangial volume expansion occur as the GFR returns to normal. After 5–10 years of type 1 DM, ~40% of individuals begin to excrete small amounts of albumin in the urine. Microalbuminuria is defined as 30–300 mg/d in a 24-h collection or 30–300 μg/mg creatinine in a spot collection (preferred method). Although the appearance of microalbuminuria in type 1 DM is an important risk factor for progression to overt proteinuria (>300 mg/d), only ~50% of individuals progress to macroalbuminuria over the next 10 years. In some individuals with type 1 diabetes and microalbuminuria of short duration, the microalbuminuria regresses. Once macroalbuminuria is present, there is a steady decline in GFR, and ~50% of individuals reach ESRD in 7–10 years. Once macroalbuminuria develops, blood pressure rises slightly and the pathologic changes are likely irreversible. Some individuals with type 1 or type 2 DM have a decline in GFR in the absence of micro- or macroalbuminuria and this is the basis for assessing the GFR on an annual basis using serum creatinine.

The nephropathy that develops in type 2 DM differs from that of type 1 DM in the following respects: (1) microalbuminuria or macroalbuminuria may be present when type 2 DM is diagnosed, reflecting its long asymptomatic period; (2) hypertension more commonly accompanies microalbuminuria or macroalbuminuria in type 2 DM; and (3) microalbuminuria may be less predictive of diabetic nephropathy and progression to macroalbuminuria in type 2 DM. Finally, it should be noted that albuminuria in type 2 DM may be secondary to factors unrelated to DM, such as hypertension, congestive heart failure (CHF), prostate disease, or infection. Diabetic nephropathy and ESRD secondary to DM develop more commonly in African Americans, Native Americans, and Hispanic individuals than in Caucasians with type 2 DM.

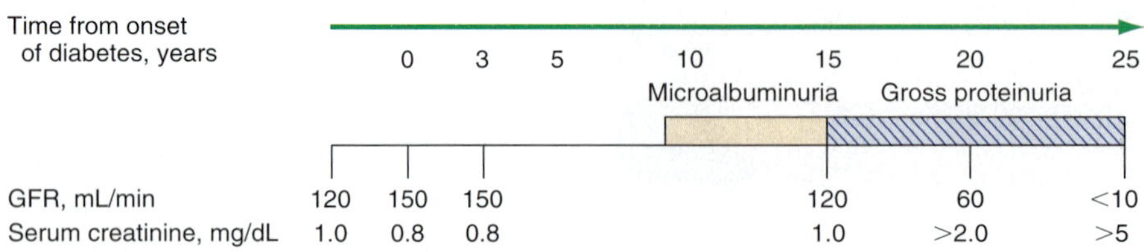

FIGURE 19-10

Time course of development of diabetic nephropathy. The relationship of time from onset of diabetes, the glomerular filtration rate (GFR), and the serum creatinine are shown. *(Adapted from RA DeFranzo, in Therapy for Diabetes Mellitus and Related Disorders, 3d ed. American Diabetes Association, Alexandria, VA, 1998.)*

Type IV renal tubular acidosis (hyporeninemic hypoaldosteronism) may occur in type 1 or 2 DM. These individuals develop a propensity to hyperkalemia, which may be exacerbated by medications [especially angiotensin-converting enzyme (ACE) inhibitors and angiotensin receptor blockers (ARBs)]. Patients with DM are predisposed to radiocontrast-induced nephrotoxicity. Risk factors for radiocontrast-induced nephrotoxicity are preexisting nephropathy and volume depletion. Individuals with DM undergoing radiographic procedures with contrast dye should be well hydrated before and after dye exposure, and the serum creatinine should be monitored for 24 h following the procedure.

℞ Treatment: DIABETIC NEPHROPATHY

The optimal therapy for diabetic nephropathy is prevention by control of glycemia. As part of comprehensive diabetes care, microalbuminuria should be detected at an early stage when effective therapies can be instituted. The recommended strategy for detecting microalbuminuria is outlined in Fig. 19-11 and includes annual measurement of the serum creatinine to estimate GFR. Interventions effective in slowing progression from microalbuminuria to macroalbuminuria include (1) normalization of glycemia, (2) strict blood pressure control, and (3) administration of ACE inhibitors or ARBs. Dyslipidemia should also be treated.

Improved glycemic control reduces the rate at which microalbuminuria appears and progresses in type 1 and type 2 DM. However, once macroalbuminuria exists, it is unclear whether improved glycemic control will slow progression of renal disease. During the phase of declining renal function, insulin requirements may fall as the kidney is a site of insulin degradation. Furthermore, many glucose-lowering medications (sulfonylureas and metformin) are contraindicated in advanced renal insufficiency.

Many individuals with type 1 or type 2 DM develop hypertension. Numerous studies in both type 1 and type 2 DM demonstrate the effectiveness of strict blood pressure control in reducing albumin excretion and slowing the decline in renal function. Blood pressure should be maintained at <130/80 mmHg in diabetic individuals without proteinuria. A slightly lower blood pressure (125/75) should be considered for individuals with microalbuminuria or macroalbuminuria (see "Hypertension" later in the chapter).

Either ACE inhibitors or ARBs should be used to reduce the progression from microalbuminuria to macroalbuminuria and the associated decline in GFR that accompanies macroalbuminuria in individuals with type 1 or type 2 DM (see "Hypertension" later in the chapter). Although direct comparisons of ACE inhibitors and ARBs are lacking, most experts believe that the two classes of drugs are equivalent in the patient with diabetes. ARBs can be used as an alternative in patients who develop ACE inhibitor–associated cough or angioedema. After 2–3 months of therapy in patients with microalbuminuria, the drug dose is increased until either the microalbuminuria disappears or the maximum dose is reached. If use of either ACE inhibitors or ARBs is not possible, then calcium channel blockers (non-dihydropyridine class), beta blockers, or diuretics should be used. However, their efficacy in slowing the fall in the GFR is not proven. Blood pressure control with any agent is extremely important, but a drug-specific benefit in diabetic nephropathy, independent of blood pressure control, has been shown only for ACE inhibitors and ARBs in patients with DM.

The ADA suggests modest restriction of protein intake in diabetic individuals with microalbuminuria (0.8 g/kg per d) or macroalbuminuria (<0.8 g/kg per d, which is the adult recommended daily allowance, or ~10% of the daily caloric intake).

Nephrology consultation should be considered when the estimated GFR is <60 mL/min per 1.743 m^2. Once macroalbuminuria ensues, the likelihood of ESRD is very high. As compared to nondiabetic individuals, hemodialysis in patients with DM is associated with more frequent complications, such as hypotension (due to autonomic neuropathy or loss of reflex tachycardia), more difficult vascular access, and accelerated progression

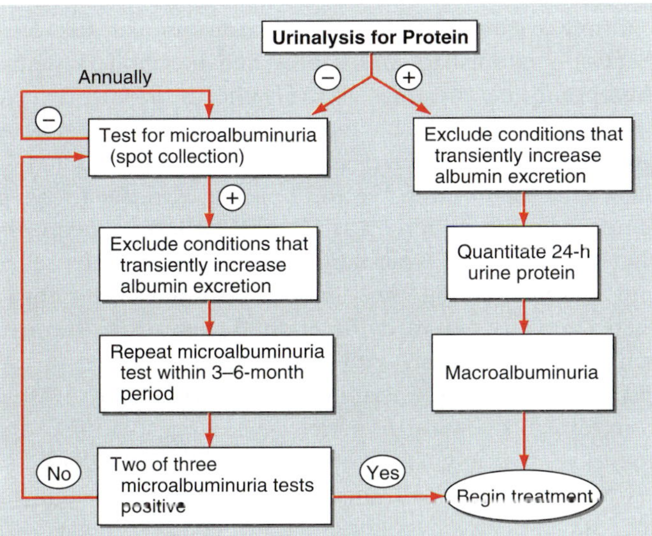

FIGURE 19-11

Screening for microalbuminuria should be performed in patients with type 1 diabetes for ≥5 years, in patients with type 2 diabetes, and during pregnancy. Non-diabetes-related conditions that might increase microalbuminuria are urinary tract infection, hematuria, heart failure, febrile illness, severe hyperglycemia, severe hypertension, and vigorous exercise. *(Adapted from RA DeFronzo, in Therapy for Diabetes Mellitus and Related Disorders, 3d ed. American Diabetes Association, Alexandria, VA, 1998.)*

of retinopathy. Survival after the onset of ESRD is shorter in the diabetic population compared to nondiabetics with similar clinical features. Atherosclerosis is the leading cause of death in diabetic individuals on dialysis, and hyperlipidemia should be treated aggressively. Renal transplantation from a living-related donor is the preferred therapy but requires chronic immunosuppression. Combined pancreas-kidney transplant offers the promise of normoglycemia and freedom from dialysis.

NEUROPATHY AND DIABETES MELLITUS

Diabetic neuropathy occurs in ~50% of individuals with longstanding type 1 and type 2 DM. It may manifest as polyneuropathy, mononeuropathy, and/or autonomic neuropathy. As with other complications of DM, the development of neuropathy correlates with the duration of diabetes and glycemic control. Additional risk factors are BMI (the greater the BMI, the greater the risk of neuropathy) and smoking. The presence of cardiovascular disease, elevated triglycerides, and hypertension is also associated with diabetic peripheral neuropathy. Both myelinated and unmyelinated nerve fibers are lost. Because the clinical features of diabetic neuropathy are similar to those of other neuropathies, the diagnosis of diabetic neuropathy should be made only after other possible etiologies are excluded. The ADA recommends screening for distal symmetric neuropathy beginning with the initial diagnosis of diabetes and screening for autonomic neuropathy 5 years after diagnosis of type 1 DM and at the time of diagnosis of type 2 DM. All individuals with diabetes should then be screened annually for both forms of neuropathy.

Polyneuropathy/Mononeuropathy

The most common form of diabetic neuropathy is distal symmetric polyneuropathy. It most frequently presents with distal sensory loss, but up to 50% of patients do not have symptoms of neuropathy. Hyperesthesia, paresthesia, and dysesthesia also may occur. Any combination of these symptoms may develop as neuropathy progresses. Symptoms may include a sensation of numbness, tingling, sharpness, or burning that begins in the feet and spreads proximally. Neuropathic pain develops in some of these individuals, occasionally preceded by improvement in their glycemic control. Pain typically involves the lower extremities, is usually present at rest, and worsens at night. Both an acute (lasting <12 months) and a chronic form of painful diabetic neuropathy have been described. As diabetic neuropathy progresses, the pain subsides and eventually disappears, but a sensory deficit in the lower extremities persists. Physical examination reveals sensory loss, loss of ankle reflexes, and abnormal position sense.

Diabetic polyradiculopathy is a syndrome characterized by severe disabling pain in the distribution of one or more nerve roots. It may be accompanied by motor weakness. Intercostal or truncal radiculopathy causes pain over the thorax or abdomen. Involvement of the lumbar plexus or femoral nerve may cause severe pain in the thigh or hip and may be associated with muscle weakness in the hip flexors or extensors (diabetic amyotrophy). Fortunately, diabetic polyradiculopathies are usually self-limited and resolve over 6–12 months.

Mononeuropathy (dysfunction of isolated cranial or peripheral nerves) is less common than polyneuropathy in DM and presents with pain and motor weakness in the distribution of a single nerve. A vascular etiology has been suggested, but the pathogenesis is unknown. Involvement of the third cranial nerve is most common and is heralded by diplopia. Physical examination reveals ptosis and ophthalmoplegia with normal pupillary constriction to light. Sometimes other cranial nerves IV, VI, or VII (Bell's palsy) are affected. Peripheral mononeuropathies or simultaneous involvement of more than one nerve (mononeuropathy multiplex) may also occur.

Autonomic Neuropathy

Individuals with longstanding type 1 or 2 DM may develop signs of autonomic dysfunction involving the cholinergic, noradrenergic, and peptidergic (peptides such as pancreatic polypeptide, substance P, etc.) systems. DM-related autonomic neuropathy can involve multiple systems, including the cardiovascular, gastrointestinal, genitourinary, sudomotor, and metabolic systems. Autonomic neuropathies affecting the cardiovascular system cause a resting tachycardia and orthostatic hypotension. Reports of sudden death have also been attributed to autonomic neuropathy. Gastroparesis and bladder-emptying abnormalities are often caused by the autonomic neuropathy seen in DM. Hyperhidrosis of the upper extremities and anhidrosis of the lower extremities result from sympathetic nervous system dysfunction. Anhidrosis of the feet can promote dry skin with cracking, which increases the risk of foot ulcers. Autonomic neuropathy may reduce counterregulatory hormone release, leading to an inability to sense hypoglycemia appropriately (hypoglycemia unawareness; Chap. 20), thereby subjecting the patient to the risk of severe hypoglycemia and complicating efforts to improve glycemic control.

℞ Treatment: DIABETIC NEUROPATHY

Treatment of diabetic neuropathy is less than satisfactory. Improved glycemic control should be aggressively pursued and will improve nerve conduction velocity, but symptoms of diabetic neuropathy may not necessarily improve. Efforts to improve glycemic control may be confounded by autonomic neuropathy and hypoglycemia unawareness. Risk factors for neuropathy such as hypertension and hypertriglyceridemia should be treated. Avoidance of neurotoxins (alcohol) and smoking, supplementation with vitamins for possible deficiencies (B_{12}, folate), and symptomatic treatment are the mainstays of therapy. Loss of sensation in the foot places the patient at risk for ulceration and its sequelae; consequently, prevention of such problems is of paramount importance. Patients with symptoms or signs of neuropathy (see "Physical Examination" later in the chapter) should check their feet daily and take precautions (footwear) aimed at preventing calluses or ulcerations. If foot deformities are present, a podiatrist should be involved.

Chronic, painful diabetic neuropathy is difficult to treat but may respond to antidepressants (tricyclic antidepressants such as amitriptyline, desipramine, nortriptyline, or imipramine or selective serotonin norepinephrine reuptake inhibitors such as duloxetine) or anticonvulsants (gabapentin, pregabalin, carbamazepine, lamotrigine). Two agents, duloxetine and pregabalin, have been approved by the U.S. Food and Drug Administration (FDA) for pain associated with diabetic neuropathy. However, pending further study, most recommend beginning with other agents such as a tricyclic antidepressant and switching if there is no response or if side effects develop. Aldose reductase inhibitors do not offer significant symptomatic relief. Referral to a pain management center may be necessary. Since the pain of acute diabetic neuropathy may resolve over time, medications may be discontinued as progressive neuronal damage from DM occurs.

Therapy of orthostatic hypotension secondary to autonomic neuropathy is also challenging. A variety of agents have limited success (fludrocortisone, midodrine, clonidine, octreotide, and yohimbine), but each has significant side effects. Nonpharmacologic maneuvers (adequate salt intake, avoidance of dehydration and diuretics, and lower extremity support hose) may offer some benefit.

GASTROINTESTINAL/GENITOURINARY DYSFUNCTION

Longstanding type 1 and 2 DM may affect the motility and function of gastrointestinal (GI) and genitourinary systems. The most prominent GI symptoms are delayed gastric emptying (gastroparesis) and altered small- and large-bowel motility (constipation or diarrhea). Gastroparesis may present with symptoms of anorexia, nausea, vomiting, early satiety, and abdominal bloating. Microvascular complications (retinopathy and neuropathy) are usually present. Nuclear medicine scintigraphy after ingestion of a radiolabeled meal is the best study to document delayed gastric emptying, but may not correlate well with symptoms. Noninvasive "breath tests" following ingestion of a radiolabeled meal are under development. Though parasympathetic dysfunction secondary to chronic hyperglycemia is important in the development of gastroparesis, hyperglycemia itself also impairs gastric emptying. Nocturnal diarrhea, alternating with constipation, is a feature of DM-related GI autonomic neuropathy. In type 1 DM, these symptoms should also prompt evaluation for celiac sprue because of its increased frequency. Esophageal dysfunction in longstanding DM may occur but is usually asymptomatic.

Diabetic autonomic neuropathy may lead to genitourinary dysfunction including cystopathy, erectile dysfunction, and female sexual dysfunction (reduced sexual desire, dyspareunia, reduced vaginal lubrication). Symptoms of diabetic cystopathy begin with an inability to sense a full bladder and a failure to void completely. As bladder contractility worsens, bladder capacity and the postvoid residual increase, leading to symptoms of urinary hesitancy, decreased voiding frequency, incontinence, and recurrent urinary tract infections. Diagnostic evaluation includes cystometry and urodynamic studies.

Erectile dysfunction and retrograde ejaculation are very common in DM and may be one of the earliest signs of diabetic neuropathy (Chap. 15). Erectile dysfunction, which increases in frequency with the age of the patient and the duration of diabetes, may occur in the absence of other signs of diabetic autonomic neuropathy.

℞ Treatment: GASTROINTESTINAL/GENITOURINARY DYSFUNCTION

Current treatments for these complications of DM are inadequate. Improved glycemic control should be a primary goal, as some aspects (neuropathy, gastric function) may improve. Smaller, more frequent meals that are easier to digest (liquid) and low in fat and fiber may minimize symptoms of gastroparesis. Agents with some efficacy include the dopamine agonists metoclopramide, 5–10 mg, and domperidone, 10–20 mg, before each meal. Erythromycin interacts with the motilin receptor and may promote gastric emptying. Diabetic diarrhea in the absence of bacterial overgrowth is treated symptomatically with loperamide and may respond to octreotide (50–75 μg three times daily, SC). Treatment of bacterial overgrowth with antibiotics is sometimes useful.

Diabetic cystopathy should be treated with timed voiding or self-catheterization, possibly with the addition of bethanechol. Drugs that inhibit type 5 phosphodiesterase are effective for erectile dysfunction, but their efficacy in individuals with DM is slightly lower than in the nondiabetic population (Chap. 15). Sexual dysfunction in women may be improved with use of vaginal lubricants, treatment of vaginal infections, and systemic or local estrogen replacement.

CARDIOVASCULAR MORBIDITY AND MORTALITY

Cardiovascular disease is increased in individuals with type 1 or type 2 DM. The Framingham Heart Study revealed a marked increase in PAD, CHF, CAD, MI, and sudden death (risk increase from one- to fivefold) in DM. The American Heart Association has designated DM as a major risk factor for cardiovascular disease (same category as smoking, hypertension, and hyperlipidemia). Type 2 diabetes patients without a prior MI have a similar risk for coronary artery–related events as nondiabetic individuals who have had a prior MI. Because of the extremely high prevalence of underlying cardiovascular disease in individuals with diabetes (especially in type 2 DM), evidence of atherosclerotic vascular disease (e.g., cardiac stress test) should be sought in an individual with diabetes who has symptoms suggestive of cardiac ischemia, peripheral or carotid arterial disease, a resting electrocardiogram indicative of prior infarction, plans to initiate an exercise program, proteinuria, or two other cardiac risk factors (ADA recommendations). Whether and how to screen asymptomatic individuals with diabetes for CAD is controversial. The absence of chest pain ("silent ischemia") is common in individuals with diabetes, and a thorough cardiac evaluation is indicated in individuals undergoing major surgical procedures. The prognosis for individuals with diabetes who have CAD or MI is worse than for nondiabetics. CAD is more likely to involve multiple vessels in individuals with DM.

The increase in cardiovascular morbidity and mortality appears to relate to the synergism of hyperglycemia with other cardiovascular risk factors. For example, after controlling for all known cardiovascular risk factors, type 2 DM increases the cardiovascular death rate twofold in men and fourfold in women. Risk factors for macrovascular disease in diabetic individuals include dyslipidemia, hypertension, obesity, reduced physical activity, and cigarette smoking. Additional risk factors more prevalent in the diabetic population include microalbuminuria, macroalbuminuria, an elevation of serum creatinine, and abnormal platelet function. Insulin resistance, as reflected by elevated serum insulin levels, is associated with an increased risk of cardiovascular complications in individuals with and without DM. Individuals with insulin resistance and type 2 DM have elevated levels of plasminogen activator inhibitors (especially PAI-1) and fibrinogen, which enhances the coagulation process and impairs fibrinolysis, thus favoring the development of thrombosis. Diabetes is also associated with endothelial, vascular smooth-muscle, and platelet dysfunction.

Evidence that improved glycemic control reduces cardiovascular complications in DM is inconclusive. In the DCCT, the number of cardiovascular events in patients with type 1 diabetes did not differ between the standard and intensively treated groups during the trial but was reduced at follow-up 17 years later. An improvement in the lipid profile of individuals in the intensive group (lower total and LDL cholesterol, lower triglycerides) during intensive diabetes management was noted. Trials to examine whether improved glycemic control reduces cardiovascular events in type 2 diabetes are underway. Concerns about the atherogenic potential of insulin remain, since in nondiabetic individuals, higher serum insulin levels (indicative of insulin resistance) are associated with a greater risk of cardiovascular morbidity and mortality. In the UKPDS, improved glycemic control did not conclusively reduce cardiovascular mortality. Importantly, treatment with insulin and the sulfonylureas did not appear to increase the risk of cardiovascular disease in individuals with type 2 DM, refuting prior claims about the atherogenic potential of these agents.

In addition to CAD, cerebrovascular disease is increased in individuals with DM (threefold increase in stroke). Individuals with DM have an increased incidence of CHF. The etiology of this abnormality is probably multifactorial and includes factors such as myocardial ischemia from atherosclerosis, hypertension, and myocardial cell dysfunction secondary to chronic hyperglycemia.

℞ Treatment: CARDIOVASCULAR DISEASE

In general, the treatment of coronary disease is not different in the diabetic individual. Revascularization procedures for CAD, including percutaneous coronary intervention (PCI) and coronary artery bypass grafting (CABG), may be less efficacious in the diabetic individual. Initial success rates of PCI in diabetic individuals are similar to those in the nondiabetic population, but diabetic patients have higher rates of restenosis and lower long-term patency and survival rates in older studies. More recently, the use of drug-eluting stents and a GPIIb/IIIa platelet inhibitor has improved the outcomes in diabetic patients, and whether there is a difference in efficacy of PCI in diabetic individuals is not clear. Although CABG may be preferred over PCI in diabetic individuals with multivessel CAD or recent Q-wave MI, PCI is preferred in patients with single-vessel CAD or two-vessel disease (no involvement of left anterior descending).

The ADA has emphasized the importance of glycemic control and aggressive cardiovascular risk modification in all individuals with DM. Past trepidation about using beta blockers in individuals who have diabetes should not prevent use of these agents since they clearly benefit diabetic patients after MI. ACE inhibitors (or ARBs) may also be particularly beneficial and should be considered in individuals with type 2 DM and other risk factors (smoking, dyslipidemia, history of cardiovascular disease, microalbuminuria). Patients with atypical chest pain or an abnormal resting ECG should be screened for CHD. Screening of asymptomatic individuals with diabetes is controversial.

Antiplatelet therapy reduces cardiovascular events in individuals with DM who have CAD. Current recommendations by the ADA include the use of aspirin for secondary prevention of coronary events. Although data demonstrating efficacy in primary prevention of coronary events in DM are lacking, antiplatelet therapy should be strongly considered, especially in diabetic individuals >30 years of age with other coronary risk factors such as hypertension, smoking, family history, or dyslipidemia. The aspirin dose (75–162 mg) is the same as that in nondiabetic individuals. Aspirin therapy does not have detrimental effects on renal function or hypertension, nor does it influence the course of diabetic retinopathy.

Cardiovascular Risk Factors

Dyslipidemia

Individuals with DM may have several forms of dyslipidemia (Chap. 21). Because of the additive cardiovascular risk of hyperglycemia and hyperlipidemia, lipid abnormalities should be assessed aggressively and treated as part of comprehensive diabetes care (**Fig. 19-12**). The most common pattern of dyslipidemia is hypertriglyceridemia and reduced HDL cholesterol levels. DM itself does not increase levels of LDL, but the small dense LDL particles found in type 2 DM are more atherogenic because they are more easily glycated and susceptible to oxidation.

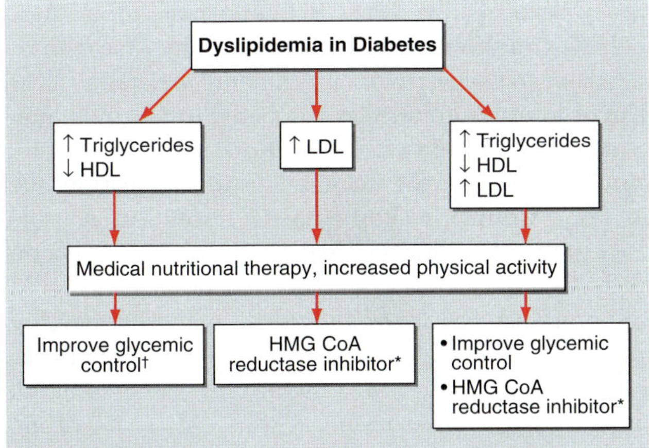

FIGURE 19-12

Dyslipidemia management in diabetes. *Second-line treatment: fibric acid derivative, ezetimibe, niacin, or bile acid–binding resin. †See text for pharmacologic treatment based on age and risk profile. LDL, low-density lipoprotein; HDL, high-density lipoprotein.

Almost all treatment studies of diabetic dyslipidemia have been performed in individuals with type 2 DM because of the greater frequency of dyslipidemia in this form of diabetes. Interventional studies have shown that the beneficial effects of LDL reduction are similar in the diabetic and nondiabetic populations. Large prospective trials of primary and secondary intervention for CHD have included some individuals with type 2 DM, and subset analyses have consistently found that reductions in LDL reduce cardiovascular events and morbidity in individuals with DM. Most clinical trials used HMG CoA reductase inhibitors, although gemfibrozil is also beneficial. No prospective studies have addressed similar questions in individuals with type 1 DM. Since the frequency of cardiovascular disease is low in children and young adults with diabetes, assessment of cardiovascular risk should be incorporated into the guidelines discussed below.

Based on the guidelines provided by the ADA and the American Heart Association, priorities in the treatment of hyperlipidemia are (1) lower the LDL cholesterol, (2) raise the HDL cholesterol, and (3) decrease the triglycerides. A treatment strategy depends on the pattern of lipoprotein abnormalities (Fig. 19-12). Initial therapy for all forms of dyslipidemia should include dietary changes, as well as the same lifestyle modifications recommended in the nondiabetic population (smoking cessation, blood pressure control, weight loss, increased physical activity). The dietary recommendations for individuals with DM are similar to those advocated by the National Cholesterol Education Program (Chap. 21) and include increased monounsaturated fat and carbohydrates and reduced saturated fats and cholesterol. Though viewed as important, the response to dietary alterations is often modest (<10% reduction in the LDL). Improvement in glycemic control will lower triglycerides and have a modest beneficial effect by raising HDL. HMG CoA reductase inhibitors are the agents of choice for lowering the LDL. According to guidelines of the ADA and the American Heart Association, the target lipid values in diabetic individuals (age >40 years) without cardiovascular disease should be LDL <2.6 mmol/L (100 mg/dL); HDL >1.1 mmol/L (40 mg/dL) in men and >1.38 mmol/L (50 mg/dL) in women, and triglycerides <1.7 mmol/L (150 mg/dL). The rationale for these goals is that the risk of CHD is similar to that in patients without diabetes who have had a prior MI. In patients >40 years, the ADA recommends addition of statin, regardless of the LDL, to reduce LDL by 30–40%.

If the patient is known to have cardiovascular disease, the ADA recommends an LDL goal of <1.8 mmol/L (70 mg/dL) as an "option" [in keeping with evidence that such a goal is beneficial in nondiabetic individuals with CAD (Chap. 21)]. Fibrates have some efficacy and should be considered when the HDL is low in the setting of a mild elevation of the LDL. Combination therapy with an HMG CoA reductase inhibitor and a fibrate or another lipid-lowering agent (ezetimibe, niacin) may be needed to reach LDL or HDL goals, but statin/fibrate combinations increase the possibility of side effects such as myositis. Nicotinic acid effectively raises HDL and can be used in patients with diabetes, but high doses (>2 g/d) may worsen glycemic control and increase insulin resistance. Bile acid–binding resins should not be used if hypertriglyceridemia is present. Pharmacologic therapy of dyslipidemia to achieve a LDL <2.6 mmol/L (100 mg/dL) should be considered in diabetic individuals <40 years of age without cardiovascular disease if the individual also has other risk factors.

Hypertension

Hypertension can accelerate other complications of DM, particularly cardiovascular disease and nephropathy. In targeting the goal of BP <130/80, therapy should first emphasize lifestyle modifications such as weight loss, exercise, stress management, and sodium restriction. Realizing that more than one agent is usually required to reach a blood pressure goal, the ADA recommends that all patients with diabetes and hypertension be treated with an ACE inhibitor or an ARB. Subsequently, agents that reduce cardiovascular risk (beta blockers, thiazide diuretics, and calcium channel blockers) should be incorporated into the regimen. While ACE inhibitors and ARBs are likely equivalent in most patients with diabetes and renal disease, the ADA recommends (1) in patients with type 1 diabetes, hypertension, and micro- or macroalbuminuria, an ACE inhibitor slowed progression of nephropathy; (2) in patients with type 2 diabetes, hypertension, and microalbuminuria, an ACE inhibitor or an ARB slowed the progression to macroalbuminuria; and (3) in patients with type 2 diabetes, hypertension, macroalbuminuria, and renal insufficiency, an ARB slowed the decline in GFR. Additional points of emphasis include:

1. ACE inhibitors are either glucose- and lipid-neutral or glucose- and lipid-beneficial and thus positively impact the cardiovascular risk profile. Calcium channel blockers, central adrenergic antagonists, and vasodilators are lipid- and glucose-neutral.
2. Beta blockers and thiazide diuretics can increase insulin resistance and negatively impact the lipid profile; beta blockers may slightly increase the risk of developing type 2 DM. Although often questioned because of the potential masking of hypoglycemic symptoms, beta blockers are safe in most patients with diabetes and reduce cardiovascular events.
3. Sympathetic inhibitors and α-adrenergic blockers may worsen orthostatic hypotension in the diabetic individual with autonomic neuropathy.
4. Equivalent reduction in blood pressure by different classes of agents may not translate into equivalent protection from cardiovascular and renal endpoints. Thiazides, beta blockers, ACE inhibitors, and ARBs positively impact cardiovascular endpoints (MI or stroke).
5. Non-dihydropyridine calcium channel blockers (verapamil and diltiazem), rather than dihydropyridine agents (amlodipine and nifedipine), are preferred in diabetics.
6. A blood pressure goal of <125/75 is suggested for individuals with macroalbuminuria, hypertension, and diabetes.
7. Serum potassium and renal function should be monitored.

Because of the high prevalence of atherosclerotic disease in individuals with DM, the possibility of renovascular hypertension should be considered when the blood pressure is not readily controlled.

LOWER EXTREMITY COMPLICATIONS

DM is the leading cause of nontraumatic lower extremity amputation in the United States. Foot ulcers and infections are also a major source of morbidity in individuals with DM. The reasons for the increased incidence of these disorders in DM involve the interaction of several pathogenic factors: neuropathy, abnormal foot biomechanics, PAD, and poor wound healing. The peripheral sensory neuropathy interferes with normal protective mechanisms and allows the patient to sustain major or repeated minor trauma to the foot, often without knowledge of the injury. Disordered proprioception causes abnormal weight bearing while walking and subsequent formation of callus or ulceration. Motor and sensory neuropathy lead to abnormal foot muscle mechanics and to structural changes in the foot (hammer toe, claw toe deformity, prominent metatarsal heads, Charcot joint). Autonomic neuropathy results in anhidrosis and altered superficial blood flow in the foot, which promote drying of the skin and fissure formation. PAD and poor wound healing impede resolution of minor breaks in the skin, allowing them to enlarge and to become infected.

Approximately 15% of individuals with DM develop a foot ulcer [great toe or metatarsophalangeal (MTP) areas are most common], and a significant subset will ultimately undergo amputation (14–24% risk with that ulcer or subsequent ulceration). Risk factors for foot ulcers or amputation include male sex, diabetes >10 years' duration, peripheral neuropathy, abnormal structure of foot (bony abnormalities, callus, thickened nails), peripheral arterial disease, smoking, history of previous ulcer or amputation, and poor glycemic control. Large calluses are often precursors to or overlie ulcerations.

℞ Treatment: LOWER EXTREMITY COMPLICATIONS

The optimal therapy for foot ulcers and amputations is prevention through identification of high-risk patients, education of the patient, and institution of measures to prevent ulceration. High-risk patients should be identified during the routine foot examination performed on all patients with DM (see "Ongoing Aspects of Comprehensive Diabetes Care" later in the chapter). Patient education should emphasize (1) careful selection of footwear, (2) daily inspection of the feet to detect early signs of poor-fitting footwear or minor trauma, (3) daily foot hygiene to keep the skin clean and moist, (4) avoidance of self-treatment of foot abnormalities and high-risk behavior (e.g., walking barefoot), and (5) prompt consultation with a health care provider if an abnormality arises. Patients at high risk for ulceration or amputation may benefit from evaluation by a foot care specialist. Interventions directed at risk factor modification include orthotic shoes and devices, callus management, nail care, and prophylactic measures to reduce increased skin pressure from abnormal bony architecture. Attention to other risk factors for vascular disease (smoking, dyslipidemia, hypertension) and improved glycemic control are also important.

Despite preventive measures, foot ulceration and infection are common and represent a serious problem. Due to the multifactorial pathogenesis of lower extremity ulcers, management of these lesions is multidisciplinary and often demands expertise in orthopedics, vascular surgery, endocrinology, podiatry, and infectious diseases. The plantar surface of the foot is the most common site of ulceration. Ulcers may be primarily neuropathic (no accompanying infection) or may have surrounding cellulitis or osteomyelitis. Cellulitis without ulceration is also frequent and should be treated with antibiotics that provide broad-spectrum coverage, including anaerobes.

An infected ulcer is a clinical diagnosis, since superficial culture of any ulceration will likely find multiple possible bacterial pathogens. The infection surrounding the foot ulcer is often the result of multiple organisms (gram-positive and -negative organisms and anaerobes), and gas gangrene may develop in the absence of clostridial infection. Cultures taken from the surface of the ulcer are not helpful; a culture from the debrided ulcer base or from purulent drainage or aspiration of the wound is the most helpful. Wound depth should be determined by inspection and probing with a blunt-tipped sterile instrument. Plain radiographs of the foot should be performed to assess the possibility of osteomyelitis in chronic ulcers that have not responded to therapy. Nuclear medicine bone scans may be helpful, but overlying subcutaneous infection is often difficult to distinguish from osteomyelitis. Indium-labeled white cell studies are more useful in determining if the infection involves bony structures or only soft tissue, but they are technically demanding. MRI of the foot may be the most specific modality, although distinguishing bony destruction due to osteomyelitis from destruction secondary to Charcot arthropathy is difficult. If surgical debridement is necessary, bone biopsy and culture may provide the answer.

Osteomyelitis is best treated by a combination of prolonged antibiotics (IV then PO) and possibly debridement of infected bone. The possible contribution of vascular insufficiency should be considered in all patients. Noninvasive blood-flow studies are often unreliable in DM, and angiography may be required, recognizing the risk of contrast-induced nephrotoxicity. Peripheral arterial bypass procedures are often effective in promoting wound healing and in decreasing the need for amputation of the ischemic limb.

A growing number of possible treatments for diabetic foot ulcers exist, but they have yet to demonstrate clear efficacy in prospective, controlled trials. A consensus statement from the ADA identified six interventions with demonstrated efficacy in diabetic foot wounds: (1) off-loading, (2) debridement, (3) wound dressings, (4) appropriate use of antibiotics, (5) revascularization, and (6) limited amputation. Off-loading is the complete avoidance of weight bearing on the ulcer, which removes the mechanical trauma that retards wound healing. Bed rest and a variety of orthotic devices or contact casting limit weight bearing on wounds or pressure points. Surgical debridement is important and effective, but clear efficacy of other modalities for wound cleaning (enzymes, soaking, whirlpools) is lacking. Dressings such as hydrocolloid dressings promote wound healing by creating a moist environment and protecting the wound. Antiseptic agents should be avoided. Topical antibiotics are of limited value. Referral for physical therapy, orthotic evaluation, and rehabilitation should occur once the infection is controlled.

Mild or non-limb-threatening infections can be treated with oral antibiotics (cephalosporin, clindamycin, amoxicillin/clavulanate, and fluoroquinolones), surgical debridement of necrotic tissue, local wound care (avoidance of weight bearing over the ulcer), and close surveillance for progression of infection. More severe ulcers may require IV antibiotics as well as bed rest and local wound care. Urgent surgical debridement may be required. Strict control of glycemia should be a goal. IV antibiotics should provide broad-spectrum coverage directed toward *Staphylococcus aureus*, streptococci, gram-negative aerobes, and anaerobic bacteria. Initial antimicrobial regimens include ertapenem, piperacillin/tazobactam, cefotetan, ampicillin/sulbactam, linezolid, or the combination of clindamycin and a fluoroquinolone. Severe infections, or infections that do not improve after

48 h of antibiotic therapy, require expansion of antimicrobial therapy to treat methicillin-resistant *S. aureus* (e.g., vancomycin) and *Pseudomonas aeruginosa.* If the infection surrounding the ulcer is not improving with IV antibiotics, reassessment of antibiotic coverage and reconsideration of the need for surgical debridement or revascularization are indicated. With clinical improvement, oral antibiotics and local wound care can be continued on an outpatient basis with close follow-up.

New information about wound biology has led to a number of new technologies (e.g., living skin equivalents and growth factors such as basic fibroblast growth factor) that may prove useful, especially in neuropathic ulcers. Recombinant platelet-derived growth factor has some benefit and complements the therapies of off-loading, debridement, and antibiotics. Hyperbaric oxygen has been used, but rigorous proof of efficacy is lacking. Negative wound pressure has been shown to accelerate wound healing of plantar wounds.

INFECTIONS

Individuals with DM have a greater frequency and severity of infection. The reasons for this include incompletely defined abnormalities in cell-mediated immunity and phagocyte function associated with hyperglycemia, as well as diminished vascularization. Hyperglycemia aids the colonization and growth of a variety of organisms (*Candida* and other fungal species). Many common infections are more frequent and severe in the diabetic population, whereas several rare infections are seen almost exclusively in the diabetic population. Examples of this latter category include rhinocerebral mucormycosis, emphysematous infections of the gallbladder and urinary tract, and "malignant" or invasive otitis externa. Invasive otitis externa is usually secondary to *P. aeruginosa* infection in the soft tissue surrounding the external auditory canal, usually begins with pain and discharge, and may rapidly progress to osteomyelitis and meningitis. These infections should be sought, in particular, in patients presenting with HHS.

Pneumonia, urinary tract infections, and skin and soft tissue infections are all more common in the diabetic population. In general, the organisms that cause pulmonary infections are similar to those found in the nondiabetic population; however, gram-negative organisms, *S. aureus*, and *Mycobacterium tuberculosis* are more frequent pathogens. Urinary tract infections (either lower tract or pyelonephritis) are the result of common bacterial agents such as *Escherichia coli*, though several yeast species (*Candida* and *Torulopsis glabrata*) are commonly observed. Complications of urinary tract infections include emphysematous pyelonephritis and emphysematous cystitis. Bacteriuria occurs frequently in individuals with diabetic cystopathy. Susceptibility to furunculosis, superficial candidal infections, and vulvovaginitis are increased. Poor glycemic control is a common denominator in individuals with these infections. Diabetic individuals have an increased rate of colonization of *S. aureus* in the skinfolds and nares. Diabetic patients also have a greater risk of postoperative wound infections. Strict glycemic control reduces postoperative infections in diabetic individuals undergoing CABG and should be the goal in all diabetic patients with an infection.

DERMATOLOGIC MANIFESTATIONS

The most common skin manifestations of DM are protracted wound healing and skin ulcerations. Diabetic dermopathy, sometimes termed *pigmented pretibial papules*, or "diabetic skin spots," begins as an erythematous area and evolves into an area of circular hyperpigmentation. These lesions result from minor mechanical trauma in the pretibial region and are more common in elderly men with DM. Bullous diseases, bullosa diabeticorum (shallow ulcerations or erosions in the pretibial region), are also seen. *Necrobiosis lipoidica diabeticorum* is a rare disorder of DM that predominantly affects young women with type 1 DM, neuropathy, and retinopathy. It usually begins in the pretibial region as an erythematous plaque or papules that gradually enlarge, darken, and develop irregular margins, with atrophic centers and central ulceration. They may be painful. Vitiligo occurs at increased frequency in individuals with type 1 diabetes. *Acanthosis nigricans* (hyperpigmented velvety plaques seen on the neck, axilla, or extensor surfaces) is sometimes a feature of severe insulin resistance and accompanying diabetes. Generalized or localized *granuloma annulare* (erythematous plaques on the extremities or trunk) and *scleredema* (areas of skin thickening on the back or neck at the site of previous superficial infections) are more common in the diabetic population. *Lipoatrophy* and *lipohypertrophy* can occur at insulin injection sites but are unusual with the use of human insulin. Xerosis and pruritus are common and are relieved by skin moisturizers.

Approach to the Patient: DIABETES MELLITUS

DM and its complications produce a wide range of symptoms and signs; those secondary to acute hyperglycemia may occur at any stage of the disease, whereas those related to chronic complications begin to appear during the second decade of hyperglycemia. Individuals with previously undetected type 2 DM may present with chronic complications of DM at the time of diagnosis. The history and physical examination should assess for symptoms or signs of acute hyperglycemia and should screen for the chronic complications and conditions associated with DM.

HISTORY A complete medical history should be obtained with special emphasis on DM-relevant aspects such as weight, family history of DM and its complications, risk factors for cardiovascular disease, exercise, smoking, and ethanol use. Symptoms of hyperglycemia include polyuria, polydipsia, weight loss, fatigue, weakness, blurry vision, frequent superficial infections (vaginitis, fungal skin infections), and slow healing of skin lesions after minor trauma. Metabolic derangements relate mostly to hyperglycemia (osmotic diuresis, reduced glucose entry into muscle) and to the catabolic state of the patient (urinary loss of glucose and calories, muscle breakdown due to protein degradation and decreased protein synthesis). Blurred vision results from changes in the water content of the lens and resolves as the hyperglycemia is controlled.

In a patient with established DM, the initial assessment should also include special emphasis on prior diabetes care, including the type of therapy, prior hemoglobin A1C levels, self-monitoring blood glucose results, frequency of hypoglycemia, presence of DM-specific complications, assessment of the patient's knowledge about diabetes, exercise, and nutrition. The chronic complications may afflict several organ systems, and an individual patient may exhibit some, all, or none of the symptoms related to the complications of DM. In addition, the presence of DM-related comorbidities should be sought (cardiovascular disease, hypertension, dyslipidemia).

PHYSICAL EXAMINATION In addition to a complete physical examination, special attention should be given to DM-relevant aspects such as weight or BMI, retinal examination, orthostatic blood pressure, foot examination, peripheral pulses, and insulin injection sites. Blood pressure >130/80 mmHg is considered hypertension in individuals with diabetes. Careful examination of the lower extremities should seek evidence of peripheral neuropathy, calluses, superficial fungal infections, nail disease, ankle reflexes, and foot deformities (such as hammer or claw toes and Charcot foot) in order to identify sites of potential skin ulceration. Vibratory sensation (128-MHz tuning fork at the base of the great toe), the ability to sense touch with a monofilament (5.07, 10-g monofilament), and pinprick sensation are useful to detect moderately advanced diabetic neuropathy. Since periodontal disease is more frequent in DM, the teeth and gums should also be examined.

CLASSIFICATION OF DM IN AN INDIVIDUAL PATIENT The etiology of diabetes in an individual with new-onset disease can usually be assigned on the basis of clinical criteria. Individuals with type 1 DM tend to have the following characteristics: (1) onset of disease prior to age 30; (2) lean body habitus; (3) requirement of insulin as the initial therapy; (4) propensity to develop ketoacidosis; and (5) an increased risk of other autoimmune disorders such as autoimmune thyroid disease, adrenal insufficiency, pernicious anemia, celiac disease, and vitiligo. In contrast, individuals with type 2 DM often exhibit the following features: (1) develop diabetes after the age of 30; (2) are usually obese (80% are obese, but elderly individuals may be lean); (3) may not require insulin therapy initially; and (4) may have associated conditions such as insulin resistance, hypertension, cardiovascular disease, dyslipidemia, or PCOS. In type 2 DM, insulin resistance is often associated with abdominal obesity (as opposed to hip and thigh obesity) and hypertriglyceridemia. Although most individuals diagnosed with type 2 DM are older, the age of diagnosis is declining, and there is a marked increase among overweight children and adolescents. Some individuals with phenotypic type 2 DM present with DKA but lack autoimmune markers and may be later treated with oral glucose-lowering agents rather than insulin (which has been termed *ketosis-prone type 2 DM*). On the other hand, some individuals (5–10%) with the phenotypic appearance of type 2 DM do not have absolute insulin deficiency but have autoimmune markers (ICA, GAD autoantibodies) suggestive of type 1 DM (termed *latent autoimmune diabetes of the adult*). Such individuals are more likely to be <50 years of age, have a normal BMI, and have a personal or family history of other autoimmune disease. They are much more likely to require insulin treatment within 5 years. However, it remains difficult to categorize some patients unequivocally. Individuals who deviate from the clinical profile of type 1 and type 2 DM, or who have other associated defects such as deafness, pancreatic exocrine disease, and other endocrine disorders, should be classified accordingly (Table 19-1).

LABORATORY ASSESSMENT The laboratory assessment should first determine whether the patient meets the diagnostic criteria for DM (Table 19-2) and then assess the degree of glycemic control (A1C, discussed later in the chapter). In addition to the standard laboratory evaluation, the patient should be screened for DM-associated conditions (e.g., microalbuminuria, dyslipidemia, thyroid dysfunction). Individuals at high risk for cardiovascular disease should be screened for asymptomatic CAD by appropriate cardiac stress testing, when indicated.

The classification of the type of DM may be facilitated by laboratory assessments. Serum insulin or C-peptide measurements do not always distinguish type 1 from type 2 DM, but a low C-peptide level confirms a patient's need for insulin. Many individuals with new-onset type 1 DM retain some C-peptide production. Measurement of islet cell antibodies at the time of diabetes onset may be useful if the type of DM is not clear based on the characteristics described above.

LONG-TERM TREATMENT

OVERALL PRINCIPLES

The goals of therapy for type 1 or type 2 DM are to (1) eliminate symptoms related to hyperglycemia, (2) reduce or eliminate the long-term microvascular and macrovascular complications of DM, and (3) allow the patient to achieve as normal a lifestyle as possible. To reach these goals, the physician should identify a target level of glycemic control for each patient, provide the patient with the educational and pharmacologic resources necessary to reach this level, and monitor/treat DM-related complications. Symptoms of diabetes usually resolve when the plasma glucose is <11.1 mmol/L (200 mg/dL), and thus most DM treatment focuses on achieving the second and third goals. The treatment goals for patients with diabetes are summarized in Table 19-8.

TABLE 19-8

TREATMENT GOALS FOR ADULTS WITH DIABETES[a]

INDEX	GOAL
Glycemic control[b]	
A1C	<7.0[c]
Preprandial capillary plasma glucose	5.0–7.2 mmol/L (90–130 mg/dL)
Peak postprandial capillary plasma glucose	<10.0 mmol/L (<180 mg/dL)[d]
Blood pressure	<130/80[e]
Lipids[f]	
Low-density lipoprotein	<2.6 mmol/L (<100 mg/dL)
High-density lipoprotein	>1.1 mmol/L (>40 mg/dL)[g]
Triglycerides	<1.7 mmol/L (<150 mg/dL)

[a]As recommended by the ADA; goals should be developed for each patient (see text). Goals may be different for certain patient populations.
[b]A1C is primary goal.
[c]While the ADA recommends an A1C <7.0% in general, in the individual patient it recommends an ". . . A1C as close to normal (<6.0%) as possible without significant hypoglycemia. . . ." Normal range for A1C—4.0–6.0 (DCCT-based assay).
[d]One to two hours after beginning of a meal.
[e]In patients with reduced GFR and macroalbuminuria, the goal is <125/75.
[f]In decreasing order of priority.
[g]For women, some suggest a goal that is 0.25 mmol/L (10 mg/dL) higher.
Source: Adapted from American Diabetes Association, 2007.

The care of an individual with either type 1 or type 2 DM requires a multidisciplinary team. Central to the success of this team are the patient's participation, input, and enthusiasm, all of which are essential for optimal diabetes management. Members of the health care team include the primary care provider and/or the endocrinologist or diabetologist, a certified diabetes educator, and a nutritionist. In addition, when the complications of DM arise, subspecialists (including neurologists, nephrologists, vascular surgeons, cardiologists, ophthalmologists, and podiatrists) with experience in DM-related complications are essential.

A number of names are sometimes applied to different approaches to diabetes care, such as intensive insulin therapy, intensive glycemic control, and "tight control." The current chapter, however, will use the term *comprehensive diabetes care* to emphasize the fact that optimal diabetes therapy involves more than plasma glucose management. Though glycemic control is central to optimal diabetes therapy, comprehensive diabetes care of both type 1 and type 2 DM should also detect and manage DM-specific complications and modify risk factors for DM-associated diseases. In addition to the physical aspects of DM, social, family, financial, cultural, and employment-related issues may impact diabetes care. The International Diabetes Federation (IDF), recognizing that resources available for diabetes care varies widely throughout the world, has issued guidelines for standard care (a well-developed service base and with health care funding systems consuming a significant part of their national wealth), minimal care (health care settings with very limited resources), and comprehensive care (health care settings with considerable resources). This chapter provides guidance for this comprehensive level of diabetes care.

PATIENT EDUCATION ABOUT DM, NUTRITION, AND EXERCISE

The patient with type 1 or type 2 DM should receive education about nutrition, exercise, care of diabetes during illness, and medications to lower the plasma glucose. Along with improved compliance, patient education allows individuals with DM to assume greater responsibility for their care. Patient education should be viewed as a continuing process with regular visits for reinforcement; it should not be a process that is completed after one or two visits to a nurse educator or nutritionist. The ADA refers to education about the individualized management plan for the patient as diabetes self-management education (DSME). More frequent contact between the patient and the diabetes management team (electronic, telephone, etc.) improves glycemic control.

Diabetes Education

The diabetes educator is a health care professional (nurse, dietician, or pharmacist) with specialized patient education skills who is certified in diabetes education (e.g., American Association of Diabetes Educators). Education topics important for optimal diabetes care include self-monitoring of blood glucose; urine ketone monitoring (type 1 DM); insulin administration; guidelines for diabetes management during illnesses; management of hypoglycemia; foot and skin care; diabetes management before, during, and after exercise; and risk factor–modifying activities.

Nutrition

Medical nutrition therapy (MNT) is a term used by the ADA to describe the optimal coordination of caloric intake with other aspects of diabetes therapy (insulin, exercise, weight loss). The ADA has issued recommendations for three types of MNT. Primary prevention measures of MNT are directed at preventing or delaying the onset of type 2 DM in high-risk individuals (obese or with pre-diabetes) by promoting weight reduction. Medical treatment of obesity is a rapidly evolving area and is discussed in Chap. 17. Secondary prevention measures of MNT are directed at preventing or delaying diabetes-related complications in diabetic individuals by improving glycemic control. Tertiary prevention measures of MNT are directed at managing diabetes-related complications (cardiovascular disease, nephropathy) in diabetic individuals. For example, in individuals with diabetes and chronic kidney disease, protein intake should be limited to 0.8 g/kg of body weight per day. MNT in patients with diabetes and cardiovascular disease should incorporate dietary principles used in nondiabetic patients with cardiovascular disease. While the recommendations for all three types of MNT overlap, this chapter emphasizes secondary prevention measures of MNT. Pharmacologic approaches that facilitate weight loss and bariatric surgery should be considered in selected patients (Chap. 17).

As for the general population, a diet that includes fruits, vegetables, fiber-containing foods, and low-fat milk is advised. Like other aspects of DM therapy, MNT must be adjusted to meet the goals of the individual patient. Furthermore, MNT education is an important component of comprehensive diabetes care and should be reinforced by regular patient education. In general, the components of optimal MNT are similar for individuals with type 1 or type 2 DM (Table 19-9). Historically, nutrition education imposed restrictive, complicated regimens on the patient. Current practices have greatly changed, though many patients and health care providers still view the diabetic diet as monolithic and static. For example, MNT now includes foods with sucrose and seeks to modify other risk factors such as hyperlipidemia and hypertension rather than focusing exclusively on weight loss in individuals with type 2 DM. The *glycemic index* is an estimate of the postprandial rise in the blood glucose when a certain amount of that food is consumed. Consumption of foods

TABLE 19-9

NUTRITIONAL RECOMMENDATIONS FOR ADULTS WITH DIABETES[a]
Fat
20–35% of total caloric intake
Saturated fat <7% of total calories
<200 mg/d of dietary cholesterol
Two or more servings of fish per week provide omega-3 polyunsaturated fatty acids
Minimal trans fat consumption
Carbohydrate
45–65% of total caloric intake (low-carbohydrate diets are not recommended)
Amount and type of carbohydrate important[b]
Sucrose-containing foods may be consumed with adjustments in insulin dose
Protein
10–35% of total caloric intake (high-protein diets are not recommended)
Other components
Fiber-containing foods may reduce postprandial glucose excursions
Nonnutrient sweeteners

[a]See text for differences for patients with type 1 or type 2 diabetes. As for the general population, a healthy diet includes fruits, vegetables, and fiber-containing foods.
[b]Amount of carbohydrate determined by estimating grams of carbohydrate in diet; glycemic index reflects how consumption of a particular food affects the blood glucose.
Source: Adapted from American Diabetes Association, 2007.

with a low glycemic index appears to reduce postprandial glucose excursions and improve glycemic control. Reduced calorie and nonnutritive sweeteners are useful. Currently, evidence does not support supplementation of the diet with vitamins, antioxidants (vitamin C and E), or micronutrients (chromium) in patients with diabetes. The goal of MNT in the individual with type 1 DM is to coordinate and match the caloric intake, both temporally and quantitatively, with the appropriate amount of insulin. MNT in type 1 DM and self-monitoring of blood glucose must be integrated to define the optimal insulin regimen. The ADA encourages patients and providers to utilize carbohydrate counting or exchange systems to estimate the nutrient content of a meal or snack. Based on the patient's estimate of the carbohydrate content of meal, an insulin-to-carbohydrate ratio determines the bolus insulin dose for a meal or snack. MNT must be flexible enough to allow for exercise, and the insulin regimen must allow for deviations in caloric intake. An important component of MNT in type 1 DM is to minimize the weight gain often associated with intensive diabetes management.

The goals of MNT in type 2 DM are slightly different and address the greatly increased prevalence of cardiovascular risk factors (hypertension, dyslipidemia, obesity) and disease in this population. The majority of these individuals are obese, and weight loss is strongly encouraged and should remain an important goal. Hypocaloric diets and modest weight loss (5–7%) often result in rapid and dramatic glucose lowering in individuals with new-onset type 2 DM. Nevertheless, numerous studies document that long-term weight loss is uncommon. MNT for type 2 DM should emphasize modest caloric reduction, reduced fat intake, increased physical activity, and reduction of hyperlipidemia and hypertension. Increased consumption of soluble, dietary fiber may improve glycemic control in individuals with type 2 DM. Weight loss and exercise improve insulin resistance.

Exercise

Exercise has multiple positive benefits including cardiovascular risk reduction, reduced blood pressure, maintenance of muscle mass, reduction in body fat, and weight loss. For individuals with type 1 or type 2 DM, exercise is also useful for lowering plasma glucose (during and following exercise) and increasing insulin sensitivity. In patients with diabetes, the ADA recommends 150 min/week (distributed over at least 3 days) of aerobic physical activity. In patients with type 2 DM, the exercise regimen should also include resistance training.

Despite its benefits, exercise presents challenges for individuals with DM because they lack the normal glucoregulatory mechanisms (normally, insulin falls and glucagon rises during exercise). Skeletal muscle is a major site for metabolic fuel consumption in the resting state, and the increased muscle activity during vigorous, aerobic exercise greatly increases fuel requirements. Individuals with type 1 DM are prone to either hyperglycemia or hypoglycemia during exercise, depending on the pre-exercise plasma glucose, the circulating insulin level, and the level of exercise-induced catecholamines. If the insulin level is too low, the rise in catecholamines may increase the plasma glucose excessively, promote ketone body formation, and possibly lead to ketoacidosis. Conversely, if the circulating insulin level is excessive, this relative hyperinsulinemia may reduce hepatic glucose production (decreased glycogenolysis, decreased gluconeogenesis) and increase glucose entry into muscle, leading to hypoglycemia.

To avoid exercise-related hyper- or hypoglycemia, individuals with type 1 DM should (1) monitor blood glucose before, during, and after exercise; (2) delay exercise if blood glucose is >14 mmol/L (250 mg/dL) and ketones are present; (3) if the blood glucose is <5.6 mmol/L (100 mg/dL), ingest carbohydrate before exercising; (3) monitor glucose during exercise and ingest carbohydrate to prevent hypoglycemia; (4) decrease insulin doses (based on previous experience) before exercise and inject insulin into a nonexercising area; and (5) learn individual glucose responses to different types of exercise and increase food intake for up to 24 h after exercise, depending on intensity and duration of exercise. In individuals with type 2 DM, exercise-related hypoglycemia is less common but can occur in individuals taking either insulin or insulin secretagogues.

Because asymptomatic cardiovascular disease appears at a younger age in both type 1 and type 2 DM, formal exercise tolerance testing may be warranted in diabetic individuals with any of the following: age >35 years, diabetes duration >15 years (type 1 DM) or >10 years (type 2 DM), microvascular complications of DM (retinopathy, microalbuminuria, or nephropathy), PAD, other risk factors of CAD, or autonomic neuropathy. Untreated proliferative retinopathy is a relative contraindication to vigorous exercise, as this may lead to vitreous hemorrhage or retinal detachment.

MONITORING THE LEVEL OF GLYCEMIC CONTROL

Optimal monitoring of glycemic control involves plasma glucose measurements by the patient and an assessment of long-term control by the physician (measurement of hemoglobin A1C and review of the patient's self-measurements of plasma glucose). These measurements are complementary: the patient's measurements provide a picture of short-term glycemic control, whereas the A1C reflects average glycemic control over the previous 2–3 months.

Self-Monitoring of Blood Glucose

Self-monitoring of blood glucose (SMBG) is the standard of care in diabetes management and allows the patient to monitor his or her blood glucose at any time. In SMBG, a small drop of blood and an easily detectable enzymatic reaction allow measurement of the capillary plasma glucose. Many glucose monitors can rapidly and accurately measure glucose (calibrated to provide plasma glucose value even though blood glucose is measured) in small amounts of blood (3–10 μL) obtained from the fingertip; alternative testing sites (e.g., forearm) are less reliable, especially when the blood glucose is changing rapidly (postprandially). A large number of blood glucose monitors are available, and the certified diabetes educator is critical in helping the patient select the optimal device and learn to use it properly. By combining glucose measurements with diet history, medication changes, and exercise history, the physician and patient can improve the treatment program.

The frequency of SMBG measurements must be individualized and adapted to address the goals of diabetes care. Individuals with type 1 DM or individuals with type 2 DM taking multiple insulin injections each day should routinely measure their plasma glucose three or more times per day to estimate and select mealtime boluses of short-acting insulin and to modify long-acting insulin doses. Most individuals with type 2 DM require less frequent monitoring, though the optimal frequency of SMBG has not been clearly defined. Individuals with type 2 DM who are taking insulin should utilize SMBG more frequently than those on oral agents. Individuals with type 2 DM who are on oral medications should utilize SMBG as a means of assessing the efficacy of their medication and the impact of diet. Since plasma glucose levels fluctuate less in these individuals, one to two SMBG measurements per day (or fewer in patients who are on oral agents or are diet-controlled) may be sufficient. Most measurements in individuals with type 1 or type 2 DM should be performed prior to a meal and supplemented with postprandial measurements to assist in reaching postprandial glucose targets (Table 19-8). Urine glucose testing does not provide an accurate assessment of glycemic control.

Devices for continuous blood glucose monitoring are the subject of intense investigation, as some systems have been approved by the FDA and others are in various stages of development. Currently, the use of these devices in routine diabetes management is limited, and they do not replace the need for a traditional glucose meter. This rapidly evolving technology requires substantial expertise on the part of the diabetes management team and the patient. Current continuous glucose monitoring systems (CGMSs) measure the glucose in interstitial fluid that is in equilibrium with the blood glucose. Alarms notify the patient if the blood glucose falls into the hypoglycemic range. The FDA refers to these as "minimally invasive" or "noninvasive" depending on how the interstitial fluid is obtained. Several devices use an indwelling SC catheter to monitor interstitial fluid glucose and provide either real-time or retrospective glucose values. Although clinical experience with these devices is limited, they appear to provide useful short-term information about the patterns of glucose changes as well as an enhanced ability to detect hypoglycemic episodes.

Ketones are an indicator of early diabetic ketoacidosis and should be measured in individuals with type 1 DM when the plasma glucose is consistently >16.7 mmol/L (300 mg/dL); during a concurrent illness; or with symptoms such as nausea, vomiting, or abdominal pain. Blood measurement of β-hydroxybutyrate is preferred over urine testing with nitroprusside-based assays that measure only acetoacetate and acetone.

Assessment of Long-Term Glycemic Control

Measurement of glycated hemoglobin is the standard method for assessing long-term glycemic control. When plasma glucose is consistently elevated, there is an increase in nonenzymatic glycation of hemoglobin; this alteration reflects the glycemic history over the previous 2–3 months, since erythrocytes have an average life span of 120 days (glycemic level in the preceding month contributes about 50% to the A1C value). There are numerous laboratory methods for measuring the various forms of glycated hemoglobin, and these have significant interassay variations. Since glycated hemoglobin measurements are usually compared to prior measurements, it is essential for the assay results to be comparable. Depending on the assay methodology, hemoglobinopathies, anemias, reticulocytosis, transfusions, and uremia may interfere with the A1C result. Measurement of A1C at the "point of care" allows for more rapid feedback and may therefore assist in adjustment of therapy.

Glycated hemoglobin or A1C should be measured in all individuals with DM during their initial evaluation and as part of their comprehensive diabetes care. As the primary predictor of long-term complications of DM, the A1C should mirror, to a certain extent, the short-term measurements of SMBG. These two measurements are complementary in that recent intercurrent illnesses may impact the SMBG measurements but not the A1C. Likewise, postprandial and nocturnal hyperglycemia may not be detected by the SMBG of fasting and preprandial capillary plasma glucose but will be reflected in the A1C. In standardized assays, the A1C approximates the following mean plasma glucose values: an A1C of 6% is 7.5 mmol/L (135 mg/dL), 7% is 9.5 mmol/L (170 mg/dL), 8% is 11.5 mmol/L (205 mg/dL), etc. [A 1% rise in the A1C translates into a 2.0-mmol/L (35 mg/dL) increase in the mean glucose.] In patients achieving their glycemic goal, the ADA recommends measurement of the A1C at least twice per year. More frequent testing (every 3 months) is warranted when glycemic control is inadequate, when therapy has changed, or in most patients with type 1 DM. The degree of glycation of other proteins, such as albumin, can be used as an alternative indicator of glycemic control when the A1C is inaccurate (hemolytic anemia, hemoglobinopathies). The fructosamine assay (measuring glycated albumin) reflects the glycemic status over the prior 2 weeks. Alternative assays of glycemic control (including the 1,5-anhydroglucitol assay) should not be routinely used since studies demonstrating that it accurately predicts the complications of DM are lacking.

℞ Treatment: TYPE 1 AND TYPE 2 DIABETES MELLITUS

ESTABLISHMENT OF TARGET LEVEL OF GLYCEMIC CONTROL Because the complications of DM are related to glycemic control, normoglycemia or near normoglycemia is the desired, but often elusive, goal for most patients. However, normalization of the plasma glucose for long periods of time is extremely difficult, as demonstrated by the DCCT. Regardless of the level of hyperglycemia, improvement in glycemic control will lower the risk of diabetes complications (Fig. 19-8).

The target for glycemic control (as reflected by the A1C) must be individualized, and the goals of therapy should be developed in consultation with the patient after considering a number of medical, social, and lifestyle issues. Some important factors to consider include the patient's age, ability to understand and implement a complex treatment regimen, presence and severity of complications of diabetes, ability to recognize hypoglycemic symptoms, presence of other medical conditions or treatments that might alter the response to therapy, lifestyle and occupation (e.g., possible consequences of experiencing hypoglycemia on the job), and level of support available from family and friends.

The ADA suggests that the glycemic goal is to achieve an A1C as close to normal as possible without significant hypoglycemia. In general, the target A1C should be <7.0% (Table 19-8) with a more stringent target (<6%) for many patients. A higher A1C goal may be appropriate for the very young or old or in individuals with limited life span or comorbid conditions. The major consideration is the frequency and severity of hypoglycemia, since this becomes more common with a more stringent A1C goal. Other groups (International Diabetes Federation and American Association of Clinical Endocrinology) have suggested that the A1C goal should be ≤6.5% in most individuals, based primarily on the observation that there is no lower limit of A1C in terms of reducing diabetes-specific complications.

TYPE 1 DIABETES MELLITUS

General Aspects The ADA recommendations for fasting and bedtime glycemic goals and A1C targets are summarized in Table 19-8. The goal is to design and implement insulin regimens that mimic physiologic insulin secretion. Because individuals with type 1 DM partially or completely lack endogenous insulin production, administration of basal, exogenous insulin is essential for regulating glycogen breakdown, gluconeogenesis, lipolysis, and ketogenesis. Likewise, insulin replacement for meals should be appropriate for the carbohydrate intake and promote normal glucose utilization and storage.

Intensive Management Intensive diabetes management has the goal of achieving euglycemia or near-normal glycemia. This approach requires multiple resources including thorough and continuing patient education, comprehensive recording of plasma glucose measurements and nutrition intake by the patient, and a variable insulin regimen that matches glucose intake and insulin dose. Insulin regimens usually include multiple-component insulin regimens, multiple daily injections (MDIs), or insulin infusion devices (each discussed later in the chapter).

The benefits of intensive diabetes management and improved glycemic control include a reduction in the microvascular complications of DM and a reduction in the macrovascular complications of DM, which persist after a period of near normoglycemia. From a psychological standpoint, the patient experiences greater control over his or her diabetes and often notes an improved sense of well-being, greater flexibility in the timing and content of meals, and the capability to alter insulin dosing with exercise. In addition, intensive diabetes management in pregnancy reduces the risk of fetal malformations and morbidity. Intensive diabetes management is strongly encouraged in newly diagnosed patients with type 1 DM because it may prolong the period of C-peptide production, which may result in better glycemic control and a reduced risk of serious hypoglycemia.

Although intensive management confers impressive benefits, it is also accompanied by significant personal and financial costs and is therefore not appropriate for all individuals.

Insulin Preparations Current insulin preparations are generated by recombinant DNA technology and consist of the amino acid sequence of human insulin or variations thereof. Animal insulin (beef or pork) is no longer used. In the United States, most insulin is formulated as U-100 (100 units/mL), whereas in some other countries it is available in other concentrations (e.g., U-40 = 40 units/mL). Human insulin has been formulated with distinctive pharmacokinetics or genetically modified to more closely mimic physiologic insulin secretion. Insulins can be classified as short-acting or long-acting (Table 19-10). For example, one short-acting insulin formulation, insulin lispro, is an insulin analogue in which the 28th and 29th amino acids (lysine and proline) on the insulin B chain have been reversed by recombinant DNA technology. Insulin aspart and insulin glulisine are other genetically modified insulin analogues with properties similar to lispro. These insulin analogues have full biologic activity but less tendency for self-aggregation, resulting in more rapid absorption and onset of action and a shorter duration of action. These characteristics are particularly advantageous for allowing entrainment of insulin injection and action to rising plasma glucose levels following meals. The shorter duration of action also appears to be associated with a decreased number of hypoglycemic episodes, primarily because the decay of insulin action corresponds to the decline in plasma glucose after a meal. Thus, insulin aspart, lispro, or glulisine is preferred over regular insulin for prandial coverage. Insulin glargine is a long-acting biosynthetic human insulin that differs from normal insulin in that asparagine is replaced by glycine at amino acid 21, and two arginine residues are added to the C-terminus of the B chain. Compared to NPH insulin, the onset of insulin glargine action is later, the duration of action is longer (~24 h), and there is no pronounced peak. A lower incidence of hypoglycemia, especially at night, has been reported with insulin glargine when compared to NPH insulin. Insulin detemir has a fatty acid side chain that prolongs its action by slowing absorption and catabolism. Regular and NPH insulin have the native

TABLE 19-10

PHARMACOKINETICS OF INSULIN PREPARATIONS

PREPARATION	TIME OF ACTION		
	ONSET, h	PEAK, h	EFFECTIVE DURATION, h
Short-acting, SC			
Lispro	<0.25	0.5–1.5	3–4
Aspart	<0.25	0.5–1.5	3–4
Glulisine	<0.25	0.5–1.5	3–4
Regular	0.5–1.0	2–3	4–6
Short-acting, inhaled			
Inhaled regular insulin	<0.25	0.5–1.5	4–6
Long-acting			
NPH	1–4	6–10	10–16
Detemir	1–4	—[a]	12–20
Glargine	1–4	—[a]	24
Insulin combinations			
75/25–75% protamine lispro, 25% lispro	<0.25	1.5 h[b]	Up to 10–16
70/30–70% protamine aspart, 30% aspart	<0.25	1.5 h[b]	Up to 10–16
50/50–50% protamine lispro, 50% lispro	<0.25	1.5 h[b]	Up to 10–16
70/30–70% NPH, 30% regular insulin	0.5–1	Dual	10–16
50/50–50% NPH, 50% regular insulin	0.5–1	Dual	10–16

[a]Glargine has minimal peak activity; detemir has some peak activity at 6–14 h.
[b]Dual: two peaks; one at 2–3 h; the second several hours later.
Source: Adapted from JS Skyler, *Therapy for Diabetes Mellitus and Related Disorders*, American Diabetes Association, Alexandria, VA, 2004.

insulin amino acid sequence. Regular insulin formulated as U-500 (500 units/mL) is available and sometimes useful in severely insulin-resistant patients.

Basal insulin requirements are provided by long-acting (NPH insulin, insulin glargine, or insulin detemir) insulin formulations. These are usually prescribed with short-acting insulin in an attempt to mimic physiologic insulin release with meals. Although mixing of NPH and short-acting insulin formulations is common practice, this mixing may alter the insulin absorption profile (especially the short-acting insulins). For example, lispro absorption is delayed by mixing with NPH. The alteration in insulin absorption when the patient mixes different insulin formulations should not discourage mixing insulins. However, the following guidelines should be followed: (1) mix the different insulin formulations in the syringe immediately before injection (inject within 2 min after mixing), (2) do not store insulin as a mixture, (3) follow the same routine in terms of insulin mixing and administration to standardize the physiologic response to injected insulin, and (4) do not mix insulin glargine or detemir with other insulins. The miscibility of human regular and NPH insulin allows for the production of combination insulins that contain 70% NPH and 30% regular (70/30), or equal mixtures of NPH and regular (50/50). Other combination insulin formulations are insulin aspart (70/30) and insulin lispro (75/25 and 50/50). By including some insulin analogue mixed with protamine, these combinations have a short-acting and long-acting profile (Table 19-10). While more convenient for the patient (only two injections per day), combination insulin formulations do not allow independent adjustment of short-acting and long-acting activity. Several insulin formulations are available as insulin "pens," which may be more convenient for some patients.

Insulin can also be delivered by inhalation by using a powder formulation of regular insulin and a delivery device. For insulin delivery, the patient uses a powdered formulation of insulin (a "blister") and a specialized inhaler to release a cloud of insulin into a reservoir from which the aerosolized insulin is inhaled. Inhaled insulin is short-acting, with an onset of action similar to insulin analogues but with a duration of action similar to regular insulin. It is therefore used for prandial coverage. Inhaled insulin must either be combined with an injected long-acting insulin to provide basal insulin coverage in type 1 or type 2 DM (Table 19-10) or used in combination with oral agents in patients with type 2 DM. Inhaled insulin appears to be similar to injected regular insulin in terms of glycemic control. It is available in 1- and 3-mg "blisters," which are equivalent to 3 and 8 units of injected regular insulin. To deliver a larger dose requires the use of more than one blister. Inhaled insulin is not approved for use in patients who smoke or have chronic lung diseases. Pulmonary function testing should be performed before starting inhaled insulin and repeated after 6 months of treatment and then annually. Side effects include cough, which improves with continued use, and hypoglycemia in a frequency similar to that seen with injected regular insulin. Long-term safety of inhaled insulin is not known. Proper use of the inhalation device requires patient education. Inhaled insulin has no physiologic advantage over injected short-acting insulin but may be considered in selected patients with type 2 DM who are unwilling to use injected insulin. Other inhaled insulin formulations are under development.

Insulin Regimens Representations of the various insulin regimens that may be utilized in type 1 DM are illustrated in Fig. 19-13. Although the insulin profiles are depicted as "smooth," symmetric curves, there is considerable patient-to-patient variation in the peak and duration. In all regimens, long-acting insulins (NPH, glargine, or detemir) supply basal insulin, whereas regular, insulin aspart, glulisine, or lispro insulin provides prandial insulin. Short-acting insulin analogues should be injected just before (<20 min) or just after a meal; regular insulin is given 30–45 min prior to a meal.

A shortcoming of current insulin regimens is that injected insulin immediately enters the systemic circulation, whereas endogenous insulin is secreted into the portal venous system. Thus, exogenous insulin administration exposes the liver to subphysiologic insulin levels. No insulin regimen reproduces the precise insulin secretory pattern of the pancreatic islet. However, the most physiologic regimens entail more frequent insulin injections, greater reliance on short-acting insulin, and more frequent capillary plasma glucose measurements. In general, individuals with type 1 DM require 0.5–1.0 U/kg per d of insulin divided into multiple doses, with ~50% of the insulin given as basal insulin.

Multiple-component insulin regimens refer to the combination of basal insulin and bolus insulin (preprandial short-acting insulin). The timing and dose of short-acting, preprandial insulin are altered to accommodate the SMBG results, anticipated food intake, and physical activity. Such regimens offer the patient with type 1 diabetes more flexibility in terms of lifestyle and the best chance for achieving near normoglycemia. One such regimen, shown in Fig. 19-13*B*, consists of basal insulin with glargine or detemir and preprandial lispro, glulisine, or insulin aspart. The insulin aspart, glulisine, or lispro dose is based on individualized algorithms that integrate the preprandial glucose and the anticipated carbohydrate intake. To determine the meal component of the preprandial insulin dose, the patient uses an insulin/carbohydrate ratio (a common ratio is 1–1.5 units/10 g of carbohydrate, but this must be determined for each individual). To this insulin dose is added the supplemental or correcting insulin based on the preprandial blood glucose [one formula uses 1 unit of insulin for every 2.7 mmol/L (50 mg/dL) over the preprandial glucose target; another formula uses (body weight in kg) × (blood glucose – desired glucose in mg/dL)/1500]. An alternative multiple-component insulin regimen consists of bedtime NPH insulin, a small dose of NPH insulin at breakfast (20–30% of bedtime dose), and preprandial short-acting insulin. Other variations of this regimen are in use but have the disadvantage that NPH

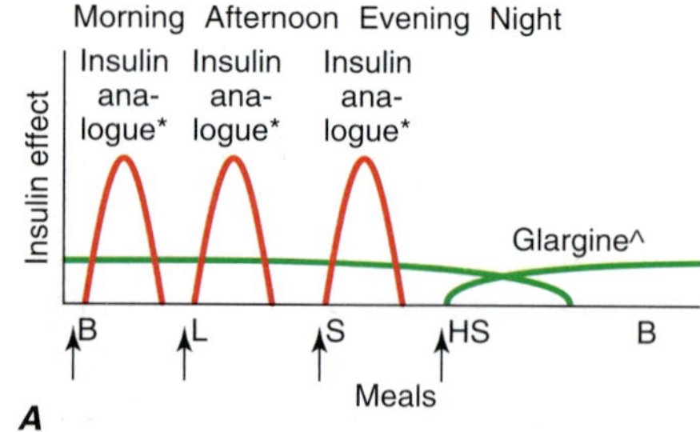

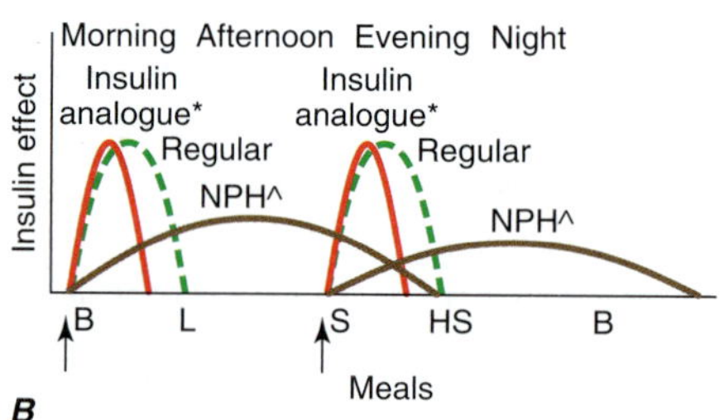

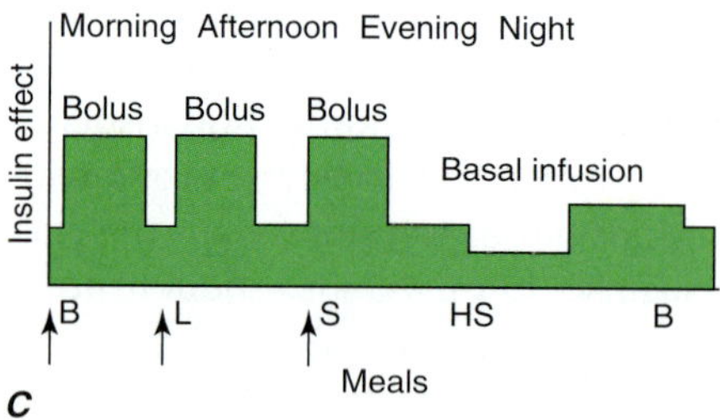

FIGURE 19-13

Representative insulin regimens for the treatment of diabetes. For each panel, the *y* axis shows the amount of insulin effect and the *x* axis shows the time of day. B, breakfast; L, lunch; S, supper; HS, bedtime; CSII, continuous subcutaneous insulin infusion. *Lispro, glulisine, or insulin aspart can be used. The time of insulin injection is shown with a vertical arrow. The type of insulin is noted above each insulin curve. ***A***. A multiple-component insulin regimen consisting of long-acting insulin (^, one shot of glargine or two shots of detemir) to provide basal insulin coverage and three shots of glulisine, lispro, or insulin aspart to provide glycemic coverage for each meal. ***B.*** The injection of two shots of long-acting insulin (^, NPH or detemir) and short-acting insulin [glulisine, lispro, insulin aspart (solid red line), or regular (green dashed line)]. Only one formulation of short-acting insulin is used. ***C.*** Insulin administration by insulin infusion device is shown with the basal insulin and a bolus injection at each meal. The basal insulin rate is decreased during the evening and increased slightly prior to the patient awakening in the morning. Glulisine, lispro, or insulin aspart is used in the insulin pump. [*Adapted from H Lebovitz (ed): Therapy for Diabetes Mellitus. American Diabetes Association, Alexandria, VA, 2004.*]

has a significant peak, making hypoglycemia more common. Frequent SMBG (more than three times per day) is absolutely essential for all types of insulin regimens.

One commonly used regimen consists of twice-daily injections of a long-acting insulin like NPH (detemir could be used instead) mixed with a short-acting insulin before the morning and evening meal (Fig. 19-13*A*). Such regimens usually prescribe two-thirds of the total daily insulin dose in the morning (with about two-thirds given as long-acting insulin and one-third as short-acting) and one-third before the evening meal (with approximately one-half given as long-acting insulin and one-half as short-acting). The drawback to such a regimen is that it enforces a rigid schedule on the patient, in terms of daily activity and the content and timing of meals. Although it is simple and effective at avoiding severe hyperglycemia, it does not generate near-normal glycemic control in most individuals with type 1 DM. Moreover, if the patient's meal pattern or content varies or if physical activity is increased, hyperglycemia or hypoglycemia may result. Moving the long-acting insulin from before the evening meal to bedtime may avoid nocturnal hypoglycemia and provide more insulin as glucose levels rise in the early morning (so-called dawn phenomenon). The insulin dose in such regimens should be adjusted based on SMBG results with the following general assumptions: (1) the fasting glucose is primarily determined by the prior evening long-acting insulin; (2) the pre-lunch glucose is a function of the morning short-acting insulin; (3) the pre-supper glucose is a function of the morning long-acting insulin; and (4) the bedtime glucose is a function of the pre-supper, short-acting insulin. This is not an optimal regimen for the patient with type 1 DM, but is sometimes used for patients with type 2 diabetes.

Continuous subcutaneous insulin infusion (CSII) is a very effective insulin regimen for the patient with type 1 diabetes (Fig. 19-13*C*). To the basal insulin infusion, a preprandial insulin ("bolus") is delivered by the insulin infusion device based on instructions from the patient, who uses an individualized algorithm incorporating the preprandial plasma glucose and anticipated carbohydrate intake. These sophisticated insulin infusion devices can accurately deliver small doses of insulin (microliters per hour) and have several advantages: (1) multiple basal infusion rates can be programmed to accommodate nocturnal versus daytime basal insulin requirement, (2) basal infusion rates can be altered during periods of exercise, (3) different waveforms of insulin infusion with meal-related bolus allow better matching of insulin depending on meal composition, and (4) programmed algorithms consider prior insulin administration and blood glucose values in calculating the insulin dose. These devices require a health professional with considerable experience with insulin infusion devices and very frequent patient interactions with the diabetes management team. Insulin infusion devices present unique challenges, such as infection at the infusion site, unexplained hyperglycemia because the infusion set becomes obstructed, or diabetic ketoacidosis if the pump becomes disconnected. Since most physicians use lispro, glulisine, or insulin aspart in CSII, the extremely short half-life of these insulins quickly leads to insulin deficiency if the delivery system is interrupted. Essential to the safe use of infusion devices is thorough patient education about pump function and frequent SMBG. Efforts to create a closed-loop system in which data from continuous glucose measurement regulates the insulin infusion rate continue.

Other Agents That Improve Glucose Control

The role of amylin, a 37-amino-acid peptide cosecreted with insulin from pancreatic beta cells, in normal glucose homeostasis is uncertain. However, based on the rationale that patients who are insulin deficient are also amylin deficient, an analogue of amylin (pramlintide) was created and found to reduce postprandial glycemic excursions in type 1 and type 2 diabetic patients taking insulin. Pramlintide injected just before a meal slows gastric emptying and suppresses glucagon but does not alter insulin levels. Pramlintide is approved for insulin-treated patients with type 1 and type 2 DM. Addition of pramlintide produces a modest reduction in the A1C and seems to dampen meal-related glucose excursions. In type 1 diabetes, pramlintide is started as a 15-μg SC injection before each meal and titrated up to a maximum of 30–60 μg as tolerated. In type 2 DM, pramlintide is started as a 60-μg SC injection before each meal and may be titrated up to a maximum of 120 μg. The major side effects are nausea and vomiting, and dose escalations should be slow to limit these side effects. Because pramlintide slows gastric emptying, it may influence absorption of other medications and should not be used in combination with other drugs that slow GI motility. The short-acting insulin given before the meal should initially be reduced to avoid hypoglycemia and then titrated as the effects of the pramlintide become evident. α-Glucosidase inhibitors are another type of agent that may be used in patients with type 1 DM.

TYPE 2 DIABETES MELLITUS

General Aspects The goals of therapy for type 2 DM are similar to those in type 1. While glycemic control tends to dominate the management of type 1 DM, the care of individuals with type 2 DM must also include attention to the treatment of conditions associated with type 2 DM (obesity, hypertension, dyslipidemia, cardiovascular disease) and detection/management of DM-related complications (Fig. 19-14). DM-specific complications may be present in up to 20–50% of

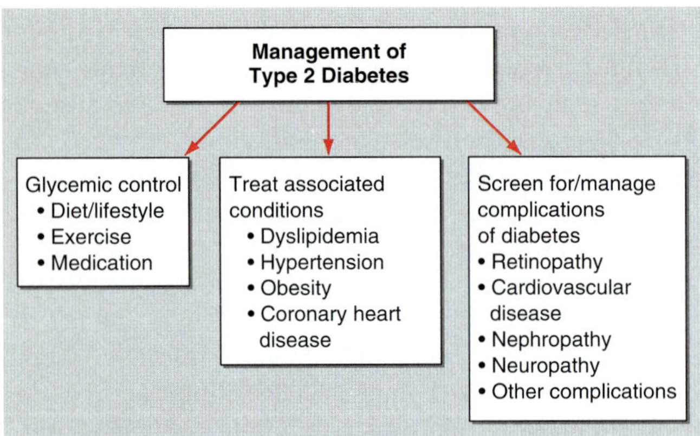

FIGURE 19-14

Essential elements in comprehensive diabetes care of type 2 diabetes.

individuals with newly diagnosed type 2 DM. Reduction in cardiovascular risk is of paramount importance as this is the leading cause of mortality in these individuals. Efforts to achieve blood pressure and lipid goals (Table 19-8) should begin in concert with glucose-lowering interventions.

Type 2 diabetes management should begin with MNT. An exercise regimen to increase insulin sensitivity and promote weight loss should also be instituted. Pharmacologic approaches to the management of type 2 DM include oral glucose-lowering agents, insulin, and other agents that improve glucose control; most physicians and patients prefer oral glucose-lowering agents as the initial choice (discussed below after review of various medications). Any therapy that improves glycemic control reduces "glucose toxicity" to the islet cells and improves endogenous insulin secretion. However, type 2 DM is a progressive disorder and ultimately requires multiple therapeutic agents and often insulin.

Glucose-Lowering Agents Advances in the therapy of type 2 DM have generated considerable enthusiasm for oral glucose-lowering agents that target different pathophysiologic processes in type 2 DM. Based on their mechanisms of action, glucose-lowering agents are subdivided into agents that increase insulin secretion, reduce glucose production, increase insulin sensitivity, and enhance GLP-1 action (Table 19-11). Glucose-lowering agents (with the exception of α-glucosidase inhibitors and an amylin analogue) are ineffective in type 1 DM and should not be used for glucose management of severely ill individuals with type 2 DM. Insulin is sometimes the initial glucose-lowering agent.

Insulin Secretagogues Insulin secretagogues stimulate insulin secretion by interacting with the ATP-sensitive potassium channel on the beta cell (Fig. 19-4). These drugs are most effective in individuals with type 2 DM of relatively recent onset (<5 years), who have residual endogenous insulin production. At maximum doses, first-generation sulfonylureas are similar in potency to second-generation agents but have a longer half-life, a greater incidence of hypoglycemia, and more frequent drug interactions (Table 19-12). Thus, second-generation sulfonylureas are generally preferred. An advantage to a more rapid onset of action is better coverage of the postprandial glucose rise, but the shorter half-life of such agents requires more than once-a-day dosing. Sulfonylureas reduce both fasting and postprandial glucose and should be initiated at low doses and increased at 1- to 2-week intervals based on SMBG. In general, sulfonylureas increase insulin acutely and thus should be taken shortly before a meal; with chronic therapy, though, the insulin release is more sustained. Glimepiride and glipizide can be given in a single daily dose and are preferred over glyburide. Repaglinide and nateglinide are not sulfonylureas but also interact with the ATP-sensitive potassium channel. Because of their short half-life, these agents are given with each meal or immediately before to reduce meal-related glucose excursions.

Insulin secretagogues are generally well tolerated. All of these agents, however, have the potential to cause profound and persistent hypoglycemia, especially in elderly individuals. Hypoglycemia is usually related to delayed meals, increased physical activity, alcohol intake, or renal insufficiency. Individuals who ingest an overdose of some agents develop prolonged and serious hypoglycemia and should be monitored closely in the hospital (Chap. 20). Most sulfonylureas are metabolized in the liver to compounds (some of which are active) that are cleared by the kidney. Thus, their use in individuals with significant hepatic or renal dysfunction is not advisable. Weight gain, a common side effect of sulfonylurea therapy, results from the increased insulin levels and improvement in glycemic control. Some sulfonylureas have significant drug interactions with alcohol and some medications including warfarin, aspirin, ketoconazole, α-glucosidase inhibitors, and fluconazole. A related isoform of ATP-sensitive potassium channels is present in the myocardium and the brain. All of these agents except glyburide have a low affinity for this isoform. Despite concerns that this agent might affect the myocardial response to ischemia and observational studies suggesting that sulfonylureas increase cardiovascular risk, the UKPDS did not show an increased cardiac mortality with glyburide.

Biguanides Metformin is representative of this class of agents. It reduces hepatic glucose production through an undefined mechanism and improves peripheral glucose utilization slightly (Table 19-11). Metformin reduces fasting plasma glucose and insulin levels, improves the

TABLE 19-11

GLUCOSE-LOWERING THERAPIES FOR TYPE 2 DIABETES

	MECHANISM OF ACTION	EXAMPLES	A1C REDUCTION (%)[a]	AGENT-SPECIFIC ADVANTAGES	AGENT-SPECIFIC DISADVANTAGES	CONTRAINDICATIONS/ RELATIVE CONTRAINDICATIONS
Oral						
Biguanides	↓ Hepatic glucose production, weight loss, glucose, utilization, insulin resistance	Metformin	1–2	Weight loss	Lactic acidosis, diarrhea, nausea	Serum creatinine >1.5 mg/dL (men), >1.4 mg/dL (women), CHF, radiographic contrast studies, seriously ill patients, acidosis
α-Glucosidase inhibitors	↓ Glucose absorption	Acarbose, miglitol	0.5–0.8	Reduce postprandial glycemia	GI flatulence, liver function tests	Renal/liver disease
Dipeptidyl peptidase IV inhibitors	Prolong endogenous GLP-1 action	Sitagliptin	0.5–1.0	Does not cause hypoglycemia		Reduce dose with renal disease
Insulin secretagogues—sulfonylureas	↑ Insulin secretion	Table 19-12	1–2	Lower fasting blood glucose	Hypoglycemia, weight gain	Renal/liver disease
Insulin secretagogues—nonsulfonylureas	↑ Insulin secretion	Table 19-12	1–2	Short onset of action, lowers postprandial glucose	Hypoglycemia	Renal/liver disease
Thiazolidinediones	↓ Insulin resistance, ↑ glucose utilization	Rosiglitazone, pioglitazone	0.5–1.4	Lower insulin requirements	Peripheral edema, CHF, weight gain, fractures, macular edema; rosiglitazone may increase risk of MI	Congestive heart failure, liver disease
Parenteral						
Insulin	↑ Glucose utilization and other anabolic actions	Table 323-11	No limit	Known safety profile	Injection, weight gain, hypoglycemia	
GLP-1 agonist	↑ Insulin, ↓ glucagon, slow gastric emptying	Exenatide	0.5–1.0	Weight loss	Injection, nausea, ↑ risk of hypoglycemia with insulin secretagogues	Renal disease, agents that also slow GI motility
Amylin agonist[b]	Slow gastric emptying, ↓ glucagon	Pramlintide	0.25–0.5	Reduce postprandial glycemia, weight loss	Injection, nausea, ↑ risk of hypoglycemia with insulin	Agents that also slow GI motility
Medical nutrition therapy and physical activity	↓ Insulin resistance, ↑ insulin secretion	Low-calorie, low-fat diet, exercise	1–2	Other health benefits	Compliance difficult, long-term success low	

[a]A1C reduction depends partly on starting A1C.
[b]Amylin agonist is approved for use in type 1 and type 2 diabetes.

TABLE 19-12

CHARACTERISTICS OF ORAL AGENTS THAT INCREASE INSULIN SECRETION

GENERIC NAME	APPROVED DAILY DOSAGE RANGE, mg	DURATION OF ACTION, h
Sulfonylurea—first generation		
Chlorpropamide	100–500	>48
Tolazamide	100–1000	12–24
Tolbutamide	500–3000	6–12
Sulfonylurea—second generation		
Glimepiride	1–8	24
Glipizide	2.5–40	12–18
Glipizide (extended release)	5–10	24
Glyburide	1.25–20	12–24
Glyburide (micronized)	0.75–12	12–24
Nonsulfonylureas		
Repaglinide	0.5–16	2–6
Nateglinide	180–360	2–4

Source: Adapted from BR Zimmerman (ed): *Medical Management of Type 2 Diabetes*, 4th ed. American Diabetes Association, Alexandria, VA, 1998.

lipid profile, and promotes modest weight loss. The initial starting dose of 500 mg once or twice a day can be increased to 1000 mg bid. An extended-release form is available and may have fewer gastrointestinal side effects (diarrhea, anorexia, nausea, metallic taste). Because of its relatively slow onset of action and gastrointestinal symptoms with higher doses, the dose should be escalated every 2–3 weeks based on SMBG measurements. The major toxicity of metformin, lactic acidosis, can be prevented by careful patient selection. Metformin should not be used in patients with renal insufficiency [serum creatinine >133 μmol/L (1.5 mg/dL) in men or >124 μmol/L (1.4 mg/dL) in women, with adjustments for age], any form of acidosis, CHF, liver disease, or severe hypoxia. Metformin should be discontinued in patients who are seriously ill, in patients who can take nothing orally, and in those receiving radiographic contrast material. Insulin should be used until metformin can be restarted.

α-Glucosidase Inhibitors α-Glucosidase inhibitors (acarbose and miglitol) reduce postprandial hyperglycemia by delaying glucose absorption; they do not affect glucose utilization or insulin secretion (Table 19-11). Postprandial hyperglycemia, secondary to impaired hepatic and peripheral glucose disposal, contributes significantly to the hyperglycemic state in type 2 DM. These drugs, taken just before each meal, reduce glucose absorption by inhibiting the enzyme that cleaves oligosaccharides into simple sugars in the intestinal lumen. Therapy should be initiated at a low dose (25 mg of acarbose or miglitol) with the evening meal and may be increased to a maximal dose over weeks to months (50–100 mg for acarbose or 50 mg for miglitol with each meal). The major side effects (diarrhea, flatulence, abdominal distention) are related to increased delivery of oligosaccharides to the large bowel and can be reduced somewhat by gradual upward dose titration. α-Glucosidase inhibitors may increase levels of sulfonylureas and increase the incidence of hypoglycemia. Simultaneous treatment with bile acid resins and antacids should be avoided. These agents should not be used in individuals with inflammatory bowel disease, gastroparesis, or a serum creatinine >177 μmol/L (2.0 mg/dL). This class of agents is not as potent as other oral agents in lowering the hemoglobin A1C but is unique because it reduces the postprandial glucose rise even in individuals with type 1 DM. If hypoglycemia from other diabetes treatments occurs while taking these agents, the patient should consume glucose since the degradation and absorption of complex carbohydrates will be retarded.

Thiazolidinediones Thiazolidinediones reduce insulin resistance. These drugs bind to the PPAR-γ (peroxisome proliferator-activated receptor-γ) nuclear receptor. The PPAR-γ receptor is found at highest levels in adipocytes but is expressed at lower levels in many other tissues. Agonists of this receptor regulate a large number of genes, promote adipocyte differentiation, reduce hepatic fat accumulation, and appear to reduce insulin resistance indirectly by enhancing fatty acid storage and possibly by increasing adiponectin levels (Table 19-11). Thiazolidinediones promote a redistribution of fat from central to peripheral locations. Circulating insulin levels decrease with use of the thiazolidinediones, indicating a reduction in insulin resistance. Although direct comparisons are not available, the two currently available thiazolidinediones appear to have similar efficacy; the therapeutic range for pioglitazone is 15–45 mg/d in a single daily dose, and for rosiglitazone the total daily dose is 2–8 mg/d administered either once daily or twice daily in divided doses. The ability of thiazolidinediones to influence cardiovascular disease or other features of the metabolic syndrome is under investigation.

The prototype of this class of drugs, troglitazone, was withdrawn from the U.S. market after reports of hepatotoxicity and an association with an idiosyncratic liver reaction that sometimes led to hepatic failure. Although rosiglitazone and pioglitazone do not appear to induce the liver abnormalities seen with troglitazone, the FDA recommends measurement of liver function tests prior to initiating therapy with a thiazolidinedione and at regular intervals (every 2 months for the first year and then periodically). Rosiglitazone raises LDL, HDL, and triglycerides slightly. Pioglitazone raises HDL to a greater degree and LDL to a lesser degree but lowers triglycerides. The clinical significance of the lipid changes with these agents is not known and may be difficult to ascertain since most patients with type 2 diabetes are also treated with a statin. Emphasis should be placed on reaching lipid, blood pressure, and glycemic targets rather than the type of therapy needed to reach those goals. Thiazolidinediones are associated with weight gain (2–3 kg), a small reduction in the hematocrit, and a mild increase in plasma volume. Peripheral edema and CHF may occur and are more common in individuals also treated with insulin. These agents are contraindicated in patients with liver disease or CHF (class III or IV). Recent meta-analyses have suggested that rosiglitazone is associated with an increased risk of myocardial infarction. The FDA has issued an alert that rare patients taking these agents may experience a worsening of diabetic macular edema. An increased risk of fractures has been noted in women taking these agents. Thiazolidinediones have been shown to induce ovulation in premenopausal women with PCOS. Women should be warned about the risk of pregnancy, since the safety of thiazolidinediones in pregnancy is not established.

Insulin Therapy in Type 2 DM Insulin should be considered as the initial therapy in type 2 DM, particularly in lean individuals or those with severe weight loss, in individuals with underlying renal or hepatic disease that precludes oral glucose-lowering agents, or in individuals who are hospitalized or acutely ill. Insulin therapy is ultimately required by a substantial number of individuals with type 2 DM because of the progressive nature of the disorder and the relative insulin deficiency that develops in patients with longstanding diabetes. Both physician and patient reluctance often delay the initiation of insulin therapy, but glucose control and patient well-being are improved by insulin therapy in patients who have not reached the glycemic target.

Because endogenous insulin secretion continues and is capable of providing some coverage of mealtime caloric intake, insulin is usually initiated in a single dose of long-acting insulin (0.3–0.4 U/kg per d), given either before breakfast and in the evening (NPH) or just before bedtime (NPH, glargine, detemir). Since fasting hyperglycemia and increased hepatic glucose production are prominent features of type 2 DM, bedtime insulin is more effective in clinical trials than a single dose of morning insulin. Glargine given at bedtime has less nocturnal hypoglycemia than NPH insulin. Some physicians prefer a relatively low, fixed starting dose of intermediate-acting insulin (15–20 units in the morning and 5–10 units at bedtime) to avoid hypoglycemia. The insulin dose may then be adjusted in 10% increments as dictated by SMBG results. Both morning and bedtime long-acting insulin may be used in combination with oral glucose-lowering agents (biguanides, α-glucosidase inhibitors, or thiazolidinediones). The combination of insulin and a thiazolidinedione promotes weight gain and edema and is a less desirable combination. Initially, basal insulin may be sufficient, but often prandial insulin coverage is needed as diabetes progresses. Other insulin formulations that have a combination of short-acting and long-acting insulin (Table 19-10) are sometimes used in patients with type 2 DM because of convenience but do not allow independent adjustment of short-acting and long-acting insulin dose. In selected patients with type 2 DM (usually insulin deficient as defined by C-peptide level), insulin infusion devices may be considered.

Agents That Enhance GLP-1 Receptor Signaling "Incretins" amplify glucose-stimulated insulin secretion. Agents that either act as a GLP-1 agonist or enhance endogenous GLP-1 activity have become available and are under development. Exenatide, a synthetic version of a peptide originally found in the saliva of the Gila monster (exendin-4), is an analogue of GLP-1. Unlike native GLP-1, which has a half-life of <5 min, differences in the exenatide amino acid sequence render it resistant to the enzyme that degrades GLP-1 (dipeptidyl peptidase IV, or DPP-IV). Thus, exenatide has prolonged GLP-1-like action by binding to GLP-1 receptors found in islets, the gastrointestinal tract, and the brain. Exenatide increases glucose-stimulated insulin secretion, suppresses glucagon, and slows gastric emptying. Exenatide does not promote weight gain; in fact, most patients experience modest weight loss. It appears that GLP-1 agonists also suppress appetite. Exenatide, approved for combination with other oral agents for type 2 DM, should be started as a 5-μg SC injection before the morning and evening meal and increased to 10 μg twice daily, depending on the response and side effects (nausea being the limiting factor). The A1C reductions with exenatide are modest compared to those with some oral agents. Exenatide is approved only for use as adjunct or combination therapy with metformin or sulfonylureas; studies of its efficacy in combination with other oral agents are underway. Exenatide should not be used in patients taking insulin. The major side effects are nausea, vomiting, and diarrhea; some patients taking insulin secretagogues may require a reduction in those agents to prevent hypoglycemia. Because it slows gastric emptying and may influence the absorption of other drugs, the timing of administration should be coordinated. Whether exenatide enhances beta cell survival, promotes beta cell proliferation, or alters the natural history of type 2 DM is not known. Other GLP-1 receptor agonists and formulations are under development. DPP-IV inhibitors represent a new class of oral agents that inhibit degradation of native GLP-1 and thus enhance incretin effect. These agents promote insulin secretion in the absence of hypoglycemia or weight gain, and appear to have a preferential effect on postprandial blood glucose. The FDA has approved the first DPP-IV inhibitor, sitagliptin, for use with diet and exercise to improve glycemic control in adult individuals with type 2 DM. It can also be used in combination with metformin or a thiazolidinedione. Sitagliptin is administered at a dose of 100 mg PO once daily. Reduced doses should be given to patients with moderate (creatinine clearance 30–50 mL/min, 50 mg once daily) or severe (creatinine clearance <30 mL/min, 25 mg once daily) renal insufficiency. Renal function should be assessed prior to initiation of sitagliptin therapy and periodically thereafter. Clinical experience with this agent is limited.

Choice of Initial Glucose-Lowering Agent The level of hyperglycemia should influence the initial choice of therapy. Assuming maximal benefit of MNT and increased physical activity has been realized, patients with mild to moderate hyperglycemia [FPG <11.1–13.9 mmol/L (200–250 mg/dL)] often respond well to a single, oral glucose-lowering agent. Patients with more severe hyperglycemia [FPG >13.9 mmol/L (250 mg/dL)] may respond partially but are unlikely to achieve normoglycemia with oral monotherapy. A stepwise approach that starts with a single agent and adds a second agent to achieve the glycemic target can be used (see "Combination Therapy" later in the chapter). Insulin can be used as initial therapy in individuals with severe hyperglycemia [FPG >13.9–16.7 mmol/L (250–300 mg/dL)] or in those who are symptomatic from the hyperglycemia. This approach is based on the rationale that more rapid glycemic control will reduce "glucose toxicity" to the islet cells, improve endogenous insulin secretion, and possibly allow oral glucose-lowering agents to be more effective. If this occurs, the insulin may be discontinued.

Insulin secretagogues, biguanides, α-glucosidase inhibitors, thiazolidinediones, and insulin are approved for monotherapy of type 2 DM. Although each class of oral glucose-lowering agents has unique advantages and disadvantages, certain generalizations apply: (1) insulin secretagogues, biguanides, DPP-IV inhibitors, and thiazolidinediones improve glycemic control to a similar degree (1–2% reduction in A1C) and are more effective than α-glucosidase inhibitors; (2) assuming a similar degree of glycemic improvement, no clinical advantage to one class of drugs has been demonstrated, and any therapy that improves glycemic control is likely beneficial; (3) insulin secretagogues and α-glucosidase inhibitors begin to lower the plasma glucose immediately, whereas the glucose-lowering effects of the biguanides and thiazolidinediones are delayed by several weeks to months; (4) not all agents are effective in all individuals with type 2 DM (primary failure); (5) biguanides, α-glucosidase inhibitors, DPP-IV inhibitors, and thiazolidinediones do not directly cause hypoglycemia; and (6) most individuals will eventually require treatment with more than one class of oral glucose-lowering agents or insulin, reflecting the progressive nature of type 2 DM.

Considerable clinical experience exists with metformin and sulfonylureas because they have been available for several decades. It is assumed that the α-glucosidase inhibitors, DPP-IV inhibitors, and thiazolidinediones, which are newer classes of oral glucose-lowering drugs, will reduce DM-related complications by improving glycemic control, although long-term data are not yet available. The thiazolidinediones are theoretically attractive because they target a fundamental abnormality in type 2 DM, namely insulin resistance. However, all of these agents are currently more costly than metformin and sulfonylureas.

A reasonable treatment algorithm for initial therapy uses metformin as initial therapy because of its efficacy, known side-effect profile, and relatively low cost (Fig. 19-15). Metformin has the advantage that it promotes mild weight loss, lowers insulin levels, and improves the lipid profile slightly. Based on SMBG results and the A1C, the dose of metformin should be increased until the glycemic target is achieved or maximum dose is reached.

Approximately one-third of individuals will reach their target glycemic goal using metformin as monotherapy.

Combination Therapy with Glucose-Lowering Agents A number of combinations of therapeutic agents are successful in type 2 DM, and the dosing of agents in combination is the same as when the agents are used alone. Because mechanisms of action of the first and second agents are different, the effect on glycemic control is usually additive. Several fixed-dose combinations of oral agents are available, but evidence that they are superior to titration of a single agent to a

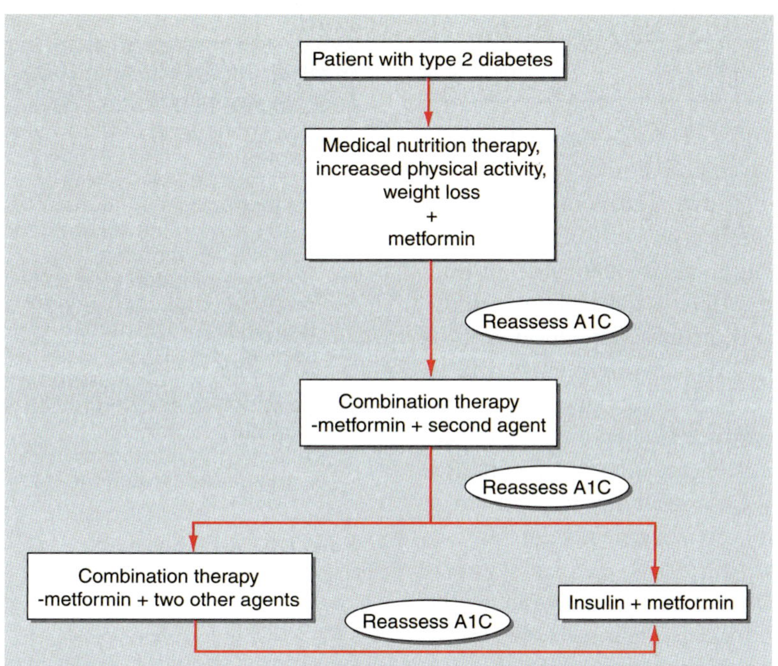

FIGURE 19-15

Glycemic management of type 2 diabetes. See text for discussion of treatment of severe hyperglycemia or symptomatic hyperglycemia. Agents that can be combined with metformin include insulin secretagogues, thiazolidinediones, α-glucosidase inhibitors, DPP-IV inhibitors, and exenatide. A1C, hemoglobin A1C.

maximum dose and then addition of a second agent is lacking. If adequate control is not achieved with the combination of two agents (based on reassessment of the A1C every 3 months), a third oral agent or basal insulin should be added (Fig. 19-15).

Treatment with insulin becomes necessary as type 2 DM enters the phase of relative insulin deficiency (as seen in longstanding DM) and is signaled by inadequate glycemic control with one or two oral glucose-lowering agents. Insulin alone or in combination should be used in patients who fail to reach the glycemic target. For example, a single dose of long-acting insulin at bedtime is effective in combination with metformin. As endogenous insulin production falls further, multiple injections of long-acting and short-acting insulin regimens are necessary to control postprandial glucose excursions. These insulin regimens are identical to the long-acting and short-acting combination regimens discussed above for type 1 DM. Since the hyperglycemia of type 2 DM tends to be more "stable," these regimens can be increased in 10% increments every 2–3 days using the fasting blood glucose results. The daily insulin dose required can become quite large (1–2 units/kg per d) as endogenous insulin production falls and insulin resistance persists. Individuals who require >1 unit/kg per d of long-acting insulin should be considered for combination therapy with metformin or a thiazolidinedione. The addition of metformin or a thiazolidinedione can reduce insulin requirements in some individuals with type 2 DM, while maintaining or even improving glycemic control. Insulin plus a thiazolidinedione promotes weight gain and is associated with peripheral edema. Addition of a thiazolidinedione to a patient's insulin regimen may necessitate a reduction in the insulin dose to avoid hypoglycemia.

EMERGING THERAPIES Whole pancreas transplantation (performed concomitantly with a renal transplant) may normalize glucose tolerance and is an important therapeutic option in type 1 DM, though it requires substantial expertise and is associated with the side effects of immunosuppression. Pancreatic islet transplantation has been plagued by limitations in pancreatic islet isolation and graft survival and remains an area of clinical investigation. Many individuals with longstanding type 1 DM still produce very small amounts of insulin or have insulin-positive cells within the pancreas. This suggests that beta cells are slowly regenerating but are quickly destroyed by the autoimmune process. Thus, efforts to suppress the autoimmune process and to stimulate beta cell regeneration are underway both at the time of diagnosis and in years after the diagnosis of type 1 DM. Closed-loop pumps that infuse the appropriate amount of insulin in response to changing glucose levels are potentially feasible now that continuous glucose-monitoring technology has been developed.

COMPLICATIONS OF THERAPY FOR DIABETES MELLITUS

As with any therapy, the benefits of efforts directed toward glycemic control must be weighed against the risks of treatment. Side effects of intensive treatment include an increased frequency of serious hypoglycemia, weight gain, increased economic costs, and greater demands on the patient. In the DCCT, quality of life was very similar in the intensive and standard therapy groups. The most serious complication of therapy for DM is hypoglycemia, and its treatment with oral glucose or glucagon injection is discussed in Chap. 20. Severe, recurrent hypoglycemia warrants examination of treatment regimen and glycemic goal for the individual patient. Weight gain occurs with most (insulin, insulin secretagogues, thiazolidinediones) but not all (metformin, α-glucosidase inhibitors, exenatide) therapies that improve glycemic control. It is partially due to the anabolic effects of insulin and the reduction in glucosuria. In the DCCT, individuals with the greatest weight gain exhibited increases in LDL cholesterol and triglycerides as well as increases in blood pressure (both systolic and diastolic) similar to those seen in individuals with type 2 DM and insulin resistance. These effects could increase the risk of cardiovascular disease. As discussed previously, transient worsening of diabetic retinopathy or neuropathy sometimes accompanies improved glycemic control.

ONGOING ASPECTS OF COMPREHENSIVE DIABETES CARE

The morbidity and mortality of DM-related complications can be greatly reduced by timely and consistent surveillance procedures (Table 19-13). These screening procedures are indicated for all individuals with DM, but numerous studies have documented that most individuals with diabetes do not receive comprehensive diabetes care. Screening for dyslipidemia and hypertension should be performed annually. In addition to routine health maintenance, individuals with diabetes should also receive the pneumococcal and tetanus vaccines (at recommended intervals) and the influenza vaccine (annually). As discussed above, aspirin therapy should be considered in many patients with diabetes.

An annual comprehensive eye examination should be performed by a qualified optometrist or ophthalmologist. If abnormalities are detected, further evaluation and treatment require an ophthalmologist skilled in diabetes-related eye disease. Because many individuals with type 2 DM have had asymptomatic diabetes for several years before diagnosis, the ADA recommends the following ophthalmologic examination schedule: (1) individuals with type 1 DM should have an initial eye examination within 3–5 years of diagnosis, (2) individuals with type 2 DM should have an initial eye examination at the time of diabetes diagnosis, (3) women with DM who are pregnant or contemplating pregnancy should have an eye examination prior to conception and during the first trimester, and (4) individuals whose eye examination is normal can have a repeat examination in 2–3 years rather than annually.

TABLE 19-13

GUIDELINES FOR ONGOING MEDICAL CARE FOR PATIENTS WITH DIABETES

- Self-monitoring of blood glucose (individualized frequency)
- A1C testing (two to four times per year)
- Patient education in diabetes management (annual)
- Medical nutrition therapy and education (annual)
- Eye examination (annual)
- Foot examination (one to two times per year by physician; daily by patient)
- Screening for diabetic nephropathy (annual; see Fig. 19-11)
- Blood pressure measurement (quarterly)
- Lipid profile and serum creatinine (estimate GFR) (annual)
- Influenza/pneumococcal immunizations
- Consider antiplatelet therapy (see text)

Note: A1C, hemoglobin A1C.

An annual foot examination should (1) assess blood flow, sensation (monofilament testing, pin prick, or tuning fork), ankle reflexes, and nail care; (2) look for the presence of foot deformities such as hammer or claw toes and Charcot foot; and (3) identify sites of potential ulceration. Calluses and nail deformities should be treated by a podiatrist; the patient should be discouraged from self-care of even minor foot problems, but should be strongly encouraged to check his or her feet daily for any early lesions. The ADA advises a visual foot inspection in patients with symptoms or signs of diabetic neuropathy at 3- or 6-month intervals.

An annual microalbuminuria measurement (albumin-to-creatinine ratio in spot urine) is advised in individuals with type 1 or type 2 DM and no protein on a routine urinalysis (Fig. 19-10). If the urinalysis detects proteinuria, the amount of protein should be quantified by standard urine protein measurements. If the urinalysis was negative for protein in the past, microalbuminuria should be the annual screening examination. Routine urine protein measurements do not detect low levels of albumin excretion. Screening should commence 5 years after the onset of type 1 DM and at the time of diagnosis of type 2 DM. Regardless of protein excretion results, the GFR should be estimated using the serum creatinine in all patients on an annual basis.

SPECIAL CONSIDERATIONS IN DIABETES MELLITUS

PSYCHOSOCIAL ASPECTS

As with any chronic, debilitating disease, the individual with DM faces a series of challenges that affect all aspects of daily life. The individual with DM must accept that he or she may develop complications related to DM. Even with considerable effort, normoglycemia can be an elusive goal, and solutions to worsening glycemic control may not be easily identifiable. The patient should view him- or herself as an essential member of the diabetes care team and not as someone who is cared for by the diabetes team. Emotional stress may provoke a change in behavior so that individuals no longer adhere to a dietary, exercise, or therapeutic regimen. This can lead to the appearance of either hyper- or hypoglycemia. Eating disorders, including binge eating disorders, bulimia, and anorexia nervosa, appear to occur more frequently in individuals with type 1 or type 2 DM.

MANAGEMENT IN THE HOSPITALIZED PATIENT

Virtually all medical and surgical subspecialties are involved in the care of hospitalized patients with diabetes. Hyperglycemia, whether in a patient with known diabetes or in someone without known diabetes, appears to be a predictor of poor outcome in hospitalized patients. General anesthesia, surgery, infection, or concurrent illness raises the levels of counterregulatory hormones (cortisol, growth hormone, catecholamines, and glucagon) and cytokines that may lead to transient insulin resistance and hyperglycemia. These factors increase insulin requirements by increasing glucose production and impairing glucose utilization and thus may worsen glycemic control. The concurrent illness or surgical procedure may lead to variable insulin absorption and also prevent the patient with DM from eating normally and may promote hypoglycemia. Glycemic control should be assessed (with A1C) and, if feasible, should be optimized prior to surgery. Electrolytes, renal function, and intravascular volume status should be assessed as well. The high prevalence of cardiovascular disease in individuals with DM (especially in type 2 DM) may require preoperative cardiovascular evaluation.

Glycemic control appears to improve the clinical outcomes in a variety of settings. In fact, many patients who do not have preexisting diabetes but who develop modest blood glucose elevations during their hospitalization appear to benefit from achieving near normoglycemia using insulin treatment. For example, maintenance of a near-normal glucose with a continuous insulin infusion reduced the risk of postoperative infection after CABG and reduced the morbidity and mortality in patients in a surgical intensive care unit. In a number of cross-sectional studies of patients with diabetes, a greater degree of hyperglycemia was associated with worse cardiac, neurologic, and infectious outcomes. The goals of diabetes management during hospitalization are near normoglycemia, avoidance of hypoglycemia, and transition back to the outpatient diabetes treatment regimen. The ADA suggests these glycemic goals for critically ill patients: ". . . as close to 6.1 mmol/L (110 mg/dL) and generally <10 mmol/L (180 mg/dL, postprandial)." In noncritically ill patients, the suggested glycemic goals are as close as possible to 5.0–7.2 mmol/L (90–130 mg/dL) preprandially and <10 mmol/L (180 mg/dL) postprandially. This process requires integrating information regarding the plasma glucose, diabetes treatment regimen, and clinical status of the patient.

The physician caring for an individual with diabetes in the perioperative period, during times of infection or serious physical illness, or simply when fasting for a diagnostic procedure must monitor the plasma glucose vigilantly, adjust the diabetes treatment regimen, and provide glucose infusion as needed. Depending on the severity of the patient's illness and the hospital setting, the physician can use either an insulin infusion or SC insulin. A "consistent carbohydrate diabetes meal plan" for hospitalized patients provides a predictable amount of carbohydrate for a particular meal each day (but not necessarily the same amount for breakfast, lunch, and supper). The hospital diet should be determined by a nutritionist; terms such as "ADA diet" or "low-sugar diet" are no longer used. Several different treatment regimens (IV or SC insulin regimens) can be employed successfully.

Insulin infusions can effectively control plasma glucose in the perioperative period and when the patient is unable to take anything PO. The absorption of SC insulin may be variable in such situations. Regular insulin is preferred over insulin analogues for IV insulin infusion since it is less expensive and equally effective. The physician must consider carefully the clinical setting in which an insulin infusion will be utilized, including whether adequate ancillary personnel are available to monitor the plasma glucose frequently and whether they can adjust the insulin infusion rate to maintain the plasma glucose within the optimal range.

Because of the short half-life of IV regular insulin, it is necessary to administer long-acting insulin prior to discontinuation of the insulin infusion to avoid a period of insulin deficiency. An alternative to an insulin infusion is basal or "scheduled" insulin provided by SC, long-acting insulin supplemented by prandial or "corrective" insulin using a short-acting insulin (insulin analogues preferred). The use of "sliding scale" insulin alone, where no insulin is given unless the blood glucose is elevated, is inadequate for in-patient glucose management and should not be used. The short-acting, preprandial insulin dose should include coverage for food consumption (based on anticipated carbohydrate intake) plus a corrective or supplemental insulin based on the patient's insulin sensitivity and the blood glucose. For example, if the patient is thin (and likely insulin sensitive), a corrective insulin supplement might be 1 unit for each 2.7 mmol/L (50 mg/dL) over the glucose target. If the patient is obese and insulin-resistant, then the insulin supplement might be 2 units for each 2.7 mmol/L (50 mg/dL) over the glucose target. It is critical to individualize the regimen and adjust the basal or "scheduled" insulin dose frequently, based on the corrective insulin required.

Individuals with type 1 DM who are undergoing general anesthesia and surgery, or who are seriously ill, should receive continuous insulin, either through an IV insulin infusion or by SC administration of a reduced dose of long-acting insulin. Short-acting insulin alone is insufficient. Prolongation of a surgical procedure or delay in the recovery room is not uncommon and may result in periods of insulin deficiency leading to DKA. Insulin infusion is the preferred method for managing patients with type 1 DM in the perioperative period or when serious concurrent illness is present (0.5–1.0 units/h of regular insulin). Insulin infusion algorithms jointly developed and implemented by nursing and physician staff are advised. If the diagnostic or surgical procedure is brief and performed under local or regional anesthesia, a reduced dose of SC, long-acting insulin may suffice (30–50% reduction, with short-acting insulin held or reduced). This approach facilitates the transition back to long-acting insulin after the procedure. Glucose may be infused to prevent hypoglycemia. The blood glucose should be monitored frequently during the illness or in the perioperative period.

Individuals with type 2 DM can be managed with either regular insulin infusion or a reduced dose of SC, long-acting insulin (25–50% reduction) plus preprandial, short-acting insulin. Oral glucose-lowering agents should be discontinued upon admission and are not useful in regulating the plasma glucose in clinical situations where the insulin requirements and glucose intake are changing rapidly. Moreover, these oral agents may be dangerous if the patient is fasting (e.g., hypoglycemia with sulfonylureas). Metformin should be withheld when radiographic contrast media will be given or if severe CHF, acidosis, or declining renal function is present.

Total Parenteral Nutrition

Total parenteral nutrition (TPN) greatly increases insulin requirements. In addition, individuals not previously known to have DM may become hyperglycemic during TPN and require insulin treatment. IV insulin infusion is the preferred treatment for hyperglycemia, and rapid titration to the required insulin dose is done most efficiently using a separate insulin infusion. After the total insulin dose has been determined, insulin may be added directly to the TPN solution or, preferably, given as a separate infusion. Often, individuals receiving either TPN or enteral nutrition receive their caloric loads continuously and not at "meal times"; consequently, SC insulin regimens must be adjusted.

Glucocorticoids

Glucocorticoids increase insulin resistance, decrease glucose utilization, increase hepatic glucose production, and impair insulin secretion. These changes lead to a worsening of glycemic control in individuals with DM and may precipitate diabetes in other individuals ("steroid-induced diabetes"). The effects of glucocorticoids on glucose homeostasis are dose-related, usually reversible, and most pronounced in the postprandial period. If the FPG is near the normal range, oral diabetes agents (e.g., sulfonylureas, metformin) may be sufficient to reduce hyperglycemia. If the FPG is >11.1 mmol/L (200 mg/dL), oral agents are usually not efficacious and insulin therapy is required. Short-acting insulin may be required to supplement long-acting insulin in order to control postprandial glucose excursions.

Reproductive Issues

Reproductive capacity in either men or women with DM appears to be normal. Menstrual cycles may be associated with alterations in glycemic control in women with DM. Pregnancy is associated with marked insulin resistance; the increased insulin requirements often precipitate DM and lead to the diagnosis of GDM. Glucose, which at high levels is a teratogen to the developing fetus, readily crosses the placenta, but insulin does not. Thus, hyperglycemia from the maternal circulation may stimulate insulin secretion in the fetus. The anabolic and growth effects of insulin may result in macrosomia. GDM complicates ~4% of pregnancies in the United States. The incidence of GDM is greatly increased in certain ethnic groups, including African Americans and Latinos, consistent with a similar increased risk of type 2 DM. Current recommendations advise screening for glucose intolerance between weeks 24 and 28 of pregnancy in women with high risk for GDM (≥25 years; obesity; family history of DM; member of an ethnic group such as Latino, Native American, Asian American, African American, or Pacific Islander). Therapy for GDM is similar to that for individuals with pregnancy-associated diabetes and involves MNT and insulin, if hyperglycemia persists. Oral glucose-lowering agents have not been approved for use during pregnancy. With current practices, the morbidity and mortality of the mother with GDM and the fetus are not different from those in the nondiabetic population. Individuals who develop GDM are at marked increased risk for developing type 2 DM in the future and should be screened periodically for DM. Most individuals with GDM revert to normal glucose tolerance after delivery, but some will continue to have overt diabetes or impairment of glucose tolerance. In addition, children of women with GDM appear to be at risk for obesity and glucose intolerance and have an increased risk of diabetes beginning in the later stages of adolescence.

Pregnancy in individuals with known DM requires meticulous planning and adherence to strict treatment regimens. Intensive diabetes management and normalization of the A1C are essential for individuals with existing DM who are planning pregnancy. The most crucial period of glycemic control is soon after fertilization. The risk of fetal malformations is increased 4–10 times in individuals with uncontrolled DM at the time of conception, and normal plasma glucose during the preconception period and throughout the periods of organ development in the fetus should be the goal.

LIPODYSTROPHIC DM

Lipodystrophy, or the loss of subcutaneous fat tissue, may be generalized in certain genetic conditions such as leprechaunism. Generalized lipodystrophy is associated with severe insulin resistance and is often accompanied by acanthosis nigricans and dyslipidemia. Localized lipodystrophy associated with insulin injections has been reduced considerably by the use of human insulin.

PROTEASE INHIBITORS AND LIPODYSTROPHY

Protease inhibitors used in the treatment of HIV disease have been associated with a centripetal accumulation of fat (visceral and abdominal area), accumulation of fat in the dorsocervical region, loss of extremity fat, decreased insulin sensitivity (elevations of the fasting insulin level and reduced glucose tolerance on IV glucose tolerance testing), and dyslipidemia. Although many aspects of the physical appearance of these individuals resemble Cushing's syndrome, increased cortisol levels do not account for this appearance. The possibility remains that this is related to HIV infection by some undefined mechanism, since some features of the syndrome were observed before the introduction of protease inhibitors. Therapy for HIV-related lipodystrophy is not well established.

FURTHER READINGS

American Diabetes Association: Clinical practice recommendations 2007. Diabetes Care 30:S4, 2007

———: Nutrition recommendations and interventions for diabetes—2006. Diabetes Care 29:2140, 2006

Bax JJ et al: Screening for coronary artery disease in patients with diabetes. Diabetes Care 30:2729, 2007

Bolen S et al: Systematic review: Comparative effectiveness and safety of oral medications for type 2 diabetes mellitus. Ann Intern Med 147:386, 2007

Chia CW et al: Incretin-based therapies in type 2 diabetes mellitus. J Clin Endocrinol Metab 93:3703, 2008

Diagnosis and classification of diabetes mellitus. Diabetes Care 31(Suppl 1):S55, 2008

Eisenbarth GS: Update in type 1 diabetes. J Clin Endocrinol Metab 92:2403, 2007

Ingelfinger JR: Aliskiren and dual therapy in type 2 diabetes mellitus. N Engl J Med 358:2503, 2008

Inzucchi SE: Management of hyperglycemia in the hospital setting. N Engl J Med 355:1903, 2006

Ryden L et al: Is glucose normalization an evidence-based treatment for patients with type 2 diabetes mellitus? Nat Clin Pract Endocrinol Metab 5:8, 2009

Saudek CD et al: A new look at screening and diagnosing diabetes mellitus. J Clin Endocrinol Metab 93:2447, 2008

_____ et al: Assessing glycemia in diabetes using self-monitoring blood glucose and hemoglobin A1c. JAMA 295:1688, 2006

Screening for gestational diabetes mellitus: U.S. Preventive Services Task Force recommendation statement. Ann Intern Med 148:759, 2008

Screening for type 2 diabetes mellitus in adults: U.S. Preventive Services Task Force recommendation statement. Ann Intern Med 148:846, 2008

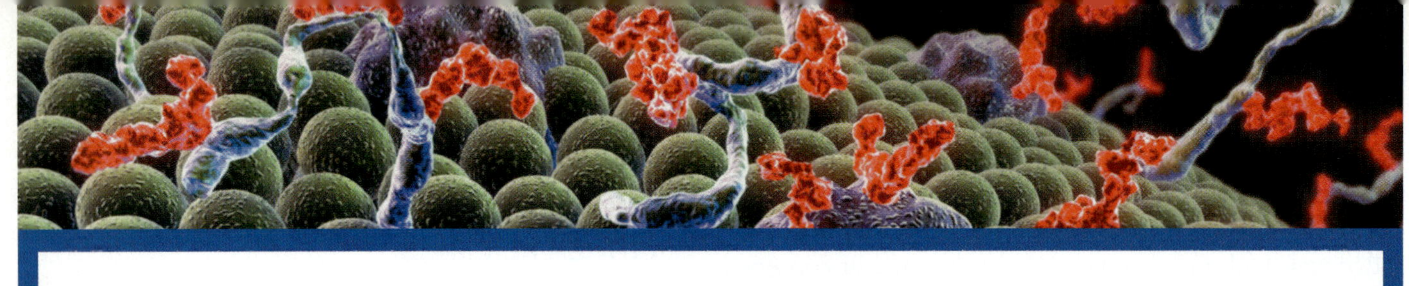

CHAPTER 20

HYPOGLYCEMIA

Philip E. Cryer

Hypoglycemia is most commonly caused by drugs used to treat diabetes mellitus or by exposure to other drugs, including alcohol. However, a number of other disorders, including insulinoma, critical organ failure, sepsis and inanition, hormone deficiencies, non–β-cell tumors, inherited metabolic disorders, and prior gastric surgery, may cause hypoglycemia (**Table 20-1**). Hypoglycemia is most convincingly documented by *Whipple's triad:* (1) symptoms consistent with hypoglycemia, (2) a low plasma glucose concentration measured with a precise method (not a glucose monitor), and (3) relief of those symptoms after the plasma glucose level is raised. The lower limit of the fasting plasma glucose concentration is normally approximately 70 mg/dL (3.9 mmol/L), but substantially lower venous glucose levels occur normally, late after a meal. Glucose levels <55 mg/dL (3.0 mmol/L) with symptoms that are relieved promptly after the glucose level is raised document hypoglycemia. Hypoglycemia can cause serious morbidity; if severe and prolonged, it can be fatal. It should be considered in any patient with episodes of confusion, an altered level of consciousness, or a seizure.

SYSTEMIC GLUCOSE BALANCE AND GLUCOSE COUNTERREGULATION

Glucose is an obligate metabolic fuel for the brain under physiologic conditions. The brain cannot synthesize glucose or store more than a few minutes' supply as glycogen and therefore requires a continuous supply of glucose from the arterial circulation. As the arterial plasma glucose concentration falls below the physiologic range, blood-to-brain glucose transport becomes insufficient to support brain energy metabolism and function. However, redundant glucose counterregulatory mechanisms normally prevent or rapidly correct hypoglycemia.

Plasma glucose concentrations are normally maintained within a relatively narrow range, roughly 70–110 mg/dL (3.9–6.1 mmol/L) in the fasting state with transient higher excursions after a meal, despite wide variations in exogenous glucose delivery from meals and in endogenous glucose utilization by, for example, exercising muscle. Between meals and during fasting, plasma glucose levels are maintained by endogenous glucose production, hepatic glycogenolysis, and hepatic (and renal) gluconeogenesis (**Fig. 20-1**). Although hepatic glycogen stores are usually sufficient to maintain plasma glucose levels for approximately 8 h, this time period can be shorter if glucose demand is increased by exercise or if glycogen stores are depleted by illness or starvation.

Gluconeogenesis requires a coordinated supply of precursors from muscle and adipose tissue to the liver (and kidneys). Muscle provides lactate, pyruvate, alanine, glutamine, and other amino acids. Triglycerides in adipose tissue are broken down into fatty acids and glycerol, which is a

TABLE 20-1

CAUSES OF HYPOGLYCEMIA

Fasting (Postabsorptive) Hypoglycemia
Drugs
Especially insulin, sulfonylureas, ethanol
Sometimes quinine, pentamidine
Rarely salicylates, sulfonamides, others
Critical illnesses
Hepatic, renal, or cardiac failure
Sepsis
Inanition
Hormone deficiencies
Cortisol, growth hormone, or both
Glucagon and epinephrine (in insulin-deficient diabetes)
Non–β-cell tumors
Endogenous hyperinsulinism
Insulinoma
Other β-cell disorders
Insulin secretagogue (sulfonylurea, other)
Autoimmune (autoantibodies to insulin or the insulin receptor)
Ectopic insulin secretion
Disorders of infancy or childhood
Transient intolerance of fasting
Congenital hyperinsulinism
Inherited enzyme deficiencies
Reactive (Postprandial) Hypoglycemia
Alimentary (postgastrectomy)
Noninsulinoma pancreatogenous hypoglycemia syndrome
In the absence of prior surgery
Following Roux-en-Y-gastric bypass
Other causes of endogenous hyperinsulinism
Hereditary fructose intolerance, galactosemia
Idiopathic

gluconeogenic precursor. Fatty acids provide an alternative oxidative fuel to tissues other than the brain (which requires glucose).

Systemic glucose balance—maintenance of the normal plasma glucose concentration—is accomplished by a network of hormones, neural signals, and substrate effects that regulate endogenous glucose production and glucose utilization by tissues other than the brain (Chap. 19). Among the regulatory factors, insulin plays a dominant role (Table 20-2; Fig. 20-1). As plasma glucose levels decline within the physiologic range in the fasting state, pancreatic β-cell insulin secretion decreases, thereby increasing hepatic glycogenolysis and hepatic (and renal) gluconeogenesis. Low insulin levels also reduce glucose utilization in peripheral tissues, inducing lipolysis and proteolysis, thereby releasing gluconeogenic precursors. Thus, a decrease in insulin secretion is the first defense against hypoglycemia.

As plasma glucose levels decline just below the physiologic range, glucose counterregulatory (plasma glucose–raising) hormones are released (Table 20-2; Fig. 20-1). Among these, pancreatic β-cell glucagon, which stimulates hepatic glycogenolysis, plays a primary role. Glucagon is the second defense against hypoglycemia. Adrenomedullary epinephrine, which stimulates hepatic glycogenolysis and gluconeogenesis (and renal gluconeogenesis), is not normally critical. However, it becomes critical when glucagon is deficient. Epinephrine is the third defense against hypoglycemia. When hypoglycemia is

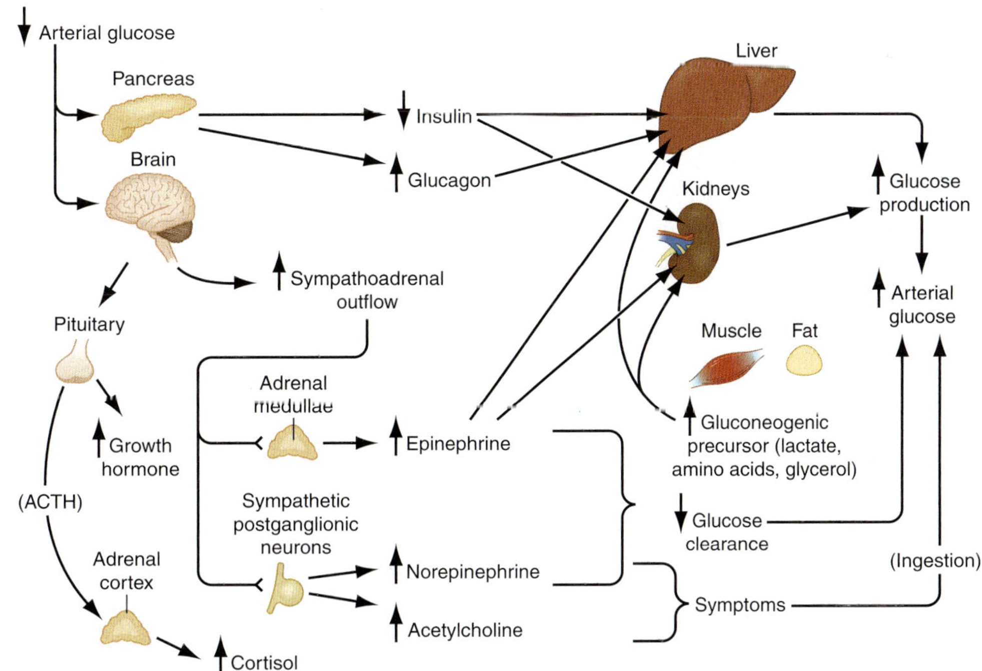

FIGURE 20-1

Physiology of glucose counterregulation—the mechanisms that normally prevent or rapidly correct hypoglycemia. In insulin-deficient diabetes, the key counterregulatory responses—suppression of insulin and increases of glucagon—are lost, and the stimulation of sympathoadrenal outflow is attenuated.

TABLE 20-2

PHYSIOLOGIC RESPONSES TO DECREASING PLASMA GLUCOSE CONCENTRATIONS

RESPONSE	GLYCEMIC THRESHOLD, mmol/L (mg/dL)	PHYSIOLOGIC EFFECTS	ROLE IN THE PREVENTION OR CORRECTION OF HYPOGLYCEMIA (GLUCOSE COUNTERREGULATION)
↓ Insulin	4.4–4.7 (80–85)	↑ R_a (↓R_d)	Primary glucose regulatory factor/first defense against hypoglycemia
↑ Glucagon	3.6–3.9 (65–70)	↑ R_a	Primary glucose counterregulatory factor/second defense against hypoglycemia
↑ Epinephrine	3.6–3.9 (65–70)	↑ R_a, ↓R_c	Third defense against hypoglycemia, critical when glucagon is deficient
↑ Cortisol and growth hormone	3.6–3.9 (65–70)	↑ R_a, ↓ R_c	Involved in defense against prolonged hypoglycemia, not critical
Symptoms	2.8–3.1 (50–55)	Recognition of hypoglycemia	Prompt behavioral defense against hypoglycemia (food ingestion)
↓ Cognition	<2.8 (<50)	—	(Compromises behavioral defense against hypoglycemia)

Note: R_a, rate of glucose appearance, glucose production by the liver and kidneys; R_c, rate of glucose clearance, glucose utilization relative to the ambient plasma glucose concentration; R_d, rate of glucose disappearance, glucose utilization by the brain (which is unaltered by the glucoregulatory hormones) and by insulin-sensitive tissues such as skeletal muscle (which is regulated by insulin, epinephrine, cortisol, and growth hormone).

prolonged, cortisol and growth hormone also support glucose production and limit glucose utilization.

As plasma glucose levels fall to lower levels, symptoms prompt the behavioral defense against hypoglycemia, including the ingestion of food (Table 20-2; Fig. 20-1).

The normal glycemic thresholds for these responses to decreasing plasma glucose concentrations are shown in Table 20-2. However, these thresholds are dynamic. They shift to higher-than-normal glucose levels in people with poorly controlled diabetes who can experience symptoms of hypoglycemia when their glucose levels decline into the normal range. On the other hand, they shift to lower-than-normal glucose levels in people with recurrent hypoglycemia, e.g., those with aggressively treated diabetes or an insulinoma. Such patients have symptoms at glucose levels lower than those that cause symptoms in healthy individuals.

CLINICAL MANIFESTATIONS

Neuroglycopenic symptoms of hypoglycemia are the direct result of central nervous system (CNS) glucose deprivation. They include behavioral changes, confusion, fatigue, seizure, loss of consciousness, and, if hypoglycemia is severe and prolonged, death. Neurogenic (or autonomic) symptoms of hypoglycemia are the result of the perception of physiologic changes caused by the CNS-mediated sympathoadrenal discharge triggered by hypoglycemia. They include adrenergic symptoms (mediated largely by norepinephrine released from sympathetic postganglionic neurons but perhaps also by epinephrine released from the adrenal medullae) such as palpitations, tremor, and anxiety. They also include cholinergic symptoms (mediated by acetylcholine released from sympathetic postganglionic neurons) such as sweating, hunger, and paresthesias. Clearly, these are nonspecific symptoms. Their attribution to hypoglycemia requires a corresponding low plasma glucose concentration and their resolution after the glucose level is raised (Whipple's triad).

Common signs of hypoglycemia include diaphoresis and pallor. Heart rate and systolic blood pressure are typically raised, but these findings may not be prominent. Neuroglycopenic manifestations are often observable. Transient focal neurologic deficits occur occasionally. Permanent neurologic deficits are rare.

ETIOLOGY AND PATHOPHYSIOLOGY

Hypoglycemia is most commonly a result of the treatment of diabetes. This topic is therefore addressed before considering other causes of hypoglycemia.

HYPOGLYCEMIA IN DIABETES

Impact and Frequency

Hypoglycemia is the limiting factor in the glycemic management of diabetes. First, it causes recurrent morbidity in most people with type 1 diabetes (T1DM) and many with type 2 diabetes (T2DM) and is sometimes fatal. Second, it precludes maintenance of euglycemia over a lifetime of diabetes and thus full realization of the well-established benefits of glycemic control. Third, it causes a vicious cycle of recurrent hypoglycemia by producing hypoglycemia-associated autonomic failure—the clinical syndromes of defective glucose counterregulation and of hypoglycemia unawareness.

Hypoglycemia is a fact of life for people with T1DM. They suffer an average of two episodes of symptomatic hypoglycemia per week and at least one episode of severe, at least temporarily disabling, hypoglycemia each year. An estimated 2–4% of people with T1DM die as a result of hypoglycemia. Overall, hypoglycemia is less frequent in T2DM. Metformin, thiazolidinediones, α-glucosidase inhibitors, glucagon-like peptide-1 (GLP-1) receptor agonists or analogues, and dipeptidyl peptidase-IV (DPP-IV) inhibitors should not cause hypoglycemia. However, they increase the risk when combined with an insulin secretagogue, such as one of the sulfonylureas, or with insulin. Notably, the frequency of hypoglycemia approaches that in T1DM as persons with T2DM develop insulin deficiency and require treatment with insulin.

Conventional Risk Factors

The conventional risk factors for hypoglycemia in diabetes are based on the premise that relative or absolute insulin excess is the sole determinant of risk. Relative or absolute insulin excess occurs when (1) insulin (or insulin secretagogue) doses are excessive, ill-timed, or of the wrong type; (2) the influx of exogenous glucose is reduced (e.g., during an overnight fast or following missed meals or snacks); (3) insulin-independent glucose utilization is increased (e.g., during exercise); (4) sensitivity to insulin is increased (e.g., with improved glycemic control, in the middle of the night, late after exercise, or with increased fitness or weight loss); (5) endogenous glucose production is reduced (e.g., following alcohol ingestion); and (6) insulin clearance is reduced (e.g., in renal failure). However, these conventional risk factors alone explain a minority of episodes; other factors are typically involved.

Hypoglycemia-Associated Autonomic Failure

While marked insulin excess alone can cause hypoglycemia, iatrogenic hypoglycemia in diabetes is typically the result of the interplay of relative or absolute insulin excess and compromised physiologic and behavioral defenses against falling plasma glucose concentrations (Table 20-2; Fig. 20-2). Defective glucose counterregulation compromises physiologic defense, and hypoglycemia unawareness compromises behavioral defense.

Defective Glucose Counterregulation

In the setting of endogenous insulin deficiency, insulin levels do not decrease as plasma glucose levels fall; the first defense against hypoglycemia is lost. Furthermore, because the decrement in intraislet insulin is normally a signal to stimulate glucagon secretion, glucagon levels do not increase as plasma glucose levels fall further; the second defense against hypoglycemia is lost. Finally, the increase in epinephrine levels, the third defense against hypoglycemia, in response to a given level of hypoglycemia is typically attenuated. The glycemic threshold for the sympathoadrenal (adrenomedullary epinephrine and sympathetic neural norepinephrine) response is shifted to lower plasma glucose concentrations. That is typically the result of recent antecedent iatrogenic hypoglycemia. In the setting of absent decrements in insulin and of absent increments in glucagon, the attenuated increment in epinephrine causes the clinical syndrome of defective glucose counterregulation. Affected patients are at 25-fold or greater increased risk of severe iatrogenic hypoglycemia during aggressive glycemic therapy of their diabetes compared with those with normal epinephrine responses.

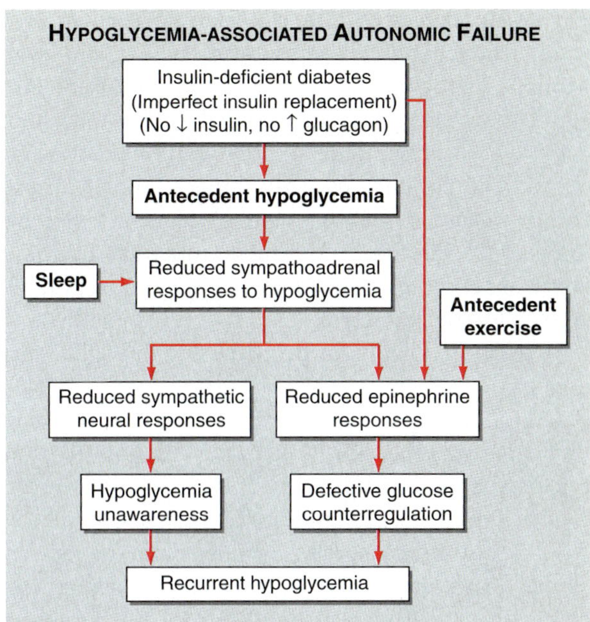

FIGURE 20-2
Hypoglycemia-associated autonomic failure in insulin-deficient diabetes. *(Adapted from Cryer PE: N Engl J Med 350:2272, 2004. Copyright Massachusetts Medical Society, 2004.)*

Hypoglycemia Unawareness

The attenuated sympathoadrenal response (largely the reduced sympathetic neural response) to hypoglycemia causes the clinical syndrome of hypoglycemia unawareness, i.e., loss of the warning adrenergic and cholinergic symptoms that previously allowed the patient to recognize developing hypoglycemia and therefore abort the episode by ingesting carbohydrates. Affected patients are at a sixfold increased risk of severe iatrogenic hypoglycemia during aggressive glycemic therapy of their diabetes.

Hypoglycemia-Associated Autonomic Failure

The concept of hypoglycemia-associated autonomic failure (HAAF) in diabetes posits that recent antecedent iatrogenic hypoglycemia (or sleep or prior exercise) causes both defective glucose counterregulation (by reducing the epinephrine response to a given level of subsequent hypoglycemia in the setting of absent insulin and glucagon responses) and hypoglycemia unawareness (by reducing the sympathoadrenal response to a given level of subsequent hypoglycemia). These impaired responses create a vicious cycle of recurrent iatrogenic hypoglycemia (Fig. 20-2). Hypoglycemia unawareness, and to some extent the reduced epinephrine component of defective glucose counterregulation, is reversible by as little as 2–3 weeks of scrupulous avoidance of hypoglycemia in most affected patients.

Based on this pathophysiology, additional risk factors for hypoglycemia in diabetes include (1) insulin deficiency that indicates that insulin levels will not decrease and glucagon levels will not increase as plasma glucose levels fall; (2) a history of severe hypoglycemia or of hypoglycemia unawareness, implying recent antecedent hypoglycemia, that indicates that the sympathoadrenal response will be attenuated; and (3) lower HbA_{1C} levels or lower glycemic goals that, all other factors being equal, increase the probability of recent antecedent hypoglycemia.

Hypoglycemia Risk Factor Reduction

It is possible to reduce the risk of hypoglycemia while maintaining a degree of glycemic control in patients with diabetes. This involves application of the principles of aggressive glycemic therapy (Chap. 19)—patient education and empowerment, frequent self-monitoring of blood glucose, flexible insulin (and other drug) regimens including the use of insulin analogues, individualized glycemic goals, and ongoing professional guidance and support—and consideration of both the conventional risk factors and those indicative of compromised glucose counterregulation. Given a history of hypoglycemia unawareness, a 2- to 3-week period of scrupulous avoidance of hypoglycemia is indicated.

FASTING HYPOGLYCEMIA

There are many causes of fasting (postabsorptive) hypoglycemia (Table 20-1). However, drugs are the most common cause by far. Those used to treat diabetes mellitus are frequent offenders, as is alcohol. Of the critical illnesses that cause hypoglycemia, sepsis is the most common. Relevant hormone deficiencies, non–β-cell tumors, and endogenous hyperinsulinism, as well as hypoglycemic disorders with their onset in infancy and childhood, are rare.

Drugs

Insulin and insulin secretagogues suppress glucose production and stimulate glucose utilization. Ethanol blocks gluconeogenesis but not glycogenolysis. Thus, alcohol-induced hypoglycemia typically occurs after a several-day ethanol binge during which the person eats little food, thereby causing glycogen depletion. Ethanol is usually measurable in blood at the time of presentation, but its levels correlate poorly with plasma glucose concentrations. Because gluconeogenesis becomes the predominant route of glucose production during prolonged hypoglycemia, alcohol can contribute to the progression of hypoglycemia in patients with insulin-treated diabetes.

Salicylates in large doses can cause hypoglycemia by inhibiting glucose production. Sulfonamides also rarely cause hypoglycemia by stimulating insulin secretion.

Pentamidine is toxic to pancreatic β cells. It causes insulin release initially, with hypoglycemia in about 10% of treated patients, and can cause diabetes later. Quinine also stimulates insulin secretion. However, the relative contribution of hyperinsulinemia to the pathogenesis of hypoglycemia in critically ill patients with malaria treated with quinine is debated. Quinolone antibiotics, particularly gatifloxacin, have been reported to cause hypoglycemia, often in the setting of drug-treated diabetes. Among the antiarrhythmic drugs, quinidine, disopyramide, and cibenzoline have been reported to cause hypoglycemia.

Hypoglycemia has been attributed to many other drugs, including the nonselective β-adrenergic antagonist propranolol. Since the glycemic actions of epinephrine and the adrenergic symptoms of hypoglycemia (but not the cholinergic symptoms such as sweating) are mediated by β_2-adrenergic receptors, it is reasonable to use a relatively selective β_1-adrenergic antagonist (e.g., atenolol or metoprolol) in a setting in which hypoglycemia might occur.

Critical Illness

Among hospitalized patients, serious illnesses such as renal, hepatic, or cardiac failure; sepsis; and inanition are second only to drugs as causes of hypoglycemia.

Rapid and extensive hepatic destruction (e.g., toxic hepatitis) causes fasting hypoglycemia because the liver is the major site of endogenous glucose production. The mechanism of hypoglycemia in patients with cardiac failure is unknown. It may involve hepatic congestion and hypoxia. Although the kidneys are a source of glucose production, hypoglycemia in patients with renal failure is also caused by the reduced clearance of insulin and reduced mobilization of gluconeogenic precursors in renal failure.

Sepsis is a relatively common cause of hypoglycemia. Increased glucose utilization is induced by cytokine production in macrophage-rich tissues such as the liver, spleen, and lung. Hypoglycemia develops if glucose production fails to keep pace. Cytokine-induced inhibition of gluconeogenesis in the setting of nutritional glycogen depletion, in combination with hepatic and renal hypoperfusion, may also contribute to hypoglycemia.

Hypoglycemia can be seen with starvation, perhaps because of loss of whole-body fat stores and subsequent depletion of gluconeogenic precursors (e.g., amino acids), necessitating increased glucose utilization.

Hormone Deficiencies

Neither cortisol nor growth hormone is critical to the prevention of hypoglycemia, at least in adults. Nonetheless, hypoglycemia can occur with prolonged fasting in patients with primary adrenocortical failure (Addison's disease) or hypopituitarism. Anorexia and weight loss are typical features of chronic cortisol deficiency and likely result in glycogen depletion. Cortisol deficiency is associated with impaired gluconeogenesis and low levels of gluconeogenic precursors, suggesting that substrate-limited gluconeogenesis, in the setting of glycogen depletion, is the cause of hypoglycemia. Growth hormone deficiency can cause hypoglycemia in young children. In addition to extended fasting, high rates of glucose utilization (e.g., during exercise or in pregnancy) or low rates of glucose production (e.g., following alcohol ingestion) can precipitate hypoglycemia in adults with previously unrecognized hypopituitarism.

Hypoglycemia is not a feature of the epinephrine-deficient state that results from bilateral adrenalectomy, when glucocorticoid replacement is adequate, nor does it occur during pharmacologic adrenergic blockade when other glucoregulatory systems are intact. Combined deficiencies of glucagon and epinephrine play a key role in the pathogenesis of iatrogenic hypoglycemia in people with insulin-deficient diabetes. Otherwise, deficiencies of these hormones are not usually considered in the differential diagnosis of a hypoglycemic disorder.

Non–β-Cell Tumors

Fasting hypoglycemia, often termed non–islet cell tumor hypoglycemia, occurs occasionally in patients with large mesenchymal or epithelial tumors (e.g., hepatomas, adrenocortical carcinomas, carcinoids). The glucose kinetic patterns resemble those of hyperinsulinism, but insulin secretion is suppressed appropriately during hypoglycemia. In most instances, hypoglycemia is due to overproduction of an incompletely processed form of insulin-like growth factor II ("big IGF-II") that does not complex normally with circulating binding proteins and thus more readily gains access to target tissues. The tumors are usually apparent clinically, and free IGF-II levels [and levels of pro-IGF-II (E1-21)] are elevated. Curative surgery is seldom possible, but reduction of tumor bulk may ameliorate hypoglycemia. Therapy with a glucocorticoid, growth hormone, or both has also been reported to alleviate hypoglycemia.

Endogenous Hyperinsulinism

Hypoglycemia due to endogenous hyperinsulinism can be caused by (1) a primary β-cell disorder, typically a β-cell tumor (insulinoma), sometimes multiple insulinomas, or, especially in infants and young children, a functional β-cell disorder with β-cell hypertrophy or hyperplasia; (2) a β-cell secretagogue such as a sulfonylurea; (3) an autoantibody to insulin; or (4) rarely, ectopic insulin secretion. None of these causes is common. Endogenous hyperinsulinism is more likely in an overtly healthy individual without clues to other potential causes of hypoglycemia. Accidental, surreptitious, or even malicious administration of an insulin secretagogue or insulin also should be considered in such an individual.

The fundamental pathophysiologic feature of endogenous hyperinsulinism caused by a primary β-cell disorder or an insulin secretagogue is the failure of insulin secretion to fall to very low levels during hypoglycemia. This is assessed by measuring plasma insulin, C peptide (the connecting peptide that is cleaved from proinsulin to produce insulin), and glucose concentrations during hypoglycemia; proinsulin levels also can be measured. Insulin, C peptide, and proinsulin levels need not be high relative to normal, euglycemic values; they are often inappropriately high in the setting of a low plasma glucose concentration. Critical diagnostic findings are a plasma insulin concentration ≥3 μU/mL (≥18 pmol/L) and a plasma C-peptide concentration ≥0.6 ng/mL (≥0.2 nmol/L) (with a plasma proinsulin concentration ≥5.0 pmol/L) when the plasma glucose concentration is <55 mg/dL (<3.0 mmol/L) with symptoms of hypoglycemia.

Most primary β-cell disorders, such as an insulinoma, cause fasting hypoglycemia. The diagnostic strategy is to make the above measurements during spontaneous, symptomatic hypoglycemia, i.e., after an overnight fast, an extended outpatient fast, or, if necessary, an inpatient prolonged (48- or 72-h) fast. It is necessary to screen the plasma for sulfonylureas and other insulin secretagogues (repaglinide, nateglinide) at the time of hypoglycemia since these produce an insulin, C-peptide, proinsulin, and glucose pattern indistinguishable from that produced by an insulinoma. Autoantibodies to insulin also should be sought but need not be measured at the time of hypoglycemia. The noninsulinoma pancreatogenous hypoglycemia syndrome, which also causes postprandial hyperinsulinemic hypoglycemia, is discussed later. The rare autoantibodies to the insulin receptor are sometimes agonists; insulin secretion is suppressed during hypoglycemia but insulin levels tend to be inappropriately high, perhaps because of decreased clearance of insulin via the receptor. Ectopic insulin secretion has been reported, but it must be quite rare and is usually not considered in the differential diagnosis of a hypoglycemic disorder. Finally, the finding of inappropriately high insulin levels but low C-peptide levels during hypoglycemia indicates exogenous insulin administration. A diagnostic algorithm for a patient with suspected endogenous hyperinsulinism is shown in Fig. 20-3.

Insulinomas are uncommon—the yearly incidence is estimated to be 1 in 250,000—but because more than

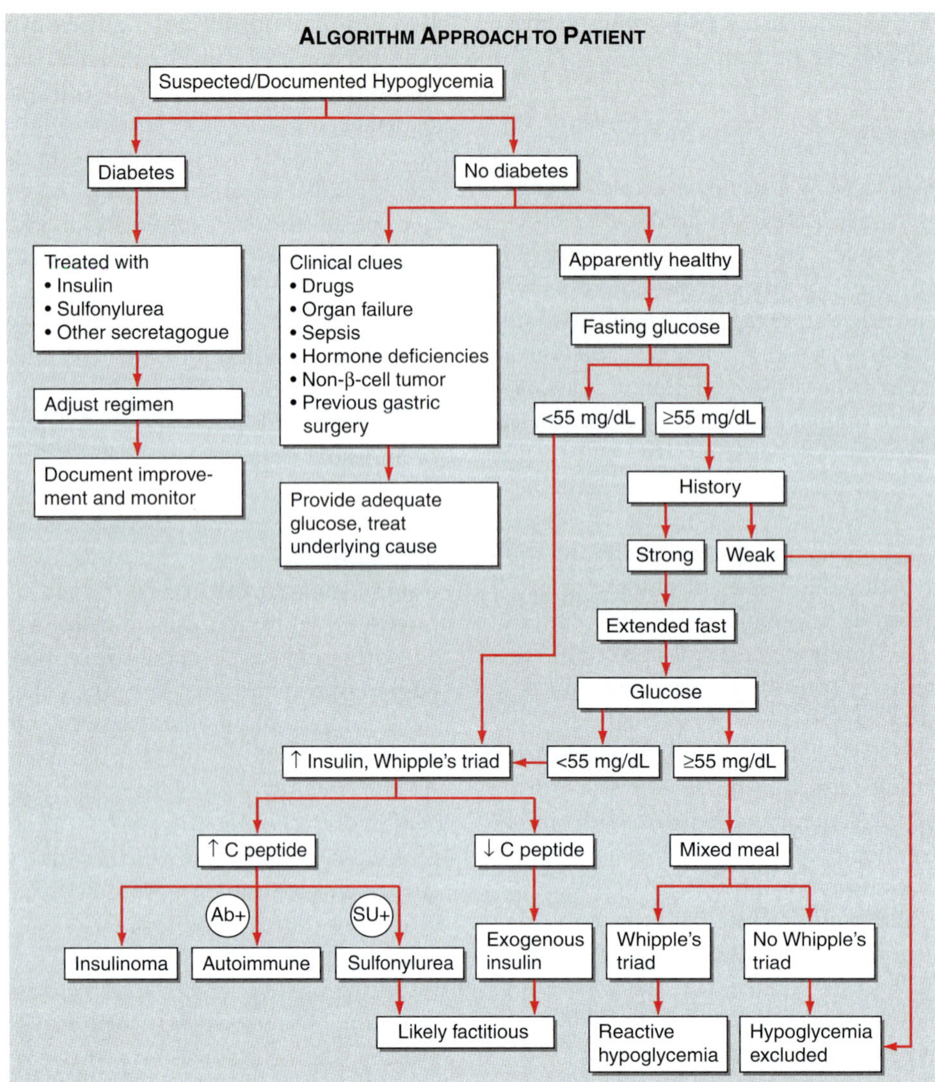

FIGURE 20-3

Diagnostic approach to a patient with documented hypoglycemia or suspected hypoglycemia based on a history of suggestive symptoms, a low plasma glucose concentration, or both. Ab+, positive for antibody to insulin; SU+, positive for sulfonylurea (or other secretagogue).

90% are benign, they are a treatable cause of potentially fatal hypoglycemia. The median age at presentation is 50 years in sporadic cases, but it usually presents in the third decade when it is a component of multiple endocrine neoplasia type 1 (Chap. 23). More than 99% of insulinomas are within the substance of the pancreas and they are usually small (90% <2.0 cm). Therefore, they come to clinical attention because of hypoglycemia rather than mass effects. Computed tomography detects approximately 70–80% of insulinomas, and magnetic resonance imaging detects about 85%. These methods detect metastases in the roughly 10% of patients with a malignant insulinoma. Transabdominal ultrasound will often identify insulinomas, and endoscopic ultrasound has a sensitivity of about 90%. Somatostatin receptor scintigraphy is thought to detect insulinomas in about half of patients. Selective pancreatic arterial calcium injections, with the endpoint of a sharp increase in hepatic venous insulin levels, regionalize insulinomas with high sensitivity, but this invasive procedure is seldom necessary. The same is true of transhepatic portal venous sampling. Intraoperative pancreatic ultrasonography almost invariably localizes insulinomas that are not readily palpable by the surgeon. Surgical resection of a solitary insulinoma is generally curative. Diazoxide, which inhibits insulin secretion, or the somatostatin analogue octreotide can be used to treat hypoglycemia in patients with unresectable tumors.

DISORDERS OF INFANCY AND CHILDHOOD

Discussion of the various disorders that cause hypoglycemia in infancy and childhood, including multiple causes of transient intolerance of fasting, congenital hyperinsulinism, and inherited enzyme deficiencies, is beyond the scope of this chapter.

REACTIVE HYPOGLYCEMIA

Reactive (postprandial) hypoglycemia occurs exclusively after meals. Its diagnosis requires documentation of Whipple's triad after a mixed meal. The diagnosis should not be made on the basis of seemingly low venous plasma glucose concentrations after an oral glucose load. It can occur following gastrectomy. Termed *alimentary hypoglycemia*, this is thought to be the result of early hyperinsulinemia caused by rapid increments in plasma glucose and enhanced secretion of the gut incretin GLP-1 coupled with suppression of glucagon secretion by GLP-1. Administration of an α-glucosidase inhibitor (e.g., acarbose or miglitol) is a conceptually attractive treatment, although controlled clinical trials documenting its efficacy are lacking.

Reactive hypoglycemia also occurs in patients with autoantibodies to insulin and in the noninsulinoma pancreatogenous hypoglycemia syndrome. Affected patients have symptomatic hyperinsulinemic postprandial hypoglycemia (but negative 72-h fasts) that remits following partial pancreatectomy. Histologic findings include β-cell hypertrophy with or without hyperplasia. A similar syndrome following Roux-en-Y gastric bypass surgery for obesity has been described.

The existence of a clinically relevant idiopathic reactive hypoglycemia syndrome is debated. The issue is whether symptoms are caused by hypoglycemia, an exaggerated sympathoadrenal response to declining glucose levels late after a meal, or some glucose-independent mechanism. In any event, caution should be exercised before labeling a person with a diagnosis of hypoglycemia. Frequent feedings, avoidance of simple sugars, and high-protein diets are commonly recommended to patients thought to have idiopathic reactive hypoglycemia. The efficacy of these approaches has not been established by controlled clinical trials.

FACTITIOUS AND ARTIFACTUAL HYPOGLYCEMIA

Factitious hypoglycemia, caused by surreptitious or even malicious administration of insulin or an insulin secretagogue, shares many clinical and laboratory features with insulinoma. It is most common among health care workers, patients with diabetes or their relatives, and people with a history of other factitious illnesses. However, it should be considered in all patients being evaluated for hypoglycemia of obscure cause. Accidental ingestion of an insulin secretagogue (e.g., the result of a pharmacy error) also occurs.

Analytical error in the measurement of plasma glucose concentrations is rare. On the other hand, glucose monitors used to guide treatment of diabetes are not quantitative instruments, particularly at low glucose levels, and these should not be used for the definitive diagnosis of hypoglycemia. Even with a quantitative method, low measured glucose concentrations can be artifactual, e.g., the result of continued glucose metabolism by the formed elements of the blood ex vivo, particularly in the presence of leukocytosis, erythrocytosis, or thrombocytosis, or if separation of the serum from the formed elements is delayed (pseudohypoglycemia).

Approach to the Patient: HYPOGLYCEMIA

In addition to recognition and documentation of hypoglycemia, and often urgent treatment, diagnosis of the hypoglycemic mechanism is critical for choosing a treatment that prevents, or at least minimizes, recurrent hypoglycemia. A diagnostic algorithm is shown in Fig. 20-3.

RECOGNITION AND DOCUMENTATION Hypoglycemia is suspected in patients with typical symptoms; in the presence of confusion, an altered level of consciousness, or a seizure; or in a clinical setting in which hypoglycemia is known to occur. Urgent treatment is often necessary in patients with suspected hypoglycemia. Blood should be drawn, whenever possible, before the administration of glucose to allow documentation of a low plasma glucose concentration. Convincing documentation of hypoglycemia requires the fulfillment of Whipple's triad. Thus, the ideal time to measure the plasma glucose level is during a symptomatic episode. A normal glucose level excludes hypoglycemia as the cause of the symptoms. A low glucose level confirms that hypoglycemia is the cause of the symptoms, provided the latter resolve after the glucose level is raised. When the cause of the hypoglycemic episode is obscure, additional measurements, while the glucose level is low and before treatment, should include plasma insulin, C-peptide, and ethanol concentrations, as well as levels of insulin secretagogues.

When the history suggests prior hypoglycemia, and a potential mechanism is not apparent, the diagnostic strategy is to measure the plasma glucose, insulin, and C-peptide levels under conditions when hypoglycemia would be expected, typically during fasting. On the other hand, while it cannot be ignored, a distinctly low plasma glucose concentration measured in a patient without corresponding symptoms raises the possibility of an artifact (pseudohypoglycemia).

DIAGNOSIS OF THE HYPOGLYCEMIC MECHANISM In a patient with documented hypoglycemia, a plausible hypoglycemic mechanism can often be deduced from the history, physical examination, and available laboratory data (Table 20-1; Fig. 20-3). Drugs, particularly those used to treat diabetes or alcohol, should be the first consideration, even in the absence of known use of a relevant drug, given the possibility of surreptitious, accidental, or malicious drug administration. Other considerations include evidence of a relevant critical illness, less commonly hormone deficiencies, and rarely a non–β-cell tumor that can be pursued diagnostically. Absent one of these mechanisms, in an otherwise overtly well individual, one should consider endogenous hyperinsulinism and proceed with measurements and assessment of symptoms under fasting conditions of sufficient duration to elicit or exclude fasting hypoglycemia.

URGENT TREATMENT Oral treatment with glucose tablets or glucose- containing fluids, candy, or food is appropriate if the patient is able and willing to take these. A reasonable initial dose is 20 g of glucose. If the patient is unable or unwilling, because of neuroglycopenia, to take carbohydrates orally, parenteral therapy is necessary. IV glucose (25 g) should be given and followed by a glucose infusion guided by serial plasma glucose measurements. If IV therapy is not practical, SC or IM glucagon (1.0 mg in adults) can be used, particularly in patients with T1DM. Because it acts by stimulating glycogenolysis, glucagon is ineffective in glycogen-depleted individuals (e.g., those with alcohol-induced hypoglycemia). It also stimulates insulin secretion and is therefore less useful in T2DM. These treatments raise plasma glucose concentrations only transiently, and patients should therefore be urged to eat as soon as is practical to replete glycogen stores.

PREVENTION OF RECURRENT HYPOGLYCEMIA Prevention of recurrent hypoglycemia requires an understanding of the hypoglycemic mechanism. Offending drugs can be discontinued or their doses reduced. Hypoglycemia caused by a sulfonylurea can persist for hours, or even days. Underlying critical illnesses can often be treated. Cortisol and growth hormone can be replaced if they are deficient. Surgical, radiotherapeutic, or chemotherapeutic reduction of a non–β-cell tumor can alleviate hypoglycemia even if the tumor cannot be cured; glucocorticoid or growth hormone administration also may reduce hypoglycemic episodes in such patients. Surgical resection of an insulinoma is curative; medical therapy with diazoxide or octreotide can be used if resection is not possible and in patients with a nontumor β-cell disorder. Partial pancreatectomy may be necessary in the latter patients. The treatment of autoimmune hypoglycemia (e.g., with a glucocorticoid or immunosuppressive drugs) is problematic, but the disorders are often self-limited. Failing these treatments, frequent feedings and avoidance of fasting may be required. Administration of uncooked cornstarch at bedtime or even an overnight intragastric infusion of glucose may be necessary in some patients.

FURTHER READINGS

Boyle PJ, Zrebiec J: Management of diabetes-related hypoglycemia. South Med J 100(2):183, 2007

Cryer PE: Glucose homeostasis and hypoglycemia, in *Williams Textbook of Endocrinology*, 11th ed, H Kronenberg et al (eds). Philadelphia, Saunders, an imprint of Elsevier, Inc 2008, pp 1503-1533

Davis SN et al: Effects of intensive therapy and antecedent hypoglycemia on counterregulatory responses to hypoglycemia in type 2 diabetes. Diabetes 58:701, 2009

Dodek P: ACP Journal Club. Review: Tight glucose control reduces septicemia, but not death, and increases hypoglycemia in critically ill adults. Ann Intern Med 150:JC1, 2009

Fatourechi MM et al: Clinical review: Hypoglycemia with intensive insulin therapy: A systematic review and meta-analyses of randomized trials of continuous subcutaneous insulin infusion versus multiple daily injections. J Clin Endocrinol Metab 94:729, 2009

Kapoor RR et al: Advances in the diagnosis and management of hyperinsulinemic hypoglycemia. Nat Clin Pract Endocrinol Metab 5:101, 2009

Service FJ: Hypoglycemic disorders. Endocrinol Metab Clin North Am 28:467, 1999

Smith CB et al: Hypoglycemia unawareness is associated with reduced adherence to therapeutic decisions in patients with type 1 diabetes: Evidence from a clinical audit. Diabetes Care 32:1196, 2009

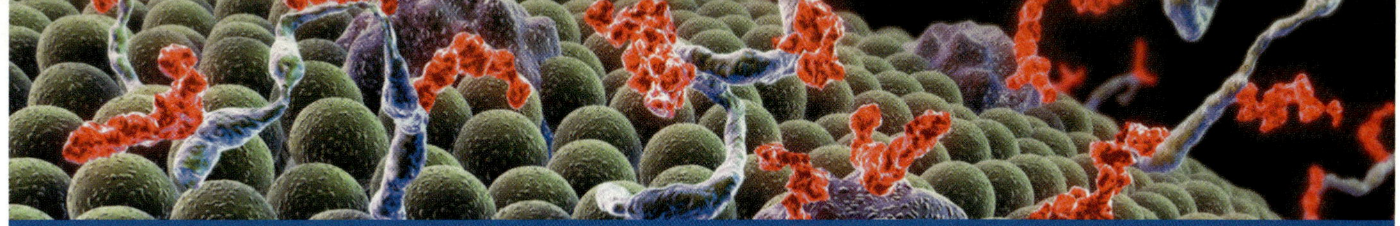

CHAPTER 21

DISORDERS OF LIPOPROTEIN METABOLISM

Daniel J. Rader ■ Helen H. Hobbs

Lipoproteins are complexes of lipids and proteins that are essential for the transport of cholesterol, triglycerides, and fat-soluble vitamins. Previously, lipoprotein disorders were the purview of specialized lipidologists, but the demonstration that lipid-lowering therapy significantly reduces the clinical complications of atherosclerotic cardiovascular disease (ASCVD) has brought the diagnosis and treatment of these disorders into the domain of the internist. The number of individuals who are candidates for lipid-lowering therapy has continued to increase. The development of safe, effective, and well-tolerated pharmacologic agents has greatly expanded the therapeutic armamentarium available to the physician to treat disorders of lipid metabolism. Therefore, the appropriate diagnosis and management of lipoprotein disorders is of critical importance in the practice of medicine. This chapter will review normal lipoprotein physiology, the pathophysiology of primary (inherited) disorders of lipoprotein metabolism, the diseases and environmental factors that cause secondary disorders of lipoprotein metabolism, and the practical approaches to their diagnosis and management.

LIPOPROTEIN METABOLISM

LIPOPROTEIN CLASSIFICATION AND COMPOSITION

Lipoproteins are large macromolecular complexes that transport hydrophobic lipids (primarily triglycerides, cholesterol, and fat-soluble vitamins) through body fluids (plasma, interstitial fluid, and lymph) to and from tissues. Lipoproteins play an essential role in the absorption of dietary cholesterol, long-chain fatty acids, and fat-soluble vitamins; the transport of triglycerides, cholesterol, and fat-soluble vitamins from the liver to peripheral tissues; and the transport of cholesterol from peripheral tissues to the liver.

Lipoproteins contain a core of hydrophobic lipids (triglycerides and cholesteryl esters) surrounded by hydrophilic lipids (phospholipids, unesterified cholesterol) and proteins that interact with body fluids. The plasma lipoproteins are divided into five major classes based on their relative density (Fig. 21-1 and Table 21-1): chylomicrons, very low density lipoproteins (VLDLs),

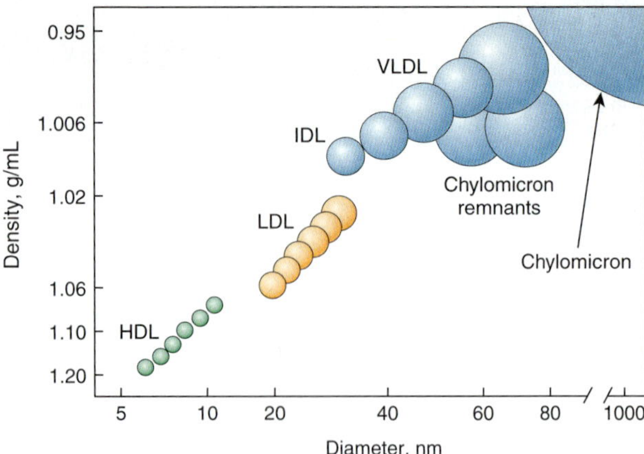

FIGURE 21-1

The density and size distribution of the major classes of lipoprotein particles. Lipoproteins are classified by density and size, which are inversely related. VLDL, very low density lipoprotein; IDL, intermediate-density lipoprotein; LDL, low-density lipoprotein; HDL, high-density lipoprotein.

intermediate-density lipoproteins (IDLs), low-density lipoproteins (LDLs), and high-density lipoproteins (HDLs). Each lipoprotein class comprises a family of particles that vary slightly in density, size, migration during electrophoresis, and protein composition. The density of a lipoprotein is determined by the amount of lipid per particle. HDL is the smallest and most dense lipoprotein, whereas chylomicrons and VLDLs are the largest and least dense lipoprotein particles. Most plasma triglyceride is transported in chylomicrons or VLDLs, and most plasma cholesterol is carried as cholesteryl esters in LDLs and HDLs.

The proteins associated with lipoproteins, called *apolipoproteins* (Table 21-2), are required for the assembly, structure, and function of lipoproteins. Apolipoproteins activate enzymes important in lipoprotein metabolism and act as ligands for cell-surface receptors. ApoA-I, which is synthesized in the liver and intestine, is found on virtually all HDL particles. ApoA-II is the second most abundant HDL apolipoprotein and is on approximately two-thirds of all HDL particles. ApoB is the major structural protein of chylomicrons, VLDLs, IDLs, and LDLs; one molecule of apoB, either apoB48 (chylomicron) or apoB100 (VLDL, IDL, or LDL), is present on each lipoprotein particle. The human liver synthesizes apoB100, and the intestine makes apoB48, which is derived from the same gene by mRNA editing. ApoE is present in multiple copies on chylomicrons, VLDLs, and IDLs, and it plays a critical role in the metabolism and clearance of triglyceride-rich particles. Three apolipoproteins of the C series (apoC-I, apoC-II, and apoC-III) also participate in the metabolism of triglyceride-rich lipoproteins. The other apolipoproteins are listed in Table 21-2.

TRANSPORT OF DIETARY LIPIDS (EXOGENOUS PATHWAY)

The exogenous pathway of lipoprotein metabolism permits efficient transport of dietary lipids (Fig. 21-2). Dietary triglycerides are hydrolyzed by lipases within the intestinal lumen and emulsified with bile acids to form micelles. Dietary cholesterol, fatty acids, and fat-soluble vitamins are absorbed in the proximal small intestine. Cholesterol and retinol are esterified (by the addition of a fatty acid) in the enterocyte to form cholesteryl esters and retinyl esters, respectively. Longer-chain

TABLE 21-1

MAJOR LIPOPROTEIN CLASSES

				APOLIPOPROTEINS		
LIPOPROTEIN	DENSITY, g/mL[a]	SIZE, nm[b]	ELECTROPHORETIC MOBILITY[c]	MAJOR	OTHER	OTHER CONSTITUENTS
Chylomicrons	0.930	75–1200	Origin	ApoB48	A-I, A-IV, C-I, C-II, C-III	Retinyl esters
Chylomicron remnants	0.930–1.006	30–80	Slow pre-β	ApoB48	E, A-I, A-IV, C-I, C-II, C-III	Retinyl esters
VLDL	0.930–1.006	30–80	Pre-β	ApoB100	E, A-I, A-II, A-V, C-I, C-II, C-III	Vitamin E
IDL	1.006–1.019	25–35	Slow pre-β	ApoB100	E, C-I, C-II, C-III	Vitamin E
LDL	1.019–1.063	18–25	β	ApoB100		Vitamin E
HDL	1.063–1.210	5–12	α	ApoA-I	A-II, A-IV, E, C-III	LCAT, CETP paraoxonase
Lp(a)	1.050–1.120	25	Pre-β	ApoB100	Apo(a)	

Note: All of the lipoprotein classes contain phospholipids, esterified and unesterified cholesterol, and triglycerides to varying degrees.

[a]The density of the particle is determined by ultracentrifugation.

[b]The size of the particle is measured using gel electrophoresis.

[c]The electrophoretic mobility of the particle on agarose gel electrophores reflects the size and surface charge of the particle, with β being the position of LDL and α being the position of HDL.

VLDL, very low density lipoprotein; IDL, intermediate-density lipoprotein; LDL, low-density lipoprotein; HDL, high-density lipoprotein; Lp(a), lipoprotein A; LCAT, lecithin-cholesterol acyltransferase; CETP, cholesteryl ester transfer protein.

TABLE 21-2

MAJOR APOLIPOPROTEINS

APOLIPOPROTEIN	PRIMARY SOURCE	LIPOPROTEIN ASSOCIATION	FUNCTION
ApoA-I	Intestine, liver	HDL, chylomicrons	Structural protein for HDL Activates LCAT
ApoA-II	Liver	HDL, chylomicrons	Structural protein for HDL
ApoA-IV	Intestine	HDL, chylomicrons	Unknown
ApoA-V	Liver	VLDL, chylomicrons	Promotes LPL-mediated triglyceride lipolysis
ApoB48	Intestine	Chylomicrons	Structural protein for chylomicrons
ApoB100	Liver	VLDL, IDL, LDL, Lp(a)	Structural protein for VLDL, LDL, IDL, Lp(a) Ligand for binding to LDL receptor
ApoC-I	Liver	Chylomicrons, VLDL, HDL	Unknown
ApoC-II	Liver	Chylomicrons, VLDL, HDL	Cofactor for LPL
ApoC-III	Liver	Chylomicrons, VLDL, HDL	Inhibits lipoprotein binding to receptors
ApoD	Spleen, brain, testes, adrenals	HDL	Unknown
ApoE	Liver	Chylomicron remnants, IDL, HDL	Ligand for binding to LDL receptor
ApoH	Liver	Chylomicrons, VLDL, LDL, HDL	B_2 glycoprotein I
ApoJ	Liver	HDL	Unknown
ApoL	Unknown	HDL	Unknown
ApoM	Liver	HDL	Unknown
Apo(a)	Liver	Lp(a)	Unknown

Note: HDL, high-density lipoprotein; LCAT, lecithin-cholesterol acyltransferase; VLDL, very low density lipoprotein; IDL, intermediate-density lipoprotein; LDL, low-density lipoprotein; Lp(a), lipoprotein A; LPL, lipoprotein lipase.

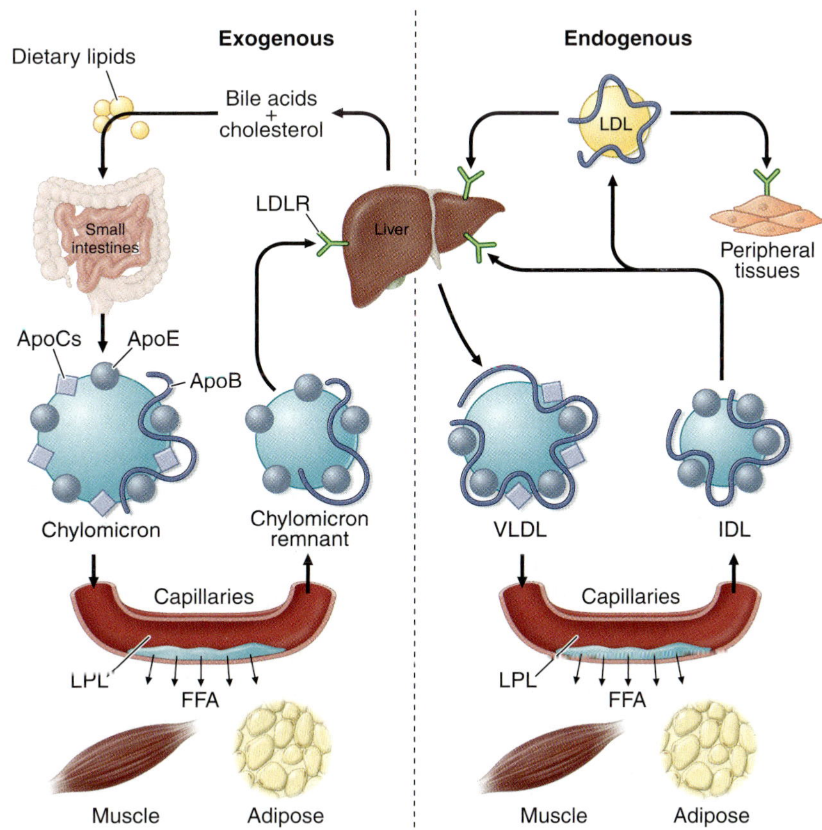

FIGURE 21-2

The exogenous and endogenous lipoprotein metabolic pathways. The exogenous pathway transports dietary lipids to the periphery and the liver. The endogenous pathway transports hepatic lipids to the periphery. LPL, lipoprotein lipase; FFA, free fatty acid; VLDL, very low density lipoprotein; IDL, intermediate-density lipoprotein; LDL, low-density lipoprotein; LDLR, low-density lipoprotein receptor.

fatty acids (>12 carbons) are incorporated into triglycerides and packaged with apoB48, cholesteryl esters, retinyl esters, phospholipids, and cholesterol to form chylomicrons. Nascent chylomicrons are secreted into the intestinal lymph and delivered via the thoracic duct directly to the systemic circulation, where they are extensively processed by peripheral tissues before reaching the liver. The particles encounter lipoprotein lipase (LPL), which is anchored to proteoglycans that decorate the capillary endothelial surfaces of adipose tissue, heart, and skeletal muscle (Fig. 21-2). The triglycerides of chylomicrons are hydrolyzed by LPL, and free fatty acids are released. ApoC-II, which is transferred to circulating chylomicrons from HDL, acts as a cofactor for LPL in this reaction. The released free fatty acids are taken up by adjacent myocytes or adipocytes and either oxidized to generate energy or reesterified and stored as triglyceride. Some of the released free fatty acids bind albumin before entering cells and are transported to other tissues, especially the liver. The chylomicron particle progressively shrinks in size as the hydrophobic core is hydrolyzed and the hydrophilic lipids (cholesterol and phospholipids) and apolipoproteins on the particle surface are transferred to HDL, creating chylomicron remnants. Chylomicron remnants are rapidly removed from the circulation by the liver through a process that requires apoE as a ligand for receptors in the liver. Consequently, few, if any, chylomicrons or chylomicron remnants are present in the blood after a 12-h fast, except in patients with disorders of chylomicron metabolism.

TRANSPORT OF HEPATIC LIPIDS (ENDOGENOUS PATHWAY)

The endogenous pathway of lipoprotein metabolism refers to the hepatic secretion of apoB-containing lipoproteins and their metabolism (Fig. 21-2). VLDL particles resemble chylomicrons in protein composition but contain apoB100 rather than apoB48 and have a higher ratio of cholesterol to triglyceride (~1 mg of cholesterol for every 5 mg of triglyceride). The triglycerides of VLDL are derived predominantly from the esterification of long-chain fatty acids in the liver. The packaging of hepatic triglycerides with the other major components of the nascent VLDL particle (apoB100, cholesteryl esters, phospholipids, and vitamin E) requires the action of the enzyme microsomal triglyceride transfer protein (MTP). After secretion into the plasma, VLDL acquires multiple copies of apoE and apolipoproteins of the C series by transfer from HDL. As with chylomicrons, the triglycerides of VLDL are hydrolyzed by LPL, especially in muscle and adipose tissue. After the VLDL remnants dissociate from LPL, they are referred to as IDLs, which contain roughly similar amounts of cholesterol and triglyceride. The liver removes approximately 40–60% of IDL by LDL receptor–mediated endocytosis via binding to apoE. The remainder of IDL is remodeled by hepatic lipase (HL) to form LDL. During this process, most of the triglyceride in the particle is hydrolyzed, and all apolipoproteins except apoB100 are transferred to other lipoproteins. The cholesterol in LDL accounts for over half of the plasma cholesterol in most individuals. Approximately 70% of circulating LDL is cleared by LDL receptor–mediated endocytosis in the liver. *Lipoprotein(a)* [Lp(a)] is a lipoprotein similar to LDL in lipid and protein composition, but it contains an additional protein called *apolipoprotein(a)* [apo(a)]. Apo(a) is synthesized in the liver and attached to apoB100 by a disulfide linkage. The major site of clearance of Lp(a) is the liver, but the uptake pathway is not known.

HDL METABOLISM AND REVERSE CHOLESTEROL TRANSPORT

All nucleated cells synthesize cholesterol, but only hepatocytes and enterocytes can effectively excrete cholesterol from the body, into either the bile or the gut lumen. In the liver, cholesterol is excreted into the bile, either directly or after conversion to bile acids. Cholesterol in peripheral cells is transported from the plasma membranes of peripheral cells to the liver and intestine by a process termed *reverse cholesterol transport* that is facilitated by HDL (**Fig. 21-3**).

Nascent HDL particles are synthesized by the intestine and the liver. Newly secreted apoA-I rapidly acquires phospholipids and unesterified cholesterol from its site of synthesis (intestine or liver) via efflux promoted by the membrane protein ATP-binding cassette protein A1 (ABCA1). This process results in the formation of discoidal HDL particles, which then recruit additional unesterified cholesterol from the periphery. Within the HDL particle, the cholesterol is esterified by lecithin-cholesterol acyltransferase (LCAT), a plasma enzyme associated with HDL, and the more hydrophobic cholesteryl ester moves to the core of the HDL particle. As HDL acquires more cholesteryl ester it becomes spherical, and additional apolipoproteins and lipids are transferred to the particles from the surfaces of chylomicrons and VLDLs during lipolysis.

HDL cholesterol is transported to hepatocytes by both an indirect and a direct pathway. HDL cholesteryl esters can be transferred to apoB-containing lipoproteins in exchange for triglyceride by the cholesteryl ester transfer protein (CETP). The cholesteryl esters are then removed from the circulation by LDL receptor–mediated endocytosis. HDL cholesterol can also be taken up directly by hepatocytes via the scavenger receptor class BI (SR-BI), a cell-surface receptor that mediates the selective transfer of lipids to cells.

HDL particles undergo extensive remodeling within the plasma compartment by a variety of lipid transfer proteins and lipases. The phospholipid transfer protein has the net effect of transferring phospholipids from

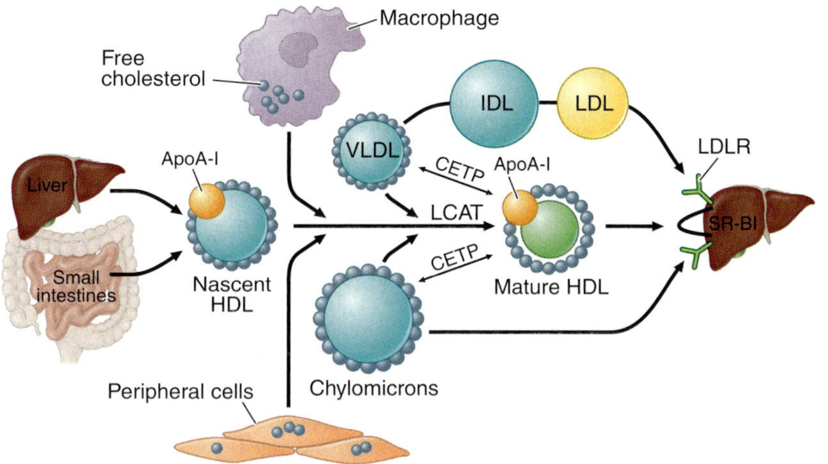

FIGURE 21-3

HDL metabolism and reverse cholesterol transport. This pathway transports excess cholesterol from the periphery back to the liver for excretion in the bile. The liver and the intestine produce nascent HDLs. Free cholesterol is acquired from macrophages and other peripheral cells and esterified by LCAT, forming mature HDLs. HDL cholesterol can be selectively taken up by the liver via SR-BI (scavenger receptor class BI). Alternatively, HDL cholesteryl ester can be transferred by CETP from HDLs to VLDLs and chylomicrons, which can then be taken up by the liver. LCAT, lecithin-cholesterol acyltransferase; CETP, cholesteryl ester transfer protein; VLDL, very low density lipoprotein; IDL, intermediate-density lipoprotein; LDL, low-density lipoprotein; HDL, high-density lipoprotein; LDLR, low-density lipoprotein receptor; TG, triglyceride.

other lipoproteins to HDL. After CETP-mediated lipid exchange, the triglyceride-enriched HDL becomes a much better substrate for HL, which hydrolyzes the triglycerides and phospholipids to generate smaller HDL particles. A related enzyme called *endothelial lipase* hydrolyzes HDL phospholipids, generating smaller HDL particles that are catabolized faster. Remodeling of HDL influences the metabolism, function, and plasma concentrations of HDL.

DISORDERS OF LIPOPROTEIN METABOLISM

Frederickson and Levy classified hyperlipoproteinemias according to the type of lipoprotein particles that accumulate in the blood (Type I to Type V) (Table 21-3). A classification scheme based on the molecular etiology and pathophysiology of the lipoprotein disorders complements this system and forms the basis for this chapter. The identification and characterization of genes responsible for the genetic forms of hyperlipidemia have provided important molecular insights into the critical roles of structural apolipoproteins, enzymes, and receptors in lipid metabolism (Table 21-4).

PRIMARY DISORDERS OF ELEVATED ApoB-CONTAINING LIPOPROTEINS

A variety of genetic conditions are associated with the accumulation in plasma of specific classes of lipoprotein particles. In general, these can be divided into those causing elevated LDL cholesterol (LDL-C) with normal triglycerides and those causing elevated triglycerides (Table 21-4).

Lipid Disorders Associated with Elevated LDL-C with Normal Triglycerides

Familial Hypercholesterolemia (FH)

FH is an autosomal codominant disorder characterized by elevated plasma levels of LDL-C with normal triglycerides, tendon xanthomas, and premature coronary atherosclerosis. FH is caused by a large number (>900) of mutations in the LDL receptor gene. It has a higher incidence in certain founder populations, such as Afrikaners, Christian Lebanese, and French Canadians. The elevated levels of LDL-C in FH are due to an increase in the production of LDL from IDL and a delayed catabolism of LDL from the blood. There is a gene dose effect, in that individuals with two mutated LDL receptor alleles (FH homozygotes) are much more affected than those with one mutant allele (FH heterozygotes).

Homozygous FH occurs in approximately 1 in 1 million persons worldwide. Patients with homozygous FH can be classified into one of two groups based on the amount of LDL receptor activity measured in their skin fibroblasts: those patients with <2% of normal LDL receptor activity (receptor negative) and those patients with 2–25% of normal LDL receptor activity (receptor defective). Most patients with homozygous FH present in childhood with cutaneous xanthomas on the hands,

TABLE 21-3

FREDERICKSON CLASSIFICATION OF HYPERLIPOPROTEINEMIAS

PHENOTYPE	I	IIa	IIb	III	IV	V
Lipoprotein, elevated	Chylomicrons	LDL	LDL and VLDL	Chylomicron and VLDL remnants	VLDL	Chylomicrons and VLDL
Triglycerides	++++	–	++	++ to +++	++	++++
Cholesterol	+ to ++	+++	++ to +++	++ to +++	– to +	++ to +++
LDL-cholesterol	↓	↑	↑	↓	↓	↓
HDL-cholesterol	+++	+	++	++	++	+++
Plasma appearance	Lactescent	Clear	Clear	Turbid	Turbid	Lactescent
Xanthomas	Eruptive	Tendon, tuberous	None	Palmar, tuberoeruptive	None	Eruptive
Pancreatitis	+++	0	0	0	0	+++
Coronary atherosclerosis	0	+++	+++	+++	+/–	+/–
Peripheral atherosclerosis	0	+	+	++	+/–	+/–
Molecular defects	LPL and apoC-II	LDL receptor, apoB100, PCSK9, ARH, ABCG5 and ABCG8	Unknown	ApoE	ApoA-V and unknown	ApoA-V and unknown
Genetic nomenclature	FCS	FH, FDB, ADH, ARH, sitosterolemia	FCHL	FDBL	FHTG	FHTG

Note: LPL, lipoprotein lipase; apo, apolipoprotein; FCS, familial chylomicronemia syndrome; FH, familial hypercholesterolemia; FDB, familial defective apoB; ARH, autosomal recessive hypercholesterolemia; ADH, autosomal dominant hypercholesterolemia; FCHL, familial combined hyperlipidemia; FDBL, familial dysbetalipoproteinemia; FHTG, familial hypertriglyceridemia.

wrists, elbows, knees, heels, or buttocks. Total cholesterol levels are usually >500 mg/dL and can be higher than 1000 mg/dL. The devastating complication of homozygous FH is accelerated atherosclerosis, which can result in disability and death in childhood. Atherosclerosis often develops first in the aortic root, where it can cause aortic valvular or supravalvular stenosis, and typically extends into the coronary ostia, which become stenotic. Children with homozygous FH often develop symptomatic coronary atherosclerosis before puberty; symptoms can be atypical, and sudden death is common. Untreated, receptor-negative patients with homozygous FH rarely survive beyond the second decade; patients with receptor-defective LDL receptor defects have a better prognosis but almost invariably develop clinically apparent atherosclerotic vascular disease by age 30, and often much sooner. Carotid and femoral disease develops later in life and is usually not clinically significant.

A careful family history should be taken, and plasma lipid levels should be measured in the parents and other first-degree relatives of patients with homozygous FH. The diagnosis of homozygous FH can be confirmed by obtaining a skin biopsy and measuring LDL receptor activity in cultured skin fibroblasts, or by quantifying the number of LDL receptors on the surfaces of lymphocytes using cell-sorting technology. Molecular assays are also available to define the mutations in the LDL receptor by DNA sequencing.

Combination therapy with an HMG-CoA reductase inhibitor and a cholesterol absorption inhibitor sometimes results in relatively modest reductions in plasma LDL-C in the FH homozygote. Patients with homozygous FH invariably require additional lipid-lowering therapy. Since the liver is quantitatively the most important tissue for removing circulating LDLs via the LDL receptor, liver transplantation is effective in decreasing plasma LDL-C levels in this disorder. Liver transplantation, however, is associated with substantial risks, including the requirement for long-term immunosuppression. The current treatment of choice for homozygous FH is LDL apheresis (a process by which the LDL particles are selectively removed from the circulation), which can promote regression of xanthomas and may slow the progression of atherosclerosis. Initiation of LDL apheresis should generally be delayed until approximately 5 years of age, except when evidence of atherosclerotic vascular disease is present.

Heterozygous FH is caused by the inheritance of one mutant LDL receptor allele and occurs in approximately 1 in 500 persons worldwide, making it one of the most common single-gene disorders. It is characterized by elevated plasma levels of LDL-C (usually 200–400 mg/dL) and normal levels of triglyceride. Patients with heterozygous FH have hypercholesterolemia from birth, although the disease is often not detected until adulthood, usually due to the detection of hypercholesterolemia on routine

TABLE 21-4

PRIMARY HYPERLIPOPROTEINEMIAS CAUSED BY KNOWN SINGLE GENE MUTATIONS

GENETIC DISORDER	GENE DEFECT	LIPOPROTEINS ELEVATED	CLINICAL FINDINGS	GENETIC TRANSMISSION	ESTIMATED INCIDENCE
Lipoprotein lipase deficiency	LPL (*LPL*)	Chylomicrons	Eruptive xanthomas, hepatosplenomegaly, pancreatitis	AR	1/1,000,000
Familial apolipoprotein C-II deficiency	ApoC-II (*APOC2*)	Chylomicrons	Eruptive xanthomas, hepatosplenomegaly, pancreatitis	AR	<1/1,000,000
ApoA-V deficiency	ApoA-V (*APOAV*)	Chylomicrons, VLDL	Eruptive xanthomas, hepatosplenomegaly, pancreatitis	AD	<1/1,000,000
Familial hepatic lipase deficiency	Hepatic lipase (*LIPC*)	VLDL remnants	Premature atherosclerosis, pancreatitis	AR	<1/1,000,000
Familial dysbetalipoproteinemia	ApoE (*APOE*)	Chylomicron and VLDL remnants	Palmar and tuberoeruptive xanthomas, CHD, PVD	AR AD	1/10,000
Familial hypercholesterolemia	LDL receptor (*LDLR*)	LDL	Tendon xanthomas, CHD	AD	1/500
Familial defective apoB100	ApoB100 (*APOB*) ($Arg_{3500} \rightarrow Gln$)	LDL	Tendon xanthomas, CHD	AD	<1/1000
Autosomal dominant hypercholesterolemia	PCSK9 (*PCSK9*)	LDL	Tendon xanthomas, CHD	AD	<1/1,000,000
Autosomal recessive hypercholesterolemia	ARH (*ARH*)	LDL	Tendon xanthomas, CHD	AR	<1/1,000,000
Sitosterolemia	*ABCG5* or *ABCG8*	LDL	Tendon xanthomas, CHD	AR	<1/1,000,000

Note: LPL, lipoprotein lipase; LDL, low-density lipoprotein; VLDL, very low density lipoprotein; ARH, autosomal recessive hypercholesterolemia; CHD, coronary heart disease; PVD, peripheral vascular disease; AR, autosomal recessive; AD, autosomal dominant.

screening, the appearance of tendon xanthomas, or the development of symptomatic coronary atherosclerotic disease (CAD). Since the disease is codominant in inheritance and has a high penetrance (>90%), one parent and ~50% of the patient's siblings usually also have hypercholesterolemia. The family history is frequently positive for premature CAD on one side of the family. Corneal arcus is common, and tendon xanthomas involving the dorsum of the hands, the elbows, the knees, and especially the Achilles tendons are present in ~75% of patients. The age of onset of CAD is highly variable and depends in part on the molecular defect in the LDL receptor gene and also on coexisting cardiac risk factors. FH heterozygotes with elevated plasma levels of Lp(a) appear to be at greater risk for cardiovascular complications. Untreated men with heterozygous FH have a ~50% chance of having a myocardial infarction before age 60. Although the age of onset of atherosclerotic heart disease is later in women with FH, coronary heart disease (CHD) is significantly more common in women with FH than in the general female population.

No definitive diagnostic test for heterozygous FH is available. Although FH heterozygotes tend to have reduced levels of LDL receptor function in skin fibroblasts, significant overlap with the LDL receptor activity levels in normal fibroblasts exists. Molecular assays have recently become available to identify the mutation in the DNA sequence, but the clinical utility of pinpointing the mutation has not been demonstrated. The clinical diagnosis is usually not problematic, but it is critical that hypothyroidism, nephrotic syndrome, and obstructive liver disease be excluded before initiating therapy.

FH patients should be aggressively treated to lower plasma levels of LDL-C. Initiation of a low-cholesterol, low-fat diet is recommended, but almost all heterozygous FH patients require lipid-lowering drug therapy. Statins are effective in heterozygous FH, but combination drug therapy with the addition of a cholesterol absorption inhibitor is frequently required, and even a third drug, such as a bile acid sequestrant or nicotinic acid, is sometimes needed. Heterozygous FH patients who cannot be adequately controlled on combination drug therapy are candidates for LDL apheresis.

Familial Defective ApoB-100 (FDB)

This is a dominantly inherited disorder that clinically resembles heterozygous FH. FDB is a rare cause of hypercholesterolemia, except in populations with significant numbers of individuals of German descent where the frequency can be as high as 1 in 1000. The disease is characterized by elevated plasma LDL-C levels with normal triglycerides, tendon xanthomas, and an increased incidence of premature ASCVD. FDB is caused by mutations in the LDL receptor–binding domain of apoB100. Most patients with FDB have a substitution of glutamine for arginine at position 3500 in apoB100, although other rarer mutations have been reported to cause this disease. As a consequence of the mutation in apoB100, LDL binds the LDL receptor with reduced affinity, and LDL is removed from the circulation at a reduced rate. Patients with FDB cannot be clinically distinguished from patients with heterozygous FH, although patients with FDB tend to have lower plasma levels of LDL-C than FH heterozygotes. The apoB100 gene mutation can be detected directly, but genetic diagnosis is not currently encouraged since the recommended management of FDB and heterozygous FH is identical.

Autosomal Recessive Hypercholesterolemia (ARH)

ARH is a rare disorder (except on Sardinia, Italy) due to mutations in a protein (ARH, also called *LDLR adaptor protein*) involved in LDL receptor–mediated endocytosis in the liver. ARH clinically resembles homozygous FH and is characterized by hypercholesterolemia, tendon xanthomas, and premature coronary artery disease. The hypercholesterolemia tends to be intermediate between the levels seen in FH homozygotes and FH heterozygotes. LDL receptor function in cultured fibroblasts is normal or only modestly reduced in ARH, whereas LDL receptor function in lymphocytes and the liver is negligible. Unlike FH homozygotes, the hyperlipidemia responds partially to treatment with HMG-CoA reductase inhibitors, but these patients usually require LDL apheresis to lower plasma LDL-C to recommended levels.

Autosomal Dominant Hypercholesterolemia (ADH)

ADH is a rare disorder caused by gain-of-function mutations in proprotein convertase subtilisin/kexin type 9 (PCSK9). Increased activity of PCSK9 appears to cause dominant hypercholesterolemia by promoting the degradation of LDL receptors in the liver, thus reducing the clearance of circulating LDL. Interestingly, loss-of-function mutations in this gene cause low LDL-C levels.

Sitosterolemia

This is a rare autosomal recessive disease caused by mutations in one of two members of the ATP-binding cassette (ABC) transporter family, ABCG5 and ABCG8. These genes are expressed in the intestine and liver, where they form a functional complex and pump plant sterols, such as sitosterol and campesterol, and animal sterols, predominantly cholesterol, from enterocytes into the gut lumen and from hepatocytes into the bile. In normal individuals, <5% of dietary plant sterols are absorbed by the proximal small intestine and delivered to the liver. Plant sterols that are carried to the liver on chylomicrons are preferentially secreted into the bile such that the plant sterol levels in plasma and tissues are normally very low. In sitosterolemia, the intestinal absorption of plant sterols is increased and biliary excretion of the sterols is reduced, resulting in increased plasma and tissue levels of sitosterol and other plant sterols.

The trafficking of cholesterol is also impaired in sitosterolemia. Patients with sitosterolemia usually have elevated plasma levels of LDL cholesterol. Patients develop tendon xanthomas as well as premature atherosclerosis and can be mistaken for FH patients. Episodes of hemolysis, presumably secondary to the incorporation of plant sterols into the red blood cell membrane, are a distinctive clinical feature of this disease. The hypercholesterolemia in subjects with sitosterolemia is unusually responsive to reductions in dietary cholesterol content. Sitosterolemia should be suspected in patients in whom the plasma cholesterol level falls more than 40% on a low-cholesterol diet.

Sitosterolemia is confirmed by demonstrating an increase in the plasma level of sitosterol using gas chromatography. The hypercholesterolemia does not respond to HMG-CoA reductase inhibitors; however, bile acid sequestrants and cholesterol-absorption inhibitors, such as ezetimibe, are effective in reducing plasma sterol levels in these patients.

Polygenic Hypercholesterolemia

This condition is characterized by hypercholesterolemia due to elevated LDL-C with a normal plasma level of triglyceride in the absence of secondary causes of hypercholesterolemia. Plasma LDL-C levels are generally not as elevated as they are in FH and FDB. Family studies are useful to differentiate polygenic hypercholesterolemia from the single-gene disorders described above; half of the first-degree relatives of patients with FH and FDB are hypercholesterolemic, whereas <10% of first-degree relatives of patients with polygenic hypercholesterolemia have hypercholesterolemia. Treatment of polygenic hypercholesterolemia is identical to that of other forms of hypercholesterolemia.

Lipid Disorders Associated with Elevated Triglycerides

Familial Chylomicronemia Syndrome (Type I Hyperlipoproteinemia; Lipoprotein Lipase and ApoC-II Deficiency)

As noted above, LPL is required for the hydrolysis of triglycerides in chylomicrons and VLDLs, and apoC-II is a cofactor for LPL (Fig. 21-2). Genetic deficiency or inactivity of either protein results in impaired lipolysis and profound elevations in plasma chylomicrons. These patients can also have elevated plasma levels of VLDL, but chylomicronemia predominates. The fasting plasma is turbid, and if left at 4°C (39.2°F) for a few hours, the chylomicrons float to the top and form a creamy supernatant. In these disorders, called *familial chylomicronemia syndromes*, fasting triglyceride levels are almost invariably >1000 mg/dL. Fasting cholesterol levels are also usually elevated but to a much lesser degree.

LPL deficiency has autosomal recessive inheritance and has a frequency of approximately 1 in 1 million in the population. *ApoC-II deficiency* is also recessive in inheritance pattern and is even less common than LPL deficiency. Multiple different mutations in the LPL and apoC-II genes cause these diseases. Obligate LPL heterozygotes have normal or mild to moderate elevations in plasma triglyceride levels, whereas individuals heterozygous for mutation in apoC-II do not have hypertriglyceridemia.

Both LPL and apoC-II deficiency usually present in childhood with recurrent episodes of severe abdominal pain due to acute pancreatitis. On funduscopic examination the retinal blood vessels are opalescent (lipemia retinalis). Eruptive xanthomas, which are small, yellowish-white papules, often appear in clusters on the back, buttocks, and extensor surfaces of the arms and legs. These typically painless skin lesions may become pruritic. Hepatosplenomegaly results from the uptake of circulating chylomicrons by reticuloendothelial cells in the liver and spleen. For unknown reasons, some patients with persistent and pronounced chylomicronemia never develop pancreatitis, eruptive xanthomas, or hepatosplenomegaly. Premature ASCVD is not generally a feature of familial chylomicronemia syndromes.

The diagnoses of LPL and apoC-II deficiency are established enzymatically in specialized laboratories by assaying triglyceride lipolytic activity in postheparin plasma. Blood is sampled after an IV heparin injection to release the endothelial-bound LPL. LPL activity is profoundly reduced in both LPL and apoC-II deficiency; in patients with apoC-II deficiency, it normalizes after the addition of normal plasma (providing a source of apoC-II).

The major therapeutic intervention in familial chylomicronemia syndromes is dietary fat restriction (to as little as 15 g/d) with fat-soluble vitamin supplementation. Consultation with a registered dietician familiar with this disorder is essential. Caloric supplementation with medium-chain triglycerides, which are absorbed directly into the portal circulation, can be useful but may be associated with hepatic fibrosis if used for prolonged periods. If dietary fat restriction alone is not successful in resolving the chylomicronemia, fish oils have been effective in some patients. In patients with apoC-II deficiency, apoC-II can be provided by infusing fresh-frozen plasma to resolve the chylomicronemia. Management of patients with familial chylomicronemia syndrome is particularly challenging during pregnancy when VLDL production is increased and may require plasmapheresis to remove the circulating chylomicrons.

ApoA-V Deficiency

A newly discovered apolipoprotein called *ApoA-V* circulates at much lower concentrations than most other apolipoproteins. Individuals who are compound heterozygotes for a mutation that causes premature truncation of ApoA-V and a sequence variant associated with increased triglyceride levels have late-onset chylomicronemia. The exact mechanism of action of ApoA-V is not known, but it appears to be required for the association of VLDL and chylomicrons with LPL.

Hepatic Lipase Deficiency

HL is a member of the same gene family as LPL and hydrolyzes triglycerides and phospholipids in remnant lipoproteins and HDLs. HL deficiency is a very rare autosomal recessive disorder characterized by elevated plasma levels of cholesterol and triglycerides (mixed hyperlipidemia) due to the accumulation of circulating lipoprotein remnants and either a normal or elevated plasma level of HDL-C. The diagnosis is confirmed by measuring HL activity in postheparin plasma. Due to the small number of patients with HL deficiency, the association of this genetic defect with ASCVD is not clearly known, but lipid-lowering therapy is recommended.

Familial Dysbetalipoproteinemia (Type III Hyperlipoproteinemia)

Like HL deficiency, familial dysbetalipoproteinemia (FDBL) (also known as *type III hyperlipoproteinemia* or *familial broad β disease*) is characterized by a mixed hyperlipidemia due to the accumulation of remnant lipoprotein particles. ApoE is present in multiple copies on chylomicron and VLDL remnants and mediates their removal via hepatic lipoprotein receptors (Fig. 21-2). FDBL is due to genetic variations in apoE that interfere with its ability to bind lipoprotein receptors. The *APOE* gene is polymorphic in sequence, resulting in the expression of three common isoforms: apoE3, which is the most common; and apoE2 and apoE4, both differ from apoE3 by a single amino acid. Although associated with slightly higher LDL-C levels and increased CHD risk, the apoE4 allele is not associated with FDBL. Patients with apoE4 have an increased incidence of late-onset Alzheimer's disease. ApoE2 has a lower affinity for the LDL receptor; therefore, chylomicron and VLDL remnants containing apoE2 are removed from plasma at a slower rate. Individuals who are homozygous for the E2 allele (the E2/E2 genotype) comprise the most common subset of patients with FDBL.

Approximately 0.5% of the general population are apoE2/E2 homozygotes, but only a small minority of these individuals develop FDBL. In most cases an additional, identifiable factor precipitates the development of hyperlipoproteinemia. The most common precipitating factors are a high-fat diet, diabetes mellitus, obesity, hypothyroidism, renal disease, estrogen deficiency, alcohol use, or certain drugs. Other mutations in apoE can cause a dominant form of FDBL where the hyperlipidemia is fully manifest in the heterozygous state, but these mutations are rare.

Patients with FDBL usually present in adulthood with xanthomas, premature coronary disease, and peripheral vascular disease. The disease seldom presents in women before menopause. Two distinctive types of xanthomas, tuberoeruptive and palmar, are seen in FCBL patients. Tuberoeruptive xanthomas begin as clusters of small papules on the elbows, knees, or buttocks and can grow to the size of small grapes. Palmar xanthomas (alternatively called *xanthomata striata palmaris*) are orange-yellow discolorations of the creases in the palms and wrists. In FDBL, the plasma levels of cholesterol and triglyceride are often elevated to a similar degree, the directly measured LDL-C is low, and the HDL-C is usually normal (in contrast to the low HDL-C usually seen in patients with elevated triglyceride levels).

The traditional approaches to diagnosis of this disorder are lipoprotein electrophoresis (broad β band) or ultracentrifugation (ratio of VLDL-C to total plasma triglyceride >0.30). Protein methods (apoE phenotyping) or DNA-based methods (apoE genotyping) can be performed to confirm homozygosity for apoE2. However, absence of the apoE2/2 genotype does not rule out the diagnosis of FDBL, since other mutations in apoE can cause this condition.

Since FDBL is associated with increased risk of premature ASCVD, it should be treated aggressively. Subjects with FDBL have more peripheral vascular disease than is typically seen in FH. Other metabolic conditions that can worsen the hyperlipidemia should be actively treated. Patients with FDBL are typically very diet-responsive and can respond favorably to weight reduction and to low-cholesterol, low-fat diets. Alcohol intake should be curtailed. HMG-CoA reductase inhibitors, fibrates, and niacin are all generally effective in the treatment of FDBL, and sometimes combination drug therapy is required.

Familial Hypertriglyceridemia (FHTG)

FHTG is a relatively common (~1 in 500) autosomal dominant disorder of unknown etiology characterized by moderately elevated plasma triglycerides accompanied by more modest elevations in cholesterol. Since the major class of lipoproteins elevated in this disorder is VLDL, patients with this disorder are often referred to as having *Type IV hyperlipoproteinemia* (Frederickson classification, Table 21-3). The elevated plasma levels of VLDL are due to increased production of VLDL, impaired catabolism of VLDL, or a combination of these mechanisms. Some patients with FHTG have a more severe form of hyperlipidemia in which both VLDLs and chylomicrons are elevated (Type V hyperlipidemia), since these two classes of lipoproteins compete for the same lipolytic pathway. Increased intake of simple carbohydrates, obesity, insulin resistance, alcohol use, and estrogen treatment, all of which increase VLDL synthesis, can exacerbate this syndrome. FHTG appears not to be associated with increased risk of ASCVD in many families.

The diagnosis of FHTG is suggested by the triad of elevated levels of plasma triglycerides (250–1000 mg/dL), normal or only mildly increased cholesterol levels (<250 mg/dL), and reduced plasma levels of HDL-C.

Plasma LDL-C levels are generally not increased and are often reduced due to defective metabolism of the triglyceride-rich particles. The identification of other first-degree relatives with hypertriglyceridemia is useful in making the diagnosis. FDBL and familial combined hyperlipidemia (FCHL) should also be ruled out since these two conditions are associated with a significantly increased risk of ASCVD. The plasma apoB levels are lower and the ratio of plasma triglycerides (TGs) to cholesterol is higher in FHTG than in either FDBL or FCHL.

It is important to consider and rule out secondary causes of the hypertriglyceridemia (Table 21-5) before making the diagnosis of FHTG. Lipid-lowering drug therapy can frequently be avoided with appropriate dietary and lifestyle changes. Patients with plasma triglyceride levels >500 mg/dL after a trial of diet and exercise should be considered for drug therapy to avoid the development of chylomicronemia and pancreatitis. Fibrate drugs or fish oils (omega-3 fatty acids) are reasonable first-line approaches for FHTG, and niacin can also be considered in this condition.

Familial Combined Hyperlipidemia

FCHL is generally characterized by moderate elevations in plasma levels of triglycerides (VLDL) and cholesterol (LDL) and reduced plasma levels of HDL-C. It is the most common inherited lipid disorder, occurring in approximately 1 in 200 persons. Approximately 20% of patients who develop CHD under age 60 have FCHL. The disease is autosomal dominant in inheritance, and affected family members typically have one of three possible phenotypes: (1) elevated plasma levels of LDL-C, (2) elevated plasma levels of triglycerides due to elevation in VLDL-C, or (3) elevated plasma levels of both LDL-C and VLDL-C. A classic feature of FCHL is that the lipoprotein profile can switch among these three phenotypes over time and may depend on factors such as diet. FCHL can manifest in childhood but is usually not fully expressed until adulthood. A cluster of other metabolic risk factors is often found in association with this hyperlipidemia, including obesity, glucose intolerance, insulin resistance, and hypertension (the so-called metabolic syndrome, Chap. 18). These patients do not develop xanthomas.

Patients with FCHL almost always have significantly elevated plasma levels of apoB. The levels of apoB are disproportionately high relative to the plasma LDL-C concentration, indicating the presence of small, dense LDL particles, which are characteristic of this syndrome. *Hyperapobetalipoproteinemia*, which has been used to describe the state of elevated plasma levels of apoB with normal plasma LDL-C levels, is probably a form of FCHL. Individuals with FCHL generally share the same metabolic defect, which is overproduction of VLDL by the liver. The molecular etiology of FCHL remains poorly understood, and it is likely that defects in several different genes can cause the phenotype of FCHL.

The presence of a mixed dyslipidemia (plasma triglyceride levels between 200 and 800 mg/dL and total cholesterol levels between 200 and 400 mg/dL, usually with HDL-C levels <40 mg/dL in men or <50 mg/dL in women) and a family history of hyperlipidemia and/or premature CHD strongly suggests the diagnosis of FCHL. The finding of an elevated plasma level of apoB level or the finding of an increased number of small, dense LDL particles in the plasma through advanced lipoprotein testing supports this diagnosis. FDBL should be considered and ruled out by β quantification in suspected patients with a mixed hyperlipidemia.

Individuals with FCHL should be treated aggressively due to significantly increased risk of premature CHD. Decreased dietary intake of saturated fat and simple carbohydrates, aerobic exercise, and weight loss can all have beneficial effects on the lipid profile. Patients with diabetes should be aggressively treated to maintain good glucose control. Most patients with FCHL require lipid-lowering drug therapy to reduce lipoprotein levels to the recommended range and reduce the high risk of ASCVD. Statins are effective in this condition, but many patients will need a second drug (cholesterol absorption inhibitor, niacin, or fibrate) for optimal control of lipoprotein levels.

INHERITED CAUSES OF LOW LEVELS OF ApoB-CONTAINING LIPOPROTEINS

Abetalipoproteinemia

The synthesis and secretion of apoB-containing lipoproteins in the enterocytes of the proximal small bowel and in the hepatocytes of the liver involve a complex series of events that coordinate the coupling of various lipids with apoB48 and apoB100, respectively. Abetalipoproteinemia is a rare autosomal recessive disease caused by loss-of-function mutations in the gene encoding MTP, a protein that transfers lipids to nascent chylomicrons and VLDLs in the intestine and liver, respectively. Plasma levels of cholesterol and triglyceride are extremely low in this disorder, and chylomicrons, VLDLs, LDLs, and apoB are undetectable in plasma. The parents of patients with abetalipoproteinemia (obligate heterozygotes) have normal plasma lipid and apoB levels. Abetalipoproteinemia usually presents in early childhood with diarrhea and failure to thrive and is characterized clinically by fat malabsorption, spinocerebellar degeneration, pigmented retinopathy, and acanthocytosis. The initial neurologic manifestations are loss of deep-tendon reflexes, followed by decreased distal lower extremity vibratory and proprioceptive sense, dysmetria, ataxia, and the development of a spastic gait, often by the third or fourth decade. Patients with abetalipoproteinemia also develop a progressive pigmented retinopathy presenting with decreased night and color vision, followed by reductions in daytime visual acuity and ultimately progressing to

TABLE 21-5

SECONDARY FORMS OF HYPERLIPIDEMIA

LDL		HDL		VLDL	IDL	CHYLOMICRONS	Lp(a)
ELEVATED	**REDUCED**	**ELEVATED**	**REDUCED**	**ELEVATED**	**ELEVATED**	**ELEVATED**	**ELEVATED**
Hypothyroidism Nephrotic syndrome Cholestasis Acute intermittent porphyria Anorexia nervosa Hepatoma Drugs: thiazides, cyclosporin, tegretol	Severe liver disease Malabsorption Malnutrition Gaucher's disease Chronic infectious disease Hypothyroidism Drugs: niacin toxicity	Alcohol Exercise Exposure to chlorinated hydrocarbons Drugs: estrogen	Smoking DM type 2 Obesity Malnutrition Gaucher's disease Drugs: anabolic steroids, beta blockers	Obesity DM type 2 Glycogen storage disease Hepatitis Alcohol Renal failure Sepsis Stress Cushing's syndrome Pregnancy Acromegaly Lipodystrophy Drugs: estrogen, beta blockers, glucocorticoids, bile acid–binding resins, retinoic acid	Multiple myeloma Monoclonal gammopathy Autoimmune disease Hypothyroidism	Autoimmune disease DM type 2	Renal insufficiency Inflammation Menopause Orchidectomy Hyperthyroidism Acromegaly Nephrosis Drugs: growth hormone, isotretinoin

Note: LDL, low-density lipoprotein; HDL, high-density lipoprotein; VLDL, very low density lipoprotein; IDL, intermediate-density lipoprotein; Lp(a), lipoprotein A; DM, diabetes mellitus.

near-blindness. The presence of spinocerebellar degeneration and pigmented retinopathy in this disease has resulted in some patients with abetalipoproteinemia being misdiagnosed as having Friedreich's ataxia. Rarely, patients with abetalipoproteinemia develop a cardiomyopathy with associated life-threatening arrhythmias.

Most clinical manifestations of abetalipoproteinemia result from defects in the absorption and transport of fat-soluble vitamins. Vitamin E and retinyl esters are normally transported from enterocytes to the liver by chylomicrons, and vitamin E is dependent on VLDL for transport out of the liver and into the circulation. As a consequence of the inability of these patients to secrete apoB-containing particles, patients with abetalipoproteinemia are markedly deficient in vitamin E and are also mildly to moderately deficient in vitamin A and vitamin K. Patients with abetalipoproteinemia should be referred to specialized centers for confirmation of the diagnosis and appropriate therapy. Treatment consists of a low-fat, high-caloric, vitamin-enriched diet accompanied by large supplemental doses of vitamin E. It is imperative that treatment be initiated as soon as possible to help forestall the development of the neurologic sequelae, which generally eventually progress even with appropriate therapy. New therapies for this serious disease are needed.

Familial Hypobetalipoproteinemia

Low plasma levels of LDL-C (the "β-lipoprotein") with a genetic or inherited basis are referred to generically as *familial hypobetalipoproteinemia*. Traditionally this term has been used to refer to the condition of low total cholesterol and LDL-C due to mutations in apoB. There is a range of mostly nonsense mutations in apoB that result in the translation of a truncated protein that has reduced secretion and/or accelerated catabolism. Individuals heterozygous for these mutations usually have LDL-C levels <80 mg/dL. They may be protected from the development of atherosclerotic vascular disease, though this has not been rigorously demonstrated. Some of these patients have evidence of increased hepatic fat. There are rare patients who have mutations in both apoB alleles and have plasma lipids similar to those in abetalipoproteinemia, but usually with a less severe neurologic phenotype. Patients with homozygous hypobetalipoproteinemia can be distinguished from individuals with abetalipoproteinemia by measuring the levels of LDL-C in the parents, which will also be low.

PCSK9 Deficiency

A phenocopy of familial hypobetalipoproteinemia has recently been shown to result from loss-of-function mutations in PCSK9, a protein that circulates in the blood and regulates LDL receptor levels. This condition is more common in people of African descent. Individuals bearing these mutations have lower plasma levels of LDL-C and have a substantial reduction in lifetime risk of CHD with no apparent adverse consequences. The mechanism of the low LDL-C appears to involve upregulation of the hepatic LDL receptor and thus increased catabolism of LDL.

GENETIC DISORDERS OF HDL METABOLISM

Mutations in certain genes encoding critical proteins in HDL synthesis and catabolism cause marked variations in plasma levels of HDL-C. Unlike the genetic forms of hypercholesterolemia, which are invariably associated with premature coronary atherosclerosis, genetic forms of hypoalphalipoproteinemia (low HDL-C) are not always associated with accelerated atherosclerosis.

INHERITED CAUSES OF LOW LEVELS OF HDL-C

ApoA-I Deficiency and Structural Mutations

Complete genetic deficiency of apoA-I due to deletion of the apoA-I gene results in the virtual absence of HDL from the plasma. The genes encoding apoA-I, apoC-III, apoA-IV, and apoA-V are clustered together on chromosome 11, and some of the patients with complete absence of apoA-I have deletions that include more than one of these genes in the complex. ApoA-I is required for LCAT function. Thus, plasma and tissue levels of free cholesterol are increased in this disease, resulting in the development of corneal opacities and planar xanthomas. Premature CHD is generally seen in the apoA-I–deficient patients.

Missense and nonsense mutations in the apoA-I gene have been identified in selected patients with low plasma HDL levels (usually 15–30 mg/dL), but these are very rare causes of low HDL-C levels in the general population. Patients heterozygous for the apoA-I_{Milano} Arg173Cys substitution have very low plasma levels of HDL due to the rapid catabolism of the mutant apolipoprotein, but they do not appear to have an increased risk of premature CHD. Most individuals with low plasma HDL-C levels due to missense mutations in apoA-I do not appear to have premature CHD or other clinical sequelae, though the disorder is too rare to study systematically. A few specific missense mutations in apoA-I cause systemic amyloidosis, and the mutant apoA-I has been found as the major component of the amyloid plaque.

Tangier Disease (ABCA1 Deficiency)

Tangier disease is a very rare autosomal codominant form of low plasma HDL-C caused by mutations in the gene encoding ABCA1, a cellular transporter that facilitates efflux of unesterified cholesterol and phospholipids from cells to apoA-I (Fig. 21-3). ABCA1 plays a critical role in the generation and stabilization of the mature HDL particle.

In its absence, HDL is rapidly cleared from the circulation. Patients with Tangier disease have plasma HDL-C levels <5 mg/dL and extremely low circulating levels of apoA-I. The disease is associated with cholesterol accumulation in the reticuloendothelial system, resulting in hepatosplenomegaly and pathognomonic enlarged, grayish-yellow or orange tonsils. An intermittent peripheral neuropathy (mononeuritis multiplex) or a sphingomyelia-like neurologic disorder can also be seen. Tangier disease is associated with increased risk of premature atherosclerotic disease, although not as great as might be anticipated, given the markedly decreased plasma levels of HDL-C and apoA-I. Patients with Tangier disease have low plasma levels of LDL-C, which may attenuate the atherosclerotic risk. Obligate heterozygotes for ABCA1 mutations have moderately reduced plasma HDL-C levels (15–30 mg/dL) and are also at increased risk of premature CHD. ABCA1 mutations may be a cause of low HDL-C in a nontrivial minority of low HDL-C patients.

LCAT Deficiency

This is a very rare autosomal recessive disorder caused by mutations in the gene encoding the plasma enzyme lecithin-cholesterol acyltransferase (Fig. 21-3). LCAT is synthesized in the liver and secreted into the plasma, where it circulates associated with lipoproteins. The enzyme mediates the esterification of cholesterol. Consequently, the proportion of free cholesterol in circulating lipoproteins is greatly increased (from ~25% to over 70% of total plasma cholesterol) in this disorder. Lack of normal cholesterol esterification impairs the formation of mature HDL particles and therefore results in rapid catabolism of circulating apoA-I. Two genetic forms of LCAT deficiency have been described in humans: complete deficiency (also called *classic LCAT deficiency*) and partial deficiency (also called *fish-eye disease*). Progressive corneal opacification due to the deposition of free cholesterol in the lens, very low plasma levels of HDL-C (usually <10 mg/dL), and variable hypertriglyceridemia are characteristic of both types. In partial LCAT deficiency, there are no other known clinical sequelae. In contrast, complete LCAT deficiency is characterized by a hemolytic anemia and progressive renal insufficiency that eventually leads to end-stage renal disease (ESRD). Remarkably, despite the extremely low plasma levels of HDL-C and apoA-I, premature ASCVD is not a consistent feature of either complete or partial LCAT deficiency, once again exemplifying the complex relationship between low plasma levels of HDL-C and the development of ASCVD. The diagnosis can be confirmed in a specialized laboratory by assaying plasma LCAT activity.

Primary Hypoalphalipoproteinemia

Low plasma levels of HDL-C (the "α-lipoprotein") is referred to as *hypoalphalipoproteinemia*. Primary hypoalphalipoproteinemia is defined as a plasma HDL-C level below the tenth percentile in the setting of relatively normal cholesterol and triglyceride levels, no apparent secondary causes of low plasma HDL-C, and no clinical signs of LCAT deficiency or Tangier disease. This syndrome is often referred to as *isolated low HDL*. A family history of low HDL-C facilitates the diagnosis of an inherited condition, which usually follows an autosomal dominant pattern. The metabolic etiology of this disease appears to be primarily accelerated catabolism of HDL and its apolipoproteins. Some of these patients may have ABCA1 mutations and therefore technically have heterozygous Tangier disease. Several kindreds with primary hypoalphalipoproteinemia have been described in association with an increased incidence of premature CHD, although this is not an invariant association. Association of hypoalphalipoproteinemia with premature CHD may depend on the specific nature of the gene defect or the underlying metabolic defect responsible for the low plasma HDL-C level.

INHERITED CAUSES OF HIGH LEVELS OF HDL-C

CETP Deficiency

Loss-of-function mutations in both alleles of the gene encoding cholesteryl ester transfer protein (CETP) cause substantially elevated HDL-C levels (usually >150 mg/dL). As noted above, CETP facilitates the transfer of cholesteryl esters from HDL to apoB-containing lipoproteins (Fig. 21-3). The absence of this transfer results in reduced catabolism of HDL and increased plasma concentrations of large, cholesterol-rich HDL particles. CETP deficiency occurs almost exclusively in persons of Japanese descent. The relationship of CETP deficiency to risk of ASCVD has not been definitively resolved and remains a matter of substantial debate. Heterozygotes for CETP deficiency have only modestly elevated HDL-C levels. Based on the phenotype of high HDL-C in CETP deficiency, pharmacologic inhibition of CETP is under development as a new therapeutic approach to the treatment of low HDL-C and ASCVD.

Familial Hyperalphalipoproteinemia

The condition of high plasma levels of HDL-C is referred to as *hyperalphalipoproteinemia* and is defined as a plasma HDL-C level above the 90th percentile. This trait runs in families, and outside of Japan it is unlikely to be due to CETP deficiency. Most, but not all, persons with this condition appear to have a reduced risk of CHD and increased longevity. Other than CETP deficiency, the genetic basis of primary hyperalphalipoproteinemia is not known.

SECONDARY DISORDERS OF LIPOPROTEIN METABOLISM

Significant changes in plasma levels of lipoproteins are seen in a variety of diseases. It is critical that secondary causes of hyperlipidemias (Table 21-5) are considered prior to initiation of lipid-lowering therapy.

Obesity

(See also Chaps. 16 and 17) Obesity is frequently accompanied by hyperlipidemia. The increase in adipocyte mass and accompanying decreased insulin sensitivity associated with obesity has multiple effects on lipid metabolism. More free fatty acids are delivered from the expanded adipose tissue to the liver, where they are reesterified in hepatocytes to form triglycerides, which are packaged into VLDLs for secretion into the circulation. The increased insulin levels promote fatty acid synthesis in the liver. Increased dietary intake of simple carbohydrates also drives hepatic production of VLDLs, resulting in elevations in VLDL and/or LDL in some obese subjects. Plasma levels of HDL-C tend to be low in obesity, due in part to reduced lipolysis. Weight loss is often associated with reductions in plasma levels of circulating apoB-containing lipoproteins and increases in the plasma levels of HDL-C.

Diabetes Mellitus

(See also Chap. 19) Patients with type 1 diabetes mellitus generally do not have hyperlipidemia if they remain under good glycemic control. Diabetic ketoacidosis is frequently accompanied by hypertriglyceridemia due to an increased hepatic influx of free fatty acids from adipose tissue. Patients with type 2 diabetes mellitus are usually dyslipidemic, even when under relatively good glycemic control. The high levels of insulin and insulin resistance associated with type 2 diabetes has multiple effects on fat metabolism: (1) a decrease in LPL activity resulting in reduced catabolism of chylomicrons and VLDLs, (2) an increase in the release of free fatty acid from the adipose tissue, (3) an increase in fatty acid synthesis in the liver, and (4) an increase in hepatic VLDL production. Patients with type 2 diabetes mellitus have several lipid abnormalities, including elevated plasma triglycerides (due to increased VLDL and lipoprotein remnants), elevated levels of dense LDL, and decreased plasma levels of HDL-C. In some diabetic patients, especially those with a genetic defect in lipid metabolism, the triglycerides can be extremely elevated, resulting in the development of pancreatitis. Elevated plasma LDL-C levels usually are not a feature of diabetes mellitus and suggest the presence of an underlying lipoprotein abnormality or may indicate the development of diabetic nephropathy. Patients with lipodystrophy, who have profound insulin resistance, have markedly elevated levels of VLDL and chylomicrons.

Thyroid Disease

(See also Chap. 4) Hypothyroidism is associated with elevated plasma LDL-C levels due primarily to a reduction in hepatic LDL receptor function and delayed clearance of LDL. Conversely, plasma levels of LDL-C are often reduced in the hyperthyroid patient. Hypothyroid patients also frequently have increased levels of circulating IDLs, and some patients with hypothyroidism also have mild hypertriglyceridemia. Because hypothyroidism is easily overlooked, all patients presenting with elevated plasma levels of LDL-C or IDL should be screened for hypothyroidism. Thyroid replacement therapy usually ameliorates the hypercholesterolemia; if not, the patient probably has a primary lipoprotein disorder and may require lipid-lowering drug therapy.

Renal Disorders

Nephrotic syndrome is often associated with pronounced hyperlipoproteinemia, which is usually mixed but can manifest as hypercholesterolemia or hypertriglyceridemia. The hyperlipidemia of nephrotic syndrome appears to be due to a combination of increased hepatic production and decreased clearance of VLDLs, with increased LDL production. Effective treatment of the underlying renal disease normalizes the lipid profile, but most patients with chronic nephrotic syndrome require lipid-lowering drug therapy.

ESRD is often associated with mild hypertriglyceridemia (<300 mg/dL) due to the accumulation of VLDLs and remnant lipoproteins in the circulation. Triglyceride lipolysis and remnant clearance are both reduced in patients with renal failure. Because the risk of ASCVD is increased in ESRD subjects with hyperlipidemia, they should be aggressively treated with lipid-lowering agents.

Patients with renal transplants usually have increased lipid levels due to the effect of the drugs required for immunosuppression (cyclosporine and glucocorticoids) and present a difficult management problem since HMG-CoA reductase inhibitors must be used cautiously in these patients.

Liver Disorders

Because the liver is the principal site of formation and clearance of lipoproteins, it is not surprising that liver diseases can profoundly affect plasma lipid levels in a variety of ways. Hepatitis due to infection, drugs, or alcohol is often associated with increased VLDL synthesis and mild to moderate hypertriglyceridemia. Severe hepatitis and liver failure are associated with dramatic reductions in plasma cholesterol and triglycerides due to reduced lipoprotein biosynthetic capacity. Cholestasis is associated with hypercholesterolemia, which can be very severe. A major pathway by which cholesterol is excreted from the body is via secretion into bile, either directly or after conversion to bile acids, and cholestasis blocks this critical excretory pathway. In cholestasis, free cholesterol, coupled with phospholipids, is secreted into the plasma as a constituent of a lamellar particle called *LP-X*. The particles can deposit in skinfolds, producing lesions resembling those seen in patients with FDBL (xanthomata strata palmaris). Planar and eruptive xanthomas can also be seen in patients with cholestasis.

Alcohol

Regular alcohol consumption has a variable effect on plasma lipid levels. The most common effect of alcohol is to increase plasma triglyceride levels. Alcohol consumption stimulates hepatic secretion of VLDLs, possibly by inhibiting the hepatic oxidation of free fatty acids, which then promote hepatic triglyceride synthesis and VLDL secretion. The usual lipoprotein pattern seen with alcohol consumption is Type IV (increased VLDLs), but persons with an underlying primary lipid disorder may develop severe hypertriglyceridemia (Type V) if they drink alcohol. Regular alcohol use also raises plasma levels of HDL-C.

Estrogen

Estrogen administration is associated with increased VLDL and HDL synthesis, resulting in elevated plasma levels of both triglycerides and HDL-C. This lipoprotein pattern is distinctive since the levels of plasma triglyceride and HDL-C are typically inversely related. Plasma triglyceride levels should be monitored when birth control pills or postmenopausal estrogen therapy is initiated to ensure that the increase in VLDL production does not lead to severe hypertriglyceridemia. Use of low-dose preparations of estrogen or the estrogen patch can minimize the effect of exogenous estrogen on lipids.

Lysosomal Storage Diseases

Cholesteryl ester storage disease (due to deficiency in lysosomal acid lipase) and glycogen storage diseases such as von Gierke's disease (caused by mutations in glucose-6-phosphatase) are rare causes of secondary hyperlipidemias.

Cushing's Syndrome

(See also Chap. 5) Glucocorticoid excess is associated with increased VLDL synthesis and hypertriglyceridemia. Patients with Cushing's syndrome can also have mild elevations in plasma levels of LDL-C.

Drugs

Many drugs have an impact on lipid metabolism and can result in significant alterations in the lipoprotein profile (Table 21-5).

SCREENING

(See also Chap. 18) Guidelines for the screening and management of lipid disorders have been provided by an expert Adult Treatment Panel (ATP) convened by the National Cholesterol Education Program (NCEP) of the National Heart Lung and Blood Institute. The NCEP ATPIII guidelines published in 2001 recommend that all adults over age 20 should have plasma levels of cholesterol, triglyceride, LDL-C, and HDL-C measured after a 12-hour overnight fast. In most clinical laboratories, the total cholesterol and triglycerides in the plasma are measured enzymatically, and then the cholesterol in the supernatant is measured after precipitation of apoB-containing lipoproteins to determine the HDL-C. The LDL-C is estimated using the following equation:

$$LDL\text{-}C = \textit{total cholesterol} - (\textit{triglycerides}/5) - HDL\text{-}C.$$

(The VLDL-C is estimated by dividing the plasma triglyceride by 5, reflecting the ratio of cholesterol to triglyceride in VLDL particles.) This formula is reasonably accurate if test results are obtained on fasting plasma and if the triglyceride level does not exceed ~300 mg/dL; by convention it cannot be used if the TGs are >400 mg/dL. The accurate determination of LDL-C levels in patients with triglyceride levels >300 mg/dL requires application of ultracentrifugation techniques or other direct assays for LDL-C. Further evaluation and treatment is based primarily on the plasma LDL-C level and the assessment of overall cardiovascular risk.

DIAGNOSIS

The critical first step in managing a lipid disorder is to determine the class or classes of lipoproteins that are increased or decreased in the patient. The Frederickson classification scheme for hyperlipoproteinemias (Table 21-3), though less commonly used now than in the past, can be helpful in this regard. Once the hyperlipidemia is accurately classified, efforts should be directed to rule out any possible secondary causes of the hyperlipidemia (Table 21-5). Although many patients with hyperlipidemia have a primary or genetic cause of their lipid disorder, secondary factors frequently contribute to the hyperlipidemia. A fasting glucose should be obtained in the initial workup of all subjects with an elevated triglyceride level. Nephrotic syndrome and chronic renal insufficiency should be excluded by obtaining urine protein and serum creatinine. Liver function tests should be performed to rule out hepatitis and cholestasis. Hypothyroidism should be ruled out by measuring serum thyroid-stimulating hormone. Patients with hyperlipidemia, especially hypertriglyceridemia, who drink alcohol or are obese should be encouraged to decrease their intake. Sedentary lifestyle, obesity, and smoking are all associated with low HDL-C levels, and patients should be counseled about these issues.

Once secondary causes for the elevated lipoprotein levels have been ruled out, attempts should be made to diagnose the primary lipid disorder since the underlying etiology has a significant effect on the risk of developing CHD, on the response to drug therapy, and on the management of other family members. Often, determining the correct diagnosis requires a detailed family medical history and, in some cases, lipid analyses in family members.

If the fasting plasma triglyceride level is >1000 mg/dL, the patient almost always has chylomicronemia and either has Type I or Type V hyperlipoproteinemia (Table 21-3). The plasma triglyceride-to-cholesterol ratio helps distinguish between these two possibilities and is higher in Type I than Type V hyperlipoproteinemia. If the patient has Type I hyperlipoproteinemia, a postheparin lipolytic assay should be performed to determine if the patient has LPL or apoC-II deficiency. Type V is a much more frequent form of chylomicronemia in the adult patient. Often treatment of secondary factors contributing to the hyperlipidemia (diet, obesity, glucose intolerance, alcohol ingestion, estrogen therapy) will change a Type V into a Type IV pattern, reducing the risk of developing acute pancreatitis.

If the levels of LDL-C are very high (>95th percentile), it is likely the patient has a genetic form of hyperlipidemia. The presence of severe hypercholesterolemia, tendon xanthomas, and an autosomal dominant pattern of inheritance are consistent with the diagnosis of either FH, FDB, or ADH due to mutations in PCSK9. At the present time there is no compelling reason to perform molecular studies to further refine the molecular diagnosis, since the treatment of FH and FDB is identical. Patients with more moderate hypercholesterolemia that does not segregate in families as a monogenic trait likely have polygenic hypercholesterolemia. Recessive forms of severe hypercholesterolemia are rare; a clue to the diagnosis of sitosterolemia is the response of the hypercholesterolemia to reductions in dietary cholesterol content and to bile acid resins.

The most common error in the diagnosis and treatment of lipid disorders is in patients with a mixed hyperlipidemia without chylomicronemia. Elevations in the plasma levels of both cholesterol and triglycerides are seen in patients with increased plasma levels of IDL (Type III) and of LDL and VLDL (Type IIB) and in patients with increased levels of VLDL (Type IV). The ratio of triglyceride to cholesterol is higher in Type IV than the other two disorders. A β quantification to determine the VLDL-C to triglyceride ratio in plasma (see discussion of FDBL) or a direct measurement of the plasma LDL-C should be performed at least once prior to initiation of lipid-lowering therapy to determine if the hyperlipidemia is due to the accumulation of remnants or to an increase in both LDL and VLDL.

℞ Treatment: LIPOPROTEIN DISORDERS

CLINICAL EVIDENCE THAT TREATMENT OF DYSLIPIDEMIA REDUCES RISK OF CHD

Multiple epidemiologic studies have demonstrated a strong relationship between serum cholesterol and CHD. A direct connection between plasma cholesterol levels and the atherosclerotic process was made in humans when aortic fatty streaks in young persons were shown to be strongly correlated with serum cholesterol levels. The elucidation of homozygous familial hypercholesterolemia was proof that high cholesterol itself caused atherosclerotic vascular disease. Moreover, PCSK9 deficiency proves that very low LDL-C levels are associated with substantial lifetime reduction in cardiovascular risk.

LDL-C Reduction Early clinical trials of cholesterol (mostly LDL-C) reduction utilized niacin, bile acid sequestrants, and even the surgical approach of partial ileal bypass to reduce serum cholesterol levels. Although most of these studies found a small but significant reduction in cardiac events, no decrease in total mortality was seen, which tempered enthusiasm for aggressive, population-based treatment of hypercholesterolemia. The discovery of more potent and well-tolerated cholesterol-lowering agents, namely HMG-CoA reductase inhibitors (statins), ushered in a series of large cholesterol reduction trials that unequivocally established the benefit of cholesterol reduction. Some of these trials were performed in patients with preexisting stable CHD. The Scandinavian Simvastatin Survival Study in hypercholesterolemic men with CHD showed reduced major coronary events by 44% and total mortality by 30% with simvastatin. The Cholesterol and Recurrent Events (CARE) study and the Long-Term Intervention with Pravastatin in Ischemic Heart Disease (LIPID) study demonstrated reduced cardiac events and cardiovascular deaths in women and men with established CHD and normal to only mildly elevated LDL-C levels. Some of the early statin trials were in individuals without preexisting CHD. In the West of Scotland Coronary Prevention Study (WOSCOPS) with pravastatin, subjects had significantly elevated baseline LDL-C levels, whereas in the Air Force/Texas Coronary Atherosclerosis Study (AFCAPS/TexCAPS) with lovastatin, baseline LDL-C levels were only modestly elevated. Both trials demonstrated significant reductions in cardiovascular events and clearly established that drug therapy for hypercholesterolemia is an effective method of decreasing risk of cardiovascular events even in persons who do not have preexisting symptomatic CHD.

More recent studies have enrolled subjects with average or subaverage LDL-C levels and have involved targeting the on-treatment LDL-C to ever lower levels. The Heart Protection Study (HPS) included 20,536 men and women, ages 40–80 years, who had either established ASCVD or were at high risk for the development of CHD (primarily diabetes); the only lipid entry criterion was a total plasma cholesterol level of >135 mg/dL. Treatment with simvastatin for an average of 5 years resulted in a 24% reduction in major coronary events and a highly significant 13% reduction in all-cause mortality. Importantly, the relative benefit of statin therapy was similar across tertiles of baseline LDL-C, and even the large subgroup of individuals with an LDL-C <100 mg/dL at baseline experienced significant benefit from therapy. This study demonstrated that statin therapy is beneficial in high-risk subjects, even if the baseline LDL-C level is below the currently recommended targeted goal; it also helped to shift the emphasis from simply treating elevated cholesterol to treating patients at high risk of CHD.

The Anglo-Scandinavian Cardiac Outcomes Trial Lipid-Lowering Arm (ASCOT-LLA) involved 19,342 hypertensive patients with at least three other cardiovascular risk factors and with total cholesterol levels <242 mg/dL. The lipid-lowering arm involved the intervention of atorvastatin 10 mg vs. placebo, and was terminated after 3.3 years due to a highly significant 36% relative risk reduction in major cardiovascular events. In the Collaborative Atorvastatin Diabetes Study (CARDS), 2838 patients with type 2 diabetes were randomized to atorvastatin 10 mg or placebo; this study was also terminated early due to a significant 37% reduction in major cardiovascular events. Both of these studies involved on-treatment LDL-C levels well below recommended targets for the patients, but still involved comparison to placebo.

The most compelling data supporting the concept that "lower is better" come from studies in which different statin regimens were directly compared. In the Treat to New Targets (TNT) trial, 10,001 patients with CHD and LDL-C <130 mg/dL were randomized to atorvastatin 80 mg vs. 10 mg daily. Atorvastatin 80 mg was associated with a significant 22% reduction in major cardiovascular events and a mean on-treatment LDL-C level of 77 mg/dL (compared with 101 mg/dL for the 10-mg dose). In the Pravastatin or Atorvastatin Evaluation and Infection Therapy (PROVE-IT) study, patients presenting with acute coronary syndromes were randomized to atorvastatin 80 mg (more intensive) or pravastatin 40 mg (less intensive). Atorvastatin 80 mg was associated with a significant 16% relative risk reduction in major cardiovascular events compared with the less-intensive pravastatin 40-mg regimen. The mean on-treatment LDL-C levels were 62 mg/dL in the atorvastatin 80-mg group and 95 mg/dL in the pravastatin 40-mg group. Based on several of these studies, a white paper was issued by the NCEP in 2004 establishing an "optional" LDL-C goal of <70 mg/dL in high-risk patients with CHD and of <100 mg/dL in very-high-risk patients without known CHD. These optional targets have been widely embraced, and clinical practice is clearly evolving to treating CHD and high-risk patients more aggressively for LDL reduction.

Treatment of the TG-HDL Axis Abnormalities of the TG-HDL axis are more common in patients with CHD or at risk for it than is elevated LDL-C. Yet the data supporting pharmacologic intervention in the TG-HDL axis is less abundant and compelling than the data supporting LDL-C reduction. Fibric acid derivatives (fibrates), nicotinic acid (niacin), and omega-3 fatty acids (fish oils) are the primary agents currently available for intervention regarding the TG-HDL axis. Fibrates have been used as lipid-lowering drugs for several decades and are more effective in reducing plasma TG levels and relatively less effective in increasing plasma HDL-C levels. The overall body of data with fibrates regarding cardiovascular outcomes trends is positive but mixed. The Helsinki Heart Study (HHS) compared gemfibrozil to placebo in hypercholesterolemic patients with no CHD and demonstrated a significant 36% reduction in coronary events. The Veteran Affairs High-Density Lipoprotein Cholesterol Intervention Trial (VA-HIT) examined the benefit of gemfibrozil in men with CHD, normal plasma levels of LDL-C levels, and low plasma levels of HDL-C levels and demonstrated a significant 22% reduction in nonfatal myocardial infarction and coronary death with gemfibrozil therapy. However, the Bezafibrate Infarction Prevention (BIP) trial of bezafibrate vs. placebo in CHD patients with low HDL-C failed to demonstrate a statistically significant reduction in coronary events, though there was a positive trend. Similarly, the Fenofibrate Intervention and Event Lowering in Diabetes (FIELD) trial of fenofibrate in 9795 patients with type 2 diabetes also failed to show a significant reduction in its primary endpoint of nonfatal myocardial infarction and coronary death, though there was a positive trend (11% relative risk reduction) and significant reductions in total cardiovascular disease events. There was significantly greater "drop-in" of the placebo group into lipid-lowering therapy, mostly statins, making the interpretation complicated. Nevertheless, the overall body of data with fibrates and CVD risk reduction is mixed. Interestingly, despite the fact that fibrates are most effective in lowering triglycerides, no fibrate trial has ever been performed specifically in subjects with hypertriglyceridemia; in addition, the benefit of the addition of a fibrate to baseline statin therapy has never been tested.

While niacin is the most effective HDL-raising drug currently available, it has never been tested for its ability to reduce cardiovascular risk in a trial in subjects with low HDL-C patients. The Coronary Drug Project showed that niacin modestly reduced cardiovascular events, but this was performed in hypercholesterolemic men with CHD. The AIM-HIGH trial is an ongoing study of the effect of niacin added to baseline statin therapy in patients with CHD and low HDL-C. Finally, while low-dose fish oils have been shown to reduce cardiovascular events, higher doses that reduce triglyceride levels have not been tested for their ability to reduce cardiovascular events. Definitive proof that treating the TG-HDL axis reduces cardiovascular events is likely to come from new therapies that are more effective in targeting these abnormalities.

LIPID-MODIFYING THERAPY The major goal of lipid-modifying therapy in most patients with disorders of lipid metabolism is to prevent ASCVD and its complications. Management of lipid disorders should be based on clinical trial data demonstrating that treatment reduces cardiovascular morbidity and mortality, although reasonable extrapolation of these data to specific subgroups is sometimes required. Clearly, elevated plasma levels of LDL-C are strongly associated with increased risk of ASCVD, and treatment to lower the levels of plasma LDL-C decreases risk of clinical cardiovascular events in both secondary and primary prevention. Although the proportional benefit accrued from reducing plasma LDL-C appears to be similar over the entire range of LDL-C values, the absolute risk reduction depends on the baseline level of cardiovascular risk. The treatment guidelines developed by the NCEP ATPIII incorporate these principles. As noted above, abnormalities in the TG-HDL axis (elevated TG, low HDL-C, or both) are commonly seen in patients with CHD or at high risk for developing it, but clinical trial data supporting the treatment of these abnormalities is much less compelling, and the pharmacologic tools for their management are more limited. Importantly, the NCEP ATPIII guidelines promote the use of the "non-HDL-C" as a secondary target of therapy in patients with TG levels >200 mg/dL. The goals for non-HDL-C are 30 mg/dL higher than the goals for LDL-C. Thus, many patients with abnormalities of the TG-HDL axis require additional therapy for reduction of non-HDL-C to recommended goals.

NONPHARMACOLOGIC TREATMENT

Diet Dietary modification is an important component in the management of dyslipidemia. The physician should assess the content of the patient's diet and provide suggestions for dietary modifications. In the patient with elevated LDL-C, dietary saturated fat and cholesterol should be restricted. For individuals with hypertriglyceridemia, the intake of simple carbohydrates should be curtailed. For severe hypertriglyceridemia (>1000 mg/dL), restriction of total fat intake is critical. The most widely used diet to lower the LDL-C level is the "Step I diet" developed by the American Heart Association. Most patients have a relatively modest (<10%) decrease in plasma levels of LDL-C on a step I diet in the absence of any associated weight loss. Almost all persons experience a decrease in plasma HDL-C levels with a reduction in the amount of total and saturated fat in their diet.

Foods and Additives Certain foods and dietary additives are associated with modest reductions in plasma cholesterol levels. Plant stanol and sterol esters are available in a variety of foods such as spreads, salad dressings, and snack bars. Plant sterol and sterol esters interfere with cholesterol absorption and reduce plasma LDL-C levels by ~10% when taken three times per day. The addition to the diet of psyllium, soy protein, or Chinese red yeast rice (which contains lovastatin) can have modest cholesterol-lowering effects. Other herbal approaches such as guggulipid have not been shown to reduce LDL-C. No controlled studies have been performed in which several of these nonpharmacologic options have been combined to address their additive or synergistic effects.

Weight Loss and Exercise The treatment of obesity, if present, can have a favorable impact on plasma lipid levels and should be actively encouraged. Plasma triglyceride levels tend to fall and HDL-C levels tend to increase in obese subjects after weight reduction. Regular aerobic exercise can also have a positive effect on lipids, in large measure due to the associated weight reduction. Aerobic exercise has a very modest elevating effect on plasma levels of HDL-C in most individuals but also has cardiovascular benefits that extend beyond the effects on plasma lipid levels.

PHARMACOLOGIC TREATMENT The decision to use drug therapy depends on the level of cardiovascular risk. Drug therapy for hypercholesterolemia in patients with established CHD is well supported by clinical trial data, as reviewed above. Even patients with CHD or risk factors who have "average" LDL-C levels benefit from treatment. Drug treatment to lower LDL-C levels in patients with CHD is also highly cost-effective. Patients with diabetes mellitus without known CHD have similar cardiovascular risk to those without diabetes but with preexisting CHD. An effective way to estimate absolute risk of a cardiovascular event over 10 years is to use a scoring system based on the Framingham Heart Study database. Patients with a 10-year absolute CHD risk of >20% are considered "CHD risk equivalents." Current NCEP ATPIII guidelines call for drug therapy to reduce LDL-C to <100 mg/dL in patients with established CHD, other ASCVD (aortic aneurysm, peripheral vascular disease, or cerebrovascular disease), diabetes mellitus, or CHD risk equivalents; and "optionally" to reduce LDL-C to <70 mg/dL in high-risk CHD patients. Based on these guidelines, virtually all CHD and CHD risk-equivalent patients require cholesterol-lowering drug therapy. Moderate-risk patients with two or more risk factors and a 10-year absolute risk of 10–20% should be treated to a goal LDL-C of <130 mg/dL or "optionally" to LDL-C <100 mg/dL.

Persons with markedly elevated plasma levels of LDL-C levels (>190 mg/dL) should be strongly considered for drug therapy even if their 10-year absolute CHD risk is not particularly elevated. The decision of whether to initiate drug treatment in individuals with plasma LDL-C levels between 130 and 190 mg/dL can be difficult. Although it is desirable to avoid drug treatment in patients who are unlikely to develop CHD, a very high proportion of patients who eventually develop CHD have plasma LDL-C levels that are in this range. Other clinical information can assist in the decision-making process. For example, a low plasma level of HDL-C (<40 mg/dL) supports a decision in favor of more aggressive therapy. Diagnosis of the metabolic syndrome also identifies a higher-risk individual who should be targeted for therapeutic lifestyle changes and might be a candidate for more aggressive drug therapy (Chap. 18). Other laboratory tests, such as an elevated plasma level of apoB, Lp(a), or high-sensitivity C-reactive protein, may help to identify additional high-risk individuals who should be considered for drug therapy when their LDL-C is in a "gray zone."

Drug treatment is also indicated in patients with triglycerides >1000 mg/dL who have been screened and treated for secondary causes of chylomicronemia. The goal is to reduce plasma triglycerides to below 500 mg/dL to prevent the risk of acute pancreatitis. When triglycerides are 500–1000 mg/dL, the decision to use drug therapy depends on the assessment of cardiovascular risk. Most major clinical endpoint trials with statins have excluded persons with triglyceride levels >350–450 mg/dL, and there are therefore few data regarding the effectiveness of statins in reducing cardiovascular risk in persons with triglycerides higher than this threshold. More data are needed regarding the relative effectiveness of statins, fibrates, niacin, and fish oils for reducing cardiovascular risk in this setting. Combination therapy is often required for optimal control of mixed dyslipidemia.

HMG-CoA Reductase Inhibitors (Statins) HMG-CoA reductase is the rate-limiting step in cholesterol biosynthesis, and inhibition of this enzyme decreases cholesterol synthesis. By inhibiting cholesterol biosynthesis, statins lead to increased hepatic LDL receptor activity and accelerated clearance of circulating LDL, resulting in a dose-dependent reduction in plasma levels of LDL-C. There is wide interindividual variation in the initial response to a statin, but once a patient is on a statin, the doubling of the statin dose produces a 6% further reduction in the level of plasma LDL-C. The statins currently available differ in their LDL-C reducing effects (Table 21-6). Statins also reduce plasma triglycerides in a dose-dependent fashion, which is proportional to their LDL-C lowering effects (if the triglycerides are <400 mg/dL). Statins have a modest HDL-raising effect (5–10%), and this effect is not dose-dependent.

Statins are well tolerated and can be taken in tablet form once a day. Potential side effects include dyspepsia, headaches, fatigue, and muscle or joint pains. Severe myopathy and even rhabdomyolysis occur rarely with statin treatment. The risk of statin-associated myopathy is increased by the presence of older age, frailty, renal insufficiency, and coadministration of drugs that interfere with the metabolism of statins, such as erythromycin and related antibiotics, antifungal agents, immunosuppressive drugs, and fibric acid derivatives (particularly gemfibrozil). Severe myopathy can usually be avoided by careful patient selection, avoidance of interacting drugs, and instructing the patient to contact the physician immediately in the event of unexplained muscle pain. In the event of muscle symptoms, the plasma creatine phosphokinase (CK) level should be obtained to document the myopathy. Serum CK levels need not be monitored on a routine basis in patients taking statins, as an elevated CK in the absence of symptoms does not predict the development of myopathy and does not necessarily suggest the need for discontinuing the drug.

Another consequence of statin therapy can be elevation in liver transaminases (ALT and AST). They should be checked before starting therapy, at 2–3 months, and then annually. Substantial (greater than three times upper limit of normal) elevation in transaminases is relatively rare, and mild to moderate (one to three times normal) elevation in transaminases in the absence of symptoms need not mandate discontinuing the medication. Severe clinical hepatitis associated with statins is exceedingly rare, and the trend is toward less frequent monitoring of transaminases in patients taking statins. The statin-associated elevation in liver enzymes resolves upon discontinuation of the medication.

Statins appear to be remarkably safe. Meta-analyses of large randomized controlled clinical trials with statins do not suggest an increase in any major noncardiac diseases. Statins are the drug class of choice for LDL-C reduction and are by far the most widely used class of lipid-lowering drugs.

Cholesterol Absorption Inhibitors Cholesterol within the lumen of the small intestine is derived from the diet (about one-third) and the bile (about two-thirds) and is actively absorbed by the enterocyte through a process that involves the protein NPC1L1. Ezetimibe (Table 21-6) is a cholesterol absorption inhibitor that binds directly to and inhibits NPC1L1 and blocks the intestinal absorption of cholesterol. In humans, ezetimibe at a dose of 10 mg was shown to inhibit cholesterol absorption by almost 60%. The result of inhibition of intestinal cholesterol absorption is likely to be reduction in hepatic cholesterol and an increased hepatic LDL receptor expression. The mean reduction in plasma LDL-C on ezetimibe (10 mg) is 18%, and the effect is additive when used in combination with a statin. Effects on TG and HDL-C levels are negligible, and no cardiovascular outcome data have been reported. When used in combination with a statin, monitoring of liver transaminases is recommended. Ezetimibe has become the preferred drug to add to a statin in patients who require further LDL-C reduction and is also widely used in patients who are statin-intolerant.

TABLE 21-6

SUMMARY OF THE MAJOR DRUGS USED FOR THE TREATMENT OF HYPERLIPIDEMIA

DRUG	MAJOR INDICATIONS	STARTING DOSE	MAXIMAL DOSE	MECHANISM	COMMON SIDE EFFECTS
HMG-CoA reductase inhibitors (statins)	Elevated LDL-C			↓ Cholesterol synthesis, ↑ Hepatic LDL receptors, ↓ VLDL production	Myalgias, arthralgias, elevated transaminases, dyspepsia
Lovastatin		20 mg daily	80 mg daily		
Pravastatin		40 mg qhs	80 mg qhs		
Simvastatin		20 mg qhs	80 mg qhs		
Fluvastatin		20 mg qhs	80 mg qhs		
Atorvastatin		10 mg qhs	80 mg qhs		
Rosuvastatin		10 mg qhs	40 mg qhs		
Cholesterol absorption inhibitors				↓ Intestinal cholesterol absorption	Elevated transaminases
Ezetimibe	Elevated LDL-C	10 mg daily	10 mg daily		
Bile acid sequestrants	Elevated LDL-C			↑ Bile acid excretion and ↑ LDL receptors	Bloating, constipation, elevated triglycerides
Cholestyramine		4 g daily	32 g daily		
Colestipol		5 g daily	40 g daily		
Colesevelam		3750 mg daily	4375 mg daily		
Nicotinic acid	Elevated LDL-C, low HDL-C, elevated TG			↓ VLDL hepatic synthesis	Cutaneous flushing, GI upset, elevated glucose, uric acid, and liver function tests
Immediate-release		100 mg tid	1 g tid		
Sustained-release		250 mg bid	1.5 g bid		
Extended-release		500 mg qhs	2 g qhs		
Fibric acid derivatives	Elevated TG, elevated remnants			↑ LPL, ↓ VLDL synthesis	Dyspepsia, myalgia, gallstones, elevated transaminases
Gemfibrozil		600 mg bid	600 mg bid		
Fenofibrate		145 mg qd	145 mg qd		
Omega-3 fatty acids	Elevated TG	3 g daily	6 g daily	↑ TG catabolism	Dyspepsia, diarrhea, fishy odor to breath

Note: LDL, low-density lipoprotein; VLDL, very low density lipoprotein; HDL, high-density lipoprotein; LDL-C, LDL cholesterol; HDL-C, HDL cholesterol; TG, triglyceride; LPL, lipoprotein lipase; GI, gastrointestinal.

Bile Acid Sequestrants (Resins) Bile acid sequestrants bind bile acids in the intestine and promote their excretion in the stool. To maintain the bile acid pool size, the liver diverts cholesterol to bile acid synthesis. The decreased hepatic intracellular cholesterol content results in upregulation of the LDL receptor and enhanced LDL clearance from the plasma. Bile acid sequestrants, including cholestyramine, colestipol, and colesevelam (Table 21-6), primarily reduce plasma LDL-C levels and can cause an increase in plasma triglycerides. Therefore, patients with hypertriglyceridemia should not be treated with bile acid–binding resins. Cholestyramine and colestipol are insoluble resins that must be suspended in liquids. Colesevelam is available as tablets but generally requires up to six to seven tablets per day for effective LDL-C lowering. Most side effects of resins are limited to the gastrointestinal tract and include bloating and constipation. Since bile acid sequestrants are not systemically absorbed, they are very safe and the cholesterol-lowering drug of choice in children and in women of childbearing age who are lactating, are pregnant, or could become pregnant. They are effective in combination with statins as well as in combination with ezetimibe and are particularly useful with one or both of these drugs for difficult-to-treat patients or those with statin intolerance.

Nicotinic Acid (Niacin) Nicotinic acid, or niacin, is a B-complex vitamin that has been used as a lipid-modifying agent for decades. It was previously shown to reduce the flux of nonesterified fatty acids (NEFAs) to the liver, resulting in reduced hepatic TG synthesis and VLDL secretion. Recently a receptor for nicotinic acid called GPR109A was discovered; it is expressed in adipocytes and, when activated, suppresses the release of NEFA by adipose. Niacin reduces plasma triglyceride and LDL-C levels and raises the plasma concentration of HDL-C (Table 21-6). Niacin is also the only currently available lipid-lowering drug that significantly reduces plasma levels of Lp(a). If properly prescribed and monitored, niacin is a safe and effective lipid-lowering agent.

The most frequent side effect of niacin is cutaneous flushing, which is mediated by activation of the same receptor GPR109A in the skin, leading to local generation of prostaglandin D_2 production. Flushing can be reduced by formulations that slow the absorption and by taking aspirin prior to dosing. In addition, there is tachyphylaxis to the flushing. Niacin therapy is generally started at lower doses and titrated over time. Immediate-release crystalline niacin is generally administered three times per day, over-the-counter sustained-release niacin is taken twice a day, and a prescription form of extended release niacin is taken once a day. Mild elevations in transaminases occur in up to 15% of patients treated with any form of niacin, but these elevations may require stopping the medication. Niacin potentiates the effect of warfarin, and these two drugs should be prescribed together with caution. Acanthosis nigricans, a dark-colored coarse skin lesion, and maculopathy are infrequent side effects of niacin. Niacin is contraindicated in patients with peptic ulcer disease and can exacerbate the symptoms of esophageal reflux. It can also raise plasma levels of uric acid and precipitate gouty attacks in susceptible patients.

Niacin can raise fasting plasma glucose levels. However, in one study in type 2 diabetics, niacin treatment was associated with only a slight increase in fasting glucose and no significant change from baseline in the HbA_{1C}. In another, low-dose niacin was found to effectively reduce triglycerides and raise HDL-C without adversely impacting on glycemic control. Thus, niacin can be used in diabetic patients, but every effort should be made to optimize the diabetes management before initiating niacin, and glucose should be carefully monitored in nondiabetic patients with impaired fasting glucose after initiation of niacin therapy.

Successful therapy with niacin requires careful education and motivation on the part of the patient. Its advantages are its low cost and long-term safety. It is the most effective drug currently available for raising HDL-C levels. It is particularly useful in patients with combined hyperlipidemia and low plasma levels of HDL-C and is effective in combination with statins.

Fibric Acid Derivatives (Fibrates) Fibric acid derivatives are agonists of PPARα, a nuclear receptor involved in the regulation of carbohydrate and lipid metabolism. Fibrates stimulate LPL activity (enhancing triglyceride hydrolysis), reduce apoC-III synthesis (enhancing lipoprotein remnant clearance), and may reduce VLDL production. Fibrates are the most effective drugs available for reducing triglyceride levels and also raise HDL-C levels modestly (Table 21-6). They have variable effects on LDL-C and in hypertriglyceridemic patients can sometimes be associated with increases in plasma LDL-C levels.

Fibrates are generally very well tolerated. The most common side effect is dyspepsia. Myopathy and hepatitis occur rarely in the absence of other lipid-lowering agents. Fibrates promote cholesterol secretion into bile and are associated with an increased risk of gallstones. Importantly, fibrates can potentiate the effect of warfarin and certain oral hypoglycemic agents, so the anticoagulation status and plasma glucose levels should be closely monitored in patients on these agents.

Fibrates are the drug class of choice in patients with severe hypertriglyceridemia (>1000 mg/dL) and are a reasonable consideration for first-line therapy in patients with moderate hypertriglyceridemia (500–1000 mg/dL) and FDBL. As noted above, the clinical trial data with fibrates overall suggests cardiovascular benefit, but the results are mixed. In patients with TG <500 mg/dL, the role of fibrates is primarily in combination with statins in selected patients with mixed dyslipidemia. In this setting, the risk of myopathy must be carefully weighed against the clinical benefit of the therapy.

Omega-3 Fatty Acids (Fish Oils) N-3 polyunsaturated fatty acids (n-3 PUFAs) are present in high concentration in fish and in flax seeds. The most widely used n-3 PUFAs for the treatment of hyperlipidemias are the two active molecules in fish oil: eicosapentaenoic acid (EPA) and decohexanoic acid (DHA). N-3 PUFAs have been concentrated into tablets and decrease fasting triglycerides in doses of 3–4 g/d. Fish oils can result in an increase in plasma LDL-C levels in some patients. Fish oil supplements can be used in combination with fibrates, niacin, or statins to treat hypertriglyceridemia. In general, fish oils are well tolerated and appear to be safe, at least at doses up to 3–4 g. Although fish oil administration is associated with a prolongation in the bleeding time, no increase in bleeding has been seen in clinical trials. A lower dose of omega-3 (about 1 g) has been associated with reduction in cardiovascular events in CHD patients and is used by some clinicians for this purpose.

Combination Drug Therapy This type of therapy is often required in patients who do not reach lipid targets on monotherapy. Combination drug therapy is frequently used for (1) patients unable to reach LDL-C and non-HDL-C goals on statin monotherapy, (2) patients with combined elevated LDL-C and abnormalities of the TG-HDL axis, and (3) patients with severe hypertriglyceridemia who do not achieve non-HDL-C goals on a fibrate or fish oils alone. Inability to achieve LDL-C (and non-HDL-C) goals is not uncommon on statin monotherapy. In this setting, a cholesterol absorption inhibitor or bile acid sequestrant can be added. Combination of niacin with a statin is an attractive option for high-risk patients who do not attain their target LDL-C level on statin monotherapy and who have a low HDL-C as their primary lipid abnormality. Conversely, in high-risk patients on statin therapy who have elevated TG levels as their primary remaining lipid abnormality, addition of a fibrate or fish oils is a reasonable consideration. Hypertriglyceridemic patients treated with a fibrate often fail to reach LDL-C and non-HDL-C goals and are therefore candidates for the addition of a statin. Coadministration of statins and fibrates has obvious appeal in patients with combined hyperlipidemia, but no clinical trials have assessed the effectiveness of a statin-fibrate combination compared with either a statin or a fibrate alone in reducing cardiovascular events, and the long-term safety of this combination is not known. Statin-fibrate combinations are known to be associated with an increased incidence of severe myopathy (up to 2.5%) and rhabdomyolysis, and therefore patients treated with these two drugs must be carefully counseled and monitored. This combination of drugs should be used cautiously in patients with underlying renal or hepatic insufficiency; in the elderly, frail, and chronically ill; and in those on multiple medications.

OTHER APPROACHES Occasionally, patients cannot tolerate any of the existing lipid-lowering drugs at doses required for adequate control of their lipid levels. A larger group of patients, most of whom have genetic lipid disorders, remain significantly hypercholesterolemic despite combination drug therapy. These patients are at high risk for development or progression of CHD and clinical CHD events. The preferred option for management of patients with severe refractory hypercholesterolemia is LDL apheresis. In this process, the patient's plasma is passed over a column that selectively removes the LDL, and the LDL-depleted plasma is returned to the patient. Patients on maximally tolerated combination drug therapy who have CHD and a plasma LDL-C level >200 mg/dL or no CHD and a plasma LDL-C level >300 mg/dL are candidates for every-other-week LDL apheresis and should be referred to a specialized lipid center.

Management of Low HDL-C Severely reduced plasma levels of HDL-C (<20 mg/dL) accompanied by triglycerides <400 mg/dL usually indicate the presence of a genetic disorder, such as a mutation in apoA-I, LCAT deficiency, or Tangier disease. HDL-C levels <20 mg/dL are common in the setting of severe hypertriglyceridemia, in which case the primary focus should be on the management of the triglycerides. HDL-C levels <20 mg/dL also occur in individuals using anabolic steroids. Secondary causes of more moderate reductions in plasma HDL (20–40 mg/dL) should be considered (Table 21-5). Smoking should be discontinued, obese persons should be encouraged to lose weight, sedentary persons should be encouraged to exercise, and diabetes should be optimally controlled. When possible, medications associated with reduced plasma levels of HDL-C should be discontinued. The presence of an isolated low plasma level of HDL-C in a patient with a borderline plasma level of LDL-C should prompt consideration of LDL-lowering drug therapy in high-risk individuals. Statins increase plasma levels of HDL-C only modestly (~5–10%). Fibrates also have only a modest effect on plasma HDL-C levels (increasing levels ~5–15%), except in patients with coexisting hypertriglyceridemia, where they can be more effective. Niacin is the most effective available HDL-C–raising therapeutic agent and can be associated with increases in plasma HDL-C by up to ~30%, although some patients do not respond to niacin therapy.

The issue of whether pharmacologic intervention should be used to specifically raise HDL-C levels has not been adequately addressed in clinical trials. In persons with established CHD and low HDL-C levels whose plasma LDL-C levels are at or below the goal, it may be reasonable to initiate therapy (with a fibrate or niacin) directed specifically at reducing plasma triglyceride levels and raising the level of plasma HDL-C. More data are required before broad recommendations are made to use drug therapy to specifically raise HDL-C levels to prevent cardiovascular events. New HDL-raising approaches are under development that may help to address this important issue.

FURTHER READINGS

Baigent C et al: Efficacy and safety of cholesterol-lowering treatment: Prospective meta-analysis of data from 90,056 participants in 14 randomised trials of statins. Lancet 366:1267, 2005

Brunzell JD: Clinical practice. Hypertriglyceridemia. N Engl J Med 357(10):1009, 2007

Carlson LA: Nicotinic acid: The broad-spectrum lipid drug. A 50th anniversary review. J Intern Med 258:94, 2005

Duffy D, Rader DJ: Emerging therapies targeting high-density lipoprotein metabolism and reverse cholesterol transport. Circulation 113:1140, 2006

Grundy SM: The issue of statin safety: Where do we stand? Circulation 111:3016, 2005

——— et al: Implications of recent clinical trials for the National Cholesterol Education Program Adult Treatment Panel III guidelines. Circulation 110:227, 2004

Kearney PM et al: Efficacy of cholesterol-lowering therapy in 18,686 people with diabetes in 14 randomised trials of statins: A meta-analysis. Lancet 371:117, 2008

LaRosa JC et al: Intensive lipid lowering with atorvastatin in patients with stable coronary disease. N Engl J Med 352:1425, 2005

Li SG: Images in clinical medicine. Familial hypercholesterolemia. N Engl J Med 360:1885, 2009

National Cholesterol Education Program: Executive summary of the third report of the National Cholesterol Education Program (NCEP) Expert Panel on Detection, Evaluation, and Treatment of High Blood Cholesterol in Adults (Adult Treatment Panel III). JAMA 285:2486, 2001

Rader DJ et al: Monogenic hypercholesterolemia: New insights in pathogenesis and treatment. J Clin Invest 111:1795, 2003

Singh IM et al: High-density lipoprotein as a therapeutic target: A systematic review. JAMA 298(7):786, 2007

Steinberg D: The statins in preventive cardiology. N Engl J Med 359:1426, 2008

SECTION IV

DISORDERS AFFECTING MULTIPLE ENDOCRINE SYSTEMS

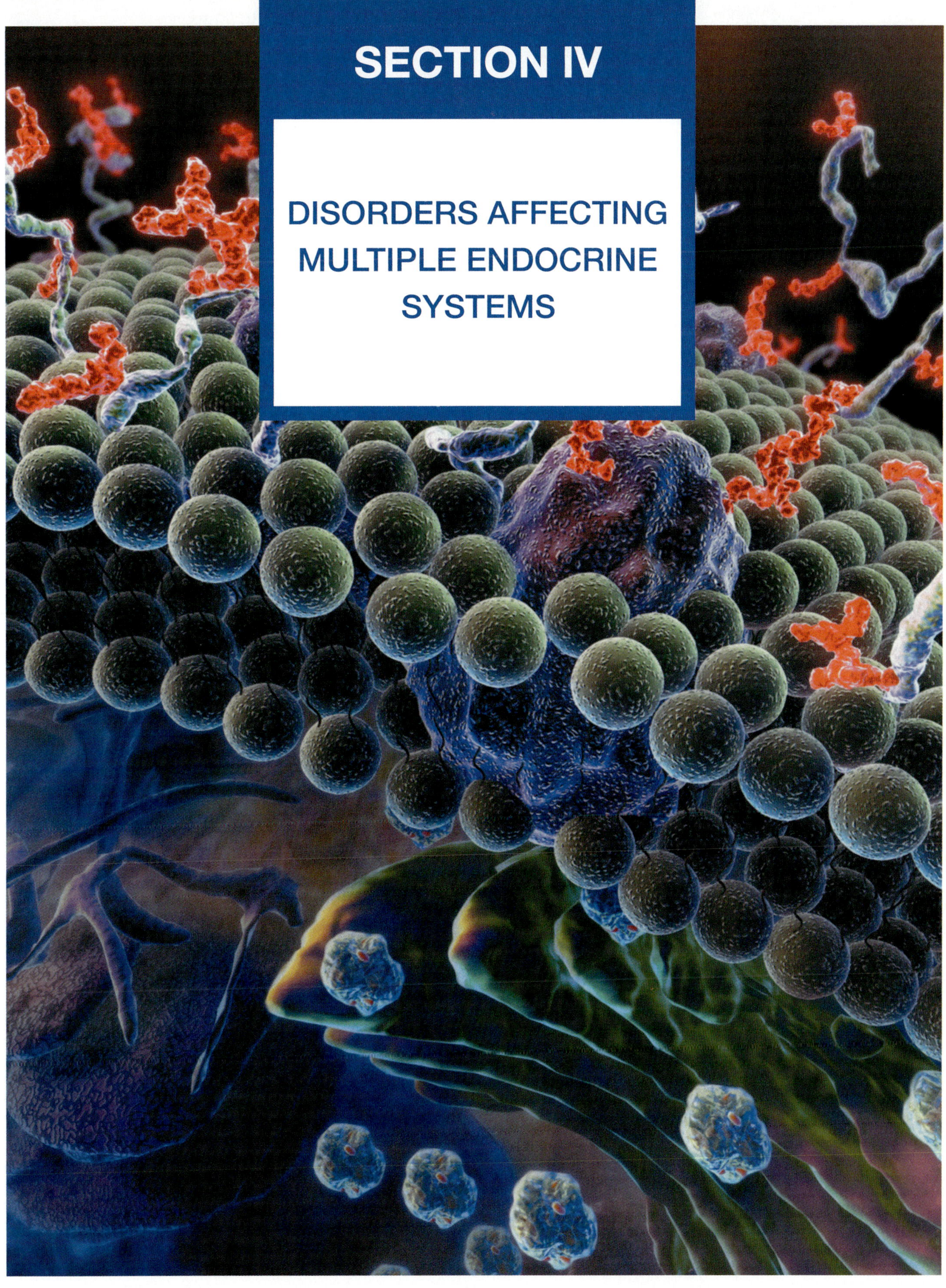

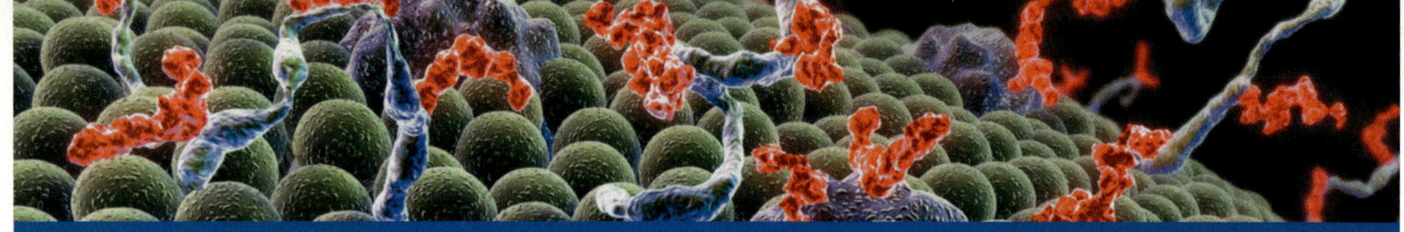

CHAPTER 22

ENDOCRINE TUMORS OF THE GASTROINTESTINAL TRACT AND PANCREAS

Robert T. Jensen

GENERAL FEATURES OF GASTROINTESTINAL NEUROENDOCRINE TUMORS

Gastrointestinal (GI) neuroendocrine tumors (NETs) are derived from the diffuse neuroendocrine system of the GI tract, which is composed of amine- and acid-producing cells with different hormonal profiles, depending on the site of origin. The tumors they produce can be divided into carcinoid tumors and pancreatic endocrine tumors (PETs). These tumors were originally classified as APUDomas (for *a*mine *p*recursor *u*ptake and *d*ecarboxylation), as were pheochromocytomas, melanomas, and medullary thyroid carcinomas because they share certain cytochemical features as well as various pathologic, biologic, and molecular features (**Table 22-1**). It was originally proposed that APUDomas had a similar embryonic origin from neural crest cells, but it is now known the peptide-secreting cells are not of neuroectodermal origin. Nevertheless, the concept is useful because the tumors have important similarities as well as some differences (Table 22-1).

CLASSIFICATION/PATHOLOGY/TUMOR BIOLOGY OF NETs

NETs are generally composed of monotonous sheets of small round cells with uniform nuclei; mitoses are uncommon. They can be tentatively identified on routine histology; however, these tumors are now principally recognized by their histologic staining patterns due to shared cellular proteins. Historically, silver staining was used and tumors were classified as showing an argentaffin reaction if they took up and reduced silver, or as being argyrophilic if they did not reduce it. More recently immunocytochemical localization of chromogranins (A, B, C), neuron-specific enolase, or synaptophysin, which are all neuroendocrine cell markers, are used (Table 22-1). Chromogranin A is currently the most widely used.

Ultrastructurally, these tumors possess electron-dense neurosecretory granules and frequently contain small clear vesicles that correspond to synaptic vesicles of neurons. NETs synthesize numerous peptides, growth factors, and bioactive amines that may be ectopically secreted, giving rise to a specific clinical syndrome

TABLE 22-1

GENERAL CHARACTERISTICS OF GI NEUROENDOCRINE TUMORS [CARCINOIDS, PANCREATIC ENDOCRINE TUMORS (PETs)]

I. Share general neuroendocrine cell markers
   A. Chromogranins (A, B, C) are acidic monomeric soluble proteins found in the large secretory granules; chromogranin A is most widely used.
   B. Neuron-specific enolase (NSE) is the γ-γ dimer of the enzyme enolase and is a cytosolic marker of neuroendocrine differentiation.
   C. Synaptophysin is an integral membrane glycoprotein of 38,000 molecular weight found in small vesicles of neurons and neuroendocrine tumors.

II. Pathologic similarities
   A. All are APUDomas showing *a*mine *p*recursor *u*ptake and *d*ecarboxylation.
   B. Ultrastructurally have dense-core secretory granules (>80 nm).
   C. Histologically appear similar with few mitoses and uniform nuclei.
   D. Frequently synthesize multiple peptides/amines, which can be detected immunocytochemically but may not be secreted.
   E. Presence or absence of clinical syndrome or type cannot be predicted by immunocytochemical studies.
   F. Histologic classifications do not predict biologic behavior; only invasion or metastases establishes malignancy.

III. Similarities of biologic behavior
   A. Generally slow growing, but a proportion is aggressive.
   B. Secrete biologically active peptides/amines, which can cause clinical symptoms.
   C. Generally have high densities of somatostatin receptors, which are used for both localization and treatment.

IV. Similarities/differences in molecular abnormalities
   A. Similarities
      1. Uncommon—alterations in common oncogenes (*ras, jun, fos,* etc.).
      2. Uncommon—alterations in common tumor-suppressor genes (p53, retinoblastoma).
      3. Alterations at MEN-1 locus (11q13) and $p16^{INK4a}$ (9p21) occur in a proportion (10–30%).
      4. Methylation of various genes occurs in 40–87% (*ras*-associated domain family I, p14, p16, O^6 methyl guanosine methyltransferase, retinoic acid receptor β).
   B. Differences
      1. PETs—loss of 3p (8–47%), 3q (8–41%), 11q (21–62%), 6q (18–68%). Gains at 17q (10–55%), 7q (16–68%).
      2. Carcinoids—loss of 18q (38–67%) > 18p (33–43%) > 9p, 16q21 (21–23%). Gains at 17q, 19p (57%).

(Table 22-2). The diagnosis of the specific syndrome requires the clinical features of the disease and cannot be made from the immunocytochemistry results alone. Furthermore, pathologists cannot distinguish between benign and malignant NETs unless metastases or invasion is present.

Carcinoid tumors are frequently classified according to their anatomic area of origin (i.e., foregut, midgut, hindgut) because tumors with similar embryonic origin share functional manifestations, histochemistry, and secretory products (Table 22-3). Foregut tumors generally have a low serotonin (5-HT) content, are argentaffin-negative but argyrophilic, occasionally secrete adrenocorticotropic hormone (ACTH) or 5-hydroxytryptophan (5-HTP) causing an atypical carcinoid syndrome (Fig. 22-1), are often multihormonal, and may metastasize to bone. They uncommonly produce a clinical syndrome due to the secreted products. Midgut carcinoids are argentaffin-positive, have a high 5-HT content, most frequently cause the typical carcinoid syndrome when they metastasize (Table 22-3, Fig. 22-1), release 5-HT and tachykinins (substance P, neuropeptide K, substance K), rarely secrete 5-HTP or ACTH, and uncommonly metastasize to bone. Hindgut carcinoids (rectum, transverse and descending colon) are argentaffin-negative, often argyrophilic, rarely contain 5-HT or cause the carcinoid syndrome (Fig. 22-1, Table 22-3), rarely secrete 5-HTP or ACTH, contain numerous peptides, and may metastasize to bone.

PETs can be classified into nine well-established specific functional syndromes (Table 22-2), four possible specific functional syndromes (PETs secreting calcitonin, renin, luteinizing hormone, or erythropoietin), and nonfunctional PETs [pancreatic polypeptide (PP)-secreting tumors, PPomas]. Each of the functional syndromes is associated with symptoms due to the specific hormone released. In contrast, nonfunctional PETs release no products that cause a specific clinical syndrome. "Nonfunctional" is a misnomer in the strict sense because they frequently ectopically secrete a number of peptides [PP, chromogranin A, ghrelin, neurotensin, α subunits of human chorionic gonadotropin (hCG), neuron-specific enolase]; however, they cause no specific clinical syndrome. The symptoms caused by nonfunctional PETs are entirely due to the tumor per se.

Carcinoid tumors can occur in almost any GI tissue (Table 22-3); however, at present most (70%) take origin from one of three sites: bronchus, jejunoileum, or colon/rectum. In the past, carcinoid tumors most frequently were reported in the appendix (i.e., 40%); however, the bronchus/lung and small intestine are now the most common sites. Overall, GI carcinoids are the most common site for these tumors, comprising 64%, with the respiratory tract second at 28%.

TABLE 22-2

GI NEUROENDOCRINE TUMOR SYNDROMES

NAME	BIOLOGICALLY ACTIVE PEPTIDE(S) SECRETED	INCIDENCE (NEW CASES/10^6 POPULATION/YEAR)	TUMOR LOCATION	MALIGNANT, %	ASSOCIATED WITH MEN 1, %	MAIN SYMPTOMS/SIGNS
Established Specific Functional Syndrome						
Carcinoid tumor						
Carcinoid syndrome	Serotonin, possibly tachykinins, motilin, prostaglandins	0.5–2	Midgut (75–87%) Foregut (2–33%) Hindgut (1–8%) Unknown (2–15%)	95–100	Rare	Diarrhea (32–84%) Flushing (63–75%) Pain (10–34%) Asthma (4–18%) Heart disease (11–41%)
Pancreatic endocrine tumor						
Zollinger-Ellison syndrome	Gastrin	0.5–1.5	Duodenum (70%) Pancreas (25%) Other sites (5%)	60–90	20–25	Pain (79–100%) Diarrhea (30–75%) Esophageal symptoms (31–56%)
Insulinoma	Insulin	1–2	Pancreas (>99%)	<10	4–5	Hypoglycemic symptoms (100%)
VIPoma (Verner-Morrison syndrome, pancreatic cholera, WDHA)	Vasoactive intestinal peptide	0.05–0.2	Pancreas (90%, adult) Other (10%, neural, adrenal, periganglionic)	40–70	6	Diarrhea (90–100%) Hypokalemia (80–100%) Dehydration (83%)
Glucagonoma	Glucagon	0.01–0.1	Pancreas (100%)	50–80	1–20	Rash (67–90%) Glucose intolerance (38–87%) Weight loss (66–96%)
Somatostatinoma	Somatostatin	Rare	Pancreas (55%) Duodenum/jejunum (44%)	>70	45	Diabetes mellitus (63–90%) Cholelithiasis (65–90%) Diarrhea (35–90%)
GRFoma	Growth hormone–releasing hormone	Unknown	Pancreas (30%) Lung (54%) Jejunum (7%) Other (13%)	>60	16	Acromegaly (100%)
ACTHoma	ACTH	Rare	Pancreas (4–16% all ectopic Cushing's)	>95	Rare	Cushing's syndrome (100%)
PET causing carcinoid syndrome	Serotonin, ? tachykinins	Rare (43 cases)	Pancreas (<1% all carcinoids)	60–88	Rare	Same as carcinoid syndrome above
PET causing hypercalcemia	PTHrP, others unknown	Rare	Pancreas (rare cause of hypercalcemia)	84	Rare	Abdominal pain due to hepatic metastases

Possible Specific Functional Syndrome						
PET secreting calcitonin	Calcitonin	Rare	Pancreas (rare cause of hypercalcitoninemia)	>80	16	Diarrhea (50%)
PET secreting renin	Renin	Rare	Pancreas	Unknown	No	Hypertension
PET secreting luteinizing hormone	Luteinizing hormone	Rare	Pancreas	Unknown	No	Anovulation, virilization (female); reduced libido (male)
PET secreting erythropoietin	Erythropoietin	Rare	Pancreas	100	No	Polycythemia
No Functional Syndrome						
PPoma/nonfunctional	None	1–2	Pancreas (100%)	>60	18–44	Weight loss (30–90%) Abdominal mass (10–30%) Pain (30–95%)

Note: MEN, multiple endocrine neoplasia; VIPoma, tumor secreting vasoactive intestinal peptide; WDHA, watery diarrhea, hypokalemia, and achlorhydria syndrome; ACTH, adrenocorticotropic hormone; PET, pancreatic endocrine tumor; PTHrP, parathyroid hormone–related peptide; PPoma, tumor secreting pancreatic polypeptide.

TABLE 22-3

CARCINOID TUMOR LOCATION, FREQUENCY OF METASTASES, AND ASSOCIATION WITH THE CARCINOID SYNDROME

	LOCATION (% OF TOTAL)	INCIDENCE OF METASTASES	INCIDENCE OF CARCINOID SYNDROME
Foregut			
Esophagus	<0.1	—	—
Stomach	4.6	10	9.5
Duodenum	2.0	—	3.4
Pancreas	0.7	71.9	20
Gallbladder	0.3	17.8	5
Bronchus, lung, trachea	27.9	5.7	13
Midgut			
Jejunum	1.8	{58.4	9
Ileum	14.9		9
Meckel's diverticulum	0.5	—	13
Appendix	4.8	38.8	<1
Colon	8.6	51	5
Liver	0.4	32.2	—
Ovary	1.0	32	50
Testis	<0.1	—	50
Hindgut			
Rectum	13.6	3.9	—

Source: Location is from the PAN-SEER data (1973–1999), and incidence of metastases from the SEER data (1992–1999), reported by IM Modlin et al: Cancer 97:934, 2003. Incidence of carcinoid syndrome is from 4349 cases studied from 1950–1971, reported by JD Godwin, Cancer 36:560, 1975.

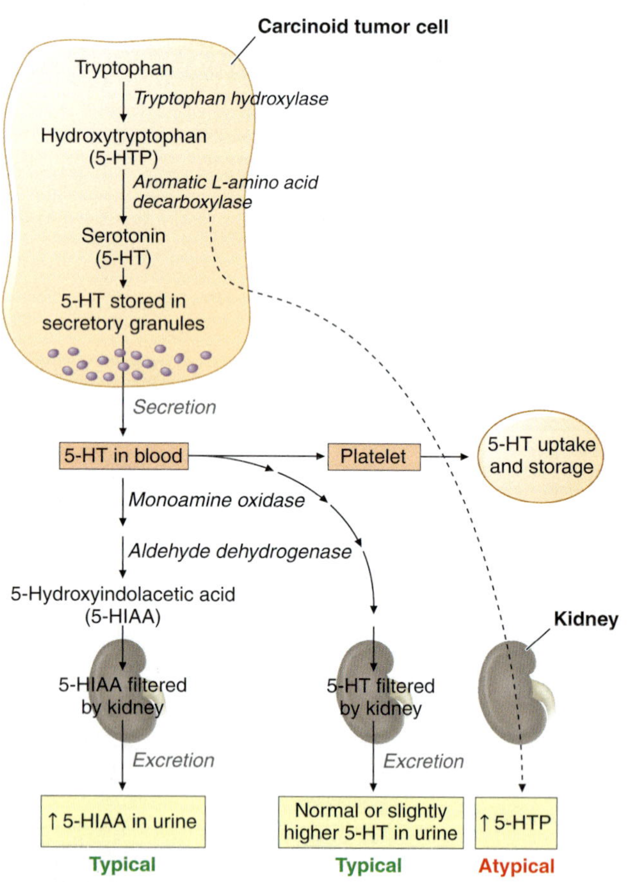

FIGURE 22-1

Synthesis, secretion, and metabolism of serotonin (5-HT) in patients with typical and atypical carcinoid syndromes. 5-HIAA, 5-hydroxyindolacetic acid.

The term *pancreatic endocrine tumor*, although widely used and therefore retained here, is also a misnomer, strictly speaking, because these tumors can occur either almost entirely in the pancreas (insulinomas, glucagonomas, nonfunctional PETs, PETs causing hypercalcemia) or at both pancreatic and extrapancreatic sites [gastrinomas, VIPomas (VIP, vasoactive intestinal peptide), somatostatinomas, GRFomas (GRF, growth hormone–releasing factor)]. PETs are also called *islet cell tumors*; however, this term is discouraged because it is not established that they originate from the islets, and many can occur at extrapancreatic sites.

A uniform World Health Organization (WHO) classification for all GI NETs (including carcinoids and PETs) divides them into three general categories: (1a) well-differentiated NETs, (1b) well-differentiated neuroendocrine carcinomas of low-grade malignancy, and (2) poorly differentiated neuroendocrine carcinomas that are usually small cell neuroendocrine carcinomas of high-grade malignancy. The term *carcinoid* is synonymous with *well-differentiated NETs* (1a). This classification is further divided on the basis of tumor location and biology. Furthermore, for the first time a standard TNM classification has been proposed for the GI foregut NETs. The availability of this WHO classification and the TNM classification should greatly facilitate the comparison of clinical, pathologic, and prognostic features and results of treatment in GI NETs from different studies.

The exact incidence of carcinoid tumors or PETs varies according to whether only symptomatic or all tumors are considered. The incidence of clinically significant carcinoids is 7–13 cases/million population per year, whereas any malignant carcinoids at autopsy are reported in 21–84 cases/million population per year. Clinically significant PETs have a prevalence of 10 cases/million population, with insulinomas, gastrinomas, and nonfunctional PETs having an incidence of 0.5–2 cases/million population per year (Table 22-2). VIPomas are two- to eightfold less common, glucagonomas are seventeen- to thirtyfold less common, and somatostatinomas the least common. In autopsy studies 0.5–1.5% of all cases have a PET; however, in <1 in 1000 cases was a functional tumor thought to occur.

Both carcinoid tumors and PETs commonly show malignant behavior (Tables 22-2 and 22-3). With PETs, except for insulinomas in which <10% are malignant, 50–100% in different series are malignant. With carcinoid tumors, the percentage showing malignant behavior varies in different locations. For the three most common sites of occurrence, the incidence of metastases varies greatly from jejunoileum (58%) > lung/bronchus (6%) > rectum (4%). With both carcinoid tumors and PETs, a number of factors influence survival and the aggressiveness of the tumor (**Table 22-4**). The presence of liver metastases is the single most important prognostic factor in single and multivariate analyses for both carcinoid tumors and PETs. Particularly important in the development of liver metastases is the size of the primary tumor. For example, with small-intestinal carcinoids, the most frequent cause of the carcinoid syndrome due to metastatic disease in the liver (Table 22-2), metastases occur in 15–25% if the tumor diameter is <1 cm, 58–80% if it is 1–2 cm, and >75% if it is >2 cm. Similar data exist for gastrinomas and other PETs, where the size of the primary tumor has been shown to be an independent predictor of the development of liver metastases. The presence of lymph node metastases, the depth of invasion, various histologic features [differentiation, mitotic rates, growth indices, vessel density, vascular endothelial growth factor (VEGF), and CD10 metalloproteinase expression], elevated serum alkaline phosphatase levels, and flow cytometric results (such as the presence of aneuploidy) are all important prognostic factors for the development of metastatic disease (Table 22-4). For patients with carcinoid tumors, additional poor prognostic factors include the development of the carcinoid syndrome, older age, male sex, the presence of a symptomatic tumor, or higher levels of a number of tumor markers [5-hydroxyindolacetic acid (5-HIAA), neuropeptide K, chromogranin A]. With PETs or gastrinomas, the best studied PET, a worse prognosis is associated with female sex, overexpression of the *ha-ras* oncogene or p53, the absence of multiple endocrine neoplasia type 1 (MEN 1), and higher levels of various tumor markers (i.e., chromogranin A, gastrin).

A number of genetic disorders are associated with an increased incidence of NETs (**Table 22-5**). Each one is caused by a loss of a possible tumor-suppressor gene. The most important is MEN 1, an autosomal dominant disorder due to a defect in a 10-exon gene on 11q13, which encodes for a 610-amino-acid nuclear protein, menin (Chap. 23). Patients with MEN 1 develop hyperparathyroidism due to parathyroid hyperplasia in 95–100%, PETs in 80–100%, pituitary adenomas in 54–80%, bronchial carcinoids in 8%, thymic carcinoids in 8%, and gastric carcinoids in 13–30% of the patients with Zollinger-Ellison syndrome (ZES). In patients with MEN 1, 80–100% develop nonfunctional PETs; functional PETs occur in 80%, with 54% developing ZES, 21% insulinomas,

TABLE 22-4

PROGNOSTIC FACTORS IN NEUROENDOCRINE TUMORS

Both carcinoid tumors and PETs
Presence of liver metastases (p <.001)
Extent of liver metastases (p <.001)
Presence of lymph node metastases (p <.001)
Depth of invasion (p <.001)
Elevated serum alkaline phosphatase levels (p = .003)
Primary tumor site (p <.001)
Primary tumor size (p <.005)
Various histologic features
Tumor differentiation (p <.001)
High growth indices (high Ki-67 index, PCNA expression)
High mitotic counts (p <.001)
Vascular or perineural invasion
Vessel density (low microvessel density, increased lymphatic density)
Low VEGF, high CD10 metalloproteinase expression)
Flow cytometric features (i.e., aneuploidy)
Carcinoid tumors
Presence of carcinoid syndrome
Laboratory results [urinary 5-HIAA level (p <.01), plasma neuropeptide K (p <.05), serum chromogranin A (p <.01)]
Presence of a second malignancy
Male sex (p <.001)
Older age (p <.01)
Mode of discovery (incidental > symptomatic)
Molecular findings [TGF-α expression (p <.05), chr 16q LOH or gain chr 4p (p <.05)]
PETs
Ha-Ras oncogene or p53 overexpression
Female sex
MEN 1 syndrome absent
Laboratory findings (increased chromogranin A in some studies; gastrinomas—increased gastrin level)
Molecular findings [increased HER2/neu expression (p = .032), chr 1q, 3p, 3q, or 6q LOH (p = .0004), EGF receptor overexpression (p = .034), gains in chr 7q, 17q, 17p, 20q]

Note: PET, pancreatic endocrine tumor; Ki-67, proliferation-associated nuclear antigen recognized by Ki-67 monoclonal antibody; PCNA, proliferating cell nuclear antigen; 5-HIAA, 5-hydroxyindoleacetic acid; TGF-α, transforming growth factor α; chr, chromosome; LOH, loss of heterozygosity; MEN, multiple endocrine neoplasia; EGF, epidermal growth factor.

TABLE 22-5

GENETIC SYNDROMES ASSOCIATED WITH AN INCREASED INCIDENCE OF NEUROENDOCRINE TUMORS [NETs (CARCINOIDS OR PANCREATIC ENDOCRINE TUMORS) (PETs)]

SYNDROME	LOCATION OF GENE MUTATION AND GENE PRODUCT	NETs SEEN/FREQUENCY
Multiple endocrine neoplasia type 1 (MEN 1)	11q13 (encodes 610-amino-acid protein, menin)	80–100% develop PETs: (nonfunctional > gastrinoma > insulinoma) Carcinoids: gastric (13–30%), bronchial/thymic (8%)
von Hippel–Lindau disease	3q25 (encodes 213-amino-acid protein)	12–17% develop PETs (almost always nonfunctional)
von Recklinghausen's disease [neurofibromatosis 1 (NF 1)]	17q11.2 (encodes 2485-amino-acid protein, neurofibromin)	Duodenal somatostatinomas (usually nonfunctional) Rarely insulinoma, gastrinoma
Tuberous sclerosis	9q34 (TSCI) encodes 1164-amino-acid protein, hamartin) 16p13 (TSC2) (encodes 1807-amino-acid protein, tuberin)	Uncommonly develop PETs [nonfunctional and functional (insulinoma, gastrinoma)]

3% glucagonomas, and 1% VIPomas. MEN 1 is present in 20–25% of all patients with ZES, in 4% with insulinomas, and in a low percentage (<5%) of the other PETs.

Three phacomatoses associated with NETs are von Hippel–Lindau disease (VHL), von Recklinghausen's disease [neurofibromatosis (NF) type 1], and tuberous sclerosis (Bourneville's disease). VHL is an autosomal dominant disorder due to defects in a gene on chromosome 3p25, which encodes a 213-amino-acid protein that interacts with the elongin family of proteins as a transcriptional regulator (Chaps. 6, 23). In addition to cerebellar hemangioblastomas, renal cancer, and pheochromocytomas, 10–17% of these patients develop a PET. Most are nonfunctional, although insulinomas and VIPomas are reported. Patients with NF 1 have defects in a gene on chromosome 17q11.2 encoding for a 2845-amino-acid protein, neurofibromin, which functions in normal cells as a suppressor of the *ras* signaling cascade. Up to 12% of these patients develop an upper GI carcinoid tumor, characteristically in the periampullary region (54%). Many are classified as somatostatinomas because they contain somatostatin immunocytochemically; however, they uncommonly secrete somatostatin or produce a clinical somatostatinoma syndrome. NF 1 has rarely been associated with insulinomas and ZES. Tuberous sclerosis is caused by mutations that alter either the 1164-amino-acid protein, hamartin (TSC1), or the 1807-amino-acid protein, tuberin (TSC2). Both hamartin and tuberin interact in a pathway related to cytosolic G protein regulation. A few cases including nonfunctional and functional PETs (insulinomas and gastrinomas) have been reported in these patients (Table 22-5).

In contrast to most common nonendocrine tumors such as carcinoma of the breast, colon, lung, or stomach, alterations in common oncogenes (*ras, myc, fos, src, jun*) or tumor-suppressor genes (p53, retinoblastoma susceptibility gene) have not been found in PETs or carcinoid tumors. Alterations that may be important in their pathogenesis include changes in the *MEN-1* gene, p16/MTS1 tumor-suppressor gene, and DPC 4/*Smad* 4 gene; amplification of the HER-2/*neu* protooncogene and growth factors and their receptors; methylation of a number of genes likely resulting in their inactivation; and deletions of unknown tumor-suppressor genes as well as gains in other unknown genes (Table 22-1). Comparative genomic hybridization and genome-wide allelotyping studies have shown differences in chromosomal losses and gains between PETs and carcinoids, some of which have prognostic significance (Table 22-4). Mutations in the *MEN-1* gene are likely particularly important. Loss of heterozygosity at the MEN-1 locus on chromosome 11q13 is seen in 93% of sporadic PETs (i.e., in patients without MEN 1) and in 26–75% of sporadic carcinoid tumors. Mutations in the *MEN-1* gene are reported in 31–34% of sporadic gastrinomas. The presence of a number of these molecular alterations (PET or carcinoid) correlates with tumor growth, tumor size, disease extent, or invasiveness and may have prognostic significance.

CARCINOID TUMORS AND CARCINOID SYNDROME

CHARACTERISTICS OF THE MOST COMMON GI CARCINOID TUMORS

Appendiceal Carcinoids

These occur in 1 in every 200–300 appendectomies, usually in the appendiceal tip. In older studies, most (i.e., >90%) are reported as <1 cm in diameter without metastases, but more recent reports find that 2–35% have metastases (Table 22-3). In the Surveillance, Epidemiology, and End Results (SEER) data of 1570 appendiceal carcinoids, 62% were localized and 27% had regional and 8% had distant metastases; half of those between 1 and 2 cm metastasized to lymph nodes. Their percentage of the total number of carcinoids has decreased from 43.9% (1950–1969) to 2.4% (1992–1999).

Small-Intestinal Carcinoids

These are frequently multiple; 70–80% are present in the ileum and 70% within 6 cm (24 in.) of the ileocecal valve. Some 40% are <1 cm in diameter, 32% are 1–2 cm, and 29% are >2 cm. Between 35 and 70% are associated with metastases (Table 22-3). They characteristically cause a marked fibrotic reaction, which can lead to intestinal obstruction. Distant metastases occur to the liver in 36–60%, to bone in 3%, and to lung in 4%. Tumor size affects the frequency of metastases. However, even small carcinoid tumors of the small intestine (<1 cm) have metastases in 15–25%, whereas it increases to 58–100% for tumors 1–2 cm in diameter. Carcinoids also occur in the duodenum, with 31% having metastases. No duodenal tumor <1 cm in two series metastasized, whereas 33% of those >2 cm had metastases. Small-intestinal carcinoids are the most common cause (60–87%) of the carcinoid syndrome and are discussed below.

Rectal Carcinoids

Rectal carcinoids are found in ~1 of every 2500 proctoscopies. Nearly all occur between 4 and 13 cm above the dentate line. Most are small, with 66–80% being <1 cm in diameter, and they rarely metastasize (5%). Tumors between 1 and 2 cm can metastasize in 5–30% and tumors >2 cm, which are uncommon, in >70%.

Bronchial Carcinoids

The frequency of bronchial carcinoids is not related to smoking. A number of different classifications of bronchial carcinoid tumors are proposed. In some studies, lung NETs are classified into four categories: typical carcinoid [also called bronchial carcinoid tumor, Kulchitsky cell carcinoma (KCC)-I]; atypical carcinoid (also called well-differentiated neuroendocrine carcinoma, KCC-II); intermediate small cell neuroendocrine carcinoma; and small cell neuroendocarcinoma (KCC-III). Another proposed classification includes three categories of lung NETs: benign or low-grade malignant (typical carcinoid), low-grade malignant (atypical carcinoid), and high-grade malignant (poorly differentiated carcinoma of the large cell or small cell type). These different categories of lung NETs have different prognoses, varying from excellent for typical carcinoid to poor for small cell neuroendocrine carcinomas.

Gastric Carcinoids

These account for 3 of every 1000 gastric neoplasms. It is thought that three different subtypes of gastric carcinoids occur. Each originates from gastric enterochromaffin-like (ECL) cells in the gastric mucosa. Two subtypes are associated with hypergastrinemic states, either chronic atrophic gastritis (type I) (80% of all gastric carcinoids) or ZES, almost always as part of the MEN 1 syndrome (type II) (6% of all cases). These tumors generally pursue a benign course, with 9–30% associated with metastases. They are usually multiple and small and infiltrate only to the submucosa. The third subtype of gastric carcinoid (type III) (sporadic) occurs without hypergastrinemia (14% of all carcinoids) and pursues an aggressive course, with 54–66% developing metastases. Sporadic carcinoids are usually single, large tumors, 50% have atypical histology, and they can be a cause of the carcinoid syndrome. Gastric carcinoids as a percentage of all carcinoids are increasing in frequency [1.96% (1969–1971), 3.6% (1973–1991), 5.8% (1991–1999)].

CARCINOID TUMORS WITHOUT THE CARCINOID SYNDROME

The age of patients at diagnosis ranges from 10–93 years with a mean of 63 years for the small intestine and 66 years for the rectum. The presentation is diverse and related to the site of origin and extent of malignant spread. In the appendix, carcinoid tumors are usually found incidentally during surgery for suspected appendicitis. Small-intestinal carcinoids in the jejunoileum present with periodic abdominal pain (51%), intestinal obstruction with ileus/invagination (31%), an abdominal tumor (17%), or GI bleeding (11%). Because of the vagueness of the symptoms, the diagnosis is usually delayed ~2 years from onset of the symptoms, ranging up to 20 years. Duodenal, gastric, and rectal carcinoids are most frequently found by chance at endoscopy. The most common symptoms of rectal carcinoids are melena/bleeding (39%), constipation (17%), and diarrhea (12%). Bronchial carcinoids are frequently discovered as a lesion on a chest radiograph, and 31% of the patients are asymptomatic. Thymic carcinoids present as anterior mediastinal masses on chest radiograph or CT scan. Ovarian and testicular carcinoids usually present as masses discovered on physical examination or ultrasound. Metastatic carcinoid tumor in the liver frequently presents as hepatomegaly in a patient who may have minimal symptoms and near-normal liver function tests.

CARCINOID TUMORS WITH SYSTEMIC SYMPTOMS DUE TO SECRETED PRODUCTS

Carcinoid tumors can contain numerous GI peptides: gastrin, insulin, somatostatin, motilin, neurotensin, tachykinins (substance K, substance P, neuropeptide K), glucagon, gastrin-releasing peptide, VIP, PP, other biologically active peptides (ACTH, calcitonin, growth hormone), prostaglandins, and bioactive amines (5-HT). These substances may or may not be released in sufficient amounts to cause symptoms. In various studies of patients with carcinoid tumors, elevated serum levels of PP were found in 43%, motilin in 14%, gastrin in 15%, and VIP in 6%. Foregut carcinoids are more likely to produce various GI peptides than midgut carcinoids. Ectopic ACTH production causing Cushing's syndrome is increasingly seen with foregut carcinoids (respiratory tract primarily) and in some series was the most common cause of the ectopic ACTH syndrome, accounting for 64% of all cases. Acromegaly due to GRF release occurs with foregut carcinoids, as does the somatostatinoma syndrome, but rarely occurs with duodenal carcinoids. The most common systemic syndrome with carcinoid tumors is the carcinoid syndrome.

TABLE 22-6

CLINICAL CHARACTERISTICS IN PATIENTS WITH CARCINOID SYNDROME

	AT PRESENTATION	DURING COURSE OF DISEASE
Symptoms/signs		
Diarrhea	32–73%	68–84%
Flushing	23–65%	63–74%
Pain	10%	34%
Asthma/wheezing	4–8%	3–18%
Pellagra	2%	5%
None	12%	22%
Carcinoid heart disease present	11%	14–41%
Demographics		
Male	46–59%	46–61%
Age		
Mean	57 yrs	52–54 yrs
Range	25–79 yrs	9–91 yrs
Tumor location		
Foregut	5–9%	2–33%
Midgut	78–87%	60–87%
Hindgut	1–5%	1–8%
Unknown	2–11%	2–15%

CARCINOID SYNDROME

Clinical Features

The cardinal features at presentation as well as during the disease course are shown in Table 22-6. Flushing and diarrhea are the two most common symptoms, occurring in up to 73% initially and in up to 89% during the course of the disease. The characteristic flush is of sudden onset; it is a deep red or violaceous erythema of the upper body, especially the neck and face, often associated with a feeling of warmth, and occasionally associated with pruritus, lacrimation, diarrhea, or facial edema. Flushes may be precipitated by stress, alcohol, exercise, certain foods such as cheese, or certain agents such as catecholamines, pentagastrin, and serotonin reuptake inhibitors. Flushing episodes may be brief, lasting 2–5 min, especially initially, or may last hours, especially later in the disease course. Flushing is usually seen with midgut carcinoids but can also occur with foregut carcinoids. With bronchial carcinoids, the flushes are frequently prolonged for hours to days, reddish in color, and associated with salivation, lacrimation, diaphoresis, diarrhea, and hypotension. The flush associated with gastric carcinoids is also reddish in color but patchy in distribution over the face and neck. It may be provoked by food and have accompanying pruritus.

Diarrhea is present in 32–73% initially and 68–84% at some time in their disease course. Diarrhea usually occurs with flushing (85% of cases). The diarrhea is usually described as watery, with 60% having <1 L/d of diarrhea. Steatorrhea is present in 67%, and in 46% it is >15 g/d (normal <7 g). Abdominal pain may be present with the diarrhea or independently in 10–34% of cases.

Cardiac manifestations occur in 11% initially and in 14–41% at some time in the disease course. The cardiac disease is due to fibrosis involving the endocardium, primarily on the right side, although left-side lesions can occur also. The dense fibrous deposits are most commonly on the ventricular aspect of the tricuspid valve and less commonly on the pulmonary valve cusps. They can result in constriction of the valves and pulmonic stenosis is usually predominant, whereas the tricuspid valve is often fixed open, resulting in regurgitation predominating. Up to 80% of patients with cardiac lesions develop heart failure. Lesions on the left side are much less extensive, occur in 30% at autopsy, and most frequently affect the mitral valve.

Other clinical manifestations include wheezing or asthma-like symptoms (8–18%) and pellagra-like skin lesions (2–25%). A variety of noncardiac problems due to increased fibrous tissue have been reported including retroperitoneal fibrosis causing urethral obstruction, Peyronie's disease of the penis, intraabdominal fibrosis, and occlusion of the mesenteric arteries or veins.

Pathobiology

In different studies, carcinoid syndrome occurred in 8% of 8876 patients with carcinoid tumors with a rate of

1.4–18.4%. It only occurs when sufficient concentrations of secreted products by the tumor reach the systemic circulation. In 91% of cases this occurs after distant metastases to the liver. Rarely, primary gut carcinoids with nodal metastases with extensive retroperitoneal invasion, pancreatic carcinoids with retroperitoneal lymph nodes, or carcinoids of the lung or ovary with direct access to the systemic circulation can cause the carcinoid syndrome without hepatic metastases. All carcinoid tumors do not have the same propensity to metastasize and cause the carcinoid syndrome. Midgut carcinoids account for 60–67% of the cases of carcinoid syndrome, foregut tumors for 2–33%, hindgut for 1–8%, and an unknown primary location for 2–15% (Tables 22-2 and 22-3).

One of the main secretory products of carcinoid tumors involved in the carcinoid syndrome is 5-HT (Fig. 22-1), which is synthesized from tryptophan. Up to 50% of dietary tryptophan can be used in this synthetic pathway by tumor cells, which can result in inadequate supplies for conversion to niacin; hence, some patients (2.5%) develop pellagra-like lesions. 5-HT has numerous biologic effects including stimulating intestinal secretion with inhibition of absorption, stimulating increases in intestinal motility, and stimulating fibrogenesis. In various studies 56–88% of all carcinoid tumors were associated with 5-HT overproduction; however, 12–26% of patients did not have the carcinoid syndrome. In one study, platelet 5-HT was elevated in 96% of patients with midgut carcinoids, in 43% with foregut tumors, and in 0% with hindgut tumors. In 90–100% of patients with the carcinoid syndrome, evidence of 5-HT overproduction is noted. 5-HT is thought to be predominantly responsible for the diarrhea by its effects on gut motility and intestinal secretion, primarily through 5-HT_3 and, to a lesser degree, 5-HT_4 receptors. Serotonin receptor antagonists (especially 5-HT_3 antagonists) relieve the diarrhea in most patients. Additional studies suggest prostaglandin E_2 and tachykinins may be important mediators of the diarrhea in some patients. 5-HT does not appear to be involved in the flushing because flushing is not relieved by serotonin receptor antagonists. In patients with gastric carcinoids the red, patchy pruritic flush is likely due to histamine release, because it can be prevented by H_1 and H_2 receptor antagonists. Numerous studies show tachykinins are stored in carcinoid tumors and released during flushing. However, octreotide can relieve the flushing induced by pentagastrin in these patients without altering the stimulated increase in plasma substance P, suggesting that other mediators must be involved in the flushing. Both histamine and 5-HT may be responsible for the wheezing as well as the fibrotic reactions involving the heart, causing Peyronie's disease and intraabdominal fibrosis. The exact mechanism of the heart disease is unclear. The valvular heart disease caused by the appetite-suppressant drug dexfenfluramine is histologically indistinguishable from that observed in carcinoid disease. Furthermore, ergot-containing dopamine receptor agonists used for Parkinson's disease (pergolide, cabergoline) cause valvular heart disease that closely resembles that seen in the carcinoid syndrome. Metabolites of fenfluramine, as well as the dopamine receptor agonists, have high affinity for 5-HT_{2B} receptors, activation of which is known to cause fibroblast mitogenesis. High levels of 5-HT_{2B} receptors are known to occur in heart valves. Studies on cultured interstitial cells from human cardiac valves demonstrate that these valvulopathic drugs induce mitogenesis by activating 5-HT_{2B} receptors and stimulating upregulation of transforming growth factor β and collagen biosynthesis. These observations support the conclusion that 5-HT overproduction by carcinoid tumors is important in mediating the valvular changes, possibly by activating 5-HT_{2B} receptors in the endocardium. Both the magnitude of serotonin overproduction and prior chemotherapy are important predictors of progression of the heart disease. Atrial natriuretic peptide overproduction is also reported in patients with cardiac disease, but its role in the pathogenesis is unknown.

Patients may develop either a typical or atypical carcinoid syndrome. In patients with the typical form, characteristically caused by a midgut carcinoid tumor, the conversion of tryptophan to 5-HTP is the rate-limiting step (Fig. 22-1). Once 5-HTP is formed it is rapidly converted to 5-HT and stored in secretory granules of the tumor or in platelets. A small amount remains in plasma that is converted to 5-HIAA, which appears in large amounts in the urine. These patients have an expanded 5-HT pool size, increased blood and platelet 5-HT, and increased urinary 5-HIAA. Some carcinoid tumors cause an atypical carcinoid syndrome thought due to a deficiency in the enzyme dopa decarboxylase, and thus, 5-HTP cannot be converted to 5-HT and instead is secreted into the bloodstream. In these patients, plasma 5-HT levels are normal but urinary levels may be increased because some 5-HTP is converted to 5-HT in the kidney. Characteristically, urinary 5-HTP and 5-HT are increased, but urinary 5-HIAA levels are only slightly elevated. Foregut carcinoids are most likely to cause an atypical carcinoid syndrome.

One of the most immediate life-threatening complications of the carcinoid syndrome is the development of a carcinoid crisis. This is more frequent in patients who have intense symptoms or have greatly increased urinary 5-HIAA levels (i.e., >200 mg/d). The crises may occur spontaneously or be provoked by stress, anesthesia, chemotherapy, or a biopsy. Patients develop intense flushing, diarrhea, abdominal pain, cardiac abnormalities including tachycardia, hypertension, or hypotension. If not adequately treated, it can be a terminal event.

DIAGNOSIS OF THE CARCINOID SYNDROME AND CARCINOID TUMORS

The diagnosis of carcinoid syndrome relies on measurement of urinary or plasma serotonin or its metabolites in the urine. The measurement of 5-HIAA is most frequently used. False-positive elevations may occur if the patient is eating serotonin-rich foods such as bananas, pineapple, walnuts, pecans, avocados, or hickory nuts or is taking certain medications (cough syrup containing guaifenesin, acetaminophen, salicylates, or l-dopa). The normal range in daily urinary 5-HIAA excretion is 2–8 mg/d. In one study, 92% of patients with carcinoid syndrome had 5-HT overproduction; in another, 5-HIAA had a 73% sensitivity and 100% specificity for carcinoid syndrome.

Most physicians use only the urinary 5-HIAA excretion rate; however, plasma and platelet serotonin levels, if available, may give additional information. Platelet serotonin levels are more sensitive than urinary 5-HIAA but are not generally available. Because patients with foregut carcinoids may produce an atypical carcinoid syndrome, if this syndrome is suspected and urinary 5-HIAA is minimally elevated or normal, other urinary metabolites of tryptophan, such as 5-HTP or 5-HT, should be measured.

Flushing occurs in a number of other conditions, such as systemic mastocytosis, chronic myeloid leukemia with increased histamine release, and menopause; as a reaction to alcohol or glutamate; and as a side effect of chlorpropamide, calcium channel blockers, and nicotinic acid. None of these conditions cause an increased urinary 5-HIAA.

The diagnosis of carcinoid tumor can be suggested by the carcinoid syndrome, by recurrent abdominal symptoms in a healthy-appearing individual, or by discovering hepatomegaly or hepatic metastases associated with minimal symptoms. Ileal carcinoids, which are 25% of all clinically detected carcinoids, should be suspected in patients with bowel obstruction, abdominal pain, flushing, or diarrhea.

Serum chromogranin A levels are elevated in 56–100% of patients with carcinoid tumors, and the level correlates with tumor bulk. Serum chromogranin A levels are not specific for carcinoid tumors because they are also elevated in patients with PETs and other NETs. Plasma neuron-specific enolase levels are also used as a marker of carcinoid tumors but are less sensitive than chromogranin A, being increased in only 17–47% of patients.

℞ Treatment: CARCINOID SYNDROME AND NON-METASTATIC CARCINOID TUMORS

CARCINOID SYNDROME Treatment includes avoiding conditions that precipitate flushing, dietary supplementation with nicotinamide, treatment of heart failure with diuretics, treatment of wheezing with oral bronchodilators, and controlling the diarrhea with antidiarrheal agents such as loperamide or diphenoxylate. If patients still have symptoms, serotonin receptor antagonists or somatostatin analogues are the drugs of choice.

There are 14 subclasses of 5-HT receptors, and antagonists for most are not available. The 5-HT_1 and 5-HT_2 receptor antagonists methysergide, cyproheptadine, and ketanserin have all been used to control the diarrhea but usually do not decrease flushing. Methysergide use is limited because it can cause retroperitoneal fibrosis. Ketanserin diminishes diarrhea in 30–100% of patients. 5-HT_3 receptor antagonists (ondansetron, tropisetron, alosetron) can control diarrhea and nausea in up to 100% of patients and occasionally ameliorate the flushing. A combination of H_1 and H_2 receptor antagonists (i.e., diphenhydramine and cimetidine or ranitidine) may control flushing in patients with foregut carcinoids.

Synthetic analogues of somatostatin (octreotide, lanreotide) are the most widely used agents to control the symptoms of patients with carcinoid syndrome (Fig. 22-2). These drugs are effective at relieving symptoms and decreasing urinary 5-HIAA levels in patients with carcinoid syndrome. Octreotide controls symptoms in >80% of patients, including the diarrhea and flushing, and 70% of patients have a >50% decrease in urinary 5-HIAA excretion. Patients with mild to moderate symptoms should initially be treated with 100 μg SC every 8 h. Individual responses vary, and some patients have received as much as 3000 μg/d. Some 40% of patients escape control after a median of 4 months, and the dose may need to be increased. Similar results are reported with lanreotide.

In patients with carcinoid crises, somatostatin analogues are effective at both treating the condition and preventing symptoms during known precipitating events such as surgery, anesthesia, chemotherapy, or stress. It is recommended that octreotide, 150–250 μg SC every 6–8 h, be used 24–48 h before anesthesia and then continued throughout the procedure.

Sustained-release preparations of both octreotide [octreotide-LAR (long-acting release)] and lanreotide [lanreotide-PR (prolonged release, lanreotide autogel)] permit infrequent injections. Octreotide-LAR (30 mg/month) gives a plasma level ≥1 ng/mL for 25 days, whereas this requires 3–6 injections per day of the non-sustained-release form. Lanreotide-PR is given IM every 10–14 days, and the lanreotide autogel every 4–6 weeks. Each of the sustained-release forms is highly effective at controlling the symptoms of the carcinoid syndrome (61–85% of patients).

Short-term side effects occur in 40–60% of patients receiving SC somatostatin analogues. Pain at the injection site and side effects related to the GI tract (59% discomfort; 15% nausea, diarrhea) are the most common. They are usually short-lived and do not interrupt

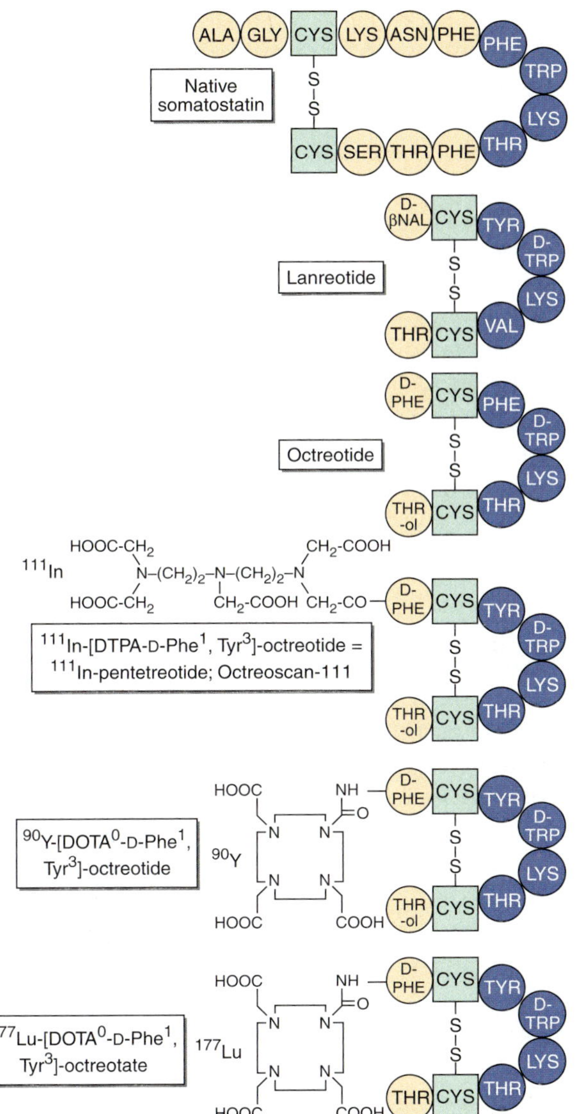

FIGURE 22-2

Structure of somatostatin and synthetic analogues used for diagnostic or therapeutic indications.

treatment. Important long-term side effects include gallstone formation, steatorrhea, and deterioration in glucose tolerance. The overall incidence of gallstones/biliary sludge in one study was 52%, with 7% having symptomatic disease requiring surgical treatment.

Interferon α (IFN-α) is effective in controlling symptoms of the carcinoid syndrome, either alone or combined with hepatic artery embolization. With IFN-α alone the response rate is 42%, and with IFN-α with hepatic artery embolization, diarrhea was controlled for 1 year in 43% and flushing in 86%.

Hepatic artery embolization alone or with chemotherapy (chemoembolization) has been used to control the symptoms of carcinoid syndrome. Embolization alone is reported to control symptoms in up to 76% of patients and chemoembolization (5-fluorouracil, doxorubicin, cisplatin, mitomycin) in 60–75% of patients. Hepatic artery embolization can have major side effects including nausea, vomiting, pain, and fever. In two studies, 5–7% of patients died from complications of hepatic artery occlusion.

Other drugs have been used successfully in small numbers of patients to control the symptoms of carcinoid syndrome. Parachlorophenylalanine can inhibit tryptophan hydroxylase and the conversion of tryptophan to 5-HTP. However, its severe side effects, including psychiatric disturbances, make it intolerable for long-term use. α-Methyldopa inhibits the conversion of 5-HTP to 5-HT; however, its effects are only partial.

CARCINOID TUMORS (NONMETASTATIC)

Surgery is the only potentially curative therapy. The extent of surgical resection is determined by the size of the primary tumor. With appendiceal carcinoids, appendectomy was curative in 103 patients followed for up to 35 years. With rectal carcinoids <1 cm, local resection is curative. With small-intestinal carcinoids <1 cm, consensus had not been reached. Because 15–69% of small-intestinal carcinoids this size have metastases, some recommend a wide resection with en bloc resection of the adjacent lymph-bearing mesentery. If the carcinoid tumor is >2 cm in rectal, appendiceal, or small-intestinal sites, a full cancer operation should be done. This includes a right hemicolectomy for appendiceal carcinoid, an abdominoperineal resection or low anterior resection for rectal carcinoids, and an en bloc resection of adjacent lymph nodes for small-intestinal carcinoids. For carcinoids 1–2 cm in diameter, a simple appendectomy is proposed by some for appendiceal tumors, whereas others favor a formal right hemicolectomy. For 1- to 2-cm rectal carcinoids, a wide local full-thickness excision is performed.

With type I or II gastric carcinoids, which are usually <1 cm, endoscopic removal is recommended. In type I or II gastric carcinoids >2 cm or if there is local invasion, some recommend total gastrectomy, whereas others recommend antrectomy in type I to reduce the hypergastrinemia; antrectomy produced regression of the carcinoids in a number of studies. For types I and III gastric carcinoids of 1 to 2 cm, there is no agreement, with some recommending endoscopic treatment, others surgical treatment. With type III gastric carcinoids >2 cm, excision and regional lymph node clearance is recommended. Most tumors <1 cm are treated endoscopically.

Resection of isolated or limited hepatic metastases may be beneficial.

PANCREATIC ENDOCRINE TUMORS

Functional PETs usually present clinically with symptoms due to the hormone excess state. Only late in the course of the disease does the tumor per se cause prominent symptoms such as abdominal pain. In contrast, all of the symptoms due to nonfunctional PETs are due to the tumor per se. The overall result of this is that some functional PETs may present with severe symptoms with a small or undetectable primary tumor, whereas nonfunctional tumors almost always present late in their disease course with large tumors, which are usually metastatic. The mean delay between onset of continuous symptoms and diagnosis of a functional PET syndrome is 4–7 years. Therefore, the diagnoses are frequently missed for extended periods of time.

Rx Treatment: PANCREATIC ENDOCRINE TUMOR

Treatment of PETs requires two different strategies. (1) Treatment must be directed at the hormone excess state, such as the gastric acid hypersecretion in gastrinomas or hypoglycemia in insulinomas. Ectopic hormone secretion usually causes the presenting symptoms and can cause life-threatening complications. (2) With all of the tumors except insulinomas, >50% are malignant (Table 22-2); therefore, treatment must also be directed against the tumor itself. Because these tumors are frequently widespread, surgical resection for cure, which addresses both treatment aspects, is not possible.

GASTRINOMA (ZOLLINGER-ELLISON SYNDROME)

A gastrinoma is a NET that secretes gastrin; the resultant hypergastrinemia causes gastric acid hypersecretion (ZES). The chronic gastric acid hypersecretion leads to growth of the gastric mucosa with increased numbers of parietal cells and proliferation of gastric ECL cells. The gastric acid hypersecretion characteristically causes peptic ulcer disease (PUD), often refractory and severe, as well as diarrhea. The most common presenting symptoms are abdominal pain (70–100%), diarrhea (37–73%), and gastroesophageal reflux disease (GERD) (30–35%); 10–20% have diarrhea only. Although peptic ulcers may occur in unusual locations, most patients have a typical duodenal ulcer. Important observations that should suggest this diagnosis include PUD with diarrhea; PUD in an unusual location or with multiple ulcers; and PUD refractory to treatment, associated with prominent gastric folds, associated with findings suggestive of MEN 1 (endocrinopathy, family history of ulcer or endocrinopathy, nephrolithiases), or without *Helicobacter pylori* present. *H. pylori* is present in >90% of idiopathic peptic ulcers but is present in <50% of patients with gastrinomas. Chronic unexplained diarrhea should also suggest gastrinoma.

About 20–25% of patients have MEN 1, and in most cases hyperparathyroidism is present prior to the gastrinoma. These patients are treated differently from those without MEN 1; therefore, MEN 1 should be sought in all patients by family history, by measuring plasma ionized calcium and prolactin levels and plasma hormone levels (parathormone, growth hormone).

Most gastrinomas (50–70%) are present in the duodenum, followed by the pancreas (20–40%) and other intraabdominal sites (mesentery, lymph nodes, biliary tract, liver, stomach, ovary). Three cases with two extraabdominal sites have been described: gastrinomas of the left ventricular septum of the heart and non-small cell lung cancer. In MEN 1, the gastrinomas are also usually in the duodenum (70–90%) or the pancreas (10–30%), and they are almost always multiple. About 60–90% of gastrinomas are malignant (Table 22-2) with metastatic spread to lymph nodes and liver. Distant metastases to bone occur in 12–30% of patients with liver metastases.

Diagnosis

The diagnosis of gastrinoma requires the demonstration of fasting hypergastrinemia and an increased basal gastric acid output (BAO) (hyperchlorhydria). Greater than 98% of patients with gastrinomas have fasting hypergastrinemia, although in 40–60% the level may be less than tenfold elevated. Therefore, when the diagnosis is suspected, a fasting gastrin level should be determined first. Potent gastric acid–suppressant drugs such as proton pump inhibitors (e.g., omeprazole, esomeprazole) can suppress acid secretion sufficiently to cause hypergastrinemia; because of their prolonged duration of action, the drugs need to be discontinued for a week before the gastrin determination. If the gastrin level is elevated, it is important to show it is increased when gastric pH is ≤2.0; physiologic hypergastrinemia secondary to achlorhydria (atrophic gastritis, pernicious anemia) is one of the most common causes of hypergastrinemia. Nearly all gastrinoma patients have a fasting pH ≤2 when off antisecretory drugs. If the fasting gastrin is >1000 ng/L (10 times increased) and the pH is ≤2.0, which occurs in 40–60% of patients with gastrinoma, the diagnosis is established after ruling out the possibility of retained antrum syndrome by history. In patients with hypergastrinemia with fasting gastrin <1000 ng/L and gastric pH ≤2.0, other conditions such as *H. pylori* infections, antral G cell hyperplasia/hyperfunction, gastric outlet obstruction, or, rarely, renal failure can masquerade as a gastrinoma. To establish the diagnosis in this group, a determination of BAO and a secretin stimulation test should be done. In patients with gastrinomas without previous gastric acid–reducing surgery, the BAO is usually (>90%) elevated (i.e., >15 meq/h). The secretin stimulation test is usually positive, with the criterion of >120 ng/L increase over the basal level having the highest sensitivity (94%) and specificity (100%).

Treatment: GASTRINOMAS

Gastric acid hypersecretion in patients with gastrinomas can be controlled in almost every case by oral gastric antisecretory drugs. Because of their long duration of action and potency, allowing once- or twice-a-day dosing, the proton pump inhibitors are the drugs of choice. H_2 receptor antagonists are also effective, although more frequent dosing (every 4–8 h) and high doses are frequently required. In patients with MEN 1 with hyperparathyroidism, correction of the hyperparathyroidism increases the sensitivity to gastric antisecretory drugs and decreases the basal acid output.

With the increased ability to control acid hypersecretion, >50% of the patients who are not cured (>60% of patients) will die from tumor-related causes. At presentation, careful imaging studies are essential to localize the extent of the tumor. One-third of patients present with hepatic metastases, and in <15% of those with hepatic metastases the disease is limited, so that surgical resection may be possible. Surgical cure is possible in 30% of patients without MEN 1 or liver metastases (40% of all patients). In patients with MEN 1, long-term surgical cure is rare because the tumors are multiple, frequently with lymph node metastases. Therefore, all patients with gastrinomas without MEN 1 or a medical condition limiting life expectancy should undergo surgery by an experienced surgeon.

INSULINOMAS

An insulinoma is an endocrine tumor of the pancreas derived from beta cells that ectopically secretes insulin, which results in hypoglycemia. The average age of occurrence is 40–50 years. The most common clinical symptoms are due to the effect of the hypoglycemia on the central nervous system (neuroglycemic symptoms) and include confusion, headache, disorientation, visual difficulties, irrational behavior, or even coma. Also, most patients have symptoms due to excess catecholamine release secondary to the hypoglycemia including sweating, tremor, and palpitations. Characteristically, these attacks are associated with fasting.

Insulinomas are generally small (>90% <2 cm) and usually not multiple (90%), and only 5–15% are malignant; they almost invariably occur only in the pancreas, distributed equally in the pancreatic head, body, and tail.

Insulinomas should be suspected in all patients with hypoglycemia, especially with a history suggesting attacks provoked by fasting or with a family history of MEN 1. Insulin is synthesized as proinsulin, a 21-amino-acid α chain and a 30-amino-acid β chain connected by a 33-amino-acid connecting peptide (C peptide). In insulinomas, in addition to elevated plasma insulin levels, elevated plasma proinsulin levels are found and C-peptide levels can be elevated.

Diagnosis

The diagnosis of insulinoma requires the demonstration of an elevated plasma insulin level at the time of hypoglycemia. A number of other conditions may cause fasting hypoglycemia, such as the inadvertent or surreptitious use of insulin or oral hypoglycemic agents, severe liver disease, alcoholism, poor nutrition, or other extrapancreatic tumors. The most reliable test to diagnose insulinoma is a fast up to 72 h with serum glucose, C-peptide, and insulin measurements every 4–8 h. If at any point the patient becomes symptomatic or glucose levels are persistently <2.2 mmol/L (40 mg/dL), the test should be terminated and repeat samples for the above studies obtained before glucose is given. Some 70–80% of patients will develop hypoglycemia during the first 24 h and 98% by 48 h. In nonobese normal subjects, serum insulin levels should decrease to <43 pmol/L (<6 μU/mL) when blood glucose decreases to ≤2.2 mmol/L (≤40 mg/dL) and the ratio of insulin to glucose is <0.3 (in mg/dL). In addition to having an insulin level >6 μU/mL when blood glucose is ≤40 mg/dL, some investigators also require an elevated C-peptide and serum proinsulin level, an insulin/glucose ratio >0.3, and a decreased plasma β-hydroxybutyrate level for the diagnosis of insulinomas. Surreptitious use of insulin or hypoglycemic agents may be difficult to distinguish from insulinomas. The combination of proinsulin levels (normal in exogenous insulin/hypoglycemic agent users), C-peptide levels (low in exogenous insulin users), antibodies to insulin (positive in exogenous insulin users), and measurement of sulfonylurea levels in serum or plasma will allow the correct diagnosis to be made. The diagnosis of insulinoma has been complicated by the introduction of specific insulin assays that do not also interact with proinsulin, as do many of the older radioimmunoassays (RIAs), and therefore give lower plasma insulin levels. The increased use of these specific insulin assays has resulted in increased numbers of patients with insulinomas having lower plasma insulin values than the 43 pmol/L (6 μU/mL) levels proposed to be characteristic of insulinomas by RIA. In these patients the assessment of proinsulin and C-peptide levels at the time of hypoglycemia are particularly helpful for establishing the correct diagnosis.

Treatment: INSULINOMAS

Only 5–15% of insulinomas are malignant; therefore, after appropriate imaging, surgery should be performed. In different studies, 75–95% of patients are cured by surgery. Before surgery, the hypoglycemia can be controlled by frequent small meals and the use of diazoxide (150–800 mg/d). Diazoxide is a benzothiadiazide whose hyperglycemic effect is attributed to inhibition of insulin release. Its side effects are sodium retention and GI symptoms such as nausea. Approximately 50–60% of patients respond to diazoxide. Other agents effective in some patients to control the hypoglycemia include verapamil and diphenylhydantoin. Long-acting somatostatin analogues such as octreotide are acutely effective in 40% of patients. However, octreotide needs to be used with care because it inhibits growth hormone secretion and can alter plasma glucagon levels; therefore, in some patients it can worsen the hypoglycemia.

For the 5–15% of patients with malignant insulinomas, the above drugs or somatostatin analogues are used initially. If they are not effective, various antitumor treatments such as hepatic arterial embolization, chemoembolization, or chemotherapy have been used (see below).

GLUCAGONOMAS

A glucagonoma is an endocrine tumor of the pancreas that secretes excessive amounts of glucagon, which causes a distinct syndrome characterized by dermatitis, glucose intolerance or diabetes, and weight loss. Glucagonomas principally occur between 45 and 70 years of age. The tumor is clinically heralded by a characteristic dermatitis (migratory necrolytic erythema) (67–90%), accompanied by glucose intolerance (40–90%), weight loss (66–96%), anemia (33–85%), diarrhea (15–29%), and thromboembolism (11–24%). The rash starts usually as an annular erythema at intertriginous and periorificial sites, especially in the groin or buttock. It subsequently becomes raised and bullae form; when the bullae rupture, eroded areas form. The lesions can wax and wane. A characteristic laboratory finding is hypoaminoacidemia, which occurs in 26–100% of patients.

Glucagonomas are generally large tumors (5–10 cm) at diagnosis. Some 50–80% occur in the pancreatic tail. From 50–82% have evidence of metastatic spread at presentation, usually to the liver. Glucagonomas are rarely extrapancreatic and usually occur singly.

Diagnosis

The diagnosis is confirmed by demonstrating an increased plasma glucagon level (normal is <150 ng/L). Plasma glucagon levels are >1000 ng/L in 90%, between 500 and 1000 ng/L in 7%, and <500 ng/L in 3%. A plasma glucagon level >1000 ng/L is considered diagnostic of glucagonoma. Other diseases causing increased plasma glucagon levels include renal insufficiency, acute pancreatitis, hypercorticism, hepatic insufficiency, prolonged fasting, or familial hyperglucagonemia. With the exception of cirrhosis, these disorders do not increase plasma glucagon to >500 ng/L.

℞ Treatment: GLUCAGONOMAS

In 50–80% of patients, metastases are present, so curative surgical resection is not possible. Surgical debulking in patients with advanced disease or other antitumor treatments may be beneficial (see below). Long-acting somatostatin analogues such as octreotide or lanreotide improve the skin rash in 75% of patients and may improve the weight loss, pain, and diarrhea but usually do not improve the glucose intolerance.

SOMATOSTATINOMA SYNDROME

The somatostatinoma syndrome is due to a NET that secretes excessive amounts of somatostatin, which causes a distinct syndrome characterized by diabetes mellitus, gallbladder disease, diarrhea, and steatorrhea. There is no general distinction in the literature between a tumor that contains somatostatin-like immunoreactivity (somatostatinoma) and does (11–45%) or does not (55–89%) produce a clinical syndrome (somatostatinoma syndrome) by secreting somatostatin. In one review of 173 cases of somatostatinomas, only 11% were associated with the somatostatinoma syndrome. The mean age of patients is 51 years. Somatostatinomas occur primarily in the pancreas and small intestine, and the frequency of the symptoms differs in each. Each of the usual symptoms is more frequent in pancreatic than intestinal somatostatinomas: diabetes mellitus (95% vs 21%), gallbladder disease (94% vs 43%), diarrhea (92% vs 38%), steatorrhea (83% vs 12%), hypochlorhydria (86% vs 12%), and weight loss (90% vs 69%). Somatostatinomas occur in the pancreas in 56–74% of cases, with the primary location being in the pancreatic head. The tumors are usually solitary (90%) and large, with a mean size of 4.5 cm. Liver metastases are frequent, being present in 69–84% of patients.

Somatostatin is a tetradecapeptide that is widely distributed in the central nervous system and GI tract, where it functions as a neurotransmitter or has paracrine and autocrine actions. It is a potent inhibitor of many processes including release of almost all hormones, acid secretion, intestinal and pancreatic secretion, and intestinal absorption. Most of the clinical manifestations are directly related to these inhibitory actions.

Diagnosis

In most cases somatostatinomas have been found by accident either at the time of cholecystectomy or during endoscopy. The presence of psammoma bodies in a duodenal tumor should particularly raise suspicion. Duodenal somatostatin-containing tumors are increasingly associated with von Recklinghausen's disease. Most of these do not cause the somatostatinoma syndrome. The diagnosis of the somatostatinoma syndrome requires the demonstration of elevated plasma somatostatin levels.

℞ Treatment: SOMATOSTATINOMAS

Pancreatic tumors are frequently (70–92%) metastatic at presentation, whereas 30–69% of small-intestinal somatostatinomas have metastases. Surgery is the treatment of choice for those without widespread hepatic metastases. Symptoms in patients with the somatostatinoma syndrome are improved by octreotide treatment.

VIPomas

VIPomas are endocrine tumors that secrete excessive amounts of VIP, which causes a distinct syndrome characterized by large-volume diarrhea, hypokalemia, and dehydration. This syndrome is also called Verner-Morrison syndrome, pancreatic cholera, and WDHA syndrome for *w*atery *d*iarrhea, *h*ypokalemia, and *a*chlorhydria, which some patients develop. The mean age of patients with this syndrome is 49 years; however, it can occur in children and when it does, it is usually caused by a ganglioneuroma or ganglioneuroblastoma.

The principal symptoms are large-volume diarrhea (100%) severe enough to cause hypokalemia (80–100%), dehydration (83%), hypochlorhydria (54–76%), and flushing (20%). The diarrhea is secretory in nature, persists during fasting, and is almost always >1 L/d and >3 L/d in 70%. Most patients do not have accompanying steatorrhea (16%), and the increased stool volume is due to increased excretion of sodium and potassium, which, with the anions, account for the osmolality of the stool. Patients frequently have hyperglycemia (25–50%) and hypercalcemia (25–50%).

VIP is a 28-amino-acid peptide important as a neurotransmitter, ubiquitously present in the central nervous system and GI tract. Its known actions include stimulation of small-intestinal chloride secretion, effects on smooth-muscle contractility, inhibition of acid secretion, and vasodilatory effects, which explain most features of the clinical syndrome.

In adults, 80–90% of VIPomas are pancreatic in location, with the rest due to VIP-secreting pheochromocytomas, intestinal carcinoids, and, rarely, ganglioneuromas. These tumors are usually solitary, 50–75% are in the pancreatic tail, and 37–68% have hepatic metastases at diagnosis. In children <10 years old, the syndrome is usually due to ganglioneuromas or ganglioblastomas and is less often malignant (10%).

Diagnosis

The diagnosis requires the demonstration of an elevated plasma VIP level and the presence of large-volume diarrhea. A stool volume of <700 mL/d is proposed to exclude the diagnosis of VIPoma. By fasting the patient, a number of causes can be excluded that cause marked diarrhea. Other diseases that can give a secretory large-volume diarrhea include gastrinomas, chronic laxative abuse, carcinoid syndrome, systemic mastocytosis, rarely medullary thyroid cancer, diabetes, and AIDS. Of these conditions, only VIPomas cause a marked increase in plasma VIP.

℞ Treatment: VASOACTIVE INTESTINAL PEPTIDOMAS

The most important initial treatment in these patients is to correct their dehydration, hypokalemia, and electrolyte losses with fluid and electrolyte replacement. These patients may require 5 L/d of fluid and >350 meq/d of potassium. Because 37–68% of adults with VIPomas have metastatic disease in the liver at presentation, a significant number of patients cannot be cured surgically. In these patients long-acting somatostatin analogues such as octreotide or lanreotide are the drugs of choice.

Octreotide will control the diarrhea in 87% of patients. In nonresponsive patients the combination of glucocorticoids and octreotide has proved helpful in a small number of patients. Other drugs reported to be helpful in small numbers of patients include prednisone (60–100 mg/d), clonidine, indomethacin, phenothiazines, loperamide, lidamidine, lithium, propranolol, and metoclopramide. Treatment of advanced disease with embolization, chemoembolization, and chemotherapy may also be helpful.

NONFUNCTIONAL PANCREATIC ENDOCRINE TUMORS

Nonfunctional PETs are endocrine tumors that originate in the pancreas and either secrete no products or their products do not cause a specific clinical syndrome. The symptoms are due entirely to the tumor per se. Nonfunctional PETs secrete chromogranin A (90–100%), chromogranin B (90–100%), PP (58%), α-hCG (40%), and β-hCG (20%). Because the symptoms are due to the tumor alone, patients with nonfunctional PETs usually present late in their disease course with invasive tumors and hepatic metastases (64–92%), and the tumors are usually large (72% >5 cm). The tumors are usually solitary except in patients with MEN 1, where they are multiple. They occur primarily in the pancreatic head. Even though these tumors do not cause a functional syndrome, immunocytochemical studies show they synthesize numerous peptides and cannot be distinguished from functional tumors by immunocytochemistry.

The most common symptoms are abdominal pain (30–80%); jaundice (20–35%); and weight loss, fatigue, or bleeding; 10–15% are found incidentally. The average time from the beginning of symptoms to diagnosis is 5 years.

Diagnosis

The diagnosis is established by histologic confirmation in a patient without either clinical symptoms or elevated plasma hormone levels. Even though chromogranin A levels are elevated in almost every patient, this is not specific for this disease as it can be found in functional PETs, carcinoids, and other neuroendocrine disorders. Plasma PP is increased in 22–71% of patients and should strongly suggest the diagnosis in a patient with a pancreatic mass because it is usually normal in patients with pancreatic adenocarcinomas. Elevated plasma PP is not diagnostic of this tumor because it is elevated in a number of other conditions such as chronic renal failure, old age, inflammatory conditions, and diabetes.

℞ Treatment: NONFUNCTIONAL PANCREATIC ENDOCRINE TUMORS

Unfortunately, surgical curative resection can be considered only in the minority of the patients because 64–92% present with metastatic disease. Treatment is directed against the tumor per se using chemotherapy, embolization, chemoembolization, or hormonal therapy.

GRFomas

GRFomas are endocrine tumors that secrete excessive amounts of GRF that causes acromegaly. The true frequency of this syndrome is not known. GRF is a 44-amino-acid peptide, and 25–44% of PETs have GRF immunoreactivity, although it is uncommonly secreted. GRFomas are lung tumors in 47–54% of cases, PETs in 29–30%, and small-intestinal carcinoids in 8–10%; up to 12% occur at other sites. Patients have a mean age of 38 years, and the symptoms are usually due to either acromegaly or the tumor itself. The acromegaly caused by GRFomas is indistinguishable from classic acromegaly. The pancreatic tumors are usually large (>6 cm), and liver metastases are present in 39%. They should be suspected in any patient with acromegaly and an abdominal tumor, in a patient with MEN 1 with acromegaly, or in a patient without a pituitary adenoma with acromegaly or associated with hyperprolactinemia, which occurs in 70% of GRFomas. GRFomas are an uncommon cause of acromegaly. The diagnosis is established by performing plasma assays for GRF and growth hormone. The normal level for GRF is <5 μg/L in men and <10 μg/L in women. Most GRFomas have a plasma GRF level ≥300 μg/L. Patients with GRFomas also have increased plasma insulin-like growth factor I levels similar to those in classic acromegaly. Surgery is the treatment of choice if diffuse metastases are not present. Long-acting somatostatin analogues such as octreotide or lanreotide are the agents of choice, with 75–100% of patients responding.

OTHER RARE PANCREATIC ENDOCRINE TUMOR SYNDROMES

Cushing's syndrome (ACTHoma) due to a PET occurs in 4–16% of all ectopic Cushing's syndrome cases. It occurs in 5% of cases of sporadic gastrinomas, almost invariably in patients with hepatic metastases, and is an independent poor prognostic factor. Paraneoplastic hypercalcemia due to PETs releasing parathyroid hormone–related peptide (PTHrP), a PTH-like material, or unknown factor is rarely reported. The tumors are usually large, and liver metastases are usually present. Most (88%) appear to be due to release of PTHrP. PETs can occasionally cause the carcinoid syndrome. PETs secreting calcitonin have been proposed as a specific clinical syndrome. Half of the patients have diarrhea, which disappears with resection of the tumor. The proposal that this could be a discrete syndrome is supported by finding that 25–42% of patients with medullary thyroid cancer with hypercalcitoninemia develop diarrhea, likely secondary to a motility disorder. A renin-producing PET has been described in a patient presenting with hypertension; PETs secreting luteinizing hormone, resulting in masculinization or decreased libido, and PETs secreting erythropoietin, resulting in polycythemia, have also been reported (Table 22-2). Ghrelin is a 28-amino-acid peptide with a number of metabolic and immunologic functions. Although it is detectable immunohistochemically in most PETs, only 1 in 24 patients (4%) with a PET had elevated plasma ghrelin levels in one study and the patient was asymptomatic. Release of ghrelin by a PET may be clinically silent.

TUMOR LOCALIZATION

Localization of the primary tumor and defining the extent of disease are essential to the proper management of all carcinoids and PETs. Numerous tumor localization methods are used in both types of NETs, including conventional imaging studies (CT, MRI, transabdominal ultrasound, selective angiography), somatostatin receptor scintigraphy (SRS), and positron emission tomographic scanning. In PETs, endoscopic ultrasound (EUS) and functional localization by measuring venous hormonal gradients are also reported useful. Bronchial carcinoids are usually detected by a standard chest radiograph and assessed by CT. Rectal, duodenal, colonic, and gastric carcinoids are usually detected by GI endoscopy.

PETs, as well as carcinoid tumors, frequently overexpress high-affinity somatostatin receptors in both their primary tumors and their metastases. Of the five types of somatostatin receptors (sst_{1-5}), radiolabeled octreotide binds with high affinity to sst_2 and sst_5, lower for sst_3, and has a very low affinity for sst_1 and sst_4. Between 90 and 100% of carcinoid tumors and PETs possess sst_2, and many also have the other four sst subtypes. Interaction with these receptors can be used to localize NETs using $[^{111}$In-DTPA-d-Phe$^1]$octreotide and radionuclide scanning (SRS) as well as for treatment of the hormone excess state with octreotide or lanreotide, as discussed earlier. Because of its sensitivity and ability to localize tumor throughout the body, SRS is now the initial imaging modality of choice for localizing both primary and metastatic NETs. SRS localizes tumor in 73–89% of patients with carcinoids and in 56–100% of patients with PETs, except for insulinomas. Insulinomas are usually small and have low densities of sst receptors, resulting in SRS being positive in only 12–50% of patients with insulinomas. Figure 22-3 shows an example of the increased sensitivity of SRS in a patient with a carcinoid tumor. The CT scan (Fig. 22-3*A*) shows a single liver metastasis, whereas the SRS demonstrates three metastases in the liver in multiple locations (Fig. 22-3*B*). Occasional false-positive responses with SRS can occur (12% in one study) because numerous other normal tissues and diseases can have high densities of sst receptors, including granulomas (sarcoid, tuberculosis, etc.), thyroid diseases (goiter, thyroiditis), and activated lymphocytes (lymphomas, wound infections). For PETs located in the pancreas, EUS is highly sensitive, localizing 77–93% of insulinomas, which occur almost exclusively within the pancreas. EUS is less sensitive for extrapancreatic tumors. If liver metastases are identified by SRS, either a CT or MRI is then recommended to assess the size and exact location of the metastases because SRS does not give information on tumor size. Functional localization measuring hormone gradients after intraarterial calcium injections in insulinomas (insulin) or gastrin gradients after secretin injections in gastrinoma is a sensitive method, being positive in 80–100% of patients. However, this method gives only regional localization and therefore is reserved for cases where other imaging modalities are negative. Positron emission tomographic scanning with ^{18}F-fluoro-DOPA in patients with carcinoids or with ^{11}C-5-HTP in patients with PETs or carcinoids has greater sensitivity than conventional imaging studies or SRS and will likely be used increasingly in the future.

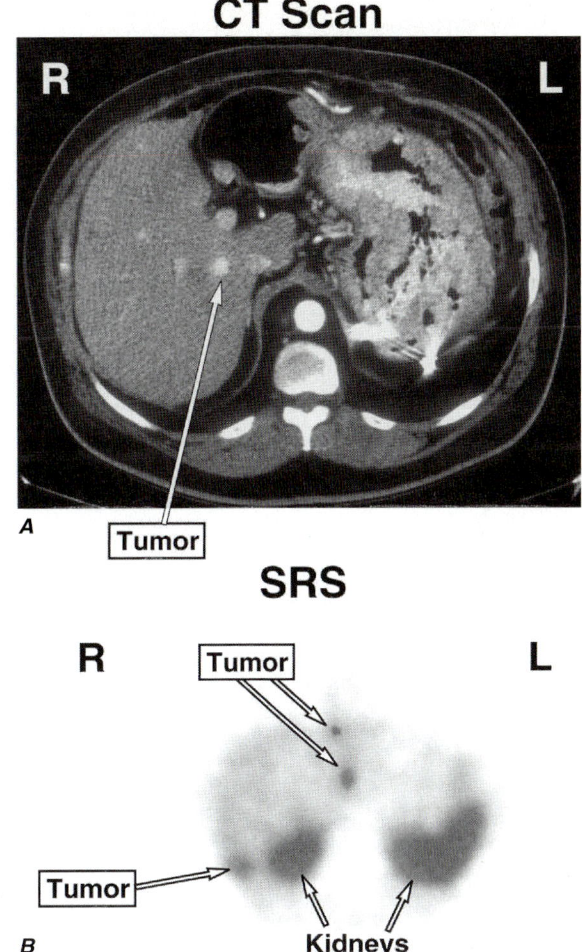

FIGURE 22-3

Ability of CT scanning (*A*) or somatostatin receptor scintigraphy (SRS) (*B*) to localize metastatic carcinoid in the liver.

℞ Treatment: ADVANCED DISEASE (DIFFUSE METASTATIC DISEASE)

The single most important prognostic factor for survival is the presence of liver metastases (Fig. 22-4). For patients with foregut carcinoids without hepatic metastases, the 5-year survival in one study was 95% and with distant metastases, 20%. With gastrinomas, the 5-year survival without liver metastases is 98%, with limited metastases in one hepatic lobe it is 78%, and with diffuse metastases it is 16%. A number of different modalities are reported to be effective in advanced disease including cytoreductive surgery (removal of all visible tumor), treatment with chemotherapy, somatostatin analogues, IFN-α, hepatic embolization alone or with chemotherapy (chemoembolization), radiotherapy, and liver transplantation.

SPECIFIC ANTITUMOR TREATMENTS Cytoreductive surgery, unfortunately, is only possible in the

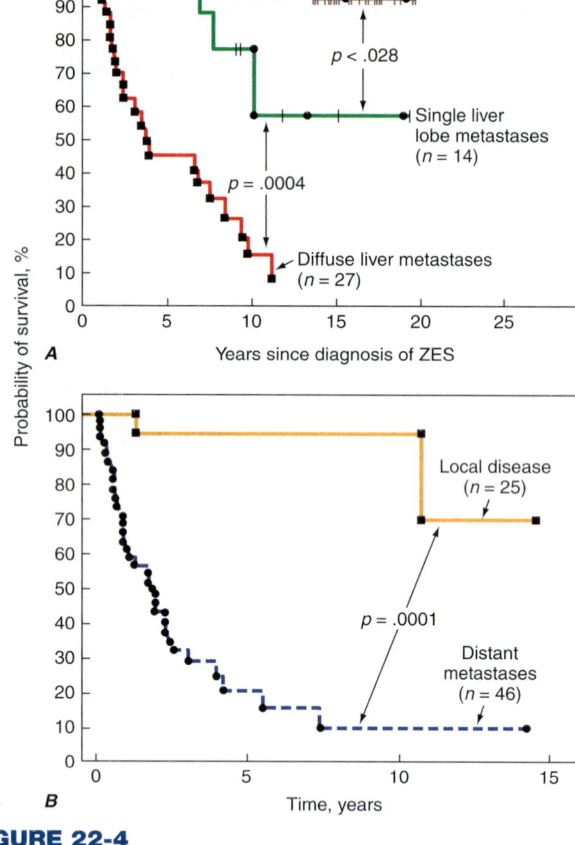

FIGURE 22-4

Effect of the presence and extent of liver metastases on survival in patients with gastrinomas (***A***) or carcinoid tumors (***B***). ZES, Zollinger-Ellison syndrome. (*A is drawn from data from 199 patients with gastrinomas modified from F Yu et al: J Clin Oncol 17:615, 1999. B is drawn from data from 71 patients with foregut carcinoid tumors from EW McDermott et al: Br J Surg 81:1007, 1994.*)

9–22% of patients who have limited hepatic metastases. Although no randomized studies have proven that hepatic resection extends life, results from a number of studies suggest it likely increases survival and therefore is recommended, if possible.

Chemotherapy for metastatic carcinoid tumors has generally been disappointing, with response rates of 0–40% with various two- or three-drug combinations. Chemotherapy for PETs has been more successful, with tumor shrinkage reported in 30–70% of patients. The current regimen of choice is streptozotocin and doxorubicin.

Long-acting somatostatin analogues such as octreotide, lanreotide, and IFN-α rarely decrease tumor size (i.e., 0–17%); however, these drugs have tumorostatic effects, stopping additional growth in 26–95% of patients with NETs. How long tumor stabilization lasts or whether it prolongs survival has not been established.

Hepatic embolization and chemoembolization (with dacarbazine, cisplatin, doxorubicin, 5-fluorouracil, or streptozotocin) have been reported to decrease tumor bulk and to help control the symptoms of the hormone excess state. These modalities are generally reserved for cases in which treatment with somatostatin analogues, IFN-α (carcinoids), or chemotherapy (PETs) fails. Embolization, when combined with treatment with octreotide and IFN-α, significantly reduces tumor progression ($p = .008$) over treatment with embolization and octreotide alone in patients with advanced midgut carcinoids.

Radiotherapy with radiolabeled somatostatin analogues that are internalized by the tumors is an approach under investigation. Three different radionuclides are being used: (1) high doses of [^{111}In-DTPA-d-Phe^{1}] octreotide (Fig. 22-2), which emits γ rays, internal conversion, and Auger electrons; yttrium-90, which emits high-energy β particles coupled by a DOTA chelating group to octreotide or octreotate; and (3) ^{177}lutetium-coupled analogues, which emit both β and γ rays. All are being tested. Tumor stabilization is reported in 41–81%, 44–88%, and 23–40%, respectively, and a decrease in tumor size in 8–30%, 6–37%, and 38%, respectively, of patients with advanced metastatic NETs. These results suggest this novel therapy may be helpful, especially in patients with advanced metastatic disease.

The use of liver transplantation has been abandoned for treatment of most metastatic tumors to the liver. However, for metastatic NETs it is still a consideration. In a review of 103 cases of malignant NETs (48 PETs, 43 carcinoids), the 2- and 5-year survival rates were 60% and 47%, respectively. However, recurrence-free survival was low (<24%). It was concluded that for younger patients with metastatic NETs limited to the liver, liver transplantation may be justified.

FURTHER READINGS

Berna MJ et al: A prospective study of gastric carcinoids and enterochromaffin-like cell changes in multiple endocrine neoplasia type 1 and Zollinger-Ellison syndrome: Identification of risk factors. J Clin Endocrinol Metab 93:1582, 2008

Forrer F et al: Peptide receptor radiotherapy. Best Pract Res Clin Endocrinol Metab 21:111, 2007

Jensen RT, Doherty GM: Carcinoid tumors and the carcinoid syndrome, in *Cancer: Principles and Practice of Oncology*, 7th ed, VT DeVita Jr, S Hellman, SA Rosenberg (eds). Philadelphia, Lippincott Williams and Wilkins, 2005, pp 1559–1574

Kulke MH et al: Glycemic control in patients with insulinoma treated with everolimus. N Engl J Med 360:195, 2009

Modlin IM et al: Therapeutic options for gastrointestinal carcinoids. Clin Gastrointest Hepatol 4:526, 2006

Oberg K, Eriksson B: Neuroendocrine tumors. Best Pract Res Clin Endocrinol Metabol 21:1, 2007

Placzkowski KA et al: Secular trends in the presentation and management of functioning insulinoma at the Mayo Clinic, 1987-2007. J Clin Endocrinol Metab 94:1069, 2009

Rindi G et al (ed): Consensus guidelines on the management of patients with digestive neuroendocrine tumors. Neuroendocrinology 84:151, 2006

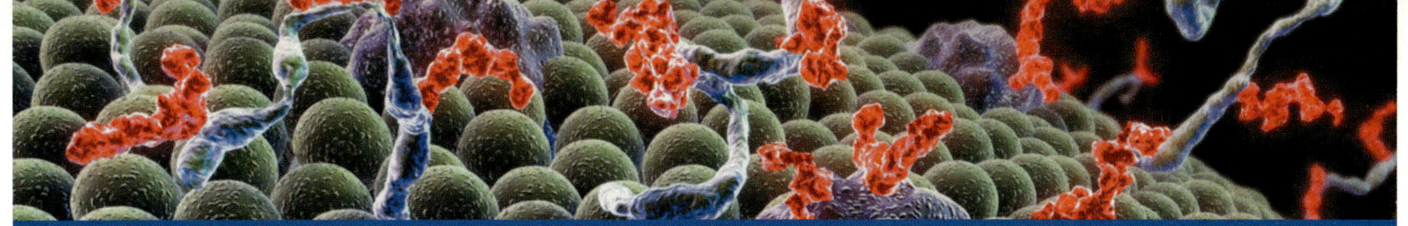

CHAPTER 23

MULTIPLE ENDOCRINE NEOPLASIAS AND AUTOIMMUNE ENDOCRINOPATHIES

Camilo Jimenez ■ Robert F. Gagel

NEOPLASTIC DISORDERS AFFECTING MULTIPLE ENDOCRINE ORGANS

Multiple endocrine neoplasia syndrome is defined as a disorder with neoplasms in two or more different hormonal tissues in several members of a family. Several distinct genetic disorders predispose to endocrine gland neoplasia and cause hormone excess syndromes (**Table 23-1**). DNA-based genetic testing is now available for these disorders, but effective management requires an understanding of endocrine neoplasia and the range of clinical features that may be manifested in an individual patient.

MULTIPLE ENDOCRINE NEOPLASIA (MEN) TYPE 1

MEN 1, or Wermer's syndrome, is inherited as an autosomal dominant trait. This syndrome is characterized by neoplasia of the parathyroid glands, enteropancreatic tumors, anterior pituitary adenomas, and other neuroendocrine tumors with variable penetrance (Table 23-1). Although rare, MEN 1 is the most common multiple endocrine neoplasia syndrome with an estimated prevalence of 2–20 per 100,000 in the general population. This syndrome is caused by inactivating mutations of the tumor suppressor gene *MEN1* located at chromosome 11q13. The *MEN1* gene codes for a nuclear protein called Menin. Menin interacts with JunD, suppressing the JunD-dependent transcriptional activation. It is unclear how this accounts for Menin growth regulatory activity, since JunD is associated with inhibition of cell growth. Each child born to an affected parent has a 50% probability of inheriting the gene. The variable penetrance of the several neoplastic components can make the differential diagnosis and treatment challenging.

Clinical Manifestations

Primary hyperparathyroidism is the most common manifestation of MEN 1, with an estimated penetrance of 95–100%. Hypercalcemia may develop during the teenage years, and most individuals are affected by age 40 (**Fig. 23-1**). Hyperparathyroidism is the earliest manifestation of the syndrome in most MEN 1 patients. The neoplastic changes in hyperparathyroidism provide a specific example of one

TABLE 23-1

DISEASE ASSOCIATIONS IN THE MULTIPLE ENDOCRINE NEOPLASIA (MEN) SYNDROMES

MEN 1	MEN 2	MIXED SYNDROMES
Parathyroid hyperplasia or adenoma Islet cell hyperplasia, adenoma, or carcinoma Pituitary hyperplasia or adenoma Other less common manifestations: foregut carcinoid, pheochromocytoma, subcutaneous or visceral lipomas	**MEN 2A** MTC Pheochromocytoma Parathyroid hyperplasia or adenoma **MEN 2A with cutaneous lichen amyloidosis** **MEN 2A with Hirschsprung disease** **Familial MTC** **MEN 2B** MTC Pheochromocytoma Mucosal and gastrointestinal neuromas Marfanoid features	**Von Hippel–Lindau syndrome** Pheochromocytoma Islet cell tumor Renal cell carcinoma Hemangioblastoma of central nervous system Retinal angiomas **Neurofibromatosis with features of MEN 1 or 2** **Carney complex** Myxomas of heart, skin, and breast Spotty cutaneous pigmentation Testicular, adrenal, and GH-producing pituitary tumors Peripheral nerve schwannomas

Note: GH, growth hormone; MTC, medullary thyroid carcinoma.

of the cardinal features of endocrine tumors in MEN 1—multicentricity. The neoplastic changes inevitably affect multiple parathyroid glands, making surgical cure difficult. Screening for hyperparathyroidism involves measurement of either an albumin-adjusted or ionized serum calcium level. The diagnosis is established by demonstrating elevated levels of serum calcium and

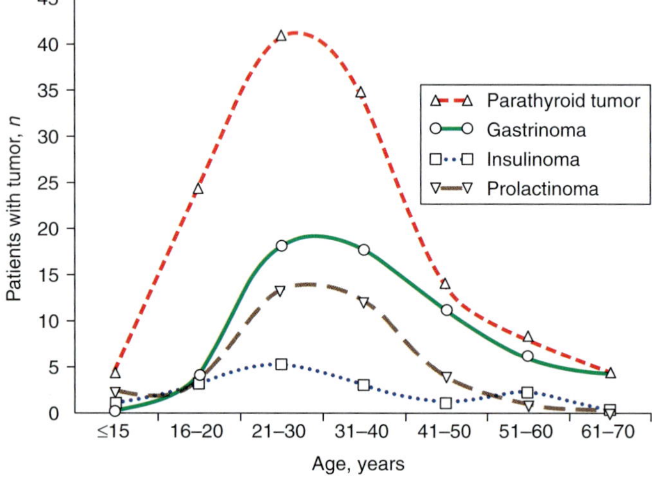

FIGURE 23-1

Age at onset of endocrine tumor expression in multiple endocrine neoplasia type 1 (MEN 1). Data derived from retrospective analysis for each endocrine organ hyperfunction in 130 cases of MEN 1. Age at onset is the age at first symptom or, with tumors not causing symptoms, age at the time of the first abnormal finding on a screening test. The rate of diagnosis of hyperparathyroidism increased sharply between ages 16 and 20 years. (*Reprinted with permission from S Marx et al: Ann Intern Med 129:484, 1998.*)

intact parathyroid hormone. Manifestations of hyperparathyroidism of MEN 1 do not differ substantially from those in sporadic hyperparathyroidism and include calcium-containing kidney stones, kidney failure, nephrocalcinosis, bone abnormalities (i.e., osteoporosis, osteitis fibrosa cystica), and gastrointestinal and musculoskeletal complaints. Management is challenging because of early onset, significant recurrence rates, and the multiplicity of parathyroid gland involvement. Differentiation of hyperparathyroidism of MEN 1 from other forms of familial primary hyperparathyroidism is usually based on family history, histologic features of resected parathyroid tissue, the presence of a *MEN1* mutation, and, sometimes, long-term observation to determine whether other manifestations of MEN 1 develop. Parathyroid hyperplasia is the most common cause of hyperparathyroidism in MEN 1, although single and multiple adenomas have been described. Hyperplasia of one or more parathyroid glands is common in younger patients; adenomas are usually found in older patients or those with longstanding disease.

Enteropancreatic tumors are the second most common manifestation of MEN 1, with an estimated penetrance of 50%. They tend to occur in parallel with hyperparathyroidism (Fig. 23-1); 30% are malignant. Most of these tumors secrete peptide hormones that cause specific clinical syndromes. These syndromes, however, may have an insidious onset and a slow progression, making their diagnosis difficult and in many cases delayed. Some enteropancreatic tumors do not secrete hormones. These "silent" tumors are usually found during radiographic screening. Metastasis, most commonly to the liver, is not uncommon.

Gastrinomas are the most common enteropancreatic tumors observed in MEN 1 patients and result in the Zollinger-Ellison syndrome (ZES). ZES is caused by excessive gastrin production and occurs in more than one-half of MEN 1 patients with small carcinoid-like tumors in the duodenal wall or, less often, by pancreatic islet cell tumors. There may be more than one gastrin-producing tumor, making localization difficult. The robust acid production may cause esophagitis, duodenal ulcers throughout the duodenum, ulcers involving the proximal jejunum, and diarrhea. The ulcer diathesis is commonly refractory to conservative therapy such as antacids. The diagnosis is made by finding increased gastric acid secretion, elevated basal gastrin levels in the serum [generally >115 pmol/L (200 pg/mL)], and an exaggerated response of serum gastrin to either secretin or calcium. Other causes of elevated serum gastrin levels, such as achlorhydria, treatment with H_2 receptor antagonists or proton pump inhibitors, retained gastric antrum, small-bowel resection, gastric outlet obstruction, and hypercalcemia, should be excluded (Fig. 23-1). High-resolution early-phase CT scanning, abdominal MRI with contrast, octreotide scan, and/or endoscopic ultrasound provide the best preoperative techniques for identification of the primary and metastatic gastrinoma; intraoperative ultrasonography is the most sensitive method for detection of small tumors. Approximately one-fourth of all ZES occurs in the context of MEN 1.

Insulinomas are the second most common enteropancreatic tumors in patients who suffer from MEN 1. Unlike gastrinomas, most insulinomas originate in the pancreas bed, becoming the most common pancreatic tumor in MEN 1. Hypoglycemia caused by insulinomas is observed in about one-third of MEN 1 patients with pancreatic islet cell tumors (Fig. 23-1). The tumors may be benign or malignant (25%). The diagnosis can be suggested by documenting hypoglycemia during a short fast with simultaneous inappropriate elevation of serum insulin and C-peptide levels. More commonly, it is necessary to subject the patient to a supervised 12- to 72-h fast to provoke hypoglycemia (Chap. 20). Large insulinomas may be identified by CT or MRI scanning; small tumors not detected by conventional radiographic techniques may be localized by endoscopic ultrasound or by selective arteriographic injection of calcium into each of the arteries that supply the pancreas and sampling the hepatic vein for insulin to determine the anatomic region containing the tumor. Intraoperative ultrasonography is frequently used to localize these tumors. The trend to earlier diagnosis of, hence, smaller tumors has reduced the usefulness of octreotide scanning, which is positive in a minority of these patients.

Glucagonoma, seen occasionally in MEN 1, causes a syndrome of hyperglycemia, skin rash (necrolytic migratory erythema), anorexia, glossitis, anemia, depression, diarrhea, and venous thrombosis. In about half of these patients the plasma glucagon level is high, leading to its designation as the *glucagonoma syndrome*, although elevation of the plasma glucagon level in MEN 1 patients is not necessarily associated with these symptoms. Some patients with this syndrome also have elevated plasma ghrelin levels. The glucagonoma syndrome may represent a complex interaction between glucagon and ghrelin overproduction and the nutritional status of the patient.

The *Verner-Morrison*, or *watery diarrhea, syndrome* consists of watery diarrhea, hypokalemia, hypochlorhydria, and metabolic acidosis. The diarrhea can be voluminous and is almost always found in association with an islet cell tumor, prompting use of the term *pancreatic cholera*. However, the syndrome is not restricted to pancreatic islet tumors and has been observed with carcinoids or other tumors. This syndrome is believed to be due to overproduction of vasoactive intestinal peptide (VIP), although plasma VIP levels may not be elevated. Hypercalcemia may be induced by the effects of VIP on bone as well as by hyperparathyroidism. Other disorders that should be considered in the differential diagnosis of chronic diarrhea include infectious or parasitic diseases, inflammatory bowel disease, sprue, or other endocrine causes such as ZES, carcinoid, or medullary thyroid carcinoma.

The pancreatic neoplasms differ from the other components of MEN 1 in that approximately one-third of the tumors display malignant features, including hepatic metastases. The pancreatic neoplasms can also be used to highlight another characteristic of MEN 1, the specific impact of a hormone produced by one component of MEN 1 on another neoplastic component of this syndrome. Specific examples include the effects of either corticotropin-releasing hormone (CRH) or growth hormone–releasing hormone (GHRH) production by an islet cell tumor to cause a syndrome of excess adrenocorticotropin (ACTH) (Cushing's disease) or GH (acromegaly) production by the pituitary gland. These secondary interactions add complexity to the diagnosis and management of these tumor syndromes. Pancreatic islet cell tumors are diagnosed by identification of a characteristic clinical syndrome, hormonal assays with or without provocative stimuli, or radiographic techniques. One approach involves annual screening of individuals at risk with measurement of basal and meal-stimulated levels of pancreatic polypeptide to identify the tumors as early as possible; the rationale of this screening strategy is the concept that surgical removal of islet cell tumors at an early stage will be curative. Other approaches to screening include measurement of serum gastrin and pancreatic polypeptide levels every 2–3 years, with the rationale that pancreatic neoplasms will be detected at a later stage but can be managed medically, if possible, or by surgery. High-resolution early-phase CT scanning or endoscopic ultrasound provides the best preoperative technique for identification of these tumors; intraoperative ultrasonography is the most sensitive method for detection of small tumors.

Pituitary tumors occur in 20–30% of patients with MEN 1 and tend to be multicentric. These tumors can exhibit aggressive behavior and local invasiveness that make them difficult to resect (Chap. 2). Prolactinomas are most common (Fig. 23-1) and are diagnosed by finding serum prolactin levels >200 μg/L, with or without a pituitary mass evident by MRI. Values <200 μg/L may be due to a prolactin-secreting neoplasm or to compression of the pituitary stalk by a different type of pituitary tumor. Acromegaly due to excessive GH production is the second most common syndrome caused by pituitary tumors in MEN 1 and can rarely be due to production of GHRH by an islet cell tumor. Cushing's disease can be caused by ACTH-producing pituitary tumors or by ectopic production of ACTH or CRH by other components of the MEN 1 syndrome including islet cell or carcinoid tumors or adrenal adenomas. Diagnosis of pituitary Cushing's disease is generally best accomplished by a high-dose dexamethasone suppression test or by petrosal venous sinus sampling for ACTH after IV injection of CRH. Differentiation of a primary pituitary tumor from an ectopic CRH-producing tumor may be difficult because the pituitary is the source of ACTH in both disorders; documentation of CRH production by a pancreatic islet or carcinoid tumor may be the only method of proving ectopic CRH production.

Adrenal cortical tumors are found in almost one-half of gene carriers but are rarely functional; malignancy in the cortical adenomas is uncommon. Rare cases of pheochromocytoma have been described in the context of MEN 1. Due to its rarity, screening for these tumors is only indicated when there are suggestive symptoms.

Carcinoid tumors in MEN 1 are of the foregut type and are derived from thymus, lung, stomach, or duodenum; they may metastasize or be locally invasive. These tumors usually produce serotonin, calcitonin, or CRH; the typical carcinoid syndrome with flushing, diarrhea, and bronchospasm is rare (Chap. 22). Mediastinal carcinoid tumors (an upper mediastinal mass) are more common in men; bronchial carcinoid tumors are more common in women. Carcinoid tumors are a late manifestation of MEN 1; some reports have emphasized the importance of routine chest CT screening for mediastinal carcinoid tumors because of their high rate of malignant transformation and aggressive behavior.

Unusual Manifestations of MEN1

Subcutaneous or visceral lipomas and cutaneous leiomyomas may also be present but rarely undergo malignant transformation. Skin angiofibromas or collagenomas are seen in most patients with MEN 1 when carefully sought.

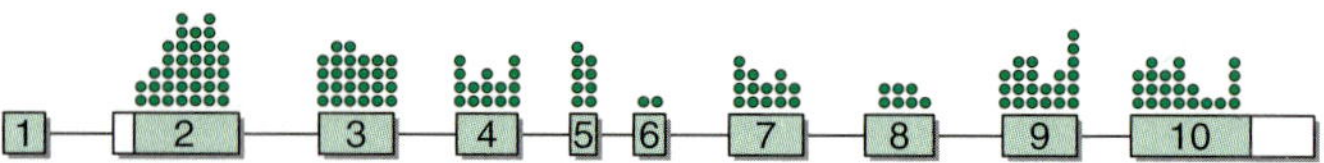

FIGURE 23-2

Schematic depiction of the *MEN1* gene and the distribution of mutations. The shaded areas show coding sequence. The closed circles show the relative distribution of mutations, mostly inactivating, in each exon. Mutation data are derived from the Human Gene Mutation Database from which more detailed information can be obtained (*www.uwcm.ac.uk/uwcm/mg/hgmd0.html*). (*From M Krawczak, DN Cooper: Trends Genet 13:1321, 1998.*)

GENETIC CONSIDERATIONS

MEN1 gene mutations are found in >90% of families with the syndrome (Fig. 23-2). Genetic testing can be performed in individuals at risk for the development of MEN 1 and is now commercially available in the United States and Europe. The major value of genetic testing in a kindred with an identifiable mutation is the assignment or exclusion of gene carrier status. In those identified as carrying the mutant gene, routine screening for individual manifestations of MEN 1 should be performed as outlined above. Those with negative genetic test results in a kindred with a known germline mutation can be excluded from further screening for MEN 1. A significant percentage of sporadic parathyroid, islet cell, and carcinoid tumors also have loss or mutation of *MEN1*. It is presumed that these mutations are somatic and occur in a single cell, leading to subsequent transformation.

Rx Treatment: MULTIPLE ENDOCRINE NEOPLASIA TYPE 1

Almost everyone who inherits a mutant *MEN1* gene develops at least one clinical manifestation of the syndrome. Most develop hyperparathyroidism, 80% develop pancreatic islet cell tumors, and more than half develop pituitary tumors. For most of these tumors, initial surgery is not curative and patients frequently require multiple surgical procedures and surgery on two or more endocrine glands during a lifetime. For this reason, it is essential to establish clear goals for management of these patients rather than to recommend surgery casually each time a tumor is discovered. Ranges for acceptable management are discussed below.

HYPERPARATHYROIDISM Individuals with serum calcium levels >3.0 mmol/L (12 mg/dL), evidence of calcium nephrolithiasis or renal dysfunction, neuropathic or muscular symptoms, or bone involvement (including osteopenia) or individuals <50 years of age should undergo parathyroid exploration. There is less agreement regarding the necessity for parathyroid exploration in individuals who do not meet these criteria, and observation may be appropriate in the MEN 1 patient with asymptomatic hyperparathyroidism.

When parathyroid surgery is indicated in MEN 1, there are two approaches. In the first, all parathyroid tissue is identified and removed at the time of primary operation, and parathyroid tissue is implanted in the nondominant forearm. Thymectomy should also be performed because of the potential for later development of malignant carcinoid tumors. If reoperation for hyperparathyroidism is necessary at a later date, transplanted parathyroid tissue can be resected from the forearm with titration of tissue removal to lower the intact parathyroid hormone (PTH) to <50% of basal.

Another approach is to remove 3–3.5 parathyroid glands from the neck (leaving ~50 mg of parathyroid tissue), carefully marking the location of residual tissue so that the remaining tissue can be located easily during subsequent surgery. If this approach is utilized, intraoperative PTH measurements should be utilized to monitor adequacy of removal of parathyroid tissue with a goal of reducing postoperative serum intact PTH to ≤50% of basal values.

The use of high-resolution CT scanning (1 mm) and imaging during three phases of contrast flow has substantially improved the ability to identify aberrantly located parathyroid tissue. As this issue arises with some frequency in the context of parathyroid disease in MEN 1, this technique should be utilized to locate parathyroid tissue before reoperation for a failed exploration, and it may be useful prior to the initial operation.

PANCREATIC ISLET CELL TUMORS (See Chap. 22 for discussion of pancreatic islet cell tumors not associated with MEN1.) Two features of pancreatic islet cell tumors in MEN 1 complicate the management. First, the pancreatic islet cell tumors are multicentric, are malignant about a third of the time, and cause death in 10–20% of patients. Second, performance of a total pancreatectomy to prevent malignancy causes diabetes mellitus, a disease with significant long-term complications that include neuropathy, retinopathy, and nephropathy. These features make it difficult to formulate clear-cut guidelines, but some general concepts appear to be valid. (1) Islet cell tumors producing insulin, glucagon, VIP, GHRH, or CRH should be resected because medical therapy for the hormonal effects of these tumors is generally ineffective. (2) Gastrin-producing islet cell tumors that cause ZES are frequently multicentric. Recent experience suggests that a high percentage of ZES in MEN 1 is caused by duodenal wall carcinoid tumors and that resection of these tumors improves the cure rate. Treatment with H_2 receptor antagonists (cimetidine or ranitidine) or proton pump inhibitors (omeprazole, lansoprazole, esomeprazole, etc.) provides an alternative, and some think preferable, therapy to surgery for control of ulcer disease in patients with multicentric tumors or with hepatic metastases. (3) In families in which there is a high incidence of malignant islet cell tumors that cause death, total pancreatectomy at an early age may be considered to prevent malignancy.

Management of metastatic islet cell carcinoma is unsatisfactory. Hormonal abnormalities can sometimes be controlled. For example, ZES can be treated with H_2 receptor antagonists or proton pump inhibitors; the somatostatin analogues, octreotide or lanreotide, are useful in the management of carcinoid, glucagonoma, and the watery diarrhea syndrome. Bilateral adrenalectomy may be required for ectopic ACTH syndrome if medical therapy is ineffective (Chap. 5). Islet cell carcinomas frequently metastasize to the liver but may grow slowly. Hepatic artery embolization, radiofrequency ablation, or chemotherapy (5-fluorouracil, streptozocin, chlorozotocin, doxorubicin, or dacarbazine) may reduce tumor mass, control symptoms of hormone excess, and prolong life; however, these treatments are never curative. Consideration should be given to participation in clinical trials of new agents that target specific molecular pathways.

PITUITARY TUMORS Treatment of prolactinomas with dopamine agonists (bromocriptine, cabergoline, or quinagolide) usually returns the serum prolactin level to normal and prevents further tumor growth (Chap. 2). Surgical resection of a prolactinoma is rarely curative but may relieve mass effects. Transsphenoidal resection is appropriate for neoplasms that secrete ACTH, GH, or the α subunit of the pituitary glycoprotein hormones. Octreotide reduces tumor mass in one-third of GH-secreting tumors and reduces GH and insulin-like growth factor I levels in >75% of patients. Pegvisomant, a GH antagonist, rapidly lowers insulin-like growth factor levels in patients with acromegaly (Chap. 2). Radiation therapy may be useful for large or recurrent tumors.

Improvements in the management of MEN 1, particularly the earlier recognition of islet cell and pituitary tumors, have improved outcomes in these patients. As a result, other neoplastic manifestations that develop later in the course of this disorder, such as carcinoid syndrome, are now seen with increased frequency.

MULTIPLE ENDOCRINE NEOPLASIA TYPE 2

Clinical Manifestations

Medullary thyroid carcinoma (MTC) and pheochromocytoma are associated in two major syndromes: MEN type 2A and MEN type 2B (Table 23-1). MEN 2A is the combination of MTC, hyperparathyroidism, and pheochromocytoma. Three subvariants of MEN 2A are familial medullary thyroid carcinoma (FMTC), MEN 2A with cutaneous lichen amyloidosis, and MEN 2A with Hirschsprung disease. MEN 2B is the combination of MTC, pheochromocytoma, mucosal neuromas, intestinal ganglioneuromatosis, and marfanoid features.

Multiple Endocrine Neoplasia Type 2A

MTC is the most common manifestation. This tumor usually develops in childhood, beginning as hyperplasia of the calcitonin-producing cells (C cells) of the thyroid. MTC is typically located at the junction of the upper one-third and lower two-thirds of each lobe of the thyroid, reflecting the high density of C cells in this location; tumors >1 cm in size are frequently associated with local or distant metastases. Measurement of the serum calcitonin level after calcium or pentagastrin injection makes it possible to diagnose this disorder at an early stage in its development (see below).

Pheochromocytoma occurs in ~50% of patients with MEN 2A and causes palpitations, nervousness, headaches, and sometimes sweating (Chap. 6). About half of the tumors are bilateral, and >50% of patients who have had unilateral adrenalectomy develop a pheochromocytoma in the contralateral gland within a decade. A second feature of these tumors is a disproportionate increase in the secretion of epinephrine relative to norepinephrine. This characteristic differentiates the MEN 2 pheochromocytomas from sporadic pheochromocytoma and those associated with von Hippel–Lindau (VHL) syndrome, hereditary paraganglioma, or neurofibromatosis. Capsular invasion is common, but metastasis is uncommon. Finally, the pheochromocytomas are almost always found in the adrenal gland, differentiating the pheochromocytomas in MEN 2 from the extraadrenal tumors more commonly found in hereditary paraganglioma syndromes.

Hyperparathyroidism occurs in 15–20% of patients, with the peak incidence in the third or fourth decade. The manifestations of hyperparathyroidism do not differ from those in other forms of primary hyperparathyroidism (Chap. 27). Diagnosis is established by finding hypercalcemia, hypophosphatemia, hypercalciuria, and an inappropriately high serum level of intact parathyroid hormone. Multiglandular parathyroid hyperplasia is the most common histologic finding, although with longstanding disease adenomatous changes may be superimposed on hyperplasia.

The most common subvariant of MEN 2A is familial MTC, an autosomal dominant syndrome in which MTC is the only manifestation (Table 23-1). The clinical diagnosis of FMTC is established by the identification of MTC in multiple generations without a pheochromocytoma. Since the penetrance of pheochromocytoma is 50% in MEN 2A, it is possible that MEN 2A could masquerade as FMTC in small kindreds. It is important to consider this possibility carefully before classifying a kindred as having FMTC; failure to do so could lead to death or serious morbidity from pheochromocytoma in an affected kindred member. The difficulty of differentiating MEN 2A and FMTC is discussed further below.

Multiple Endocrine Neoplasia Type 2B

The association of MTC, pheochromocytoma, mucosal neuromas, and a marfanoid habitus is designated MEN 2B. MTC in MEN 2B develops earlier and is more aggressive than in MEN 2A. Metastatic disease has been described prior to 1 year of age, and death may occur in the second or third decade of life. However, the prognosis is not invariably bad even in patients with metastatic disease, as evidenced by a number of multigenerational families with this disease.

Pheochromocytoma occurs in more than half of MEN 2B patients and does not differ from that in MEN 2A. Hypercalcemia is rare in MEN 2B, and there are no well-documented examples of hyperparathyroidism.

The mucosal neuromas and marfanoid body habitus are the most distinctive features and are recognizable in childhood. Neuromas are present on the tip of the tongue, under the eyelids, and throughout the gastrointestinal tract and are true neuromas, distinct from neurofibromas. The most common presentation in children relates to gastrointestinal symptomatology including intermittent colic, pseudoobstruction, and diarrhea.

GENETIC CONSIDERATIONS

Mutations of the *RET* proto-oncogene have been identified in most patients with MEN 2 (Fig. 23-3). *RET* encodes a tyrosine kinase receptor that, in combination with a co-receptor, GFRα, is normally activated by glial cell–derived neurotrophic factor (GDNF) or other members of this transforming growth factor β–like family of peptides including artemin, persephin, and neurturin. In the C cell there is evidence that persephin normally activates the *RET*/GFRα-4 receptor complex and is partially responsible for migration of the C cells into the thyroid gland, whereas in the gastrointestinal tract, GDNF activates the *RET*/GFRα-1 complex. *RET* mutations induce constitutive activity of the receptor, explaining the autosomal dominant transmission of the disorder.

Naturally occurring mutations localize to two regions of the *RET* tyrosine kinase receptor. The first is a cysteine-rich extracellular domain; point mutations in the coding sequence for one of six cysteines (codons 609, 611, 618, 620, 630, or 634) cause amino acid substitutions that induce receptor dimerization and activation in the absence of its ligand. Codon 634 mutations occur in 80% of MEN 2A kindreds and are most commonly associated with classic MEN 2A features (Figs. 23-2 and 23-3); an arginine substitution at this codon accounts for half of all MEN 2A mutations. All reported families with

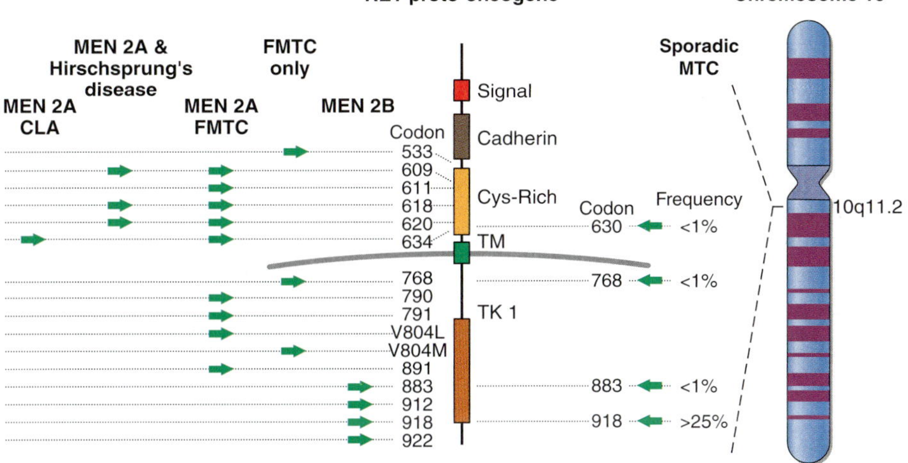

FIGURE 23-3

Schematic diagram of the *RET* proto-oncogene showing mutations found in MEN type 2 and sporadic medullary thyroid carcinoma (MTC). The *RET* proto-oncogene is located on the proximal arm of chromosome 10q (10q11.2). Activating mutations of two functional domains of RET tyrosine kinase receptor have been identified. The first affects a cysteine-rich (Cys-Rich) region in the extracellular portion of the receptor. Each germline mutation changes a cysteine at codons 609, 611, 618, 620, or 634 to another amino acid. The second region is the intracellular tyrosine kinase (TK) domain. Codon 634 mutations account for ~80% of all germline mutations. Mutations of codons 630, 768, 883, and 918 have been identified as somatic (non-germline) mutations that occur in a single parafollicular or C cell within the thyroid gland in sporadic MTC. A codon 918 mutation is the most common somatic mutation. MEN 2, multiple endocrine neoplasia type 2; CLA, cutaneous lichen amyloidosis; FMTC, familial medullary thyroid carcinoma; Signal, the signal peptide; Cadherin, a cadherin-like region in the extracellular domain; TM, transmembrane domain; TK, tyrosine kinase domain.

MEN 2A and cutaneous lichen amyloidosis have a codon 634 mutation. Mutations of codons 609, 611, 618, or 620 occur in 10–15% of MEN 2A kindreds and are more commonly associated with FMTC (Fig. 23-3). Mutations in codons 609, 618, and 620 have also been identified in a variant of MEN 2A that includes Hirschsprung disease (Fig. 23-3). The second region of the *RET* tyrosine kinase that is mutated in MEN 2 is in the substrate recognition pocket at codon 918 (Fig. 23-3). This activating mutation is present in ~95% of patients with MEN 2B and accounts for 5% of all *RET* proto-oncogene mutations in MEN 2. Mutations of codon 883 and 922 have also been identified in a few patients with MEN 2B.

Uncommon mutations (<5% of the total) include those of codons 533 (exon 8), 666, 768, 777, 790, 791, 804, 891, and 912. Mutations associated with only FMTC include codons 533, 768, and 912. With greater experience, mutations that were once associated with FMTC only (666, 791, V804L, V804M, and 891) have since been found in MEN 2A as there have been occasional descriptions of pheochromocytoma. At present it is reasonable to conclude that only kindreds with codon 533, 768, or 912 mutations are consistently associated with FMTC; in kindreds with all other *RET* mutations, pheochromocytoma is a possibility. The recognition that germline mutations occur in at least 6% of patients with apparently sporadic MTC has led to the firm recommendation that all patients with MTC should be screened for these mutations. The effort to screen patients with sporadic MTC when combined with the fact that new kindreds with classic MEN 2A are being recognized less frequently has led to a shift in the mutation frequencies. These findings mirror results in other malignancies where germline mutations of cancer-causing genes contribute to a greater percentage of apparently sporadic cancer than previously considered. The recognition of new *RET* mutations suggests that more will be identified in the future.

Somatic mutations (found only in the tumor and not transmitted in the germline) of the *RET* proto-oncogene have been identified in sporadic MTC; 25–35% of sporadic tumors have codon 918 mutations, and somatic mutations in codons 630, 768, and 804 have also been identified (Fig. 23-3).

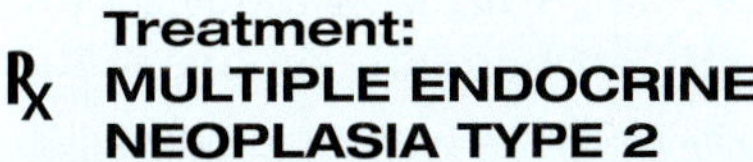

Treatment: MULTIPLE ENDOCRINE NEOPLASIA TYPE 2

SCREENING FOR MULTIPLE ENDOCRINE NEOPLASIA TYPE 2 Death from MTC can be prevented by early thyroidectomy. The identification of *RET* proto-oncogene mutations and the application of DNA-based molecular diagnostic techniques to identify these mutations has simplified the screening process. During the initial evaluation of a kindred, a *RET* proto-oncogene analysis should be performed on an individual with proven MEN 2A. Establishment of the specific germline mutation facilitates the subsequent analysis of other family members. Each family member at risk should be tested twice for the presence of the specific mutation; the second analysis should be performed on a new DNA sample and, ideally, in a second laboratory to exclude sample mix-up or technical error (see *www.genetests.org* for an up-to-date list of laboratory testing sites). Both false-positive and false-negative analyses have been described; a false-negative test result is of the greatest concern because calcitonin testing is now rarely performed as a diagnostic backup study; if there is a genetic test error, a child may present in the second or third decade with metastatic MTC. Individuals in a kindred with a known mutation who have two normal analyses can be excluded from further screening.

There is general consensus that children with codon 883, 918, and 922 mutations, those associated with MEN 2B, should have a total thyroidectomy and central lymph node dissection (level VI) performed during the first months of life or soon after identification of the syndrome. If local metastasis is discovered, a more extensive lymph node dissection (levels II to V) is generally indicated. In children with codon 611, 618, 620, 630, 634, and 891 mutations, thyroidectomy should be performed before the age of 6 years because of reports of local metastatic disease in children this age. Finally, there are kindreds with codon 609, 768, 790, 791, 804, and 912 mutations where the phenotype of MTC appears to be less aggressive. The clinician caring for children with one of these mutations faces a dilemma. In many kindreds there has never been a death from MTC caused by one of these mutations. However, in other kindreds there are examples of metastatic disease occurring early in life. For example, metastatic disease prior to the age of 6 years has been described with codon 609 and 804 mutations and before the age of 14 years in a patient with a codon 912 mutation. In kindreds with these mutations, two management approaches have been suggested: (1) perform a total thyroidectomy with or without central node dissection at some arbitrary age (perhaps 6–10 years of age), or (2) continue annual or biannual calcitonin provocative testing with performance of total thyroidectomy with or without central neck dissection when the test becomes abnormal. The pentagastrin test involves measurement of serum calcitonin basally and at 2, 5, 10, and 15 min after a bolus injection of 5 μg pentagastrin per kilogram body weight. Patients should be warned before pentagastrin injection of epigastric tightness, nausea, warmth, and tingling of extremities and reassured that the symptoms will last ~2 min. If pentagastrin is unavailable, an alternative is a short calcium infusion, performed by obtaining a baseline serum calcitonin and then infusing 150 mg calcium salt IV over 10 min with measurement of serum calcitonin at 5, 10, 15, 30 min after initiation of the infusion.

The *RET* proto-oncogene analysis should be performed in patients with suspected MEN 2B to detect codon 883, 918, and 922 mutations, especially in newborn children where the diagnosis is suspected but the clinical phenotype is not fully developed. Other family members at risk for MEN 2B should also be tested because the mucosal neuromas can be subtle. Most MEN 2B mutations represent de novo mutations derived from the paternal allele. In the rare families with proven germline transmission of MTC but no identifiable *RET* proto-oncogene mutation (sequencing of the entire *RET* gene should be performed), annual pentagastrin or calcium testing should be performed on members at risk.

Annual screening for pheochromocytoma in patients with germline *RET* mutations should be performed by measuring basal plasma or 24-h urine catecholamines and metanephrines. The goal is to identify a pheochromocytoma before it causes significant symptoms or is likely to cause sudden death, an event most commonly associated with large tumors. Although there are kindreds with FMTC and specific *RET* mutations in which no pheochromocytomas have been identified (Fig. 23-3), clinical experience is insufficient to exclude pheochromocytoma screening in these individuals. Radiographic studies, such as MRI or CT scans, are generally reserved for individuals with abnormal screening tests or with symptoms suggestive of pheochromocytoma (Chap. 6). Women should be tested during pregnancy because undetected pheochromocytoma can cause maternal death during childbirth.

Measurement of serum calcium and parathyroid hormone levels every 2–3 years provides an adequate screen for hyperparathyroidism, except in those families in which hyperparathyroidism is a prominent component, where measurements should be made annually.

MEDULLARY THYROID CARCINOMA Hereditary MTC is a multicentric disorder. Total thyroidectomy with a central lymph node dissection should be performed in children who carry the mutant gene. Incomplete thyroidectomy leaves the possibility of later transformation of residual C cells. The goal of early therapy is cure, and a strategy that does not accomplish this goal is short-sighted. Long-term follow-up studies indicate an excellent outcome, with ~90% of children free of disease 15–20 years after surgery. In contrast, 15–25% of patients in whom the diagnosis is made on the basis of a palpable thyroid nodule die from the disease within 15–20 years.

In adults with MTC >1 cm in size, metastases to regional lymph nodes are common (>75%). Total thyroidectomy with central lymph node dissection and selective dissection of other regional chains provide the best chance for cure. In patients with extensive local metastatic disease in the neck, external radiation may prevent local recurrence or reduce tumor mass but is not curative. Chemotherapy with combinations of Adriamycin, vincristine, cyclophosphamide, and dacarbazine may provide palliation. Clinical trials with small compounds that interact with the ATP-binding pocket of the RET receptor and prevent phosphorylation of tyrosine (tyrosine kinase inhibitors) have shown promise for treatment of hereditary MTC. Some of these agents will be entering phase II and III trials and should be considered in patients with metastatic disease. Phase I and II studies of some of these agents have documented tumor regression and lowering of calcitonin and carcinoembryonic antigen in some patients.

PHEOCHROMOCYTOMA The long-term goal for management of pheochromocytoma is to prevent death and cardiovascular complications. Improvements in radiographic imaging of the adrenals make direct examination of the apparently normal contralateral gland during surgery less important, and the rapid evolution of laparoscopic abdominal or retroperitoneal surgery has simplified management of early pheochromocytoma. The major question is whether to remove both adrenal glands or to remove only the affected adrenal at the time of primary surgery. Issues to be considered in making this decision include the possibility of malignancy (<15 reported cases), the high probability of developing pheochromocytoma in the apparently unaffected gland over an 8- to 10-year period, and the risks of adrenal insufficiency caused by removal of both glands (at least two deaths related to adrenal insufficiency have occurred in MEN 2 patients). Most clinicians recommend removing only the affected gland. If both adrenals are removed, glucocorticoid and mineralocorticoid replacement is mandatory. An alternative approach is to perform a cortical-sparing adrenalectomy, removing the pheochromocytoma and adrenal medulla, leaving the adrenal cortex behind. This approach is usually successful and eliminates the necessity for steroid hormone replacement in most patients, although the pheochromocytoma recurs in a small percentage.

HYPERPARATHYROIDISM Hyperparathyroidism has been managed by one of two approaches. Removal of 3.5 glands with maintenance of the remaining half gland in the neck is the usual procedure. In families in whom hyperparathyroidism is a prominent manifestation (almost always associated with a codon 634 *RET* mutation) and recurrence is common, total parathyroidectomy with transplantation of parathyroid tissue into the nondominant forearm is preferred. This approach is discussed above in the context of hyperparathyroidism associated with MEN 1.

OTHER GENETIC ENDOCRINE TUMOR SYNDROMES

A number of mixed syndromes exist in which the neoplastic associations differ from those in MEN 1 or 2 (Table 23-1).

The cause of VHL syndrome, the association of central nervous system tumors, renal cell carcinoma, pheochromocytoma, and islet cell neoplasms, is a mutation in the *VHL* tumor-suppressor gene. Germline-inactivating mutations of the *VHL* gene cause tumor formation when there is additional loss or somatic mutation of the normal *VHL* allele in brain, kidney, pancreatic islet, or adrenal medullary cells. Missense mutations been identified in >40% of VHL families with pheochromocytoma, suggesting that families with this type of mutation should be surveyed routinely for pheochromocytoma. A point that may be useful in differentiating VHL from MEN 1 (overlapping features include islet cell tumor and rare pheochromocytoma) or MEN 2 (overlapping feature is pheochromocytoma) is that hyperparathyroidism rarely occurs in VHL.

The molecular defect in type 1 neurofibromatosis inactivates neurofibromin, a cell membrane–associated protein that normally activates a GTPase. Inactivation of this protein impairs GTPase and causes continuous activation of p21 Ras and its downstream tyrosine kinase pathway. Endocrine tumors also form in less common neoplastic genetic syndromes. These include Cowden's disease, Carney complex, familial acromegaly, and familial carcinoid syndrome. Carney complex consists of myxomas of the heart, skin, and breast; peripheral nerve schwannomas; spotty skin pigmentation; and testicular, adrenal, and GH-secreting pituitary tumors. Linkage analysis has identified two loci: chromosome 2p in half of families and 17q in the others. The 17q gene has been identified as the regulatory subunit (type IA) of protein kinase A (*PRKA1A*).

IMMUNOLOGIC SYNDROMES AFFECTING MULTIPLE ENDOCRINE ORGANS

When immune dysfunction affects two or more endocrine glands and other nonendocrine immune disorders are present, the *polyglandular autoimmune* (PGA) *syndromes* should be considered. The PGA syndromes are classified as two main types: the type I syndrome starts in childhood and is characterized by mucocutaneous candidiasis, hypoparathyroidism, and adrenal insufficiency; the type II, or Schmidt, syndrome is more likely to present in adults and most commonly consists of adrenal insufficiency, thyroiditis, or type 1 diabetes mellitus. Some authors have attempted to subdivide PGA II on the basis of association with some autoimmune disorders but not others (i.e., type II and type III). The type III syndrome is heterogeneous and may consist of autoimmune thyroid

TABLE 23-2

FEATURES OF POLYGLANDULAR AUTOIMMUNE (PGA) SYNDROMES

PGA I	PGA II
Epidemiology	
Autosomal recessive	Polygenic inheritance
Mutations in APECED gene	HLA-DR3 and HLA-DR4 associated
Childhood onset	Adult onset
Equal male/female ratio	Female predominance
Disease Associations	
Mucocutaneous candidiasis	Adrenal insufficiency
Hypoparathyroidism	Hypothyroidism
Adrenal insufficiency	Graves' disease
Hypogonadism	Type 1 diabetes
Alopecia	Hypogonadism
Hypothyroidism	Hypophysitis
Dental enamel hypoplasia	Myasthenia gravis
Malabsorption	Vitiligo
Chronic active hepatitis	Alopecia
Vitiligo	Pernicious anemia
Pernicious anemia	Celiac disease

Note: APECED, autoimmune polyendocrinopathy-candidiasis-ectodermal dystrophy.

disease along with a variety of other autoimmune endocrine disorders (Table 23-2). However, little information is gained by making this subdivision in terms of understanding pathogenesis or prevention of future endocrine complications in individual patients or in the affected families.

POLYGLANDULAR AUTOIMMUNE SYNDROME TYPE I

PGA type I is usually recognized in the first decade of life and requires two of three components for diagnosis: mucocutaneous candidiasis, hypoparathyroidism, and adrenal insufficiency. Mucocutaneous candidiasis and hypoparathyroidism present with similar high frequency (100% and 79–96%, respectively). Adrenal insufficiency is observed in 60–72% of patients. Mineralocorticoids and glucocorticoids may be lost simultaneously or sequentially. PGA type 1 is also called *autoimmune polyendocrinopathy-candidiasis-ectodermal dystrophy* (APECED). Other endocrine defects can include gonadal failure (60% female, 14% male), hypothyroidism (5%), and destruction of the beta cells of the pancreatic islets and development of insulin-dependent (type 1) diabetes mellitus (14% lifetime risk). Additional features include hypoplasia of the dental enamel, nail dystrophy, tympanic membrane sclerosis, vitiligo, keratopathy, and gastric parietal cell dysfunction resulting in pernicious anemia (13%). Some patients develop autoimmune hepatitis (12%), malabsorption (variably attributed to intestinal lymphangiectasia, bacterial overgrowth, or hypoparathyroidism), asplenism, achalasia, and cholelithiasis (Table 23-2). At the outset, only one organ may be involved, but the number increases with time so that patients eventually manifest two to five components of the syndrome.

Most patients initially present with oral candidiasis in childhood; it is poorly responsive to treatment (Chap. 27) and relapses frequently. Chronic hypoparathyroidism usually occurs before adrenal insufficiency develops. More than 60% of postpubertal women develop premature hypogonadism. The endocrine components, including adrenal insufficiency and hypoparathyroidism, may not develop until the fourth decade, making continued surveillance necessary.

Type I PGA syndrome is not associated with a particular HLA type and is usually inherited as an autosomal recessive trait. It may occur sporadically. The responsible gene, designated as either *APECED* or *AIRE*, encodes a transcription factor that is expressed in thymus and lymph nodes; a variety of different mutations have been reported. The mechanism by which these mutations lead to the diverse manifestations of type I PGA is still unknown.

POLYGLANDULAR AUTOIMMUNE SYNDROME TYPE II

PGA type II is characterized by two or more of the endocrinopathies listed in Table 23-2. Most often these include primary adrenal insufficiency, Graves' disease or autoimmune hypothyroidism, type 1 diabetes mellitus, or primary hypogonadism. Because adrenal insufficiency is relatively rare, it is frequently used to define the presence of the syndrome. Among patients with adrenal insufficiency, type 1 diabetes mellitus coexists in 52% and autoimmune thyroid disease occurs in 69%. However, many patients with antimicrosomal and antithyroglobulin antibodies never develop abnormalities of thyroid function. Thus, increased antibody titers alone are poor predictors of future disease. Other associated conditions include hypophysitis, celiac disease (2–3%), atrophic gastritis, and pernicious anemia (13%). Vitiligo, caused by antibodies against the melanocyte, and alopecia are less common than in the type I syndrome. Mucocutaneous candidiasis does not occur. A few patients develop a late-onset, usually transient hypoparathyroidism caused by antibodies that compete with parathyroid hormone for binding to the parathyroid hormone receptor. Up to 25% of patients with myasthenia gravis, and an even higher percentage who have myasthenia and a thymoma, have PGA type II.

The type II syndrome is familial in nature, often transmitted as an autosomal dominant trait with incomplete penetrance. Like many of the individual autoimmune endocrinopathies, certain HL-DR3 and -DR4 alleles increase disease susceptibility; several different genes probably contribute to the expression of this syndrome.

A variety of autoantibodies are seen in PGA type II, including antibodies directed against (1) thyroid antigens such as thyroid peroxidase, thyroglobulin, or the thyroid-stimulating hormone (TSH) receptor; (2) adrenal side chain cleavage enzyme, steroid 21-hydroxylase, or ACTH receptor; and (3) pancreatic islet glutamic acid decarboxylase or the insulin receptor, among others. The roles of cytokines such as interferon and cell-mediated immunity are unclear.

DIAGNOSIS

The clinical manifestations of adrenal insufficiency often develop slowly, may be difficult to detect, and can be fatal if not diagnosed and treated appropriately. Thus, prospective screening should be performed routinely in all patients and family members at risk for PGA types I and II. The most effective screening test for adrenal disease is a cosyntropin stimulation test (Chap. 5). A fasting blood glucose level can be obtained to screen for hyperglycemia. Additional screening tests should include measurements of TSH, luteinizing hormone, follicle-stimulating hormone, and, in men, testosterone levels. In families with suspected type I PGA syndrome, calcium and phosphorus levels should be measured. These screening studies should be performed every 1–2 years up to about age 50 in families with PGA type II syndrome and until about age 40 in patients with type I syndrome. Screening measurements of autoantibodies against potentially affected endocrine organs are of uncertain prognostic value. The differential diagnosis of PGA syndrome should include the DiGeorge syndrome (hypoparathyroidism due to glandular agenesis and mucocutaneous candidiasis), Kearns-Sayre syndrome (hypoparathyroidism, primary hypogonadism, type 1 diabetes mellitus, and panhypopituitarism), Wolfram's syndrome (congenital diabetes insipidus and diabetes mellitus), IPEX syndrome (*i*mmunodysregulation, *p*olyendocrinopathy, and *e*nteropathy, *X*-linked), and congenital rubella (type 1 diabetes mellitus and hypothyroidism).

℞ Treatment: POLYGLANDULAR AUTOIMMUNE SYNDROME

With the exception of Graves' disease, the management of each of the endocrine components of the disease involves hormone replacement and is covered in detail in the chapters on adrenal, thyroid, gonadal, and parathyroid disease (Chaps. 4, 5, 8, 10, 27). Some aspects of therapy deserve special emphasis. Primary hypothyroidism can mask adrenal insufficiency by prolonging the half-life of cortisol; consequently, administration of thyroid hormone to a patient with unsuspected adrenal insufficiency can precipitate adrenal crisis. Thus, all patients with hypothyroidism in the context of PGA syndrome should be screened for adrenal disease and, if it is present, be treated with glucocorticoids prior to or concurrently with thyroid hormone therapy. Hypoglycemia or decreasing insulin requirements in a patient with diabetes mellitus type 1 may be the earliest symptom of adrenal insufficiency. Consequently, such patients should be screened for adrenal disease. Treatment of mucocutaneous candidiasis with ketoconazole may induce adrenal insufficiency. This drug may also elevate liver enzymes, making the diagnosis of autoimmune hepatitis more difficult. Hypocalcemia in PGA type II is more commonly due to malabsorption associated with celiac disease than to hypoparathyroidism.

OTHER AUTOIMMUNE ENDOCRINE SYNDROMES

Insulin Resistance Caused by Antibodies

Rare insulin-resistance syndromes occur in patients who develop antibodies that block the interaction of insulin with its receptor. Conversely, other classes of anti-insulin receptor antibodies can activate the receptor and can cause hypoglycemia; this disorder should be considered in the differential diagnosis of fasting hypoglycemia (Chap. 20).

Patients with insulin receptor antibodies and acanthosis nigricans are often middle-aged women who acquire insulin resistance in association with other autoimmune disorders such as systemic lupus erythematosus or Sjögren's syndrome. Vitiligo, alopecia, Raynaud's phenomenon, and arthritis may also be seen. Other autoimmune endocrine disorders, including thyrotoxicosis, hypothyroidism, and hypogonadism, occur rarely. Acanthosis nigricans, a velvety, hyperpigmented, thickened skin lesion, is prominent on the dorsum of the neck and other skinfold areas in the axillae or groin and often heralds the diagnosis in these patients. However, acanthosis nigricans also occurs in patients with obesity or polycystic ovarian syndrome, in which insulin resistance appears to be due to a postreceptor defect; thus, acanthosis nigricans itself is not diagnostic of the immunologic form of insulin resistance.

Some patients with acanthosis nigricans have mild glucose intolerance, with a compensatory increase in insulin secretion that is only detected when insulin levels are measured. Others have severe diabetes mellitus requiring massive doses of insulin (several thousand units per day) to lower the blood glucose levels. The nature of the antibodies determines the manifestations; though insulin resistance is more common, fasting hypoglycemia can result from insulinomimetic antibodies.

Insulin-resistant diabetes mellitus associated with anti-insulin antibodies occurs in patients with ataxia telangiectasia. This is an autosomal recessive disorder caused by mutations in *ATM*, a gene involved in cellular responses to ionizing radiation and oxidative damage. This disorder is characterized by ataxia, telangiectasia, immune abnormalities, and an increased incidence of malignancies.

Autoimmune Insulin Syndrome with Hypoglycemia

This disorder typically occurs in patients with other autoimmune disorders and is caused by polyclonal autoantibodies that bind to endogenously synthesized insulin. If the insulin dissociates from the antibodies several hours or more after a meal, hypoglycemia can result. Most cases of the syndrome have been described from Japan, and there may be a genetic component. In plasma cell dyscrasias such as multiple myeloma, the plasma cells may produce monoclonal antibodies against insulin and cause hypoglycemia by a similar mechanism.

Antithyroxine Antibodies and Hypothyroidism

Circulating autoantibodies against thyroid hormones in patients with both immune thyroid disease and plasma cell dyscrasias such as Waldenström's macroglobulinemia can bind thyroid hormones, decrease their biologic activity, and result in primary hypothyroidism. In other patients the antibodies simply interfere with thyroid hormone immunoassays and cause false elevations or decreases in measured hormone levels.

Crow-Fukase Syndrome

The features of this syndrome are highlighted by an acronym that emphasizes its important features: *p*olyneuropathy, *o*rganomegaly, *e*ndocrinopathy, *M* proteins, and *s*kin changes (POEMS). The most important feature is a severe, progressive sensorimotor polyneuropathy associated with a plasma cell dyscrasia. Localized collections of plasma cells (plasmacytomas) can cause sclerotic bone lesions and produce monoclonal IgG or IgA proteins. Endocrine manifestations in men or women include hyperprolactinemia, diabetes mellitus type 2, primary hypothyroidism, and adrenal insufficiency. Additional findings include ovarian failure and amenorrhea in women and testicular failure, impotence, and gynecomastia in men. Skin changes include hyperpigmentation, thickening of the dermis, hirsutism, and hyperhidrosis. Hepatomegaly and lymphadenopathy occur in about two-thirds of patients, and splenomegaly is seen in about one-third. Other manifestations include increased cerebrospinal fluid pressure with papilledema, peripheral edema, ascites, pleural effusions, glomerulonephritis, and fever. Median survival may be >10 years, though shorter in patients with extravascular volume overload or clubbing.

The systemic nature of the disorder may cause confusion with other connective tissue diseases. The endocrine manifestations suggest an autoimmune basis of the disorder, but circulating antibodies against endocrine cells have not been demonstrated. Increased serum and tissue levels of interleukin 6, interleukin 1β, vascular endothelial growth factor, matrix metalloproteins, and tumor necrosis factor α are present, but the pathophysiologic basis for the POEMS syndrome is uncertain. Therapy directed against the plasma cell dyscrasia such as local radiation of bony lesions, chemotherapy, thalidomide, plasmapheresis, bone marrow or stem cell transplantation, and treatment with all-*trans* retinoic acid may improve the endocrine manifestations.

FURTHER READINGS

Agarwal SK et al: Rare germline mutations in cyclin-dependent kinase inhibitor genes in multiple endocrine neoplasia type 1 and related states. J Clin Endocrinol Metab 94:1826, 2009

Asari R et al: Estimated risk of pheochromocytoma recurrence after adrenal-sparing surgery in patients with multiple endocrine neoplasia type 2A. Arch Surg 141:1199, 2006

Berna MJ et al: A prospective study of gastric carcinoids and enterochromaffin-like cell changes in multiple endocrine neoplasia type 1 and Zollinger-Ellison syndrome: Identification of risk factors. J Clin Endocrinol Metab 93:1582, 2008

DeGroot JW et al: RET as a diagnostic and therapeutic target in sporadic and hereditary endocrine tumors. Endocr Rev 27:535, 2006

Dittmar M et al: Polyglandular autoimmune syndromes: Immunogenetics and long-term follow-up. J Clin Endocrinol Metab 88:2983, 2003

Falchetti A et al: Multiple endocrine neoplasia type I variants and phenocopies: More than a nosological issue? J Clin Endocrinol Metab 94:1518, 2009

Igreja S et al: Assessment of p27 (cyclin-dependent kinase inhibitor 1B) and aryl hydrocarbon receptor-interacting protein (AIP) genes in multiple endocrine neoplasia (MEN1) syndrome patients without any detectable MEN1 gene mutations. Clin Endocrinol (Oxf) 70:259, 2009

Learoyd DL et al: Routine screening for germline RET mutations is recommended for all patients with medullary thyroid cancer. Nat Clin Pract Endocrinol Metab 5:6, 2009

Ozawa A et al: The parathyroid/pituitary variant of MEN1 usually has causes other than p27kip1 mutations. J Clin Endocrinol Metab 92(5):1948, 2007

Pellegata NS et al: Germ-line mutations in p27Kip1 cause a multiple endocrine neoplasia syndrome in rats and humans. Proc Natl Acad Sci USA 103:15558, 2006

Plaza-Menacho I et al: Current concepts in RET-related genetics, signaling and therapeutics. Trends Genet 22:627, 2006

Schlumberger M et al: New therapeutic approaches to treat medullary thyroid carcinoma. Nat Clin Pract Endocrinol Metab 4:22, 2008

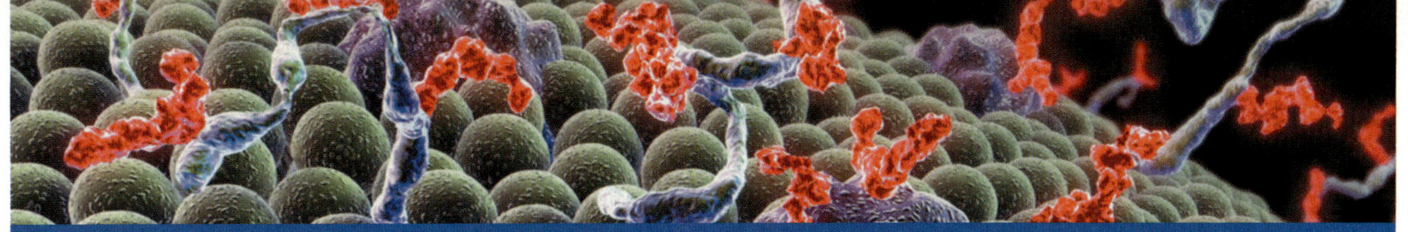

CHAPTER 24

ENDOCRINE PARANEOPLASTIC SYNDROMES

J. Larry Jameson

In addition to local tissue invasion and metastasis, neoplastic cells can produce a variety of peptides that can stimulate hormonal, hematologic, dermatologic, or neurologic responses. *Paraneoplastic syndromes* refer to the disorders that accompany benign or malignant tumors but are not directly related to mass effects or invasion. Tumors of neuroendocrine origin, such as small cell lung carcinoma (SCLC) and carcinoids, produce a wide array of peptide hormones and are common causes of paraneoplastic syndromes. However, almost every type of malignancy has the potential to produce hormones or cytokines, or to induce immunologic responses. Careful studies of the prevalence of paraneoplastic syndromes indicate that they are more common than is generally appreciated. The signs, symptoms, and metabolic alterations associated with paraneoplastic disorders may be overlooked in the context of a malignancy and its treatment. Consequently, atypical clinical manifestations in a patient with cancer should prompt consideration of a paraneoplastic syndrome. The most common endocrinologic and hematologic syndromes associated with underlying neoplasia will be discussed here.

ENDOCRINE PARANEOPLASTIC SYNDROMES

ETIOLOGY

Hormones can be produced from eutopic or ectopic sources. *Eutopic* refers to the expression of a hormone from its normal tissue of origin, whereas *ectopic* refers to hormone production from an atypical tissue source. For example, adrenocorticotropic hormone (ACTH) is expressed eutopically by the corticotrope cells of the anterior pituitary, but it can be expressed ectopically in SCLC. Many hormones are produced at low levels from a wide array of tissues, in addition to the classic endocrine source. Thus, ectopic expression is often a quantitative change rather than an absolute change in tissue expression. Nevertheless, the term *ectopic expression* is firmly entrenched and conveys the abnormal physiology associated with neoplastic hormone production. In addition to high levels of hormones, ectopic expression is typically characterized by abnormal regulation of hormone production (e.g., defective feedback control) and peptide processing (resulting in large, unprocessed precursors).

A diverse array of molecular mechanisms has been suggested to cause ectopic hormone production, but this process remains incompletely understood. In rare instances, genetic rearrangements explain aberrant hormone expression. For example, translocation of the *parathyroid hormone* (*PTH*) gene resulted in high levels of PTH expression in an ovarian carcinoma, presumably because the genetic rearrangement brings the *PTH* gene under the control of ovary-specific regulatory elements. A related phenomenon is well documented in many forms of leukemia and lymphoma, in which somatic genetic rearrangements confer a growth advantage and alter cellular differentiation and function. Although genetic rearrangements may cause selected cases of ectopic hormone production, this mechanism is probably unusual, as many tumors are associated with excessive production of numerous peptides. It is likely that cellular dedifferentiation underlies most cases of ectopic hormone production. In support of this idea, many cancers are poorly differentiated histologically, and certain tumor products, such as human chorionic gonadotropin (hCG), parathyroid hormone–related protein (PTHrP), and α-fetoprotein, are characteristic of gene expression at earlier developmental stages. On the other hand, the propensity of certain cancers to produce particular hormones (e.g., squamous cell carcinomas produce PTHrP) suggests that dedifferentiation is partial or that selective pathways are derepressed. These expression profiles are likely to be driven by alterations in transcriptional repression, changes in DNA methylation, or other factors that govern cell differentiation. Consistent with this idea, many solid tumors harbor poorly differentiated "cancer stem cells," a subpopulation of cells that are capable of initiating new tumors.

In SCLC, the pathway of differentiation has been defined. The neuroendocrine phenotype is dictated in part by the basic helix-loop-helix (bHLH) transcription factor human achaete-scute homologue 1 (hASH-1), which is expressed at abnormally high levels in SCLC associated with ectopic ACTH. The activity of hASH-1 is inhibited by hairy enhancer of split 1 (HES-1) and by Notch proteins, which are also capable of inducing growth arrest. Thus, abnormal expression of these developmental transcription factors appears to provide a link between cell proliferation and differentiation.

Ectopic hormone production would only be an epiphenomenon associated with cancer if it did not result in clinical manifestations. Excessive and unregulated production of hormones such as ACTH, PTHrP, or vasopressin can lead to substantial morbidity and can complicate the cancer treatment plan. Moreover, the paraneoplastic endocrinopathies are sometimes the presenting feature of underlying malignancy and may prompt the search for an unrecognized tumor.

A large number of paraneoplastic endocrine syndromes have been described, linking overproduction of particular hormones with specific types of tumors. However, certain recurring syndromes emerge from this group (Table 24-1). The most common paraneoplastic endocrine syndromes include hypercalcemia from overproduction of PTHrP and other factors, hyponatremia from excess vasopressin, and Cushing's syndrome from ectopic ACTH.

HYPERCALCEMIA CAUSED BY ECTOPIC PRODUCTION OF PTHrP

(See also Chap. 27)

Etiology

Humoral hypercalcemia of malignancy (HHM) occurs in up to 20% of patients with cancer. HHM is most common in cancers of the lung, head and neck, skin, esophagus, breast, and genitourinary tract, and in multiple myeloma and lymphomas. Several distinct humoral causes of HHM occur, most commonly overproduction of PTHrP. In addition to acting as a circulating humoral factor, bone metastases (e.g., breast, multiple myeloma) may produce PTHrP, leading to local osteolysis and hypercalcemia.

PTHrP is structurally related to PTH and it binds to the PTH receptor, explaining the similar biochemical features of HHM and hyperparathyroidism. PTHrP plays a key role in skeletal development and regulates cellular proliferation and differentiation in other tissues including skin, bone marrow, breast, and hair follicles. The mechanism of PTHrP induction in malignancy is incompletely understood; however, tumor-bearing tissues commonly associated with HHM normally produce PTHrP during development or cell renewal. Mutations in certain oncogenes, such as *Ras*, can activate PTHrP expression. In adult T cell lymphoma, the transactivating Tax protein produced by human T cell lymphotropic virus I (HTLV-I) stimulates PTHrP promoter activity. Metastatic lesions to bone are more likely to produce PTHrP than are metastases in other tissues, suggesting that bone produces factors that enhance PTHrP production, or that PTHrP-producing metastases have a selective growth advantage in bone. Thus, PTHrP production can be stimulated by mutations in oncogenes, by altered expression of viral or cellular transcription factors, and by local growth factors.

Another relatively common cause of HHM is excess production of 1,25-dihydroxyvitamin D. Like granulomatous disorders associated with hypercalcemia, lymphomas can produce an enzyme that converts 25-hydroxyvitamin D to the more active 1,25-dihydroxyvitamin D, leading to enhanced gastrointestinal calcium absorption. Other causes of HHM include tumor-mediated production of osteolytic cytokines and inflammatory mediators.

Clinical Manifestations

The typical presentation of HHM is a patient with a known malignancy who is found to be hypercalcemic on routine laboratory tests. Less often, hypercalcemia is the initial presenting feature of malignancy. Particularly when calcium levels are markedly increased [>3.5 mmol/L (>14 mg/dL)], patients may experience fatigue, mental status changes, dehydration, or symptoms of nephrolithiasis.

Diagnosis

Features that favor HHM, as opposed to primary hyperparathyroidism, include known malignancy, recent onset of hypercalcemia, and very high serum calcium levels.

TABLE 24-1

PARANEOPLASTIC SYNDROMES CAUSED BY ECTOPIC HORMONE PRODUCTION

PARANEOPLASTIC SYNDROME	ECTOPIC HORMONE	TYPICAL TUMOR TYPES[a]
Common		
Hypercalcemia of malignancy	Parathyroid hormone-related protein (PTHrP)	Squamous cell (head and neck, lung, skin), breast, genitourinary, gastrointestinal
	1,25-Dihydroxyvitamin D	Lymphomas
	Parathyroid hormone (PTH) (rare)	Lung, ovary
	Prostaglandin E_2 (PGE_2) (rare)	Renal, lung
Syndrome of inappropriate antidiuretic hormone secretion (SIADH)	Vasopressin	Lung (squamous, small cell), gastrointestinal, genitourinary, ovary
Cushing's syndrome	Adrenocorticotropic hormone (ACTH)	Lung (small cell, bronchial carcinoid, adenocarcinoma, squamous), thymus, pancreatic islet, medullary thyroid carcinoma
	Corticotropin-releasing hormone (CRH) (rare)	Pancreatic islet, carcinoid, lung, prostate
	Ectopic expression of gastric inhibitory peptide (GIP), luteinizing hormone (LH)/human chorionic gonadotropin (hCG), other G protein–coupled receptors (rare)	Macronodular adrenal hyperplasia
Less Common		
Non-islet cell hypoglycemia	Insulin-like growth factor II (IGF-II)	Mesenchymal tumors, sarcomas, adrenal, hepatic, gastrointestinal, kidney, prostate
	Insulin (rare)	Cervix (small cell carcinoma)
Male feminization	hCG[b]	Testis (embryonal, seminomas), germinomas, choriocarcinoma, lung, hepatic, pancreatic islet
Diarrhea or intestinal hypermotility	Calcitonin[c]	Lung, colon, breast, medullary thyroid carcinoma
	Vasoactive intestinal peptide (VIP)	Pancreas, pheochromocytoma, esophagus
Rare		
Oncogenic osteomalacia	Phosphatonin [fibroblast growth factor 23 (FGF23)]	Hemangiopericytomas, osteoblastomas, fibromas, sarcomas, giant cell tumors, prostate, lung
Acromegaly	Growth hormone–releasing hormone (GHRH)	Pancreatic islet, bronchial and other carcinoids
	Growth hormone (GH)	Lung, pancreatic islet
Hyperthyroidism	Thyroid-stimulating hormone (TSH)	Hydatidiform mole, embryonal tumors, struma ovarii
Hypertension	Renin	Juxtaglomerular tumors, kidney, lung, pancreas, ovary

[a]Only the most common tumor types are listed. For most ectopic hormone syndromes, an extensive list of tumors has been reported to produce one or more hormones.
[b]hCG is produced eutopically by trophoblastic tumors. Certain tumors produce disproportionate amounts of the hCG α or hCG β subunits. High levels of hCG rarely cause hyperthyroidism because of weak binding to the TSH receptor.
[c]Calcitonin is produced eutopically by medullary thyroid carcinoma and is used as a tumor marker.

Like hyperparathyroidism, hypercalcemia caused by PTHrP is accompanied by hypercalciuria and hypophosphatemia. Measurement of PTH is useful to exclude primary hyperparathyroidism; the PTH level should be suppressed in HHM. An elevated PTHrP level confirms the diagnosis, and it is increased in ~80% of hypercalcemic patients with cancer. 1,25-Dihydroxyvitamin D levels may be increased in patients with lymphoma.

℞ Treatment: HUMORAL HYPERCALCEMIA OF MALIGNANCY

The management of HHM begins with removal of excess calcium in the diet, medications, or IV solutions. Oral phosphorus (e.g., 250 mg Neutra-Phos three to four times daily) should be given until serum phosphorus is

>1.0 mmol/L (>3 mg/dL). Saline rehydration is used to dilute serum calcium and promote calciuresis. Forced diuresis with furosemide or other loop diuretics can enhance calcium excretion but provides relatively little value except in life-threatening hypercalcemia. When used, loop diuretics should be administered only after complete rehydration and with careful monitoring of fluid balance. Bisphosphonates such as pamidronate (30–90 mg IV), zoledronate (4–8 mg IV), or etidronate (7.5 mg/kg per day PO for 3–7 consecutive days) can reduce serum calcium within 1–2 days and suppress calcium release for several weeks. Bisphosphonate infusions can be repeated or oral bisphosphonates can be used for chronic treatment. Dialysis should be considered in severe hypercalcemia when saline hydration and bisphosphonate treatments are not possible or are too slow in onset. Previously used agents, such as calcitonin and mithramycin, have little utility now that bisphosphonates are available. Calcitonin (2–8 U/kg SC every 6–12 h) should be considered when rapid correction of severe hypercalcemia is needed. Hypercalcemia associated with lymphomas, multiple myeloma, or leukemia may respond to glucocorticoid treatment (e.g., prednisone 40–100 mg PO in four divided doses).

ECTOPIC VASOPRESSIN: TUMOR-ASSOCIATED SIADH

Etiology

Vasopressin is an antidiuretic hormone normally produced by the posterior pituitary gland. Ectopic vasopressin production by tumors is a common cause of the syndrome of inappropriate antidiuretic hormone (SIADH), occurring in at least half of patients with SCLC. Compensatory mechanisms, such as decreased thirst, suppression of aldosterone, and production of atrial natriuretic peptide (ANP), may mitigate the development of hyponatremia in patients who produce excessive vasopressin. Tumors with neuroendocrine features, such as SCLC and carcinoids, are the most common sources of ectopic vasopressin production, but it also occurs in other forms of lung cancer and with central nervous system (CNS) lesions, head and neck cancer, and genitourinary, gastrointestinal, and ovarian cancers. The mechanism of activation of the vasopressin gene in these tumors is unknown but often involves concomitant expression of the adjacent oxytocin gene, suggesting derepression of this locus.

Clinical Manifestations

Most patients with ectopic vasopressin secretion are asymptomatic and are identified because of the presence of hyponatremia on routine chemistry testing. Symptoms may include weakness, lethargy, nausea, confusion, depressed mental status, and seizures. The severity of symptoms reflects the rapidity of onset as well as the extent of hyponatremia. Hyponatremia usually develops slowly but may be exacerbated by the administration of IV fluids or the institution of new medications. Thirst is typically suppressed.

Diagnosis

The diagnostic features of ectopic vasopressin production are the same as those of other causes of SIADH (Chap. 3). Hyponatremia and reduced serum osmolality occur in the setting of an inappropriately normal or increased urine osmolality. Urine sodium excretion is normal or increased unless volume depletion is present. Other causes of hyponatremia should be excluded, including renal, adrenal, or thyroid insufficiency. Physiologic sources of vasopressin stimulation (CNS lesions, pulmonary disease, nausea), adaptive circulatory mechanisms (hypotension, heart failure, hepatic cirrhosis), and medications, including many chemotherapeutic agents, should also be considered as possible causes of hyponatremia. Vasopressin assay is not usually necessary to make the diagnosis.

℞ Treatment: ECTOPIC VASOPRESSIN: TUMOR-ASSOCIATED SIADH

Most patients with ectopic vasopressin production develop hyponatremia over several weeks or months. The disorder should be corrected gradually unless mental status is altered or there is risk of seizures. Treatment of the underlying malignancy may reduce ectopic vasopressin production but this response is slow, if it occurs at all. Fluid restriction to less than urine output, plus insensible losses, is often sufficient to partially correct hyponatremia. However, strict monitoring of the amount and types of liquids consumed or administered IV is required for fluid restriction to be effective. Salt tablets or saline are not helpful unless volume depletion is also present. Demeclocycline (150–300 mg PO three to four times daily) can be used to inhibit vasopressin action on the renal distal tubule but its onset of action is relatively slow (1–2 weeks). Conivaptan, a nonpeptide V_2 receptor antagonist, can be administered either PO (20–120 mg bid) or IV (10–40 mg), and is particularly effective when used in combination with fluid restriction in euvolemic hyponatremia. Severe hyponatremia (Na <115 meq/L) or mental status changes may require treatment with hypertonic (3%) or normal saline infusion together with furosemide, to enhance free-water clearance. The rate of sodium correction should be slow (0.5–1 meq/L per h) to prevent rapid fluid shifts and the possible development of central pontine myelinolysis.

CUSHING'S SYNDROME CAUSED BY ECTOPIC ACTH PRODUCTION

(See also Chap. 5)

Etiology

Ectopic ACTH production accounts for 10–20% of Cushing's syndrome. The syndrome is particularly common in neuroendocrine tumors. SCLC (>50%) is by far the most common cause of ectopic ACTH, followed by thymic carcinoid (15%), islet cell tumors (10%), bronchial carcinoid (10%), other carcinoids (5%), and pheochromocytomas (2%). Ectopic ACTH production is caused by increased expression of the proopiomelanocortin (POMC) gene, which encodes ACTH, along with melanocyte-stimulating hormone (MSH), β-lipotropin, and several other peptides. In many tumors, there is abundant but aberrant expression of the POMC gene from an internal promoter, proximal to the third exon, which encodes ACTH. However, because this product lacks the signal sequence necessary for protein processing, it is not secreted. Increased production of ACTH arises instead from less abundant, but unregulated, POMC expression from the same promoter site used in the pituitary. However, because the tumors lack many of the enzymes needed to process the POMC polypeptide, it is typically released as multiple large, biologically inactive fragments along with relatively small amounts of fully processed, active ACTH.

Rarely, corticotropin-releasing hormone (CRH) is produced by pancreatic islet tumors, SCLC, medullary thyroid cancer, carcinoids, or prostate cancer. When levels are high enough, CRH can cause pituitary corticotrope hyperplasia and Cushing's syndrome. Tumors that produce CRH sometimes also produce ACTH, raising the possibility of a paracrine mechanism for ACTH production.

A distinct mechanism for ACTH-independent Cushing's syndrome involves ectopic expression of various G protein–coupled receptors in the adrenal nodules. Ectopic expression of the gastric inhibitory peptide (GIP) receptor is the best-characterized example of this mechanism. In this case, meals induce GIP secretion, which inappropriately stimulates adrenal growth and glucocorticoid production.

Clinical Manifestations

The clinical features of hypercortisolemia are detected in only a small fraction of patients with documented ectopic ACTH production. Patients with ectopic ACTH syndrome generally exhibit less marked weight gain and centripetal fat redistribution, probably because the exposure to excess glucocorticoids is relatively short and because cachexia reduces the propensity for weight gain and fat deposition. The ectopic ACTH syndrome is associated with several clinical features that distinguish it from other causes of Cushing's syndrome (e.g., pituitary adenomas, adrenal adenomas, iatrogenic glucocorticoid excess). The metabolic manifestations of ectopic ACTH syndrome are dominated by fluid retention and hypertension, hypokalemia, metabolic alkalosis, glucose intolerance, and, often, steroid psychosis. The very high ACTH levels often cause increased pigmentation, and melanotrope-stimulating hormone (MSH) activity derived from the POMC precursor peptide is also increased. The extraordinarily high glucocorticoid levels in patients with ectopic sources of ACTH can lead to marked skin fragility and easy bruising. In addition, the high cortisol levels often overwhelm the renal 11β-hydroxysteroid dehydrogenase type II enzyme, which normally inactivates cortisol and prevents it from binding to renal mineralocorticoid receptors. Consequently, in addition to the excess mineralocorticoids produced by ACTH stimulation of the adrenal gland, high levels of cortisol exert activity through the mineralocorticoid receptor, leading to severe hypokalemia.

Diagnosis

The diagnosis of ectopic ACTH syndrome is usually not difficult in the setting of a known malignancy. Urine free cortisol levels fluctuate but are typically greater than two to four times normal and the plasma ACTH level is usually >22 pmol/L (>100 pg/mL). A suppressed ACTH level excludes this diagnosis and indicates an ACTH-independent cause of Cushing's syndrome (e.g., adrenal or exogenous glucocorticoid). In contrast to pituitary sources of ACTH, most ectopic sources of ACTH do not respond to glucocorticoid suppression. Therefore, high-dose dexamethasone (8 mg PO) suppresses 8:00 A.M. serum cortisol (50% decrease from baseline) in ~80% of pituitary ACTH-producing adenomas but fails to suppress ectopic ACTH in ~90% of cases. Bronchial and other carcinoids are well-documented exceptions to these general guidelines, as these ectopic sources of ACTH may exhibit feedback regulation indistinguishable from pituitary adenomas, including suppression by high-dose dexamethasone, and ACTH responsiveness to adrenal blockade with metyrapone. If necessary, petrosal sinus catheterization can be used to evaluate a patient with ACTH-dependent Cushing's syndrome when the source of ACTH is unclear. After CRH stimulation, a 3:1 petrosal sinus/peripheral ACTH ratio strongly suggests a pituitary ACTH source. Imaging studies are also useful in the evaluation of suspected carcinoid lesions, allowing biopsy and characterization of hormone production using special stains.

Treatment: CUSHING'S SYNDROME CAUSED BY ECTOPIC ACTH PRODUCTION

The morbidity associated with the ectopic ACTH syndrome can be substantial. Patients may experience depression or personality changes because of extreme cortisol excess. Metabolic derangements including diabetes mellitus and hypokalemia can worsen fatigue. Poor wound healing and predisposition to infections can complicate the surgical management of tumors, and opportunistic infections, caused by organisms such as *Pneumocystis carinii* and mycoses, are often the cause of death in patients with ectopic ACTH production. Depending on prognosis and treatment plans for the underlying malignancy, measures to reduce cortisol levels are often indicated. Treatment of the underlying malignancy may reduce ACTH levels but is rarely sufficient to reduce cortisol levels to normal. Adrenalectomy is not practical for most of these patients but should be considered if the underlying tumor is not resectable and the prognosis is otherwise favorable (e.g., carcinoid). Medical therapy with ketoconazole (200–400 mg PO bid), metyrapone (250–500 mg PO every 6 h), mitotane (3–6 g PO in four divided doses, tapered to maintain low cortisol production), or other agents that block steroid synthesis or action is often the most practical strategy for managing the hypercortisolism associated with ectopic ACTH production (Chap. 2). Glucocorticoid replacement should be provided to avoid adrenal insufficiency. Unfortunately, many patients will eventually progress despite medical blockade.

TUMOR-INDUCED HYPOGLYCEMIA CAUSED BY EXCESS PRODUCTION OF IGF-II

(See also Chap. 20)

Mesenchymal tumors, hemangiopericytomas, hepatocellular tumors, adrenal carcinomas, and a variety of other large tumors have been reported to produce excessive amounts of insulin-like growth factor type II (IGF-II) precursor, which binds weakly to insulin receptors and strongly to IGF-I receptors, leading to insulin-like actions. The gene encoding IGF-II resides on a chromosome 11p15 locus that is normally imprinted (that is, expression is exclusively from a single parental allele). Biallelic expression of the IGF-II gene occurs in a subset of tumors, suggesting loss of methylation and loss of imprinting as a mechanism for gene induction. In addition to increased IGF-II production, IGF-II bioavailability is increased due to complex alterations in circulating binding proteins. Increased IGF-II suppresses growth hormone (GH) and insulin, resulting in reduced IGF-binding protein 3 (IGFBP-3), IGF-I, and acid-labile subunit (ALS). The reduction in ALS and IGFBP-3, which normally sequester IGF-II, causes it to be displaced to a small circulating complex that has greater access to insulin target tissues. For this reason, circulating IGF-II levels may not be markedly increased, despite causing hypoglycemia. In addition to IGF-II–mediated hypoglycemia, tumors may occupy enough of the liver to impair gluconeogenesis.

In most cases, the tumor causing hypoglycemia is clinically apparent and hypoglycemia develops in association with fasting. The diagnosis is made by documenting low serum glucose and suppressed insulin levels in association with symptoms of hypoglycemia. Serum IGF-II levels may not be increased (IGF-II assays may not detect IGF-II precursors). Increased IGF-II mRNA expression is found in most of these tumors. Any medications associated with hypoglycemia should be eliminated. Treatment of the underlying malignancy, if possible, may reduce the predisposition to hypoglycemia. Frequent meals and IV glucose, especially during sleep or fasting, are often necessary to prevent hypoglycemia. Glucagon, GH, and glucocorticoids have also been used to enhance glucose production.

HUMAN CHORIONIC GONADOTROPIN

hCG is composed of α and β subunits and can be produced as intact hormone, which is biologically active, or as uncombined biologically inert subunits. Ectopic production of intact hCG occurs most often in association with testicular embryonal tumors, germ cell tumors, extragonadal germinomas, lung cancer, hepatoma, and pancreatic islet tumors. Eutopic production of hCG occurs with trophoblastic malignancies. Low levels of hCG or its uncombined α or β subunits have been reported in a wide array of tumors. hCG α-subunit production is particularly common in lung cancer and pancreatic islet cancer. In men, high hCG levels stimulate steroidogenesis and aromatase activity in testicular Leydig cells, resulting in increased estrogen production and the development of gynecomastia. Precocious puberty in boys or gynecomastia in men should prompt measurement of hCG and consideration of a testicular tumor or another source of ectopic hCG production. Most women are asymptomatic. hCG is easily measured. Treatment should be directed at the underlying malignancy.

ONCOGENIC OSTEOMALACIA

Hypophosphatemic oncogenic osteomalacia, also called tumor-induced osteomalacia (TIO), is characterized by markedly reduced serum phosphorus and renal phosphate wasting, leading to muscle weakness, bone pain, and osteomalacia. Serum calcium and PTH levels are normal and 1,25-dihydroxyvitamin D is low. Oncogenic osteomalacia is usually caused by benign mesenchymal tumors, such as hemangiopericytomas, fibromas, or giant cell tumors, often of the skeletal extremities or head. It has also been described in sarcomas and in patients with prostate and lung cancer. Resection of the tumor reverses the disorder, confirming its humoral basis. The circulating phosphaturic factor is called *phosphatonin*—a factor that inhibits renal tubular reabsorption of phosphate and renal conversion of 25-hydroxyvitamin D to 1,25-dihydroxyvitamin D. Phosphatonin has been identified as fibroblast growth factor 23 (FGF23). FGF23 levels are increased in some, but not all, patients with osteogenic osteomalacia. The disorder exhibits biochemical features similar to those seen with inactivating mutations in the *PHEX* gene, the cause of hereditary X-linked hypophosphatemia. The *PHEX* gene encodes a protease that inactivates FGF23. Treatment involves removal of the tumor, if possible, and supplementation with phosphate and vitamin D. Octreotide treatment reduces phosphate wasting in some patients with tumors that express somatostatin receptor subtype 2. Octreotide scans may also be useful to detect these tumors.

FURTHER READINGS

DeLellis RA, Xia L: Paraneoplastic endocrine syndromes: A review. Endocr Pathol 14:303, 2003

Emel EA et al: Sensitivity of fibroblast growth factor 23 measurements in tumor-induced osteomalacia. J Clin Endocrinol Metab 91:2055, 2006

Gabrilovich M et al: Paraneoplastic polymyositis associated with squamous cell carcinoma of the lung. Chest 129(6):1721, 2006

Jan de Beur SM: Tumor-induced osteomalacia. JAMA 294:1260, 2005

Jones PA, Baylin SB: The fundamental role of epigenetic events in cancer. Nat Rev Genet 3:415, 2002

Mundy GR et al: PTH-related peptide (PTHrP) in hypercalcemia. J Am Soc Nephrol 19:672, 2008

Rikhof B et al: The insulin-like growth factor system and sarcomas. J Pathol 217:469, 2009

Shaikh A et al: Regulation of phosphate homeostasis by the phosphatonins and other novel mediators. Pediatr Nephrol 23:1203, 2008

Stewart AF: Clinical practice. Hypercalcemia associated with cancer. N Engl J Med 352:373, 2005

Zemskova MS et al: Diagnostic accuracy of chromogranin A and calcitonin precursors measurements for the discrimination of ectopic ACTH secretion from Cushing's disease. J Clin Endocrinol Metab, 2009

SECTION V

DISORDERS OF BONE AND CALCIUM METABOLISM

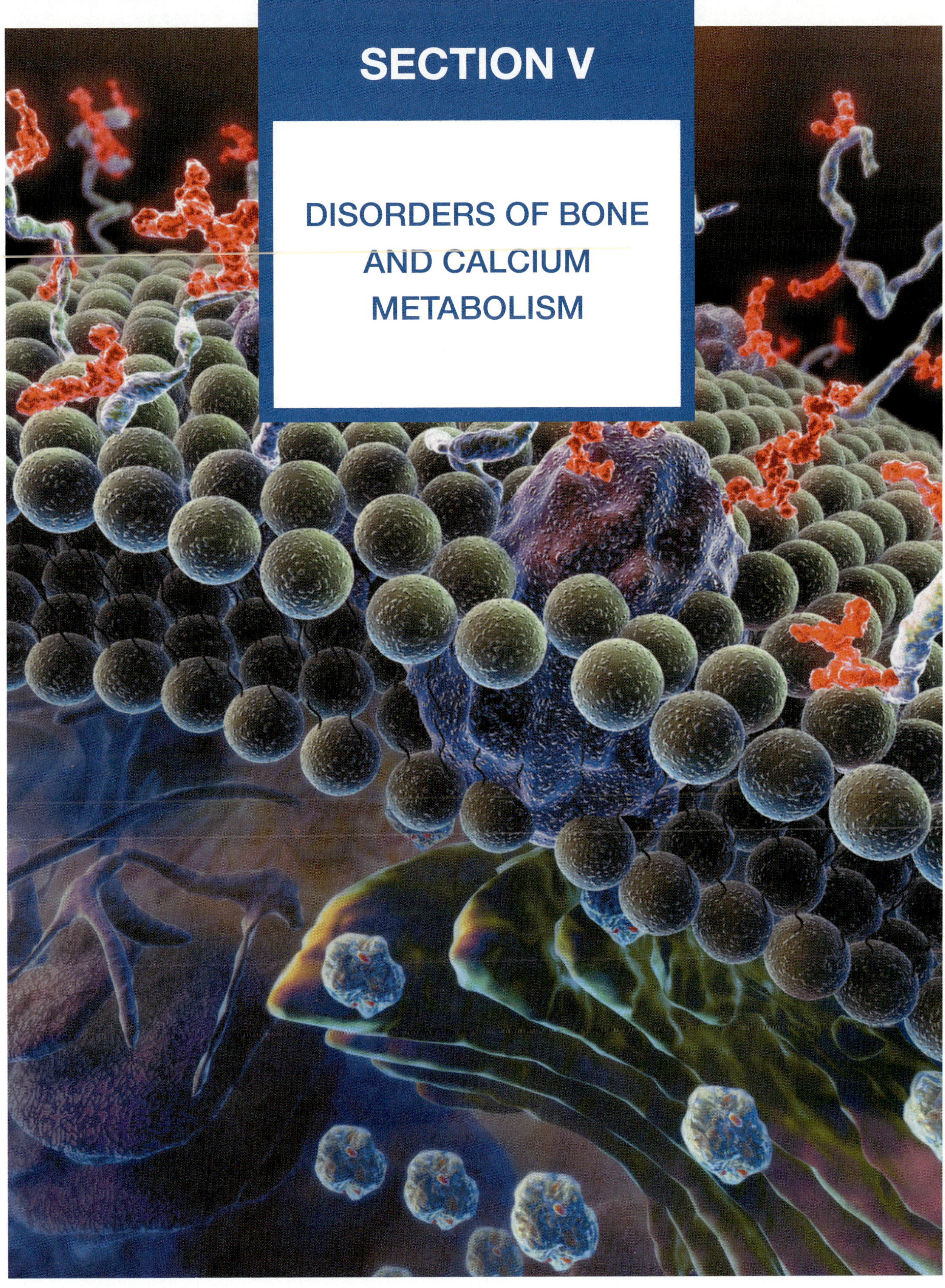

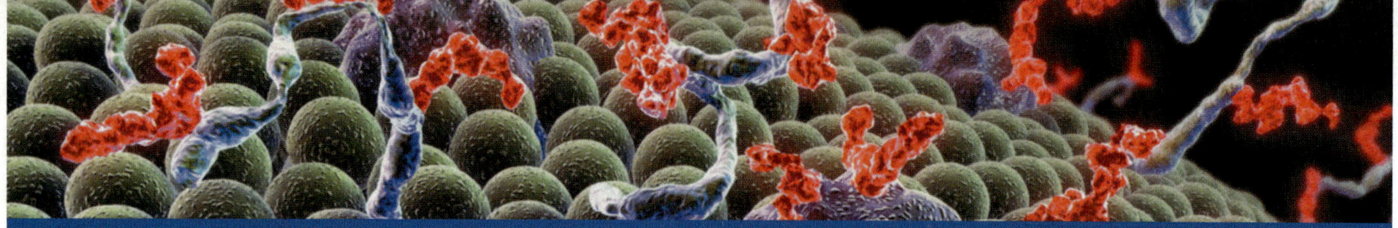

CHAPTER 25

BONE AND MINERAL METABOLISM IN HEALTH AND DISEASE

F. Richard Bringhurst ■ Marie B. Demay ■ Stephen M. Krane ■ Henry M. Kronenberg

BONE STRUCTURE AND METABOLISM

Bone is a dynamic tissue that is remodeled constantly throughout life. The arrangement of compact and cancellous bone provides a strength and density suitable for both mobility and protection. In addition, bone provides a reservoir for calcium, magnesium, phosphorus, sodium, and other ions necessary for homeostatic functions. The skeleton is highly vascular and receives about 10% of the cardiac output. Remodeling of bone is accomplished by two distinct cell types: osteoblasts produce bone matrix and osteoclasts resorb the matrix.

The extracellular components of bone consist of a solid mineral phase in close association with an organic matrix, of which 90–95% is type I collagen. The noncollagenous portion of the organic matrix is heterogeneous and contains serum proteins, such as albumin, as well as many locally produced proteins, whose functions are incompletely understood. These proteins include cell attachment/signaling proteins, such as thrombospondin, osteopontin, and fibronectin; calcium-binding proteins such as matrix gla protein and osteocalcin; and proteoglycans such as biglycan and decorin. Some of these proteins organize collagen fibrils; others influence mineralization and binding of the mineral phase to the matrix.

The mineral phase is made up of calcium and phosphate and is best characterized as a poorly crystalline hydroxyapatite. The mineral phase of bone is deposited initially in intimate relation to the collagen fibrils and is found in specific locations in the "holes" between the collagen fibrils. This architectural arrangement of mineral and matrix results in a two-phase material well suited to withstand mechanical stresses. The organization of collagen influences the amount and type of mineral phase formed in bone. Although the primary structures of type I collagen in skin and bone tissues are similar, there are differences in posttranslational modifications and distribution of intermolecular cross-links. The holes in the packing structure of the collagen are larger in mineralized collagen of bone and dentin than in unmineralized collagens such as tendon. Single amino-acid substitutions in the helical portion of either the α1 (*COL1A1*) or α2 (*COL1A2*) chains of type I collagen disrupt the organization of bone in osteogenesis imperfecta. The severe skeletal fragility associated with these disorders highlights the importance of the fibrillar matrix in the structure of bone.

Osteoblasts synthesize and secrete the organic matrix. They are derived from cells of mesenchymal origin (**Fig. 25-1*A***). Active osteoblasts are found on the surface

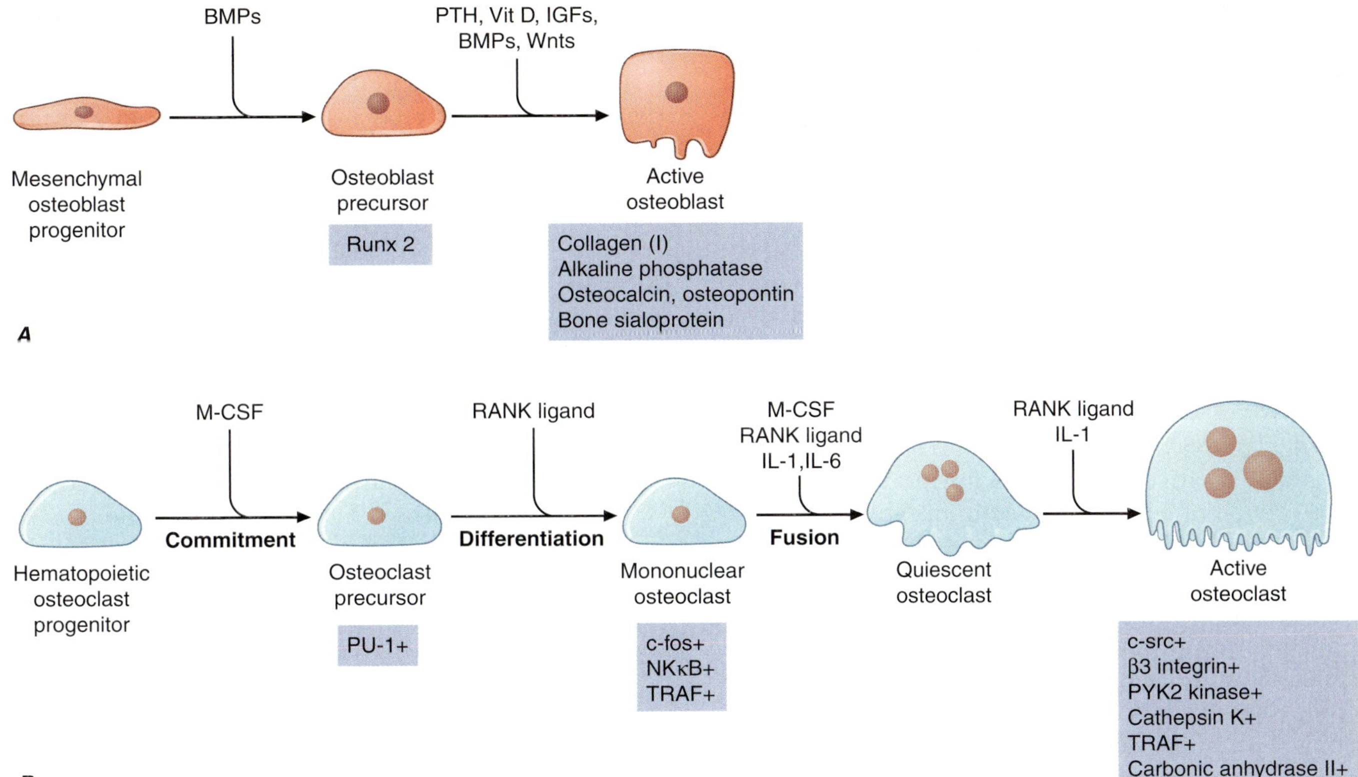

FIGURE 25-1

Pathways regulating development of (*A*) osteoblasts and (*B*) osteoclasts. Hormones, cytokines, and growth factors that control cell proliferation and differentiation are shown above the arrows. Transcription factors and other markers specific for various stages of development are depicted below the arrows. BMPs, bone morphogenic proteins; Wnts, wingless-type, mouse mammary tumor virus integration site; PTH, parathyroid hormone; Vit D, vitamin D; IGFs, insulin-like growth factors; Runx2, Runt-related transcription factor 2; M-CSF, macrophage colony-stimulating factor; PU-1, a monocyte- and B lymphocyte–specific ets family transcription factor; NFκB, nuclear factor κB; TRAF, tumor necrosis factor receptor–associated factors; RANK ligand, receptor activator of NFκB ligand; IL-1, interleukin-1; IL-6, interleukin-6. (*Modified from T Suda et al: Endocr Rev 20:345, 1999; with permission.*)

of newly forming bone. As an osteoblast secretes matrix, which is then mineralized, the cell becomes an *osteocyte*, still connected with its blood supply through a series of canaliculi. Osteocytes comprise the vast majority of the cells in bone. They are thought to be the mechanosensors in bone that communicate signals to surface osteoblasts and their progenitors through the canalicular network. Mineralization of the matrix, both in trabecular bone and in osteones of compact cortical bone (*haversian systems*), begins soon after the matrix is secreted (primary mineralization) but is not completed for several weeks or even longer (secondary mineralization). While this mineralization takes advantage of the high concentrations of calcium and phosphate already near saturation in serum, mineralization is a carefully regulated process dependent on the activity of osteoblast-derived alkaline phosphatase, which probably works by hydrolyzing inhibitors of mineralization.

Genetic studies in humans and mice have identified several key genes that control osteoblast development. Core-binding factor A1 (*CBFA1*, also called *Runx2*) is a transcription factor expressed specifically in chondrocyte (cartilage cells) and osteoblast progenitors, as well as in hypertrophic chondrocytes and mature osteoblasts. *Runx2* regulates the expression of several important osteoblast proteins including osterix (another transcription factor needed for osteoblast maturation), osteopontin, bone sialoprotein, type I collagen, osteocalcin, and the receptor activator of NFκB (RANK) ligand. *Runx2* expression is regulated, in part, by bone morphogenic proteins (BMPs). *Runx2*-deficient mice are devoid of osteoblasts, whereas mice with a deletion of only one allele (*Runx2* +/–) exhibit a delay in formation of the clavicles and some cranial bones. The latter abnormalities are similar to those in the human disorder *cleidocranial dysplasia*, which is also caused by heterozygous inactivating mutations in *Runx2*.

The paracrine signaling molecule, Indian hedgehog (Ihh), also plays a critical role in osteoblast development, as evidenced by Ihh-deficient mice that lack osteoblasts in bone formed on a cartilage mold (endochondral ossification). Signals originating from members of the wnt (wingless-type mouse mammary tumor virus integration site) family of paracrine factors are also important. Humans and mice missing a wnt-family co-receptor, LRP5 (lipoprotein receptor–related protein 5), have osteoporosis. Remarkably, humans with an overactive form of LRP5 have increased bone mass. Numerous other growth-regulatory factors affect osteoblast function, including the three closely related transforming growth factors β, fibroblast growth factors (FGFs) 2 and 18, platelet-derived growth factor, and insulin-like growth factors (IGFs) I and II. Hormones such as parathyroid hormone (PTH) and 1,25-dihydroxyvitamin D [$1,25(OH)_2D$] activate receptors expressed by osteoblasts to ensure mineral homeostasis and to influence a variety of bone cell functions.

Resorption of bone is carried out mainly by *osteoclasts*, multinucleated cells that are formed by fusion of cells derived from the common precursor of macrophages and osteoclasts. Multiple factors regulating osteoclast development have been identified (**Fig. 25-1*B***). Factors produced by osteoblasts or marrow stromal cells allow osteoblasts to control osteoclast development and activity. Macrophage colony-stimulating factor (M-CSF) plays a critical role during several steps in the pathway and ultimately leads to fusion of osteoclast progenitor cells to form multinucleated, active osteoclasts. RANK ligand, a member of the tumor necrosis factor (TNF) family, is expressed on the surface of osteoblast progenitors and stromal fibroblasts. In a process involving cell-cell interactions, RANK ligand binds to the RANK receptor on osteoclast progenitors, stimulating osteoclast differentiation and activation. Alternatively, a soluble decoy receptor, referred to as osteoprotegerin, can bind RANK ligand and inhibit osteoclast differentiation. Several growth factors and cytokines (including interleukins 1, 6, and 11; TNF; and interferon γ) modulate osteoclast differentiation and function. Most hormones that influence osteoclast function do not directly target this cell but instead influence M-CSF and RANK ligand signaling by osteoblasts. Both PTH and $1,25(OH)_2D$ increase osteoclast number and activity, whereas estrogen decreases osteoclast number and activity by this indirect mechanism. Calcitonin, in contrast, binds to its receptor on the basal surface of osteoclasts and directly inhibits osteoclast function.

Osteoclast-mediated resorption of bone takes place in scalloped spaces (*Howship's lacunae*) where the osteoclasts are attached through a specific $\alpha_v\beta_3$ integrin to components of the bone matrix such as osteopontin. The osteoclast forms a tight seal to the underlying matrix and secretes protons, chloride, and proteinases into a confined space likened to an extracellular lysosome. The active osteoclast surface forms a ruffled border that contains a specialized proton pump ATPase, which secretes acid and solubilizes the mineral phase. Carbonic anhydrase (type II isoenzyme) within the osteoclast generates the needed protons. The bone matrix is resorbed in the acid environment adjacent to the ruffled border by proteases that act at low pH, such as cathepsin K.

In the embryo and in the growing child, bone develops by remodeling and replacing previously calcified cartilage (endochondral bone formation) or is formed without a cartilage matrix (intramembranous bone formation). Chondrocytes proliferate, secrete, and mineralize a matrix; enlarge (hypertrophy); and then die, thereby enlarging bone and providing the matrix and factors that stimulate endochondral bone formation. This program is regulated by both local factors, such as IGF-I and -II, parathyroid hormone–related peptide (PTHrP), and FGFs, and by systemic hormones such as growth hormone, glucocorticoids, and estrogen.

New bone, whether formed in infants or in adults during repair, has a relatively high ratio of cells to matrix and is characterized by coarse fiber bundles of collagen that are interlaced and randomly dispersed (woven bone). In adults, the more mature bone is organized with fiber bundles regularly arranged in parallel or concentric sheets (lamellar bone). In long bones, deposition of lamellar bone in a concentric arrangement around blood vessels forms the haversian systems. Growth in length of bones is dependent on proliferation of cartilage cells and on the endochondral sequence at the growth plate. Growth in width and thickness is accomplished by formation of bone at the periosteal surface and by resorption at the endosteal surface, with the rate of formation exceeding that of resorption. In adults, after the growth plates close, growth in length and endochondral bone formation cease, except for some activity in the cartilage cells beneath the articular surface. Even in adults, however, remodeling of bone (within haversian systems as well as trabecular bone) continues throughout life. In adults, ~4% of the surface of trabecular bone (such as iliac crest) is involved in active resorption, whereas 10–15% of trabecular surfaces is covered with osteoid. Radioisotope studies indicate that as much as 18% of the total skeletal calcium is deposited and removed each year. Thus, bone is an active metabolizing tissue that requires an intact blood supply. The cycle of bone resorption and formation is a highly orchestrated process carried out by the basic multicellular unit, composed of a group of osteoclasts and osteoblasts (**Fig. 25-2**).

The response of bone to fractures, infection, and interruption of blood supply and to expanding lesions is relatively limited. Dead bone must be resorbed, and new bone must be formed, a process carried out in association with growth of new blood vessels into the involved area. In injuries that disrupt the organization of the tissue, such as a fracture in which apposition of fragments is poor or when motion exists at the fracture site, the progenitor stromal cells differentiate into cells with functional capacities different from those of osteoblasts, and varying amounts of fibrous tissue and cartilage are formed. When there is good apposition with fixation and little motion at

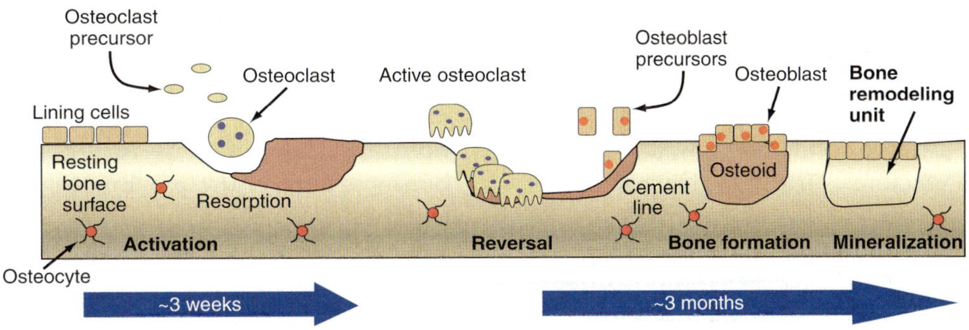

Osteoclast precursor
Osteoclast
Active osteoclast
Osteoblast precursors
Osteoblast
Bone remodeling unit
Lining cells
Resting bone surface
Resorption
Osteoid
Cement line
Activation
Reversal
Bone formation
Mineralization
Osteocyte
~3 weeks
~3 months

FIGURE 25-2

Schematic representation of bone remodeling. The cycle of bone remodeling is carried out by the basic multicellular unit (BMU), composed of a group of osteoclasts and osteoblasts. In cortical bone, the BMUs tunnel through the tissue, whereas in cancellous bone, they move across the trabecular surface. The process of bone remodeling is initiated by contraction of the lining cells and the recruitment of osteoclast precursors. These precursors fuse to form multinucleated, active osteoclasts that mediate bone resorption. Osteoclasts adhere to bone and subsequently remove it by acidification and proteolytic digestion. As the BMU advances, osteoclasts leave the resorption site and osteoblasts move in to cover the excavated area and begin the process of new bone formation by secreting osteoid, which is eventually mineralized into new bone. After osteoid mineralization, osteoblasts flatten and form a layer of lining cells over new bone.

the fracture site, repair occurs predominantly by formation of new bone without other scar tissue.

Remodeling of bone occurs along lines of force generated by mechanical stress. The signals from these mechanical stresses are sensed by osteocytes, which transmit signals to osteoclasts or osteoblasts, or their precursors. A bowing deformity increases new bone formation at the concave surface and resorption at the convex surface, seemingly designed to produce the strongest mechanical structure. Expanding lesions in bone, such as tumors, induce resorption at the surface in contact with the tumor, by producing ligands, such as PTHrP, that stimulate osteoclast differentiation and function. Even in a disorder as architecturally disruptive as Paget's disease, remodeling is dictated by mechanical forces. Thus, bone plasticity reflects the interaction of cells with each other and with the environment.

Measurement of the products of osteoblast and osteoclast activity can assist in the diagnosis and management of bone diseases. Osteoblast activity can be assessed by measuring serum bone-specific alkaline phosphatase. Similarly, osteocalcin, a protein secreted from osteoblasts, is made virtually only by osteoblasts. Osteoclast activity can be assessed by measurement of products of collagen degradation. Collagen molecules are covalently linked to each other in the extracellular matrix through the formation of hydroxypyridinium cross-links. These cross-linked peptides can be measured both in urine and in blood.

CALCIUM METABOLISM

Over 99% of the 1–2 kg of calcium present normally in the adult human body resides in the skeleton, where it provides mechanical stability and serves as a reservoir sometimes needed to maintain extracellular fluid (ECF) calcium concentration (Fig. 25-3). Skeletal calcium accretion first becomes significant during the third trimester of fetal life, accelerates throughout childhood and adolescence, reaches a peak in early adulthood, and gradually declines thereafter at rates that rarely exceed

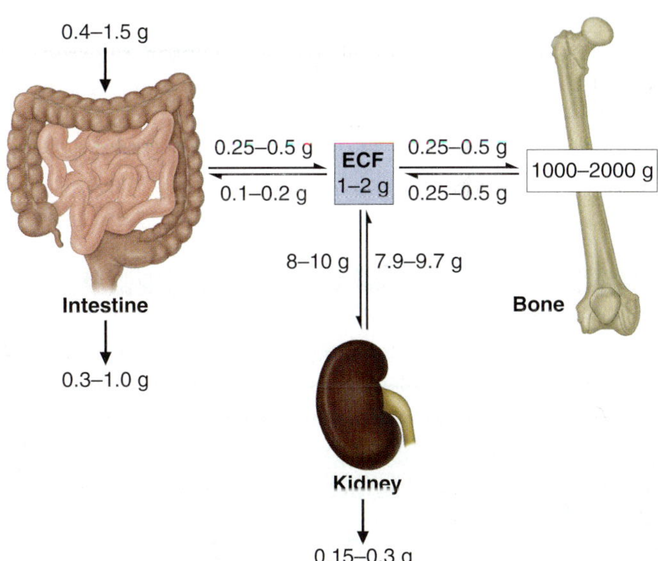

FIGURE 25-3

Calcium homeostasis. Schematic illustration of calcium content of extracellular fluid (ECF) and bone as well as of diet and feces; magnitude of calcium flux per day as calculated by various methods is shown at sites of transport in intestine, kidney, and bone. Ranges of values shown are approximate and chosen to illustrate certain points discussed in text. In conditions of calcium balance, rates of calcium release from and uptake into bone are equal.

1–2% per year. These slow changes in total skeletal calcium content contrast with relatively high daily rates of closely matched fluxes of calcium into and out of bone (~250–500 mg each), a process mediated by coupled osteoblastic and osteoclastic activity. Another 0.5–1% of skeletal calcium is freely exchangeable (e.g., in chemical equilibrium) with that in the ECF.

The concentration of ionized calcium in the ECF must be maintained within a narrow range because of the critical role it plays in a wide array of cellular functions, especially those involved in neuromuscular activity, secretion, and signal transduction. Intracellular cytosolic free calcium levels are ~100 nmol/L and are 10,000-fold lower than ionized calcium concentration in the blood and ECF (1.1–1.3 mmol/L). This steep chemical gradient promotes rapid calcium influx through various membrane calcium channels that can be activated by hormones, metabolites, or neurotransmitters, swiftly changing cellular function. In blood, total calcium concentration is normally 2.2–2.6 m*M* (8.5–10.5 mg/dL), of which ~50% is ionized. The remainder is bound ionically to negatively charged proteins (predominantly albumin and immunoglobulins) or loosely complexed with phosphate, citrate, sulfate, or other anions. Alterations in serum protein concentrations directly affect the total blood calcium concentration, even if the ionized calcium concentration remains normal. An algorithm to correct for protein changes adjusts the total serum calcium (in mg/dL) upward by 0.8 times the deficit in serum albumin (g/dL) or by 0.5 times the deficit in serum immunoglobulin (in g/dL). Such corrections provide only rough approximations of actual free calcium concentrations, however, and may be misleading, particularly during acute illness. Acidosis also alters ionized calcium by reducing its association with proteins. The best practice is to measure blood ionized calcium directly by a method that employs calcium-selective electrodes in acute settings during which calcium abnormalities might occur.

Control of the ionized calcium concentration in the ECF ordinarily is accomplished by adjusting the rates of calcium movement across intestinal and renal epithelia. These adjustments are mediated mainly via changes in blood levels of the hormones PTH and 1,25$(OH)_2$D.

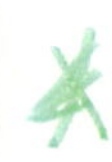

Blood ionized calcium directly suppresses PTH secretion by activating parathyroid calcium-sensing receptors (CaSRs). Also, ionized calcium indirectly affects PTH secretion via effects on 1,25$(OH)_2$D production. This active vitamin D metabolite inhibits PTH production by an incompletely understood mechanism of negative feedback (Chap. 27).

Normal dietary calcium intake in the United States varies widely, ranging from 10–37 mmol/d (400–1500 mg/d). Many individuals, in an effort to prevent osteoporosis, routinely supplement this further with oral calcium salts to a total intake of 37–50 mmol/d (1500–2000 mg/d). Intestinal absorption of ingested calcium involves both active (transcellular) and passive (paracellular) mechanisms. Passive calcium absorption is nonsaturable and approximates 5% of daily calcium intake, whereas the active mechanism, controlled principally by 1,25$(OH)_2$D, normally ranges from 20–70%. Active calcium transport occurs mainly in the proximal small bowel (duodenum and proximal jejunum), although some active calcium absorption occurs in most segments of the small intestine. Optimal rates of calcium absorption require gastric acid. This is especially true for weakly dissociable calcium supplements such as calcium carbonate. In fact, large boluses of calcium carbonate are poorly absorbed because of their neutralizing effect upon gastric acid. In achlorhydric subjects or for those taking drugs that inhibit gastric acid secretion, supplements should be taken with meals to optimize their absorption. Use of calcium citrate may be preferable in these circumstances. Calcium absorption may also be blunted in disease states such as pancreatic or biliary insufficiency, in which ingested calcium remains bound to unabsorbed fatty acids or other food constituents. At high levels of calcium intake, synthesis of 1,25$(OH)_2$D is reduced, which decreases the rate of active intestinal calcium absorption. The opposite occurs with dietary calcium restriction. Some calcium, ~2.5–5.0 mmol/d (100–200 mg/d), is excreted as an obligate component of intestinal secretions and is not regulated by calciotropic hormones.

The feedback-controlled hormonal regulation of intestinal absorptive efficiency results in a relatively constant daily net calcium absorption of ~5–7.5 mmol/d (200–400 mg/d), despite large changes in daily dietary calcium intake. This daily load of absorbed calcium is excreted by the kidneys in a manner that is also tightly regulated by the concentration of ionized calcium in the blood. Approximately 8–10 g/d of calcium is filtered by the glomeruli, of which only 2–3% appears in the urine. Most filtered calcium (65%) is reabsorbed in the proximal tubules via a passive, paracellular route that is coupled to concomitant NaCl reabsorption and not specifically regulated. The cortical thick ascending limb of Henle's loop (cTAL) reabsorbs roughly another 20% of filtered calcium, also via a paracellular mechanism. Calcium reabsorption in the cTAL requires a tight-junctional protein called paracellin-1 and is inhibited by increased blood concentrations of calcium or magnesium, acting via the CaSR, which is highly expressed on basolateral membranes in this nephron segment. Operation of the renal CaSR provides a mechanism, independent of those engaged directly by PTH or 1,25$(OH)_2$D, whereby serum ionized calcium can control renal calcium reabsorption. Finally, ~10% of filtered calcium is reabsorbed in the distal convoluted tubules (DCT) by a transcellular mechanism. Calcium enters the luminal surface of the cell through specific apical calcium channels, whose number is regulated. It then moves across the cell in association with a specific calcium-binding protein (calbindin-D28k) that buffers cytosolic calcium concentrations from the large mass of transported calcium. Ca^{2+}-ATPases and Na^+/Ca^{2+} exchangers actively extrude calcium across the basolateral surface and thereby maintain the transcellular calcium gradient. All of these processes are stimulated, directly or indirectly, by PTH. The DCT is also the site of action of thiazide diuretics, which lower urinary calcium excretion. Conversely, dietary sodium loads, or increased distal sodium delivery caused by loop diuretics or saline infusion, reduce DCT calcium reabsorption.

The homeostatic mechanisms that normally maintain a constant serum ionized calcium concentration may fail at extremes of calcium intake or when the hormonal systems or organs involved are compromised. Thus, even with maximal activity of the vitamin D–dependent intestinal active transport system, sustained calcium intakes <5 mmol/d (<200 mg/d) cannot provide enough net calcium absorption to replace obligate losses via the intestine, kidney, sweat, or other secretions. In this case, increased blood levels of PTH and $1,25(OH)_2D$ activate osteoclastic bone resorption to obtain needed calcium from bone, which leads to progressive bone loss and negative calcium balance. Increased PTH and $1,25(OH)_2D$ also enhance renal calcium reabsorption, and $1,25(OH)_2D$ enhances calcium absorption in the gut. At very high calcium intakes [>100 mmol/d; >4 g/d], passive intestinal absorption continues to deliver calcium into the ECF, despite maximally downregulated intestinal active transport and renal tubular calcium reabsorption. This can cause severe hypercalciuria, nephrocalcinosis, progressive renal failure, and hypercalcemia (e.g., "milk alkali syndrome"). Deficiency or excess of PTH or vitamin D, intestinal disease, and renal failure represent other commonly encountered challenges to normal calcium homeostasis (Chap. 27).

PHOSPHORUS METABOLISM

Although 85% of the ~600 g of body phosphorus is present in bone mineral, phosphorus is also a major intracellular constituent, both as the free anion(s) and as a component of numerous organophosphate compounds including structural proteins, enzymes, transcription factors, carbohydrate and lipid intermediates, high-energy stores (ATP, creatine phosphate), and nucleic acids. Unlike calcium, phosphorus exists intracellularly at concentrations close to those present in ECF (e.g., 1–2 mmol/L). In cells and in the ECF, phosphorus exists in several forms, predominantly as $H_2PO_4^-$ or $NaHPO_4^-$, with perhaps 10% as HPO_4^{2-}. This mixture of anions will be referred to here as "phosphate." In serum, about 12% of phosphorus is bound to proteins. Concentrations of phosphates in blood and ECF are generally expressed in terms of elemental phosphorus, the normal range in adults being 0.75–1.45 mmol/L (2.5–4.5 mg/dL). Because the volume of the intracellular fluid compartment is twice that of the ECF, measurements of ECF phosphate may not accurately reflect phosphate availability within cells that follows even modest shifts of phosphate from one compartment to the other.

Phosphate is widely available in foods and is efficiently absorbed (65%) by the small intestine, even in the absence of vitamin D. On the other hand, phosphate absorptive efficiency may be further enhanced (to 85–90%) via active transport mechanisms that are stimulated by $1,25(OH)_2D$. These involve activation of Na^+/PO_4^{2-} co-transporters that move phosphate into intestinal cells against an unfavorable electrochemical gradient. Daily net intestinal phosphate absorption varies widely according to the composition of the diet but is generally in the range of 500–1000 mg/d. Phosphate absorption can be inhibited by large doses of calcium salts or by sevelamer hydrochloride (Renagel), strategies commonly used to control levels of serum phosphate in renal failure. Aluminum hydroxide antacids also reduce phosphate absorption but are less commonly used because of the potential for aluminum toxicity. Low serum phosphate directly stimulates renal proximal tubular synthesis of $1,25(OH)_2D$.

Serum phosphate levels vary by as much as 50% on a normal day. This reflects the effect of food intake but also an underlying circadian rhythm that produces a nadir between 7 and 10 A.M. Carbohydrate administration, especially as IV dextrose solutions in fasting subjects, can decrease serum phosphate by >0.7 mmol/L (2 mg/dL) due to rapid uptake into, and utilization by, cells. A similar response is observed in the treatment of diabetic ketoacidosis and during metabolic or respiratory alkalosis. Because of this wide variation in serum phosphate, it is best to perform measurements in the basal, fasting state.

Control of serum phosphate is determined mainly by the rate of renal tubular reabsorption of the filtered load, which is ~4–6 g/d. Because intestinal phosphate absorption is highly efficient, urinary excretion is not constant but varies directly with dietary intake. The fractional excretion of phosphate (ratio of phosphate to creatinine clearance) is generally in the range of 10–15%. The proximal tubule is the principal site at which renal phosphate reabsorption is regulated. This is accomplished by changes in the apical expression and activity of a specific Na^+/PO_4^{2-} co-transporter (NaPi-2) in the proximal tubule. Apical expression of NaPi-2 is rapidly reduced by PTH, the major known hormonal regulator of renal phosphate excretion. FGF23 can dramatically impair phosphate reabsorption (see below). Activating *FGF23* mutations cause the rare disorder autosomal dominant hypophosphatemic rickets. In contrast to PTH, this molecule also leads to reduced synthesis of $1,25(OH)_2D$, which may worsen the resulting hypophosphatemia by lowering intestinal phosphate absorption. Renal reabsorption of phosphate is responsive to changes in dietary intake, such that experimental dietary phosphate restriction leads to a dramatic lowering of urinary phosphate within hours, preceding any decline in serum phosphate (e.g., filtered load). This physiologic renal adaptation to changes in dietary phosphate availability occurs independently of PTH. Findings in *FGF23*-knockout mice suggest that FGF23 normally acts to lower blood phosphate and $1,25(OH)_2D$ levels. In turn, elevations of blood phosphate increases blood levels of FGF23.

Renal phosphate reabsorption is impaired by hypocalcemia, hypomagnesemia, and severe hypophosphatemia. Phosphate clearance is enhanced by ECF volume expansion and impaired by dehydration. Phosphate retention is an important pathophysiologic feature of renal insufficiency.

HYPOPHOSPHATEMIA

Causes

Hypophosphatemia can occur by one or more of three primary mechanisms: (1) inadequate intestinal phosphate absorption, (2) excessive renal phosphate excretion, or (3) rapid redistribution of phosphate from the ECF into bone or soft tissue (Table 25-1). Because phosphate is so abundant in foods, inadequate intestinal absorption is almost never observed now that aluminum hydroxide antacids, which bind phosphate in the gut, are no longer commonly used. Fasting or starvation, however, may result in depletion of body phosphate and predispose to subsequent hypophosphatemia during refeeding, especially if this is accomplished with IV glucose alone.

Chronic hypophosphatemia usually signifies a persistent renal tubular phosphate-wasting disorder. Excessive activation of PTH/PTHrP receptors in the proximal tubule, because of primary or secondary hyperparathyroidism or because of the PTHrP-mediated hypercalcemia syndrome in malignancy (Chap. 27), is among the more common causes of renal hypophosphatemia, especially because of the high prevalence of vitamin D deficiency in older Americans. Familial hypocalciuric hypercalcemia and Jansen's chondrodystrophy are rare examples of genetic disorders in this category (Chap. 27).

Several genetic and acquired diseases cause PTH/PTHrP-independent tubular phosphate wasting, with associated rickets and osteomalacia. All of these diseases manifest severe hypophosphatemia; renal phosphate wasting, sometimes accompanied by aminoaciduria; low blood levels of $1,25(OH)_2D$; low-normal serum levels of calcium; and evidence of impaired cartilage or bone mineralization. Analysis of these diseases has led to the discovery of a "new" hormone, FGF23, that is an important physiologic regulator of phosphate metabolism. FGF23 decreases phosphate reabsorption in the proximal tubule and also suppresses the 1-hydroxylase responsible for synthesis of $1,25(OH)_2D$. FGF23 is synthesized by cells of the osteoblast lineage. High-phosphate diets increase FGF23 levels, and low-phosphate diets decrease them. Autosomal

TABLE 25-1

CAUSES OF HYPOPHOSPHATEMIA

- I. Reduced renal tubular phosphate reabsorption
  - A. PTH/PTHrP-dependent
    - 1. Primary hyperparathyroidism
    - 2. Secondary hyperparathyroidism
      - a. Vitamin D deficiency/resistance
      - b. Calcium starvation/malabsorption
      - c. Bartter syndrome
      - d. Autosomal recessive renal hypercalciuria with hypomagnesemia
    - 3. PTHrP-dependent hypercalcemia of malignancy
    - 4. Familial hypocalciuric hypercalcemia
  - B. PTH/PTHrP-independent
    - 1. Genetic hypophosphatemia
      - a. X-linked hypophosphatemic rickets
      - b. Dent disease
      - c. Autosomal dominant hypophosphatemic rickets
      - d. Fanconi syndrome(s)
      - e. Cystinosis
      - f. Wilson disease
      - g. McCune-Albright syndrome (fibrous dysplasia)
      - h. Idiopathic hypercalciuria (absorptive subtype)
      - i. Hereditary hypophosphatemia with hypercalciuria (Bedouins)
    - 2. Tumor-induced osteomalacia
    - 3. Other systemic disorders
      - a. Poorly controlled diabetes mellitus
      - b. Alcoholism
      - c. Hyperaldosteronism
      - d. Hypomagnesemia
      - e. Amyloidosis
      - f. Hemolytic uremic syndrome
      - g. Renal transplantation or partial liver resection
      - h. Rewarming or induced hyperthermia
    - 4. Drugs or toxins
      - a. Ethanol
      - b. Acetazolamide, other diuretics
      - c. High-dose estrogens or glucocorticoids
      - d. Heavy metals (lead, cadmium)
      - e. Toluene, *N*-methyl formamide
      - f. Cisplatin, ifosfamide, foscarnet, rapamycin
      - g. Calcitonin, pamidronate
- II. Impaired intestinal phosphate absorption
  - A. Aluminum-containing antacids
  - B. Sevelamer
- III. Shifts of extracellular phosphate into cells
  - A. IV glucose
  - B. Insulin therapy of prolonged hyperglycemia or diabetic ketoacidosis
  - C. Catecholamines (epinephrine, dopamine, albuterol)
  - D. Acute respiratory alkalosis
  - E. Gram-negative sepsis, toxic shock syndrome
  - F. Recovery from starvation or acidosis
  - G. Rapid cellular proliferation
    - 1. Leukemic blast crisis
    - 2. Intensive erythropoietin, other CSF therapy
- IV. Accelerated net bone formation
  - A. Following parathyroidectomy
  - B. Treatment of vitamin D deficiency, Paget's disease
  - C. Osteoblastic metastases

Note: CSF, cerebrospinal fluid; PTH, parathyroid hormone; PTHrP, parathyroid hormone–related peptide.

dominant hypophosphatemic rickets (ADHR) was the first disease linked to abnormalities in FGF23. ADHR results from activating mutations in the gene encoding FGF23. The most common inherited cause of hypophosphatemia is X-linked hypophosphatemic rickets (XLHR), which results from inactivating mutations in an endopeptidase termed *PHEX* (*p*hosphate-regulating gene with *h*omologies to *e*ndopeptidases on the *X* chromosome) that is most abundantly expressed on the surface of mature osteoblasts. Patients with XLH usually have high FGF23 levels, and ablation of the FGF23 gene reverses the hypophosphatemia found in the mouse version of XLH. How inactivation of PHEX leads to increased levels of FGF23 has not yet been determined. A third hypophosphatemic disorder, tumor-induced osteomalacia (TIO), is an acquired disorder in which tumors, usually of mesenchymal origin and generally histologically benign, secrete molecules that induce renal phosphate wasting. The hypophosphatemic syndrome resolves completely within hours to days following successful resection of the responsible tumor. Such tumors express large amounts of FGF23 mRNA, and patients with TIO usually exhibit elevations of FGF23 in their blood.

Dent's disease is an X-linked recessive disorder caused by inactivating mutations in CLCN5, a chloride transporter expressed in endosomes of the proximal tubule; features include hypercalciuria, hypophosphatemia, and recurrent kidney stones. Renal phosphate wasting is common among poorly controlled diabetics and alcoholics, who therefore are at risk for iatrogenic hypophosphatemia when treated with insulin or IV glucose, respectively. Diuretics and certain other drugs and toxins can cause defective renal tubular phosphate reabsorption (Table 25-1).

In hospitalized patients, hypophosphatemia is often attributable to massive redistribution of phosphate from the ECF into cells. Insulin therapy of diabetic ketoacidosis is a paradigm for this phenomenon, in which the severity of the hypophosphatemia is related to the extent of antecedent depletion of phosphate and other electrolytes (Chap. 19). The hypophosphatemia is usually greatest at a point many hours after initiation of insulin therapy and is difficult to predict from baseline measurements of serum phosphate at the time of presentation, when prerenal azotemia can obscure significant phosphate depletion. Other factors that may contribute to such acute redistributive hypophosphatemia include antecedent starvation or malnutrition, administration of IV glucose without other nutrients, elevated blood catecholamines (endogenous or exogenous), respiratory alkalosis, and recovery from metabolic acidosis.

Hypophosphatemia can also occur transiently (over weeks to months) during the phase of accelerated net bone formation following parathyroidectomy for severe primary hyperparathyroidism or during treatment of vitamin D deficiency or lytic Paget's disease. This is usually most prominent in patients who preoperatively have evidence of high bone turnover (e.g., high serum levels of alkaline phosphatase). Osteoblastic metastases can also lead to this syndrome.

Clinical and Laboratory Findings

The clinical manifestations of severe hypophosphatemia reflect a generalized defect in cellular energy metabolism because of ATP depletion, a shift from oxidative phosphorylation toward glycolysis, and associated tissue or organ dysfunction. Acute, severe hypophosphatemia occurs mainly or exclusively in hospitalized patients with underlying serious medical or surgical illness and preexisting phosphate depletion due to excessive urinary losses, severe malabsorption, or malnutrition. Chronic hypophosphatemia tends to be less severe, with a clinical presentation dominated by musculoskeletal complaints such as bone pain, pseudofractures, and proximal muscle weakness or, in children, rickets and short stature.

Neuromuscular manifestations of severe hypophosphatemia are variable but may include muscle weakness, lethargy, confusion, disorientation, hallucinations, dysarthria, dysphagia, oculomotor palsies, anisocoria, nystagmus, ataxia, cerebellar tremor, ballismus, hyporeflexia, impaired sphincter control, distal sensory deficits, paresthesia, hyperesthesia, generalized or Guillain Barré–like ascending paralysis, seizures, coma, and death. Serious sequelae such as paralysis, confusion, and seizures are likely only at phosphate concentrations <0.25 mmol/L (<0.8 mg/dL). Rhabdomyolysis may develop during rapidly progressive hypophosphatemia. The diagnosis of hypophosphatemia-induced rhabdomyolysis may be overlooked, as up to 30% of patients with acute hypophosphatemia (<0.7 m*M*) have creatine phosphokinase elevations that peak 1–2 days after the nadir in serum phosphate, when the release of phosphate from injured myocytes may have led to a near-normalization of circulating levels of phosphate.

Respiratory failure and cardiac dysfunction, reversible with phosphate treatment, may occur at serum phosphate levels of 0.5–0.8 mmol/L (1.5–2.5 mg/dL). Renal tubular defects, including tubular acidosis, glycosuria, and impaired reabsorption of sodium and calcium, may occur. Hematologic abnormalities correlate with reductions in intracellular ATP and 2,3-diphosphoglycerate and may include erythrocyte microspherocytosis and hemolysis; impaired oxyhemoglobin dissociation; defective leukocyte chemotaxis, phagocytosis, and bacterial killing; and platelet dysfunction with spontaneous gastrointestinal hemorrhage.

Rx Treatment: HYPOPHOSPHATEMIA

Severe hypophosphatemia [<0.75 mmol/L (<2 mg/dL)], particularly in the setting of underlying phosphate depletion, constitutes a dangerous electrolyte abnormality that should be corrected promptly. Unfortunately, the cumulative deficit in body phosphate cannot be easily predicted from knowledge of the circulating level of phosphate, and therapy must be approached empirically. The threshold for IV phosphate therapy and the dose administered should reflect consideration of renal function, the likely severity and duration of the underlying phosphate depletion, and the presence and severity of symptoms consistent with those of hypophosphatemia. In adults, phosphate may be safely administered IV as neutral mixtures of sodium and potassium phosphate salts at initial doses of 0.2–0.8 mmol/kg of elemental phosphorus over 6 h (e.g., 10–50 mmol over 6 h), with doses >20 mmol/6 h reserved for those who have serum levels <0.5 mmol/L (1.5 mg/dL) and normal renal function. A suggested approach is presented in Table 25-2. Serum levels of phosphate and calcium must be monitored closely (every 6–12 h) throughout treatment. It is necessary to avoid a serum calcium-phosphorus product >50 to reduce the risk of heterotopic calcification. Hypocalcemia, if present, should be corrected before administering IV phosphate. Less severe hypophosphatemia, in the range of 0.5–0.8 mmol/L (1.5–2.5 mg/dL), can usually be treated with oral phosphate in divided doses of 750–2000 mg/d, as elemental phosphorus; higher doses can cause bloating and diarrhea.

Management of chronic hypophosphatemia requires knowing the cause(s) of the disorder. Hypophosphatemia related to the secondary hyperparathyroidism of vitamin D deficiency usually responds to treatment with vitamin D and calcium alone. XLHR, ADHR, TIO, and related renal tubular disorders are usually managed with divided oral doses of phosphate, often with calcium and $1,25(OH)_2D$ supplements to bypass the block in renal $1,25(OH)_2D$ synthesis and prevent secondary hyperparathyroidism caused by suppression of ECF calcium levels. Thiazide diuretics may be used to prevent nephrocalcinosis in patients who are managed this way. Complete normalization of hypophosphatemia is generally not possible in these conditions. Optimal therapy of TIO is extirpation of the responsible tumor, which may be localized by radiographic skeletal survey or bone scan (many are located in bone) or by radionuclide scanning using sestamibi or labeled octreotide. Successful treatment of TIO-induced hypophosphatemia with octreotide has been reported in a small number of patients.

TABLE 25-2

INTRAVENOUS THERAPY OF HYPOPHOSPHATEMIA

CONSIDER

Likely severity of underlying phosphate depletion
Concurrent parenteral glucose administration
Presence of neuromuscular, cardiopulmonary, or hematologic complications of hypophosphatemia
Renal function [reduce dose by 50% if serum creatinine >220 μmol/L (>2.5 mg/dL)]
Serum calcium level (correct hypocalcemia first; reduce dose by 50% in hypercalcemia)

GUIDELINES

Serum Phosphorus, m*M* (mg/dL)	Rate of Infusion, mmol/h	Duration, h	Total Administered, mmol
<0.8 (<2.5)	2.0	6	12
<0.5 (<1.5)	4.0	6	24
<0.3 (<1.0)	8.0	6	48

Note: Rates shown are calculated for a 70-kg person; levels of serum calcium and phosphorus must be measured every 6–12 h during therapy; infusions can be repeated to achieve stable serum phosphorus levels >0.8 mmol/L (>2.5 mg/dL); most formulations available in the United States provide 3 mmol/mL of sodium or potassium phosphate.

HYPERPHOSPHATEMIA

Causes

When the filtered load of phosphate and glomerular filtration rate (GFR) are normal, control of serum phosphate levels is achieved by adjusting the rate at which phosphate is reabsorbed by the proximal tubular NaPi-2 co-transporter. The principal hormonal regulator of NaPi-2 activity is PTH. Hyperphosphatemia, defined in adults as a fasting serum phosphate concentration >1.8 mmol/L (5.5 mg/dL), usually results from impaired glomerular filtration, hypoparathyroidism, excessive delivery of phosphate into the ECF (from bone, gut, or parenteral phosphate therapy), or some combination of these factors (Table 25-3). The upper limit of normal serum phosphate concentrations is higher in children and neonates [2.4 mmol/L (7 mg/dL)]. It is useful to distinguish hyperphosphatemia caused by impaired renal phosphate excretion from that which results from excessive delivery of phosphate into the ECF (Table 25-3).

In chronic renal insufficiency, reduced GFR leads to phosphate retention. Hyperphosphatemia, in turn, further impairs renal synthesis of $1,25(OH)_2D$ and stimulates PTH secretion and hypertrophy, both directly and indirectly (by lowering blood ionized calcium levels). Thus, hyperphosphatemia is a major cause of the secondary hyperparathyroidism of renal failure and must be addressed early in the course of the disease (Chap. 27).

TABLE 25-3

CAUSES OF HYPERPHOSPHATEMIA

I. Impaired renal phosphate excretion
  A. Renal insufficiency
  B. Hypoparathyroidism
    1. Developmental
    2. Autoimmune
    3. After neck surgery or radiation
    4. Activating mutations of the calcium-sensing receptor
  C. Parathyroid suppression
    1. Parathyroid-independent hypercalcemia
      a. Vitamin D or vitamin A intoxication
      b. Sarcoidosis, other granulomatous diseases
      c. Immobilization, osteolytic metastases
      d. Milk-alkali syndrome
    2. Severe hypermagnesemia or hypomagnesemia
  D. Pseudohypoparathyroidism
  E. Acromegaly
  F. Tumoral calcinosis
  G. Heparin therapy
II. Massive extracellular fluid phosphate loads
  A. Rapid administration of exogenous phosphate (IV, PO, rectal)
  B. Extensive cellular injury or necrosis
    1. Crush injuries
    2. Rhabdomyolysis
    3. Hyperthermia
    4. Fulminant hepatitis

Hypoparathyroidism leads to hyperphosphatemia via increased expression of NaPi-2 co-transporters in the proximal tubule. Hypoparathyroidism, or parathyroid suppression, has multiple potential causes including autoimmune disease; developmental, surgical, or radiation-induced absence of functional parathyroid tissue; vitamin D intoxication or other causes of PTH-independent hypercalcemia; cellular PTH resistance (pseudohypoparathyroidism or hypomagnesemia); infiltrative disorders such as Wilson disease and hemochromatosis; and impaired PTH secretion caused by hypermagnesemia, severe hypomagnesemia, or activating mutations in the CaSR. Hypocalcemia may also contribute directly to impaired phosphate clearance, as calcium infusion can induce hyperphosphaturia in hypoparathyroid subjects. Increased tubular phosphate reabsorption also occurs in acromegaly, during heparin administration, and in tumoral calcinosis. Tumoral calcinosis is caused by a rare group of genetic disorders in which the *FGF23* gene is either inactivated directly or in which FGF23 is processed in a way that leads to low levels of active FGF23 in the bloodstream. These abnormalities cause elevated serum $1,25(OH)_2D$, parathyroid suppression, increased intestinal calcium absorption, and focal hyperostosis with large, lobulated periarticular heterotopic ossifications (especially at shoulders or hips) and are accompanied by hyperphosphatemia. In some forms of tumoral calcinosis serum phosphorus levels are normal.

When large amounts of phosphate are rapidly delivered into the ECF, hyperphosphatemia can occur despite normal renal function. Examples include overzealous IV phosphate therapy, oral or rectal administration of large amounts of phosphate-containing laxatives or enemas (especially in children), extensive soft tissue injury or necrosis (crush injuries, rhabdomyolysis, hyperthermia, fulminant hepatitis, cytotoxic chemotherapy), extensive hemolytic anemia, or transcellular phosphate shifts induced by severe metabolic or respiratory acidosis.

Clinical Findings

The clinical consequences of acute, severe hyperphosphatemia are due mainly to the formation of widespread calcium phosphate precipitates and resulting hypocalcemia. Thus, tetany, seizures, accelerated nephrocalcinosis (with renal failure, hyperkalemia, hyperuricemia, and metabolic acidosis), and pulmonary or cardiac calcifications (including development of acute heart block) may occur. The severity of these complications relates to the elevation of serum phosphate levels, which can reach concentrations as high as 7 mmol/L (20 mg/dL) in instances of massive soft tissue injury or tumor lysis syndrome.

℞ Treatment: HYPERPHOSPHATEMIA

Therapeutic options for management of severe hyperphosphatemia are limited. Volume expansion may enhance renal phosphate clearance. Aluminum hydroxide antacids or sevelamer may be helpful in chelating and limiting absorption of offending phosphate salts present in the intestine. Hemodialysis is the most effective therapeutic strategy and should be considered early in the course of severe hyperphosphatemia, especially in the setting of renal failure and symptomatic hypocalcemia.

MAGNESIUM METABOLISM

Magnesium is the major intracellular divalent cation. Normal concentrations of extracellular magnesium and calcium are crucial for normal neuromuscular activity. Intracellular magnesium forms a key complex with ATP and is an important co-factor for a wide range of enzymes, transporters, and nucleic acids required for normal cellular function, replication, and energy metabolism. The concentration of magnesium in serum is closely regulated within the range of 0.7–1.0 mmol/L (1.5–2.0 meq/L; 1.7–2.4 mg/dL), of which 30% is protein-bound and another 15% is loosely complexed to phosphate and other anions. Half of the 25 g (1000 mmol) of total body magnesium is located in bone, only half of which is insoluble in the mineral phase. Almost all extraskeletal magnesium is present within cells, where the total concentration is 5 m*M*, 95% of which is bound to proteins and other macromolecules. Because only 1% of body magnesium resides in the ECF, measurements of serum magnesium levels may not accurately reflect the level of total body magnesium stores.

Dietary magnesium content normally ranges from 6–15 mmol/d (140–360 mg/d), of which 30–40% is absorbed, mainly in the jejunum and ileum. Intestinal magnesium absorptive efficiency is stimulated by $1,25(OH)_2D$ and can reach 70% during magnesium deprivation. Urinary magnesium excretion normally matches net intestinal absorption and is ~4 mmol/d (100 mg/d). Regulation of serum magnesium concentrations is achieved mainly by control of renal magnesium reabsorption. Only 20% of filtered magnesium is reabsorbed in the proximal tubule, whereas 60% is reclaimed in the cTAL and another 5–10% in the DCT. Magnesium reabsorption in the cTAL occurs via a paracellular route that requires both a lumen-negative potential, created by NaCl reabsorption, and the tight-junction protein, paracellin-1. Magnesium reabsorption in the cTAL is increased by PTH but inhibited by hypercalcemia or hypermagnesemia, both of which activate the CaSR in this nephron segment.

HYPOMAGNESEMIA

Causes

Hypomagnesemia usually signifies substantial depletion of body magnesium stores (0.5–1 mmol/kg). Hypomagnesemia can result from intestinal malabsorption; protracted vomiting, diarrhea, or intestinal drainage; defective renal tubular magnesium reabsorption; or rapid shifts of magnesium from the ECF into cells, bone, or third spaces (Table 25-4). Dietary magnesium deficiency is unlikely except possibly in the setting of alcoholism. A rare genetic disorder causing selective intestinal magnesium malabsorption has been described (primary infantile hypomagnesemia). Another rare inherited disorder (hypomagnesemia with secondary hypocalcemia) is caused by mutations in the gene encoding TRPM6, a protein that, along with TRPM7, forms a channel important for both intestinal and renal magnesium transport. Malabsorptive states, often compounded by vitamin D deficiency, can critically limit magnesium absorption and produce hypomagnesemia, despite the compensatory effects of secondary hyperparathyroidism and of hypocalcemia and hypomagnesemia to enhance cTAL magnesium reabsorption. Diarrhea or surgical drainage fluid may contain ≥5 mmol/L of magnesium.

Several genetic magnesium-wasting syndromes are described, including inactivating mutations of genes encoding the DCT NaCl co-transporter (Gitelman syndrome), proteins required for cTAL Na-K-2Cl transport (Bartter syndrome), paracellin-1 (autosomal recessive renal hypomagnesemia with hypercalciuria), a DCT Na^+,K^+-ATPase γ subunit (autosomal dominant renal hypomagnesemia with hypocalciuria), the FXYD2 γ subunit of the distal tubular basolateral Na^+,K^+-ATPase, and a mitochondrial DNA gene encoding a mitochondrial tRNA. ECF

TABLE 25-4

CAUSES OF HYPOMAGNESEMIA

I. Impaired intestinal absorption
  A. Primary infantile hypomagnesemia
  B. Malabsorption syndromes
  C. Vitamin D deficiency
II. Increased intestinal losses
  A. Protracted vomiting/diarrhea
  B. Intestinal drainage, fistulae
III. Impaired renal tubular reabsorption
  A. Genetic magnesium-wasting syndromes
    1. Gitelman syndrome
    2. Bartter syndrome
    3. Paracellin-1 mutations
    4. Na^+,K^+-ATPase g-subunit mutations (FXYD2)
    5. Autosomal dominant, with low bone mass
  B. Acquired renal disease
    1. Tubulointerstitial disease
    2. Postobstruction, ATN (diuretic phase)
    3. Renal transplantation
  C. Drugs and toxins
    1. Ethanol
    2. Diuretics (loop, thiazide, osmotic)
    3. Cisplatin
    4. Pentamidine, foscarnet
    5. Cyclosporine
    6. Aminoglycosides, amphotericin B
  D. Other
IV. Extracellular fluid volume expansion
  A. Hyperaldosteronism
  B. SIADH
  C. Diabetes mellitus
  D. Hypercalcemia
  E. Phosphate depletion
  F. Metabolic acidosis
  G. Hyperthyroidism
V. Rapid shifts from extracellular fluid
  A. Intracellular redistribution
    1. Recovery from diabetic ketoacidosis
    2. Refeeding syndrome
    3. Correction of respiratory acidosis
    4. Catecholamines
  B. Accelerated bone formation
    1. Post parathyroidectomy
    2. Treatment of vitamin D deficiency
    3. Osteoblastic metastases
  C. Other
    1. Pancreatitis, burns, excessive sweating
    2. Pregnancy (third trimester) and lactation

Note: ATN, acute tubular necrosis; SIADH, syndrome of inappropriate antidiuretic hormone.

expansion, hypercalcemia, and severe phosphate depletion may impair magnesium reabsorption, as can various forms of renal injury, including those caused by drugs such as cisplatin, cyclosporine, aminoglycosides, and pentamidine (Table 25-4). A rising blood concentration of ethanol directly impairs tubular magnesium reabsorption, and persistent glycosuria with osmotic diuresis leads to magnesium wasting and likely contributes to the high frequency of hypomagnesemia in poorly controlled diabetics. Magnesium depletion is aggravated by metabolic acidosis, which causes intracellular losses as well.

Hypomagnesemia due to rapid shifts of magnesium from ECF into the intracellular compartment can occur during recovery from diabetic ketoacidosis, from starvation, or from respiratory acidosis. Less acute shifts may be seen during rapid bone formation after parathyroidectomy, with treatment of vitamin D deficiency, or with osteoblastic metastases. Large amounts of magnesium may be lost with acute pancreatitis, with extensive burns, with protracted and severe sweating, and during pregnancy and lactation.

Clinical and Laboratory Findings

Hypomagnesemia may cause generalized alterations in neuromuscular function, including tetany, tremor, seizures, muscle weakness, ataxia, nystagmus, vertigo, apathy, depression, irritability, delirium, and psychosis. Patients are usually asymptomatic when serum magnesium concentrations are >0.5 mmol/L (1 meq/L; 1.2 mg/dL), although the severity of symptoms may not correlate with serum magnesium levels. Cardiac arrhythmias may occur, including sinus tachycardia, other supraventricular tachycardias, and ventricular arrhythmias. Electrocardiographic abnormalities may include prolonged PR or QT intervals, T-wave flattening or inversion, and ST straightening. Sensitivity to digitalis toxicity may be enhanced.

Other electrolyte abnormalities often seen with hypomagnesemia, including hypocalcemia (with hypocalciuria) and hypokalemia, may not be easily corrected unless magnesium is administered as well. The hypocalcemia may be a result of concurrent vitamin D deficiency, although hypomagnesemia can cause impaired synthesis of $1,25(OH)_2D$, cellular resistance to PTH, and, at very low serum magnesium [<0.4 mmol/L (<0.8 meq/L; <1 mg/dL)], a defect in PTH secretion; these abnormalities are reversible with therapy.

℞ Treatment: HYPOMAGNESEMIA

Mild, asymptomatic hypomagnesemia may be treated with oral magnesium salts [$MgCl_2$, MgO, $Mg(OH)_2$] in divided doses totaling 20–30 mmol/d (40–60 meq/d). Diarrhea may occur with larger doses. More severe hypomagnesemia should be treated parenterally, preferably with IV $MgCl_2$, which can be administered safely as a continuous infusion of 50 mmol/d (100 meq Mg^{2+}/d) if renal function is normal. If GFR is reduced, the infusion rate should be lowered by 50–75%. Use of IM $MgSO_4$ is discouraged; the injections are painful and provide relatively little magnesium (2 mL of 50% $MgSO_4$ supplies only 4 mmol). $MgSO_4$ may be given IV instead of $MgCl_2$, although the sulfate anions may bind calcium in serum and urine and aggravate hypocalcemia. Serum magnesium should be monitored at intervals of 12–24 h during therapy, which may continue for several days because of impaired renal conservation of magnesium (only 50–70% of the daily IV magnesium dose is retained) and delayed repletion of intracellular deficits, which may be as high as 1–1.5 mmol/kg (2–3 meq/kg).

It is important to consider the need for calcium, potassium, and phosphate supplementation in patients with hypomagnesemia. Vitamin D deficiency frequently coexists and should be treated with oral or parenteral vitamin D or 25(OH)D [but not $1,25(OH)_2D$, which may impair tubular magnesium reabsorption, possibly via PTH suppression]. In severely hypomagnesemic patients with concomitant hypocalcemia and hypophosphatemia, administration of IV magnesium alone may worsen hypophosphatemia, provoking neuromuscular symptoms or rhabdomyolysis, due to rapid stimulation of PTH secretion. This is avoided by administering both calcium and magnesium.

HYPERMAGNESEMIA

Causes

Hypermagnesemia is rarely seen in the absence of renal insufficiency, as normal kidneys can excrete large amounts (250 mmol/d) of magnesium. Mild hypermagnesemia due to excessive reabsorption in the cTAL occurs with calcium-sensing receptor mutations in familial hypocalciuric hypercalcemia and has been described in some patients with adrenal insufficiency, hypothyroidism, or hypothermia. Massive exogenous magnesium exposures, usually via the gastrointestinal tract, can overwhelm renal excretory capacity and cause life-threatening hypermagnesemia (Table 25-5). A notable example of this is prolonged retention of even normal amounts of magnesium-containing cathartics in patients with intestinal ileus, obstruction, or perforation. Extensive soft tissue injury or necrosis can also deliver large amounts of magnesium into the ECF in patients who have suffered trauma, shock, sepsis, cardiac arrest, or severe burns.

Clinical and Laboratory Findings

The most prominent clinical manifestations of hypermagnesemia are vasodilation and neuromuscular blockade, which

TABLE 25-5

CAUSES OF HYPERMAGNESEMIA

Impaired Mg excretion Renal failure Familial hypocalciuric hypercalcemia Excessive Mg intake Cathartics Intestinal obstruction/perforation following magnesium ingestion Parenteral magnesium administration Magnesium-rich urologic irrigants	Rapid Mg mobilization from soft tissues Trauma Extensive burns Shock, sepsis Post cardiac arrest Other disorders Adrenal insufficiency Hypothyroidism Hypothermia

may appear at serum magnesium concentrations >2 mmol/L (>4 meq/L; >4.8 mg/dL). Hypotension, refractory to vasopressors or volume expansion, may be an early sign. Nausea, lethargy, and weakness may progress to respiratory failure, paralysis, and coma, with hypoactive tendon reflexes, at serum magnesium levels >4 mmol/L. Other findings may include gastrointestinal hypomotility or ileus; facial flushing; pupillary dilation; paradoxical bradycardia; prolongation of PR, QRS, and QT intervals; heart block; and, at serum magnesium levels approaching 10 mmol/L, asystole.

Hypermagnesemia, acting via the CaSR, causes hypocalcemia and hypercalciuria due to both parathyroid suppression and impaired cTAL calcium reabsorption.

℞ Treatment: HYPERMAGNESEMIA

Successful treatment of hypermagnesemia generally involves identifying and interrupting the source of magnesium and employing measures to increase magnesium clearance from the ECF. Use of magnesium-free cathartics or enemas may be helpful in clearing ingested magnesium from the gastrointestinal tract. Vigorous IV hydration should be attempted, if appropriate. Hemodialysis is effective and may be required in patients with significant renal insufficiency. Calcium, administered IV in doses of 100–200 mg over 1–2 h, has been reported to provide temporary improvement in signs and symptoms of hypermagnesemia.

VITAMIN D

SYNTHESIS AND METABOLISM

1,25-Dihydroxyvitamin D [1,25$(OH)_2$D] is the major steroid hormone involved in mineral ion homeostasis regulation. Vitamin D and its metabolites are hormones and hormone precursors rather than vitamins, since in the proper biologic setting, they can be synthesized endogenously (Fig. 25-4). In response to ultraviolet radiation of the skin, a photochemical cleavage results in the formation of vitamin D from 7-dehydrocholesterol. Cutaneous production of vitamin D is decreased by melanin and high solar protection factor sunblocks, which effectively impair skin penetration of ultraviolet light. The increased use of sunblocks in North America and Western Europe and a reduction in the magnitude of solar exposure of the general population over the past several decades has led to an increased reliance on dietary sources of vitamin D. In the United States and Canada, these sources largely consist of fortified cereals and dairy products, in addition to fish oils and egg yolks. Vitamin D from plant sources is in the form of vitamin D_2, whereas that from animal sources is vitamin D_3.

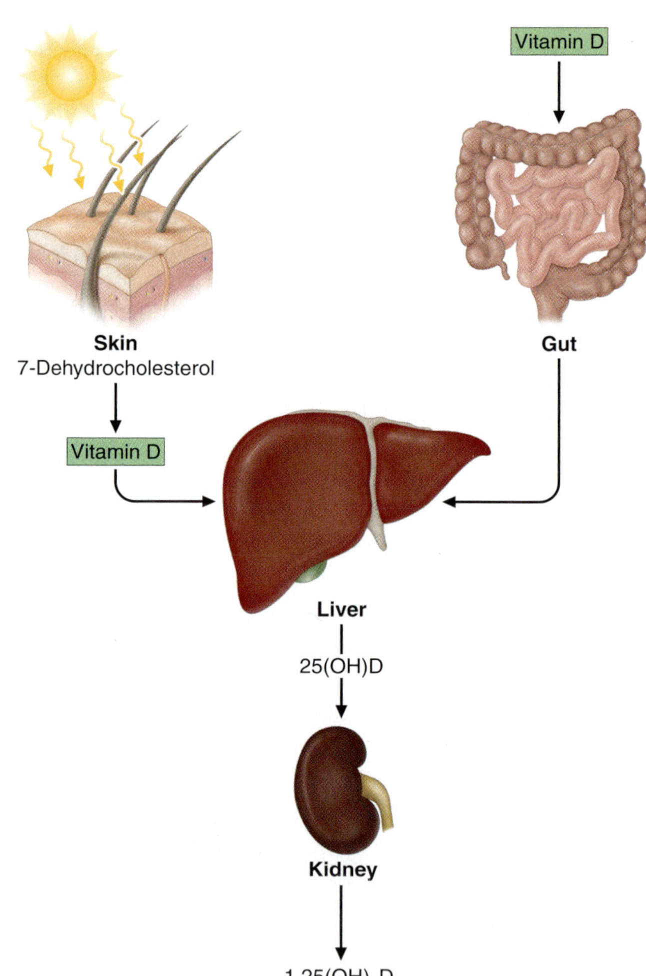

FIGURE 25-4

Vitamin D synthesis and activation. Vitamin D is synthesized in the skin in response to ultraviolet radiation and is also absorbed from the diet. It is then transported to the liver, where it undergoes 25-hydroxylation. This metabolite is the major circulating form of vitamin D. The final step in hormone activation, 1α-hydroxylation, occurs in the kidney.

These two forms have equivalent biologic activity and are activated equally well by the vitamin D hydroxylases in humans. Vitamin D enters the circulation, whether absorbed from the intestine or synthesized cutaneously, bound to vitamin D–binding protein, an α-globulin synthesized in the liver. Vitamin D is subsequently 25-hydroxylated in the liver by cytochrome P450–like enzymes in the mitochondria and microsomes. The activity of this hydroxylase is not tightly regulated, and the resultant metabolite, 25-hydroxyvitamin D [25(OH)D], is the major circulating and storage form of vitamin D. Approximately 88% of 25(OH)D circulates bound to the vitamin D–binding protein, 0.03% is free, and the rest circulates bound to albumin. The half-life of 25(OH)D is approximately 2–3 weeks; however, it is dramatically shortened when vitamin D–binding protein levels are reduced, as can occur with increased urinary losses in the nephrotic syndrome.

The second hydroxylation, required for the formation of the mature hormone, occurs in the kidney (Fig. 25-5). The 25-hydroxyvitamin D-1α-hydroxylase is a tightly regulated cytochrome P450–like mixed function oxidase expressed in the proximal convoluted tubule cells of the kidney. PTH and hypophosphatemia are the major inducers of this microsomal enzyme, whereas calcium, FGF23, and the enzyme's product, $1,25(OH)_2D$, repress it. The 25-hydroxyvitamin D-1α-hydroxylase is also present in epidermal keratinocytes, but keratinocyte production of $1,25(OH)_2D$ is not thought to contribute to circulating levels of this hormone. In addition to being present in the trophoblastic layer of the placenta, the 1α-hydroxylase is produced by macrophages associated with granulomata and lymphomas. In these latter pathologic states, the activity of the enzyme is induced by interferon γ and TNF-α but is not regulated by calcium or $1,25(OH)_2D$; therefore, hypercalcemia, associated with elevated levels of $1,25(OH)_2D$, may be observed. Treatment of sarcoidosis-associated hypercalcemia with glucocorticoids, ketoconazole, or chloroquine reduces $1,25(OH)_2D$ production and effectively lowers serum calcium. In contrast, chloroquine has not been shown to lower the elevated serum $1,25(OH)_2D$ levels in patients with lymphoma.

The major pathway for inactivation of vitamin D metabolites is an additional hydroxylation step by the vitamin D 24-hydroxylase, an enzyme that is expressed in most tissues. $1,25(OH)_2D$ is the major inducer of this enzyme; therefore, this hormone promotes its own inactivation, thereby limiting its biologic effects. Polar metabolites of $1,25(OH)_2D$ are secreted into the bile and reabsorbed via the enterohepatic circulation. Impairment of this recirculation, seen with diseases of the terminal ileum, leads to accelerated losses of vitamin D metabolites.

ACTIONS OF $1,25(OH)_2D$

$1,25(OH)_2D$ mediates its biologic effects by binding to a member of the nuclear receptor superfamily, the vitamin D receptor (VDR). This receptor belongs to the subfamily that includes the thyroid hormone receptors, the retinoid receptors, and the peroxisome proliferator–activated receptors; however, in contrast to the other members of this subfamily, only one VDR isoform has been isolated. The VDR binds to target DNA sequences as a heterodimer with the retinoid X receptor, recruiting a series of coactivators that modify chromatin and approximate the VDR to the basal transcriptional apparatus, resulting in the induction of target gene expression. The mechanism of transcriptional repression by the VDR varies with different target genes but has been shown to involve either interference

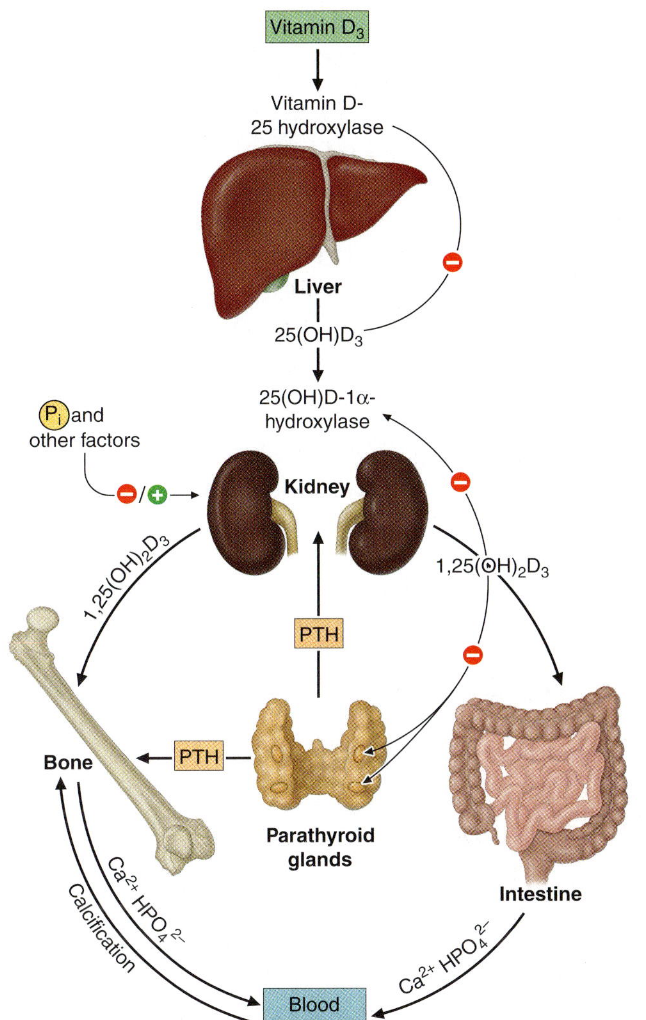

FIGURE 25-5

Schematic representation of the hormonal control loop for vitamin D metabolism and function. A reduction in the serum calcium below ~2.2 mmol/L (8.8 mg/dL) prompts a proportional increase in the secretion of parathyroid hormone (PTH) and so mobilizes additional calcium from the bone. PTH promotes the synthesis of $1,25(OH)_2D$ in the kidney, which, in turn, stimulates the mobilization of calcium from bone and intestine and regulates the synthesis of PTH by negative feedback.

with the action of activating transcription factors or the recruitment of novel proteins to the VDR complex, resulting in transcriptional repression.

The affinity of the VDR for 1,25$(OH)_2$D is approximately three orders of magnitude higher than that for other vitamin D metabolites. Under normal physiologic circumstances, these other metabolites are not thought to stimulate receptor-dependent actions. However, in states of vitamin D toxicity, the markedly elevated levels of 25(OH)D may lead to hypercalcemia by interacting directly with the VDR and by displacing 1,25$(OH)_2$D from vitamin D–binding protein, resulting in increased bioavailability of the active hormone.

The VDR is expressed in a wide range of cells and tissues. The molecular actions of 1,25$(OH)_2$D have been most extensively studied in tissues involved in the regulation of mineral ion homeostasis. This hormone is a major inducer of calbindin 9K, a calcium-binding protein expressed in the intestine, which is thought to play an important role in the active transport of calcium across the enterocyte. The two major calcium transporters expressed by intestinal epithelia, TRPV5 and TRPV6 (transient receptor potential vanilloid), are also vitamin D responsive. By inducing the expression of these and other genes in the small intestine, 1,25$(OH)_2$D increases the efficiency of intestinal calcium absorption, and it has also been shown to have several important actions in the skeleton. The VDR is expressed in osteoblasts and regulates the expression of several genes in this cell. These genes include the bone matrix proteins, osteocalcin and osteopontin, which are upregulated by 1,25$(OH)_2$D, in addition to type I collagen, which is transcriptionally repressed by 1,25$(OH)_2$D. Both 1,25$(OH)_2$D and parathyroid hormone induce the expression of RANK ligand, which promotes osteoclast differentiation and increases osteoclast activity, by binding to RANK on osteoclast progenitors and mature osteoclasts. This is the mechanism by which 1,25$(OH)_2$D induces bone resorption. However, the skeletal features associated with VDR-knockout mice (rickets, osteomalacia) are largely corrected by increasing calcium and phosphorus intake, underscoring the importance of vitamin D action in the gut.

The VDR is expressed in the parathyroid gland, and 1,25$(OH)_2$D has been shown to have antiproliferative effects on parathyroid cells and to suppress the transcription of the parathyroid hormone gene. These effects of 1,25$(OH)_2$D on the parathyroid gland are an important part of the rationale for current therapies directed at preventing and treating hyperparathyroidism associated with renal insufficiency.

The VDR is also expressed in tissues and organs that do not play a role in mineral ion homeostasis. Notable in this respect is the observation that 1,25$(OH)_2$D has an antiproliferative effect on several cell types, including keratinocytes, breast cancer cells, and prostate cancer cells. The effects of 1,25$(OH)_2$D and the VDR on keratinocytes are particularly intriguing. Alopecia is seen in humans and mice with mutant VDRs but is not a feature of vitamin D deficiency; thus, the effects of the VDR on the hair follicle are ligand-independent.

VITAMIN D DEFICIENCY

The mounting concern about the relationship between solar exposure and the development of skin cancer has led to increased reliance on dietary sources of vitamin D. Although the prevalence of vitamin D deficiency varies, the third National Health and Nutrition Examination Survey (NHANES III) revealed that vitamin D deficiency is prevalent throughout the United States. The clinical syndrome of vitamin D deficiency can be a result of deficient production of vitamin D in the skin, lack of dietary intake, accelerated losses of vitamin D, impaired vitamin D activation, or resistance to the biologic effects of 1,25$(OH)_2$D (**Table 25-6**). The elderly and nursing home residents are particularly at risk for vitamin D deficiency, since both the efficiency of vitamin D synthesis in the skin and the absorption of vitamin D from the intestine decline with age. Similarly, intestinal malabsorption of dietary fats leads to vitamin D deficiency. This is further exacerbated in the presence of terminal ileal disease, which results in impaired enterohepatic circulation of vitamin D metabolites. In addition to intestinal diseases, accelerated inactivation of vitamin D metabolites can be seen with drugs that induce hepatic cytochrome P450 mixed function oxidases, such as barbiturates, phenytoin, and rifampin. Impaired 25-hydroxylation, associated with severe liver disease or isoniazid, is an infrequent cause of vitamin D deficiency. Impaired 1α-hydroxylation is prevalent in the population with profound renal dysfunction, due to an increase in circulating FGF23 levels and a decrease in functional renal mass. Thus, therapeutic interventions should be considered in patients whose creatinine clearance is <0.5 mL/s

TABLE 25-6

CAUSES OF IMPAIRED VITAMIN D ACTION	
Vitamin D deficiency	Impaired 1α-hydroxylation
Impaired cutaneous production	Hypoparathyroidism
Dietary absence	Renal failure
Malabsorption	Ketoconazole
Accelerated loss of vitamin D	1α-Hydroxylase mutation
Increased metabolism (barbiturates, phenytoin, rifampin)	Oncogenic osteomalacia
Impaired enterohepatic circulation	X-linked hypophosphatemic rickets
Impaired 25-hydroxylation	Target organ resistance
Liver disease	Vitamin D receptor mutation
Isoniazid	Phenytoin

(30 mL/min). Mutations in the renal 1α-hydroxylase are the basis for the genetic disorder, pseudo-vitamin D–deficiency rickets. This autosomal recessive disorder presents with the syndrome of vitamin D deficiency in the first year of life. Patients present with growth retardation, rickets, and hypocalcemic seizures. Serum $1,25(OH)_2D$ levels are low, despite normal 25(OH)D levels and elevated PTH levels. Treatment with vitamin D metabolites that do not require 1α-hydroxylation results in disease remission, although lifelong therapy is required. A second autosomal recessive disorder, hereditary vitamin D–resistant rickets, a consequence of vitamin D receptor mutations, is a greater therapeutic challenge. These patients present in a similar fashion during the first year of life, but alopecia often accompanies the disorder, demonstrating a functional role of the VDR in postnatal hair regeneration. Serum levels of $1,25(OH)_2D$ are dramatically elevated in these individuals, both because of increased production due to stimulation of 1α-hydroxylase activity as a consequence of secondary hyperparathyroidism and because of impaired inactivation, since induction of 24-hydroxylase by $1,25(OH)_2D$ requires an intact VDR. Since the receptor mutation results in hormone resistance, daily calcium and phosphorus infusions may be required to bypass the defect in intestinal mineral ion absorption.

Regardless of the cause, the clinical manifestations of vitamin D deficiency are largely a consequence of impaired intestinal calcium absorption. Mild to moderate vitamin D deficiency is asymptomatic, whereas longstanding vitamin D deficiency results in hypocalcemia accompanied by secondary hyperparathyroidism, impaired mineralization of the skeleton (osteopenia on x-ray or decreased bone mineral density), and proximal myopathy. In the absence of an intercurrent illness, the hypocalcemia associated with longstanding vitamin D deficiency rarely presents with acute symptoms of hypocalcemia, such as numbness, tingling, or seizures. However, the concurrent development of hypomagnesemia, which impairs parathyroid function, or the administration of potent bisphosphonates, which impair bone resorption, can lead to acute symptomatic hypocalcemia in vitamin D–deficient individuals.

RICKETS AND OSTEOMALACIA

In children, prior to epiphyseal fusion, vitamin D deficiency results in growth retardation associated with an expansion of the growth plate known as *rickets*. Three layers of chondrocytes are present in the normal growth plate: the reserve zone, the proliferating zone, and the hypertrophic zone. Rickets associated with impaired vitamin D action is characterized by expansion of the hypertrophic chondrocyte layer. The proliferation and differentiation of the chondrocytes in the rachitic growth plate are normal, and the expansion of the growth plate is a consequence of impaired apoptosis of the late hypertrophic chondrocytes, an event that precedes replacement of these cells by osteoblasts during endochondral bone formation. Investigations in murine models demonstrate that hypophosphatemia, which in vitamin D deficiency is a consequence of secondary hyperparathyroidism, is a key etiologic factor in the development of the rachitic growth plate.

The hypocalcemia and hypophosphatemia that accompany vitamin D deficiency result in impaired mineralization of bone matrix proteins, a condition known as *osteomalacia*. Osteomalacia is also a feature of longstanding hypophosphatemia, which may be a consequence of renal phosphate wasting or chronic use of etidronate or phosphate-binding antacids. This hypomineralized matrix is biomechanically inferior to normal bone; as a result, patients with vitamin D deficiency are prone to bowing of weight-bearing extremities and skeletal fractures. Vitamin D and calcium supplementation have been shown to decrease the incidence of hip fracture among ambulatory nursing home residents in France, suggesting that undermineralization of bone contributes significantly to morbidity in the elderly. Proximal myopathy is a striking feature of severe vitamin D deficiency, both in children and in adults. Rapid resolution of the myopathy is observed upon vitamin D treatment.

Though vitamin D deficiency is the most common cause of rickets and osteomalacia, many disorders lead to inadequate mineralization of the growth plate and bone. Calcium deficiency without vitamin D deficiency, the disorders of vitamin D metabolism previously discussed, and hypophosphatemia can all lead to inefficient mineralization. Even in the presence of normal calcium and phosphate levels, chronic acidosis and drugs such as bisphosphonates can lead to osteomalacia. The inorganic calcium/phosphate mineral phase of bone cannot form at low pH, and bisphosphonates bind to and prevent mineral crystal growth. Since alkaline phosphatase is necessary for normal mineral deposition, probably because the enzyme can hydrolyze inhibitors of mineralization such as inorganic pyrophosphate, genetic inactivation of the alkaline phosphatase gene (hereditary hypophosphatasia) can also lead to osteomalacia in the setting of normal calcium and phosphate levels.

DIAGNOSIS OF VITAMIN D DEFICIENCY, RICKETS, AND OSTEOMALACIA

The most specific screening test for vitamin D deficiency in otherwise healthy individuals is a serum 25(OH)D level. While the normal ranges vary, levels of 25(OH)D <37 nmol/L (<15 ng/mL) are associated with increasing PTH levels and lower bone density; optimal vitamin D levels are >62 nmol/L (>25 ng/mL). Vitamin D deficiency leads to impaired intestinal absorption of calcium, resulting in decreased serum total and ionized calcium values. This hypocalcemia results in secondary hyperparathyroidism, a homeostatic response that initially maintains serum calcium levels at the expense of the skeleton. Due to the PTH-induced increase in bone turnover, alkaline phosphatase levels are often increased. In addition to increasing bone resorption, PTH decreases urinary calcium excretion, while promoting phosphaturia. This results in hypophosphatemia, which exacerbates the mineralization defect in the skeleton. With prolonged vitamin D deficiency resulting in osteomalacia, calcium stores in the skeleton become relatively inaccessible, since osteoclasts cannot resorb unmineralized osteoid, and frank hypocalcemia ensues. Since PTH is a major stimulus for the renal 25(OH)D 1α-hydroxylase, there is increased synthesis of the active hormone, $1,25(OH)_2D$. Paradoxically, levels of this hormone are often normal in severe vitamin D deficiency. Therefore, measurements of $1,25(OH)_2D$ are not an accurate reflection of vitamin D stores and should not be used to diagnose vitamin D deficiency in patients with normal renal function.

Radiologic features of vitamin D deficiency in children include a widened, expanded growth plate, characteristic of rickets. These findings are not only apparent in the long bones but are also present at the costochondral junction, where the expansion of the growth plate leads to swellings known as the "rachitic rosary." Impairment of intramembranous bone mineralization leads to delayed fusion of the calvarial sutures and a decrease in the radio-opacity of cortical bone in the long bones. If vitamin D deficiency occurs after epiphyseal fusion, the main radiologic finding is a decrease in cortical thickness and relative radiolucency of the skeleton. A specific radiologic feature of osteomalacia, whether associated with phosphate wasting or vitamin D deficiency, is pseudofractures, or Looser's zones (**Fig. 25-6**). These are radiolucent lines that occur where large arteries are in contact with the underlying skeletal elements; it is thought that the arterial pulsations lead to the radiolucencies. As a result, these pseudofractures are usually a few millimeters wide and several centimeters long, and are seen particularly in the scapula, the pelvis, and the femoral neck.

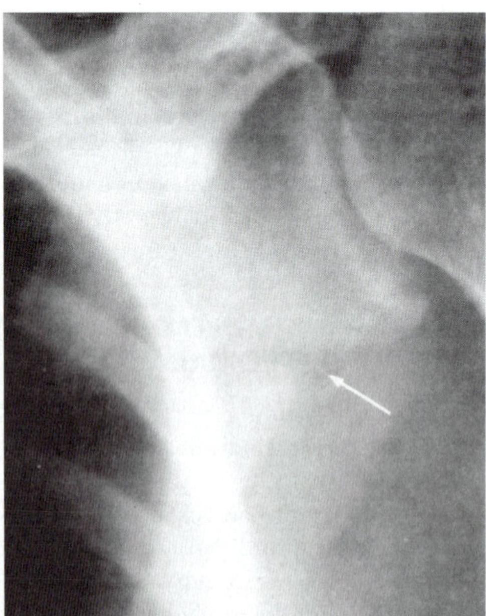

FIGURE 25-6
Radiograph of the scapula of a 58-year-old woman with phosphaturia as a cause of osteomalacia. The presence of a pseudofracture, or Looser's zone, is indicated by an arrow.

℞ Treatment: VITAMIN D DEFICIENCY

Daily intake of a multivitamin (400 IU) is often insufficient to prevent vitamin D deficiency. Based on the observation that 800 IU of vitamin D, with calcium supplementation, decreases the risk of hip fractures in elderly women, this higher dose is thought to be an appropriate daily intake for prevention of vitamin D deficiency in adults. The safety margin for vitamin D is large, and vitamin D toxicity is usually observed only in patients taking doses in the range of 40,000 IU daily. Treatment of vitamin D deficiency should be directed at the underlying disorder, if possible, and should also be tailored to the severity of the condition. Vitamin D should always be repleted in conjunction with calcium supplementation since most, if not all, of the consequences of vitamin D deficiency are a result of impaired mineral ion homeostasis. In patients in whom 1α-hydroxylation is impaired, metabolites not requiring this activation step are the treatment of choice. These include $1,25(OH)_2D_3$ [calcitriol (Rocaltrol), 0.25–0.5 μg/d] and 1,25-dihydroxyvitamin D_2 (Hectorol, 2.5–5 μg/d). If the pathway required for activation of vitamin D is intact, severe vitamin D deficiency can be treated with pharmacologic repletion initially (50,000 IU weekly for 3–12 weeks), followed by maintenance therapy (800 IU daily). Pharmacologic doses may be required for maintenance therapy in patients who are taking medications, such as barbiturates or phenytoin, that accelerate metabolism of or cause resistance to $1,25(OH)_2D$. If intestinal malabsorption is a contributing factor, repletion can be performed with IM vitamin D (250,000 IU biannually). Calcium supplementation should include 1.5–2.0 g/d of elemental calcium. Normocalcemia is usually observed within 1 week of institution of therapy, although increases in PTH and alkaline phosphatase levels may persist for 3–6 months. The most efficacious methods to monitor treatment and resolution of vitamin D deficiency are serum and urinary calcium measurements. In patients who are vitamin D replete and taking adequate calcium supplementation, the 24-h urinary calcium excretion should be in the range of 100–250 mg/24 h. Lower levels suggest problems with adherence to the treatment regimen or with absorption of calcium or vitamin D supplements. Levels >250 mg/24 h predispose to nephrolithiasis and should lead to a reduction in vitamin D dosage and/or calcium supplementation.

FURTHER READINGS

ADAMS JS et al: Unexpected actions of vitamin D: New perspectives on the regulation of innate and adaptive immunity. Nat Clin Pract Endocrinol Metab 4:80, 2008

DELUCA HF: Overview of general physiologic features and functions of vitamin D. Am J Clin Nutr 80:1689S, 2004

GIOVANNUCCI E: Expanding roles of vitamin D. J Clin Endocrinol Metab 94:418, 2009

HEANEY RP: Bone health. Am J Clin Nutr 85(1):300S, 2007

HOLICK MF: Vitamin D deficiency. N Engl J Med 357(3):266, 2007

KARSENTY G: The complexities of skeletal biology. Nature 316, 2003

KOBAYASHI T et al: Minireview: Transcriptional regulation in development of bone. Endocrinology 146:1012, 2005

LEE P et al: Vitamin D deficiency in critically ill patients. N Engl J Med 360:1912, 2009

TEITELBAUM SL, ROSS SP: Genetic regulation of osteoclast development and function. Nat Rev Genet 4:638, 2003

YU X, WHITE KE: FGF23 and disorders of phosphate homeostasis. Cytokine Growth Factor Rev 16:221, 2005

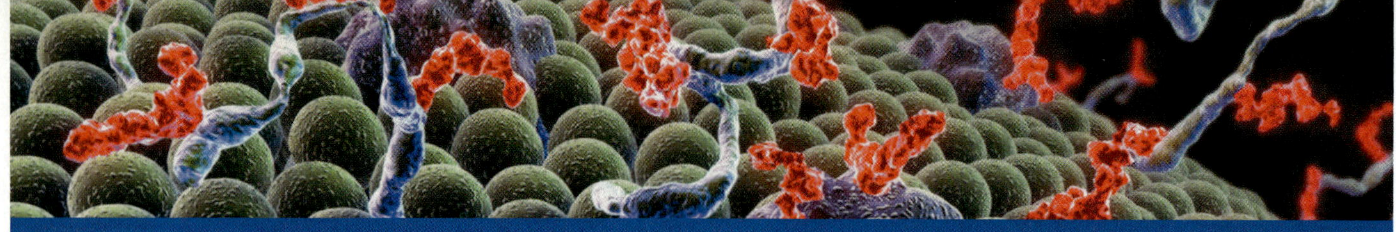

CHAPTER 26

APPROACH TO HYPERCALCEMIA AND HYPOCALCEMIA

Sundeep Khosla

The calcium ion plays a critical role in normal cellular function and signaling, regulating diverse physiologic processes such as neuromuscular signaling, cardiac contractility, hormone secretion, and blood coagulation. Thus, extracellular calcium concentrations are maintained within an exquisitely narrow range through a series of feedback mechanisms that involve parathyroid hormone (PTH) and the active vitamin D metabolite 1,25-dihydroxyvitmin D [1,25$(OH)_2$D]. These feedback mechanisms are orchestrated by integrating signals between the parathyroid glands, kidney, intestine, and bone (**Fig. 26-1**) (Chap. 25).

Disorders of serum calcium concentration are relatively common and often serve as a harbinger of underlying disease. This chapter provides a brief summary of the approach to patients with altered serum calcium levels. See Chap. 27 for a detailed discussion of this topic.

HYPERCALCEMIA

ETIOLOGY

The causes of hypercalcemia can be understood and classified based on derangements in the normal feedback mechanisms that regulate serum calcium (**Table 26-1**). Excess PTH production, which is not appropriately suppressed by increased serum calcium concentrations, occurs in primary neoplastic disorders of the parathyroid glands (parathyroid adenomas, hyperplasia, or, rarely, carcinoma) that are associated with increased parathyroid cell mass and impaired feedback inhibition by calcium. Inappropriate PTH secretion for the ambient level of serum calcium also occurs with heterozygous inactivating calcium sensor receptor (CaSR) mutations, which impair extracellular calcium sensing by the parathyroid glands and the kidneys, resulting in familial hypocalciuric hypercalcemia (FHH). Although PTH secretion by tumors is extremely rare, many solid tumors produce PTH-related peptide (PTHrP), which shares homology with PTH in the first 13 amino acids and binds the PTH receptor, thus mimicking effects of PTH on bone and the kidney. In PTHrP-mediated hypercalcemia of malignancy, PTH levels are suppressed by the high serum calcium levels. Hypercalcemia associated with granulomatous disease (e.g., sarcoidosis) or lymphomas is caused by enhanced conversion of 25(OH)D to the potent 1,25$(OH)_2$D. In these disorders, 1,25$(OH)_2$D enhances intestinal calcium absorption, resulting in hypercalcemia and suppressed PTH. Disorders that directly increase calcium mobilization from bone, such as hyperthyroidism

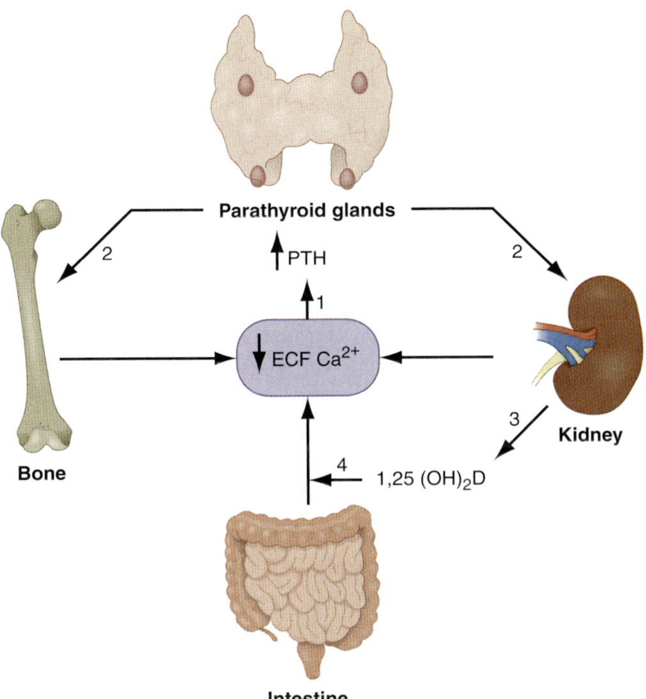

FIGURE 26-1

Feedback mechanisms maintaining extracellular calcium concentrations within a narrow, physiologic range [8.9–10.1 mg/dL (2.2–2.5 m*M*)]. A decrease in extracellular (ECF) calcium (Ca^{2+}) triggers an increase in parathyroid hormone (PTH) secretion (1) via activation of the calcium sensor receptor on parathyroid cells. PTH, in turn, results in increased tubular reabsorption of calcium by the kidney (2) and resorption of calcium from bone (2) and also stimulates renal $1,25(OH)_2D$ production (3). $1,25(OH)_2D$, in turn, acts principally on the intestine to increase calcium absorption (4). Collectively, these homeostatic mechanisms serve to restore serum calcium levels to normal.

or osteolytic metastases, also lead to hypercalcemia with suppressed PTH secretion, as does exogenous calcium overload, as in milk-alkali syndrome, or total parenteral nutrition with excessive calcium supplementation.

CLINICAL MANIFESTATIONS

Mild hypercalcemia (up to 11–11.5 mg/dL) is usually asymptomatic and recognized only on routine calcium measurements. Some patients may complain of vague neuropsychiatric symptoms, including trouble concentrating, personality changes, or depression. Other presenting symptoms may include peptic ulcer disease or nephrolithiasis, and fracture risk may be increased. More severe hypercalcemia (>12–13 mg/dL), particularly if it develops acutely, may result in lethargy, stupor, or coma, as well as gastrointestinal symptoms (nausea, anorexia, constipation, or pancreatitis). Hypercalcemia decreases renal concentrating ability, which may cause polyuria and polydipsia. With longstanding hyperparathyroidism, patients may present with bone pain or pathologic fractures. Finally, hypercalcemia can result in significant electrocardiographic changes, including bradycardia, AV block, and short QT interval; changes in serum calcium can be monitored by following the QT interval.

TABLE 26-1

CAUSES OF HYPERCALCEMIA
Excessive PTH production
Primary hyperparathyroidism (adenoma, hyperplasia, rarely carcinoma)
Tertiary hyperparathyroidism (long-term stimulation of PTH secretion in renal insufficiency)
Ectopic PTH secretion (very rare)
Inactivating mutations in the CaSR (FHH)
Alterations in CaSR function (lithium therapy)
Hypercalcemia of malignancy
Overproduction of PTHrP (many solid tumors)
Lytic skeletal metastases (breast, myeloma)
Excessive $1,25(OH)_2D$ production
Granulomatous diseases (sarcoidosis, tuberculosis, silicosis)
Lymphomas
Vitamin D intoxication
Primary increase in bone resorption
Hyperthyroidism
Immobilization
Excessive calcium intake
Milk-alkali syndrome
Total parenteral nutrition
Other causes
Endocrine disorders (adrenal insufficiency, pheochromocytoma, VIPoma)
Medications (thiazides, vitamin A, antiestrogens)

Note: CaSR, calcium sensor receptor; FHH, familial hypocalciuric hypercalcemia; PTH, parathyroid hormone; PTHrP, PTH-related peptide; VIP, vasoactive intestinal peptide.

DIAGNOSTIC APPROACH

The first step in the diagnostic evaluation of hyper- or hypocalcemia is to ensure that the alteration in serum calcium levels is not due to abnormal albumin concentrations. About 50% of total calcium is ionized, and the rest is bound principally to albumin. Although direct measurements of ionized calcium are possible, they are easily influenced by collection methods and other artifacts; thus, it is generally preferable to measure total calcium and albumin to "correct" the serum calcium. When serum albumin concentrations are reduced, a corrected calcium concentration is calculated by adding 0.2 m*M* (0.8 mg/dL) to the total calcium level for every decrement in serum albumin of 1.0 g/dL below the reference value of 4.1 g/dL for albumin, and conversely for elevations in serum albumin.

A detailed history may provide important clues regarding the etiology of the hypercalcemia (Table 26-1). Chronic hypercalcemia is most commonly caused by primary hyperparathyroidism, as opposed to the second most common etiology of hypercalcemia, an underlying malignancy. The history should include medication use, previous neck surgery, and systemic symptoms suggestive of sarcoidosis or lymphoma.

Once true hypercalcemia is established, the second most important laboratory test in the diagnostic evaluation is a PTH level using a two-site assay for the intact hormone. Increases in PTH are often accompanied by hypophosphatemia. In addition, serum creatinine should be measured to assess renal function; hypercalcemia may impair renal function, and renal clearance of PTH may be altered depending on the fragments detected by the assay. If the PTH level is increased (or "inappropriately normal") in the setting of an elevated calcium and low phosphorus, the diagnosis is almost always primary hyperparathyroidism. Since individuals with familial hypocalciuric hypercalcemia (FHH) may also present with mildly elevated PTH levels and hypercalcemia, this diagnosis should be considered and excluded because parathyroid surgery is ineffective in this condition. A calcium/creatinine clearance ratio (calculated as urine calcium/serum calcium divided by urine creatinine/serum creatinine) of <0.01 is suggestive of FHH, particularly when there is a family history of mild, asymptomatic hypercalcemia. Ectopic PTH secretion is extremely rare.

A suppressed PTH level in the face of hypercalcemia is consistent with non-parathyroid-mediated hypercalcemia, most often due to underlying malignancy. Although a tumor that causes hypercalcemia is generally overt, a PTHrP level may be needed to establish the diagnosis of hypercalcemia of malignancy. Serum 1,25(OH)$_2$D levels are increased in granulomatous disorders, and clinical evaluation in combination with laboratory testing will generally provide a diagnosis for the various disorders listed in Table 26-1.

℞ Treatment: HYPERCALCEMIA

Mild, asymptomatic hypercalcemia does not require immediate therapy, and management should be dictated by the underlying diagnosis. By contrast, significant, symptomatic hypercalcemia usually requires therapeutic intervention independent of the etiology of hypercalcemia. Initial therapy of significant hypercalcemia begins with volume expansion since hypercalcemia invariably leads to dehydration; 4–6 L of IV saline may be required over the first 24 h, keeping in mind that underlying comorbidities (e.g., congestive heart failure) may require the use of loop diuretics to enhance sodium and calcium excretion. However, loop diuretics should not be initiated until the volume status has been restored to normal. If there is increased calcium mobilization from bone (as in malignancy or severe hyperparathyroidism), drugs that inhibit bone resorption should be considered. Zoledronic acid (e.g., 4 mg IV over ~30 min), pamidronate (e.g., 60–90 mg IV over 2–4 h), and etidronate (e.g., 7.5 mg/kg per d for 3–7 consecutive days) are approved by the U.S. Food and Drug Administration for the treatment of hypercalcemia of malignancy in adults. Onset of action is within 1–3 days, with normalization of serum calcium levels occurring in 60–90% of patients. Bisphosphonate infusions may need to be repeated if hypercalcemia relapses. Because of their effectiveness, bisphosphonates have replaced calcitonin and plicamycin, which are rarely used in current practice for the management of hypercalcemia. In rare instances, dialysis may be necessary. Finally, while IV phosphate chelates calcium and decreases serum calcium levels, this therapy can be toxic because calcium-phosphate complexes may deposit in tissues and cause extensive organ damage.

In patients with 1,25(OH)$_2$D-mediated hypercalcemia, glucocorticoids are the preferred therapy, as they decrease 1,25(OH)$_2$D production. IV hydrocortisone (100–300 mg daily) or PO prednisone (40–60 mg daily) for 3–7 days is used most often. Other drugs, such as ketoconazole, chloroquine, and hydroxychloroquine, may also decrease 1,25(OH)$_2$D production and are used occasionally.

HYPOCALCEMIA

ETIOLOGY

The causes of hypocalcemia can be differentiated according to whether serum PTH levels are low (hypoparathyroidism) or high (secondary hyperparathyroidism). Although there are many potential causes of hypocalcemia, impaired PTH or vitamin D production is the most common etiology (**Table 26-2**) (Chap. 27). Because PTH is the main defense against hypocalcemia, disorders associated with deficient PTH production or secretion may be associated with profound, life-threatening hypocalcemia. In adults, hypoparathyroidism most commonly results from inadvertent damage to all four glands during thyroid or parathyroid gland surgery. Hypoparathyroidism is a cardinal feature of autoimmune endocrinopathies (Chap. 23); rarely, it may be associated with infiltrative diseases such as sarcoidosis. Impaired PTH secretion may be secondary to magnesium deficiency or to activating mutations in the CaSR, which suppress PTH, leading to effects that are opposite to those that occur in FHH.

Vitamin D deficiency, impaired 1,25(OH)$_2$D production (primarily secondary to renal insufficiency), or, rarely, vitamin D resistance also cause hypocalcemia. However, the degree of hypocalcemia in these disorders is generally not as severe as that seen with hypoparathyroidism

TABLE 26-2

CAUSES OF HYPOCALCEMIA

Low Parathyroid Hormone Levels (Hypoparathyroidism)
Parathyroid agenesis
Isolated
DiGeorge syndrome
Parathyroid destruction
Surgical
Radiation
Infiltration by metastases or systemic diseases
Autoimmune
Reduced parathyroid function
Hypomagnesemia
Activating CaSR mutations
High Parathyroid Hormone Levels (Secondary Hyperparathyroidism)
Vitamin D deficiency or impaired 1,25(OH)$_2$D production/action
Nutritional vitamin D deficiency (poor intake or absorption)
Renal insufficiency with impaired 1,25(OH)$_2$D production
Vitamin D resistance, including receptor defects
Parathyroid hormone resistance syndromes
PTH receptor mutations
Pseudohypoparathyroidism (G protein mutations)
Drugs
Calcium chelators
Inhibitors of bone resorption (bisphosphonates, plicamycin)
Altered vitamin D metabolism (phenytoin, ketoconazole)
Miscellaneous causes
Acute pancreatitis
Acute rhabdomyolysis
Hungry bone syndrome after parathyroidectomy
Osteoblastic metastases with marked stimulation of bone formation (prostate cancer)

Note: CaSR, calcium sensor receptor; PTH, parathyroid hormone.

because the parathyroids are capable of mounting a compensatory increase in PTH secretion. Hypocalcemia may also occur in conditions associated with severe tissue injury such as burns, rhabdomyolysis, tumor lysis, or pancreatitis. The cause of hypocalcemia in these settings may include a combination of low albumin, hyperphosphatemia, tissue deposition of calcium, and impaired PTH secretion.

CLINICAL MANIFESTATIONS

Patients with hypocalcemia may be asymptomatic if the decreases in serum calcium are relatively mild and chronic, or they may present with life-threatening complications. Moderate to severe hypocalcemia is associated with paresthesias, usually of the fingers, toes, and circumoral regions, and is caused by increased neuromuscular irritability. On physical examination, a Chvostek's sign (twitching of the circumoral muscles in response to gentle tapping of the facial nerve just anterior to the ear) may be elicited, although it is also present in ~10% of normal individuals. Carpal spasm may be induced by inflation of a blood pressure cuff to 20 mmHg above the patient's systolic blood pressure for 3 min (Trousseau's sign). Severe hypocalcemia can induce seizures, carpopedal spasm, bronchospasm, laryngospasm, and prolongation of the QT interval.

DIAGNOSTIC APPROACH

In addition to measuring serum calcium, it is useful to determine albumin, phosphorus, and magnesium levels. As for the evaluation of hypercalcemia, determining the PTH level is central to the evaluation of hypocalcemia. A suppressed (or "inappropriately low") PTH level in the setting of hypocalcemia establishes absent or reduced PTH secretion (hypoparathyroidism) as the cause of the hypocalcemia. Further history will often elicit the underlying cause (i.e., parathyroid agenesis vs destruction). By contrast, an elevated PTH level (secondary hyperparathyroidism) should direct attention to the vitamin D axis as the cause of the hypocalcemia. Nutritional vitamin D deficiency is best assessed by obtaining serum 25-hydroxyvitamin D levels, which reflect vitamin D stores. In the setting of renal insufficiency or suspected vitamin D resistance, serum 1,25(OH)$_2$D levels are informative.

℞ Treatment: HYPOCALCEMIA

The approach to treatment depends on the severity of the hypocalcemia, the rapidity with which it develops, and the accompanying complications (e.g., seizures, laryngospasm). Acute, symptomatic hypocalcemia is initially managed with calcium gluconate, 10 mL 10% wt/vol (90 mg or 2.2 mmol), diluted in 50 mL of 5% dextrose or 0.9% sodium chloride, given IV over 5 min. Continuing hypocalcemia often requires a constant IV infusion (typically 10 ampuls of calcium gluconate or 900 mg of calcium in 1 L of 5% dextrose or 0.9% sodium chloride administered over 24 h). Accompanying hypomagnesemia, if present, should be treated with appropriate magnesium supplementation.

Chronic hypocalcemia due to hypoparathyroidism is treated with calcium supplements (1000 1500 mg/d elemental calcium in divided doses) and either vitamin D$_2$ or D$_3$ (25,000–100,000 U daily) or calcitriol [1,25(OH)$_2$D, 0.25–2 μg/d]. Other vitamin D metabolites (dihydrotachysterol, alfacalcidol) are now used less frequently. Vitamin D deficiency, however, is best treated using vitamin D supplementation, with the dose depending on the severity of the deficit and the underlying cause. Thus, nutritional vitamin D deficiency generally responds to relatively low doses of vitamin D (50,000 U two to three times per week for several months), while vitamin D deficiency due to malabsorption may require much higher doses (100,000 U/d or more). The treatment goal is to bring serum calcium into the low-normal range and to avoid hypercalciuria, which may lead to nephrolithiasis.

FURTHER READINGS

Bilezikian JP, Silverberg SJ: Asymptomatic primary hyperparathyroidism. N Engl J Med 350:1746, 2004

Farford B et al: Nonsurgical management of primary hyperparathyroidism. Mayo Clin Proc 82(3):351, 2007

Finkelstein JS, Potts JT Jr: Medical management of hypercalcemia, in *Endocrinology*, 5th ed, LJ DeGroot, JL Jameson (eds). Philadelphia, Elsevier, 2006

Kifor O et al: Activating antibodies to the calcium-sensing receptor in two patients with autoimmune hypoparathyroidism. J Clin Endocrinol Metab 89:548, 2004

LeGrand SB et al: Narrative review: Furosemide for hypercalcemia: An unproven yet common practice. Ann Intern Med 149:259, 2008

Stewart AF: Hypercalcemia associated with cancer. N Engl J Med 352:373, 2005

Thakker RV: Genetics of endocrine and metabolic disorders: Parathyroid. Rev Endocr Metab Disord 5:37, 2004

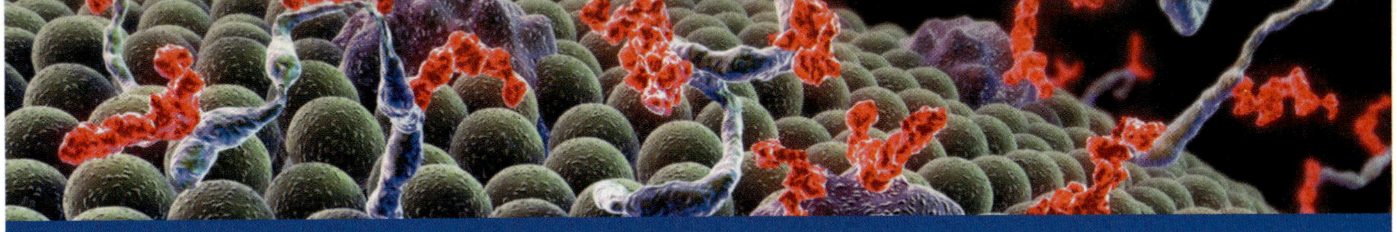

CHAPTER 27

DISEASES OF THE PARATHYROID GLAND

John T. Potts, Jr.

The four parathyroid glands are located posterior to the thyroid gland. They produce parathyroid hormone (PTH), which is the primary regulator of calcium physiology. PTH acts directly on bone, where it induces calcium resorption, and on the kidney, where it stimulates calcium reabsorption and synthesis of 1,25-dihydroxyvitamin D [$1,25(OH)_2D$], a hormone that stimulates gastrointestinal calcium absorption. Serum PTH levels are tightly regulated by a negative feedback loop. Calcium, acting through the calcium-sensing receptor, and vitamin D, acting through its nuclear receptor, inhibit PTH release and synthesis. Understanding the hormone pathways that regulate calcium levels and bone metabolism is essential for effective diagnosis and management of a wide array of hyper- and hypocalcemic disorders.

Hyperparathyroidism (HPT), characterized by excess production of PTH, is a common cause of hypercalcemia and is usually the result of autonomously functioning adenomas or hyperplasia. Surgery for this disorder is highly effective and has been shown to reverse some of the deleterious effects of long-standing PTH excess on bone density. Hypercalcemia of malignancy is also common and is usually due to the overproduction of parathyroid hormone–related peptide (PTHrP) by cancer cells. The similarities in the biochemical characteristics of hyperparathyroidism and hypercalcemia of malignancy, first noted by Albright in 1941, are now known to reflect the actions of PTH and PTHrP through the same G protein–coupled PTH/PTHrP receptor.

The genetic basis of multiple endocrine neoplasia (MEN) types 1 and 2, familial hypocalciuric hypercalcemia (FHH), the different forms of pseudohypoparathyroidism (PHP), Jansen's syndrome, disorders of vitamin D synthesis and action, and the molecular events associated with parathyroid gland neoplasia have provided new insights into calcium metabolism. The advent of new drugs, including bisphosphonates and selective estrogen receptor modulators (SERMs), offers new avenues for the treatment and prevention of metabolic bone disease. PTH analogues are promising therapeutic agents for the treatment of postmenopausal or senile osteoporosis, and calcimimetic agents, which act through the calcium-sensing receptor, may provide new approaches for PTH suppression.

PARATHYROID HORMONE

PHYSIOLOGY

The primary function of PTH is to maintain the extracellular fluid (ECF) calcium concentration within a narrow normal range. The hormone acts directly on bone and kidney and indirectly on intestine through its effects on synthesis of 1,25$(OH)_2$D to increase serum calcium concentrations; in turn, PTH production is closely regulated by the concentration of serum ionized calcium. This feedback system is the critical homeostatic mechanism for maintenance of ECF calcium. Any tendency toward hypocalcemia, as might be induced by calcium-deficient diets, is counteracted by an increased secretion of PTH. This in turn (1) increases the rate of dissolution of bone mineral, thereby increasing the flow of calcium from bone into blood; (2) reduces the renal clearance of calcium, returning more of the calcium filtered at the glomerulus into ECF; and (3) increases the efficiency of calcium absorption in the intestine by stimulating the production of 1,25$(OH)_2$D. Immediate control of blood calcium is due to PTH effects on bone and, to a lesser extent, on renal calcium clearance. Maintenance of steady-state calcium balance, on the other hand, probably results from the effects of 1,25$(OH)_2$D on calcium absorption (Chap. 25). The renal actions of the hormone are exerted at multiple sites and include inhibition of phosphate transport (proximal tubule), increased reabsorption of calcium (distal tubule), and stimulation of the renal 25(OH)D-1α-hydroxylase. As much as 12 mmol (500 mg) calcium is transferred between the ECF and bone each day (a large amount in relation to the total ECF calcium pool), and PTH has a major effect on this transfer. The homeostatic role of the hormone can preserve calcium concentration in blood at the cost of bone destruction.

PTH has multiple actions on bone, some direct and some indirect. PTH-mediated changes in bone calcium release can be seen within minutes. The chronic effects of PTH are to increase the number of bone cells, both osteoblasts and osteoclasts, and to increase the remodeling of bone; these effects are apparent within hours after the hormone is given and persist for hours after PTH is withdrawn. Continuous exposure to elevated PTH (as in hyperparathyroidism or long-term infusions in animals) leads to increased osteoclast-mediated bone resorption. However, the intermittent administration of PTH, elevating hormone levels for 1–2 h each day, leads to a net stimulation of bone formation rather than bone breakdown. Striking increases, especially in trabecular bone in the spine and hip, have been reported with the use of PTH in combination with estrogen. PTH as monotherapy caused a highly significant reduction in fracture incidence in a worldwide placebo-controlled trial.

Osteoblasts (or stromal cell precursors), which have PTH receptors, are crucial to this bone-forming effect of PTH; osteoclasts, which mediate bone breakdown, lack PTH receptors. PTH-mediated stimulation of osteoclasts is believed to be indirect, acting in part through cytokines released from osteoblasts to activate osteoclasts; in experimental studies of bone resorption in vitro, osteoblasts must be present for PTH to activate osteoclasts to resorb bone (Chap. 25).

STRUCTURE

PTH is an 84-amino-acid single-chain peptide. The amino acid portion, PTH(1–34), is highly conserved and is critical for the biologic actions of the molecule. Modified synthetic fragments of the amino-terminal sequence as small as PTH(1–11) are sufficient to activate the major receptor (see below). The carboxyl-terminal region of PTH binds to a separate receptor (cPTH-R), but it has not yet been cloned. Fragments shortened at the amino terminus bind to cPTH-R and inhibit the actions of the full-length PTH(1–84) or the PTH(1–34) active fragments.

BIOSYNTHESIS, SECRETION, AND METABOLISM

Synthesis

Parathyroid cells have multiple methods of adapting to increased needs for PTH production. Most rapid (within minutes) is secretion of preformed hormone in response to hypocalcemia. Second, within hours, PTH mRNA expression is induced by sustained hypocalcemia. Finally, protracted challenge leads within days to cellular replication to increase gland mass.

PTH is initially synthesized as a larger molecule (preproparathyroid hormone, consisting of 115 amino acids), which is then reduced in size by a second cleavage (proparathyroid hormone, 90 amino acids) before secretion as the 84-amino-acid peptide. In one kindred with hypoparathyroidism, a mutation in the preprotein region of the gene interferes with hormone transport and secretion.

Transcriptional suppression of the PTH gene by calcium is nearly maximal at physiologic calcium concentrations. Hypocalcemia increases transcriptional activity within hours. 1,25$(OH)_2D_3$ strongly suppresses PTH gene transcription. In patients with renal failure, IV administration of supraphysiologic levels of 1,25$(OH)_2D_3$ or analogues of the active metabolite can dramatically suppress PTH overproduction, which is sometimes difficult to control due to severe secondary HPT. Regulation of proteolytic destruction of preformed hormone (posttranslational regulation of hormone production) is an important mechanism for mediating rapid (minutes) changes in hormone availability. High calcium increases and low calcium inhibits the proteolytic destruction of hormone stores.

Regulation of PTH Secretion

PTH secretion increases steeply to a maximum value of five times the basal rate of secretion as calcium concentration falls from normal to the range of 1.9–2.0 mmol/L (7.5–8.0 mg/dL) (measured as total calcium). The ionized fraction of blood calcium is the important determinant of hormone secretion. Severe intracellular magnesium deficiency impairs PTH secretion (see below).

ECF calcium controls PTH secretion by interaction with a calcium sensor, a G protein–coupled receptor (GPCR) for which Ca^{2+} ions act as the ligand. This receptor is a member of a distinctive subfamily of the GPCR superfamily that is characterized by a large extracellular domain suitable for "clamping" the small-molecule ligand. Stimulation of the receptor by high calcium levels suppresses PTH secretion. The receptor is present in parathyroid glands and the calcitonin-secreting cells (C cells) of the thyroid, as well as in other sites such as brain and kidney. Genetic evidence has revealed a key biologic role for the calcium-sensing receptor in parathyroid gland responsiveness to calcium and in renal calcium clearance. Point mutations associated with loss of function cause a syndrome, FHH, resembling hyperparathyroidism but with hypocalciuria. On the other hand, gain-of-function mutations cause a form of hypocalcemia resembling hypoparathyroidism.

Metabolism

The secreted form of PTH is indistinguishable by immunologic criteria and by molecular size from the 84-amino-acid peptide [PTH(1–84)] extracted from glands. However, much of the immunoreactive material found in the circulation is smaller than the extracted or secreted hormone. The principal circulating fragments of immunoreactive hormone lack a portion of the critical amino-terminal sequence required for biologic activity and, hence, are biologically inactive fragments (so-called middle- and carboxyl-terminal fragments). Much of the proteolysis of hormone occurs in the liver and kidney. Peripheral metabolism of PTH does not appear to be regulated by physiologic states (high versus low calcium, etc.); hence, peripheral metabolism of hormone, although responsible for rapid clearance of secreted hormone, appears to be a high-capacity, metabolically invariant catabolic process.

The rate of clearance of the secreted 84-amino-acid peptide from blood is more rapid than the rate of clearance of the biologically inactive fragment(s) corresponding to the middle- and carboxyl-terminal regions of PTH. Consequently, the interpretation of PTH immunoassays is influenced by the nature of the peptide fragments detected by the antibodies.

Although the problems inherent in PTH measurements have been largely circumvented by use of double-antibody assays that detect only the intact molecule, more recent evidence revealed larger PTH fragments that may affect the interpretation of most currently available double-antibody assays. Large amino-terminally truncated forms of PTH are present in normal and uremic individuals in addition to PTH(1–84). The concentration of these fragments relative to that of intact PTH(1–84) is higher with induced hypercalcemia than in eucalcemic or hypocalcemic conditions and is higher in patients with renal failure. These fragments have limited portions of the amino-terminal portion of the hormone degraded; PTH(7–84) has been identified as a major component of these amino-terminally truncated fragments. Growing evidence suggests that the PTH(7–84)-related amino-terminally truncated fragments can act as an inhibitor of PTH action and may be of clinical significance, particularly in renal failure. Efforts to prevent secondary HPT by a variety of measures (vitamin D analogues, higher calcium intake, and phosphate-lowering strategies) may have led to oversuppression of biologically active intact PTH since the amino-terminally truncated PTH reacts in many first-generation double-antibody PTH assays. The role, if any, of excessive PTH suppression due to inaccurate measurement of PTH in adynamic bone disease in renal failure is unknown. Newer assays with extreme amino-terminal epitopes that detect only full-length PTH(1–84) are being studied intensively.

PARATHYROID HORMONE–RELATED PROTEIN

The paracrine factor termed *PTHrP* is responsible for most instances of hypercalcemia of malignancy (Chap. 24), a syndrome that resembles HPT. Many different cell types produce PTHrP, including brain, pancreas, heart, lung, mammary tissue, placenta, endothelial cells, and smooth muscle. In fetal animals, PTHrP directs transplacental calcium transfer, and high concentrations of PTHrP are produced in mammary tissue and secreted into milk. Human and bovine milk contain very high concentrations of the hormone, the biologic significance of which is unknown. PTHrP may also play a role in uterine contraction and other biologic functions.

PTH and PTHrP, although distinctive products of different genes, exhibit considerable functional and structural homology (**Fig. 27-1**) and may have evolved from a shared ancestral gene. The structure of the gene for human PTHrP, however, is more complex than that of PTH, containing multiple exons and multiple sites for alternate splicing patterns during formation of the mature mRNA. Protein products of 141, 139, and 173 amino acids are produced, and other molecular forms may result from tissue-specific degradation at accessible internal cleavage sites. The biologic roles of these various molecular species and the nature of the circulating forms of PTHrP are unclear. It is uncertain whether PTHrP circulates at any significant level in adults; as a paracrine factor, PTHrP may be produced, act, and be destroyed locally within tissues. In adults, PTHrP appears to have little influence on calcium homeostasis, except in disease states, when large tumors, especially of the squamous cell type, lead to massive overproduction of the hormone.

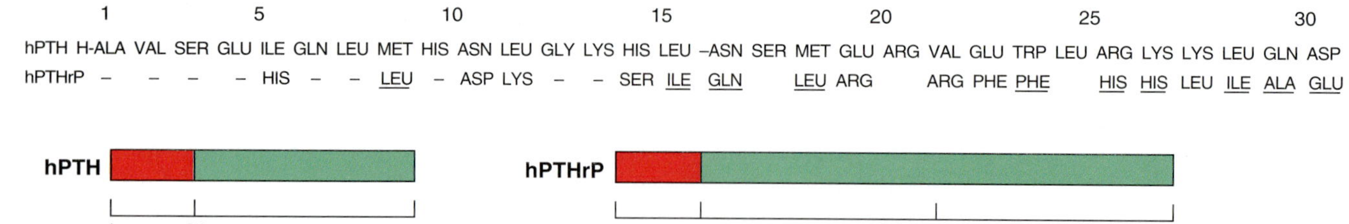

FIGURE 27-1

Schematic diagram to illustrate similarities and differences in structure of human parathyroid hormone (hPTH) and human PTH-related peptide (hPTHrP). Close structural (and functional) homology exists between the first 30 amino acids of hPTH and hPTHrP. The PTHrP sequence may be ≥144-amino-acid residues in length. PTH is only 84 residues long; after residue 30, there is little structural homology between the two. Dashed lines in the PTHrP sequence indicate identity; underlined residues, although different from those of PTH, still represent conservative changes (charge or polarity preserved). Eleven amino acids are identical, and a total of 21 of 30 are homologues.

PTH AND PTHrP HORMONE ACTION

Both PTH and PTHrP bind to and activate the PTH/PTHrP receptor. The 500-amino-acid PTH/PTHrP receptor (also known as the PTH-1 receptor, PTH1R) belongs to a subfamily of GPCRs that includes those for glucagon, secretin, and vasoactive intestinal peptide. The extracellular regions are involved in hormone binding, and the intracellular domains, after hormone activation, bind G protein subunits to transduce hormone signaling into cellular responses through stimulation of second messengers. A second receptor that binds PTH, originally termed the *PTH-2 receptor* (PTH2R), is expressed in brain, pancreas, and several other tissues. PTH1R responds equivalently to PTH and PTHrP, whereas PTH2R responds only to PTH. The endogenous ligand of this receptor is now believed to be a peptide distinct from PTH, a 39-amino-acid hypothalamic peptide (*tubular infundibular peptide*, TIP-39). PTH1R and PTH2R can be traced backward in evolutionary time to fish. Zebrafish PTH1R and PTH2R exhibit the same selective responses to PTH and PTHrP as do human PTH1R and PTH2R. The evolutionary conservation of structure and function suggests important biologic roles for these receptors, even in fish (which lack discrete parathyroid glands).

Studies using cloned PTH1R confirm that it can be coupled to more than one G protein and second-messenger kinase pathway, apparently explaining the multiplicity of pathways stimulated by PTH. Stimulation of protein kinases (A and C) and calcium transport channels is associated with a variety of hormone-specific tissue responses. These responses include inhibition of phosphate and bicarbonate transport, stimulation of calcium transport, and activation of renal 1α-hydroxylase in the kidney. The responses in bone include effects on collagen synthesis; increased alkaline phosphatase, ornithine decarboxylase, citrate decarboxylase, and glucose-6-phosphate dehydrogenase activities; DNA, protein, and phospholipid synthesis; and calcium and phosphate transport. Ultimately, these biochemical events lead to an integrated hormonal response in bone turnover and calcium homeostasis. PTH also activates Na^+/Ca^{2+} exchanges in renal distal tubular sites and stimulates translocation of preformed calcium transport channels, moving them from the interior to the apical surface to mediate increased tubular uptake of calcium. PTH-dependent stimulation of phosphate excretion (blocking reabsorption—the opposite effect from actions on calcium in the kidney) involves the sodium-dependent phosphate cotransporter, NPT-2, lowering its apical membrane content (and therefore function). Similar shifts may be involved in other renal tubular transport effects of PTH.

PTHrP exerts important developmental influences on fetal bone development and in adult physiology. A homozygous knockout of the PTHrP gene (or the gene for the PTH receptor) in mice causes a lethal deformity in which animals are born with severe skeletal deformities resembling chondrodysplasia (Fig. 27-2). The heterozygous

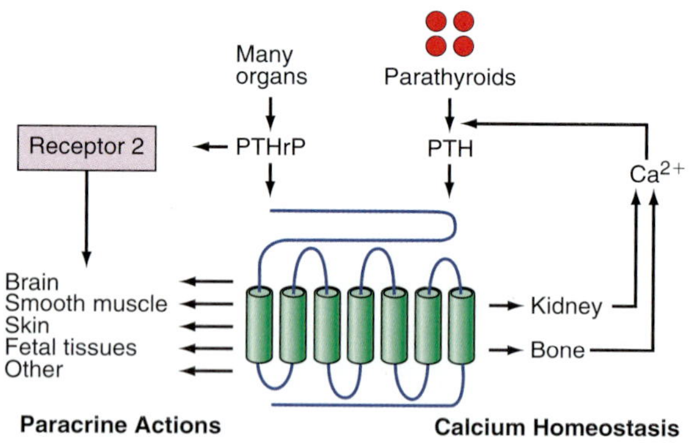

FIGURE 27-2

Dual role for the actions of the PTH/PTHrP receptor (PTH1R). Parathyroid hormone (PTH; endocrine-calcium homeostasis) and PTH-related peptide (PTHrP; paracrine–multiple tissue actions including growth plate cartilage in developing bone) use the single receptor for their disparate functions mediated by the amino-terminal 30 residues of either peptide. Other regions of both ligands interact with other receptors (not shown).

PTHrP gene knockout animals display reduced mineral density consistent with osteoporosis. Experiments with these mouse models point to a hitherto unappreciated role of PTHrP as a paracrine/autocrine factor that modulates bone metabolism in adults as well as during bone development.

CALCITONIN

(See also Chap. 23) Calcitonin is a hypocalcemic peptide hormone that in several mammalian species acts as an antagonist to PTH. Calcitonin seems to be of limited physiologic significance in humans, however, at least in calcium homeostasis. It is of medical significance because of its role as a tumor marker in sporadic and hereditary cases of medullary carcinoma and its medical use as an adjunctive treatment in severe hypercalcemia and in Paget's disease of bone.

The hypocalcemic activity of calcitonin is accounted for primarily by inhibition of osteoclast-mediated bone resorption and secondarily by stimulation of renal calcium clearance. These effects are mediated by receptors on osteoclasts and renal tubular cells. Calcitonin exerts additional effects through receptors present in the brain, gastrointestinal tract, and immune system. The hormone, for example, exerts analgesic effects directly on cells in the hypothalamus and related structures, possibly by interacting with receptors for related peptide hormones, such as calcitonin gene–related peptide (CGRP) or amylin. The latter ligands have specific high-affinity receptors and can also bind to and trigger calcitonin receptors. The calcitonin receptors are homologous in structure to PTH1R.

The thyroid is the major source of the hormone, and the cells involved in calcitonin synthesis arise from neural crest tissue. During embryogenesis, these cells migrate into the ultimobranchial body, derived from the last branchial pouch. In submammalian vertebrates, the ultimobranchial body constitutes a discrete organ, anatomically separate from the thyroid gland; in mammals, the ultimobranchial gland fuses with and is incorporated into the thyroid gland.

The naturally occurring calcitonins consist of a peptide chain of 32 amino acids. There is considerable sequence variability among species. Calcitonin from salmon, which is used therapeutically, is 10–100 times more potent than mammalian forms in lowering serum calcium.

There are two calcitonin genes, α and β; the transcriptional control of these genes is complex. Two different mRNA molecules are transcribed from the α gene; one is translated into the precursor for calcitonin, and the other message is translated into an alternative product, CGRP. CGRP is synthesized wherever the calcitonin mRNA is expressed, e.g., in medullary carcinoma of the thyroid. The β, or CGRP-2, gene is transcribed into the mRNA for CGRP in the central nervous system (CNS); this gene does not produce calcitonin, however. CGRP has cardiovascular actions and may serve as a neurotransmitter or play a developmental role in the CNS.

The circulating level of calcitonin in humans is lower than that in many other species. In humans, even extreme variations in calcitonin production do not change calcium and phosphate metabolism; no definite effects are attributable to calcitonin deficiency (totally thyroidectomized patients receiving only replacement thyroxine) or excess (patients with medullary carcinoma of the thyroid, a calcitonin-secreting tumor) (Chap. 23). Calcitonin has been a useful pharmacologic agent to suppress bone resorption in Paget's disease (Chap. 29) and osteoporosis (Chap. 28) and in the treatment of hypercalcemia of malignancy (see below). However, the physiologic role, if any, of calcitonin in humans is uncertain. However, a knockout of the calcitonin gene in mice leads to *increased* bone mineral density, suggesting that its biologic role is still not fully understood.

HYPERCALCEMIA

(See also Chap. 26) Hypercalcemia can be a manifestation of a serious illness such as malignancy or can be detected coincidentally by laboratory testing in a patient with no obvious illness. The number of patients recognized with asymptomatic hypercalcemia, usually hyperparathyroidism, increased in the late twentieth century.

Whenever hypercalcemia is confirmed, a definitive diagnosis must be established. Although hyperparathyroidism, a frequent cause of asymptomatic hypercalcemia, is a chronic disorder in which manifestations, if any, may be expressed only after months or years, hypercalcemia can also be the earliest manifestation of malignancy, the second most common cause of hypercalcemia in the adult. The causes of hypercalcemia are numerous (**Table 27-1**), but hyperparathyroidism and cancer account for 90% of cases.

Before undertaking a diagnostic workup, it is essential to be sure that true hypercalcemia, not a false-positive laboratory test, is present. A false-positive diagnosis of hypercalcemia is usually the result of inadvertent hemoconcentration during blood collection or elevation in serum proteins such as albumin. Hypercalcemia is a chronic problem, and it is cost-effective to obtain several serum calcium measurements; these tests need not be in the fasting state.

Clinical features are helpful in differential diagnosis. Hypercalcemia in an adult who is asymptomatic is usually due to primary hyperparathyroidism. In malignancy-associated hypercalcemia the disease is usually not occult; rather, symptoms of malignancy bring the patient to the physician, and hypercalcemia is discovered during the evaluation. In such patients the interval between detection of hypercalcemia and death, especially without vigorous treatment, is often <6 months. Accordingly, if

TABLE 27-1

CLASSIFICATION OF CAUSES OF HYPERCALCEMIA

I. Parathyroid-related
  A. Primary hyperparathyroidism
    1. Solitary adenomas
    2. Multiple endocrine neoplasia
  B. Lithium therapy
  C. Familial hypocalciuric hypercalcemia
II. Malignancy-related
  A. Solid tumor with metastases (breast)
  B. Solid tumor with humoral mediation of hypercalcemia (lung, kidney)
  C. Hematologic malignancies (multiple myeloma, lymphoma, leukemia)
III. Vitamin D–related
  A. Vitamin D intoxication
  B. ↑ $1,25(OH)_2D$; sarcoidosis and other granulomatous diseases
  C. Idiopathic hypercalcemia of infancy
IV. Associated with high bone turnover
  A. Hyperthyroidism
  B. Immobilization
  C. Thiazides
  D. Vitamin A intoxication
V. Associated with renal failure
  A. Severe secondary hyperparathyroidism
  B. Aluminum intoxication
  C. Milk-alkali syndrome

an asymptomatic individual has had hypercalcemia or some manifestation of hypercalcemia, such as kidney stones, for >1 or 2 years, it is unlikely that malignancy is the cause. Nevertheless, differentiating primary hyperparathyroidism from *occult* malignancy can occasionally be difficult, and careful evaluation is required, particularly when the duration of the hypercalcemia is unknown. Hypercalcemia not due to hyperparathyroidism or malignancy can result from excessive vitamin D action, high bone turnover from any of several causes, or renal failure (Table 27-1). Dietary history and a history of ingestion of vitamins or drugs are often helpful in diagnosing some of the less frequent causes. PTH immunoassays based on double-antibody methods serve as the principal laboratory test in differential diagnosis.

Hypercalcemia from any cause can result in fatigue, depression, mental confusion, anorexia, nausea, vomiting, constipation, reversible renal tubular defects, increased urination, a short QT interval in the electrocardiogram, and, in some patients, cardiac arrhythmias. There is a variable relation from one patient to the next between the severity of hypercalcemia and the symptoms. Generally, symptoms are more common at calcium levels >2.9–3 mmol/L (11.5–12.0 mg/dL), but some patients, even at this level, are asymptomatic. When the calcium level is >3.2 mmol/L (13 mg/dL), calcification in kidneys, skin, vessels, lungs, heart, and stomach occurs and renal insufficiency may develop, particularly if blood phosphate levels are normal or elevated due to impaired renal function. Severe hypercalcemia, usually defined as ≥3.7–4.5 mmol/L (15–18 mg/dL), can be a medical emergency; coma and cardiac arrest can occur.

Acute management of the hypercalcemia is usually successful. The type of treatment is based on the severity of the hypercalcemia and the nature of associated symptoms, as outlined below.

PRIMARY HYPERPARATHYROIDISM

Natural History and Incidence

Primary hyperparathyroidism is a generalized disorder of calcium, phosphate, and bone metabolism due to an increased secretion of PTH. The elevation of circulating hormone usually leads to hypercalcemia and hypophosphatemia. There is great variation in the manifestations. Patients may present with multiple signs and symptoms, including recurrent nephrolithiasis, peptic ulcers, mental changes, and, less frequently, extensive bone resorption. However, with greater awareness of the disease and wider use of multiphasic screening tests, including measurements of blood calcium, the diagnosis is frequently made in patients who have no symptoms and minimal, if any, signs of the disease other than hypercalcemia and elevated levels of PTH. The manifestations may be subtle, and the disease may have a benign course for many years or a lifetime. This milder form of the disease is usually termed *asymptomatic HPT*. Rarely, hyperparathyroidism develops or worsens abruptly and causes severe complications, such as marked dehydration and coma, so-called hypercalcemic parathyroid crisis.

The annual incidence of the disease is calculated to be as high as 0.2% in patients >60, with an estimated prevalence, including undiscovered asymptomatic patients, of ≥1%; some reports suggest the incidence may be declining. If confirmed, these changing estimates may reflect less frequent routine testing of serum calcium in recent years, earlier overestimates in incidence, or unknown factors. The disease has a peak incidence between the third and fifth decades but occurs in young children and in the elderly.

Etiology

Parathyroid tumors are most often encountered as isolated adenomas without other endocrinopathy. They may also arise in hereditary syndromes, such as MEN syndromes. Parathyroid tumors may also arise as secondary to underlying disease (excessive stimulation in secondary hyperparathyroidism, especially chronic renal failure), or after other forms of excessive stimulation, such as lithium therapy. These etiologies are discussed below.

Solitary Adenomas

A single abnormal gland is the cause in ~80% of patients; the abnormality in the gland is usually a benign neoplasm or adenoma and rarely a parathyroid carcinoma. Some surgeons and pathologists report that the enlargement of multiple glands is common; double adenomas are reported. In ~15% of patients, all glands are hyperfunctioning; *chief cell parathyroid hyperplasia* is usually hereditary and frequently associated with other endocrine abnormalities.

Hereditary Syndromes and Multiple Parathyroid Tumors

Hereditary hyperparathyroidism can occur without other endocrine abnormalities but is usually part of a *multiple endocrine neoplasia* syndrome (Chap. 23). MEN 1 (Wermer's syndrome) consists of hyperparathyroidism and tumors of the pituitary and pancreas, often associated with gastric hypersecretion and peptic ulcer disease (Zollinger-Ellison syndrome). MEN 2A is characterized by pheochromocytoma and medullary carcinoma of the thyroid, as well as hyperparathyroidism; MEN 2B has additional associated features such as multiple neuromas but usually lacks hyperparathyroidism. Each of these MEN syndromes is transmitted in an apparent autosomal dominant manner, although, as noted below, the genetic basis of MEN 1 does not involve a dominant allele.

The *hyperparathyroidism jaw tumor* (HPT-JT) syndrome occurs in families with parathyroid tumors (sometimes carcinoma) in association with benign jaw tumors.

Some kindred exhibit hereditary hyperparathyroidism without other endocrinopathies. This disorder is often termed *nonsyndromic familial isolated hyperparathyroidism* (FIHP). There is speculation that these families may be examples of variable expression of the other syndromes, such as MEN 1, MEN 2, or the HPT-JT syndrome, but they may also have distinctive, still unidentified genetic causes.

Pathology

Adenomas are most often located in the inferior parathyroid glands, but in 6–10% of patients, parathyroid adenomas may be located in the thymus, the thyroid, or the pericardium or behind the esophagus. Adenomas are usually 0.5–5 g in size but may be as large as 10–20 g (normal glands weigh 25 mg on average). Chief cells are predominant in both hyperplasia and adenoma. With chief cell hyperplasia, the enlargement may be so asymmetric that some involved glands appear grossly normal. If generalized hyperplasia is present, however, histologic examination reveals a uniform pattern of chief cells and disappearance of fat even in the absence of an increase in gland weight. Thus, microscopic examination of biopsy specimens of several glands is essential to interpret findings at surgery.

Parathyroid carcinoma is often not aggressive. Long-term survival without recurrence is common if at initial surgery the entire gland is removed without rupture of the capsule. Recurrent parathyroid carcinoma is usually slow-growing with local spread in the neck, and surgical correction of recurrent disease may be feasible. Occasionally, however, parathyroid carcinoma is more aggressive, with distant metastases (lung, liver, and bone) found at the time of initial operation. It may be difficult to appreciate initially that a primary tumor is carcinoma; increased numbers of mitotic figures and increased fibrosis of the gland stroma may precede invasion. The diagnosis of carcinoma is often made in retrospect. Hyperparathyroidism from a parathyroid carcinoma may be indistinguishable from other forms of primary hyperparathyroidism but is usually more severe clinically. A potential clue to the diagnosis is offered by the degree of calcium elevation. Calcium values of 3.5–3.7 mmol/L (14–15 mg/dL) are frequent with carcinoma and may alert the surgeon to remove the abnormal gland with care to avoid capsular rupture. Recent findings concerning the genetic basis of parathyroid carcinoma (distinct from that of benign adenomas) indicate the need, in these kindreds, for family screening.

GENETIC DEFECTS ASSOCIATED WITH HYPERPARATHYROIDISM

As in many other types of neoplasia, two fundamental types of genetic defects have been identified in parathyroid gland tumors: (1) overactivity of protooncogenes and (2) loss of function of tumor-suppressor genes. The former, by definition, can lead to uncontrolled cellular growth and function by activation (gain-of-function mutation) of a single allele of the responsible gene, whereas the latter requires loss of function of both allelic copies. Biallelic loss of function of a tumor-suppressor gene is usually characterized by a germ-line defect (all cells) and an additional somatic deletion/mutation in the excised tumor (Fig. 27-3).

Mutations in the *MEN1* gene locus, encoding the protein MENIN, on chromosome 11q13 are responsible for causing MEN 1; the normal allele of this gene fits the definition of a tumor-suppressor gene. Inheritance of one mutated allele in this hereditary syndrome, followed by loss of the other allele via somatic cell mutation, leads to monoclonal expansion and tumor development. Also, in ~15–20% of sporadic parathyroid adenomas, both alleles of the *MEN1* locus on chromosome 11 are somatically deleted, implying that the same defect responsible for MEN 1 can also cause the sporadic disease (Fig. 27-3*A*). Consistent with the Knudson hypothesis for two-step neoplasia in certain inherited cancer syndromes, the earlier onset of hyperparathyroidism in the hereditary syndromes reflects the need for only one mutational event to trigger the monoclonal outgrowth. In sporadic adenomas, typically occurring later in life, two different somatic events must occur before the *MEN1* gene is silenced.

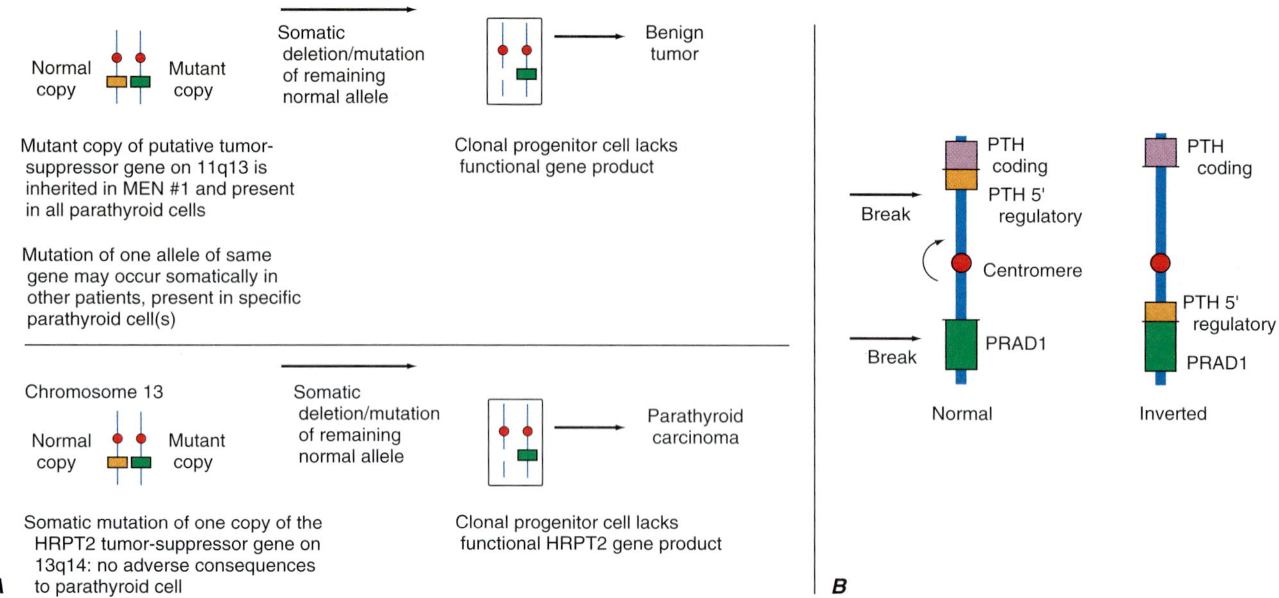

FIGURE 27-3

***A.* Schematic diagram indicating molecular events** in tumor susceptibility. The patient with the hereditary abnormality (multiple endocrine neoplasia, or MEN) is envisioned as having one defective gene inherited from the affected parent on chromosome 11, but one copy of the normal gene is present from the other parent. In the monoclonal tumor (benign tumor), a somatic event, here partial chromosomal deletion, removes the remaining normal gene from a cell. In nonhereditary tumors, two successive somatic mutations must occur, a process that takes a longer time. By either pathway, the cell, deprived of growth-regulating influence from this gene, has unregulated growth and becomes a tumor. A different genetic locus also involving loss of a tumor-suppressor gene termed HRPT2 is involved in the pathogenesis of parathyroid carcinoma. [*From A Arnold: J Clin Endocrine Metab 77(5):1108, 1993. Copyright 1993, The Endocrine Society.*] ***B.* Schematic illustration of the mechanism and consequences of gene rearrangement** and overexpression of the PRAD 1 protooncogene (pericentromeric inversion of chromosome 11) in parathyroid adenomas. The excessive expression of PRAD 1 (a cell cycle control protein, cyclin D1) by the highly active PTH gene promoter in the parathyroid cell contributes to excess cellular proliferation. [*From J Habener et al, in L DeGroot, JL Jameson (eds): Endocrinology, 4th ed. Philadelphia, Saunders, 2001; with permission.*]

Other presumptive antioncogenes involved in hyperparathyroidism include a still unidentified gene mapped to chromosome 1p seen in 40% of sporadic parathyroid adenomas and a gene mapped to chromosome Xp11 in patients with secondary hyperparathyroidism and renal failure, who progressed to "tertiary" hyperparathyroidism, now known to reflect monoclonal outgrowths within previously hyperplastic glands.

A more complex pattern, still incompletely resolved, arises with genetic defects and carcinoma of the parathyroids seen in MEN 2. This appears to be due to biallelic loss of a functioning copy of a gene, *HRPT2* (or CDC73), originally identified as the cause of the HPT-JT syndrome. Several inactivating mutations have been identified in *HRPT2* (located on chromosome 1q25), which encodes a 531-amino-acid protein called parafibromin. A protooncogene, *RET*, is mutated in all cases of MEN 2. With both types of genetically determined carcinoma syndromes (as with the loss of the *MEN1* in parathyroid adenomas), the responsible genetic mutations in *HRPT2* or *RET* appear to be necessary, but not sufficient, for the malignancies outlined below.

In general, the detection of additional genetic defects in these parathyroid tumor–related syndromes and the variations seen in phenotypic expression/penetrance indicate the multiplicity of the genetic factors responsible. Nonetheless, the ability to detect the presence of the major genetic contributors has greatly aided a more informed management of family members of patients identified in the hereditary syndromes such as MEN 1, MEN 2, and HPT-JT.

An important contribution from studies on the genetic origin of parathyroid carcinoma has been the realization that the mutations involve a different pathway than that involved with the benign gland enlargements. Unlike the pathogenesis of genetic alterations seen in colon cancer, where lesions evolve from benign adenomas to malignant disease by progressive genetic changes, the alterations commonly seen in most parathyroid cancers (*HRPT2* mutations) are infrequently seen in sporadic parathyroid adenomas.

Abnormalities at the *Rb* gene were first noted in parathyroid cancer. The *Rb* gene, a tumor-suppressor gene located on chromosome 13q14, was initially associated with retinoblastoma but has since been implicated in other neoplasias, including parathyroid carcinoma. Early studies implicated allelic deletions of the *Rb* gene in many parathyroid carcinomas and decreased or absent expression of the Rb protein. However, because there are often large deletions in chromosome 13 that include many genes in addition to the *Rb* locus (with similar findings in some pituitary carcinomas), it remains possible that other tumor-suppressor genes on chromosome 13 may be playing a role in parathyroid carcinoma.

Study of the parathyroid cancers found in some patients with the HPT-JT syndrome has led to identification of a much larger role for mutations in the *HRPT2* gene in most parathyroid carcinomas, including those that arise sporadically, without apparent association with the HPT-JT syndrome. Mutations in the coding region have been identified in 75–80% of all parathyroid cancers analyzed, leading to the conclusion that, with addition of presumed mutations in the noncoding regions, this genetic defect may be seen in essentially all parathyroid carcinomas. Of special importance was the discovery that, in some sporadic parathyroid cancers, germ-line mutations have been found; this, in turn, has led to careful investigation of the families of these patients and a new clinical indication for genetic testing in this setting.

Hypercalcemia occurring in family members (who are also found to have the germ-line mutations) can lead to the finding, at parathyroid surgery, of premalignant parathyroid tumors.

Overall, it seems there are multiple factors in parathyroid cancer, in addition to the *HRPT2* gene, although the *HRPT2* gene mutation is the most invariant abnormality. Deletions in the *Rb* gene locus may play an additional role in pathogenesis of parathyroid cancer, as well as other still uncharacterized genetic defects.

RET encodes a tyrosine kinase–type receptor; specific inherited germ-line mutations lead to a constitutive activation of the receptor, thereby explaining the autosomal dominant mode of transmission and the relatively early onset of neoplasia. In the MEN 2 syndrome, the *RET* protooncogene may be responsible for the earliest disorder detected, the polyclonal disorder (C cell hyperplasia, which then is transformed into a clonal outgrowth—a medullary carcinoma with the participation of other, still uncharacterized genetic defects).

In some parathyroid adenomas, activation of a protooncogene has been identified (Fig. 27-3*B*). A reciprocal translocation involving chromosome 11 has been identified that juxtaposes the *PTH* gene promoter upstream of a gene product termed *PRAD-1*, encoding a cyclin D protein that plays a key role in normal cell division. This translocation plus other mechanisms that cause an equivalent overexpression of cyclin D1 are found in 20–40% of parathyroid adenomas.

Mouse models have confirmed the role of several of the major identified genetic defects in parathyroid disease and the MEN syndromes. Loss of the *MEN1* gene locus, or overexpression of the *PRAD-1* protooncogene or the mutated *RET* protooncogene, has been analyzed by genetic manipulation in mice, with the expected onset of parathyroid tumors or medullary carcinoma, respectively.

Signs and Symptoms

Half or more of patients with hyperparathyroidism are asymptomatic. In series in which patients are followed without operation, as many as 80% are classified as without symptoms. Manifestations of hyperparathyroidism involve primarily the kidneys and the skeletal system. Kidney involvement, due either to deposition of calcium in the renal parenchyma or to recurrent nephrolithiasis, was present in 60–70% of patients prior to 1970. With earlier detection, renal complications occur in <20% of patients in many large series. Renal stones are usually composed of either calcium oxalate or calcium phosphate. In occasional patients, repeated episodes of nephrolithiasis or the formation of large calculi may lead to urinary tract obstruction, infection, and loss of renal function. Nephrocalcinosis may also cause decreased renal function and phosphate retention.

The distinctive bone manifestation of hyperparathyroidism is *osteitis fibrosa cystica*, which occurred in 10–25% of patients in series reported 50 years ago. Histologically, the pathognomonic features are an increase in the giant multinucleated osteoclasts in scalloped areas on the surface of the bone (Howship's lacunae) and a replacement of the normal cellular and marrow elements by fibrous tissue. X-ray changes include resorption of the phalangeal tufts and replacement of the usually sharp cortical outline of the bone in the digits by an irregular outline (subperiosteal resorption). In recent years, osteitis fibrosa cystica has been very rare in primary hyperparathyroidism, probably due to the earlier detection of the disease.

With the use of multiple markers of bone turnover, such as formation indices (bone-specific alkaline phosphatase, osteocalcin, and type I procollagen peptides) and bone resorption indices (including hydroxypyridinium collagen cross-links and telopeptides of type I collagen), increased skeletal turnover is detected in essentially all patients with established hyperparathyroidism.

Dual-energy x-ray absorptiometry (DEXA) of the spine provides reproducible quantitative estimates (within a few percent) of spinal bone density. Similarly, bone density in the extremities can be quantified by densitometry of the hip or of the distal radius at a site chosen to be primarily cortical. CT is a very sensitive technique for estimating spinal bone density, but reproducibility of standard CT is no better than 5%. Newer CT techniques (spiral, "extreme" CT) are more reproducible but are currently available in a limited number of medical centers. Cortical bone density is reduced while cancellous bone density, especially in the spine, is relatively preserved. Serial studies in patients who choose to be followed without surgery have indicated that in the majority of patients there is little further change over a number of years, consistent with laboratory data indicating relatively unchanged blood calcium and PTH levels. After an initial loss of bone mass in patients with mild asymptomatic hyperparathyroidism, a new equilibrium may be reached, with bone density and biochemical manifestations of the disease remaining relatively unchanged. However, some evidence suggests that there may be an increased fracture risk, including the spine, despite the relative preservation of spinal bone density; thus, some uncertainty about optimal management continues, even in asymptomatic patients.

In symptomatic patients, dysfunctions of the CNS, peripheral nerve and muscle, gastrointestinal tract, and joints also occur. It has been reported that severe neuropsychiatric manifestations may be reversed by parathyroidectomy; it remains unclear, in the absence of controlled studies, whether this improvement has a defined cause-and-effect relationship. Generally, the fact that hyperparathyroidism is common in elderly patients, in whom there are often other problems, suggests the possibility that such coexisting problems as hypertension, renal deterioration, and depression may not be parathyroid-related and suggests caution in recommending parathyroid surgery as a cure for these manifestations.

When present, neuromuscular manifestations may include proximal muscle weakness, easy fatigability, and atrophy of muscles and may be so striking as to suggest a primary neuromuscular disorder. The distinguishing feature is the complete regression of neuromuscular disease after surgical correction of the hyperparathyroidism.

Gastrointestinal manifestations are sometimes subtle and include vague abdominal complaints and disorders of the stomach and pancreas. Again, cause and effect are unclear. In MEN 1 patients with hyperparathyroidism, duodenal ulcer may be the result of associated pancreatic tumors that secrete excessive quantities of gastrin (Zollinger-Ellison syndrome). Pancreatitis has been reported in association with hyperparathyroidism, but the incidence and the mechanism are not established.

In reports from European centers, the frequency of pathophysiologic deterioration, especially cardiovascular (as well as other systems), is more frequent than the U.S. experience with milder disease. The differences are not fully explained, but greater severity at initial diagnosis (fewer cases determined by routine screening) and vitamin D deficiency are possible explanations for the different manifestations of disease.

DIAGNOSIS

The diagnosis is typically made by detecting an elevated immunoreactive PTH level in a patient with asymptomatic hypercalcemia (see "Differential Diagnosis: Special Tests" later in the chapter). Serum phosphate is usually low but may be normal, especially if renal failure has developed.

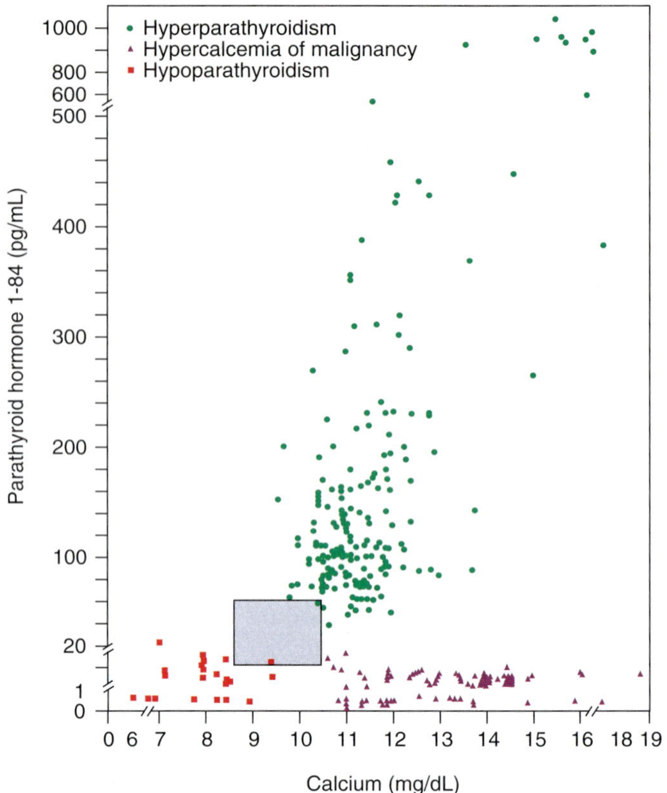

FIGURE 27-4

Levels of immunoreactive parathyroid hormone (PTH) detected in patients with primary hyperparathyroidism, hypercalcemia of malignancy, and hypoparathyroidism. Boxed area represents the upper and normal limits of blood calcium and/or immunoreactive PTH. [*From SR Nussbaum, JT Potts, Jr, in L DeGroot, JL Jameson (eds): Endocrinology, 4th ed. Philadelphia, Saunders, 2001; with permission.*]

Many tests based on renal responses to excess PTH (renal calcium and phosphate clearance; blood phosphate, chloride, magnesium; urinary or nephrogenous cyclic AMP) were used in earlier decades. These tests have low specificity for hyperparathyroidism and are therefore not cost-effective; they have been replaced by PTH immunoassays combined with simultaneous blood calcium measurements (**Fig. 27-4**).

℞ Treatment: HYPERPARATHYROIDISM

MEDICAL SURVEILLANCE VERSUS SURGICAL TREATMENT The critical management question is whether the disease should be treated surgically. If severe hypercalcemia [3.7–4.5 mmol/L (15–18 mg/dL)] is present, surgery is mandatory as soon as the diagnosis can be confirmed by a PTH immunoassay. However, in most patients with hyperparathyroidism, hypercalcemia is mild and does not require urgent surgical or medical treatment.

The National Institutes of Health (NIH) held a Consensus Conference on Management of Asymptomatic Hyperparathyroidism in 1990. *Asymptomatic hyperparathyroidism* was defined as documented (presumptive) hyperparathyroidism without signs or symptoms attributable to the disease. The consensus was that patients <50 should undergo surgery, given the long surveillance that would be required. Other considerations that favored surgery included concern that consistent follow-up would be unlikely or that coexistent illness would complicate management. Patients >50 were deemed appropriate for medical monitoring if certain criteria were met, the patients wished to avoid surgery, or the guidelines for recommending surgery were not present (**Table 27-2**). Careful evaluation of patients over the subsequent 12 years provided reassurance that in some patients medical monitoring rather than surgery was still prudent yet promoted new questions about the natural history of the disease with or without surgery.

Data developed since the Consensus Conference indicated that a subgroup of patients had selective vertebral osteopenia out of proportion to bone loss at other sites and responded to surgery with striking restoration of bone mass (average >20%). Given reports of increased fracture risk by some centers, plus the advent of newer medical therapies and less invasive surgical procedures, the NIH convened a Workshop on Asymptomatic Hyperparathyroidism in 2002, and an independent (non-NIH) panel offered a revised set of recommendations. The changes reflect both practical considerations (such as the difficulty in creatinine clearance measurements and therefore substituting calculations based on serum creatinine) and concerns regarding potential deleterious skeletal effects in untreated patients (Tables 27-2 and **27-3**). Accordingly, indications for surgical intervention were lowered (i.e., stricter serum calcium and bone density criteria). As before, it was emphasized that asymptomatic patients should be monitored regularly and that surgical correction of hyperparathyroidism can always be undertaken when indicated, if medically feasible, since the success rate is high (>90%), mortality is low, and morbidity is minimal. The goals of monitoring are early detection of worsening hypercalcemia, deteriorating bone or renal status, or other complications of hyperparathyroidism. No specific recommendations about medical therapy were made, but early data showed the promise of the newer agents, with the prediction that they would be used in future clinical practice to increase bone mass in patients not electing surgery as further experience is gained. Neither panel recommended estrogen use in patients for whom surgery was not elected because there was insufficient cumulative experience with such therapy to balance theoretical risks (breast and endometrial cancer) versus benefits. Raloxifene (Evista), the first of the SERMs, has been shown to have many of the bone-protective effects of estrogen in osteoporotic subjects yet at the same time lowers the incidence of breast cancer; preliminary use of this agent in a small series of hyperparathyroid patients led to increased bone density. As much as a 5% increase in bone mineral density in the spine and hip was reported with alendronate use in asymptomatic patients. Experience with calcimimetics, drugs that selectively stimulate the calcium sensor and suppress

TABLE 27-2

GUIDELINES FOR PARATHYROID SURGERY IN ASYMPTOMATIC PRIMARY HYPERPARATHYROIDISM[a]

MEASUREMENT	GUIDELINES, 1990	GUIDELINES, 2002
Serum calcium (above upper limit of normal)	0.3–0.4 mmol/L (1–1.5 mg/dL) above normal	0.3 mmol/L (1.0 mg/dL) above normal
24-h urinary calcium	>400 mg	>400 mg
Creatinine clearance	Reduced by 30%	Reduced by 30%
Bone mineral density	Z-score <–2.0 (forearm)	T-score <–2.5 at any site
Age	<50	<50

[a]Surgery is also indicated in patients for whom medical surveillance is neither desired nor possible.
Source: From JP Bilezikian et al: J Clin Endocrinol Metab 87:5353, 2002.

TABLE 27-3

MANAGEMENT GUIDELINES FOR PATIENTS WITH ASYMPTOMATIC PRIMARY HYPERPARATHYROIDISM WHO DO NOT UNDERGO PARATHYROID SURGERY

MEASUREMENT	OLDER GUIDELINES	NEW GUIDELINES
Serum calcium	Biannually	Biannually
24-h urinary calcium	Annually	Not recommended[a]
Creatinine clearance	Annually	Not recommended[a]
Serum creatinine	Annually	Annually[b]
Bone density	Annually (forearm)	Annually (lumbar spine, hip, forearm)
Abdominal x-ray (+/– ultrasound)	Annually	Not recommended[a]

[a]Except at the time of initial evaluation.
[b]If the serum creatinine concentration suggests a change in the creatinine clearance when the Cockroft-Gault equation is applied, further, more direct assessments of the creatinine clearance are recommended.
Source: From JP Bilezikian et al: J Clin Endocrinol Metab 87:5353, 2002.

PTH secretion, indicates that these agents decrease calcium levels to normal over 2 years of continuous use. Effects on PTH are less marked but significant.

SURGICAL TREATMENT Parathyroid exploration is challenging and should be undertaken by an experienced surgeon. Certain features help in predicting the pathology (e.g., multiple abnormal glands in familial cases). However, some critical decisions regarding management can be made only during the operation.

Increasingly, minimally invasive surgical procedures are being practiced. With conventional surgery, one approach is still based on the view that typically only one gland (the adenoma) is abnormal. If an enlarged gland is found, a normal gland should be sought. In this view, if a biopsy of a normal-sized second gland confirms its histologic (and presumed functional) normality, no further exploration, biopsy, or excision is needed. At the other extreme is the minority viewpoint that all four glands be sought and that most of the total parathyroid tissue mass should be removed. The concern with the former approach is that the recurrence rate of hyperparathyroidism may be high if a second abnormal gland is missed; the latter approach could involve unnecessary surgery and an unacceptable rate of hypoparathyroidism. When normal glands are found in association with one enlarged gland, excision of the single adenoma usually leads to cure or at least years free of symptoms. Long-term follow-up studies to establish true rates of recurrence are limited.

Recently, there has been growing experience with new surgical strategies that feature a minimally invasive approach guided by improved preoperative localization and intraoperative monitoring by PTH assays. Preoperative ^{99m}Tc sestamibi scans with single photon emission CT (SPECT) are used to predict the location of an abnormal gland and intraoperative sampling of PTH before and at 5-min intervals after removal of a suspected adenoma to confirm a rapid fall (>50%) to normal levels of PTH. In several centers, a combination of preoperative sestamibi imaging, cervical block anesthesia, minimal surgical incision, and intraoperative PTH measurements has allowed successful outpatient surgical management with a clear-cut cost benefit compared to general anesthesia and more extensive neck surgery. The use of these minimally invasive approaches requires clinical judgment to select patients unlikely to have multiple gland disease (e.g., MEN or secondary hyperparathyroidism). The growing acceptance of the technique and its relative ease for the patient has lowered the threshold for surgery.

Usually the severity of the hypercalcemia provides a preoperative clue to parathyroid carcinoma. In such cases, when neck exploration is undertaken, the tissue should be widely excised; care is taken to avoid rupture of the capsule to prevent local seeding of tumor cells.

Multiple gland hyperplasia, as predicted in familial cases, poses more difficult questions of surgical management. Once a diagnosis of hyperplasia is established, all the glands must be identified. Two schemes have been proposed for surgical management. One is to totally remove three glands with partial excision of the fourth gland; care is taken to leave a good blood supply for the remaining gland. Other surgeons advocate total parathyroidectomy with immediate transplantation of a portion of a removed, minced parathyroid gland into the muscles of the forearm, with the view that surgical excision is easier from the ectopic site in the arm if there is recurrent hyperfunction.

In a minority of cases, if no abnormal parathyroid glands are found in the neck, the issue of further exploration must be decided. There are documented cases of five or six parathyroid glands and of unusual locations for adenomas, such as in the mediastinum.

When a second parathyroid exploration is indicated, the minimally invasive techniques for preoperative localization such as ultrasound, CT scan, and isotope scanning are combined with venous sampling and/or selective digital arteriography in one of the centers specializing in these procedures. Intraoperative monitoring of PTH levels by rapid PTH immunoassays may be useful in guiding the surgery. At one center, long-term cures have been achieved with selective embolization or injection of large amounts of contrast material into the end-arterial circulation feeding the parathyroid tumor.

A decline in serum calcium occurs within 24 h after successful surgery; usually blood calcium falls to low-normal values for 3–5 days until the remaining parathyroid tissue resumes full hormone secretion. Acute postoperative hypocalcemia is likely only if severe bone mineral deficits are present or if injury to all the normal parathyroid glands occurs during surgery. In general, there are few problems encountered in patients with uncomplicated disease such as a single adenoma (the clear majority), who do not have symptomatic bone disease nor a large deficit in bone mineral, who are vitamin D and magnesium sufficient, and who have good renal and gastrointestinal function. The extent of postoperative hypocalcemia varies with the surgical approach. If all glands are biopsied, hypocalcemia may be transiently symptomatic and more prolonged. Hypocalcemia is more likely to be symptomatic after second parathyroid explorations, particularly when normal parathyroid tissue was removed at the initial operation and when the manipulation and/or biopsy of the remaining normal glands is more extensive in the search for the missing adenoma.

Patients with hyperparathyroidism have efficient intestinal calcium absorption due to the increased levels of $1,25(OH)_2D$ stimulated by PTH excess. Once hypocalcemia signifies successful surgery, patients can be put on a high-calcium intake or be given oral calcium supplements. Despite mild hypocalcemia, most patients do not require parenteral therapy. If the serum calcium falls to <2 mmol/L (8 mg/dL), *and if the phosphate level rises simultaneously*, the possibility that surgery has caused hypoparathyroidism must be considered. With unexpected hypocalcemia, coexistent hypomagnesemia should be considered, as it interferes with PTH secretion and causes functional hypoparathyroidism (Chap. 25).

Signs of hypocalcemia include symptoms such as muscle twitching, a general sense of anxiety, and positive Chvostek and Trousseau signs coupled with serum calcium consistently <2 mmol/L (8 mg/dL). Parenteral calcium replacement at a low level should be instituted when hypocalcemia is symptomatic. The rate and duration of IV therapy are determined by the severity of the symptoms and the response of the serum calcium to treatment. An infusion of 0.5–2 (mg/kg)/h or 30–100 mL/h of a 1-mg/mL solution usually suffices to relieve symptoms. Usually, parenteral therapy is required for only a few days. If symptoms worsen or if parenteral calcium is needed for >2–3 days, therapy with a vitamin D analogue and/or oral calcium (2–4 g/d) should be started. It is cost-effective to use calcitriol (doses of 0.5–1.0 μg/d) because of the rapidity of onset of effect and prompt cessation of action when stopped, in comparison to other forms of vitamin D. A rise in blood calcium after several months of vitamin D replacement may indicate restoration of parathyroid function to normal. It is also appropriate to monitor serum PTH serially to estimate gland function in such patients.

If magnesium deficiency was present, it can complicate the postoperative course. Magnesium deficiency impairs the secretion of PTH, and so hypomagnesemia should be corrected whenever detected. Magnesium replacement can be effective orally (e.g., $MgCl_2$, $MgOH_2$), but parenteral repletion is usual to ensure postoperative recovery, if magnesium deficiency is suspected due to low blood magnesium levels. Because the depressant effect of magnesium on central and peripheral nerve functions does not occur at levels <2 mmol/L (normal range 0.8–1.2 mmol/L), parenteral replacement can be given rapidly. A cumulative dose as great as 0.5–1 mmol/kg of body weight can be administered if severe hypomagnesemia is present; often, however, total doses of 20–40 mmol are sufficient.

OTHER PARATHYROID-RELATED CAUSES OF HYPERCALCEMIA

Lithium Therapy

Lithium, used in the management of bipolar depression and other psychiatric disorders, causes hypercalcemia in ~10% of treated patients. The hypercalcemia is dependent on continued lithium treatment, remitting and recurring when lithium is stopped and restarted. The parathyroid adenomas reported in some hypercalcemic patients with lithium therapy may reflect the presence of an independently occurring parathyroid tumor; a permanent effect of lithium on parathyroid gland growth need not be implicated as most patients have complete reversal of hypercalcemia when lithium is stopped. However, longstanding stimulation of parathyroid cell replication by lithium may predispose to development of adenomas (as is documented in secondary hyperparathyroidism and renal failure).

At the levels achieved in blood in treated patients, lithium can be shown in vitro to shift the PTH secretion curve to the right in response to calcium; i.e., higher calcium levels are required to lower PTH secretion, probably acting at the calcium sensor (see below). This effect can cause elevated PTH levels and consequent hypercalcemia in otherwise normal individuals. Fortunately, there are usually alternative medications for the underlying psychiatric illness. Parathyroid surgery should not be recommended unless hypercalcemia and elevated PTH levels persist after lithium is discontinued.

GENETIC DISORDERS CAUSING HYPERPARATHYROID-LIKE SYNDROMES

Familial Hypocalciuric Hypercalcemia

FHH (also called *familial benign hypercalcemia*) is inherited as an autosomal dominant trait. Affected individuals are discovered because of asymptomatic hypercalcemia. This disorder and Jansen's disease are variants of hyperparathyroidism. FHH involves excessive secretion of PTH, whereas Jansen's disease is caused by excessive biologic activity of the PTH receptor in target tissues. Neither disorder, however, involves a primary growth disorder of the parathyroids.

The pathophysiology of FHH is now understood. The primary defect is abnormal sensing of the blood calcium by the parathyroid gland and renal tubule, causing inappropriate secretion of PTH and excessive renal reabsorption of calcium. The calcium sensor is a member of the third family of GPCRs (type C, or III). The receptor responds to the ECF calcium concentration, suppressing PTH secretion through second-messenger signaling, thereby providing negative-feedback regulation of PTH secretion. Many different mutations in the calcium-sensing receptor have been identified in patients with FHH (Fig. 27-5). These mutations lower the capacity of the sensor to bind calcium, and the mutant receptors function as though blood calcium levels were low; excessive secretion of PTH occurs from an otherwise normal gland. Approximately two-thirds of patients with FHH have mutations within the protein-coding region of the gene. The remaining one-third of kindreds may have mutations in the gene promoter or may involve still

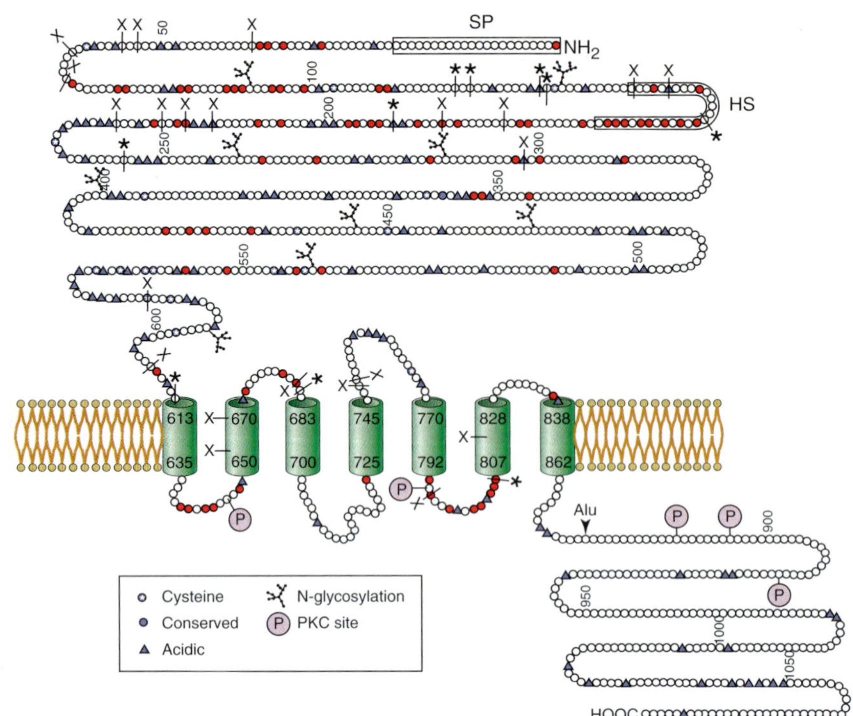

FIGURE 27-5

Mutations in the calcium sensor receptor. The extracellular domain binds calcium, leading to conformational changes that stimulate Gq-coupled activation of the phospholipase C and suppression of PTH. The identified sequence alterations (X) cause loss of function and lead to inadequate suppression of parathyroid hormone release and, therefore, mild hypercalcemia (FHH). *, a gain-of-function mutation that causes hypocalcemia; •, conserved residues; ◆, acidic residues. *(From EM Brown et al: J Nutr 125:1965S, 1995; with permission.)*

unknown mechanisms in other regions of the genome identified through mapping studies (e.g., chromosome 19).

Even before elucidation of the pathophysiology of FHH, abundant clinical evidence served to separate the disorder from primary hyperparathyroidism; these clinical features are still useful in differential diagnosis. Patients with primary hyperparathyroidism have <99% renal calcium reabsorption, whereas most patients with FHH have >99% reabsorption. The hypercalcemia in FHH is often detectable in affected members of the kindreds in the first decade of life, whereas hypercalcemia rarely occurs in patients with primary hyperparathyroidism or the MEN syndromes who are <10. PTH may be elevated in FHH, but the values are usually normal or lower for the same degree of calcium elevation than in patients with primary hyperparathyroidism. Parathyroid surgery performed in a few patients with FHH before the nature of the syndrome was understood led to permanent hypoparathyroidism; nevertheless, hypocalciuria persisted, establishing that hypocalciuria is not PTH-dependent (now known to be due to the abnormal calcium sensor in the kidney).

Few clinical signs or symptoms are present in patients with FHH, and other endocrine abnormalities are not present. Most patients are detected as a result of family screening after hypercalcemia is detected in a proband. In those patients inadvertently operated on, the parathyroids appeared normal or moderately hyperplastic. Parathyroid surgery is not appropriate, nor, in view of the lack of symptoms, does medical treatment seem needed to lower the calcium. Calcimimetic agents that bind to the calcium sensor and elevate the set point are under investigation.

One striking exception to the rule against parathyroid surgery in this syndrome is the occurrence, usually in consanguineous marriages (due to the rarity of the gene mutation), of a homozygous or compound heterozygote state, resulting in complete loss of the calcium sensor function. In this condition, neonatal severe hypercalcemia, total parathyroidectomy is mandatory. Rare but well-documented cases of acquired hypocalciuric hypercalcemia are reported due to antibodies against the calcium sensor. They appear to be a complication of an underlying autoimmune disorder and respond to therapies directed against the underlying disorder.

Jansen's Disease

Mutations in the PTH1R have been identified as responsible for this rare autosomal dominant syndrome. Because the mutations lead to constitutive receptor function, one abnormal copy of the mutant receptor is sufficient to cause the disease, thereby accounting for its dominant mode of transmission. The disorder leads to short-limbed dwarfism due to abnormal regulation of the bone growth plate. In adult life, there are numerous abnormalities in bone, including multiple cystic resorptive areas resembling those seen in severe hyperparathyroidism. Hypercalcemia and hypophosphatemia with undetectable or low PTH levels are typically seen. The pathogenesis of the disease has been confirmed by transgenic experiments in which targeted expression of the mutant receptor to the growth plate emulated several features of the disorder.

MALIGNANCY-RELATED HYPERCALCEMIA

Clinical Syndromes and Mechanisms of Hypercalcemia

Hypercalcemia due to malignancy is common (occurring in as many as 20% of cancer patients, especially with certain types of tumor, such as lung carcinoma), often severe and difficult to manage, and, on rare occasions, difficult to distinguish from primary hyperparathyroidism. Although malignancy is often clinically obvious or readily detectable by medical history, hypercalcemia can occasionally be due to an occult tumor. Previously, hypercalcemia associated with malignancy was thought to be due to local invasion and destruction of bone by tumor cells; many cases are now known to result from the elaboration by the malignant cells of humoral mediators of hypercalcemia. PTHrP is the responsible humoral agent in most solid tumors that cause hypercalcemia.

The histologic character of the tumor is more important than the extent of skeletal metastases in predicting hypercalcemia. Small cell carcinoma (oat cell) and adenocarcinoma of the lung, although the most common lung tumors associated with skeletal metastases, rarely cause hypercalcemia. By contrast, many patients with squamous cell carcinoma of the lung develop hypercalcemia. Histologic studies of bone in patients with squamous cell or epidermoid carcinoma of the lung, in sites invaded by tumor as well as areas remote from tumor invasion, reveal increased bone resorption.

Two main mechanisms of hypercalcemia are operative in cancer hypercalcemia. Many solid tumors associated with hypercalcemia, particularly squamous cell and renal tumors, produce and secrete PTHrP that causes increased bone resorption and mediate the hypercalcemia through systemic actions on the skeleton. Alternatively, direct bone marrow invasion occurs with hematologic malignancies such as leukemia, lymphoma, and multiple myeloma. Lymphokines and cytokines (including PTHrP) produced by cells involved in the marrow response to the tumors promote resorption of bone through local destruction. Several hormones, hormone analogues, cytokines, and growth factors have been implicated as the result of clinical assays, in vitro tests, or chemical isolation. The etiologic factor produced by activated normal lymphocytes and by myeloma and lymphoma cells, originally termed *osteoclast activation factor*, now appears to represent the biologic action of several different cytokines, probably interleukin 1 and lymphotoxin or tumor necrosis factor. In some lymphomas, there is a third mechanism, caused by an increased blood level of $1,25(OH)_2D$, produced by the abnormal lymphocytes.

In the more common mechanism, usually termed *humoral hypercalcemia of malignancy*, solid tumors (cancers of the lung and kidney, in particular), in which bone metastases are absent, minimal, or not detectable clinically, secrete PTHrP measurable by immunoassay. Secretion by the tumors of the PTH-like factor, PTHrP, activates the PTH1R, resulting in a pathophysiology closely resembling hyperparathyroidism. The clinical picture resembles primary hyperparathyroidism (hypophosphatemia accompanies hypercalcemia), and elimination or regression of the primary tumor leads to disappearance of the hypercalcemia.

As in hyperparathyroidism, patients with the humoral hypercalcemia of malignancy have elevated urinary nephrogenous cyclic AMP excretion, hypophosphatemia, and increased urinary phosphate clearance. However, in humoral hypercalcemia of malignancy, immunoreactive PTH is undetectable or suppressed, making the differential diagnosis easier. Other features of the disorder differ from those of true hyperparathyroidism. The biologic actions of PTH and PTHrP are exerted through the same receptor, but subtle differences in responses must account for the discordance. Other cytokines elaborated by the malignancy may contribute to the variations from hyperparathyroidism in these patients. Patients may have low to normal levels of $1,25(OH)_2D$ instead of elevated levels as in true hyperparathyroidism. In some patients with the humoral hypercalcemia of malignancy, osteoclastic resorption is unaccompanied by an osteoblastic or bone-forming response, implying inhibition of the normal coupling of bone formation and resorption.

Several different assays (single- or double-antibody, different epitopes) have been developed to detect PTHrP. Most data indicate that circulating PTHrP levels are undetectable (or low) in normal individuals, elevated in most cancer patients with the humoral syndrome, and high in human milk. The etiologic mechanisms in cancer hypercalcemia may be multiple in the same patient. For example, in breast carcinoma (metastatic to bone) and in a distinctive type of T cell lymphoma/leukemia initiated by human T cell lymphotropic virus I, hypercalcemia is caused by direct local lysis of bone as well as by a humoral mechanism involving excess production of PTHrP. Hyperparathyroidism has been reported to coexist with the humoral cancer syndrome and, rarely, ectopic hyperparathyroidism due to tumor elaboration of true PTH is reported.

Levels of PTH measured by the double-antibody technique are undetectable or extremely low in tumor hypercalcemia, as would be expected with the mediation of the hypercalcemia by a factor other than PTH (the hypercalcemia suppresses the normal parathyroid glands). In a patient with minimal symptoms referred for hypercalcemia, low or undetectable PTH levels would focus attention on a possible occult malignancy.

Ordinarily, the diagnosis of cancer hypercalcemia is not difficult because tumor symptoms are prominent when hypercalcemia is detected. Indeed, hypercalcemia may be noted incidentally during the workup of a patient with known or suspected malignancy. Clinical suspicion that malignancy is the cause of the hypercalcemia is heightened when there are other paraneoplastic signs or symptoms, such as weight loss, fatigue, muscle weakness, or unexplained skin rash, or when symptoms specific for a particular tumor are present. Squamous cell tumors are most frequently associated with hypercalcemia, particularly tumors of the lung, kidney, head and neck, and urogenital tract. Radiologic examinations can focus on these areas when clinical evidence is unclear. Bone scans with technetium-labeled bisphosphonate are useful for detection of osteolytic metastases; the sensitivity is high, but specificity is low. Results must be confirmed by conventional x-rays to be certain that areas of increased uptake are due to osteolytic metastases per se. Bone marrow biopsies are helpful in patients with anemia or abnormal peripheral blood smears.

℞ Treatment: MALIGNANCY-RELATED HYPERCALCEMIA

Treatment of the hypercalcemia of malignancy is first directed to control of tumor; reduction of tumor mass usually corrects hypercalcemia. If a patient has severe hypercalcemia yet has a good chance for effective tumor therapy, treatment of the hypercalcemia should be vigorous while awaiting the results of definitive therapy. If hypercalcemia occurs in the late stages of a tumor that is resistant to antitumor therapy, the treatment of the hypercalcemia should be judicious as high calcium levels can have a mild sedating effect. Standard therapies for hypercalcemia are applicable to patients with malignancy.

VITAMIN D–RELATED HYPERCALCEMIA

Hypercalcemia caused by vitamin D can be due to excessive ingestion or abnormal metabolism of the vitamin. Abnormal metabolism of the vitamin is usually acquired in association with a widespread granulomatous disorder. Vitamin D metabolism is carefully regulated, particularly the activity of renal 1α-hydroxylase, the enzyme responsible for the production of $1,25(OH)_2D$ (Chap. 25). The regulation of 1α-hydroxylase and the normal feedback suppression by $1,25(OH)_2D$ seem to work less well in infants than in adults and to operate poorly, if at all, in sites other than the renal tubule; these phenomena explain the occurrence of hypercalcemia secondary to excessive $1,25(OH)_2D_3$ production in infants with Williams syndrome and in adults with sarcoidosis or lymphoma.

Vitamin D Intoxication

Chronic ingestion of 40–100 times the normal physiologic requirement of vitamin D (amounts >40,000–100,000 U/d) is usually required to produce significant hypercalcemia in normal individuals. Nonetheless, an upper limit of dietary intake of 2000 U/d (50 μg/d) in adults is now recommended because of concerns about potential toxic effects of cumulative supraphysiologic doses. Vitamin D excess increases intestinal calcium absorption and, if severe, also increases bone resorption.

Hypercalcemia in vitamin D intoxication is due to an excessive biologic action of the vitamin, perhaps the consequence of increased levels of 25(OH)D rather than merely increased levels of the active metabolite $1,25(OH)_2D$ (the latter may not be elevated in vitamin D intoxication). 25(OH)D has definite, if low, biologic activity in intestine and bone. The production of 25(OH)D is less tightly regulated than is the production of $1,25(OH)_2D$. Hence, concentrations of 25(OH)D are elevated several fold in patients with excess vitamin D intake.

The diagnosis is substantiated by documenting elevated levels of 25(OH)D. Hypercalcemia is usually controlled by restriction of dietary calcium intake and appropriate attention to hydration. These measures, plus discontinuation of vitamin D, usually lead to resolution of hypercalcemia. However, vitamin D stores in fat may be substantial, and vitamin D intoxication may persist for weeks after vitamin D ingestion is terminated. Such patients are responsive to glucocorticoids, which, in doses of 100 mg/d of hydrocortisone or its equivalent, usually return serum calcium levels to normal over several days; severe intoxication may require intensive therapy.

Sarcoidosis and Other Granulomatous Diseases

In patients with sarcoidosis and other granulomatous diseases, such as tuberculosis and fungal infections, excess $1,25(OH)_2D$ is synthesized in macrophages or other cells in the granulomas. Indeed, increased $1,25(OH)_2D$ levels have been reported in anephric patients with sarcoidosis and hypercalcemia. Macrophages obtained from granulomatous tissue convert 25(OH)D to $1,25(OH)_2D$ at an increased rate. There is a positive correlation in patients with sarcoidosis between 25(OH)D levels (reflecting vitamin D intake) and the circulating concentrations of 1,25(OH)$_2$D, whereas normally there is no increase in 1,25(OH)$_2$D with increasing 25(OH)D levels due to multiple feedback controls on renal 1-hydroxylase (Chap. 25). The usual regulation of active metabolite production by calcium phosphate or PTH does not operate in these patients. Clearance of 1,25(OH)$_2$D from blood may be decreased in sarcoidosis as well. PTH levels are usually low and 1,25(OH)$_2$D levels are elevated, but primary hyperparathyroidism and sarcoidosis may coexist in some patients.

Management of the hypercalcemia can often be accomplished by avoiding excessive sunlight exposure and limiting vitamin D and calcium intake. Presumably, however, the abnormal sensitivity to vitamin D and abnormal regulation of 1,25(OH)$_2$D synthesis will persist as long as the disease is active. Alternatively, glucocorticoids in the equivalent of ≤100 mg/d of hydrocortisone control hypercalcemia. Glucocorticoids appear to act by blocking excessive production of 1,25(OH)$_2$D as well as the response to it in target organs.

Idiopathic Hypercalcemia of Infancy

This rare disorder, usually referred to as *Williams syndrome*, is an autosomal dominant disorder characterized by multiple congenital development defects, including supravalvular aortic stenosis, mental retardation, and an elfin facies, in association with hypercalcemia due to abnormal sensitivity to vitamin D. The syndrome was first recognized in England after the fortification of milk with vitamin D. Levels of 1,25(OH)$_2$D are elevated, ranging from 46–120 nmol/L (150–500 pg/mL). The mechanism of the abnormal sensitivity to vitamin D and of the increased circulating levels of 1,25(OH)$_2$D is still unclear. Studies suggest that genetic mutations involving microdeletions at the elastin locus and perhaps other genes on chromosome 7 may play a role in the pathogenesis.

HYPERCALCEMIA ASSOCIATED WITH HIGH BONE TURNOVER

Hyperthyroidism

As many as 20% of hyperthyroid patients have high-normal or mildly elevated serum calcium concentrations; hypercalciuria is even more common. The hypercalcemia is due to increased bone turnover, with bone resorption exceeding bone formation. Severe calcium elevations are not typical, and the presence of such suggests a concomitant disease such as hyperparathyroidism. Usually, the diagnosis is obvious, but signs of hyperthyroidism may occasionally be occult, particularly in the elderly (Chap. 4). Hypercalcemia is managed by treatment of the hyperthyroidism. Reports that thyroid-stimulating hormone (TSH) itself normally has a bone protective effect suggest that suppressed TSH levels also play a role in hypercalcemia.

Immobilization

Immobilization is a rare cause of hypercalcemia in adults in the absence of an associated disease but may cause hypercalcemia in children and adolescents, particularly after spinal cord injury and paraplegia or quadriplegia. With resumption of ambulation, the hypercalcemia in children usually returns to normal.

The mechanism appears to involve a disproportion between bone formation and bone resorption. Hypercalciuria and increased mobilization of skeletal calcium can develop in normal volunteers subjected to extensive bed rest, although hypercalcemia is unusual. Immobilization of an adult with a disease associated with high bone turnover, however, such as Paget's disease, may cause hypercalcemia.

Thiazides

Administration of benzothiadiazines (thiazides) can cause hypercalcemia in patients with high rates of bone turnover, such as patients with hypoparathyroidism treated with high doses of vitamin D. Traditionally, thiazides are associated with aggravation of hypercalcemia in primary hyperparathyroidism, but this effect can be seen in other high-bone-turnover states as well. The mechanism of thiazide action is complex. Chronic thiazide administration leads to reduction in urinary calcium; the hypocalciuric effect appears to reflect the enhancement of proximal tubular resorption of sodium and calcium in response to sodium depletion. Some of this renal effect is due to augmentation of PTH action and is more pronounced in individuals with intact PTH secretion. However, thiazides cause hypocalciuria in hypoparathyroid patients on high-dose vitamin D and oral calcium replacement if sodium intake is restricted. This finding is the rationale for the use of thiazides as an adjunct to therapy in hypoparathyroid patients, as discussed below. Thiazide administration to normal individuals causes a transient increase in blood calcium (usually within the high-normal range) that reverts to preexisting levels after a week or more of continued administration. If hormonal function and calcium and bone metabolism are normal, homeostatic controls are reset to counteract the calcium-elevating effect of the thiazides. In the presence of hyperparathyroidism or increased bone turnover from another cause, homeostatic mechanisms are ineffective. The abnormal effects of the thiazide on calcium metabolism disappear within days of cessation of the drug.

Vitamin A Intoxication

Vitamin A intoxication is a rare cause of hypercalcemia and is most commonly a side effect of dietary faddism. Calcium levels can be elevated into the 3–3.5-mmol/L (12–14-mg/dL) range after the ingestion of 50,000–100,000 units of vitamin A daily (10–20 times the minimum daily requirement). Typical features of severe hypercalcemia include fatigue, anorexia, and, in some, severe muscle and bone pain. Excess vitamin A intake is presumed to increase bone resorption.

The diagnosis can be established by history and by measurement of vitamin A levels in serum. Occasionally, skeletal x-rays reveal periosteal calcifications, particularly in the hands. Withdrawal of the vitamin is usually associated with prompt disappearance of the hypercalcemia and reversal of the skeletal changes. As in vitamin D intoxication, administration of 100 mg/d hydrocortisone or its equivalent leads to a rapid return of the serum calcium to normal.

HYPERCALCEMIA ASSOCIATED WITH RENAL FAILURE

Severe Secondary Hyperparathyroidism

Secondary hyperparathyroidism occurs when partial resistance to the metabolic actions of PTH leads to excessive production of the hormone. Parathyroid gland hyperplasia occurs because resistance to the normal level of PTH leads to hypocalcemia, which, in turn, is a stimulus to parathyroid gland enlargement.

Secondary hyperparathyroidism occurs not only in patients with renal failure but also in those with osteomalacia due to multiple causes (Chap. 25), including deficiency of vitamin D action, and PHP (deficient response to PTH at the level of the receptor). Hypocalcemia seems to be the common denominator in initiating secondary hyperparathyroidism. Primary (1°) and secondary (2°) hyperparathyroidism can be distinguished conceptually by the autonomous growth of the parathyroid glands in primary hyperparathyroidism (presumably irreversible) and the adaptive response of the parathyroids in secondary hyperparathyroidism (typically reversible). In fact, reversal over weeks from an abnormal pattern of secretion, presumably accompanied by involution of parathyroid gland mass to normal, occurs in patients who have been treated effectively to reverse the resistance to PTH (such as with calcium and vitamin D in osteomalacia). However, it is now recognized that a true clonal outgrowth (irreversible) can arise in longstanding, inadequately treated chronic renal failure [e.g., tertiary (3°) hyperparathyroidism].

Patients with secondary hyperparathyroidism may develop bone pain, ectopic calcification, and pruritus. The bone disease seen in patients with secondary hyperparathyroidism and renal failure is termed *renal osteodystrophy*. Osteomalacia (predominantly due to vitamin D and calcium deficiency) and/or osteitis fibrosa cystica (excessive PTH action on bone) may occur.

Two other skeletal disorders are associated with long-term dialysis in patients with renal failure. Aluminum deposition (see below) is associated with an osteomalacia-like picture. The other entity is a low-bone-turnover state termed "aplastic" or "adynamic" bone disease; PTH levels are lower than in typical secondary hyperparathyroidism. It is believed that the condition is caused, at least in part, by excessive PTH suppression, which may be even greater than previously appreciated in light of evidence that some of the immunoreactive PTH detected by most commercially available PTH assays is not the full-length biologically active molecule but may consist of amino-terminally truncated fragments that do not activate the PTH1R.

℞ Treatment: SECONDARY HYPERPARATHYROIDISM

Medical therapy to reverse secondary hyperparathyroidism includes reduction of excessive blood phosphate by restriction of dietary phosphate, the use of nonabsorbable antacids, and careful, selective addition of calcitriol (0.25–2.0 μg/d); calcium carbonate had been preferred over aluminum-containing antacids to prevent aluminum toxicity. However, synthetic gels that also bind phosphate (such as sevelamer) are widely used, with the advantage of avoiding not only aluminum retention but also excess calcium elevation. IV calcitriol, administered as several pulses each week, helps control secondary hyperparathyroidism. Aggressive but carefully administered medical therapy can often, but not always, reverse hyperparathyroidism and its symptoms and manifestations.

Occasional patients develop severe manifestations of secondary hyperparathyroidism, including hypercalcemia, pruritus, extraskeletal calcifications, and painful bones, despite aggressive medical efforts to suppress the hyperparathyroidism. PTH hypersecretion no longer responsive to medical therapy, a state of severe hyperparathyroidism in patients with renal failure that requires surgery, has been referred to as *tertiary hyperparathyroidism*. Parathyroid surgery is necessary to control this condition. Based on genetic evidence from examination of tumor samples in these patients, the emergence of autonomous parathyroid function is due to a monoclonal outgrowth of one or more previously hyperplastic parathyroid glands. The adaptive response has become an independent contributor to disease; this finding seems to emphasize the importance of optimal medical management to reduce the proliferative response of the parathyroid cells that enables the irreversible genetic change.

Aluminum Intoxication

Aluminum intoxication (and often hypercalcemia as a complication of medical treatment) may occur in patients on chronic dialysis; manifestations include acute dementia and unresponsive and severe osteomalacia. Bone pain; multiple nonhealing fractures, particularly of the ribs and pelvis; and a proximal myopathy may occur. Hypercalcemia develops when these patients are treated with vitamin D or calcitriol because of impaired skeletal responsiveness. Aluminum is present at the site of osteoid mineralization, osteoblastic activity is minimal, and calcium incorporation into the skeleton is impaired. Prevention is accomplished by avoidance of aluminum excess in the dialysis regimen; treatment of established disease involves mobilizing aluminum through the use of the chelating agent deferoxamine.

Milk-Alkali Syndrome

The milk-alkali syndrome is due to excessive ingestion of calcium and absorbable antacids such as milk or calcium carbonate. It is much less frequent since nonabsorbable antacids and other treatments became available for peptic ulcer disease. However, the increased use of calcium carbonate in the management of osteoporosis has led to reappearance of the syndrome. Several clinical presentations—acute, subacute, and chronic—have been described, all of which feature hypercalcemia, alkalosis, and renal failure. The chronic form of the disease, termed *Burnett's syndrome*, is associated with irreversible renal damage. The acute syndromes reverse if the excess calcium and absorbable alkali are stopped.

Individual susceptibility is important in the pathogenesis, as some patients are treated with calcium carbonate and alkali regimens without developing the syndrome. One variable is the fractional calcium absorption as a function of calcium intake. Some individuals absorb a high fraction of calcium, even with intakes ≥2 g of elemental calcium per day, instead of reducing calcium absorption with high intake, as occurs in most normal individuals. Resultant mild hypercalcemia after meals in such patients is postulated to contribute to the generation of alkalosis. Development of hypercalcemia causes increased sodium excretion and some depletion of total-body water. These phenomena and perhaps some suppression of endogenous PTH secretion due to mild hypercalcemia lead to increased bicarbonate resorption and to alkalosis in the face of continued calcium carbonate ingestion. Alkalosis per se selectively enhances calcium resorption in the distal nephron, thus aggravating the hypercalcemia. The cycle of mild hypercalcemia → bicarbonate retention → alkalosis → renal calcium retention → severe hypercalcemia perpetuates and aggravates hypercalcemia and alkalosis as long as calcium and absorbable alkali are ingested.

DIFFERENTIAL DIAGNOSIS: SPECIAL TESTS

Differential diagnosis of hypercalcemia is best achieved by using clinical criteria, but the immunoassay for PTH is especially useful in distinguishing among major causes (Fig. 27-6). The clinical features that deserve emphasis are the presence or absence of symptoms or signs of disease and evidence of chronicity. If one discounts fatigue or depression, >90% of patients with primary hyperparathyroidism have *asymptomatic hypercalcemia*; symptoms of malignancy are usually present in cancer-associated hypercalcemia. Disorders other than hyperparathyroidism and malignancy cause <10% of cases of hypercalcemia,

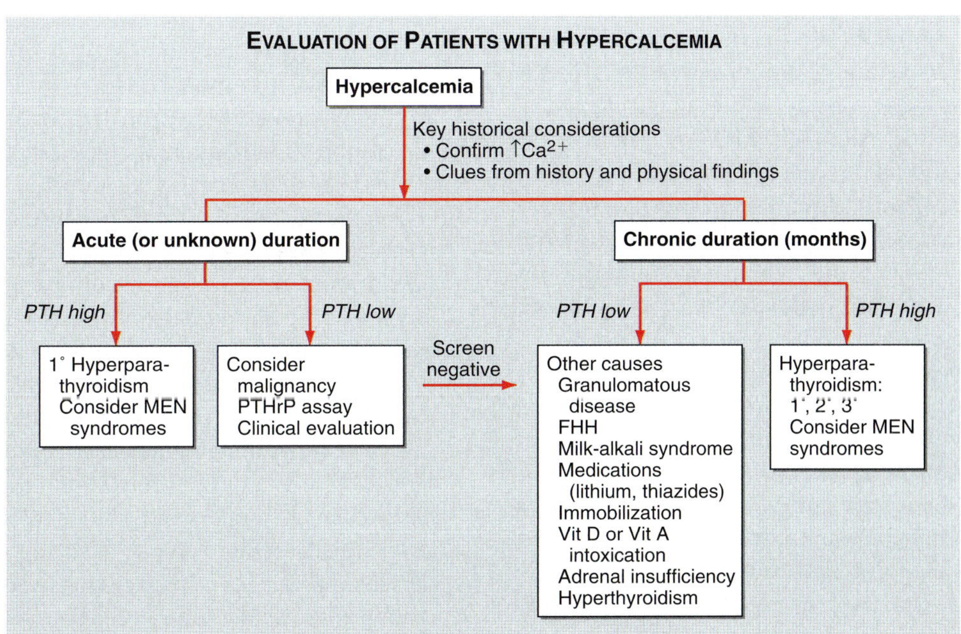

FIGURE 27-6

Algorithm for the evaluation of patients with hypercalcemia. See text for details. FHH, familial hypocalciuric hypercalcemia; MEN, multiple endocrine neoplasia; PTH, parathyroid hormone; PTHrP, parathyroid hormone–related peptide.

and some of the nonparathyroid causes are associated with clear-cut manifestations such as renal failure.

Hyperparathyroidism is the likely diagnosis in patients with *chronic hypercalcemia*. If hypercalcemia has been manifest for >1 year, malignancy can usually be excluded as the cause. A striking feature of malignancy-associated hypercalcemia is the rapidity of the course, whereby signs and symptoms of the underlying malignancy are evident within months of the detection of hypercalcemia. Although clinical considerations are helpful in arriving at the correct diagnosis of the cause of hypercalcemia, appropriate laboratory testing is essential for definitive diagnosis. The immunoassay for PTH should separate hyperparathyroidism from all other causes of hypercalcemia. Patients with hyperparathyroidism have elevated PTH levels despite hypercalcemia, whereas patients with malignancy and the other causes of hypercalcemia (except for disorders mediated by PTH such as lithium-induced hypercalcemia) have levels of hormone below normal or undetectable. Assays based on the double-antibody method for PTH exhibit very high sensitivity (especially if serum calcium is simultaneously evaluated) and specificity for the diagnosis of primary hyperparathyroidism (Fig. 27-4).

In summary, PTH values are elevated in >90% of parathyroid-related causes of hypercalcemia, undetectable or low in malignancy-related hypercalcemia, and undetectable or normal in vitamin D–related and high-bone-turnover causes of hypercalcemia. In view of the specificity of the PTH immunoassay and the high frequency of hyperparathyroidism in hypercalcemic patients, it is cost-effective to measure the PTH level in all hypercalcemic patients unless malignancy or a specific nonparathyroid disease is obvious. False-positive PTH assay results are rare. There are very rare reports of ectopic production of excess PTH by nonparathyroid tumors. Immunoassays for PTHrP are helpful in diagnosing certain types of malignancy-associated hypercalcemia. Although FHH is parathyroid-related, the disease should be managed distinctively from hyperparathyroidism. Clinical features and the low urinary calcium excretion can help make the distinction. Because the incidence of malignancy and hyperparathyroidism both increase with age, they can coexist as two independent causes of hypercalcemia.

$1,25(OH)_2D$ levels are elevated in many (but not all) patients with primary hyperparathyroidism. In other disorders associated with hypercalcemia, concentrations of $1,25(OH)_2D$ are low or, at the most, normal. However, this test is of low specificity and is not cost-effective, as not all patients with hyperparathyroidism have elevated $1,25(OH)_2D$ levels, and not all nonparathyroid hypercalcemic patients have suppressed $1,25(OH)_2D$. Measurement of $1,25(OH)_2D$ is, however, critically valuable in establishing the cause of hypercalcemia in sarcoidosis and certain lymphomas.

A useful general approach is outlined in Fig. 27-6. If the patient is *asymptomatic* and there is evidence of *chronicity* to the hypercalcemia, hyperparathyroidism is almost certainly the cause. If PTH levels (usually measured at least twice) are elevated, the clinical impression is confirmed and little additional evaluation is necessary. If there is only a short history or no data as to the duration of the hypercalcemia, *occult malignancy* must be considered; if the PTH levels are not elevated, then a thorough workup must be undertaken for malignancy, including chest x-ray, CT of chest and abdomen, and bone scan. Immunoassays for PTHrP may be especially useful in such situations. Attention should also be paid to clues for underlying hematologic disorders such as anemia, increased plasma globulin, and abnormal serum immunoelectrophoresis; bone scans can be negative in some patients with metastases, such as in multiple myeloma. Finally, if a patient with chronic hypercalcemia is asymptomatic and malignancy therefore seems unlikely on clinical grounds, but PTH values are not elevated, it is useful to search for other chronic causes of hypercalcemia, such as occult sarcoidosis. A careful history of dietary supplements and drug use may suggest intoxication with vitamin D or vitamin A or the use of thiazides.

℞ Treatment: HYPERCALCEMIC STATES

The approach to medical treatment of hypercalcemia varies with its severity (Table 27-4). Mild hypercalcemia, <3.0 mmol/L (12 mg/dL), can be managed by hydration. More severe hypercalcemia [levels of 3.2–3.7 mmol/L (13–15 mg/dL)] must be managed aggressively; above that level, hypercalcemia can be life-threatening and requires emergency measures. By using a combination of approaches in severe hypercalcemia, the serum calcium concentration can be decreased by 0.7–2.2 mmol/L (3–9 mg/dL) within 24–48 h in most patients, enough to relieve acute symptoms, prevent death from hypercalcemic crisis, and permit diagnostic evaluation. Therapy can then be directed at the underlying disorder—the second priority.

Hypercalcemia develops because of excessive skeletal calcium release, increased intestinal calcium absorption, or inadequate renal calcium excretion. Understanding the particular pathogenesis helps guide therapy. For example, hypercalcemia in patients with malignancy is primarily due to excessive skeletal calcium release and is, therefore, minimally improved by restriction of dietary calcium. On the other hand, patients with vitamin D hypersensitivity or vitamin D intoxication have excessive intestinal calcium absorption, and restriction of dietary calcium is beneficial. Decreased renal function or ECF depletion decreases urinary calcium excretion. In such situations, rehydration may rapidly reduce or reverse the hypercalcemia, even though increased bone resorption persists. As outlined below, the more severe the hypercalcemia, the greater the number of combined therapies that should be used. Rapid-acting (hours) approaches—rehydration, forced

TABLE 27-4

THERAPIES FOR SEVERE HYPERCALCEMIA

TREATMENT	ONSET OF ACTION	DURATION OF ACTION	ADVANTAGES	DISADVANTAGES
Most Useful Therapies				
Hydration with saline	Hours	During infusion	Rehydration invariably needed	Volume overload, cardiac decompensation, intensive monitoring, electrolyte disturbance, inconvenience
Forced diuresis; saline plus loop diuretic	Hours	During treatment	Rapid action	
Bisphosphonates 1st generation: etidronate	1–2 days	5–7 days in doses used	First available bisphosphonate; intermediate onset of action	Less effective than other bisphosphonates
2d generation: pamidronate	1–2 days	10–14 days to weeks	High potency; intermediate onset of action	Fever in 20% hypophosphatemia, hypocalcemia, hypomagnesemia
3d generation: zoledronate	1–2 days	>3 weeks	High potency; rapid infusion; prolonged duration of action	Minor; fever, rarely hypocalcemia or hypophosphatemia
Calcitonin	Hours	1–2 days	Rapid onset of action; useful as adjunct in severe hypercalcemia	Rapid tachyphylaxis
Special Use Therapies				
Phosphate Oral	24 h	During use	Chronic management (with hypophosphatemia); low toxicity if P <4 mg/dL	Limited use except as adjuvant or chronic therapy
Intravenous	Hours	During use and 24–48 h afterward	Rapid action, highly potent but *rarely used* except with severe hypercalcemia and cardiac and renal decompensation present	Ectopic calcification; renal damage, fatal hypocalcemia
Glucocorticoids	Days	Days, weeks	Oral therapy, antitumor agent	Active only in certain malignancies; glucocorticoid side effects
Dialysis	Hours	During use and 24–48 h afterward	Useful in renal failure; onset of effect in hours; can immediately reverse life-threatening hypercalcemia	Complex procedure, reserved for extreme or special circumstances

diuresis, and calcitonin—can be used with the most effective antiresorptive agents, such as bisphosphonates (since severe hypercalcemia usually involves excessive bone resorption).

HYDRATION, INCREASED SALT INTAKE, MILD AND FORCED DIURESIS The first principle of treatment is to restore normal hydration. Many hypercalcemic patients are dehydrated because of vomiting, inanition, and/or hypercalcemia-induced defects in urinary concentrating ability. The resultant drop in glomerular filtration rate is accompanied by an additional decrease in renal tubular sodium and calcium clearance. Restoring a normal ECF volume corrects these abnormalities and increases urine calcium excretion by 2.5–7.5 mmol/d (100–300 mg/d). Increasing urinary sodium excretion to 400–500 mmol/d increases urinary calcium excretion even further than simple rehydration. After rehydration has been achieved, saline can be administered or furosemide or ethacrynic acid can be given twice daily to depress the tubular reabsorptive mechanism for calcium (care must be taken to prevent dehydration). The combined use of these therapies can increase urinary calcium excretion to ≥12.5 mmol/d (500 mg/d) in most hypercalcemic patients. Since this is a substantial percentage of the exchangeable calcium pool, the serum calcium concentration usually falls 0.25–0.75 mmol/L (1–3 mg/dL) within 24 h. Precautions should be taken to prevent potassium and magnesium depletion; calcium-containing renal calculi are a potential complication.

Under life-threatening circumstances, the preceding approach can be pursued more aggressively, giving as much as 6 L isotonic saline (900 mmol sodium) daily plus furosemide or equivalent in doses up to 100 mg every 1–2 h or ethacrynic acid in doses up to 40 mg every 1–2 h. Urinary calcium excretion may exceed 25 mmol/d (1000 mg/d), and the serum calcium may decrease by ≥1 mmol/L (4 mg/dL) within 24 h. Depletion of potassium and magnesium is inevitable unless replacements are given; pulmonary edema can be precipitated. The potential complications can be reduced by careful monitoring of central venous pressure and plasma or urine electrolytes; catheterization of the bladder may be necessary. This treatment approach should be supplemented with agents to block bone resorption. Though these agents do not become effective for several days, forced diuresis is difficult to sustain even in patients with good cardiopulmonary and renal function.

BISPHOSPHONATES The bisphosphonates are analogues of pyrophosphate, with high affinity for bone, especially in areas of increased bone turnover, where they are powerful inhibitors of bone resorption. These bone-seeking compounds are stable in vivo because phosphatase enzymes cannot hydrolyze the central carbon-phosphorus-carbon bond. The bisphosphonates are concentrated in areas of high bone turnover and are taken up by and inhibit osteoclast action; the mechanism of action is complex. Bisphosphonates alter osteoclast proton pump function or impair the release of acid hydrolases into the extracellular lysosomes contiguous with mineralized bone. They may also inhibit the differentiation of monocyte-macrophage precursors into osteoclasts and possibly have effects on osteoblasts as well. The bisphosphonate molecules that contain amino groups in the side chain structure (see below) interfere with prenylation of proteins and can lead to cellular apoptosis. The highly active non-amino-group–containing bisphosphonates are also metabolized to cytotoxic products.

The initial bisphosphonate widely used in clinical practice, etidronate, was effective but had several disadvantages, including the capacity to inhibit bone formation as well as blocking resorption. Subsequently, a number of second-generation compounds have become the mainstays of antiresorptive therapy for treatment of hypercalcemia and osteoporosis. The newer bisphosphonates have a highly favorable ratio of blocking resorption versus inhibiting bone formation; they inhibit osteoclast-mediated skeletal resorption yet do not cause mineralization defects at ordinary doses. Though the bisphosphonates have similar structures, the routes of administration, efficacy, toxicity, and side effects vary. The potency of the compounds for inhibition of bone resorption varies over 10,000-fold, increasing in the order of etidronate, tiludronate, pamidronate, alendronate, risedronate, and zoledronate. Oral alendronate and risedronate are approved for the therapy of osteoporosis in the United States and elsewhere. The IV use of pamidronate and zoledronate is approved for the treatment of hypercalcemia in the United States; between 30 and 90 mg pamidronate, given as a single IV dose over a few hours, returns serum calcium to normal within 24–48 h with an effect that lasts for weeks in 80–100% of patients. Zoledronate given in doses of 4 or 8 mg/5-min infusion has a more rapid and more sustained effort than pamidronate in direct comparison.

These drugs are used extensively in cancer patients. Absolute survival improvements are noted with pamidronate and zoledronate in multiple myeloma, for example. However, though still rare, there are increasing reports of jaw necrosis, especially after dental surgery, mainly in cancer patients treated with multiple doses of the more potent bisphosphonates.

CALCITONIN Calcitonin acts within a few hours of its administration, through receptors on osteoclasts, to block bone resorption and, in addition, to increase urinary calcium excretion by inhibition of renal tubular calcium reabsorption. If administered as a single agent, calcitonin, after 24 h of use, results in minimal lowering of calcium. Tachyphylaxis, a known phenomenon with this drug, seems to explain the results, since the drug is effective in the first hours of use. However, in life-threatening hypercalcemia, calcitonin can be used effectively within the first 24 h in combination with rehydration and saline diuresis while waiting for more sustained effects from a simultaneously administered bisphosphonate, such as pamidronate. Usual doses of calcitonin are 2–8 U/kg of body weight IV, SC, or IM every 6–12 h.

OTHER THERAPIES *Plicamycin* (formerly mithramycin), which inhibits bone resorption, has been a useful therapeutic agent but is now seldom used because of its toxicity and the effectiveness of bisphosphonates. Plicamycin must be given IV, either as a bolus or by slow infusion; the usual dose is 25 μg/kg of body weight. *Gallium nitrate* exerts a hypocalcemic action by inhibiting bone resorption and altering the structure of bone crystals. It is not often used now because of superior alternatives.

Glucocorticoids have utility, especially in hypercalcemia complicating certain malignancies. They increase urinary calcium excretion and decrease intestinal calcium absorption when given in pharmacologic doses, but they also cause negative skeletal calcium balance. In normal individuals and in patients with primary hyperparathyroidism, glucocorticoids neither increase nor decrease the serum calcium concentration. In patients with hypercalcemia due to certain osteolytic malignancies, however, glucocorticoids may be effective as a result of antitumor effects. The malignancies in which hypercalcemia responds to glucocorticoids include multiple myeloma, leukemia, Hodgkin's disease, other lymphomas, and carcinoma of the breast, at least early in the course of the disease. Glucocorticoids are also effective in treating hypercalcemia due to vitamin D intoxication and sarcoidosis. Glucocorticoids are also useful in the rare form of hypercalcemia, now recognized in certain autoimmune disorders in which inactivating antibodies against the receptor imitate FHH. Elevated PTH and calcium levels are effectively lowered by the glucocorticoids. In all the preceding situations, the hypocalcemic effect develops over several days, and the usual glucocorticoid dosage is 40–100 mg prednisone (or its equivalent) daily in four divided doses. The side effects of chronic glucocorticoid therapy may be acceptable in some circumstances.

Dialysis is often the treatment of choice for severe hypercalcemia complicated by renal failure, which is difficult to manage medically. Peritoneal dialysis with calcium-free dialysis fluid can remove 5–12.5 mmol (200–500 mg) of calcium in 24–48 h and lower the serum calcium concentration by 0.7–3 mmol/L (3–12 mg/dL). Large quantities of phosphate are lost during dialysis, and serum inorganic phosphate concentrations usually fall, thus aggravating hypercalcemia. Therefore, the serum inorganic phosphate concentration should be measured after dialysis, and phosphate supplements should be added to the diet or to dialysis fluids if necessary.

Phosphate therapy, PO or IV, has a limited role in certain circumstances (Chap. 25). Correcting hypophosphatemia lowers the serum calcium concentration by several mechanisms, including bone/calcium exchange. The usual oral treatment is 1–1.5 g phosphorus per day for several days, given in divided doses. It is generally believed, but not established, that toxicity does not occur if therapy is limited to restoring serum inorganic phosphate concentrations to normal.

Raising the serum inorganic phosphate concentration above normal decreases serum calcium levels, sometimes strikingly. IV phosphate is one of the most dramatically effective treatments available for severe hypercalcemia but is toxic and even dangerous (fatal hypocalcemia). For these reasons, it is used rarely and only in severely hypercalcemic patients with cardiac or renal failure where dialysis, the preferable alternative, is not feasible or is unavailable.

SUMMARY The various therapies for hypercalcemia are listed in Table 27-4. The choice depends on the underlying disease, the severity of the hypercalcemia, the serum inorganic phosphate level, and the renal, hepatic, and bone marrow function. Mild hypercalcemia [≤3 mmol/L (12 mg/dL)] can usually be managed by hydration. Severe hypercalcemia [≥3.7 mmol/L (15 mg/dL)] requires rapid correction. Calcitonin should be given for its rapid, albeit short-lived, blockade of bone resorption, and IV pamidronate or zoledronate should be administered, although its onset of action is delayed for 1–2 days. In addition, for the first 24–48 h, aggressive sodium-calcium diuresis with IV saline and, following rehydration, large doses of furosemide or ethacrynic acid can be used, but only if appropriate monitoring is available and cardiac and renal function are adequate. Otherwise, dialysis may be necessary. Intermediate degrees of hypercalcemia between 3.0 and 3.7 mmol/L (12 and 15 mg/dL) should be approached with vigorous hydration and then the most appropriate selection for the patient of the combinations used with severe hypercalcemia.

HYPOCALCEMIA

(See also Chap. 26)

PATHOPHYSIOLOGY OF HYPOCALCEMIA: CLASSIFICATION BASED ON MECHANISM

Chronic hypocalcemia is less common than hypercalcemia; causes include chronic renal failure, hereditary and acquired hypoparathyroidism, vitamin D deficiency, PHP, and hypomagnesemia.

Acute rather than chronic hypocalcemia is seen in critically ill patients or as a consequence of certain medications and often does not require specific treatment. Transient hypocalcemia is seen with severe sepsis, burns, acute renal failure, and extensive transfusions with citrated blood. Although as many as half of patients in an intensive care setting are reported to have calcium concentrations <2.1 mmol/L (8.5 mg/dL), most do not have a reduction in ionized calcium. Patients with severe sepsis may have a decrease in ionized calcium (true hypocalcemia), but in other severely ill individuals, hypoalbuminemia is the primary cause of the reduced total calcium concentration. Alkalosis increases calcium binding to proteins, and in this setting direct measurements of ionized calcium should be made.

Medications such as protamine, heparin, and glucagon may cause transient hypocalcemia. These forms of hypocalcemia are usually not associated with tetany and resolve with improvement in the overall medical condition. The hypocalcemia after repeated transfusions of citrated blood usually resolves quickly.

Patients with *acute pancreatitis* have hypocalcemia that persists during the acute inflammation and varies in degree with the severity of the pancreatitis. The cause of hypocalcemia remains unclear. PTH values are reported to be low, normal, or elevated, and both resistance to PTH and impaired PTH secretion have been postulated. Occasionally, a chronic low total calcium and low ionized calcium concentration are detected in an elderly patient without obvious cause and with a paucity of symptoms; the pathogenesis is unclear.

Chronic hypocalcemia, however, is usually symptomatic and requires treatment. Neuromuscular and neurologic manifestations of chronic hypocalcemia include muscle spasms, carpopedal spasm, facial grimacing, and, in extreme cases, laryngeal spasm and convulsions. Respiratory arrest may occur. Increased intracranial pressure occurs in some patients with longstanding hypocalcemia, often in association with papilledema. Mental changes include irritability, depression, and psychosis. The QT interval on the electrocardiogram is prolonged, in contrast to its shortening with hypercalcemia. Arrhythmias occur, and digitalis effectiveness may be reduced. Intestinal cramps and chronic malabsorption may occur. Chvostek's or Trousseau's sign can be used to confirm latent tetany.

The classification of hypocalcemia shown in Table 27-5 is based on an organizationally useful premise that PTH is responsible for minute-to-minute regulation of plasma calcium concentration and, therefore, that the occurrence of hypocalcemia must mean a failure of the homeostatic action of PTH. Failure of the PTH response can occur if there is hereditary or acquired parathyroid gland failure, if PTH is ineffective in target organs, or if the action of the hormone is overwhelmed by the loss of calcium from the ECF at a rate faster than it can be replaced.

PTH ABSENT

Whether hereditary or acquired, hypoparathyroidism has a number of common components. Symptoms of untreated hypocalcemia are shared by both types of hypoparathyroidism, although the onset of hereditary hypoparathyroidism is more gradual and is often associated with other developmental defects. Basal ganglia calcification and extrapyramidal syndromes are more common and earlier in onset in hereditary hypoparathyroidism. In earlier decades, acquired hypoparathyroidism secondary to surgery in the neck was more common than hereditary hypoparathyroidism, but the frequency of surgically induced parathyroid failure has diminished as a result of improved surgical techniques that spare the parathyroid glands and increased use of nonsurgical therapy for hyperthyroidism. PHP, an example of ineffective PTH action rather than a failure of parathyroid gland production, may share several features with hypoparathyroidism, including extraosseous calcification and extrapyramidal manifestations such as choreoathetotic movements and dystonia.

TABLE 27-5

FUNCTIONAL CLASSIFICATION OF HYPOCALCEMIA (EXCLUDING NEONATAL CONDITIONS)

PTH Absent	
Hereditary hypoparathyroidism Acquired hypoparathyroidism	Hypomagnesemia
PTH Ineffective	
Chronic renal failure Active vitamin D lacking ↓ Dietary intake or sunlight Defective metabolism: Anticonvulsant therapy Vitamin D–dependent rickets type I	Active vitamin D ineffective Intestinal malabsorption Vitamin D–dependent rickets type II Pseudohypoparathyroidism
PTH Overwhelmed	
Severe, acute hyperphosphatemia Tumor lysis Acute renal failure Rhabdomyolysis	Osteitis fibrosa after parathyroidectomy

Note: PTH, parathyroid hormone.

Papilledema and raised intracranial pressure may occur in both hereditary and acquired hypoparathyroidism, as do chronic changes in fingernails and hair and lenticular cataracts, the latter usually reversible with treatment of hypocalcemia. Certain skin manifestations, including alopecia and candidiasis, are characteristic of hereditary hypoparathyroidism associated with autoimmune polyglandular failure (Chap. 23).

Hypocalcemia associated with hypomagnesemia is associated with both deficient PTH release and impaired responsiveness to the hormone. Patients with hypocalcemia secondary to hypomagnesemia have absent or low levels of circulating PTH, indicative of diminished hormone release despite maximum physiologic stimulus by hypocalcemia. Plasma PTH levels return to normal with correction of the hypomagnesemia. Thus, hypoparathyroidism with low levels of PTH in blood can be due to hereditary gland failure, acquired gland failure, or acute but reversible gland dysfunction (hypomagnesemia).

Genetic Abnormalities and Hereditary Hypoparathyroidism

Hereditary hypoparathyroidism can occur as an isolated entity without other endocrine or dermatologic manifestations (idiopathic hypoparathyroidism). More typically, it occurs in association with other abnormalities such as defective development of the thymus or failure of other endocrine organs such as the adrenal, thyroid, or ovary (Chap. 23). Idiopathic and hereditary hypoparathyroidism are often manifest within the first decade but may appear later.

Genetic defects associated with hypoparathyroidism are rare but serve to illuminate the complexity of organ development, hormonal biosynthesis and secretion, and tissue-specific patterns of endocrine effector function. Often, the hypoparathyroidism is isolated, signifying a highly specific functional disturbance. When the hypoparathyroidism is associated with other developmental or organ defects, treatment of the hypocalcemia can still be effective.

A rare form of hypoparathyroidism associated with defective development of both the thymus and the parathyroid glands is termed *DiGeorge syndrome*, or the *velocardiofacial syndrome*. Congenital cardiovascular, facial, and other developmental defects are present, and most patients die in early childhood with severe infections, hypocalcemia and seizures, or cardiovascular complications. Some survive into adulthood, and milder, incomplete forms occur. Most cases are sporadic, but an autosomal dominant form involving microdeletions of chromosome 22q11.2 has been described. Smaller deletions in chromosome 22 are seen in incomplete forms of DiGeorge syndrome, appearing in childhood or adolescence, that are manifest primarily by parathyroid gland failure. The chromosome 22 defect is now termed *DSG1*; more recently, a defect in chromosome 10p was also recognized—now called *DSG2*. The phenotypes seem similar. Studies on the chromosome 22 defect have pinpointed a transcription factor, TBX1. Deletions of the orthologous mouse gene show a phenotype similar to the human syndrome.

Another autosomal dominant developmental defect, featuring hypoparathyroidism, deafness, and renal dysplasia (HDR), has been studied at a genetic level. Cytogenic abnormalities in some, but not all, kindreds point to translocation defects on chromosome 10, as in DiGeorge syndrome. However, the lack of immunodeficiency and heart defects distinguishes the two syndromes. Mouse models, as well as deletional analysis in some HDR patients, has pointed to transcription factor GATA3, which is important in embryonic development and is expressed in developing kidney, ear structures, and the parathyroids.

Another pair of linked developmental disorders involving the parathyroids is recognized. *Kenney-Caffey syndrome* features hypoparathyroidism, short stature, osteosclerosis, and thick cortical bones. A defect seen in Middle Eastern patients, including Bedouin kindreds, termed *Sanjad-Sakati syndrome*, also exhibits growth failure and other dysmorphic features. This syndrome, which is clearly autosomal recessive, involves a gene on chromosome 1q42-q43. Both syndromes apparently involve a chaperone protein, called *TBCE*, relevant to tubulin function.

Hypoparathyroidism can occur in association with a complex hereditary autoimmune syndrome involving failure of the adrenals, the ovaries, the immune system, and the parathyroids in association with recurrent mucocutaneous candidiasis, alopecia, vitiligo, and pernicious anemia (Chap. 23). The responsible gene on chromosome 21q22.3 has been identified. The protein product, which resembles a transcription factor, has been termed the *autoimmune regulator*, or AIRE. A stop codon mutation occurs in many Finnish families with the disorder, commonly referred to as *polyglandular autoimmune type 1 deficiency*.

Hypoparathyroidism is seen in two disorders associated with mitochondrial dysfunction and myopathy, one termed *Kearns-Sayre syndrome* (KSS), with ophthalmoplegia and pigmentary retinopathy, and the other termed *MELAS syndrome*, *m*itochondrial *e*ncephalopathy, *l*actic *a*cidosis, and *s*trokelike episodes. Mutations or deletions in mitochondrial genes have been identified.

Several forms of hypoparathyroidism, each rare in frequency, are seen as isolated defects; the genetic mechanisms are varied. The inheritance includes autosomal dominant, autosomal recessive, and X-linked modes. Three separate autosomal defects involving the parathyroid gene have been recognized: one is dominant; the other two are recessive. The dominant form has a point mutation in the signal sequence, a critical region involved in intracellular transport of the hormone precursor. An Arg for Cys mutation interferes with processing of the precursor and seems to block the processing of the product of the normal allele. The other two forms are recessive. One point mutation also blocks cleavage of the PTH precursor but requires both alleles to cause hypoparathyroidism. The third involves a single nucleotide base change that results in an exon splicing defect; the lost exon contains the promoter—hence, the gene is silenced. An X-linked recessive form of hypoparathyroidism has been described in males and the defect has been localized to chromosome Xq26-q27, perhaps involving the *SOX3* gene.

Abnormalities in the calcium-sensing receptor (CaSR) are detected in three distinctive hypocalcemic disorders. All are rare but at least 10 different gain-of-function mutations have been found in one form of hypocalcemia termed *autosomal dominant hypocalcemic hypercalciuria (ADHH)*. The receptor senses the ambient calcium level as excessive and suppresses PTH secretion, leading to hypocalcemia. The hypocalcemia is aggravated by constitutive receptor activity in the renal tubule causing renal calcium wasting. Recognition of the syndrome is important because efforts to treat the hypocalcemia with vitamin D analogues and increased oral calcium exacerbate the already excessive urinary calcium secretion (several grams or more per 24 h), leading to irreversible renal damage from stones and ectopic calcification.

Bartter syndrome is a group of disorders associated with disturbances in electrolyte and acid/base balance, sometimes with nephrocalcinosis and other features. Several types of ion channels or transporters are involved. Curiously, *Bartter syndrome type V* has the electrolyte and pH disturbances seen in the other syndromes but appears to be due to a gain-of-function in the CaSR. The defect may be more severe than in ADHH and explains the additional features seen beyond hypocalcemia and hypercalciuria.

As with autoimmune disorders that block the CaSR (discussed above under hypercalcemic conditions), there are autoantibodies that at least transiently activate the CaSR, leading to suppressed PTH secretion and hypocalcemia. This disorder, which may wax and wane, could be classified as an acquired form of hypoparathyroidism but is listed here with other disorders involving the CaSR.

Acquired Hypoparathyroidism

Acquired chronic hypoparathyroidism is usually the result of inadvertent surgical removal of all the parathyroid glands; in some instances, not all the tissue is removed, but the remainder undergoes vascular supply compromise secondary to fibrotic changes in the neck after surgery. In the past, the most frequent cause of acquired hypoparathyroidism was surgery for hyperthyroidism. Hypoparathyroidism now usually occurs after surgery for hyperparathyroidism when the surgeon, facing the dilemma of removing too little tissue and thus not curing the hyperparathyroidism, removes too much. Parathyroid function may not be totally absent in all patients with postoperative hypoparathyroidism.

Even rarer causes of acquired chronic hypoparathyroidism include radiation-induced damage subsequent to radioiodine therapy of hyperthyroidism and glandular damage in patients with hemochromatosis or hemosiderosis after repeated blood transfusions. Infection may involve one or more of the parathyroids but usually does not cause hypoparathyroidism because all four glands are rarely involved.

Transient hypoparathyroidism is frequent following surgery for hyperparathyroidism. After a variable period of hypoparathyroidism, normal parathyroid function may return due to hyperplasia or recovery of remaining tissue. Occasionally, recovery occurs months after surgery.

℞ Treatment: ACQUIRED AND HEREDITARY HYPOPARATHYROIDISM

Treatment involves replacement with vitamin D or $1,25(OH)_2D_3$ (calcitriol) combined with a high oral calcium intake. In most patients, blood calcium and phosphate levels are satisfactorily regulated, but some patients show resistance and a brittleness, with a tendency to alternate between hypocalcemia and hypercalcemia. For many patients, vitamin D in doses of 40,000–120,000 U/d (1–3 mg/d) combined with ≥1 g elemental calcium is satisfactory. The wide dosage range reflects the variation encountered from patient to patient; precise regulation of each patient is required. Compared to typical daily requirements in euparathyroid patients of 200 U/d (or in older patients as high as 800 U/d), the high dose of vitamin D (as much as 100-fold higher) reflects the reduced conversion of vitamin D to $1,25(OH)_2D$. Many physicians now use 0.5–1.0 μg of calcitriol in management of such patients, especially if they are difficult to control. Because of its storage in fat, when vitamin D is withdrawn, weeks are required for the disappearance of the biologic effects, compared with a few days for calcitriol, which has a rapid turnover.

Oral calcium and vitamin D restore the overall calcium-phosphate balance but do not reverse the lowered urinary calcium reabsorption typical of hypoparathyroidism. Therefore, care must be taken to avoid excessive urinary calcium excretion after vitamin D and calcium replacement therapy; otherwise, kidney stones can develop. Thiazide diuretics lower urine calcium by as much as 100 mg/d in hypoparathyroid patients on vitamin D, provided they are maintained on a low-sodium diet. Use of thiazides seems to be of benefit in mitigating hypercalciuria and easing the daily management of these patients.

Hypomagnesemia

Severe hypomagnesemia (<0.4 mmol/L; <0.8 meq/L) is associated with hypocalcemia (Chap. 25). Restoration of the total-body magnesium deficit leads to rapid reversal of hypocalcemia. There are at least two causes of the hypocalcemia—impaired PTH secretion and reduced responsiveness to PTH.

The effects of magnesium on PTH secretion are similar to those of calcium; hypermagnesemia suppresses and hypomagnesemia stimulates PTH secretion. The effects of magnesium on PTH secretion are normally of little significance, however, because the calcium effects dominate. Greater change in magnesium than in calcium is needed to influence hormone secretion. Nonetheless, hypomagnesemia might be expected to increase hormone secretion. It is therefore surprising to find that severe hypomagnesemia is associated with blunted secretion of PTH. The explanation for the paradox is that severe, chronic hypomagnesemia leads to intracellular magnesium deficiency, which interferes with secretion and peripheral responses to PTH. The mechanism of the cellular abnormalities caused by hypomagnesemia is unknown, although effects on adenylate cyclase (for which magnesium is a cofactor) have been proposed.

PTH levels are undetectable or inappropriately low in severe hypomagnesemia despite the stimulus of severe hypocalcemia, and acute repletion of magnesium leads to a rapid increase in PTH level. Serum phosphate levels are often not elevated, in contrast to the situation with acquired or idiopathic hypoparathyroidism, probably because phosphate deficiency is a frequent accompaniment of hypomagnesemia.

Diminished peripheral responsiveness to PTH also occurs in some patients, as documented by subnormal response in urinary phosphorus and urinary cyclic AMP excretion after administration of exogenous PTH to patients who are hypocalcemic and hypomagnesemic. Both blunted PTH secretion and lack of renal response to administered PTH can occur in the same patient. When acute magnesium repletion is undertaken, the restoration of PTH levels to normal or supranormal may precede restoration of normal serum calcium by several days.

℞ Treatment: HYPOMAGNESEMIA

Repletion of magnesium cures the condition. Repletion should be parenteral. Attention must be given to restoring the intracellular deficit, which may be considerable. After IV magnesium administration, serum magnesium may return transiently to the normal range, but unless replacement therapy is adequate, serum magnesium will again fall. If the cause of the hypomagnesemia is renal magnesium wasting, magnesium may have to be given chronically to prevent recurrence.

PTH INEFFECTIVE

PTH is ineffective when the hormone receptor–guanyl nucleotide–binding protein complex is defective (PHP, discussed later in the chapter), when PTH action to promote calcium absorption from the diet is impaired because of vitamin D deficiency or because vitamin D is ineffective (receptor or synthesis defects), or in chronic renal failure in which the calcium-elevating action of PTH is impaired.

Typically, hypophosphatemia is more severe than hypocalcemia in vitamin D deficiency states because of the increased secretion of PTH, which, although only partly effective in elevating blood calcium, is capable of promoting phosphaturia.

PHP, on the other hand, has a pathophysiology different from the other disorders of ineffective PTH action. PHP resembles hypoparathyroidism (in which PTH synthesis is deficient) and is manifested by hypocalcemia and hyperphosphatemia, yet elevated PTH levels. The cause of the disorder is defective hormone activation of guanyl nucleotide–binding proteins, resulting in failure of PTH to increase intracellular cyclic AMP.

Chronic Renal Failure

Improved medical management of chronic renal failure now allows many patients to survive for years and hence time enough to develop features of renal osteodystrophy, which must be controlled to avoid its morbidity. Phosphate retention and impaired production of $1,25(OH)_2D$ are the principal factors that cause calcium deficiency, secondary hyperparathyroidism, and bone disease. Low levels of $1,25(OH)_2D$ due to hyperphosphatemia and destruction of renal tissue are critical in the development of hypocalcemia. The uremic state also causes impairment of intestinal absorption by mechanisms other than defects in vitamin D metabolism. Nonetheless, treatment with supraphysiologic amounts of vitamin D or calcitriol corrects the impaired calcium absorption.

Hyperphosphatemia in renal failure lowers blood calcium levels by several mechanisms, including extraosseous deposition of calcium and phosphate, impairment of the bone-resorbing action of PTH, and reduction in $1,25(OH)_2D$ production by remaining renal tissue.

℞ Treatment: CHRONIC RENAL FAILURE

Therapy of chronic renal failure involves appropriate management of patients prior to dialysis and adjustment of regimens once dialysis is initiated. Attention should be paid to restriction of phosphate in the diet; avoidance of aluminum-containing phosphate-binding antacids to prevent the problem of aluminum intoxication; provision of an adequate calcium intake by mouth, usually 1–2 g/d; and supplementation with 0.25–1.0 μg/d calcitriol. Each patient must be monitored closely. The aim of therapy is to restore normal calcium balance to prevent osteomalacia and secondary hyperparathyroidism and, in light of evidence of genetic changes and monoclonal outgrowths of parathyroid glands in renal failure patients, to prevent secondary from becoming autonomous hyperparathyroidism. Reduction of hyperphosphatemia and restoration of normal intestinal calcium absorption by calcitriol can improve blood calcium levels and reduce the manifestations of secondary hyperparathyroidism. Since adynamic bone disease can occur in association with low PTH levels, it is important to avoid excessive suppression of the parathyroid glands while recognizing the beneficial effects of controlling the secondary hyperparathyroidism. These patients should probably be closely monitored with PTH assays that detect only the full-length PTH(1–84) to ensure that biologically active PTH and not inactive, inhibitory PTH fragments are measured.

Vitamin D Deficiency Due to Inadequate Diet and/or Sunlight

Vitamin D deficiency due to inadequate intake of dairy products enriched with vitamin D, lack of vitamin supplementation, and reduced sunlight exposure in the elderly, particularly during winter in northern latitudes, is more common in the United States than previously recognized. Biopsies of bone in elderly patients with hip fracture (documenting osteomalacia) and abnormal levels of vitamin D metabolites, PTH, calcium, and phosphate indicate that vitamin D deficiency may occur in as many as 25% of elderly patients, particularly in northern latitudes in the United States. Concentrations of 25(OH)D are low or low-normal in these patients. Quantitative histomorphometry of bone biopsy specimens reveals widened osteoid seams consistent with osteomalacia (Chap. 25). PTH hypersecretion compensates for the tendency for the blood calcium to fall but also induces renal phosphate wasting and results in osteomalacia.

Treatment involves adequate replacement with vitamin D and calcium until the deficiencies are corrected. Severe hypocalcemia rarely occurs in moderately severe vitamin D deficiency of the elderly, but vitamin D deficiency must be considered in the differential diagnosis of mild hypocalcemia.

Mild hypocalcemia, secondary hyperparathyroidism, severe hypophosphatemia, and a variety of nutritional deficiencies occur with gastrointestinal diseases. Hepatocellular dysfunction can lead to reduction in 25(OH)D levels, as in portal or biliary cirrhosis of the liver, and malabsorption of vitamin D and its metabolites, including $1,25(OH)_2D$, may occur in a variety of bowel diseases, hereditary or acquired. Hypocalcemia itself can lead to steatorrhea, due to deficient production of pancreatic enzymes and bile salts. Depending on the disorder, vitamin D or its metabolites can be given parenterally, guaranteeing adequate blood levels of active metabolites.

Defective Vitamin D Metabolism

Anticonvulsant Therapy

Anticonvulsant therapy with any of several agents induces acquired vitamin D deficiency by increasing the conversion of vitamin D to inactive compounds and/or causing resistance to its action. The more marginal the vitamin D intake in the diet, the more likely that anticonvulsant therapy will lead to abnormal mineral and bone metabolism.

Vitamin D–Dependent Rickets Type I

Rickets can be due to *resistance to the action* of vitamin D as well as to vitamin D deficiency. Vitamin D–dependent rickets type I, previously termed *pseudo-vitamin D–resistant rickets*, differs from true vitamin D–resistant rickets (vitamin D–dependent rickets type II, see below) in that it is less severe and the biochemical and radiographic abnormalities can be reversed with appropriate doses of the vitamin or the active metabolite $1,25(OH)_2D_3$. Physiologic amounts of calcitriol cure the disease (Chap. 25). This finding fits with the pathophysiology of the disorder, which is autosomal recessive, and is now known to be caused by mutations in the gene encoding 25(OH)D-1α-hydroxylase. Both alleles are inactivated in all patients, and compound heterozygotes, harboring distinct mutations, are common.

Clinical features include hypocalcemia, often with tetany or convulsions; hypophosphatemia; secondary hyperparathyroidism; and osteomalacia, often associated with skeletal deformities and increased alkaline phosphatase. Treatment involves physiologic replacement doses of $1,25(OH)_2D_3$ (Chap. 25).

Vitamin D–Dependent Rickets Type II

Vitamin D–dependent rickets type II results from end-organ resistance to the active metabolite $1,25(OH)_2D_3$. The clinical features resemble those of the type I disorder and include hypocalcemia, hypophosphatemia, secondary hyperparathyroidism, and rickets but also partial or total alopecia. Plasma levels of $1,25(OH)_2D$ are at least three times normal, in keeping with the refractoriness of the end organs. All of the genetically characterized phenotypes have mutations in the gene for the vitamin D receptor. Treatment is difficult, given the receptor defect (Chap. 25).

Pseudohypoparathyroidism

PHP is a hereditary disorder characterized by symptoms and signs of hypoparathyroidism, typically in association with distinctive skeletal and developmental defects. The hypoparathyroidism is due to a deficient end-organ response to PTH. Hyperplasia of the parathyroids, a response to hormone resistance, causes elevation of PTH levels. Studies, both clinical and basic, have clarified some aspects of this syndrome, including the variable clinical spectrum, the pathophysiology, the genetic defects, and the inheritance.

A working classification of the various forms of PHP is given in **Table 27-6**. The classification scheme is based on the signs of ineffective PTH action (low calcium and high phosphate), urinary cyclic AMP response to exogenous PTH, the presence or absence of *Albright's hereditary osteodystrophy* (AHO), and assays of the concentration of the $G_s\alpha$ subunit of the adenylate cyclase enzyme. Using these criteria, there are four types: PHP type I, subdivided into a and b categories; PHP-II; and pseudopseudohypoparathyroidism (PPHP).

PHP-Ia and PHP-Ib

Individuals with PHP-I, the most common of the disorders, show a deficient urinary cyclic AMP response to administration of exogenous PTH. Patients with PHP-I are divided into type a, with AHO and reduced amounts of $G_s\alpha$ in in vitro assays with erythrocytes, and type b, lacking AHO and with normal amounts of $G_s\alpha$ in erythrocytes. There is a third type (PHP-Ic, reported in a few patients) that differs from PHP-Ia only in having normal erythrocyte levels of $G_s\alpha$ despite having AHO, hypocalcemia, and decreased urinary cyclic AMP responses to PTH (presumably with a post-$G_s\alpha$ defect in adenyl cyclase stimulation).

Most patients have PHP-Ia and reveal characteristic features of AHO, consisting of short stature, round face, skeletal anomalies (brachydactyly), and heterotopic calcification. Patients have low calcium and high phosphate levels, as with true hypoparathyroidism. PTH levels, however, are elevated, reflecting resistance to hormone action.

Amorphous deposits of calcium and phosphate are found in the basal ganglia in about half of patients. The defects in metacarpal and metatarsal bones are sometimes accompanied by short phalanges as well, possibly reflecting premature closing of the epiphyses. The typical findings

TABLE 27-6

CLASSIFICATION OF PSEUDOHYPOPARATHYROIDISM (PHP) AND PSEUDOPSEUDOHYPOPARATHYROIDISM (PPHP)

TYPE	HYPOCALCEMIA, HYPERPHOSPHATEMIA	RESPONSE OF URINARY cAMP TO PTH	SERUM PTH	$G_s\alpha$ SUBUNIT DEFICIENCY	AHO	RESISTANCE TO HORMONES IN ADDITION TO PTH
PHP-Ia	Yes	↓	↑	Yes	Yes	Yes
PHP-Ib	Yes	↓	↑	No	No	No
PHP-II	Yes	Normal	↑	No	No	No
PPHP	No	Normal	Normal	Yes	Yes	±

Note: ↓, decreased; ↑, increased; AHO, Albright's hereditary osteodystrophy; PTH, parathyroid hormone.

are short fourth and fifth metacarpals and metatarsals. The defects are usually bilateral. Exostoses and radius curvus are frequent. Impairments in olfaction and taste and unusual dermatoglyphic abnormalities have been reported.

Inheritance and Genetic Patterns

Multiple defects have now been identified in the *GNAS-1* gene in PHP-Ia and PPHP patients. This gene, which is located on chromosome 20q13, encodes the stimulatory G protein subunit $G_s\alpha$, among other products (see below). Mutations include abnormalities in splice junctions associated with deficient mRNA production and point mutations that result in a protein with defective function; these mutations can be detected, as well as a 50% reduction in $G_s\alpha$ levels in erythrocytes, reflecting loss of the protein from the mutated allele.

Detailed analyses of disease transmission in affected kindreds have clarified many features of PHP-Ia, PPHP, and PHP-Ib (Fig. 27-7). The former two entities, traced through multiple kindreds, have an inheritance pattern consistent with gene imprinting—only females, not males, can transmit the full disease with hypocalcemia—and PHP and PPHP do not coexist in the same generation. The phenomenon of gene imprinting, independent of any mutation, involves selective inactivation of either the maternal or the paternal allele. In the case of the $G_s\alpha$ transcript, it is paternally imprinted (silenced) in the renal cortex (where the disease manifestation is expressed), so that the disease PHP-Ia can never be inherited from the father carrying the defective allele but only from a mother whose allelic product is critical in the kidney. In the renal cortex, it is postulated that only the maternal allele is normally active (independent of any mutation), such that lack of activity from a defective paternal allele is not of consequence. This explains the occurrence in PHP-Ia of hypocalcemia, hyperphosphatemia, and other stigmata such as variable resistance to other hormones (since similar tissue-specific imprinting occurs in other endocrine organs). Strong evidence favoring this overall hypothesis comes from gene knockout studies in the mouse (ablating exon 2 of the gene responsible for $G_s\alpha$ synthesis). Mice inheriting the mutant allele from the female had undetectable $G_s\alpha$ protein in renal cortex and were hypocalcemic and resistant to renal actions of PTH. Offspring inheriting the mutant allele from the male showed no evidence of PTH resistance or hypercalcemia.

Imprinting is tissue selective. The defective *GNAS* allele is not imprinted or silenced in many tissues. It seems likely, therefore, that the AHO phenotype recognized in

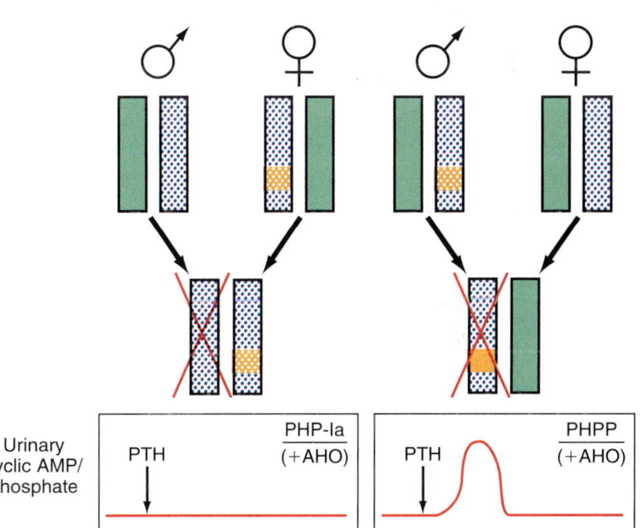

FIGURE 27-7

Paternal imprinting of renal parathyroid hormone (PTH) resistance (*GNAS-1* gene for $G_s\alpha$ subunit) in pseudohypoparathyroidism (PHPIa). An impaired excretion of urinary cyclic AMP and phosphate is observed in patients with PHP. In the renal cortex, there is selective silencing of the paternal $G_s\alpha$ gene mRNA. The disease becomes manifest only in patients who inherit the defective gene from an obligate female carrier (*left*). If the genetic defect is inherited from an obligate male gene carrier, there is no biochemical abnormality; administration of PTH causes an appropriate increase in the urinary cyclic AMP and phosphate concentration [pseudo-PHP (PPHP); *right*]. Both patterns of inheritance lead to Albright's hereditary osteodystrophy (AHO), perhaps because of haplotype insufficiency—i.e., both copies of $G_s\alpha$ must be active in the fetus for normal bone development.

PPHP as well as PHP-Ia reflects haplotype insufficiency during embryonic development.

The complex mechanisms that control the *GNAS* gene contribute to challenges involved in unraveling the pathogenesis of these disorders, especially that of PHP-1b. Much intensive work with kindreds having PHP-1b, as well as studies of the complex regulation of the *GNAS* gene locus, have now offered an explanation for the features of PHP-1b, particularly the absence of $G_s\alpha$ deficiency in erythrocytes used to determine $G_s\alpha$ subunit deficiency (Table 27-6), in the setting of defective urinary cyclic response to PTH, the absence of the AHO phenotype, and maternal inheritance of the disease.

The defect in PHP-Ib is not a mutation in the $G_s\alpha$ portion of the gene but rather upstream deletions on the maternal allele that interfere with the normal methylation patterns, such that in the renal cortex neither the paternal (normally imprinted) nor the usual maternally expressed allele is active in transcription of $G_s\alpha$. There is no $G_s\alpha$ in the renal cortex but normal expression in other tissues, hence the normal erythrocyte levels of $G_s\alpha$ and the normal development of bone (no AHO phenotype).

PHP-Ib, lacking the AHO phenotype, shares with PHP-Ia the resistance to PTH action; a blunted urinary cyclic AMP response to administered PTH, a standard test for hormone resistance (Table 27-6); and an inheritance pattern of disease transmission only from the mother. PHP-Ib patients, however, show normal levels of $G_s\alpha$ in erythrocytes. Bone responsiveness may be excessive rather than blunted in PHP-Ib compared to PHP-Ia patients, based on case reports that have emphasized an osteitis fibrosa–like pattern in some PHP patients who lack the AHO phenotype.

PHP-II refers to patients with hypocalcemia and hyperphosphatemia who have a normal urinary cyclic AMP response to PTH. These patients are assumed to have a defect in the response to PTH at a locus distal to cyclic AMP production, although at least some patients may instead have occult vitamin D deficiency.

The diagnosis of these hormone-resistant states can usually be made without difficulty when there is a positive family history for developmental defects and/or the presence of developmental anomalies, including brachydactyly, in association with the signs and symptoms of hypoparathyroidism. In both categories—PHP-Ia and -Ib—serum PTH levels are elevated, particularly when patients are hypocalcemic. However, patients with PHP-Ib or PHP-II do not have phenotypic abnormalities, only hypocalcemia with high PTH levels, confirming hormone resistance. In PHP-Ib, the response of urinary cyclic AMP to the administration of exogenous PTH is blunted. The diagnosis of PHP-II is more complex, in that cyclic AMP responses in urine are, by definition, normal. Since vitamin D deficiency itself can dissociate phosphaturic and urinary cyclic AMP responses to exogenous PTH, vitamin D deficiency must be excluded before the diagnosis of PHP-II can be entertained.

℞ Treatment: PSEUDOHYPOPARATHYROIDISM

Treatment of PHP is similar to that of hypoparathyroidism, except that the doses of vitamin D and calcium are usually lower than those required in true hypoparathyroidism, presumably because the defect in PHP is only partial because of imprinting in specific tissues and tissue sites (renal cortex vs renal medulla)—hence, urinary calcium clearance, a distal tubular function, is not affected. Variability in response makes it necessary to establish the optimal regimen for each patient, based on maintaining the appropriate blood calcium level and urinary calcium excretion.

PTH OVERWHELMED

Occasionally, loss of calcium from the ECF is so severe that PTH cannot compensate. Such situations include acute pancreatitis and severe, acute hyperphosphatemia, often in association with renal failure, conditions in which there is rapid efflux of calcium from the ECF. Severe hypocalcemia can occur quickly; PTH rises in response to hypocalcemia but does not return blood calcium to normal.

Severe, Acute Hyperphosphatemia

Severe hyperphosphatemia is associated with extensive tissue damage or cell destruction (Chap. 25). The combination of increased release of phosphate from muscle and impaired ability to excrete phosphorus because of renal failure causes moderate to severe hyperphosphatemia, the latter causing calcium loss from the blood and mild to moderate hypocalcemia. Hypocalcemia is usually reversed with tissue repair and restoration of renal function as phosphorus and creatinine values return to normal. There may even be a mild hypercalcemic period in the oliguric phase of renal function recovery. This sequence, severe hypocalcemia followed by mild hypercalcemia, reflects widespread deposition of calcium in muscle and subsequent redistribution of some of the calcium to the ECF after phosphate levels return to normal.

Other causes of hyperphosphatemia include hypothermia, massive hepatic failure, and hematologic malignancies, either because of high cell turnover of malignancy or because of cell destruction by chemotherapy.

℞ Treatment: SEVERE, ACUTE HYPERPHOSPHATEMIA

Treatment is directed toward lowering of blood phosphate by the administration of phosphate-binding antacids or dialysis, often needed for the management of renal failure. Although calcium replacement may be necessary if hypocalcemia is severe and symptomatic, calcium administration during the hyperphosphatemic period tends to increase extraosseous calcium deposition and aggravate tissue damage. The levels of 1,25$(OH)_2$D may be low during the hyperphosphatemic phase and return to normal during the oliguric phase of recovery.

Osteitis Fibrosis after Parathyroidectomy

Severe hypocalcemia after parathyroid surgery is rare now that osteitis fibrosa cystica is an infrequent manifestation of hyperparathyroidism. When osteitis fibrosa cystica is severe, however, bone mineral deficits can be large. After parathyroidectomy, hypocalcemia can persist for days if calcium replacement is inadequate. Treatment may require parenteral administration of calcium; addition of calcitriol and oral calcium supplementation is sometimes needed for weeks to a month or two until bone defects are filled (which, of course, is of therapeutic benefit in the skeleton), making it possible to discontinue parenteral calcium and/or reduce the amount.

DIFFERENTIAL DIAGNOSIS OF HYPOCALCEMIA

Care must be taken to ensure that true hypocalcemia is present; in addition, acute transient hypocalcemia can be a manifestation of a variety of severe, acute illnesses, as discussed above. *Chronic hypocalcemia*, however, can usually be ascribed to a few disorders associated with absent or ineffective PTH. Important clinical criteria include the duration of the illness, signs or symptoms of associated disorders, and the presence of features that suggest a hereditary abnormality. A nutritional history can be helpful in recognizing a low intake of vitamin D and calcium in the elderly, and a history of excessive alcohol intake may suggest magnesium deficiency.

Hypoparathyroidism and PHP are typically lifelong illnesses, usually (but not always) appearing by adolescence; hence, a recent onset of hypocalcemia in an adult is more likely due to nutritional deficiencies, renal failure, or intestinal disorders that result in deficient or ineffective vitamin D. Neck surgery, even long past, however, can be associated with a delayed onset of postoperative hypoparathyroidism. A history of seizure disorder raises the issue of anticonvulsive medication. Developmental defects may point to the diagnosis of PHP. Rickets and a variety of neuromuscular syndromes and deformities may indicate ineffective vitamin D action, either due to defects in vitamin D metabolism or to vitamin D deficiency.

A pattern of *low calcium with high phosphorus* in the absence of renal failure or massive tissue destruction almost invariably means hypoparathyroidism or PHP. A *low calcium and low phosphorus* points to absent or ineffective vitamin D, thereby impairing the action of PTH on calcium metabolism (but not phosphate clearance). The relative ineffectiveness of PTH in calcium homeostasis in vitamin D deficiency, anticonvulsant therapy, gastrointestinal disorders, and hereditary defects in vitamin D metabolism leads to secondary hyperparathyroidism as a compensation. The excess PTH on renal tubule phosphate transport accounts for renal phosphate wasting and hypophosphatemia.

Exceptions to these patterns may occur. Most forms of hypomagnesemia are due to longstanding nutritional deficiency as seen in chronic alcoholics. Despite the fact that the hypocalcemia is principally due to an acute absence of PTH, phosphate levels are usually low, rather than elevated as in hypoparathyroidism. Chronic renal failure is often associated with hypocalcemia and hyperphosphatemia, despite secondary hyperparathyroidism.

Diagnosis is usually established by application of the PTH immunoassay, tests for vitamin D metabolites, and measurements of the urinary cyclic AMP response to exogenous PTH. In hereditary and acquired hypoparathyroidism and in severe hypomagnesemia, PTH is either undetectable or in the normal range. This finding in a hypocalcemic patient is supportive of hypoparathyroidism, as distinct from ineffective PTH action, in which even mild hypocalcemia is associated with elevated PTH levels. Hence, a failure to detect elevated PTH levels establishes the diagnosis of hypoparathyroidism; elevated levels suggest the presence of secondary hyperparathyroidism, as found in many of the situations in which the hormone is ineffective due to associated abnormalities in vitamin D action. Assays for 25(OH)D can be helpful. Low or low-normal 25(OH)D indicates vitamin D deficiency due to lack of sunlight, inadequate vitamin D intake, or intestinal malabsorption. Recognition that mild hypocalcemia, rickets, and hypophosphatemia are due to anticonvulsant therapy is made by history.

℞ Treatment: HYPOCALCEMIC STATES

The management of hypoparathyroidism, PHP, chronic renal failure, and hereditary defects in vitamin D metabolism involves the use of vitamin D or vitamin D metabolites and calcium supplementation. Vitamin D itself is the least expensive form of vitamin D replacement and is frequently used in the management of uncomplicated hypoparathyroidism and some disorders associated with ineffective vitamin D action. When vitamin D is used prophylactically, as in the elderly or in those with chronic anticonvulsant therapy, there is a wider margin of safety than with the more potent metabolites. However, most of the conditions in which vitamin D is administered chronically for hypocalcemia require amounts 50–100 times the daily replacement dose because the formation of 1,25$(OH)_2$D is deficient. In such situations, vitamin D is no safer than the active metabolite because intoxication can occur with high-dose therapy (because of storage in fat). Calcitriol is more rapid in onset of action and also has a short biologic half-life.

Vitamin D [at least 2000 U/d (5 μg/d) (higher levels required in older persons)] or calcitriol (0.25–1.0 μg/d) is required to prevent rickets in normal individuals. In contrast, 40,000–120,000 U (1–3 mg) of vitamin D_2 or D_3 is typically required in hypoparathyroidism. The dose of calcitriol is unchanged in hypoparathyroidism, since the defect is in hydroxylation by the 25(OH)D-1α-hydroxylase. Calcitriol is also used in disorders of 25(OH)D-1α-hydroxylase; vitamin D receptor defects are much more difficult to treat.

Patients with hypoparathyroidism should be given 2–3 g elemental calcium PO each day. The two agents, vitamin D or calcitriol and oral calcium, can be varied independently. If hypocalcemia alternates with episodes of hypercalcemia in more brittle patients with hypoparathyroidism, administration of calcitriol and use of thiazides, as discussed above, may make management easier.

FURTHER READINGS

BASTEPE M, JÜPPNER H: *GNAS* locus and pseudohypoparathyroidism. Horm Res 63:65, 2005

BILEZIKIAN JP et al: Summary statement from a workshop on asymptomatic primary hyperparathyroidism: A perspective for the 21st century. J Bone Min Res 17(Suppl 2):N2, 2002

———, Potts JT Jr: Asymptomatic primary hyperparathyroidism: New issues and new questions—bridging the past with the future. J Bone Min Res 17(Suppl 2):N57, 2002

DEGROOT LJ, JAMESON JL (eds): *Endocrinology,* 5th ed. Philadelphia, Saunders, 2005

EASTELL R et al: Diagnosis of asymptomatic primary hyperparathyroidism: Proceedings of the third international workshop. J Clin Endocrinol Metab 94:340, 2009

FRASER WD: Hyperparathyroidism. Lancet 374:145, 2009

SHOBACK D: Clinical practice. Hypoparathyroidism. N Engl J Med 359:391, 2008

SILVERBERG SJ et al: Presentation of asymptomatic primary hyperparathyroidism: Proceedings of the third international workshop. J Clin Endocrinol Metab 94:351, 2009

STEWART AF: Clinical practice: Hypercalcemia associated with cancer. N Engl J Med 352:373, 2005

THEMAN TA et al: PTH(1-34) replacement therapy in a child with hypoparathyroidism caused by a sporadic calcium receptor mutation. J Bone Miner Res 24:964, 2009

UDELSMAN R et al: Surgery for asymptomatic primary hyperparathyroidism: Proceedings of the third international workshop. J Clin Endocrinol Metab 94:366, 2009

WEINSTEIN LS et al: Minireview: GNAS: Normal and abnormal functions. Endocrinology 145:5459, 2004

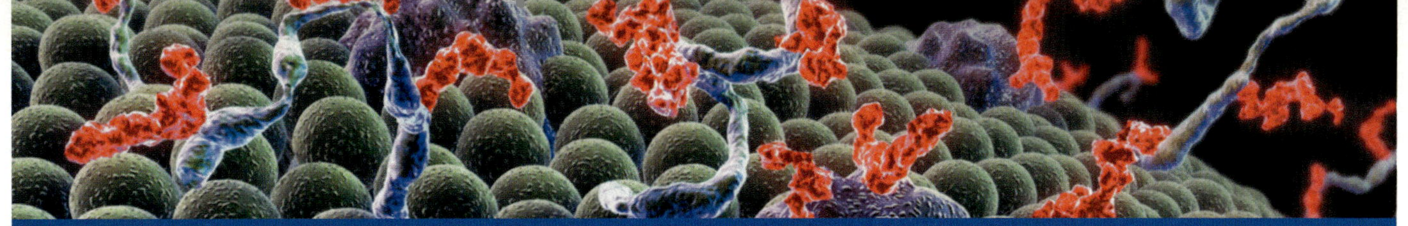

CHAPTER 28

OSTEOPOROSIS

Robert Lindsay ■ Felicia Cosman

Osteoporosis, a condition characterized by decreased bone strength, is prevalent among postmenopausal women but also occurs in men and women with underlying conditions or major risk factors associated with bone demineralization. Its chief clinical manifestations are vertebral and hip fractures, although fractures can occur at any skeletal site. Osteoporosis affects >10 million individuals in the United States, but only a small proportion are diagnosed and treated.

DEFINITION

Osteoporosis is defined as a reduction in the strength of bone leading to an increased risk of fractures. Loss of bone tissue is associated with deterioration in skeletal microarchitecture. The World Health Organization (WHO) operationally defines osteoporosis as a bone density that falls 2.5 standard deviations (SD) below the mean for young healthy adults of the same gender—also referred to as a *T-score* of –2.5. Postmenopausal women who fall at the lower end of the young normal range (a T-score of >1 SD below the mean) are defined as having low bone density and are also at increased risk of osteoporosis. More than 50% of the fractures, including hip fractures, among postmenopausal women occur in this group.

EPIDEMIOLOGY

In the United States, as many as 8 million women and 2 million men have osteoporosis (T-score < –2.5), and an additional 18 million individuals have bone mass levels that put them at increased risk of developing osteoporosis (e.g., bone mass T-score < –1.0). Osteoporosis occurs more frequently with increasing age as bone tissue is progressively lost. In women, the loss of ovarian function at menopause (typically about age 50) precipitates rapid bone loss such that most women meet the diagnostic criterion for osteoporosis by age 70–80.

The epidemiology of fractures follows the trend for bone density loss. Fractures of the distal radius increase in frequency before age 50 and plateau by age 60, with only a modest age-related increase thereafter. In contrast, incidence rates for hip fractures double every 5 years after age 70 (**Fig. 28-1**). This distinct epidemiology may be related to the way people fall as they age, with fewer falls on an outstretched hand and more falls directly on the hip. At least 1.5 million fractures occur each year in the United States as a consequence of osteoporosis. As the population continues to age, the total number of fractures will continue to escalate.

About 300,000 hip fractures occur each year in the United States, most of which require hospital admission

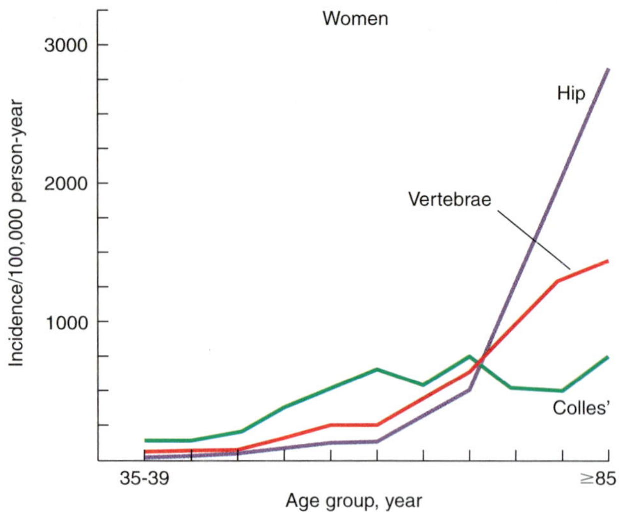

FIGURE 28-1

Epidemiology of vertebral, hip, and Colles' fractures with age. [*Adapted from C Cooper, LJ Melton III: Trends Endocrinol Metab 3:224, 1992; with permission.*]

and surgical intervention. The probability that a 50-year-old white individual will have a hip fracture during his or her lifetime is 14% for women and 5% for men; the risk for African Americans is lower (about half these rates). Hip fractures are associated with a high incidence of deep-vein thrombosis and pulmonary embolism (20–50%) and a mortality rate between 5 and 20% during the year after surgery.

There are about 700,000 vertebral crush fractures per year in the United States. Only a fraction of these are recognized clinically, since many are relatively asymptomatic and are identified incidentally during radiography for other purposes (Fig. 28-2). Vertebral fractures rarely require hospitalization but are associated with long-term morbidity and a slight increase in mortality, primarily related to pulmonary disease. Multiple vertebral fractures lead to height loss (often of several inches), kyphosis, and secondary pain and discomfort related to altered biomechanics of the back. Thoracic fractures can be associated with restrictive lung disease, whereas lumbar fractures are associated with abdominal symptoms including distention, early satiety, and constipation.

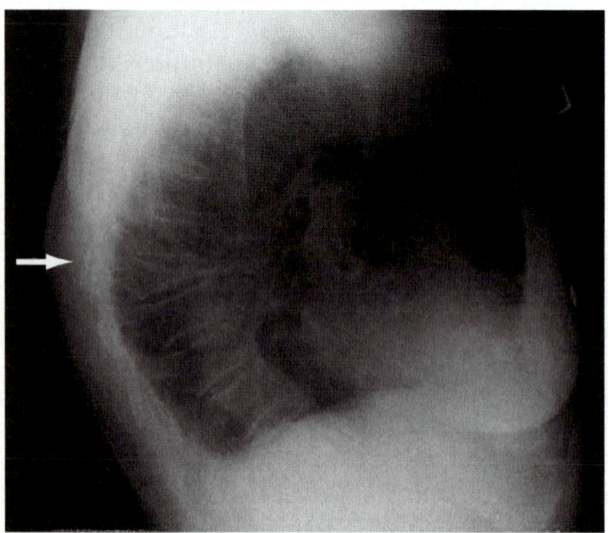

FIGURE 28-2

Lateral spine x-ray showing severe osteopenia and a severe wedge-type deformity (severe anterior compression).

Approximately 250,000 wrist fractures occur in the United States each year. Fractures of other bones (estimated to be ~300,000 per year) also occur with osteoporosis, which is not surprising given that bone loss is a systemic phenomenon. Fractures of the pelvis and proximal humerus are clearly associated with osteoporosis. Although some fractures are the result of major trauma, the threshold for fracture is reduced for an osteoporotic bone (Fig. 28-3). In addition to bone density, there are a number of risk factors for fracture; the common ones are summarized in Table 28-1. Age, prior fractures, a family history of osteoporosis-related fractures, low body weight, cigarette consumption, and excessive alcohol use are each independent predictors of fracture. Chronic diseases with inflammatory components that increase skeletal remodeling, such as rheumatoid arthritis, increase the risk of osteoporosis, as do diseases associated with malabsorption. Chronic diseases that increase the risk of falling or frailty, including dementia, Parkinson's disease, and multiple sclerosis, also increase fracture risk.

In the United States and Europe, osteoporosis-related fractures are more common among women than men, presumably due to a lower peak bone mass as well as postmenopausal bone loss in women. However, this gender difference in bone density and age-related increase in hip fractures is not as apparent in some other cultures, possibly due to genetics, physical activity level, or diet.

Fractures are themselves risk factors for future fractures (Table 28-1). Vertebral fractures increase the risk of other vertebral fractures as well as fractures of the peripheral skeleton such as hip and wrist. Wrist fractures also increase the risk of vertebral and hip fractures. Consequently,

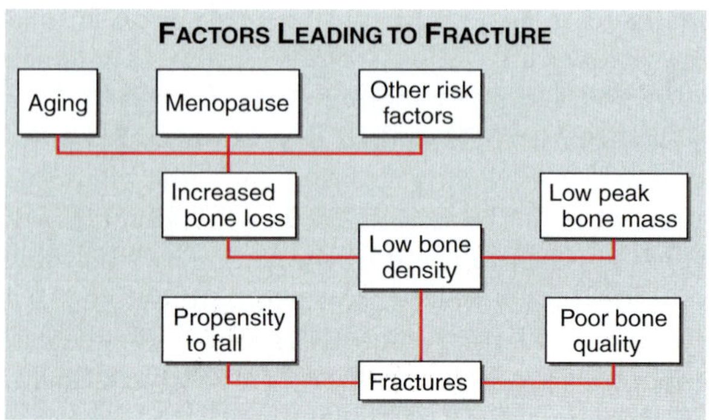

FIGURE 28-3

Factors leading to osteoporotic fractures.

TABLE 28-1

RISK FACTORS FOR OSTEOPOROSIS FRACTURE

Nonmodifiable	Estrogen deficiency
Personal history of fracture as an adult	Early menopause (<45 years) or bilateral ovariectomy
History of fracture in first-degree relative	Prolonged premenstrual amenorrhea (>1 year)
Female sex	Low calcium intake
Advanced age	Alcoholism
Caucasian race	Impaired eyesight despite adequate correction
Dementia	Recurrent falls
Potentially modifiable	Inadequate physical activity
Current cigarette smoking	Poor health/frailty
Low body weight [<58 kg (127 lb)]	

among individuals over the age of 50, any fracture should be considered as potentially related to osteoporosis, irrespective of the circumstances of fracture. Osteoporotic bone is more likely to fracture than normal bone at any level of trauma, and a fracture in a person over 50 should trigger evaluation for osteoporosis.

PATHOPHYSIOLOGY

BONE REMODELING

Osteoporosis results from bone loss due to age-related changes in bone remodeling as well as extrinsic and intrinsic factors that exaggerate this process. These changes may be superimposed on a low peak bone mass. Consequently, understanding the bone remodeling process is fundamental to understanding the pathophysiology of osteoporosis (Chap. 25). During growth, the skeleton increases in size by linear growth and by apposition of new bone tissue on the outer surfaces of the cortex (Fig. 28-4). This latter process is called *modeling*, a process that also allows the long bones to adapt in shape to the stresses placed upon them. Increased sex hormone production at puberty is required for skeletal maturation, which reaches maximum mass and density in early adulthood. It is around puberty that the sexual dimorphism in skeletal size becomes obvious, although true bone density remains similar between sexes. Nutrition and lifestyle also play an important role in growth, though genetic factors primarily determine peak skeletal mass and density. Numerous genes control skeletal growth, peak bone mass, and body size, as well as skeletal structure and density. Heritability estimates of 50–80% for bone density and size have been derived based on twin studies. Though peak bone mass is often lower among individuals with a family history of osteoporosis, association studies of candidate genes [vitamin D receptor; type I collagen, the estrogen receptor (ER), interleukin (IL) 6; and insulin-like growth factor (IGF) I] and bone mass, bone turnover, and fracture prevalence have been

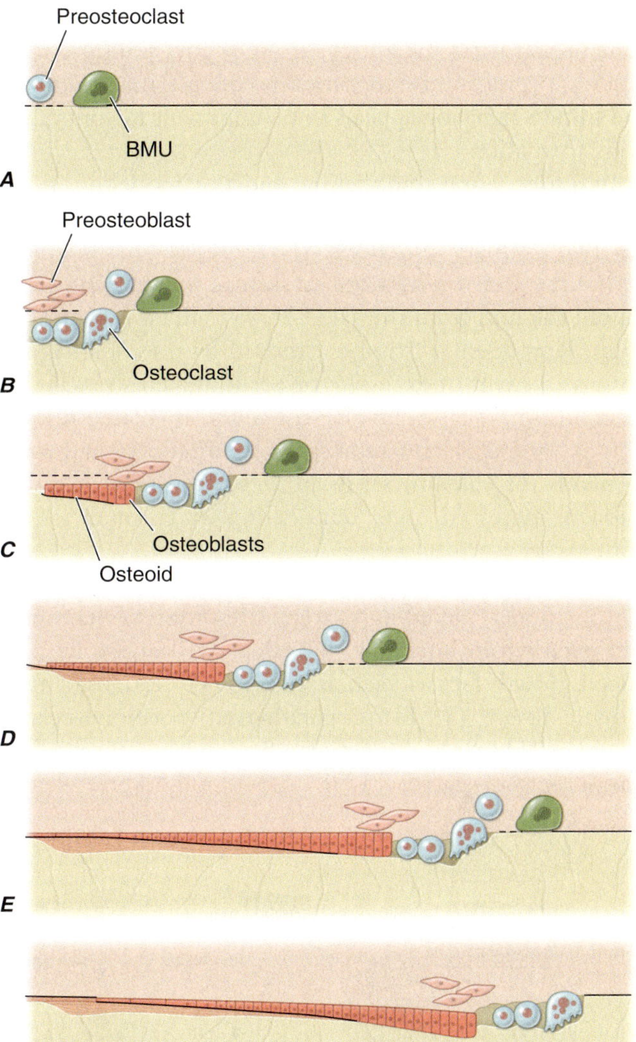

FIGURE 28-4

Mechanism of bone remodeling. The basic molecular unit (BMU) moves along the trabecular surface at a rate of about 10 μm/d. The figure depicts remodeling over ~120 days. ***A.*** Origination of BMU-lining cells contract to expose collagen and attract preosteoclasts. ***B.*** Osteoclasts fuse into multinucleated cells that resorb a cavity. Mononuclear cells continue resorption and preosteoblasts are stimulated to proliferate. ***C.*** Osteoblasts align at bottom of cavity and start forming osteoid (black). ***D.*** Osteoblasts continue formation and mineralization. Previous osteoid starts to mineralize (horizontal lines). ***E.*** Osteoblasts begin to flatten. ***F.*** Osteoblasts turn into lining cells; bone remodeling at initial surface (left of drawing) is now complete, but BMU is still advancing (to the right). [*Adapted from SM Ott, in JP Bilezikian et al (eds): Principles of Bone Biology, vol 18. San Diego, Academic Press, 1996, pp 231–241.*]

inconsistent. Linkage studies suggest that a genetic locus on chromosome 11 is associated with high bone mass. Families with high bone mass and without much apparent age-related bone loss have been shown to have a point mutation in LRP 5, a low-density lipoprotein receptor–related protein. The role of this gene in the general population is not clear, although a nonfunctional mutation results in osteoporosis-pseudoglioma syndrome, and LRP 5 signaling appears to be important in controlling bone formation.

In adults, bone remodeling, and not modeling, is the principal metabolic skeletal process. Bone remodeling has two primary functions: (1) to repair microdamage within the skeleton to maintain skeletal strength and (2) to supply calcium from the skeleton to maintain serum calcium. Remodeling may be activated by microdamage to bone as a result of excessive or accumulated stress. Acute demands for calcium involve osteoclast-mediated resorption as well as calcium transport by osteocytes. Chronic demands for calcium result in secondary hyperparathyroidism, increased bone remodeling, and overall loss of bone tissue.

Bone remodeling is also regulated by several circulating hormones, including estrogens, androgens, vitamin D, and parathyroid hormone (PTH), as well as locally produced growth factors such as IGF-I and -II, transforming growth factor (TGF) β, parathyroid hormone–related peptide (PTHrP), ILs, prostaglandins, and members of the tumor necrosis factor (TNF) superfamily. These factors primarily modulate the rate at which new remodeling sites are activated, a process that results initially in bone resorption by osteoclasts, followed by a period of repair during which new bone tissue is synthesized by osteoblasts. The cytokine responsible for communication between the osteoblasts, other marrow cells, and osteoclasts has been identified as RANK ligand (receptor activator of NF-κB; RANKL). RANKL, a member of the TNF family, is secreted by osteoblasts and certain cells of the immune system (Chap. 25). The osteoclast receptor for this protein is referred to as *RANK*. Activation of RANK by RANKL is a final common path in osteoclast development and activation. A humoral decoy for RANKL, also secreted by osteoblasts, is referred to as *osteoprotegerin* (**Fig. 28-5**). Modulation of osteoclast recruitment and activity appears to be related to the interplay among these three factors. Additional influences include nutrition (particularly calcium intake) and physical activity level.

In young adults, resorbed bone is replaced by an equal amount of new bone tissue. Thus, the mass of the skeleton remains constant after peak bone mass is achieved in adulthood. After age 30–45, however, the resorption and formation processes become imbalanced, and resorption exceeds

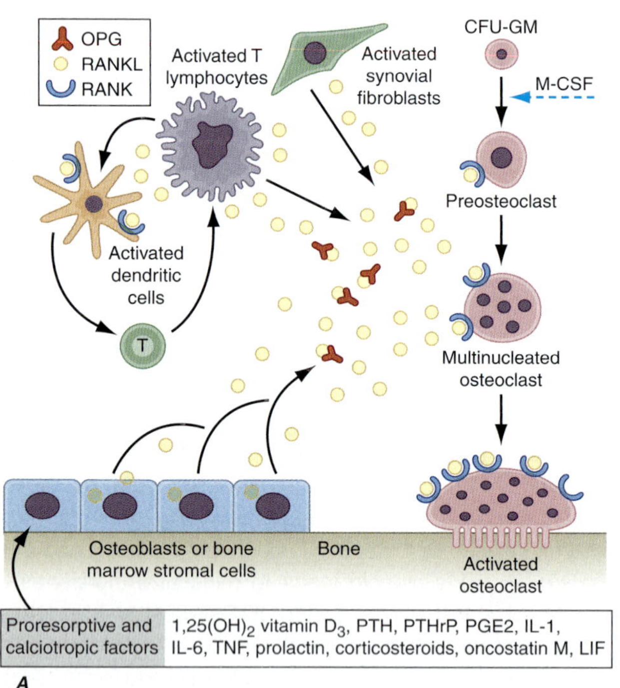

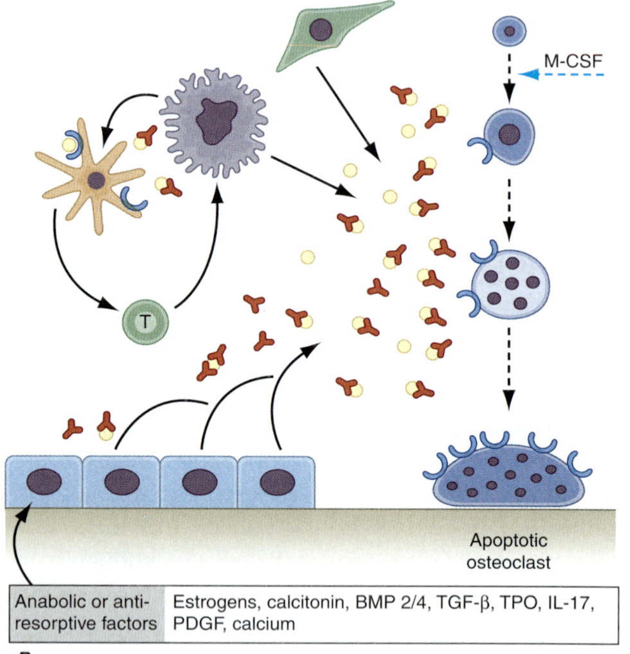

FIGURE 28-5

Hormonal control of bone resorption. *A.* Proresorptive and calciotropic factors. ***B.*** Anabolic and antiosteoclastic factors. RANKL expression is induced in osteoblasts, activated T cells, synovial fibroblasts, and bone marrow stromal cells. It binds to membrane-bound receptor RANK to promote osteoclast differentiation, activation, and survival. Conversely, osteoprotegerin (OPG) expression is induced by factors that block bone catabolism and promote anabolic effects. OPG binds and neutralizes RANKL, leading to a block in osteoclastogenesis and decreased survival of preexisting osteoclasts. RANKL, receptor activator of nuclear factor NF-κB; PTH, parathyroid hormone; PGE_2, prostaglandin E_2; TNF, tumor necrosis factor; LIF, leukemia inhibitory factor; TPO, thrombospondin; PDGF, platelet-derived growth factor; OPG-L, osteoprotegerin-ligand; IL, interleukin; TGF-β, transforming growth factor β. *(From WJ Boyle et al: Nature 423: 337, 2003.)*

formation. This imbalance may begin at different ages and varies at different skeletal sites; it becomes exaggerated in women after menopause. Excessive bone loss can be due to an increase in osteoclastic activity and/or a decrease in osteoblastic activity. In addition, an increase in remodeling activation frequency, and thus the number of remodeling sites, can magnify the small imbalance seen at each remodeling unit. Increased recruitment of bone remodeling sites produces a reversible reduction in bone tissue but can also result in permanent loss of tissue and disrupted skeletal architecture. In trabecular bone, if the osteoclasts penetrate trabeculae, they leave no template for new bone formation to occur and, consequently, rapid bone loss ensues and cancellous connectivity becomes impaired. A higher number of remodeling sites increases the likelihood of this event. In cortical bone, increased activation of remodeling creates more porous bone. The effect of this increased porosity on cortical bone strength may be modest if the overall diameter of the bone is not changed. However, decreased apposition of new bone on the periosteal surface coupled with increased endocortical resorption of bone decreases the biomechanical strength of long bones. Even a slight exaggeration in normal bone loss increases the risk of osteoporosis-related fractures, due to the architectural changes that occur.

CALCIUM NUTRITION

Peak bone mass may be impaired by inadequate calcium intake during growth among other nutritional factors (calories, protein, and other minerals), thereby leading to increased risk of osteoporosis later in life. During the adult phase of life, insufficient calcium intake contributes to relative secondary hyperparathyroidism and an increase in the rate of bone remodeling to maintain normal serum calcium levels. PTH stimulates the hydroxylation of vitamin D in the kidney, leading to increased levels of 1,25-dihydroxyvitamin D [1,25$(OH)_2$D] and enhanced gastrointestinal calcium absorption. PTH also reduces renal calcium loss. Although these are all appropriate compensatory homeostatic responses for adjusting calcium economy, the long-term effects are detrimental to the skeleton because the increased remodeling rates and the ongoing imbalance between resorption and formation at remodeling sites combine to accelerate loss of bone tissue.

Total daily calcium intakes of <400 mg are detrimental to the skeleton, and intakes in the 600–800-mg range, which is about the average intake among adults in the United States, are also likely suboptimal. The recommended daily required intake of 1000–1200 mg for adults accommodates population heterogeneity in controlling calcium balance.

VITAMIN D

(See also Chap. 25) Severe vitamin D deficiency causes rickets in children or osteomalacia in adults. However, there is accumulating evidence that vitamin D insufficiency may be more prevalent than previously thought, particularly among individuals at increased risk, such as the elderly; in those living in northern latitudes; and in individuals with poor nutrition, malabsorption, or chronic liver or renal disease. Dark-skinned individuals are also at high risk of vitamin D deficiency. An expert consensus panel has suggested that the accepted levels for serum 25-hydroxyvitamin D [25(OH)D] have been set too low, and that optimal targets for serum 25(OH)D are >75 nmol/L (30 ng/mL). To achieve this level for most adults requires intakes of 800–1000 units/d, particularly in individuals who avoid sunlight or routinely use ultraviolet-blocking lotions. Vitamin D insufficiency leads to compensatory secondary hyperparathyroidism and is an important risk factor for osteoporosis and fractures. Some studies have shown that >50% of inpatients on a general medical service exhibit biochemical features of vitamin D deficiency, including increased levels of PTH and alkaline phosphatase and lower levels of ionized calcium. In women living in northern latitudes, it has been shown that vitamin D levels decline during the winter months. This is associated with seasonal bone loss, reflecting increased bone turnover. Even among healthy ambulatory individuals, mild vitamin D deficiency is increasing in prevalence. Treatment with vitamin D can return levels to normal [>75 μmol/L (30 ng/mL)] and prevent the associated increase in bone remodeling, bone loss, and fractures. Reduced fracture rates have also been documented among individuals in northern latitudes who have greater vitamin D intake and have higher 25(OH)D levels. Vitamin D adequacy may also affect risk and/or severity of other diseases including cancers (colorectal, prostate, and breast), autoimmune diseases, and diabetes.

ESTROGEN STATUS

Estrogen deficiency probably causes bone loss by two distinct but interrelated mechanisms: (1) activation of new bone remodeling sites and (2) exaggeration of the imbalance between bone formation and resorption. The change in activation frequency causes a transient bone loss until a new steady state between resorption and formation is achieved. The remodeling imbalance, however, results in a permanent decrement in mass. In addition, the very presence of more remodeling sites in the skeleton increases the probability that trabeculae will be penetrated, thereby eliminating the template upon which new bone can be formed and accelerating the loss of bony tissue.

The most frequent estrogen-deficient state is the cessation of ovarian function at the time of menopause, which occurs on average at the age of 51 (Chap. 12). Thus, with current life expectancy, an average woman will spend about 30 years without ovarian supply of estrogen.

The mechanism by which estrogen deficiency causes bone loss is summarized in Fig. 28-5. Marrow cells (macrophages, monocytes, osteoclast precursors, mast cells) as well as bone cells (osteoblasts, osteocytes, osteoclasts) express ERs α and β. Loss of estrogen increases production of RANKL and may reduce production of osteoprotegerin, increasing osteoclast recruitment. Estrogen may also play an important role in determining the life span of bone cells by controlling the rate of apoptosis. Thus, in situations of estrogen deprivation, the life span of osteoblasts may be decreased, whereas the longevity and activity of osteoclasts are increased.

Since remodeling is initiated at the surface of bone, it follows that trabecular bone—which has a considerably larger surface area (80% of the total) than cortical bone—will be preferentially affected by estrogen deficiency. Fractures occur earliest at sites where trabecular bone contributes most to bone strength; consequently, vertebral fractures are the most common early consequence of estrogen deficiency.

PHYSICAL ACTIVITY

Inactivity, such as prolonged bed rest or paralysis, results in significant bone loss. Concordantly, athletes have higher bone mass than the general population. These changes in skeletal mass are most marked when the stimulus begins during growth and before the age of puberty. Adults are less capable than children of increasing bone mass following restoration of physical activity. Epidemiologic data support the beneficial effects on the skeleton of chronic high levels of physical activity. Fracture risk is lower in rural communities and in countries where physical activity is maintained into old age. However, when exercise is initiated during adult life, the effects of moderate exercise on the skeleton are modest, with a bone mass increase of 1–2% in short-term studies of <2 years' duration. It is argued that more active individuals are less likely to fall and are more capable of protecting themselves upon falling, thereby reducing fracture risk.

CHRONIC DISEASE

Various genetic and acquired diseases are associated with an increase in the risk of osteoporosis (Table 28-2). Mechanisms that contribute to bone loss are unique for each disease and typically result from multiple factors including nutrition, reduced physical activity levels, and factors that affect bone-remodeling rates. In most, but not all, circumstances the primary diagnosis is made before osteoporosis presents clinically.

MEDICATIONS

A large number of medications used in clinical practice have potentially detrimental effects on the skeleton (Table 28-3). *Glucocorticoids* are the most common cause of medication-induced osteoporosis. It is often not possible to determine the extent to which osteoporosis is related to the glucocorticoid or to other factors, as treatment is superimposed on the effects of the primary disease, which may in itself be associated with bone loss (e.g., rheumatoid arthritis). Excessive doses of thyroid hormone can accelerate bone remodeling and result in bone loss.

Other medications have less detrimental effects upon the skeleton than pharmacologic doses of glucocorticoids.

TABLE 28-2

DISEASES ASSOCIATED WITH AN INCREASED RISK OF GENERALIZED OSTEOPOROSIS IN ADULTS

Hypogonadal states	Hematologic disorders/ malignancy
Turner syndrome	Multiple myeloma
Klinefelter syndrome	Lymphoma and leukemia
Anorexia nervosa	Malignancy-associated parathyroid hormone (PTHrP) production
Hypothalamic amenorrhea	Mastocytosis
Hyperprolactinemia	Hemophilia
Other primary or secondary hypogonadal states	Thalassemia
Endocrine disorders	Selected inherited disorders
Cushing's syndrome	Osteogenesis imperfecta
Hyperparathyroidism	Marfan syndrome
Thyrotoxicosis	Hemochromatosis
Type 1 diabetes mellitus	Hypophosphatasia
Acromegaly	Glycogen storage diseases
Adrenal insufficiency	Homocystinuria
Nutritional and gastrointestinal disorders	Ehlers-Danlos syndrome
Malnutrition	Porphyria
Parenteral nutrition	Menkes' syndrome
Malabsorption syndromes	Epidermolysis bullosa
Gastrectomy	Other disorders
Severe liver disease, especially biliary cirrhosis	Immobilization
Pernicious anemia	Chronic obstructive pulmonary disease
Rheumatologic disorders	Pregnancy and lactation
Rheumatoid arthritis	Scoliosis
Ankylosing spondylitis	Multiple sclerosis
	Sarcoidosis
	Amyloidosis

PTHrP, parathyroid hormone–related peptide.

TABLE 28-3

DRUGS ASSOCIATED WITH AN INCREASED RISK OF GENERALIZED OSTEOPOROSIS IN ADULTS

Glucocorticoids	Excessive thyroxine
Cyclosporine	Aluminum
Cytotoxic drugs	Gonadotropin-releasing hormone agonists
Anticonvulsants	Heparin
Excessive alcohol	Lithium
Aromatase inhibitors	

Anticonvulsants are thought to increase the risk of osteoporosis, although many affected individuals have concomitant insufficiency of 1,25$(OH)_2$D, as some anticonvulsants induce the cytochrome P450 system and vitamin D metabolism. Patients undergoing transplantation are at high risk for rapid bone loss and fracture, not only from glucocorticoids but also from treatment with other *immunosuppressants*, such as cyclosporine and tacrolimus (FK506). In addition, these patients often have underlying metabolic abnormalities, such as hepatic or renal failure, that predispose to bone loss.

Aromatase inhibitors, which potently block the aromatase enzyme that converts androgens and other adrenal precursors to estrogen, reduce circulating postmenopausal estrogen levels dramatically. These agents, used in various stages for breast cancer treatment, have also been shown to have a detrimental effect on bone density and risk of fracture.

CIGARETTE CONSUMPTION

The use of cigarettes over a long period has detrimental effects on bone mass. These effects may be mediated directly, by toxic effects on osteoblasts, or indirectly by modifying estrogen metabolism. On average, cigarette smokers reach menopause 1–2 years earlier than the general population. Cigarette smoking also produces secondary effects that can modulate skeletal status, including intercurrent respiratory and other illnesses, frailty, decreased exercise, poor nutrition, and the need for additional medications (e.g., glucocorticoids for lung disease).

MEASUREMENT OF BONE MASS

Several noninvasive techniques are now available for estimating skeletal mass or density. These include dual-energy x-ray absorptiometry (DXA), single-energy x-ray absorptiometry (SXA), quantitative CT, and ultrasound.

DXA is a highly accurate x-ray technique that has become the standard for measuring bone density in most centers. Though it can be used for measurements of any skeletal site, clinical determinations are usually made of the lumbar spine and hip. Portable DXA machines have been developed that measure the heel (calcaneus), forearm (radius and ulna), or finger (phalanges). DXA can also be used to measure body composition. In the DXA technique, two x-ray energies are used to estimate the area of mineralized tissue, and the mineral content is divided by the area, which partially corrects for body size. However, this correction is only partial since DXA is a two-dimensional scanning technique and cannot estimate the depths or posteroanterior length of the bone. Thus, small people tend to have lower-than-average bone mineral density (BMD). Bone spurs, which are frequent in osteoarthritis, tend to falsely increase bone density of the spine and are a particular problem in measuring the spine of older individuals. Because DXA instrumentation is provided by several different manufacturers, the output varies in absolute terms. Consequently, it has become standard practice to relate the results to "normal" values using T-scores, which compare individual results to those in a young population that is matched for race and gender. Z-scores compare individual results to those of an age-matched population that is also matched for race and gender. Thus, a 60-year-old woman with a Z-score of –1 (1 SD below mean for age) has a T-score of –2.5 (2.5 SD below mean for a young control group) (Fig. 28-6). A T-score below –2.5 in the lumbar spine, femoral neck, or total hip is taken as a diagnosis of osteoporosis.

CT is used primarily to measure the spine and more recently the hip. Peripheral CT is used to measure bone in the forearm or tibia. The results obtained from CT are different from all others currently available since this technique is three dimensional and can provide a true density (mass of bone tissue per unit volume). CT can also specifically analyze trabecular bone and cortical bone content and volume separately. However, CT remains expensive, involves greater radiation exposure, and is less reproducible than DXA. A new technique employing high-resolution CT scanning (called *Xtreme CT*) can also provide information on skeletal architecture, including cancellous connectivity.

Ultrasound is used to measure bone mass by calculating the attenuation of the signal as it passes through bone or the speed with which it traverses the bone. It is unclear whether ultrasound assesses properties of bone other than mass (e.g., quality), but this is a potential advantage of the technique. Because of its relatively low cost and mobility, ultrasound is amenable for use as a screening procedure.

All of these techniques for measuring BMD have been approved by the U.S. Food and Drug Administration (FDA) based on their capacity to predict fracture risk. The hip is the preferred site of measurement in most individuals, since it predicts the risk of hip fracture, the most important

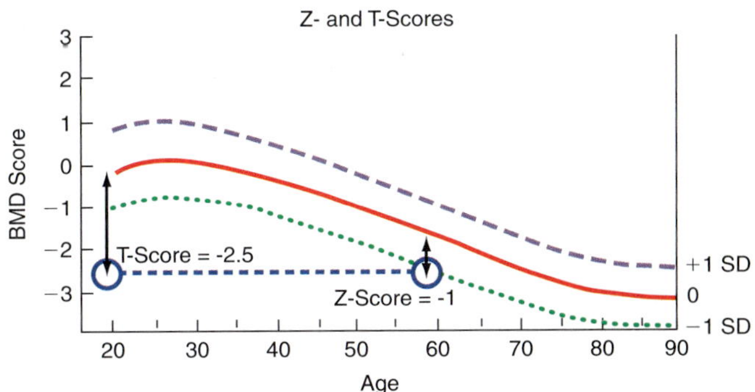

FIGURE 28-6

Relationship between Z-scores and T-scores in a 60-year-old woman. BMD, bone mineral density; SD, standard deviation.

consequence of osteoporosis, better than any other bone density measurement site. When hip measurements are performed by DXA, the spine can be measured at the same time. In younger individuals, such as perimenopausal or early postmenopausal women, spine measurements may be the most sensitive indicator of bone loss.

WHEN TO MEASURE BONE MASS

Clinical guidelines have been developed for use of bone densitometry in clinical practice. The original National Osteoporosis Foundation guidelines recommend bone mass measurements in postmenopausal women, assuming they have one or more risk factors for osteoporosis in addition to age, gender, and estrogen deficiency. The guidelines further recommend that bone mass measurement be considered in *all* women by age 65, a position ratified by the U.S. Preventive Health Services Task Force. Criteria approved for Medicare reimbursement of BMD are summarized in Table 28-4.

WHEN TO TREAT BASED ON BONE MASS RESULTS

Most guidelines suggest that patients be considered for treatment when BMD is >2.5 SD below the mean value for young adults (T-score ≤ –2.5), a level consistent with the diagnosis of osteoporosis. Treatment should also be considered in postmenopausal women with risk factors, even if BMD is not in the osteoporosis range. It is important to consider the risk of fracture for individuals, including those whose BMD is within the premenopausal range. Risk factors (age, prior fracture, family history of hip fracture, low body weight, cigarette consumption, excessive alcohol, steroid use, and rheumatoid arthritis) can be combined with BMD to assess the likelihood of a fracture over a 5- or 10-year period. Treatment thresholds depend on cost-effectiveness analyses but will likely be ~1% per year of risk in the United States.

TABLE 28-4

FDA-APPROVED INDICATIONS FOR BMD TESTS[a]
Estrogen-deficient women at clinical risk of osteoporosis
Vertebral abnormalities on x-ray suggestive of osteoporosis (osteopenia, vertebral fracture)
Glucocorticoid treatment equivalent to ≥7.5 mg of prednisone, or duration of therapy >3 months
Primary hyperparathyroidism
Monitoring response to an FDA-approved medication for osteoporosis
Repeat BMD evaluations at >23-month intervals, or more frequently, if medically justified

[a]Criteria adapted from the 1998 Bone Mass Measurement Act.
Note: FDA, U.S. Food and Drug Administration; BMD, bone mineral density.

Approach to the Patient: OSTEOPOROSIS

The perimenopausal transition is a good opportunity to initiate discussion about risk factors for osteoporosis and to consider indications for a BMD test. A careful history and physical examination should be performed to identify risk factors for osteoporosis. A low Z-score increases the suspicion of a secondary disease. Height loss >2.5–3.8 cm (>1–1.5 in.) is an indication for radiography or vertebral fracture assessment by DXA to rule out asymptomatic vertebral fractures, as is the presence of significant kyphosis or back pain, particularly if it began after menopause. For patients who present with fractures, it is important to ensure that the fractures are not caused by an underlying malignancy. Usually this is clear on routine radiography, but on occasion, CT, MRI, or radionuclide scans may be necessary.

ROUTINE LABORATORY EVALUATION There is no established algorithm for the evaluation of women presenting with osteoporosis. A general evaluation that includes complete blood count, serum and 24-h urine calcium, and renal and hepatic function tests is useful for identifying selected secondary causes of low bone mass, particularly for women with fractures or very low Z-scores. An elevated serum calcium level suggests hyperparathyroidism or malignancy, whereas a reduced serum calcium level may reflect malnutrition and osteomalacia. In the presence of hypercalcemia, a serum PTH level differentiates between hyperparathyroidism (PTH↑) and malignancy (PTH↓), and a high PTHrP level can help document the presence of humoral hypercalcemia of malignancy (Chap. 27). A low urine calcium (<50 mg/24 h) suggests osteomalacia, malnutrition, or malabsorption; a high urine calcium (>300 mg/24 h) is indicative of hypercalciuria and must be investigated further. Hypercalciuria occurs primarily in three situations: (1) a renal calcium leak, which is more frequent in males with osteoporosis; (2) absorptive hypercalciuria, which can be idiopathic or associated with increased $1,25(OH)_2D$ in granulomatous disease; or (3) hematologic malignancies or conditions associated with excessive bone turnover such as Paget's disease, hyperparathyroidism, and hyperthyroidism.

Individuals who have osteoporosis-related fractures or bone density in the osteoporotic range should have a measurement of serum 25(OH)D level, since the intake of vitamin D required to achieve a target level >32 ng/mL is very variable. Vitamin D levels should be optimized in all individuals being treated for osteoporosis. Hyperthyroidism should be evaluated by measuring thyroid-stimulating hormone (TSH).

When there is clinical suspicion of Cushing's syndrome, urinary free cortisol levels or a fasting serum cortisol should be measured after overnight dexamethasone. When bowel disease, malabsorption, or malnutrition is suspected, serum albumin, cholesterol, and a complete blood count should be checked. Asymptomatic malabsorption might be heralded by anemia (macrocytic–vitamin B_{12} or folate deficiency; or microcytic–iron deficiency) or low serum cholesterol or urinary calcium levels. If these or other features suggest malabsorption, further evaluation is required. Asymptomatic celiac disease with selective malabsorption is being found with increasing frequency; the diagnosis can be made by testing for antigliadin, antiendomysial, or transglutaminase antibodies but may require endoscopic biopsy. A trial of a gluten-free diet can be confirmatory. When osteoporosis is found associated with symptoms of rash, multiple allergies, diarrhea, or flushing, mastocytosis should be excluded using 24-h urine histamine collection or serum tryptase.

Myeloma can masquerade as generalized osteoporosis, although it more commonly presents with bone pain and characteristic "punched-out" lesions on radiography. Serum and urine electrophoresis and evaluation for light chains in urine are required to exclude this diagnosis. A bone marrow biopsy may be required to rule out myeloma (in patients with equivocal electrophoretic results) and can also be used to exclude mastocytosis, leukemia, and other marrow infiltrative disorders, such as Gaucher's disease.

BONE BIOPSY Tetracycline labeling of the skeleton allows determination of the rate of remodeling as well as evaluation for other metabolic bone diseases. The current use of BMD tests, in combination with hormonal evaluation and biochemical markers of bone remodeling, has largely replaced the clinical use of bone biopsy, although it remains an important tool in clinical research.

BIOCHEMICAL MARKERS Several biochemical tests are now available that provide an index of the overall rate of bone remodeling (Table 28-5). Biochemical markers are usually characterized as those related primarily to *bone formation* or *bone resorption*. These tests measure the overall state of bone remodeling at a single point in time. Clinical use of these tests has been hampered by biologic variability (in part related to circadian rhythm) as well as to analytical variability, although the latter is improving.

For the most part, remodeling markers do not predict rates of bone loss well enough to use this information clinically. However, markers of bone resorption may help in the prediction of fracture risk, independently of bone density, particularly in older individuals. In women ≥65 years, when bone density results are greater than the usual treatment thresholds noted above, a high level of bone resorption should prompt consideration of treatment. The primary use of biochemical markers is for monitoring the response to treatment. With the introduction of antiresorptive therapeutic agents, bone remodeling declines rapidly, with the fall in resorption occurring earlier than the fall in formation. Inhibition of bone resorption is maximal within 3–6 months. Thus, measurement of bone resorption prior to initiating therapy and 4–6 months after starting therapy provides an earlier estimate of patient response than does bone densitometry. A decline in resorptive markers can be ascertained after treatment with bisphosphonates or estrogen; this effect is less marked after treatment with either raloxifene or intranasal calcitonin. A biochemical marker response to therapy is particularly useful for asymptomatic patients and might help to ensure long-term adherence to treatment. Bone turnover markers are also useful in monitoring the effects of 1-34hPTH, or teriparatide, which rapidly increases bone formation and later bone resorption.

TABLE 28-5

BIOCHEMICAL MARKERS OF BONE METABOLISM IN CLINICAL USE
Bone formation
Serum bone-specific alkaline phosphatase
Serum osteocalcin
Serum propeptide of type I procollagen
Bone resorption
Urine and serum cross-linked N-telopeptide
Urine and serum cross-linked C-telopeptide
Urine total free deoxypyridinoline

Rx Treatment: OSTEOPOROSIS

MANAGEMENT OF OSTEOPOROTIC FRACTURES Treatment of the patient with osteoporosis frequently involves management of acute fractures as well as treatment of the underlying disease. Hip fractures almost always require surgical repair if the patient is to become ambulatory again. Depending on the location and severity of the fracture, condition of the neighboring joint, and general status of the patient, procedures may include open reduction and internal fixation with pins and plates, hemiarthroplasties, and total arthroplasties. These surgical procedures are followed by intense rehabilitation in an attempt to return patients to their prefracture functional level. Long bone fractures often require either external or internal fixation. Other fractures (e.g., vertebral, rib, and pelvic fractures) are usually managed with supportive care, requiring no specific orthopedic treatment.

Only ~25–30% of vertebral compression fractures present with sudden-onset back pain. For acutely symptomatic fractures, treatment with analgesics is required, including nonsteroidal anti-inflammatory agents and/or acetaminophen, sometimes with the addition of a narcotic agent (codeine or oxycodone). A few small, randomized clinical trials suggest that calcitonin may reduce pain related to acute vertebral compression fracture. A recently developed technique involves percutaneous injection of artificial cement (polymethylmethacrylate) into the vertebral body (vertebroplasty or kyphoplasty); this offers significant immediate pain relief in the majority of patients. Long-term effects are unknown, and conclusions are based on observational studies in patients with severe persistent back pain from acute or subacute vertebral fractures. There have been no long-term randomized controlled trials of either vertebroplasty or kyphoplasty to date. Short periods of bed rest may be helpful for pain management, but, in general, early mobilization is recommended as it helps prevent further bone loss associated with immobilization. Occasionally, use of a soft elastic-style brace may facilitate earlier mobilization. Muscle spasms often occur with acute compression fractures and can be treated with muscle relaxants and heat treatments.

Severe pain usually resolves within 6–10 weeks. Chronic pain is probably not bony in origin; instead, it is related to abnormal strain on muscles, ligaments, and tendons and to secondary facet-joint arthritis associated with alterations in thoracic and/or abdominal shape. Chronic pain is difficult to treat effectively and may require analgesics, sometimes including narcotic analgesics. Frequent intermittent rest in a supine or semireclining position is often required to allow the soft tissues, which are under tension, to relax. Back-strengthening exercises (paraspinal) may be beneficial. Heat treatments help relax muscles and reduce the muscular component of discomfort. Various physical modalities, such as ultrasound and transcutaneous nerve stimulation, may be beneficial in some patients. Pain also occurs in the neck region, not as a result of compression fractures (which almost never occur in the cervical spine as a result of osteoporosis) but because of chronic strain associated from trying to elevate the head in a person with a severe thoracic kyphosis.

Multiple vertebral fractures are often associated with psychological symptoms, not always commonly appreciated. The changes in body configuration and back pain can lead to marked loss of self-image and a secondary depression. Altered balance, precipitated by the kyphosis and the anterior movement of the body's center of gravity, leads to a fear of falling, a consequent tendency to remain indoors, and the onset of social isolation. These symptoms can sometimes be alleviated by family support and/or psychotherapy. Medication may be necessary when depressive features are present.

MANAGEMENT OF THE UNDERLYING DISEASE

Risk Factor Reduction Patients should be thoroughly educated to reduce the impact of modifiable risk factors associated with bone loss and falling. Medications should be reviewed to ensure that all are necessary. Glucocorticoid medication, if present, should be evaluated to determine that it is truly indicated and is being given in doses as low as possible. For those on thyroid hormone replacement, TSH testing should be performed to determine that an excessive dose is not being used, as thyrotoxicosis can be associated with increased bone loss. In patients who smoke, efforts should be made to facilitate smoking cessation. Reducing risk factors for falling also includes alcohol abuse treatment and a review of the medical regimen for any drugs that might be associated with orthostatic hypotension and/or sedation, including hypnotics and anxiolytics. If nocturia occurs, the frequency should be reduced, if possible (e.g., by decreasing or modifying diuretic use), as arising in the middle of sleep is a common precipitant of a fall. Patients should be instructed about environmental safety with regard to eliminating exposed wires, curtain strings, slippery rugs, and mobile tables. Avoiding stocking feet on wood floors, checking carpet condition (particularly on stairs), and providing good light in paths to bathrooms and outside the home are important preventive measures. Treatment for impaired vision is recommended, particularly a problem with depth perception, which is specifically associated with increased falling risk. Elderly patients with neurologic impairment (e.g., stroke, Parkinson's disease, Alzheimer's disease) are particularly at risk of falling and require specialized supervision and care.

Nutritional Recommendations

Calcium A large body of data indicates that optimal calcium intake reduces bone loss and suppresses bone turnover. Recommended intakes from an Institute of Medicine report are shown in **Table 28-6**. The National Health and Nutritional Evaluation Studies (NHANES) have consistently documented that average calcium intakes fall considerably short of these recommendations. The preferred source of calcium is from dairy products and other foods, but many patients require calcium supplementation. Food sources of calcium are dairy products (milk, yogurt, and cheese) and fortified foods such as certain cereals, waffles, snacks, juices, and crackers. Some of these fortified foods contain as much calcium per serving as milk.

If a calcium supplement is required, it should be taken in doses ≤600 mg at a time, as the calcium absorption fraction decreases at higher doses. Calcium supplements

TABLE 28-6

ADEQUATE CALCIUM INTAKE

LIFE STAGE GROUP	ESTIMATED ADEQUATE DAILY CALCIUM INTAKE, mg/d
Young children (1–3 years)	500
Older children (4–8 years)	800
Adolescents and young adults (9–18 years)	1300
Men and women (19–50 years)	1000
Men and women (51 and older)	1200

Note: Pregnancy and lactation needs are the same as for nonpregnant women (e.g., 1300 mg/d for adolescents/young adults and 1000 mg/d for those ≥19 years).

Source: Adapted from the Standing Committee on the Scientific Evaluation of Dietary Reference Intakes. Food and Nutrition Board. Institute of Medicine. Washington, DC, 1997, National Academy Press.

should be calculated based on the elemental calcium content of the supplement, not the weight of the calcium salt (Table 28-7). Calcium supplements containing carbonate are best taken with food since they require acid for solubility. Calcium citrate supplements can be taken at any time. To confirm bioavailability, calcium supplements can be placed in distilled vinegar. They should dissolve within 30 min.

Several controlled clinical trials of calcium plus vitamin D have confirmed reductions in clinical fractures, including fractures of the hip (~20–30% risk reduction). All recent studies of pharmacologic agents have been conducted in the context of calcium replacement (± vitamin D). Thus, it is standard practice to ensure an adequate calcium and vitamin D intake in patients with osteoporosis, whether they are receiving additional pharmacologic therapy or not. A systematic review confirmed a greater BMD response to antiresorptive therapy when calcium intake was adequate.

TABLE 28-7

ELEMENTAL CALCIUM CONTENT OF VARIOUS ORAL CALCIUM PREPARATIONS

CALCIUM PREPARATION	ELEMENTAL CALCIUM CONTENT
Calcium citrate	60 mg/300 mg
Calcium lactate	80 mg/600 mg
Calcium gluconate	40 mg/500 mg
Calcium carbonate	400 mg/g
Calcium carbonate+ 5 μg vitamin D_2 (OsCal 250)	250 mg/tablet
Calcium carbonate (Tums 500)	500 mg/tablet

Source: Adapted from SM Krane and MF Holick, Chap. 355 in HPIM, 14th ed, 1998.

Although side effects from supplemental calcium are minimal (eructation and constipation mostly with carbonate salts), individuals with a history of kidney stones should have a 24-h urine calcium determination before starting increased calcium to avoid significant hypercalciuria.

Vitamin D Vitamin D is synthesized in skin under the influence of heat and ultraviolet light (Chap. 25). However, large segments of the population do not obtain sufficient vitamin D to maintain what is now considered an adequate supply [serum 25(OH)D consistently >75 mmol/L (30 ng/mL)]. Since vitamin D supplementation at doses that would achieve these serum levels is safe and inexpensive, the Institute of Medicine recommends daily intakes of 200 IU for adults <50 years of age, 400 IU for those 50–70 years, and 600 IU for those >70 years. Multivitamin tablets usually contain 400 IU, and many calcium supplements also contain vitamin D. Some data suggest that higher doses (≥1000 IU) may be required in the elderly and chronically ill.

Other Nutrients Other nutrients such as salt, high animal protein intakes, and caffeine may have modest effects on calcium excretion or absorption. Adequate vitamin K status is required for optimal carboxylation of osteocalcin. States in which vitamin K nutrition or metabolism is impaired, such as with long-term warfarin therapy, have been associated with reduced bone mass. Research concerning cola intake is controversial but suggests a possible link to reduced bone mass through factors that are independent of caffeine.

Magnesium is abundant in foods, and magnesium deficiency is quite rare in the absence of a serious chronic disease. Magnesium supplementation may be warranted in patients with inflammatory bowel disease, celiac disease, chemotherapy, severe diarrhea, malnutrition, or alcoholism. Dietary phytoestrogens, which are derived primarily from soy products and legumes (e.g., garbanzo beans, chickpeas, and lentils), exert some estrogenic activity but are insufficiently potent to justify their use in place of a pharmacologic agent in the treatment of osteoporosis.

Patients with hip fracture are often frail and relatively malnourished. Some data suggest an improved outcome in such patients when they are provided calorie and protein supplementation. Excessive protein intake can increase renal calcium excretion, but this can be corrected by an adequate calcium intake.

Exercise Exercise in young individuals increases the likelihood that they will attain the maximal genetically determined peak bone mass. Meta-analyses of studies performed in postmenopausal women indicate that weight-bearing exercise prevents bone loss but does not appear to result in substantial gain of bone mass. This beneficial effect wanes if exercise is discontinued. Most of the studies are short-term, and a more substantial effect on bone mass is likely if exercise is continued over a long period of time. Exercise also has beneficial effects on neuromuscular function, and it improves coordination, balance, and strength, thereby reducing the risk of falling. A walking program is a practical way to start. Other activities such as dancing, racquet sports, cross-country skiing, and use of gym equipment are also recommended, depending on the patient's personal preference and general condition. Even women who cannot walk benefit from swimming or water exercises, not so much for the effects on bone, which are quite minimal, but because of effects on muscle. Exercise habits should be consistent, optimally at least three times a week.

PHARMACOLOGIC THERAPIES Until fairly recently, estrogen treatment, either by itself or in concert with a progestin, was the primary therapeutic agent for prevention or treatment of osteoporosis. However, a number of new drugs have appeared, and more are expected in the near future. Some are agents that specifically treat osteoporosis (bisphosphonates, calcitonin, PTH); others, such as selective estrogen response modulators (SERMs), have broader effects. The availability of these drugs allows therapy to be tailored to the needs of an individual patient.

Estrogens A large body of clinical trial data indicates that various types of estrogens (conjugated equine estrogens, estradiol, estrone, esterified estrogens, ethinyl estradiol, and mestranol) reduce bone turnover, prevent bone loss, and induce small increases in bone mass of the spine, hip, and total body. The effects of estrogen are seen in women with natural or surgical menopause and in late postmenopausal women with or without established osteoporosis. Estrogens are efficacious when administered orally or transdermally. For both oral and transdermal routes of administration, combined estrogen/progestin preparations are now available in many countries, obviating the problem of taking two tablets or using a patch and oral progestin. One large study, referred to as PEPI (Postmenopausal Estrogen/ Progestin Intervention Trial), indicated that C-21 progestins alone do not augment the effect of standard estrogen doses on bone mass (Fig. 28-7).

Dose of Estrogen For oral estrogens, the standard recommended doses have been 0.3 mg/d for esterified estrogens, 0.625 mg/d for conjugated equine estrogens, and 5 μg/d for ethinyl estradiol. For transdermal estrogen, the commonly used dose supplies 50 μg estradiol per day, but a lower dose may be appropriate for some individuals. Dose response data for conjugated equine estrogens indicate that lower doses (0.3 and 0.45 mg/d) are effective. Doses even lower have been associated with bone mass protection.

Fracture Data Epidemiologic databases indicate that women who take estrogen replacement have a 50% reduction, on average, of osteoporotic fractures, including hip fractures. The beneficial effect of estrogen is greatest among those who start replacement early and continue the treatment; the benefit declines after discontinuation such that there is no residual protective effect against fracture by 10 years after discontinuation. The first clinical trial evaluating fractures as secondary outcomes, the Heart and Estrogen-Progestin Replacement Study (HERS) trial, showed no effect of hormone therapy against hip or other clinical fractures in women with established coronary artery disease. These data made the results of the Women's Health Initiative (WHI) exceedingly important (Chap. 12). The estrogen-progestin arm of the WHI in >16,000 postmenopausal healthy women indicated that hormone therapy reduces the risk

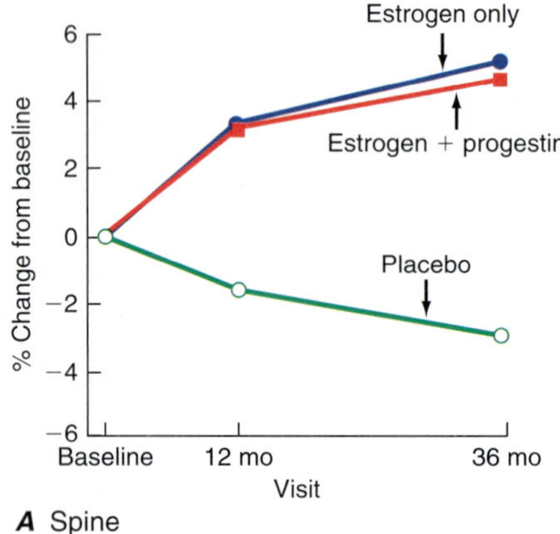

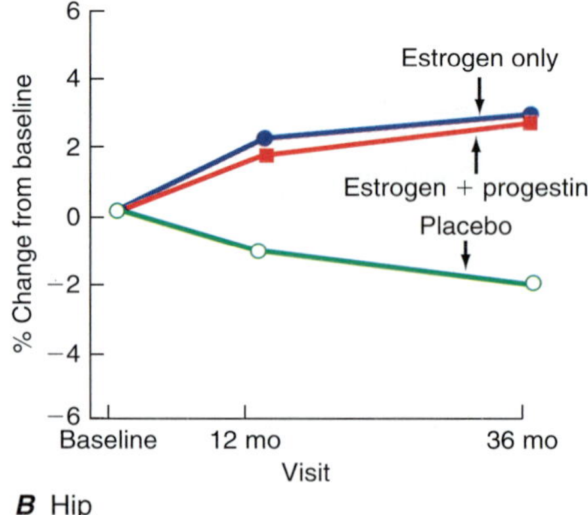

FIGURE 28-7

Results of hormone therapy regimens on bone mineral density (BMD) of the spine (***A***) and hip (***B***). Unadjusted mean percent change in BMD in the hip by treatment assignment and visit: adherent PEPI participants only. Results from the Postmenopausal Estrogen/Progestin Interventions (PEPI) Trial. Estrogen, conjugated equine estrogen 0.625 mg/d; progestin, medroxyprogesterone acetate 10 mg/d. (*Adapted from TL Bush et al: JAMA 276:1389, 1996.*)

of hip and clinical spine fracture by 34% and all clinical fractures by 24%.

A few smaller clinical trials have evaluated spine fracture occurrence as an outcome with estrogen therapy. They have consistently shown that estrogen treatment reduces the incidence of vertebral compression fracture.

The WHI has now provided a vast amount of data on the multisystemic effects of hormone therapy. Although earlier observational studies suggested that estrogen replacement might reduce heart disease, the WHI showed that combined estrogen-progestin treatment increased risk of fatal and nonfatal myocardial infarction by ~29%, confirming data from the HERS. Other important relative risks included a 40% increase in stroke, a 100% increase in venous thromboembolic disease, and a 26% increase in risk of breast cancer. Subsequent analyses have confirmed the increased risk of stroke and shown a twofold increase in dementia. Benefits other than the fracture reductions noted above included a 37% reduction in risk of colon cancer. These relative risks have to be interpreted in light of absolute risk (**Fig. 28-8**). For example, out of 10,000 women treated with estrogen-progestin for 1 year, there will be 8 excess heart attacks, 8 excess breast cancers, 18 excess venous thromboembolic events, 5 fewer hip fractures, 44 fewer clinical fractures, and 6 fewer colorectal cancers. These numbers must be multiplied by years of hormone treatment. There was no effect of hormone treatment on risk of uterine cancer or total mortality.

It is important to note that these WHI findings apply specifically to hormone treatment in the form of conjugated equine estrogen plus medroxyprogesterone acetate. The relative benefits and risks of unopposed estrogen in women who had hysterectomy vary somewhat. They still show benefits against fracture occurrence and increased

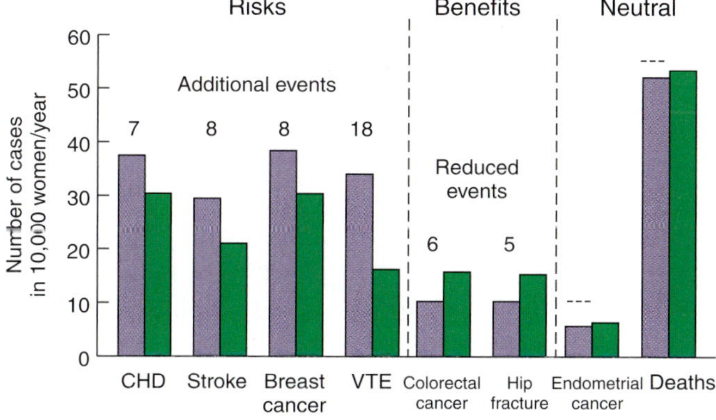

FIGURE 28-8

Effects of hormone therapy on event rates: green, placebo; purple, estrogen and progestin. CHD, coronary heart disease; VTE, venous thromboembolic events. (*Adapted from Women's Health Initiative. WHI HRT Update. Available at http://www.nhlbi.nih.gov/health/women/upd2002.htm.*)

risk of venous thrombosis and stroke, similar in magnitude to the risks for combined hormone therapy. In contrast, though, the estrogen-only arm of the WHI indicated no increased risk of heart attack or breast cancer. The data suggest that at least some of the detrimental effects of combined therapy are related to the progestin component.

Mode of Action Two subtypes of ERs, α and β, have been identified in bone and other tissues. Cells of monocyte lineage express both ERα and -β, as do osteoblasts. Estrogen-mediated effects vary depending on the receptor type. Using ER knockout mouse models, elimination of ERα produces a modest reduction in bone mass, whereas mutation of ERβ has less effect on bone. A male patient with a homozygous mutation of ERα had markedly decreased bone density as well as abnormalities in epiphyseal closure, confirming the important role of ERα in bone biology. The mechanism of estrogen action in bone is an area of active investigation (Fig. 28-5). Although data are conflicting, estrogens may inhibit osteoclasts directly. However, the majority of estrogen (and androgen) effects on bone resorption are mediated indirectly through paracrine factors produced by osteoblasts. These actions include (1) increasing IGF-I and TGF-β and (2) suppressing IL-1 (α and β), IL-6, TNF-α, and osteocalcin synthesis. The indirect estrogen actions primarily decrease bone resorption.

Progestins In women with a uterus, daily progestin or cyclical progestins at least 12 days per month are prescribed in combination with estrogens to reduce the risk of uterine cancer. Medroxyprogesterone acetate and norethindrone acetate blunt the high-density lipoprotein response to estrogen, but micronized progesterone does not. Neither medroxyprogesterone acetate nor micronized progesterone appears to have an independent effect on bone; at lower doses of estrogen, norethindrone acetate might have an additive benefit. On breast tissue, progestins may increase the risk of breast cancer.

SERMs Two SERMs are currently being used in postmenopausal women: raloxifene, which is approved for the prevention and treatment of osteoporosis, and tamoxifen, which is approved for the prevention and treatment of breast cancer.

Tamoxifen reduces bone turnover and bone loss in postmenopausal women compared to placebo groups. These findings support the concept that tamoxifen acts as an estrogenic agent in bone. There are limited data on the effect of tamoxifen on fracture risk, but the Breast Cancer Prevention study indicated a possible reduction in clinical vertebral, hip, and Colles' fractures. The major benefit of tamoxifen is on breast cancer occurrence.

The breast cancer prevention trial indicated that tamoxifen administration over 4–5 years reduced the incidence of new invasive and noninvasive breast cancer by ~45% in women at increased risk of breast cancer. The incidence of ER-positive breast cancers was reduced by 65%. Tamoxifen increases the risk of uterine cancer in postmenopausal women, limiting its use for breast cancer prevention in women at low or moderate risk.

Raloxifene (60 mg/d) has effects on bone turnover and bone mass that are very similar to those of tamoxifen, indicating that this agent is also estrogenic on the skeleton. The effect of raloxifene on bone density (+1.4–2.8% versus placebo in the spine, hip, and total body) is somewhat less than that seen with standard doses of estrogens. Raloxifene reduces the occurrence of vertebral fracture by 30–50%, depending on the population; however, there are no data confirming that raloxifene can reduce the risk of nonvertebral fractures over 8 years of observation.

Raloxifene, like tamoxifen and estrogen, has effects in other organ systems. The most beneficial effect appears to be a reduction in invasive breast cancer (mainly decreased ER-positive) occurrence of ~65% in women who take raloxifene compared to placebo. In a head-to-head study, raloxifene was as effective as tamoxifen in preventing breast cancer in high-risk women, but in a separate study had no effect on heart disease in women with increased risk for this outcome. In contrast to tamoxifen, raloxifene is not associated with an increase in the risk of uterine cancer or benign uterine disease. Raloxifene increases the occurrence of hot flashes but reduces serum total and low-density lipoprotein cholesterol, lipoprotein(a), and fibrinogen.

Mode of Action of SERMs All SERMs bind to the ER, but each agent produces a unique receptor-drug conformation. As a result, specific coactivator or co-repressor proteins are bound to the receptor (Chap. 1), resulting in differential effects on gene transcription that vary depending on other transcription factors present in the cell. Another aspect of selectivity is the affinity of each SERM for the different ERα and -β subtypes, which are expressed differentially in various tissues. These tissue-selective effects of SERMs offer the possibility of tailoring estrogen therapy to best meet the needs and risk factor profile of an individual patient.

Bisphosphonates Alendronate, risedronate, and ibandronate are approved for the prevention and treatment of postmenopausal osteoporosis. Risedronate and alendronate are approved for the treatment of steroid-induced osteoporosis, and risedronate is also approved for prevention of steroid-induced osteoporosis. Both alendronate and risedronate are approved for treatment of osteoporosis in men.

Alendronate has been shown to decrease bone turnover and increase bone mass in the spine by up to 8% versus placebo and by 6% versus placebo in the hip. Multiple trials have evaluated its effect on fracture occurrence. The Fracture Intervention Trial provided evidence in >2000 women with prevalent vertebral fractures that daily alendronate treatment (5 mg/d for 2 years and 10 mg/d for 9 months afterwards) reduces vertebral fracture risk by about 50%, multiple vertebral fractures by up to 90%, and hip fractures by up to 50% (**Fig. 28-9**). Several subsequent trials have confirmed these findings. For example, in a study of >1900 women with low bone mass treated with alendronate (10 mg/d) versus placebo, the incidence of all nonvertebral fractures was reduced by ~47% after only 1 year.

Trials comparing once-weekly alendronate, 70 mg, with daily 10-mg dosing have shown equivalence with regard to bone mass and bone turnover responses. Consequently, once-weekly therapy is generally preferred because of the low incidence of gastrointestinal side effects and ease of

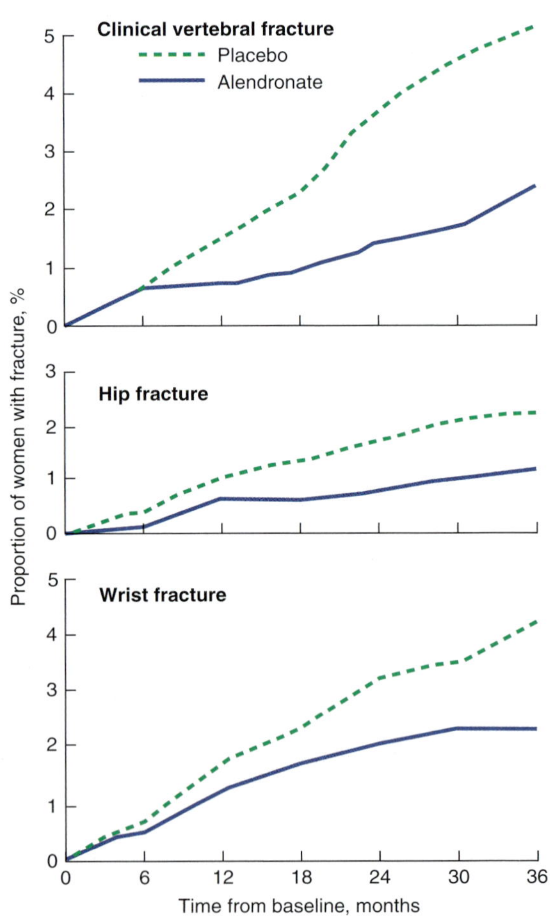

FIGURE 28-9

Cumulative proportions of women with osteoporosis who suffered clinical fracture (vertebral, hip, or wrist) during 3 years of treatment with alendronate or placebo (FIT 1). (*From DM Black et al: Lancet 348:1535, 1996.*)

administration. Alendronate should be given with a full glass of water before breakfast, as bisphosphonates are poorly absorbed. Because of the potential for esophageal irritation, alendronate is contraindicated in patients who have stricture or inadequate emptying of the esophagus. It is recommended that patients remain upright for at least 30 min after taking the medication to avoid esophageal irritation. Cases of esophagitis, esophageal ulcer, and esophageal stricture have been described, but the incidence appears to be low. In clinical trials, overall gastrointestinal symptomatology was no different with alendronate compared to placebo. Alendronate is also available in a preparation that contains vitamin D.

Risedronate also reduces bone turnover and increases bone mass. Controlled clinical trials have demonstrated 40–50% reduction in vertebral fracture risk over 3 years, accompanied by a 40% reduction in clinical nonspine fractures. The only clinical trial specifically designed to evaluate hip fracture outcome (HIP) indicated that risedronate reduced hip fracture risk in women in their seventies with confirmed osteoporosis by 40%. In contrast, risedronate was not effective at reducing hip fracture occurrence in older women (80+ years) without proven osteoporosis. Studies have shown that 35 mg of risedronate administered once weekly is therapeutically equivalent to 5 mg/d. Patients should take risedronate with a full glass of plain water, to facilitate delivery to the stomach, and should not lie down for 30 min after taking the drug. The incidence of gastrointestinal side effects in trials with risedronate was similar to that of placebo.

Etidronate was the first bisphosphonate to be approved, initially for use in Paget's disease and hypercalcemia. This agent has also been used in osteoporosis trials of smaller magnitude than those performed for alendronate and risedronate but is not approved by the FDA for treatment of osteoporosis. Etidronate probably has some efficacy against vertebral fracture when given as an intermittent cyclical regimen (2 weeks on, $2^1/_2$ months off). There has not been any study of its effectiveness against nonvertebral fractures.

Ibandronate is the third amino-bisphosphonate approved in the United States. Ibandronate (2.5 mg/d) has been shown in clinical trials to reduce vertebral fracture risk by ~40% but with no overall effect on nonvertebral fractures. In a post hoc analysis of subjects with a femoral neck T-score of –3 or below, ibandronate reduced the risk of nonvertebral fractures by ~60%. In clinical trials, ibandronate doses of 150 mg/month PO or 3 mg every 3 months IV had greater effects on turnover and bone mass than 2.5 mg/d. Patients should take oral ibandronate in the same way as other bisphosphonates, but with 1 h elapsing before other food or drink (other than plain water).

Zoledronic acid is a potent bisphosphonate with unique administration regimens (once yearly IV). Although it is not yet approved for use in osteoporosis, the data suggest that it is highly effective in fracture risk reduction. In a study of >7000 women followed for 3 years, zoledronic acid (5 mg as a single IV infusion annually) reduced the risk of vertebral fractures by 70%, nonvertebral fractures by 25%, and hip fractures by 40%. These results were associated with less height loss and disability. In the treated population, there was an increased risk of atrial fibrillation (2%) and arthralgia and a 15% risk of fever, in comparison to placebo.

Mode of Action Bisphosphonates are structurally related to pyrophosphates, compounds that are incorporated into bone matrix. Bisphosphonates specifically impair osteoclast function and reduce osteoclast number, in part by the induction of apoptosis. Recent evidence suggests that the nitrogen-containing bisphosphonates also inhibit protein prenylation, one of the end products in the mevalonic acid pathway, by inhibition of the enzyme farnesyl pyrophosphate synthase. This effect disrupts intracellular protein trafficking and may ultimately lead to apoptosis. Some bisphosphonates have very long retention in the skeleton and may exert long-term effects. The consequences of this, if any, are unknown. A phenomenon that has been called *osteonecrosis of the jaw* (ONJ) has been described, mostly in patients with cancer given high doses of zoledronic acid or pamidronate. A few cases have been described in patients with osteoporosis treated with oral bisphosphonates. The background incidence of ONJ in this population is not known, and thus the attributable risk for bisphosphonates is not clear, but it appears to be relatively rare.

Calcitonin Calcitonin is a polypeptide hormone produced by the thyroid gland (Chap. 27). Its physiologic role is unclear as no skeletal disease has been described in association with calcitonin deficiency or calcitonin excess. Calcitonin preparations are approved by the FDA for Paget's disease, hypercalcemia, and osteoporosis in women >5 years past menopause.

Injectable calcitonin produces small increments in bone mass of the lumbar spine. However, difficulty of administration and frequent reactions, including nausea and facial flushing, make general use limited. A nasal spray containing calcitonin (200 IU/d) is available for treatment of osteoporosis in postmenopausal women. One study suggests that nasal calcitonin produces small increments in bone mass and a small reduction in new vertebral fractures in calcitonin-treated patients versus those on calcium alone. There has been no proven effectiveness against nonvertebral fractures. An oral preparation of calcitonin has recently been approved for use in osteoporosis.

Calcitonin is not indicated for prevention of osteoporosis and is not sufficiently potent to prevent bone loss in early postmenopausal women. Calcitonin might have an analgesic effect on bone pain, both in the SC and possibly the nasal form.

Mode of Action Calcitonin suppresses osteoclast activity by direct action on the osteoclast calcitonin receptor. Osteoclasts exposed to calcitonin cannot maintain their active ruffled border, which normally maintains close contact with underlying bone.

Parathyroid Hormone Endogenous PTH is an 84-amino-acid peptide that is largely responsible for calcium homeostasis (Chap. 27). Although chronic elevation of PTH, as occurs in hyperparathyroidism, is associated with bone loss (particularly cortical bone), PTH can also exert anabolic effects on bone. Consistent with this, some observational studies have indicated that mild elevations in PTH are associated with maintenance of trabecular bone mass. On the basis of these findings, several clinical trials have been performed using an exogenous PTH analogue [human PTH(1–34); teriparatide], which is now approved for the treatment of established osteoporosis in both men and women. The first randomized controlled trial in postmenopausal women showed that PTH, when superimposed on ongoing estrogen therapy, produced substantial increments in bone mass (13% over a 3-year period compared to estrogen alone) and reduced the risk of vertebral compression deformity. In the pivotal study (median, 19 months' duration), 20 μg PTH(1–34) daily by SC injection reduced vertebral fractures by 65% and nonvertebral fractures by 45% (Fig. 28-10). Treatment is administered as a single daily injection given for a maximum of 2 years. Teriparatide produces increases in bone mass and mediates architectural improvements in skeletal structure. These effects are lower when patients have been previously exposed to bisphosphonates, possibly in proportion to the potency of the antiresorptive effect. When human PTH(1–34) is being considered for treatment-naïve patients, it is best administered as monotherapy and followed by an antiresorptive agent such as a bisphosphonate.

Side effects of teriparatide are generally mild and can include muscle pain, weakness, dizziness, headache, and nausea. Rodents given prolonged treatment with PTH in relatively high doses developed osteogenic sarcomas. One case of osteosarcoma has been described in a patient treated with teriparatide. At present this seems to equate to the background incidence of osteosarcoma in this population.

PTH use may be limited by its mode of administration; alternative modes of delivery are being investigated. The optimal frequency of administration also remains to be established, and it is possible that PTH might also be effective when used intermittently. Cost may also be a limiting factor.

Mode of Action Exogenously administered PTH appears to have direct actions on osteoblast activity, with biochemical and histomorphometric evidence of de novo bone formation early in response to PTH, prior to activation of bone resorption. Subsequently, PTH activates bone remodeling but still appears to favor bone formation over bone resorption. PTH stimulates IGF-I and collagen production and appears to increase osteoblast number by stimulating replication, enhancing osteoblast recruitment, and inhibiting apoptosis. Unlike

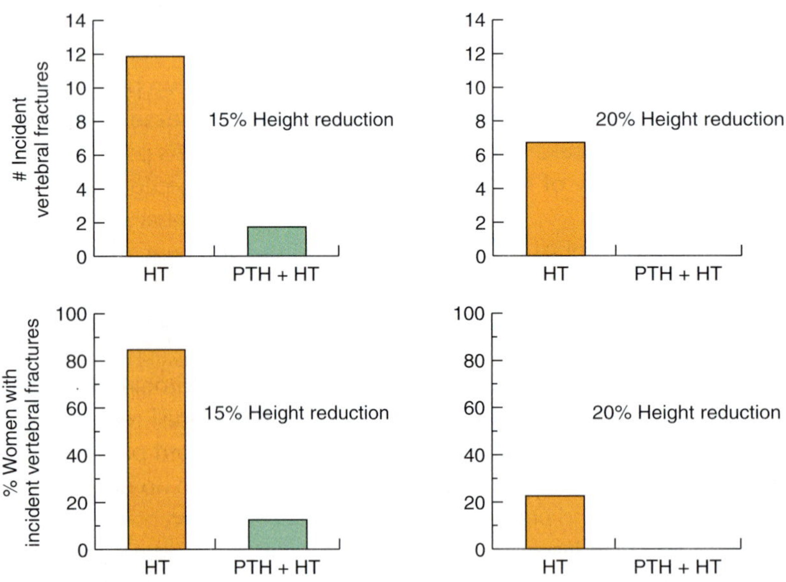

FIGURE 28-10

Number of incident vertebral deformities (15% and 20% reductions) in women with osteoporosis on HT, compared to HT + PTH over 3 years. HT, hormone therapy; PTH, parathyroid hormone. (*From F Cosman et al: J Bone Miner Res 16:925, 2001.*)

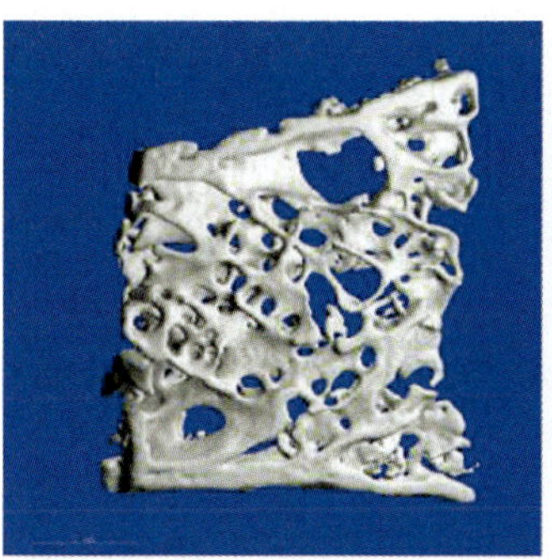
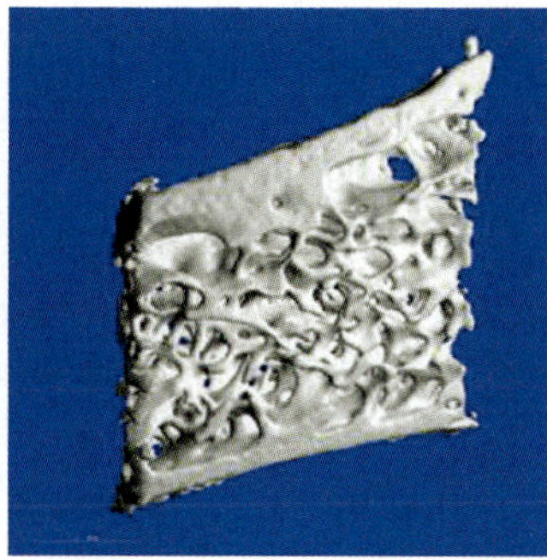

A *B*

FIGURE 28-11

Effect of parathyroid hormone (PTH) treatment on bone microarchitecture. Paired biopsy specimens from a 64-year-old woman before (***A***) and after (***B***) treatment with PTH. *(From DW Dempster et al: J Bone Miner Res 16:1846, 2001.)*

all other treatments, PTH produces a true increase in bone tissue and an apparent restoration of bone microarchitecture (Fig. 28-11).

Fluoride Fluoride has been available for many years and is a potent stimulator of osteoprogenitor cells when studied in vitro. It has been used in multiple osteoporosis studies with conflicting results, in part related to use of varying doses and preparations. Despite increments in bone mass of up to 10%, there are no consistent effects of fluoride on vertebral or nonvertebral fracture; the latter might actually increase when high doses of fluoride are used. Fluoride remains an experimental agent, despite its long history and multiple studies.

Strontium ranelate is approved in several European countries for the treatment of osteoporosis. It increases bone mass throughout the skeleton; in clinical trials, the drug reduced the risk of vertebral fractures by 37% and nonvertebral fractures by 14%. It appears to be modestly antiresorptive, while at the same time not causing as much of a decrease in bone formation (measured biochemically). Strontium is incorporated into hydroxyapatite, replacing calcium, a feature that might explain some of its fracture benefits. Small increased risks of venous thrombosis, seizures, and abnormal cognition have been seen and require further study.

Other Potential Anabolic Agents Several small studies of growth hormone (GH), alone or in combination with other agents, have not shown consistent or substantial positive effects on skeletal mass. Many of these studies are relatively short-term, and the effects of GH, growth hormone–releasing hormone, and the IGFs are still under investigation. Anabolic steroids, mostly derivatives of testosterone, act primarily as antiresorptive agents to reduce bone turnover but may also stimulate osteoblastic activity. Effects on bone mass remain unclear but appear weak, in general, and use is limited by masculinizing side effects. Several recent observational studies suggest that the statin drugs, currently used to treat hypercholesterolemia, may be associated with increased bone mass and reduced fractures, but conclusions from clinical trials are mixed.

NONPHARMACOLOGIC APPROACHES Protective pads worn around the outer thigh, which cover the trochanteric region of the hip, can prevent hip fractures in elderly residents in nursing homes. The use of hip protectors is limited largely by compliance and comfort, but new devices are being developed that may circumvent these problems and provide adjunctive treatments.

Kyphoplasty and *vertebroplasty* are also useful nonpharmacologic approaches for the treatment of painful vertebral fractures. However, no long-term data are available.

TREATMENT MONITORING There are currently no well-accepted guidelines for monitoring treatment of osteoporosis. Because most osteoporosis treatments produce small or moderate bone mass increments on average, it is reasonable to consider BMD as a monitoring tool. Changes must exceed ~4% in the spine and 6% in the hip to be considered significant in any individual. The hip is the preferred site due to larger surface area and greater reproducibility. Medication-induced increments may require several years to produce changes of this magnitude (if they do at all). Consequently, it can be argued that BMD should be repeated at intervals >2 years. Only significant BMD reductions should prompt a change in medical regimen, as it is expected that many individuals will not show responses greater than the detection limits of the current measurement techniques.

Biochemical markers of bone turnover may prove useful for treatment monitoring, but little hard evidence currently supports this concept; it remains unclear which endpoint is most useful. If bone turnover markers are used, a determination should be made before starting therapy and repeated ≥4 months after therapy is initiated. In general, a change in bone turnover markers must be 30–40% lower than the baseline to be significant because of the biologic and technical variability in these tests. A positive change in biochemical markers and/or bone density can be useful to help patients adhere to treatment regimens.

GLUCOCORTICOID-INDUCED OSTEOPOROSIS

Osteoporotic fractures are a well-characterized consequence of the hypercortisolism associated with Cushing's syndrome. However, the therapeutic use of glucocorticoids is by far the most common form of glucocorticoid-induced osteoporosis. Glucocorticoids are widely used in the treatment of a variety of disorders, including chronic lung disorders, rheumatoid arthritis and other connective tissue diseases, inflammatory bowel disease, and posttransplantation. Osteoporosis and related fractures are serious side effects of chronic glucocorticoid therapy. Because the effects of glucocorticoids on the skeleton are often superimposed upon the consequences of aging and menopause, it is not surprising that women and the elderly are most frequently affected. The skeletal response to steroids is remarkably heterogeneous, however, and even young, growing individuals treated with glucocorticoids can present with fractures.

The risk of fractures depends on the dose and duration of glucocorticoid therapy, although recent data suggest that there may be no completely safe dose. Bone loss is more rapid during the early months of treatment, and trabecular bone is more severely affected than cortical bone. As a result, fractures have been shown to increase within 3 months of steroid treatment. There is an increase in fracture risk in both the axial and appendicular skeleton, including risk of hip fracture. Bone loss can occur with any route of steroid administration including high-dose inhaled glucocorticoids and intraarticular injections. Alternate-day delivery does not appear to ameliorate the skeletal effects of glucocorticoids.

PATHOPHYSIOLOGY

Glucocorticoids increase bone loss by multiple mechanisms including (1) inhibition of osteoblast function and an increase in osteoblast apoptosis, resulting in impaired synthesis of new bone; (2) stimulation of bone resorption, probably as a secondary effect; (3) impairment of the absorption of calcium across the intestine, probably by a vitamin D–independent effect; (4) increase of urinary calcium loss and perhaps induction of some degree of secondary hyperparathyroidism; (5) reduction of adrenal androgens and suppression of ovarian and testicular secretion of estrogens and androgens; and (6) induction of glucocorticoid myopathy, which may exacerbate effects on skeletal and calcium homeostasis as well as increase the risk of falls.

EVALUATION OF THE PATIENT

Because of the prevalence of glucocorticoid-induced bone loss, it is important to evaluate the status of the skeleton in all patients starting or already receiving long-term glucocorticoid therapy. Modifiable risk factors should be identified, including those for falls. Examination should include height and muscle strength testing. Laboratory evaluation should include an assessment of 24-h urinary calcium. All patients on long-term (>3 months) glucocorticoids should have measurement of bone mass at both the spine and hip using DXA. If only one skeletal site can be measured, it is best to assess the spine in individuals <60 years and the hip for those >60 years.

PREVENTION

Bone loss caused by glucocorticoids can be prevented, and the risk of fractures significantly reduced. Strategies must include using the lowest dose of glucocorticoid for disease management. Topical and inhaled routes of administration are preferred, where appropriate. Risk factor reduction is important, including smoking cessation, limitation of alcohol consumption, and participation in weight-bearing exercise, when appropriate. All patients should receive an adequate calcium and vitamin D intake from the diet or from supplements.

℞ Treatment: GLUCOCORTICOID-INDUCED OSTEOPOROSIS

Only bisphosphonates have been demonstrated in large clinical trials to reduce the risk of fractures in patients being treated with glucocorticoids. Risedronate prevents bone loss and reduces vertebral fracture risk by ~70%. Similar beneficial effects are observed in studies of alendronate. Controlled trials of hormone therapy have shown bone-sparing effects, and calcitonin also has some protective effect in the spine. Thiazides reduce urine calcium loss, but their role in prevention of fractures is unclear. PTH has also been studied in a small group of women with glucocorticoid-induced osteoporosis, where bone mass increased substantially, and teriparatide is currently being investigated in a larger multicenter trial.

FURTHER READINGS

Barrett-Connor E et al: Effects of raloxifene on cardiovascular events and breast cancer in postmenopausal women. N Engl J Med 355:125, 2006

Black DM et al: Randomized trial of once-weekly parathyroid hormone (1-84) on bone mineral density and remodeling. J Clin Endocrinol Metab 93:2166, 2008

Boonen S et al: Effects of previous antiresorptive therapy on the bone mineral density response to two years of teriparatide treatment in postmenopausal women with osteoporosis. J Clin Endocrinol Metab 93:852, 2008

Cosman F: Anabolic therapy for osteoporosis: Parathyroid hormone. Curr Rheumatol Rep 8:63, 2006

Cummings SR et al: Denosumab for prevention of fractures in postmenopausal women with osteoporosis. N Engl J Med 361:756, 2009

Deroo BJ et al: Estrogen receptors and human disease. J Clin Invest 116:561, 2006

Heaney RP: Bone health. Am J Clin Nutr 85:300S, 2007

Lyles KW et al: Zoledronic acid and clinical fractures and mortality after hip fracture. N Engl J Med 357:1799, 2007

MAUCK KF, CLARKE BL: Diagnosis, screening, prevention, and treatment of osteoporosis. Mayo Clin Proc 81:662, 2006

MULDER JE et al: Drug insight: Existing and emerging therapies for osteoporosis. Nat Clin Pract Endocrinol Metab 2:670, 2006

POOLE KE, COMPSTON JE: Osteoporosis and its management. BMJ 333:1251, 2006

SMITH MR et al: Denosumab in men receiving androgen-deprivation therapy for prostate cancer. N Engl J Med 361:745, 2009

STYRKARSDOTTIR U et al: Multiple genetic loci for bone mineral density and fractures. N Engl J Med 358:2355, 2008

VOGEL V et al: Effects of tamoxifen vs raloxifene on the risk of developing invasive breast cancer and other disease outcomes. JAMA 295:2727, 2006

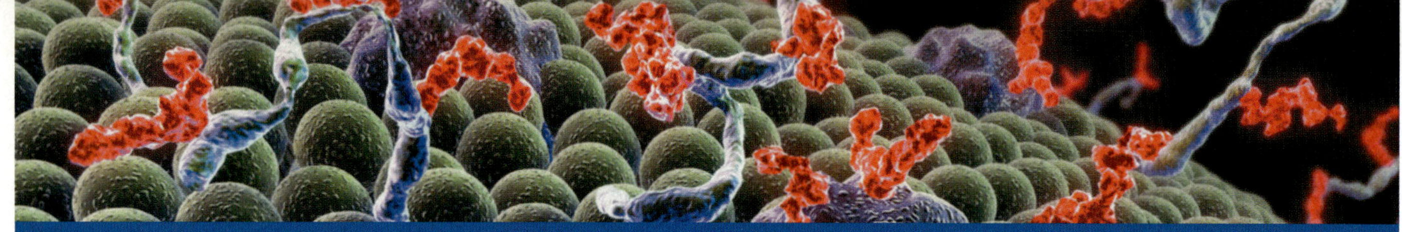

CHAPTER 29

PAGET'S DISEASE AND OTHER DYSPLASIAS OF BONE

Murray J. Favus ■ Tamara J. Vokes

PAGET'S DISEASE OF BONE

Paget's disease is a localized bone disorder that affects widespread areas of the skeleton through increased bone remodeling. The pathologic process is initiated by overactive osteoclastic bone resorption followed by a compensatory increase in osteoblastic new bone formation. New pagetic bone is structurally disorganized and more susceptible to deformities and fractures. Although most patients are asymptomatic, a variety of symptoms and complications may result directly from bony involvement or secondarily from the expansion of bone and subsequent compression of surrounding neural tissue.

EPIDEMIOLOGY

There is a marked geographic variation in the frequency of Paget's disease, with high prevalence in Western Europe (Great Britain, France, and Germany but not Switzerland or Scandinavia) and among those who have immigrated to Australia, New Zealand, South Africa, and North and South America. The disease is rare in native populations of the Americas, Africa, Asia, and the Middle East. The prevalence is greater in males and increases with age. Autopsy series reveal Paget's disease in about 3% of those over age 40. Prevalence of positive skeletal radiographs in patients over age 55 is 2.5% for men and 1.6% for women. Elevated alkaline phosphatase (ALP) levels in asymptomatic patients have an age-adjusted incidence of 12.7 and 7 per 100,000 person-years in men and women, respectively. The frequency of diagnosis by either radiographic or biochemical criteria has decreased during the past 20 years.

Etiology

The etiology of Paget's disease of bone remains unknown, but evidence supports both genetic and viral etiologies. A positive family history is found in 15–25% of patients and, when present, raises the prevalence of the disease seven- to tenfold among first-degree relatives.

A homozygous deletion of the *TNFRSF11B* gene, which encodes osteoprotegerin (**Fig. 29-1**), causes juvenile Paget's disease, a disorder characterized by uncontrolled osteoclastic differentiation and resorption. Familial patterns of disease in several large kindreds are consistent

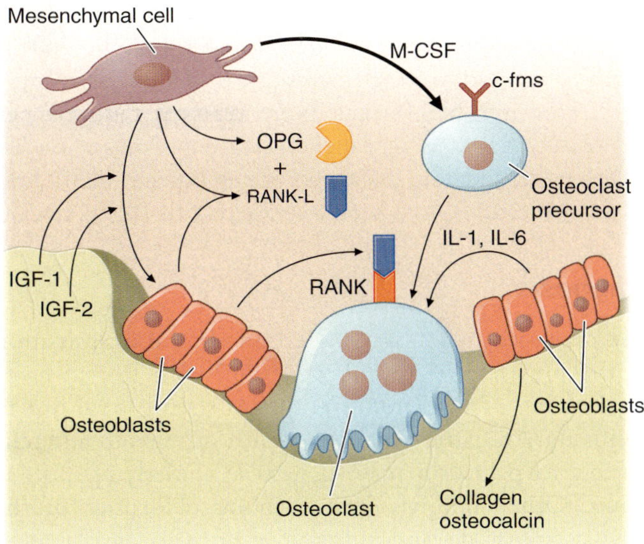

FIGURE 29-1

Diagram illustrating factors that promote differentiation and function of osteoclasts and osteoblasts and the role of the RANK pathway. Stromal bone marrow (mesenchymal) cells and differentiated osteoblasts produce multiple growth factors and cytokines, including macrophage colony-stimulating factor (M-CSF), to modulate osteoclastogenesis. RANKL (receptor activator of NF-κB ligand) is produced by osteoblast progenitors and mature osteoblasts and can bind to a soluble decoy receptor known as OPG (osteoprotegerin) to inhibit RANKL action. Alternatively, a cell-cell interaction between osteoblast and osteoclast progenitors allows RANKL to bind to its membrane-bound receptor, RANK, thereby stimulating osteoclast differentiation and function. RANK binds intracellular proteins called TRAFS (tumor necrosis factor receptor–associated factors) that mediate receptor signaling through transcription factors such as NF-κB. M-CSF binds to its receptor, c-fms, which is the cellular homologue of the *fms* oncogene. See text for the potential role of these pathways in disorders of osteoclast function such as Paget's disease and osteopetrosis.

with an autosomal dominant pattern of inheritance with variable penetrance. A susceptibility locus for Paget's disease has been mapped to chromosome 18q21-22, a region that contains a gene responsible for a rare Paget's disease–like skeletal disorder known as *familial expansile osteolysis*. The gene encodes the receptor activator of nuclear factor-κB (RANK), a member of the tumor necrosis factor superfamily critical for osteoclast differentiation (Fig. 29-1). In other families, susceptibility loci have been mapped to loci on chromosomes 18q23, 6p21.3, 5q31, and 5q35. Mutations of the *SQSTM1* gene (sequestasome-1 or p62 protein) in the C-terminal ubiquitin-binding domain have been identified in familial and sporadic cases of Paget's disease. The p62 protein is involved in NF-κB signaling and regulates osteoclastic differentiation. The phenotypic variability in patients with *SQSTM1* mutations suggests that additional factors, such as other genetic influences or viral infection, may influence clinical expression of the disease.

Several lines of evidence suggest that a viral infection may contribute to the clinical manifestations of Paget's disease, including (1) the presence of cytoplasmic and nuclear inclusions resembling paramyxoviruses (measles and respiratory syncytial virus) in pagetic osteoclasts and (2) viral mRNA in precursor and mature osteoclasts. The viral etiology is further supported by conversion of osteoclast precursors to pagetic-like osteoclasts by vectors containing the measles virus nucleocapsid or matrix genes. However, the viral etiology has been questioned by the inability to culture a live virus from pagetic bone and by failure to clone the full-length viral genes from material obtained from patients with Paget's disease.

Pathophysiology

The principal abnormality in Paget's disease is the increased number and activity of osteoclasts. Pagetic osteoclasts are large, increased 10- to 100-fold in number, and have a greater number of nuclei (as many as 100 compared to 3–5 nuclei in the normal osteoclast). The overactive osteoclasts may create a sevenfold increase in resorptive surfaces and an erosion rate of 9 μg/d (normal is 1 μg/d). Several causes for the increased number and activity of pagetic osteoclasts have been identified: (1) osteoclastic precursors are hypersensitive to $1,25(OH)_2D_3$; (2) osteoclasts are hyperresponsive to RANK ligand (RANKL), the osteoclast stimulatory factor that mediates the effects of most osteotropic factors on osteoclast formation; (3) marrow stromal cells from pagetic lesions have increased RANKL expression; (4) osteoclast precursor recruitment is increased by interleukin (IL) 6, which is increased in the blood of patients with active Paget's disease and is overexpressed in pagetic osteoclasts; (5) expression of the protooncogene *c-fos*, which increases osteoclastic activity, is increased; and (6) the antiapoptotic oncogene *Bcl-2* in pagetic bone is overexpressed. Numerous osteoblasts are recruited to active resorption sites and produce large amounts of new bone matrix. As a result, bone turnover is high and bone mass is normal or increased, not reduced.

The characteristic feature of Paget's disease is increased bone resorption accompanied by accelerated bone formation. An initial osteolytic phase involves prominent bone resorption and marked hypervascularization. Radiographically, this manifests as an advancing lytic wedge, or "blade of grass" lesion. The second phase is a period of very active bone formation and resorption that replaces normal lamellar bone with haphazard (woven) bone. The mosaic pattern of woven bone is structurally inferior and can bow and fracture more readily. At the same time, fibrous connective tissue may replace normal bone marrow. In the final sclerotic phase, bone resorption declines progressively and leads to a hard, dense, less vascular pagetic or mosaic bone, which represents the so-called burned-out phase of Paget's disease. All three phases may be present at the same time at different skeletal sites.

Clinical Manifestations

Asymptomatic patients are often diagnosed by discovery of an elevated ALP level on routine blood chemistry testing or from an abnormality on a skeletal radiograph obtained for another indication. The skeletal sites most commonly involved are the pelvis, vertebral bodies, skull, femur, and tibia. Numerous active sites of skeletal involvement are more common in familial cases with an early presentation.

Pain is the most common presenting symptom. It results from increased bony vascularity, expanding lytic lesions, fractures, bowing, or other deformities of the extremities. Bowing of the femur or tibia causes gait abnormalities and abnormal mechanical stresses with secondary osteoarthritis of the hip or knee joints. Long bone bowing also causes extremity pain by stretching the muscles attached to the bone softened by the pagetic process. Back pain results from enlarged pagetic vertebrae, vertebral compression fractures, spinal stenosis, degenerative changes of the joints, and altered body mechanics with kyphosis and forward tilt of the upper back. Rarely, spinal cord compression may result from bone enlargement or from the vascular steal syndrome. Skull involvement may cause headaches, symmetric or asymmetric enlargement of the parietal or frontal bones (frontal bossing), and increased head size. Cranial expansion may narrow cranial foramina and cause neurologic complications including hearing loss from cochlear nerve damage from temporal bone involvement, cranial nerve palsies, and softening of the base of the skull (*platybasia*) and the risk of brainstem compression. Pagetic involvement of the facial bones may cause facial deformity, loss of teeth and other dental conditions, and, rarely, airway compression.

Fractures are serious complications of Paget's disease and usually occur in long bones at areas of active or advancing lytic lesions. Common fracture sites are the femoral shaft and subtrochanteric regions. Neoplasms arising from pagetic bone are rare. The incidence of sarcoma appears to be decreasing, possibly because of earlier, more effective treatment with potent antiresorptive agents. The majority of tumors are osteosarcomas, which usually present with new pain in a longstanding pagetic lesion. Osteoclast-rich benign giant cell tumors may arise in areas adjacent to pagetic bone and respond to glucocorticoid therapy.

Cardiovascular complications may occur in patients with involvement of large (15–35%) portions of the skeleton and a high degree of disease activity (ALP four times above normal). The extensive arteriovenous shunting and marked increases in blood flow through the vascular pagetic bone lead to a high-output state and cardiac enlargement. However, high-output heart failure is relatively rare and usually develops in patients with concomitant cardiac pathology. In addition, calcific aortic stenosis and diffuse vascular calcifications have been associated with Paget's disease.

Diagnosis

The diagnosis may be suggested on clinical examination by the presence of an enlarged skull with frontal bossing, bowing of an extremity, or short stature with simian posturing. An extremity with an area of warmth and tenderness to palpation may suggest an underlying pagetic lesion. Other findings include bony deformity of the pelvis, skull, spine, and extremities; arthritic involvement of the joints adjacent to lesions; and leg length discrepancy resulting from deformities of the long bones.

Paget's disease is usually diagnosed from radiologic and biochemical abnormalities. Radiographic findings typical of Paget's disease include enlargement or expansion of an entire bone or area of a long bone, cortical thickening, coarsening of trabecular markings, and typical lytic and sclerotic changes. Skull radiographs (**Fig. 29-2**) reveal regions of "cotton wool," or osteoporosis circumscripta; thickening of diploic areas; and enlargement and sclerosis of a portion or all of one or more skull bones. Vertebral cortical thickening of the superior and inferior end plates creates a "picture frame" vertebra. Diffuse radiodense enlargement of a vertebra is referred to as "ivory vertebra." Pelvic radiographs may demonstrate disruption or fusion of the sacroiliac joints; porotic and radiodense lesions of the ilium with whorls of coarse trabeculation; a thickened and sclerotic ileopectinal line (Brim sign); and softening with protrusio acetabuli, with axial migration of the hips and functional flexion contracture. Radiographs of long bones reveal bowing deformity and typical pagetic changes of cortical thickening and expansion and areas of lucency and sclerosis (**Fig. 29-3**). Radionuclide ^{99m}Tc bone scans are less specific but are more sensitive than standard radiographs for identifying sites of active skeletal lesions. Suspected areas of malignant transformation are best distinguished from pagetic bone by CT or MRI. Definitive diagnosis of malignancy requires bone biopsy.

Biochemical evaluation is useful in the diagnosis and management of Paget's disease. The marked increase in bone turnover can be monitored using biochemical markers of bone formation and resorption. The parallel rise in serum ALP and urinary hydroxyproline levels, markers of bone formation and resorption, respectively, confirm the coupling of bone formation and resorption in Paget's disease. The degree of bone marker elevation reflects the extent and severity of the disease. Patients with the highest elevation of ALP (10 times the upper limit of normal) typically have involvement of the skull

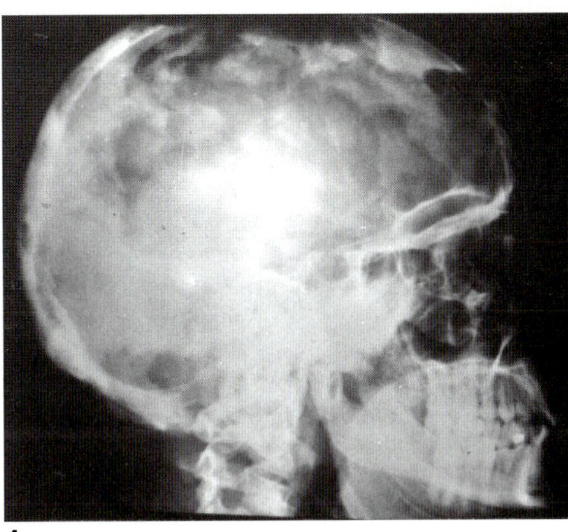

A

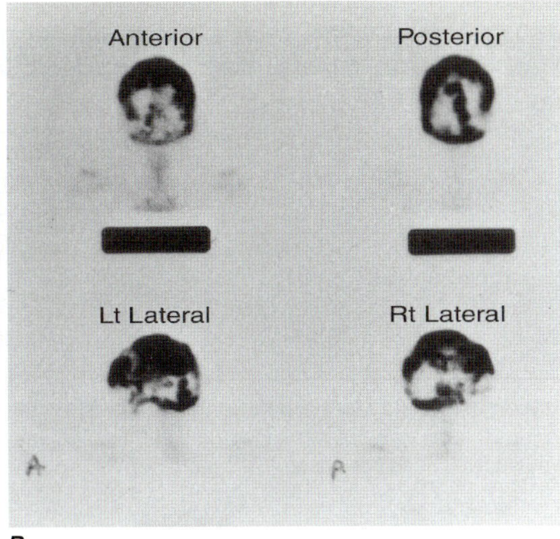

B

FIGURE 29-2

A 48-year-old woman with Paget's disease of the skull. ***A.*** Lateral radiograph showing areas of both bone resorption and sclerosis. ***B.*** ^{99m}Tc HDP bone scan with anterior, posterior, and lateral views of the skull showing diffuse isotope uptake by the frontal, parietal, occipital, and petrous bones.

and at least one other skeletal site. Lower values suggest less extensive involvement or a quiescent phase of the disease. For most patients, serum total ALP remains the test of choice for both diagnosis and assessing response to therapy. Occasionally, a symptomatic patient with evidence of progression at a single site may have a normal total ALP level but increased bone-specific ALP. Serum osteocalcin, a marker of bone formation, is not always elevated in patients with active Paget's disease and is not recommended for use in diagnosis or management.

FIGURE 29-3

Radiograph of a 73-year-old man with Paget's disease of the right proximal femur. Note the coarsening of the trabecular pattern with marked cortical thickening and narrowing of the joint space consistent with osteoarthritis secondary to pagetic deformity of the right femur.

Urinary and serum deoxypyridinoline, N-telopeptide, and C-telopeptide levels are products of type I collagen degradation and are more specific for bone resorption than hydroxyproline. These newer bone resorption markers have distinct advantages over measurement of 24-h or second-morning void hydroxyproline/creatinine ratio, which requires control of dietary gelatin intake and precise urine collection and analysis. The new resorption markers decrease more rapidly in response to therapy than does ALP.

Serum calcium and phosphate levels are normal in Paget's disease. Immobilization of a patient with active Paget's disease may rarely cause hypercalcemia and hypercalciuria and increase the risk for nephrolithiasis. However, the discovery of hypercalcemia, even in the presence of immobilization, should prompt a search for another cause of hypercalcemia. In contrast, hypocalcemia or mild secondary hyperparathyroidism may develop in Paget patients with very active bone formation and insufficient dietary calcium intake. Hypocalcemia can occur during bisphosphonate therapy when bone resorption is rapidly suppressed and active bone formation continues. Hypocalcemia may be prevented by adequate calcium and vitamin D intake.

℞ Treatment: PAGET'S DISEASE OF BONE

The development of effective and potent pharmacologic agents (Table 29-1) has changed the treatment philosophy from treating only symptomatic patients to treating asymptomatic patients who are at risk for complications. Pharmacologic therapy is indicated in the following circumstances: to control symptoms caused by

TABLE 29-1

PHARMACOLOGIC AGENTS APPROVED FOR TREATMENT OF PAGET'S DISEASE

NAME (BRAND)	POTENCY[a]	DOSE	MODE OF ADMINISTRATION
Etidronate (Didronel)	1	400 mg/d for 6 mos	Fasting PO
Tiludronate (Skelid)	10	400 mg/d for 3 mos	Fasting PO
Pamidronate (Aredia)	100	30 mg/d for 3 doses *or* 60–90 mg once	IV
Alendronate (Fosamax)	700	30 mg/d for 2 mos	Fasting PO
Risedronate (Actonel)	1000	30 mg/d for 2 mos	Fasting PO
Zoledronate (Zometa)	NK	5 mg	IV
Calcitonin (Miacalcin)	NA	100 U daily	SC

[a]Potency is relative to etidronate. For each tablet, etidronate strength is 400 mg; tiludronate is 200 mg; alendronate is 40 mg; and risedronate is 30 mg. Miacalcin nasal spray is not approved for use in Paget's disease.
Note: NK, not known; NA, does not apply.

metabolically active Paget's disease such as bone pain, fracture, headache, pain from pagetic radiculopathy or arthropathy, or neurologic complications; to decrease local blood flow and minimize operative blood loss in patients undergoing surgery at an active pagetic site; to reduce hypercalciuria that may occur during immobilization; and to decrease the risk of complications when disease activity is high (elevated ALP) and when the site of involvement involves weight-bearing bones, areas adjacent to major joints, vertebral bodies, and skull. Whether early therapy prevents late complications remains to be determined. However, the restoration of normal bone architecture following suppression of pagetic activity suggests that treatment may prevent further deformities and complications.

Agents approved for treatment of Paget's disease suppress the very high rates of bone resorption and secondarily decrease the high rates of bone formation (Table 29-1). As a result of decreasing bone turnover, pagetic structural patterns, including areas of poorly mineralized woven bone, are replaced by more normal cancellous or lamellar bone. The improvement in skeletal structure can be demonstrated on standard radiographs and ^{99m}Tc bone scans, which show decreased isotope accumulation in pagetic sites. Reduced bone turnover can be documented by a decline in urine or serum resorption markers (pyridinoline, deoxypyridinoline, N-telopeptide, C-telopeptide) and serum markers of bone formation (ALP, osteocalcin).

The potencies of various bisphosphonates are expressed relative to that of etidronate, the first clinically useful agent in this class. Etidronate use is now limited as the doses required to suppress bone resorption may impair mineralization. Thus, etidronate is administered in 6-month treatment cycles followed by a 6-month drug-free period. Failure to adhere to the cyclic regimen can produce osteomalacia manifested by bone pain and fractures. Etidronate should not be used in patients with advanced lytic lesions in weight-bearing bones. The major advantage of etidronate is that it is relatively well tolerated and only occasionally causes transient diarrhea or bone pain.

The second-generation oral bisphosphonates tiludronate, alendronate, and risedronate are more potent than etidronate in controlling bone turnover and thus induce a longer remission at a lower dose. The lower doses reduce the risks of impaired mineralization and osteomalacia. Oral bisphosphonates are poorly absorbed and have the potential to produce esophageal ulceration, reflux, and, rarely, perforation. They should be taken first thing in the morning on an empty stomach, followed by maintenance of upright posture with no food or drink for 30–60 min. Other medications, liquids, and food should be delayed for at least 30–60 min after taking bisphosphonates to optimize absorption. Tiludronate daily for 3 months normalizes ALP in 24–35% of moderately affected patients. In patients with moderate to severe disease, alendronate for 6 months normalizes ALP in >67% of patients, with an overall fall in ALP of 79% compared to 44% with etidronate. In patients with moderately active disease, risedronate daily for 2–3 months reduces serum ALP by 80% and by 6 months after treatment normalizes indices of bone turnover in 73% of patients compared to 15% of those receiving etidronate.

Pamidronate is approved for IV use in Paget's disease. The recommended dose is 30 mg dissolved in 500 mL of normal saline or dextrose IV over 4 h on 3 consecutive days. The dose can be adjusted to each patient's requirements. A single 60-mg IV dose of pamidronate may normalize bone turnover in patients with mild disease. In contrast, patients with moderate to severe disease (elevation of ALP of three to four times normal) may require two to four doses of pamidronate, 60–90 mg IV, every 1–2 weeks. Patients with very severe disease may require a total dose of pamidronate of 300–500 mg given weekly over several weeks. Although suppression of urinary bone markers occurs after a few days to weeks, normalization of serum ALP levels often requires at least 3 months. Consequently, the effects of pamidronate are best evaluated 3 months after the initial dose.

In 2006, IV zoledronate received approval by the U.S. Food and Drug Administration (FDA) for use in Paget's disease. One 5-mg infusion of zoledronate normalizes ALP in about 90% of patients by 6 months, and the therapeutic effect persists for an additional 6 months in most patients.

Pamidronate and zoledronate are generally well tolerated; however, a small number of patients experience a flulike syndrome that may begin 24 h after the first infusion. In patients with high bone turnover, vitamin D (400–800 IU daily) and calcium (500 mg three times daily) should be provided to prevent hypocalcemia and secondary hyperparathyroidism. Indications for IV therapy include mild disease and normalization of bone turnover after a single infusion; previous prevention of disease progression; refractoriness to oral therapy; need for rapid response for those with neurologic symptoms, those with severe bone pain due to a lytic lesion, or those at risk of an impending fracture; and as pretreatment prior to elective surgery in an area of active disease. Remission following pamidronate and zoledronate therapy may persist for ≥1 year.

The SC injectable form of salmon calcitonin is approved for the treatment of Paget's disease. Intranasal calcitonin spray is approved for osteoporosis at a dose of 200 U/d; however, the efficacy of this dose in Paget's disease has not been thoroughly studied. The usual starting dose of injectable calcitonin (100 U/d) reduces ALP by 50% and may relieve skeletal symptoms. The dose may be reduced to 50 U/d three times weekly after an initial favorable response to 100 U daily; however, the lower dose may require long-term use to sustain efficacy. The common side effects of calcitonin therapy are nausea and facial flushing. Secondary resistance after prolonged use may be due to either the formation of anticalcitonin antibodies or downregulation of osteoclastic cell-surface calcitonin receptors. The lower potency and injectable mode of delivery make this agent a less attractive treatment option that should be reserved for patients who either do not tolerate or do not respond to bisphosphonates.

SCLEROSING BONE DISORDERS

OSTEOPETROSIS

Osteopetrosis refers to a group of disorders caused by severe impairment of osteoclast-mediated bone resorption. Other terms that are often used include marble bone disease, which captures the solid x-ray appearance of the involved skeleton, and Albers-Schonberg disease, which refers to the milder, adult form of osteopetrosis also known as autosomal dominant osteopetrosis type II. The major types of osteopetrosis include malignant (severe, infantile, autosomal recessive) osteopetrosis and benign (adult, autosomal dominant) osteopetrosis types I and II. A rare autosomal recessive intermediate form has a more benign prognosis. Autosomal recessive carbonic anhydrase (CA) II deficiency produces osteopetrosis of intermediate severity associated with renal tubular acidosis and cerebral calcification.

Etiology and Genetics

Naturally occurring and gene knockout animal models with phenotypes similar to those of the human disorders have been used to explore the genetic basis of osteopetrosis. The primary defect in osteopetrosis is the loss of osteoclastic bone resorption and preservation of normal osteoblastic bone formation. Osteoprotegerin (OPG) is a soluble decoy receptor that binds osteoblast-derived RANK ligand, which mediates osteoclast differentiation and activation (Fig. 29-1). Transgenic mice that overexpress OPG develop osteopetrosis, presumably by blocking RANK ligand. Mice deficient in RANK lack osteoclasts and develop severe osteopetrosis.

Recessive mutations of CA II prevent osteoclasts from generating an acid environment in the clear zone between its ruffled border and the adjacent mineral surface. Absence of CA II, therefore, impairs osteoclastic bone resorption. Other forms of human disease have less clear genetic defects. About one-half of the patients with malignant infantile osteopetrosis have a mutation in the *TCIRG1* gene encoding the osteoclast-specific subunit of the vacuolar proton pump, which mediates the acidification of the interface between bone mineral and the osteoclast ruffled border. Mutations in the *CICN7* chloride channel gene cause autosomal dominant osteopetrosis type II.

Clinical Presentation

The incidence of autosomal recessive severe (malignant) osteopetrosis ranges from 1 in 200,000 to 1 in 500,000 live births. As bone and cartilage fail to undergo modeling, paralysis of one or more cranial nerves may occur due to narrowing of the cranial foramina. Failure of skeletal modeling also results in inadequate marrow space, leading to extramedullary hematopoiesis with hypersplenism and pancytopenia. Hypocalcemia due to lack of osteoclastic bone resorption may occur in infants and young children. The untreated infantile disease is fatal, often before age 5.

Adult (benign) osteopetrosis is an autosomal dominant disease that is usually diagnosed by the discovery of typical skeletal changes in young adults who undergo radiologic evaluation of a fracture. The prevalence is 1 in 100,000 to 1 in 500,000 adults. The course is not always benign, as fractures may be accompanied by loss of vision, deafness, psychomotor delay, mandibular osteomyelitis, and other complications usually associated with the juvenile form. In some kindreds, nonpenetrance results in skip generations, while in other families severely affected children are born into families with benign disease. The milder form of the disease does not usually require treatment.

Radiography

Typically, there are generalized symmetric increases in bone mass with thickening of both cortical and trabecular bone. Diaphyses and metaphyses are broadened, and alternating sclerotic and lucent bands may be seen in the iliac crests, at the ends of long bones, and in vertebral bodies. The cranium is usually thickened, particularly at the base of the skull, and the paranasal and mastoid sinuses are underpneumatized.

Laboratory Findings

The only significant laboratory findings are elevated serum levels of osteoclast-derived tartrate-resistant acid phosphatase (TRAP) and the brain isoenzyme of creatine kinase. Serum calcium may be low in severe disease, and parathyroid hormone and 1,25-dihydroxyvitamin D levels may be elevated in response to hypocalcemia.

℞ Treatment: OSTEOPETROSIS

Allogenic HLA-identical bone marrow transplantation has been successful in some children. Following transplantation, the marrow contains progenitor cells and normally functioning osteoclasts. A cure is most likely when children are transplanted before age 4. Marrow transplantation from nonidentical HLA-matched donors has a much higher failure rate. Limited studies in small numbers of patients have suggested variable benefits following treatment with interferon γ-1β, 1,25-dihydroxyvitamin D (which stimulates osteoclasts directly), methylprednisolone, and a low calcium/high-phosphate diet.

Surgical intervention is indicated to decompress optic or auditory nerve compression. Orthopedic management is required for the surgical treatment of fractures and their complications including malunion and postfracture deformity.

PYKNODYSOSTOSIS

This is an autosomal recessive form of osteosclerosis that is believed to have affected the French impressionist painter Henri de Toulouse-Lautrec. The molecular basis involves mutations in the gene that encodes cathepsin K, a lysosomal metalloproteinase highly expressed in osteoclasts and important for bone matrix degradation. Osteoclasts are present but do not function normally. Pyknodysostosis is a form of short-limb dwarfism that presents with frequent fractures but usually normal life span. Clinical features include short stature; kyphoscoliosis and deformities of the chest; high arched palate; proptosis; blue sclerae; dysmorphic features including small face and chin, frontooccipital prominence, pointed beaked nose, large cranium, and obtuse mandibular angle; and small square hands with hypoplastic nails. Radiographs demonstrate a generalized increase in bone density, but in contrast to osteopetrosis, the long bones are normally shaped. Separated cranial sutures, including the persistent patency of the anterior fontanel, are characteristic of the disorder. There may also be hypoplasia of the sinuses, mandible, distal clavicles, and terminal phalanges. Persistence of deciduous teeth and sclerosis of the calvarium and base of the skull are also common. Histologic evaluation shows normal cortical bone architecture with decreased osteoblastic and osteoclastic activities. Serum chemistries are normal, and unlike osteopetrosis, there is no anemia. There is no known treatment for this condition, and no reports of attempted bone marrow transplant.

PROGRESSIVE DIAPHYSEAL DYSPLASIA

Also known as *Camurati-Engelmann disease*, progressive diaphyseal dysplasia is an autosomal dominant disorder that is characterized radiographically by diaphyseal hyperostosis and a symmetric thickening and increased diameter of the endosteal and periosteal surfaces of the diaphyses of the long bones, particularly the femur and tibia, and, less often, the fibula, radius, and ulna. The genetic defect responsible for the disease has been localized to the area of chromosome 19q13.2 encoding tumor growth factor (TGF) β1. The mutation promotes activation of TGF-β1. The clinical severity is variable. The most common presenting symptoms are pain and tenderness of the involved areas, fatigue, muscle wasting, and gait disturbance. The weakness may be mistaken for muscular dystrophy. Characteristic body habitus includes thin limbs with little muscle mass yet prominent and palpable bones and, when the skull is involved, large head with prominent forehead and proptosis. Patients may also display signs of cranial nerve palsies, hydrocephalus, central hypogonadism, and Raynaud phenomenon. Radiographically, patchy progressive endosteal and periosteal new bone formation is observed along the diaphyses of the long bones. Bone scintigraphy shows increased radiotracer uptake in involved areas.

Treatment with low-dose glucocorticoids relieves bone pain and may reverse the abnormal bone formation. Intermittent bisphosphonate therapy has produced clinical improvement in a limited number of patients.

HYPEROSTOSIS CORTICALIS GENERALISATA

This is also known as *van Buchem disease*; it is an autosomal recessive disorder characterized by endosteal hyperostosis in which osteosclerosis involves the skull, mandible, clavicles, and ribs. The major manifestations are due to narrowed cranial foramina with neural compressions that may result in optic atrophy, facial paralysis, and deafness. Adults may have an enlarged mandible. Serum ALP levels may be elevated, which reflects the uncoupled bone remodeling with high osteoblastic formation rates and low osteoclastic resorption. As a result, there is increased accumulation of normal bone. Endosteal hyperostosis with syndactyly, known as *sclerosteosis*, is a more severe form. The genetic defects for both sclerosteosis and van Buchem disease have been assigned to the same region of the chromosome 17q12-q21. It is possible that both conditions may have deactivating mutations in the *BEER* (bone-expressed equilibrium regulator) gene.

MELORHEOSTOSIS

Melorheostosis (Greek, "flowing hyperostosis") may occur sporadically or follow a pattern consistent with an autosomal recessive disorder. The major manifestation is progressive linear hyperostosis in one or more bones of one limb, usually a lower extremity. The name comes from the radiographic appearance of the involved bone, which resembles melted wax that has dripped down a candle. Symptoms appear during childhood as pain or stiffness in the area of sclerotic bone. There may be associated ectopic soft tissue masses, composed of cartilage or osseous tissue, and skin changes overlying the involved bone, consisting of scleroderma-like areas and hypertrichosis. The disease does not progress in adults, but pain and stiffness may persist. Laboratory tests are unremarkable. No specific etiology is known. There is no specific treatment. Surgical interventions to correct contractures are often unsuccessful.

OSTEOPOIKILOSIS

The literal translation of osteopoikilosis is "spotted bones"; it is a benign autosomal dominant condition in which numerous small, variably shaped (usually round or oval) foci of bony sclerosis are seen in the epiphyses and adjacent metaphyses. The lesions may involve any bone except the skull, ribs, and vertebrae. They may be misidentified as metastatic lesions. The main differentiating points are that bony lesions of osteopoikilosis are stable over time and do not accumulate radionucleotide on bone scanning. In some kindreds, osteopoikilosis is associated with connective tissue nevi known as *dermatofibrosis lenticularis disseminata*, also known as *Buschke-Ollendorf syndrome*. Histologic inspection reveals thickened but otherwise normal trabeculae and islands of normal cortical bone. No treatment is indicated.

HEPATITIS C–ASSOCIATED OSTEOSCLEROSIS

Hepatitis C–associated osteosclerosis (HCAO) is a rare acquired diffuse osteosclerosis in adults with prior hepatitis C infection. After a latent period of several years, patients develop diffuse appendicular bone pain and a generalized increase in bone mass with elevated serum ALP. Bone biopsy and histomorphometry reveal increased rates of bone formation, decreased bone resorption with a marked decrease in osteoclasts, and dense lamellar bone. One patient had increased serum OPG levels, and bone biopsy showed large numbers of osteoblasts positive for OPG and reduced osteoclast number. Empirical therapy includes pain control and there may be beneficial response to either calcitonin or bisphosphonate.

DISORDERS ASSOCIATED WITH DEFECTIVE MINERALIZATION

HYPOPHOSPHATASIA

This is a rare inherited disorder that presents as rickets in infants and children or osteomalacia in adults with paradoxically low serum levels of ALP. The frequency of the severe neonatal and infantile forms is about 1 in 100,000 live births in Canada, where the disease is most common because of its high prevalence among Mennonites and Hutterites. It is rare in African Americans. The severity of the disease is remarkably variable, ranging from intrauterine death associated with profound skeletal hypomineralization at one extreme, to premature tooth loss as the only manifestation in some adults. Severe cases are inherited in an autosomal recessive manner, but the genetic patterns are less clear for the milder forms. The disease is caused by a deficiency of tissue nonspecific (bone/liver/kidney) ALP (TNSALP), which, although ubiquitous, results only in bone abnormalities. Protein levels and functions of the other ALP isozymes (germ cell, intestinal, placental) are normal. Defective ALP permits accumulation of its major naturally occurring substrates including phosphoethanolamine (PEA), inorganic pyrophosphate (PPi), and pyridoxal 5′-phosphate (PLP). The accumulation of PPi interferes with mineralization through its action as a potent inhibitor of hydroxyapatite crystal growth.

Perinatal hypophosphatasia becomes manifest during pregnancy and is often complicated by polyhydramnios and intrauterine death. The infantile form becomes clinically apparent before age 6 months with failure to thrive, rachitic deformities, functional craniosynostosis despite widely open fontanels (which are actually hypomineralized areas of the calvarium), raised intracranial pressure, and flail chest and predisposition to pneumonia. Hypercalcemia and hypercalciuria are common. This form has a mortality rate of about 50%. Prognosis seems to improve for the children who survive infancy. Childhood hypophosphatasia has variable clinical presentation. Premature loss of deciduous teeth (before age 5 years) is the hallmark of the disease. Rickets causes delayed walking with waddling gait, short stature, and dolichocephalic skull with frontal bossing. The disease often improves during puberty but may recur in adult life. Adult hypophosphatasia presents during middle age with painful, poorly healing metatarsal stress fractures or thigh pain due to femoral pseudofractures.

Laboratory investigation reveals low ALP levels and normal or elevated levels of serum calcium and phosphorus despite clinical and radiologic evidence of rickets or osteomalacia. Serum parathyroid hormone, 25-hydroxyvitamin D, and 1,25-dihydroxyvitamin D levels are normal. The elevation of PLP is specific for the disease and may even be present in asymptomatic parents of severely affected children. As vitamin B_6 increases PLP levels, vitamin B_6 supplements should be discontinued 1 week before testing.

There is no established medical therapy. In contrast to other forms of rickets and osteomalacia, calcium and vitamin D supplementation should be avoided as they may aggravate hypercalcemia and hypercalciuria. A low-calcium diet, glucocorticoids, and calcitonin have been used in a small number of patients with variable responses. Because fracture healing is poor, placement of intramedullary rods is best for acute fracture repair and for prophylactic prevention of fractures.

AXIAL OSTEOMALACIA

This is a rare disorder characterized by defective skeletal mineralization despite normal serum calcium and phosphate levels. Clinically, the disorder presents in middle-aged or elderly men with chronic axial skeletal discomfort. Cervical spine pain may also be present. Radiographic findings are mainly osteosclerosis due to coarsened trabecular patterns typical of osteomalacia. Spine, pelvis, and ribs are most commonly affected. Histologic changes show defective mineralization and flat, inactive osteoblasts. The primary defect appears to be an acquired defect in osteoblast function. The course is benign and there is no established treatment. Calcium and vitamin D therapies are not effective.

FIBROGENESIS IMPERFECTA OSSIUM

This is a rare condition of unknown etiology. It presents in both sexes, in middle age or later, with progressive, intractable skeletal pain and fractures, worsening immobilization, and a debilitating course. Radiographic evaluation reveals generalized osteomalacia, osteopenia, and occasional pseudofractures. Histologic features include a tangled pattern of collagen fibrils with abundant osteoblasts and osteoclasts. There is no effective treatment. Spontaneous remission has been reported in a small number of patients. Calcium and vitamin D have not been beneficial.

FIBROUS DYSPLASIA AND MCCUNE-ALBRIGHT SYNDROME

Fibrous dysplasia is a sporadic disorder characterized by the presence of one (monostotic) or more (polyostotic) expanding fibrous skeletal lesions composed of bone-forming mesenchyme. The association of the polyostotic form with café-au-lait spots and hyperfunction of an endocrine system such as pseudoprecocious puberty of ovarian origin is known as *McCune-Albright syndrome* (MAS). A spectrum of the phenotypes is caused by activating mutations in the *GNAS1* gene, which encodes the α subunit of the stimulatory G protein ($G_s\alpha$). As the postzygotic mutations occur at different stages of early development, the extent and type of tissue affected are variable and explain the mosaic pattern of skin and bone changes. GTP binding activates the $G_s\alpha$ regulatory protein and mutations in regions of $G_s\alpha$ that selectively inhibit GTPase activity, which results in constitutive stimulation of the cyclic AMP–protein kinase A signal transduction pathway. Such mutations of the $G_s\alpha$ protein–coupled receptor may cause autonomous function in bone (parathyroid hormone receptor); skin (melanocyte-stimulating hormone receptor); and various endocrine glands including ovary (follicle-stimulating hormone receptor), thyroid (thyroid-stimulating hormone receptor), adrenal (adrenocorticotropic hormone receptor), and pituitary (growth hormone–releasing hormone receptor). The skeletal lesions are composed largely of mesenchymal cells that do not differentiate into osteoblasts, resulting in the formation of imperfect bone. In some areas of bone, fibroblast-like cells develop features of osteoblasts in that they produce extracellular matrix that organizes into woven bone. Calcification may occur in some areas. In other areas, cells have features of chondrocytes and produce cartilage-like extracellular matrix.

Clinical Presentation

Fibrous dysplasia occurs with equal frequency in both sexes, whereas MAS with precocious puberty is more common (10:1) in girls. The monostotic form is the most common and is usually diagnosed in patients between 20 and 30 years of age without associated skin lesions. The polyostotic form typically manifests in children <10 years of age and may progress with age. Early-onset disease is generally more severe. Lesions may become quiescent in puberty and progress during pregnancy or with estrogen therapy. In polyostotic fibrous dysplasia, the lesions most commonly involve the maxilla and other craniofacial bones, ribs, and metaphyseal or diaphyseal portions of the proximal femur or tibia. Expanding bone lesions may cause pain, deformity, fractures, and nerve entrapment. Sarcomatous degeneration involving the facial bones or femur is infrequent (<1%). The risk of malignant transformation is increased by radiation, which has proven to be ineffective treatment. In rare patients with widespread lesions, renal phosphate wasting and hypophosphatemia may cause rickets or osteomalacia. Hypophosphatemia may be due to production of a phosphaturic factor by the abnormal fibrous tissue.

MAS patients may have café-au-lait spots, which are flat, hyperpigmented skin lesions that have rough borders ("coast of Maine") in contrast to the café-au-lait lesions of neurofibromatosis that have smooth borders ("coast of California"). The most common endocrinopathy is isosexual pseudoprecocious puberty in girls. Other less common endocrine disorders include thyrotoxicosis, Cushing's syndrome, acromegaly, hyperparathyroidism, hyperprolactinemia, and pseudoprecocious puberty in boys.

Radiographic Findings

In long bones, the fibrous dysplastic lesions are typically well-defined, radiolucent areas with thin cortices and a ground-glass appearance. Lesions may be lobulated with trabeculated areas of radiolucency (**Fig. 29-4**). Involvement of facial bones usually presents as radiodense lesions, which may create a leonine appearance (leontiasis ossea). Expansile cranial lesions may narrow foramina and cause optic lesions, reduce hearing, and create other manifestations of cranial nerve compression.

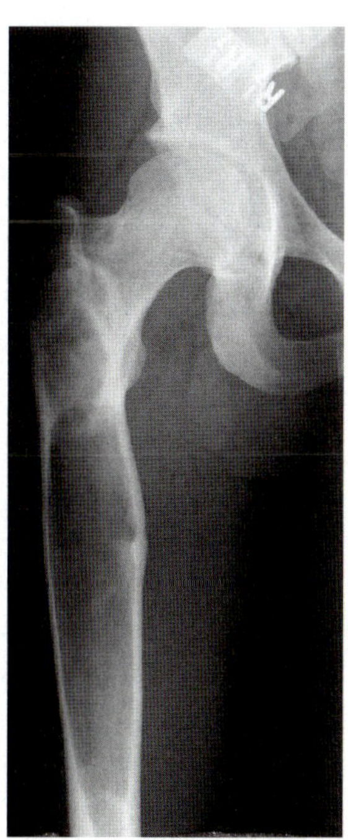

FIGURE 29-4

Radiograph of a 16-year-old male with fibrous dysplasia of the right proximal femur. Note the multiple cystic lesions, including the large lucent lesion in the proximal mid-shaft with scalloping of the interior surface. The femoral neck contains two lucent cystic lesions.

Laboratory Results

Serum ALP is occasionally elevated but calcium, parathyroid hormone, 25-hydroxyvitamin D, and 1,25-dihydroxyvitamin D levels are normal. Patients with extensive polyostotic lesions may have hypophosphatemia, hyperphosphaturia, and osteomalacia. The hypophosphatemia and phosphaturia are directly related to the levels of fibroblast growth factor 23 (FGF-23). Biochemical markers of bone turnover may be elevated.

Treatment:
℞ FIBROUS DYSPLASIA AND MCCUNE-ALBRIGHT SYNDROME

Spontaneous healing of the lesions does not occur, and there is no established effective treatment. Improvement in bone pain and partial or complete resolution of radiographic lesions have been reported after IV bisphosphonate therapy. Surgical stabilization is used to prevent pathologic fracture or destruction of a major joint space and to relieve nerve root or cranial nerve compression or sinus obstruction.

OTHER DYSPLASIAS OF BONE AND CARTILAGE

PACHYDERMOPERIOSTOSIS

Pachydermoperiostosis, or hypertrophic osteoarthropathy (primary or idiopathic), is an autosomal dominant disorder characterized by periosteal new bone formation that involves the distal extremities. The lesions present as clubbing of the digits and hyperhidrosis and thickening of the skin, primarily of the face and forehead. The changes usually appear during adolescence, progress over the next decade, and then become quiescent. During the active phase, progressive enlargement of the hands and feet produces a pawlike appearance, which may be mistaken for acromegaly. Arthralgias, pseudogout, and limited mobility may also occur. The disorder must be differentiated from secondary hypertrophic osteopathy that develops during the course of serious pulmonary disorders. The two conditions can be differentiated by standard radiography of the digits in which secondary pachydermoperiostosis has exuberant periosteal new bone formation and a smooth and undulating surface. In contrast, primary hypertrophic osteopathy has an irregular periosteal surface.

There are no diagnostic blood or urine tests. Synovial fluid does not have an inflammatory profile. There is no specific therapy, although a limited experience with colchicine suggests some benefit in controlling the arthralgias.

OSTEOCHONDRODYSPLASIAS

These include several hundred heritable disorders of connective tissue. These primary abnormalities of cartilage manifest as disturbances in cartilage and bone growth. Selected growth plate chondrodysplasias are described here.

Achondrodysplasia

This is a relatively common form of short-limb dwarfism that occurs in 1 in 15,000 to 1 in 40,000 live births. The disease is caused by a mutation of the fibroblast growth factor receptor 3 (*FGFR3*) gene that results in a gain-of-function state. Most cases are sporadic mutations. However, when the disorder appears in families, the inheritance pattern is consistent with an autosomal dominant disorder. The primary defect is abnormal chondrocyte proliferation at the growth plate that causes development of short but proportionately thick long bones. Other regions of the long bones may be relatively unaffected. The disorder is manifest by the presence of short limbs (particularly the proximal portions), normal trunk, large head, saddle nose, and an exaggerated lumbar lordosis. Severe spinal deformity may lead to cord compression. The homozygous disorder is more serious than the sporadic form and may cause neonatal death. Pseudoachondroplasia clinically resembles achondroplasia but has no skull abnormalities.

Enchondromatosis

This is also called *dyschondroplasia*, or *Ollier disease*; it is also a disorder of the growth plate in which the primary cartilage is not resorbed. Cartilage ossification proceeds normally but it is not resorbed normally, leading to cartilage accumulation. The changes are most marked at the ends of long bones where the highest growth rates occur. Chondrosarcoma develops infrequently. The association of enchondromatosis and cavernous hemangiomas of the skin and soft tissues is known as *Maffucci syndrome*. Both Ollier disease and Maffucci syndrome are associated with various malignancies, including granulosa cell tumor of the ovary and cerebral glioma.

Multiple Exostoses

This is also called *diaphyseal aclasis*, or *osteochondromatosis*; it is a genetic disorder that follows an autosomal dominant pattern of inheritance. In this condition, areas of growth plates become displaced, presumably by growing through a defect in the perichondrium. The lesion begins with vascular invasion of the growth plate cartilage, resulting in a characteristic radiographic finding of a mass that is in direct communication with the marrow cavity of the parent bone. The underlying cortex is resorbed. The disease is caused by inactivating mutations of the *EXT1* and *EXT2* genes, whose products normally regulate processing of chondrocyte cytoskeletal proteins. The products of the *EXT* gene likely function as tumor suppressors, with the loss-of-function mutation resulting in abnormal proliferation of growth plate cartilage. Solitary or multiple lesions are located in the metaphyses of long bones. Although usually asymptomatic, the lesions may interfere with joint or tendon function or compress peripheral nerves. The lesions stop growing when growth ceases but may recur during pregnancy. There is a small risk for malignant transformation into chondrosarcoma.

EXTRASKELETAL (ECTOPIC) CALCIFICATION AND OSSIFICATION

Deposition of calcium phosphate crystals (*calcification*) or formation of true bone (*ossification*) in nonosseous soft tissue may occur by one of three mechanisms: (1) metastatic calcification due to a supranormal calcium × phosphate concentration product in extracellular fluid; (2) dystrophic calcification due to mineral deposition into metabolically impaired or dead tissue despite normal serum levels of calcium and phosphate; and (3) ectopic ossification, or true bone formation. Disorders that may cause extraskeletal calcification or ossification are listed in Table 29-2.

METASTATIC CALCIFICATION

Soft tissue calcification may complicate diseases associated with significant hypercalcemia, hyperphosphatemia, or both. In addition, vitamin D and phosphate treatments or calcium administration in the presence of mild hyperphosphatemia, such as during hemodialysis, may induce ectopic calcification. Calcium phosphate precipitation may complicate any disorder when the serum calcium × phosphate concentration product is >75. The initial calcium phosphate deposition is in the form of small, poorly organized crystals, which subsequently organize into hydroxyapatite crystals. Calcifications that occur in hypercalcemic states with normal or low phosphate have a predilection for kidney, lungs, and gastric mucosa. Hyperphosphatemia with normal or low serum calcium may promote soft tissue calcification with predilection for the kidney and arteries. The disturbances of calcium and phosphate in renal failure and hemodialysis are common causes of soft tissue (metastatic) calcification.

TUMORAL CALCINOSIS

This is a rare genetic disorder characterized by masses of metastatic calcifications in soft tissues around major

TABLE 29-2

DISEASES AND CONDITIONS ASSOCIATED WITH ECTOPIC CALCIFICATION AND OSSIFICATION

Metastatic calcification	Dystrophic calcification
Hypercalcemic states	Inflammatory disorders
Primary hyperparathyroidism	Scleroderma
Sarcoidosis	Dermatomyositis
Vitamin D intoxication	Systemic lupus erythematosus
Milk-alkali syndrome	Trauma induced
Renal failure	Ectopic ossification
Hyperphosphatemia	Myositis ossificans
Tumoral calcinosis	Post surgery
Secondary hyperparathyroidism	Burns
Pseudohypoparathyroidism	Neurologic injury
Renal failure	Other trauma
Hemodialysis	Fibrodysplasia ossificans progressiva
Cell lysis following chemotherapy	
Therapy with vitamin D and phosphate	

joints, most often shoulders, hips, and ankles. Tumoral calcinosis differs from other disorders in that the periarticular masses contain hydroxyapatite crystals or amorphous calcium phosphate complexes, while in fibrodysplasia ossificans progressiva, true bone is formed in soft tissues. About one-third of tumoral calcinosis cases are familial, with both autosomal recessive and autosomal dominant modes of inheritance reported. The disease is also associated with a variably expressed abnormality of dentition marked by short bulbous roots, pulp calcification, and radicular dentin deposited in swirls. The primary defect responsible for the metastatic calcification appears to be hyperphosphatemia resulting from the increased capacity of the renal tubule to reabsorb filtered phosphate. Spontaneous soft tissue calcification is related to the elevated serum phosphate, which along with normal serum calcium exceeds the concentration product of 75.

All of the North American patients reported have been African American. The disease usually presents in childhood and continues lifelong. The calcific masses are typically painless and grow at variable rates, sometimes becoming large and bulky. The masses are often located near major joints but remain extracapsular. Joint range of motion is not usually restricted unless the tumors are very large. Complications include compression of neural structures and ulceration of the overlying skin with drainage of chalky fluid and risk of secondary infection. Small deposits not detected by standard radiographs may be detected by ^{99m}Tc bone scanning. The most common laboratory findings are hyperphosphatemia and elevated serum 1,25-dihydroxyvitamin D levels. Serum calcium, parathyroid hormone, and ALP levels are usually normal. Renal function is also usually normal. Urine calcium and phosphate excretions are low, and calcium and phosphate balances are positive.

An acquired form of the disease may occur with other causes of hyperphosphatemia, such as secondary hyperparathyroidism associated with hemodialysis, hypoparathyroidism, pseudohypoparathyroidism, and massive cell lysis following chemotherapy for leukemia. Tissue trauma from joint movement may contribute to the periarticular calcifications. Metastatic calcifications are also seen in conditions associated with hypercalcemia, such as in sarcoidosis, vitamin D intoxication, milk-alkali syndrome, and primary hyperparathyroidism. In these conditions, however, mineral deposits are more likely to occur in proton-transporting organs such as kidney, lungs, and gastric mucosa in which an alkaline milieu is generated by the proton pumps.

Rx Treatment: TUMORAL CALCINOSIS

Therapeutic successes have been achieved with surgical removal of subcutaneous calcified masses, which tend not to recur if all calcification is removed from the site. Reduction of serum phosphate by chronic phosphorus restriction may be accomplished using low dietary phosphorus intake alone or in combination with oral phosphate binders. The addition of the phosphaturic agent acetazolamide may be useful. Limited experience using the phosphaturic action of calcitonin deserves further testing.

DYSTROPHIC CALCIFICATION

Posttraumatic calcification may occur with normal serum calcium and phosphate levels and normal ion solubility product. The deposited mineral is either in the form of amorphous calcium phosphate or hydroxyapatite crystals. Soft tissue calcification complicating connective tissue disorders such as scleroderma, dermatomyositis, and systemic lupus erythematosus may involve localized areas of the skin or deeper subcutaneous tissue and is referred to as *calcinosis circumscripta*. Mineral deposition at sites of deeper tissue injury including periarticular sites is called *calcinosis universalis*.

ECTOPIC OSSIFICATION

True extraskeletal bone formation that begins in areas of fasciitis following surgery, trauma, burns, or neurologic injury is referred to as *myositis ossificans*. The bone formed is organized as lamellar or trabecular, with normal osteoblasts and osteoclasts conducting active remodeling. Well-developed haversian systems and marrow elements may be present. A second cause of ectopic bone formation occurs in an inherited disorder, *fibrodysplasia ossificans progressiva*.

FIBRODYSPLASIA OSSIFICANS PROGRESSIVA

This is also called *myositis ossificans progressiva*; it is a rare autosomal dominant disorder characterized by congenital deformities of the hands and feet and episodic soft tissue swellings that ossify. Ectopic bone formation occurs in fascia, tendons, ligaments, and connective tissue within voluntary muscles. Tender, rubbery induration, sometimes precipitated by trauma, develops in the soft tissue and gradually calcifies. Eventually, heterotopic bone forms at these sites of soft tissue trauma. Morbidity results from heterotopic bone interfering with normal movement and function of muscle and other soft tissues. Mortality is usually related to restrictive lung disease caused by an inability of the chest to expand. Laboratory tests are unremarkable.

There is no effective medical therapy. Bisphosphonates, glucocorticoids, and a low-calcium diet have largely been ineffective in halting progression of the ossification. Surgical removal of ectopic bone is not recommended, as the trauma of surgery may precipitate formation of new areas of heterotopic bone. Dental complications including frozen jaw may occur following injection of local anesthetics. Thus, CT imaging of the mandible should be undertaken to detect early sites of soft tissue ossification before they are appreciated by standard radiography.

FURTHER READINGS

Hocking LJ et al: Domain-specific mutations in sequestosome 1 (SQSTM1) cause familial and sporadic Paget's disease. Hum Mol Genet 11:2735, 2002

Langston AL et al: Randomised trial of intensive bisphosphonate treatment versus symptomatic management in Paget's disease of bone. J Bone Miner Res, 2009, in press

Matthews BG et al: Failure to detect measles virus ribonucleic acid in bone cells from patients with Paget's disease. J Clin Endocrinol Metab 93:1398, 2008

Merchant A et al: Somatic mutations in SQSTM1 detected in affected tissues from patients with sporadic Paget's disease of bone. J Bone Miner Res 24:484, 2009

Ralston SH et al: Pathogenesis and management of Paget's disease of bone. Lancet 372:155, 2008

Whyte MP: Paget's disease of bone. N Engl J Med 355:593, 2006

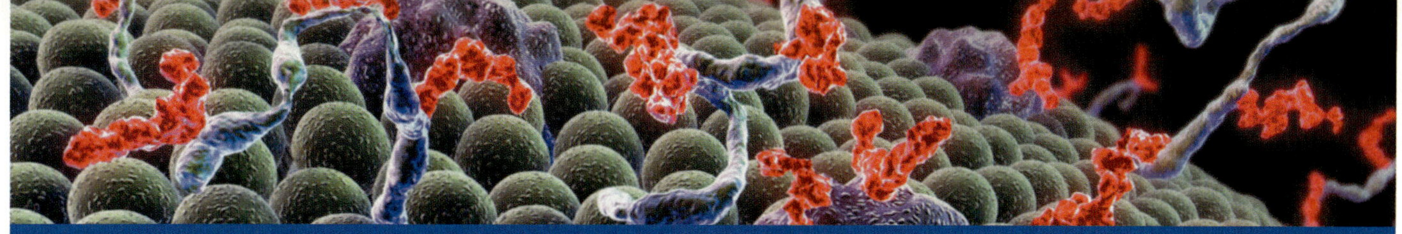

APPENDIX

LABORATORY VALUES OF CLINICAL IMPORTANCE

Alexander Kratz ■ Michael A. Pesce ■ Daniel J. Fink[†]

INTRODUCTORY COMMENTS

The following are tables of reference values for laboratory tests, special analytes, and special function tests. A variety of factors can influence reference values. Such variables include the population studied, the duration and means of specimen transport, laboratory methods and instrumentation, and even the type of container used for the collection of the specimen. The reference or "normal" ranges given in this appendix may therefore not be appropriate for all laboratories, and these values should only be used as general guidelines. Whenever possible, reference values provided by the laboratory performing the testing should be utilized in the interpretation of laboratory data. Values supplied in this Appendix reflect typical reference ranges in adults. Pediatric reference ranges may vary significantly from adult values.

In preparing the Appendix, the authors have taken into account the fact that the system of international units (SI, système international d'unités) is used in most countries and in some medical journals. However, clinical laboratories may continue to report values in "conventional" units. Therefore, both systems are provided in the Appendix. The dual system is also used in the text except for (1) those instances in which the numbers remain the same but only the terminology is changed (mmol/L for meq/L or IU/L for mIU/mL), when only the SI units are given; and (2) most pressure measurements (e.g., blood and cerebrospinal fluid pressures), when the conventional units (mmHg, mmH_2O) are used. In all other instances in the text the SI unit is followed by the traditional unit in parentheses.

[†]Deceased

REFERENCE VALUES FOR LABORATORY TESTS

TABLE A-1

HEMATOLOGY AND COAGULATION

ANALYTE	SPECIMEN[a]	SI UNITS	CONVENTIONAL UNITS
Activated clotting time	WB	70–180 s	70–180 seconds
Activated protein C resistance (Factor V Leiden)	P	Not applicable	Ratio >2.1
Alpha$_2$ antiplasmin	P	0.87–1.55	87–155%
Antiphospholipid antibody panel			
PTT-LA (Lupus anticoagulant screen)	P	Negative	Negative
Platelet neutralization procedure	P	Negative	Negative
Dilute viper venom screen	P	Negative	Negative
Anticardiolipin antibody	S		
IgG		0–15 arbitrary units	0–15 GPL
IgM		0–15 arbitrary units	0–15 MPL
Antithrombin III	P		
Antigenic		220–390 mg/L	22–39 mg/dL
Functional		0.7–1.30 U/L	70–130%
Anti-Xa assay (heparin assay)	P		
Unfractionated heparin		0.3–0.7 kIU/L	0.3–0.7 IU/mL
Low-molecular-weight heparin		0.5–1.0 kIU/L	0.5–1.0 IU/mL
Danaparoid (Organ)		0.5–0.8 kIU/L	0.5–0.8 IU/mL
Autohemolysis test	WB	0.004–0.045	0.4–4.50%
Autohemolysis test with glucose	WB	0.003–0.007	0.3–0.7%
Bleeding time (adult)		<7.1 min	<7.1 min
Clot retraction	WB	0.50–1.00/2 h	50–100%/2 h
Cryofibrinogen	P	Negative	Negative
D-Dimer	P	0.22–0.74 μg/mL	0.22–0.74 μg/mL
Differential blood count	WB		
Neutrophils		0.40–0.70	40–70%
Bands		0.0–0.05	0–5%
Lymphocytes		0.20–0.50	20–50%
Monocytes		0.04–0.08	4–8%
Eosinophils		0.0–0.6	0–6%
Basophils		0.0–0.02	0–2%
Eosinophil count	WB	150–300/μL	150–300/mm^3
Erythrocyte count	WB		
Adult males		4.30–5.60 × 10^{12}/L	4.30–5.60 × 10^6/mm^3
Adult females		4.00–5.20 × 10^{12}/L	4.00–5.20 × 10^6/mm^3
Erythrocyte life span	WB		
Normal survival		120 days	120 days
Chromium labeled, half-life ($t_{1/2}$)		25–35 days	25–35 days
Erythrocyte sedimentation rate	WB		
Females		0–20 mm/h	0–20 mm/h
Males		0–15 mm/h	0–15 mm/h
Euglobulin lysis time	P	7200–14400 s	120–240 min
Factor II, prothrombin	P	0.50–1.50	50–150%
Factor V	P	0.50–1.50	50–150%
Factor VII	P	0.50–1.50	50–150%
Factor VIII	P	0.50–1.50	50–150%
Factor IX	P	0.50–1.50	50–150%
Factor X	P	0.50–1.50	50–150%
Factor XI	P	0.50–1.50	50–150%
Factor XII	P	0.50–1.50	50–150%
Factor XIII screen	P	Not applicable	Present
Factor inhibitor assay	P	<0.5 Bethesda Units	<0.5 Bethesda Units
Fibrin(ogen) degradation products	P	0–1 mg/L	0–1 μg/mL
Fibrinogen	P	2.33–4.96 g/L	233–496 mg/dL
Glucose-6-phosphate dehydrogenase (erythrocyte)	WB	<2400 s	<40 min
Ham's test (acid serum)	WB	Negative	Negative

(Continued)

TABLE A-1 (*CONTINUED*)

HEMATOLOGY AND COAGULATION			
ANALYTE	SPECIMEN[a]	SI UNITS	CONVENTIONAL UNITS
Hematocrit	WB		
Adult males		0.388–0.464	38.8–46.4
Adult females		0.354–0.444	35.4–44.4
Hemoglobin			
Plasma	P	6–50 mg/L	0.6–5.0 mg/dL
Whole blood	WB		
Adult males		133–162 g/L	13.3–16.2 g/dL
Adult females		120–158 g/L	12.0–15.8 g/dL
Hemoglobin electrophoresis	WB		
Hemoglobin A		0.95–0.98	95–98%
Hemoglobin A_2		0.015–0.031	1.5–3.1%
Hemoglobin F		0–0.02	0–2.0%
Hemoglobins other than A, A_2, or F		Absent	Absent
Heparin-induced thrombocytopenia antibody	P	Negative	Negative
Joint fluid crystal	JF	Not applicable	No crystals seen
Joint fluid mucin	JF	Not applicable	Only type I mucin present
Leukocytes			
Alkaline phosphatase (LAP)	WB	0.2–1.6 μkat/L	13–100 μ/L
Count (WBC)	WB	$3.54–9.06 \times 10^9$/L	$3.54–9.06 \times 10^3$/mm^3
Mean corpuscular hemoglobin (MCH)	WB	26.7–31.9 pg/cell	26.7–31.9 pg/cell
Mean corpuscular hemoglobin concentration (MCHC)	WB	323–359 g/L	32.3–35.9 g/dL
Mean corpuscular hemoglobin of reticulocytes (CH)	WB	24–36 pg	24–36 pg
Mean corpuscular volume (MCV)	WB	79–93.3 fL	79–93.3 μm^3
Mean platelet volume (MPV)	WB	9.00–12.95 fL	9.00–12.95 μm^3
Osmotic fragility of erythrocytes	WB		
Direct		0.0035–0.0045	0.35–0.45%
Index		0.0030–0.0065	0.30–0.65%
Partial thromboplastin time, activated	P	26.3–39.4 s	26.3–39.4 s
Plasminogen	P		
Antigen		84–140 mg/L	8.4–14.0 mg/dL
Functional		0.70–1.30	70–130%
Plasminogen activator inhibitor 1	P	4–43 μg/L	4–43 ng/mL
Platelet aggregation	PRP	Not applicable	>65% aggregation in response to adenosine diphosphate, epinephrine, collagen, ristocetin, and arachidonic acid
Platelet count	WB	$165–415 \times 10^9$/L	$165–415 \times 10^3$/mm^3
Platelet, mean volume	WB	6.4–11 fL	6.4–11.0 μm^3
Prekallikrein assay	P	0.50–1.5	50–150%
Prekallikrein screen	P		No deficiency detected
Protein C	P		
Total antigen		0.70–1.40	70–140%
Functional		0.70–1.30	70–130%
Protein S	P		
Total antigen		0.70–1.40	70–140%
Functional		0.65–1.40	65–140%
Free antigen		0.70–1.40	70–140%
Prothrombin gene mutation G20210A	WB	Not applicable	Not present
Prothrombin time	P	12.7–15.4 s	12.7–15.4 s
Protoporphyrin, free erythrocyte	WB	0.28–0.64 μmol/L of red blood cells	16–36 μg/dL of red blood cells
Red cell distribution width	WB	<0.145	<14.5%
Reptilase time	P	16–23.6 s	16–23.6 s
Reticulocyte count	WB		
Adult males		0.008–0.023 red cells	0.8–2.3% red cells
Adult females		0.008–0.020 red cells	0.8–2.0% red cells

(*Continued*)

TABLE A-1 (*CONTINUED*)

HEMATOLOGY AND COAGULATION

ANALYTE	SPECIMEN[a]	SI UNITS	CONVENTIONAL UNITS
Reticulocyte hemoglobin content	WB	>26 pg/cell	>26 pg/cell
Ristocetin cofactor (functional von Willebrand factor)	P		
Blood group O		0.75 mean of normal	75% mean of normal
Blood group A		1.05 mean of normal	105% mean of normal
Blood group B		1.15 mean of normal	115% mean of normal
Blood group AB		1.25 mean of normal	125% mean of normal
Sickle cell test	WB	Negative	Negative
Sucrose hemolysis	WB	<0.1	<10% hemolysis
Thrombin time	P	15.3–18.5 s	15.3–18.5 s
Total eosinophils	WB	150–300 × 10^6/L	150–300/mm^3
Transferrin receptor	S, P	9.6–29.6 nmol/L	9.6–29.6 nmol/L
Viscosity			
Plasma	P	1.7–2.1	1.7–2.1
Serum	S	1.4–1.8	1.4–1.8
Von Willebrand factor (vWF) antigen (factor VIII:R antigen)	P		
Blood group O		0.75 mean of normal	75% mean of normal
Blood group A		1.05 mean of normal	105% mean of normal
Blood group B		1.15 mean of normal	115% mean of normal
Blood group AB		1.25 mean of normal	125% mean of normal
Von Willebrand factor multimers	P	Normal distribution	Normal distribution
White blood cells: see "leukocytes"			

[a]P, plasma; JF, joint fluid; PRP, platelet-rich plasma; S, serum; WB, whole blood.

TABLE A-2

CLINICAL CHEMISTRY AND IMMUNOLOGY

ANALYTE	SPECIMEN[a]	SI UNITS	CONVENTIONAL UNITS
Acetoacetate	P	20–99 μmol/L	0.2–1.0 mg/dL
Adrenocorticotropin (ACTH)	P	1.3–16.7 pmol/L	6.0–76.0 pg/mL
Alanine aminotransferase (AST, SGPT)	S	0.12–0.70 μkat/L	7–41 U/L
Albumin	S		
Female		41–53 g/L	4.1–5.3 g/dL
Male		40–50 g/L	4.0–5.0 g/L
Aldolase	S	26–138 nkat/L	1.5–8.1 U/L
Aldosterone (adult)			
Supine, normal sodium diet	S, P	55–250 pmol/L	2–9 ng/dL
Upright, normal sodium diet	S, P		2–5-fold increase over supine value
Supine, low-sodium diet	S, P		2–5-fold increase over normal sodium diet level
	U	6.38–58.25 nmol/d	2.3–21.0 μg/24 h
Alpha fetoprotein (adult)	S	0–8.5 μg/L	0–8.5 ng/mL
Alpha$_1$ antitrypsin	S	1.0–2.0 g/L	100–200 mg/dL
Ammonia, as NH_3	P	11–35 μmol/L	19–60 μg/dL
Amylase (method dependent)	S	0.34–1.6 μkat/L	20–96 U/L
Androstenedione (adult)	S	1.75–8.73 nmol/L	50–250 ng/dL
Angiotensin-converting enzyme (ACE)	S	0.15–1.1 μkat/L	9–67 U/L
Anion gap	S	7–16 mmol/L	7–16 mmol/L
Apo B/Apo A-1 ratio		0.35–0.98	0.35–0.98
Apolipoprotein A-1	S	1.19–2.40 g/L	119–240 mg/dL
Apolipoprotein B	S	0.52–1.63 g/L	52–163 mg/dL
Arterial blood gases			
$[HCO_3^-]$		22–30 mmol/L	22–30 meq/L
P_{CO2}		4.3–6.0 kPa	32–45 mmHg
pH		7.35–7.45	7.35–7.45
P_{O2}		9.6–13.8 kPa	72–104 mmHg

(*Continued*)

TABLE A-2 (*CONTINUED*)

CLINICAL CHEMISTRY AND IMMUNOLOGY

ANALYTE	SPECIMEN[a]	SI UNITS	CONVENTIONAL UNITS
Aspartate aminotransferase (AST, SGOT)	S	0.20–0.65 μkat/L	12–38 U/L
Autoantibodies			
Anti-adrenal antibody	S	Not applicable	Negative at 1:10 dilution
Anti-double-strand (native) DNA	S	Not applicable	Negative at 1:10 dilution
Anti–glomerular basement membrane antibodies	S		
Qualitative		Negative	Negative
Quantitative		<5 kU/L	<5 U/mL
Anti-granulocyte antibody	S	Not applicable	Negative
Anti-Jo-1 antibody	S	Not applicable	Negative
Anti-La antibody	S	Not applicable	Negative
Anti-mitochondrial antibody	S	Not applicable	Negative
Antineutrophil cytoplasmic autoantibodies, cytoplasmic (C-ANCA)	S		
Qualitative		Negative	Negative
Quantitative (antibodies to proteinase 3)		<2.8 kU/L	<2.8 U/mL
Antineutrophil cytoplasmic autoantibodies, perinuclear (P-ANCA)	S		
Qualitative		Negative	Negative
Quantitative (antibodies to myeloperoxidase)		<1.4 kU/L	<1.4 U/mL
Antinuclear antibody	S	Not applicable	Negative at 1:40
Anti–parietal cell antibody	S	Not applicable	Negative at 1:20
Anti-Ro antibody	S	Not applicable	Negative
Anti-platelet antibody	S	Not applicable	Negative
Anti-RNP antibody	S	Not applicable	Negative
Anti-Scl 70 antibody	S	Not applicable	Negative
Anti-Smith antibody	S	Not applicable	Negative
Anti-smooth-muscle antibody	S	Not applicable	Negative at 1:20
Anti-thyroglobulin	S	Not applicable	Negative
Anti-thyroid antibody	S	<0.3 kIU/L	<0.3 IU/mL
B-type natriuretic peptide (BNP)	P	Age and gender specific: <167 ng/L	Age and gender specific: <167 pg/mL
Bence Jones protein, serum	S	Not applicable	None detected
Bence Jones protein, urine, qualitative	U	Not applicable	None detected in 50× concentrated urine
Bence Jones Protein, urine, quantitative	U		
Kappa		<25 mg/L	<2.5 mg/dL
Lambda		<50 mg/L	<5.0 mg/dL
β_2-Microglobulin			
	S	<2.7 mg/L	<0.27 mg/dL
	U	<120 μg/d	<120 μg/day
Bilirubin	S		
Total		5.1–22 μmol/L	0.3–1.3 mg/dL
Direct		1.7–6.8 μmol/L	0.1–0.4 mg/dL
Indirect		3.4–15.2 μmol/L	0.2–0.9 mg/dL
C peptide (adult)	S, P	0.17–0.66 nmol/L	0.5–2.0 ng/mL
C1-esterase-inhibitor protein	S		
Antigenic		124–250 mg/L	12.4–24.5 mg/dL
Functional		Present	Present
CA 125	S	0–35 kU/L	0–35 U/mL
CA 19-9	S	0–37 kU/L	0–37 U/mL
CA 15-3	S	0–34 kU/L	0–34 U/mL
CA 27-29	S	0–40 kU/L	0–40 U/mL
Calcitonin	S		
Male		3–26 ng/L	3–26 pg/mL
Female		2–17 ng/L	2–17 pg/mL
Calcium	S	2.2–2.6 mmol/L	8.7–10.2 mg/dL
Calcium, ionized	WB	1.12–1.32 mmol/L	4.5–5.3 mg/dL
Carbon dioxide content (TCO_2)	P (sea level)	22–30 mmol/L	22–30 meq/L

(*Continued*)

TABLE A-2 (*CONTINUED*)

CLINICAL CHEMISTRY AND IMMUNOLOGY

ANALYTE	SPECIMEN[a]	SI UNITS	CONVENTIONAL UNITS
Carboxyhemoglobin (carbon monoxide content)	WB		
Nonsmokers		0–0.04	0–4%
Smokers		0.04–0.09	4–9%
Onset of symptoms		0.15–0.20	15–20%
Loss of consciousness and death		>0.50	>50%
Carcinoembryonic antigen (CEA)	S		
Nonsmokers		0.0–3.0 μg/L	0.0–3.0 ng/mL
Smokers	S	0.0–5.0 μg/L	0.0–5.0 ng/mL
Ceruloplasmin	S	250–630 mg/L	25–63 mg/dL
Chloride	S	102–109 mmol/L	102–109 meq/L
Cholesterol: see **Table A-4**			
Cholinesterase	S	5–12 kU/L	5–12 U/mL
Complement			
C3	S	0.83–1.77 g/L	83–177 mg/dL
C4	S	0.16–0.47 g/L	16–47 mg/dL
Total hemolytic complement (CH50)	S	50–150%	50–150%
Factor B	S	0.17–0.42 g/L	17–42 mg/dL
Coproporphyrins (types I and III)	U	150–470 μmol/d	100–300 μg/d
Cortisol			
Fasting, 8 A.M.–12 noon	S	138–690 nmol/L	5–25 μg/dL
12 noon–8 P.M.		138–414 nmol/L	5–15 μg/dL
8 P.M.–8 A.M.		0–276 nmol/L	0–10 μg/dL
Cortisol, free	U	55–193 nmol/24 h	20–70 μg/24 h
C-reactive protein	S	0.2–3.0 mg/L	0.2–3.0 mg/L
Creatine kinase (total)	S		
Females		0.66–4.0 μkat/L	39–238 U/L
Males		0.87–5.0 μkat/L	51–294 U/L
Creatine kinase-MB	S		
Mass		0.0–5.5 μg/L	0.0–5.5 ng/mL
Fraction of total activity (by electrophoresis)		0–0.04	0–4.0%
Creatinine	S		
Female		44–80 μmol/L	0.5–0.9 ng/mL
Male		53–106 μmol/L	0.6–1.2 ng/mL
Cryoproteins	S	Not applicable	None detected
Dehydroepiandrosterone (DHEA) (adult)			
Male	S	6.2–43.4 nmol/L	180–1250 ng/dL
Female		4.5–34.0 nmol/L	130–980 ng/dL
Dehydroepiandrosterone (DHEA) sulfate	S		
Male (adult)		100–6190 μg/L	10–619 μg/dL
Female (adult, premenopausal)		120–5350 μg/L	12–535 μg/dL
Female (adult, postmenopausal)		300–2600 μg/L	30–260 μg/dL
Deoxycorticosterone (DOC) (adult)	S	61–576 nmol/L	2–19 ng/dL
11-Deoxycortisol (adult) (compound S) (8:00 A.M.)	S	0.34–4.56 nmol/L	12–158 ng/dL
Dihydrotestosterone			
Male	S, P	1.03–2.92 nmol/L	30–85 ng/dL
Female		0.14–0.76 nmol/L	4–22 ng/dL
Dopamine	P	<475 pmol/L	<87 pg/mL
Dopamine	U	425–2610 nmol/d	65–400 μg/d
Epinephrine	P		
Supine (30 min)		<273 pmol/L	<50 pg/mL
Sitting		<328 pmol/L	<60 pg/mL
Standing (30 min)		<491 pmol/L	<90 pg/mL
Epinephrine	U	0–109 nmol/d	0–20 μg/d
Erythropoietin	S	4–27 U/L	4–27 U/L

(*Continued*)

CLINICAL CHEMISTRY AND IMMUNOLOGY

ANALYTE	SPECIMEN[a]	SI UNITS	CONVENTIONAL UNITS
Estradiol	S, P		
Female			
Menstruating:			
Follicular phase		74–532 pmol/L	<20–145 pg/mL
Midcycle peak		411–1626 pmol/L	112–443 pg/mL
Luteal phase		74–885 pmol/L	<20–241 pg/mL
Postmenopausal		217 pmol/L	<59 pg/mL
Male		74 pmol/L	<20 pg/mL
Estrone	S, P		
Female			
Menstruating:			
Follicular phase		55–555 pmol/L	15–150 pg/mL
Luteal phase		55–740 pmol/L	15–200 pg/mL
Postmenopausal		55–204 pmol/L	15–55 pg/mL
Male		55–240 pmol/L	15–65 pg/mL
Fatty acids, free (nonesterified)	P	<0.28–0.89 mmol/L	<8–25 mg/dL
Ferritin	S		
Female		10–150 μg/L	10–150 ng/mL
Male		29–248 μg/L	29–248 ng/mL
Follicle-stimulating hormone (FSH)	S, P		
Female			
Menstruating:			
Follicular phase		3.0–20.0 IU/L	3.0–20.0 mIU/mL
Ovulatory phase		9.0–26.0 IU/L	9.0–26.0 mIU/mL
Luteal phase		1.0–12.0 IU/L	1.0–12.0 mIU/mL
Postmenopausal		18.0–153.0 IU/L	18.0–153.0 mIU/mL
Male		1.0–12.0 IU/L	1.0–12.0 mIU/mL
Free testosterone, adult			
Female	S	2.1–23.6 pmol/L	0.6–6.8 pg/mL
Male		163–847 pmol/L	47–244 pg/mL
Fructosamine	S	<285 μmol/L	<285 μmol/L
Gamma glutamyltransferase	S	0.15–0.99 μkat/L	9–58 U/L
Gastrin	S	<100 ng/L	<100 pg/mL
Glucagon	P	20–100 ng/L	20–100 pg/mL
Glucose (fasting)	P		
Normal		4.2–6.1 mmol/L	75–110 mg/dL
Impaired glucose tolerance		6.2–6.9 mmol/L	111–125 mg/dL
Diabetes mellitus		>7.0 mmol/L	>125 mg/dL
Glucose, 2 h postprandial	P	3.9–6.7 mmol/L	70–120 mg/dL
Growth hormone (resting)	S	0.5–17.0 μg/L	0.5–17.0 ng/mL
Hemoglobin A_{lc}	WB	0.04–0.06 Hb fraction	4.0–6.0%
High-density lipoprotein (HDL) (see **Table A-4**)			
Homocysteine	P	4.4–10.8 μmol/L	4.4–10.8 μmol/L
Human chorionic gonadotropin (hCG)	S		
Nonpregnant female		<5 IU/L	<5 mIU/mL
1–2 weeks postconception		9–130 IU/L	9–130 mIU/mL
2–3 weeks postconception		75–2600 IU/L	75–2600 mIU/mL
3–4 weeks postconception		850–20,800 IU/L	850–20,800 mIU/mL
4–5 weeks postconception		4000–100,200 IU/L	4000–100,200 mIU/mL
5–10 weeks postconception		11,500–289,000 IU/L	11,500–289,000 mIU/mL
10–14 weeks postconception		18,300–137,000 IU/L	18,300–137,000 mIU/mL
Second trimester		1400–53,000 IU/L	1400–53,000 mIU/mL
Third trimester		940–60,000 IU/L	940–60,000 mIU/mL
β-Hydroxybutyrate	P	0–290 μmol/L	0–3 mg/dL
5-Hydroindoleacetic acid [5-HIAA]	U	10.5–36.6 μmol/d	2–7 mg/d
17-Hydroxyprogesterone (adult)	S		
Male		0.15–7.5 nmol/L	5–250 ng/dL
Female			
Follicular phase		0.6–3.0 nmol/L	20–100 ng/dL
Midcycle peak		3–7.5 nmol/L	100–250 ng/dL
Luteal phase		3–15 nmol/L	100–500 ng/dL
Postmenopausal		≤2.1 nmol/L	≤70 ng/dL

(Continued)

TABLE A-2 (*CONTINUED*)

CLINICAL CHEMISTRY AND IMMUNOLOGY

ANALYTE	SPECIMEN[a]	SI UNITS	CONVENTIONAL UNITS
Hydroxyproline	U, 24 hour	38–500 μmol/d	38–500 μmol/d
Immunofixation	S	Not applicable	No bands detected
Immunoglobulin, quantitation (adult)			
IgA	S	0.70–3.50 g/L	70–350 mg/dL
IgD	S	0–140 mg/L	0–14 mg/dL
IgE	S	24–430 μg/L	10–179 IU/mL
IgG	S	7.0–17.0 g/L	700–1700 mg/dL
IgG_1	S	2.7–17.4 g/L	270–1740 mg/dL
IgG_2	S	0.3–6.3 g/L	30–630 mg/dL
IgG_3	S	0.13–3.2 g/L	13–320 mg/dL
IgG_4	S	0.11–6.2 g/L	11–620 mg/dL
IgM	S	0.50–3.0 g/L	50–300 mg/dL
Insulin	S, P	14.35–143.5 pmol/L	2–20 μU/mL
Iron	S	7–25 μmol/L	41–141 μg/dL
Iron-binding capacity	S	45–73 μmol/L	251–406 μg/dL
Iron-binding capacity saturation	S	0.16–0.35	16–35%
Joint fluid crystal	JF	Not applicable	No crystals seen
Joint fluid mucin	JF	Not applicable	Only type I mucin present
Ketone (acetone)	S, U	Negative	Negative
17-Ketosteroids	U	0.003–0.012 g/d	3–12 mg/d
Lactate	P, arterial	0.5–1.6 mmol/L	4.5–14.4 mg/dL
	P, venous	0.5–2.2 mmol/L	4.5–19.8 mg/dL
Lactate dehydrogenase	S	2.0–3.8 μkat/L	115–221 U/L
Lactate dehydrogenase isoenzymes	S		
Fraction 1 (of total)		0.14–0.26	14–26%
Fraction 2		0.29–0.39	29–39%
Fraction 3		0.20–0.25	20–25%
Fraction 4		0.08–0.16	8–16%
Fraction 5		0.06–0.16	6–16%
Lipase (method dependent)	S	0.51–0.73 μkat/L	3–43 U/L
Lipids: see **Table A-4**			
Lipoprotein(a)	S	0–300 mg/L	0–30 mg/dL
Low-density lipoprotein (LDL) (see **Table A-4**)			
Luteinizing hormone (LH)	S, P		
Female			
Menstruating			
Follicular phase		2.0–15.0 U/L	2.0–15.0 U/L
Ovulatory phase		22.0–105.0 U/L	22.0–105.0 U/L
Luteal phase		0.6–19.0 U/L	0.6–19.0 U/L
Postmenopausal		16.0–64.0 U/L	16.0–64.0 U/L
Male		2.0–12.0 U/L	2.0–12.0 U/L
Magnesium	S	0.62–0.95 mmol/L	1.5–2.3 mg/dL
Metanephrine	P	<0.5 nmol/L	<100 pg/mL
Metanephrine	U	30–211 mmol/mol creatinine	53–367 μg/g creatinine
Methemoglobin	WB	0.0–0.01	0–1%
Microalbumin urine	U		
24-h urine		0.0–0.03 g/d	0–30 mg/24 h
Spot urine		0.0–0.03 g/g creatinine	0–30 μg/mg creatinine
Myoglobin	S		
Male		19–92 μg/L	19–92 μg/L
Female		12–76 μg/L	12–76 μg/L
Norepinephrine	U	89–473 nmol/d	15–80 μg/d
Norepinephrine	P		
Supine (30 min)		650–2423 pmol/L	110–410 pg/mL
Sitting		709–4019 pmol/L	120–680 pg/mL
Standing (30 min)		739–4137 pmol/L	125–700 pg/mL

(*Continued*)

TABLE A-2 (*CONTINUED*)

CLINICAL CHEMISTRY AND IMMUNOLOGY

ANALYTE	SPECIMEN[a]	SI UNITS	CONVENTIONAL UNITS
N-telopeptide (cross linked), NTx	S		
Female, premenopausal		6.2–19.0 nmol BCE	6.2–19.0 nmol BCE
Male		5.4–24.2 nmol BCE	5.4–24.2 nmol BCE
Bone collagen equivalent (BCE)			
N-telopeptide (cross linked), NTx	U		
Female, premenopausal		17–94 nmol BCE/ mmol creatinine	17–94 nmol BCE/mmol creatinine
Female, postmenopausal		26–124 nmol BCE/ mmol creatinine	26–124 nmol BCE/mmol creatinine
Male		21–83 nmol BCE/ mmol creatinine	21–83 nmol BCE/mmol creatinine
Bone collagen equivalent (BCE)			
5′ Nucleotidase	S	0.02–0.19 μkat/L	0–11 U/L
Osmolality	P	275–295 mosmol/kg serum water	275–295 mosmol/kg serum water
	U	500–800 mosmol/kg water	500–800 mosmol/kg water
Osteocalcin	S	11–50 μg/L	11–50 ng/mL
Oxygen content	WB		
Arterial (sea level)		17–21	17–21 vol%
Venous (sea level)		10–16	10–16 vol%
Oxygen percent saturation (sea level)	WB		
Arterial		0.97	94–100%
Venous, arm		0.60–0.85	60–85%
Parathyroid hormone (intact)	S	8–51 ng/L	8–51 pg/mL
Phosphatase, alkaline	S	0.56–1.63 μkat/L	33–96 U/L
Phosphorus, inorganic	S	0.81–1.4 mmol/L	2.5–4.3 mg/dL
Porphobilinogen	U	None	None
Potassium	S	3.5–5.0 mmol/L	3.5–5.0 meq/L
Prealbumin	S	170–340 mg/L	17–34 mg/dL
Progesterone	S, P		
Female			
Follicular		<3.18 nmol/L	<1.0 ng/mL
Midluteal		9.54–63.6 nmol/L	3–20 ng/mL
Male		<3.18 nmol/L	<1.0 ng/mL
Prolactin	S	0–20 μg/L	0–20 ng/mL
Prostate-specific antigen (PSA)	S		
Male			
<40 years		0.0–2.0 μg/L	0.0–2.0 ng/mL
>40 years		0.0–4.0 μg/L	0.0–4.0 ng/mL
PSA, free; in males 45–75 years, with PSA values between 4 and 20 μg/mL	S	>0.25 associated with benign prostatic hyperplasia	>25% associated with benign prostatic hyperplasia
Protein fractions	S		
Albumin		35–55 g/L	3.5–5.5 g/dL (50–60%)
Globulin		20–35 g/L	2.0–3.5 g/dL (40–50%)
$Alpha_1$		2–4 g/L	0.2–0.4 g/dL (4.2–7.2%)
$Alpha_2$		5–9 g/L	0.5–0.9 g/dL (6.8–12%)
Beta		6–11 g/L	0.6–1.1 g/dL (9.3–15%)
Gamma		7–17 g/L	0.7–1.7 g/dL (13–23%)
Protein, total	S	67–86 g/L	6.7–8.6 g/dL
Pyruvate	P, arterial	40–130 μmol/L	0.35–1.14 mg/dL
	P, venous	40–130 μmol/L	0.35–1.14 mg/dL
Rheumatoid factor	S, JF	<30 kIU/L	<30 IU/mL
Serotonin	WB	0.28–1.14 μmol/L	50–200 ng/mL
Serum protein electrophoresis	S	Not applicable	Normal pattern

(*Continued*)

TABLE A-2 (CONTINUED)

CLINICAL CHEMISTRY AND IMMUNOLOGY

ANALYTE	SPECIMEN[a]	SI UNITS	CONVENTIONAL UNITS
Sex hormone–binding globulin (adult)	S		
Male		13–71 nmol/L	13–71 nmol/L
Female		18–114 nmol/L	18–114 nmol/L
Sodium	S	136–146 mmol/L	136–146 meq/L
Somatomedin-C (IGF-1) (adult)	S		
16–24 years		182–780 μg/L	182–780 ng/mL
25–39 years		114–492 μg/L	114–492 ng/mL
40–54 years		90–360 μg/L	90–360 ng/mL
>54 years		71–290 μg/L	71–290 ng/mL
Somatostatin	P	<25 ng/L	<25 pg/mL
Testosterone, total, morning sample	S		
Female		0.21–2.98 nmol/L	6–86 ng/dL
Male		9.36–37.10 nmol/L	270–1070 ng/dL
Thyroglobulin	S	0.5–53 μg/L	0.5–53 ng/mL
Thyroid-binding globulin	S	13–30 mg/L	1.3–3.0 mg/dL
Thyroid-stimulating hormone	S	0.34–4.25 mIU/L	0.34–4.25 μIU/mL
Thyroxine, free (fT_4)	S	10.3–21.9 pmol/L	0.8–1.7 ng/dL
Thyroxine, total (T_4)	S	70–151 nmol/L	5.4–11.7 μg/dL
(Free) thyroxine index	S	6.7–10.9	6.7–10.9
Transferrin	S	2.0–4.0 g/L	200–400 mg/dL
Triglycerides (see **Table A-4**)	S	0.34–2.26 mmol/L	30–200 mg/dL
Triiodothyronine, free (fT_3)	S	3.7–6.5 pmol/L	2.4–4.2 pg/mL
Triiodothyronine, total (T_3)	S	1.2–2.1 nmol/L	77–135 ng/dL
Troponin I	S		
Normal population, 99 %tile		0–0.08 μg/L	0–0.08 ng/mL
Cut-off for MI		>0.4 μg/L	>0.4 ng/mL
Troponin T	S		
Normal population, 99 %tile		0–0.1 μg/L	0–0.01 ng/mL
Cut-off for MI		0–0.1 μg/L	0–0.1 ng/mL
Urea nitrogen	S	2.5–7.1 mmol/L	7–20 mg/dL
Uric acid	S		
Females		0.15–0.33 μmol/L	2.5–5.6 mg/dL
Males		0.18–0.41 μmol/L	3.1–7.0 mg/dL
Urobilinogen	U	0.09–4.2 μmol/d	0.05–25 mg/24 h
Vanillylmandelic acid (VMA)	U, 24 h	<30 μmol/d	<6 mg/d
Vasoactive intestinal polypeptide	P	0–60 ng/L	0–60 pg/mL

[a]P, plasma; S, serum; U, urine; WB, whole blood; JF, joint fluid.

TABLE A-3

TOXICOLOGY AND THERAPEUTIC DRUG MONITORING

	THERAPEUTIC RANGE		TOXIC LEVEL	
DRUG	SI UNITS	CONVENTIONAL UNITS	SI UNITS	CONVENTIONAL UNITS
Acetaminophen	66–199 μmol/L	10–30 μg/mL	>1320 μmol/L	>200 μg/mL
Amikacin				
Peak	34–51 μmol/L	20–30 μg/mL	>60 μmol/L	>35 μg/mL
Trough	0–17 μmol/L	0–10 μg/mL	>17 μmol/L	>10 μg/mL
Amitriptyline/Nortriptyline (Total Drug)	430–900 nmol/L	120–250 ng/mL	>1800 nmol/L	>500 ng/mL
Amphetamine	150–220 nmol/L	20–30 ng/mL	>1500 nmol/L	>200 ng/mL
Bromide	1.3–6.3 mmol/L 9.4–18.8 mmol/L	Sedation: 10–50 mg/dL Epilepsy: 75–150 mg/dL	6.4–18.8 mmol/L >18.8 mmol/L >37.5 mmol/L	51–150 mg/dL: mild toxicity >150 mg/dL: severe toxicity >300 mg/dL: lethal

(Continued)

TABLE A-3 (*CONTINUED*)

TOXICOLOGY AND THERAPEUTIC DRUG MONITORING

	THERAPEUTIC RANGE		TOXIC LEVEL	
DRUG	SI UNITS	CONVENTIONAL UNITS	SI UNITS	CONVENTIONAL UNITS
Carbamazepine	17–42 µmol/L	4–10 µg/mL	85 µmol/L	>20 µg/mL
Chloramphenicol				
Peak	31–62 µmol/L	10–20 µg/mL	>77 µmol/L	>25 µg/mL
Trough	15–31 µmol/L	5–10 µg/mL	>46 µmol/L	> 15 µg/mL
Chlordiazepoxide	1.7–10 µmol/L	0.5–3.0 µg/mL	>17 µmol/L	>5.0 µg/mL
Clonazepam	32–240 nmol/L	10–75 ng/mL	>320 nmol/L	>100 ng/mL
Clozapine	0.6–2.1 µmol/L	200–700 ng/mL	>3.7 µmol/L	>1200 ng/mL
Cocaine			>3.3 µmol/L	>1.0 µg/mL
Codeine	43–110 nmol/mL	13–33 ng/mL	>3700 nmol/mL	>1100 ng/mL (lethal)
Cyclosporine				
Renal Transplant				
0–6 months	208–312 nmol/L	250–375 ng/mL	>312 nmol/L	>375 ng/mL
6–12 months after transplant	166–250 nmol/L	200–300 ng/mL	>250 nmol/L	>300 ng/mL
>12 months	83–125 nmol/L	100–150 ng/mL	>125 nmol/L	>150 ng/mL
Cardiac Transplant				
0–6 months	208–291 nmol/L	250–350 ng/mL	>291 nmol/L	>350 ng/mL
6–12 months after transplant	125–208 nmol/L	150–250 ng/mL	>208 nmol/L	>250 ng/mL
>12 months	83–125 nmol/L	100–150 ng/mL	>125 nmol/L	150 ng/mL
Lung Transplant				
0–6 months	250–374 nmol/L	300–450 ng/mL	>374 nmol/L	>450 ng/mL
Liver Transplant				
0–7 days	249–333 nmol/L	300–400 ng/mL	>333 nmol/L	>400 ng/mL
2–4 weeks	208–291 nmol/L	250–350 ng/mL	>291 nmol/L	>350 ng/mL
5–8 weeks	166–249 nmol/L	200–300 ng/mL	>249 nmol/L	>300 ng/mL
9–52 weeks	125–208 nmol/L	150–250 ng/mL	>208 nmol/L	>250 ng/mL
>1 year	83–166 nmol/L	100–200 ng/mL	>166 nmol/L	>200 ng/mL
Desipramine	375–1130 nmol/L	100–300 ng/mL	>1880 nmol/L	>500 ng/mL
Diazepam (and Metabolite)				
Diazepam	0.7–3.5 µmol/L	0.2–1.0 µg/mL	>7.0 µmol/L	>2.0 µg/mL
Nordazepam	0.4–6.6 µmol/L	0.1–1.8 µg/mL	>9.2 µmol/L	>2.5 µg/mL
Digoxin	0.64–2.6 nmol/L	0.5–2.0 ng/mL	>3.1 nmol/L	>2.4 ng/mL
Disopyramide	>7.4 µmol/L	2.5 µg/mL	20.6 µmol/L	>7 µg/mL
Doxepin and Nordoxepin				
Doxepin	0.36–0.98 µmol/L	101–274 ng/mL	>1.8 µmol/L	>503 ng/mL
Nordoxepin	0.38–1.04 µmol/L	106–291 ng/mL	>1.9 µmol/L	>531 ng/mL
Ethanol				
Behavioral changes			>4.3 mmol/L	>20 mg/dL
Legal limit			≥17 mmol/L	≥80 mg/dL
Critical with acute exposure			>54 mmol/L	>250 mg/dL
Ethylene Glycol				
Toxic			>2 mmol/L	>12 mg/dL
Lethal			>20 mmol/L	>120 mg/dL
Ethosuximide	280–700 µmol/L	40–100 µg/mL	>700 µmol/L	>100 µg/mL
Flecainide	0.5–2.4 µmol/L	0.2–1.0 µg/mL	>3.6 µmol/L	>1.5 µg/mL
Gentamicin				
Peak	10–21 µmol/mL	5–10 µg/mL	>25 µmol/mL	>12 µg/mL
Trough	0–4.2 µmol/mL	0–2 µg/mL	>4.2 µmol/mL	>2 µg/mL
Heroin (Diacetyl Morphine)			>700 µmol/L	>200 ng/mL (as morphine)
Ibuprofen	49–243 µmol/L	10–50 µg/mL	>97 µmol/L	>200 µg/mL

(*Continued*)

TABLE A-3 (*CONTINUED*)

TOXICOLOGY AND THERAPEUTIC DRUG MONITORING

	THERAPEUTIC RANGE		TOXIC LEVEL	
DRUG	SI UNITS	CONVENTIONAL UNITS	SI UNITS	CONVENTIONAL UNITS
Imipramine (and Metabolite)				
Desimipramine	375–1130 nmol/L	100–300 ng/mL	>1880 nmol/L	>500 ng/mL
Total Imipramine + Desimipramine	563–1130 nmol/L	150–300 ng/mL	>1880 nmol/L	>500 ng/mL
Lidocaine	5.1–21.3 μmol/L	1.2–5.0 μg/mL	>38.4 μmol/L	>9.0 μg/mL
Lithium	0.5–1.3 meq/L	0.5–1.3 meq/L	>2 mmol/L	>2 meq/L
Methadone	1.3–3.2 μmol/L	0.4–1.0 μg/mL	>6.5 μmol/L	>2 μg/mL
Methamphetamine		20–30 ng/mL		0.1–1.0 μg/mL
Methanol			>6 mmol/L	>20 mg/dL
			>16 mmol/L	>50 mg/dL
			>28 mmol/L	Severe toxicity >89 mg/dL Lethal
Methotrexate				
Low-dose	0.01–0.1 μmol/L	0.01–0.1 μmol/L	>0.1 mmol/L	>0.1 mmol/L
High-dose (24 h)	<5.0 μmol/L	<5.0 μmol/L	>5.0 μmol/L	>5.0 μmol/L
High-dose (48 h)	<0.50 μmol/L	<0.50 μmol/L	>0.5 μmol/L	>0.5 μmol/L
High-dose (72 h)	<0.10 μmol/L	<0.10 μmol/L	>0.1 μmol/L	>0.1 μmol/L
Morphine	35–250 μmol/L	10–70 ng/mL	180–14000 μmol/L	50–4000 ng/mL
Nitroprusside (as Thiocyanate)	103–499 μmol/L	6–29 μg/mL	860 μmol/L	>50 μg/mL
Nortriptyline	190–569 nmol/L	50–150 ng/mL	>1900 nmol/L	>500 ng/mL
Phenobarbital	65–172 μmol/L	15–40 μg/mL	>215 μmol/L	>50 μg/mL
Phenytoin	40–79 μmol/L	10–20 μg/mL	>118 μmol/L	>30 μg/mL
Phenytoin, Free	4.0–7.9 μg/mL	1–2 μg/mL	>13.9 μg/mL	>3.5 μg/mL
% Free	0.08–0.14	8–14%		
Primidone and Metabolite				
Primidone	23–55 μmol/L	5–12 μg/mL	>69 μmol/L	>15 μg/mL
Phenobarbital	65–172 μmol/L	15–40 μg/mL	>215 μmol/L	>50 μg/mL
Procainamide				
Procainamide	17–42 μmol/L	4–10 μg/mL	>51 μmol/L	>12 μg/mL
NAPA (N-acetylprocainamide)	22–72 μmol/L	6–20 μg/mL	>126 μmol/L	>35 μg/mL
Quinidine	>6.2–15.4 μmol/L	2.0–5.0 μg/mL	>31 μmol/L	>10 μg/mL
Salicylates	145–2100 μmol/L	2–29 mg/dL	>2172 μmol/L	>30 mg/dL
Sirolimus (Trough Level)				
Kidney Transplant	4.4–13.1 nmol/L	4–12 ng/mL	>16 nmol/L	>15 ng/mL
Tacrolimus (FK506) (Trough)				
Kidney and Liver				
0–2 months post transplant	12–19 nmol/L	10–15 ng/mL	>25 nmol/L	>20 ng/mL
>2 months post transplant	6–12 nmol/L	5–10 ng/mL		
Heart				
0–2 months post transplant	19–25 nmol/L	15–20 ng/mL	>25 nmol/L	>20 ng/mL
3–6 months post transplant	12–19 nmol/L	10–15 ng/mL		
>6 months post transplant	10–12 nmol/L	8–10 ng/mL		
Theophylline	56–111 μg/mL	10–20 μg/mL	>140 μg/mL	>25 μg/mL
Thiocyanate				
After nitroprusside infusion	103–499 μmol/L	6–29 μg/mL	860 μmol/L	>50 μg/mL
Nonsmoker	17–69 μmol/L	1–4 μg/mL		
Smoker	52–206 μmol/L	3–12 μg/mL		
Tobramycin				
Peak	11–22 μg/L	5–10 μg/mL	>26 μg/L	>12 μg/mL
Trough	0–4.3 μg/L	0–2 μg/mL	>4.3 μg/L	>2 μg/mL
Valproic acid	350–700 μmol/L	50–100 μg/mL	>1000 μmol/L	>150 μg/mL
Vancomycin				
Peak	14–28 μmol/L	20–40 μg/mL	>55 μmol/L	>80 μg/mL
Trough	3.5–10.4 μmol/L	5–15 μg/mL	>14 μmol/L	>20 μg/mL

TABLE A-4

CLASSIFICATION OF LDL, TOTAL, AND HDL CHOLESTEROL	
LDL Cholesterol, mg/dL (mmol/L)	
<70 (<1.81)	Therapeutic option for very high risk patients
<100 (<2.59)	Optimal
100–129 (2.59–3.34)	Near optimal/above optimal
130–159 (3.36–4.11)	Borderline high
160–189 (4.14–4.89)	High
≥190 (≥4.91)	Very high
Total Cholesterol, mg/dL (mmol/L)	
<200 (<5.17)	Desirable
200–239 (5.17–6.18)	Borderline high
≥240 (≥6.21)	High
HDL Cholesterol, mg/dL (mmol/L)	
<40 (<1.03)	Low
≥60 (≥1.55)	High

Note: LDL, low-density lipoprotein; HDL, high-density lipoprotein
Source: Executive summary of the third report of the National Cholesterol Education Program (NCEP) expert panel on detection, evaluation, and treatment of high blood cholesterol in adults (adult treatment panel III). JAMA 285:2486, 2001; and Implications of recent clinical trials for the National Cholesterol Education Program Adult Treatment Panel III Guidelines: SM Grundy et al for the Coordinating Committee of the National Cholesterol Education Program. Circulation 110:227, 2004.

REFERENCE VALUES FOR SPECIFIC ANALYTES

TABLE A-5

URINE ANALYSIS

	REFERENCE RANGE	
	SI UNITS	**CONVENTIONAL UNITS**
Acidity, titratable	20–40 mmol/d	20–40 meq/d
Ammonia	30–50 mmol/d	30–50 meq/d
Amylase		4–400 U/L
Amylase/creatinine clearance ratio $[(Cl_{am}/Cl_{cr}) \times 100]$	1–5	1–5
Calcium (10 meq/d or 200 mg/d dietary calcium)	<7.5 mmol/d	<300 mg/d
Creatine, as creatinine		
Female	<760 µmol/d	<100 mg/d
Male	<380 µmol/d	<50 mg/d
Creatinine	8.8–14 mmol/d	1.0–1.6 g/d
Eosinophils	<100,000 eosinophils/L	<100 eosinophils/mL
Glucose (glucose oxidase method)	0.3–1.7 mmol/d	50–300 mg/d
5-Hydroxyindoleacetic acid (5-HIAA)	10–47 µmol/d	2–9 mg/d
Iodine, spot urine		
WHO classification of iodine deficiency		
Not iodine deficient	>100 µg/L	>100 µg/L
Mild iodine deficiency	50–100 µg/L	50–100 µg/L
Moderate iodine deficiency	20–49 µg/L	20–49 µg/L
Severe iodine deficiency	<20 µg/L	<20 µg/L
Microalbumin		
Normal	0.0–0.03 g/d	0–30 mg/d
Microalbuminuria	0.03–0.30 g/d	30–300 mg/d
Clinical albuminuria	>0.3 g/d	>300 mg/d
Microalbumin/creatinine ratio		
Normal	0–3.4 g/mol creatinine	0–30 µg/mg creatinine
Microalbuminuria	3.4–34 g/mol creatinine	30–300 µg/mg creatinine
Clinical albuminuria	>34 g/mol creatinine	>300 µg/mg creatinine

(Continued)

TABLE A-5 (*CONTINUED*)

URINE ANALYSIS

	REFERENCE RANGE	
	SI UNITS	CONVENTIONAL UNITS
Oxalate		
Male	80–500 μmol/d	7–44 mg/d
Female	45–350 μmol/d	4–31 mg/d
pH	5.0–9.0	5.0–9.0
Phosphate (phosphorus) (varies with intake)	12.9–42.0 mmol/d	400–1300 mg/d
Potassium (varies with intake)	25–100 mmol/d	25–100 meq/d
Protein	<0.15 g/d	<150 mg/d
Sediment		
Red blood cells	0–2/high-power field	
White blood cells	0–2/high-power field	
Bacteria	None	
Crystals	None	
Bladder cells	None	
Squamous cells	None	
Tubular cells	None	
Broad casts	None	
Epithelial cell casts	None	
Granular casts	None	
Hyaline casts	0–5/low-power field	
Red blood cell casts	None	
Waxy casts	None	
White cell casts	None	
Sodium (varies with intake)	100–260 mmol/d	100–260 meq/d
Specific gravity	1.001–1.035	1.001–1.035
Urea nitrogen	214–607 mmol/d	6–17 g/d
Uric acid (normal diet)	1.49–4.76 mmol/d	250–800 mg/d

Note: WHO, World Health Organization.

SPECIAL FUNCTION TESTS

TABLE A-6

RENAL FUNCTION TESTS

	REFERENCE RANGE	
	SI UNITS	CONVENTIONAL UNITS
Clearances (corrected to 1.72 m^2 body surface area)		
Measures of glomerular filtration rate		
Inulin clearance (Cl)		
Males (mean ± 1 SD)	2.1 ± 0.4 mL/s	124 ± 25.8 mL/min
Females (mean ± 1 SD)	2.0 ± 0.2 mL/s	119 ± 12.8 mL/min
Endogenous creatinine clearance	1.5–2.2 mL/s	91–130 mL/min
Measures of effective renal plasma flow and tubular function		
p-Aminohippuric acid clearance (Cl_{PAH})		
Males (mean ± 1 SD)	10.9 ± 2.7 mL/s	654 ± 163 mL/min
Females (mean ± 1 SD)	9.9 ± 1.7 mL/s	594 ± 102 mL/min
Concentration and dilution test		
Specific gravity of urine		
After 12-h fluid restriction	>1.025	>1.025
After 12-h deliberate water intake	≤1.003	≤1.003
Protein excretion, urine	<0.15 g/d	<150 mg/d
Specific gravity, maximal range	1.002–1.028	1.002–1.028
Tubular reabsorption, phosphorus	0.79–0.94 of filtered load	79–94% of filtered load

MISCELLANEOUS

TABLE A-7

BODY FLUIDS AND OTHER MASS DATA

	REFERENCE RANGE	
	SI UNITS	CONVENTIONAL UNITS
Ascitic fluid		
Body fluid		
Total volume (lean) of body weight	50% (in obese) to 70%	
Intracellular	0.3–0.4 of body weight	
Extracellular	0.2–0.3 of body weight	
Blood		
Total volume		
Males	69 mL per kg body weight	
Females	65 mL per kg body weight	
Plasma volume		
Males	39 mL per kg body weight	
Females	40 mL per kg body weight	
Red blood cell volume		
Males	30 mL per kg body weight	1.15–1.21 L/m^2 of body surface area
Females	25 mL per kg body weight	0.95–1.00 L/m^2 of body surface area
Body mass index	18.5–24.9 kg/m^2	18.5–24.9 kg/m^2

TABLE A-8

RADIATION-DERIVED UNITS

QUANTITY	OLD UNIT	SI UNIT	NAME FOR SI UNIT (AND ABBREVIATION)	CONVERSION
Activity	curie (Ci)	Disintegrations per second (dps)	becquerel (Bq)	1 Ci = 3.7×10^{10} Bq 1 mCi = 37 mBq 1 μCi = 0.037 MBq or 37 GBq 1 Bq = 2.703×10^{-11} Ci
Absorbed dose	rad	joule per kilogram (J/kg)	gray (Gy)	1 Gy = 100 rad 1 rad = 0.01 Gy 1 mrad = 10^{-3} cGy
Exposure	roentgen (R)	coulomb per kilogram (C/kg)	—	1 C/kg = 3876 R 1 R = 2.58×10^{-4} C/kg 1 mR = 258 pC/kg
Dose equivalent	rem	joule per kilogram (J/kg)	sievert (Sv)	1 Sv = 100 rem 1 rem = 0.01 Sv 1 mrem = 10 μSv

ACKNOWLEDGMENT

The authors acknowledge the contributions of Dr. Patrick M. Sluss, Dr. James L. Januzzi, and Dr. Kent B. Lewandrowski to this chapter in previous editions of Harrison's Principles of Internal Medicine.

FURTHER READINGS

KRATZ A et al: Case records of the Massachusetts General Hospital. Weekly clinicopathological exercises. Laboratory reference values. N Engl J Med 351(15):1548, 2004

LEHMAN HP, HENRY JB: SI units, in *Henry's Clinical Diagnosis and Management by Laboratory Methods*, 21st ed, RC McPherson, MR Pincus (eds). Philadelphia, Elsevier Saunders, 2007, pp 1404–1418

PESCE MA: Reference ranges for laboratory tests and procedures, in *Nelson's Textbook of Pediatrics*, 18th ed, RM Klegman et al (eds). Philadelphia, Elsevier Saunders, 2007, pp 2943–2949

SOLBERG HE: Establishment and use of reference values, in *Tietz Textbook of Clinical Chemistry and Molecular Diagnostics*, 4th ed, CA Burtis et al (eds). Philadelphia, Elsevier Saunders, 2006, pp 425–448

REVIEW AND SELF-ASSESSMENT*

Charles Wiener ■ Gerald Bloomfield ■ Cynthia D. Brown ■ Joshua Schiffer ■ Adam Spivak

QUESTIONS

DIRECTIONS: Choose the **one best** response to each question.

1. What is the most common cause of hypothyroidism worldwide?

A. Autoimmune disease
B. Graves' disease
C. Iatrogenic causes
D. Iodine deficiency
E. Medication side effects

2. A 23-year-old woman presents to the clinic complaining of months of weight gain, fatigue, amenorrhea, and worsening acne. She cannot identify when her symptoms began precisely, but she reports that without a change in her diet she has noted a 12.3-kg weight gain over the past 6 months. She has been amenorrheic for several months. On examination she is noted to have truncal obesity with bilateral purplish striae across both flanks. Cushing's syndrome is suspected. Which of the following tests should be used to make the diagnosis?

A. 24-h urine free cortisol
B. Basal adrenocorticotropic hormone (ACTH)
C. Corticotropin-releasing hormone (CRH) level at 8 A.M.
D. Inferior petrosal venous sampling
E. Overnight 1 mg dexamethasone suppression test

3. Secretion of gonadotropin-releasing hormone (GnRH) normally stimulates release of luteinizing hormone (LH) and follicle-stimulating hormone (FSH), which promote production and release of testosterone and estrogen. Which mechanism below best explains how long-acting gonadotropin-releasing hormone agonists (e.g., leuprolide) decrease testosterone levels in the management of prostate cancer?

A. GnRH agonists also promote production of sex hormone–binding globulin, which decreases the availability of testosterone
B. Negative feedback loop between GnRH and LH/FSH
C. Sensitivity of LH and FSH to pulse frequency of GnRH
D. Translocation of the cytoplasmic nuclear receptor into the nucleus with constitutive activation of GnRH

4. A 44-year-old woman seeks evaluation for irregular menstrual cycles with heavy menstrual bleeding. She reports that her menses had been regular with 28-day cycles since her early twenties. However, for the past 6 months, her cycles have been 22–25 days with heavy associated bleeding that is unusual for her. She has had rare hot flashes and sleep disturbance. She is requesting assistance in controlling these symptoms. You suspect she is perimenopausal, and hormonal testing on day 2 of her menses confirms this suspicion. You are considering treatment with oral contraceptives for control of her symptoms and to protect against unintended pregnancy. All of the following would be considered contraindications to use of oral contraceptive pills *except*

A. breast cancer
B. cigarette smoking
C. kidney disease
D. liver disease
E. prior history of deep-vein thrombosis

5. All of the following are risk factors for the development of osteoporotic fractures *except*

A. African-American race
B. current cigarette smoking
C. female sex
D. low body weight
E. physical inactivity

6. All of the following drugs are associated with an increased risk of osteoporosis in adults *except*

A. cyclosporine
B. Dilantin
C. heparin
D. prednisone
E. ranitidine

7. A 34-year-old woman presents to your clinic with a variety of complaints that have been worsening over the past year or so. She notes fatigue, amenorrhea, and weight gain. She states that her primary physician diagnosed her with hypothyroidism several

*Questions and answers were taken from Wiener C, et al (eds). *Harrison's Principles of Internal Medicine Self-Assessment and Board Review,* 17th ed. New York: McGraw-Hill, 2008.

7. *(Continued)*
months ago, and she has been faithfully taking thyroid hormone replacement. Her thyroid-stimulating hormone (TSH) has been in the normal range over the last two laboratory checks. When her symptoms did not improve on Synthroid, she was sent to your clinic for further evaluation. A diagnosis of panhypopituitarism is considered. All of the following are consistent with normal pituitary function *except*

A. basal elevation of follicle-stimulating hormone (FSH) and luteinizing hormone (LH) in a postmenopausal woman
B. elevation of aldosterone after infusion of cosyntropin
C. elevation of growth hormone after ingestion of a glucose load
D. elevation of cortisol after injection of regular insulin
E. elevation of TSH after infusion of thyrotropin-releasing hormone (TRH)

8. A 42-year-old woman is brought to the emergency room by ambulance for altered mental status. The glucose level by fingerstick monitoring was below the measurement capabilities of the monitor (<40 mg/dL). After 2 ampules of 50% dextrose, the patient's fingerstick glucose remains at 42 mg/dL. She remains unconscious and had a 1-min seizure while in transport. She has no history of diabetes mellitus. Her family denies that she has been recently ill, but recently she has been depressed. She works as a registered nurse on a medical floor of the hospital. Which of the following tests would confirm an overdose of exogenous insulin?

A. Plasma glucose <55 mg/dL, plasma insulin >18 pmol/L, and plasma C-peptide levels undetectable
B. Plasma glucose <55 mg/dL, plasma insulin >18 pmol/L, and plasma C-peptide levels >0.6 ng/mL
C. Plasma glucose <55 mg/dL, plasma insulin <18 pmol/L, and plasma glucagon <12 pmol/L
D. Plasma glucose <55 mg/dL, plasma insulin <18 pmol/L, and C-peptide levels undetectable

9. A 44-year-old male is involved in a motor vehicle collision. He sustains multiple injuries to the face, chest, and pelvis. He is unresponsive in the field and is intubated for airway protection. An IV line is placed. The patient is admitted to the intensive care unit (ICU) with multiple orthopedic injuries. He is stabilized medically and on hospital day 2 undergoes successful open reduction and internal fixation of the right femur and right humerus. After his return to the ICU, you review his laboratory values. Thyroid-stimulating hormone (TSH) is 0.3 mU/L, and

9. *(Continued)*
the total T_4 level is normal. T_3 is 0.6 μg/dL. What is the most appropriate next management step?

A. Initiation of levothyroxine
B. A radioiodine uptake scan
C. A thyroid ultrasound
D. Observation
E. Initiation of prednisone

10. All of the following biochemical markers are a measure of bone resorption *except*

A. serum alkaline phosphatase
B. serum cross-linked N-telopeptide
C. serum cross-linked C-telopeptide
D. urine hydroxyproline
E. urine total free deoxypyridinoline

11. A 54-year-old woman is referred to endocrinology for evaluation of osteoporosis after a recent evaluation of back pain revealed a compression fracture of the T4 vertebral body. She is perimenopausal with irregular menstrual periods and frequent hot flashes. She does not smoke. She otherwise is well and healthy. Her weight is 70 kg, and height is 168 cm. A bone mineral density scan shows a T-score of –3.5 SD and a Z-score of –2.5 SD. All of the following tests are indicated for the evaluation of osteoporosis in this patient *except*

A. 24-h urine calcium
B. follicle-stimulating hormone and luteinizing hormone levels
C. serum calcium
D. renal function panel
E. vitamin D levels (25-hydroxyvitamin D)

12. A 67-year-old woman presents to the clinic after a fall on the ice a week ago. She visited the local emergency room immediately after the fall, where hip radiographs were performed and were negative for fracture or dislocation. They did reveal fusion of the sacroiliac joints and coarse trabeculations in the ilium, consistent with Paget's disease. A comprehensive metabolic panel was also sent at that visit and is remarkable for an alkaline phosphatase of 157 U/L, with normal serum calcium and phosphate levels. She was discharged with analgesics and told to follow up with her primary care doctor for further management of her radiographic findings. She is recovering from her fall and denies any longstanding pain or immobility of her hip joints. She states that her father suffered from a bone disease that caused him headaches and hearing loss near the end of his life.

12. *(Continued)*
She is very concerned about the radiographs and wants to know what they mean. Which of the following is the best treatment strategy at this point?

A. Initiate physical therapy and non-weight-bearing exercises to strengthen the hip.
B. No treatment; she is asymptomatic. Follow radiographs and laboratory findings every 6 months.
C. Prescribe vitamin D and calcium.
D. Start an oral bisphosphonate.
E. Start high-dose prednisone with rapid taper over 1 week.

13. A 29-year-old woman presents to your clinic complaining of difficulty swallowing, sore throat, and tender swelling in her neck. She has also noted fevers intermittently over the past week. Several weeks prior to her current symptoms she experienced symptoms of an upper respiratory tract infection. She has no past medical history. On physical examination, she is noted to have a small goiter that is painful to the touch. Her oropharynx is clear. Laboratory studies are sent, and reveal a white blood cell count of 14,100 cells/μL with a normal differential, erythrocyte sedimentation rate (ESR) of 53 mm/h, and a thyroid-stimulating hormone (TSH) of 21 μIU/mL. Thyroid antibodies are negative. What is the most likely diagnosis?

A. Autoimmune hypothyroidism
B. Cat-scratch fever
C. Graves' disease
D. Ludwig's angina
E. Subacute thyroiditis

14. What is the most appropriate treatment for the patient described above?

A. Iodine ablation of the thyroid
B. Large doses of aspirin
C. Local radiation therapy
D. No treatment necessary
E. Propylthiouracil

15. The Diabetes Control and Complications Trial (DCCT) provided definitive proof that reduction in chronic hyperglycemia

A. improves microvascular complications in type 1 diabetes mellitus
B. improves macrovascular complications in type 1 diabetes mellitus
C. improves microvascular complications in type 2 diabetes mellitus

15. *(Continued)*
D. improves macrovascular complications in type 2 diabetes mellitus
E. improves both microvascular and macrovascular complications in type 2 diabetes mellitus

16. A 54-year-old woman undergoes thyroidectomy for follicular carcinoma of the thyroid. About 6 h after surgery, the patient complains of tingling around her mouth. She subsequently develops a pins-and-needles sensation in the fingers and toes. The nurse calls the physician to the bedside to evaluate the patient after she has severe hand cramps when her blood pressure is taken. Upon evaluation, the patient is still complaining of intermittent cramping of her hands. Since surgery, she has received morphine sulfate, 2 mg, for pain and Compazine, 5 mg, for nausea. She has had no change in her vital signs and is afebrile. Tapping on the inferior portion of the zygomatic arch 2 cm anterior to the ear produces twitching at the corner of the mouth. An electrocardiogram (ECG) shows a QT interval of 575 ms. What is the next step in evaluation and treatment of this patient?

A. Administration of benztropine, 2 mg IV
B. Administration of calcium gluconate, 2 g IV
C. Administration of magnesium sulphate, 4 g IV
D. Measurement of calcium, magnesium, phosphate, and potassium levels
E. Measurement of forced vital capacity

17. A 49-year-old male is brought to the hospital by his family because of confusion and dehydration. The family reports that for the last 3 weeks he has had persistent copious watery diarrhea that has not abated with the use of over-the-counter medications. The diarrhea has been unrelated to food intake and has persisted during fasting. The stool does not appear fatty and is not malodorous. The patient works as an attorney, is a vegetarian, and has not traveled recently. No one in the household has had similar symptoms. Before the onset of diarrhea, he had mild anorexia and a 5-lb weight loss. Since the diarrhea began, he has lost at least 10 pounds. The physical examination is notable for blood pressure of 100/70, heart rate of 110/min, and temperature of 36.8°C (98.2°F). Other than poor skin turgor, confusion, and diffuse muscle weakness, the physical examination is unremarkable. Laboratory studies are notable for a normal complete blood count and the following chemistry results:

Na^+	146 meq/L
K^+	3.0 meq/L

17. *(Continued)*

Cl^-	96 meq/L
HCO_3^-	36 meq/L
BUN	32 mg/dL
Creatinine	1.2 mg/dL

A 24-h stool collection yields 3 L of tea-colored stool. Stool sodium is 50 meq/L, potassium is 25 meq/L, and stool osmolality is 170 mosmol/L. Which of the following diagnostic tests is most likely to yield the correct diagnosis?

A. Serum cortisol
B Serum thyroid-stimulating hormone (TSH)
C. Serum vasoactive intestinal peptide (VIP)
D. Urinary 5-hydroxyindoleacetic acid (5-HIAA)
E. Urinary metanephrine

18. A 68-year-old woman with stage IIIB squamous cell carcinoma of the lung is admitted to the hospital because of altered mental status and dehydration. Upon admission, she is found to have a calcium level of 19.6 mg/dL and phosphate of 1.8 mg/dL. Concomitant measurement of parathyroid hormone was 0.1 pg/mL (normal 10–65 pg/mL), and a screen for parathyroid hormone–related peptide was positive. Over the first 24 h, the patient receives 4 L of normal saline with furosemide diuresis. The next morning, the patient's calcium is now 17.6 mg/dL and phosphate is 2.2 mg/dL. She continues to have delirium. What is the best approach for ongoing treatment of this patient's hypercalcemia?

A. Continue therapy with large-volume fluid administration and forced diuresis with furosemide.
B. Continue therapy with large-volume fluid administration, but stop furosemide and treat with hydrochlorothiazide.
C. Initiate therapy with calcitonin alone.
D. Initiate therapy with pamidronate alone.
E. Initiate therapy with calcitonin and pamidronate.

19. Differentiating primary dysmenorrhea from other causes of chronic cyclical pelvic pain is important because there is a specific treatment for primary dysmenorrhea. What is the pathophysiology/treatment for primary dysmenorrhea?

A. Ectopic endometrium/oral contraceptives
B. History of sexual abuse/counseling
C. Increased stores of prostaglandin precursors/anti-inflammatory medication
D. Ruptured Graafian follicle/oral contraceptives

20. A 25-year-old female notes increasing facial hair and acne for the last 4 months. She has noticed some deepening of her voice but denies changes in her libido or genitalia. She weighs 94 kg and is 5 feet 5 inches tall. Blood pressure is 126/70 mmHg. Examination is notable for moderate obesity. There is no evidence of abdominal striae or bruising. All of the following would be important initial steps in the clinical assessment of this patient *except*

A. medication history
B. family history
C. serum testosterone level
D. serum dehydroepiandrosterone sulfate (DHEAS) level
E. abdominal ultrasound

21. A patient visited a local emergency room 1 week ago with a headache. She received a head MRI, which did not reveal a cause for her symptoms, but the final report states "an empty sella is noted. Advise clinical correlation." The patient was discharged from the emergency room with instructions to follow up with her primary care physician as soon as possible. Her headache has resolved, and the patient has no complaints; however, she comes to your office 1 day later very concerned about this unexpected MRI finding. What should be the next step in her management?

A. Diagnose her with subclinical panhypopituitarism, and initiate low-dose hormone replacement.
B. Reassure her and follow laboratory results closely.
C. Reassure her and repeat MRI in 6 months.
D. This may represent early endocrine malignancy—whole-body positron emission tomography/CT is indicated.
E. This MRI finding likely represents the presence of a benign adenoma—refer to neurosurgery for resection.

22. A 16-year-old previously healthy teenage boy presents to the local emergency room with a headache that has been worsening over the course of 2 months. His parents note that "he just hasn't seemed like himself," and over the past 2 weeks has been complaining of double vision. He experienced profuse vomiting this afternoon, which prompted his visit. He also describes weight gain over the same 2-month time period and has not been sleeping well. On examination, he is drowsy, and funduscopic examination reveals papilledema. He has no fever, neck stiffness, or elevated white blood cell count. Which of the following is the most likely cause?

A. Carney syndrome
B. Congenital panhypopituitarism
C. Craniopharyngioma
D. McCune-Albright syndrome
E. Meningioma

23. At the midpoint of the menstrual cycle, a luteinizing hormone (LH) surge occurs via an estrogen-mediated pathway. Though chronic low levels of estrogen are inhibitory to LH release, gradually rising estrogen levels stimulate LH secretion. This relationship between estrogen and LH is an example of which endocrine regulatory system?

A. Autocrine regulation
B. Negative feedback control
C. Paracrine regulation
D. Positive feedback control

24. Which of the following is the most common site for a fracture associated with osteoporosis?

A. Femur
B. Hip
C. Radius
D. Vertebra
E. Wrist

25. Postmenopausal estrogen therapy has been shown to increase a female's risk of all of the following clinical outcomes *except*

A. breast cancer
B. hip fracture
C. myocardial infarction
D. stroke
E. venous thromboembolism

26. All of the following therapies have been shown to reduce the risk of hip fractures in postmenopausal women with osteoporosis *except*

A. alendronate
B. estrogen
C. parathyroid hormone
D. raloxifene
E. risedronate
F. vitamin D plus calcium

27. A 45-year-old man is diagnosed with pheochromocytoma after presentation with confusion, marked hypertension to 250/140 mmHg, tachycardia, headaches, and flushing. His fractionated plasma metanephrines show a normetanephrine level of 560 pg/mL and a metanephrine level of 198 pg/mL (normal values: normetanephrine: 18–111 pg/mL; metanephrine: 12–60 pg/mL). CT scanning of the abdomen with IV contrast demonstrates a 3-cm mass in the right adrenal gland. A brain MRI with gadolinium shows edema of the white matter near the parietooccipital junction consistent with reversible posterior

27. *(Continued)*
leukoencephalopathy. You are asked to consult regarding management. Which of the following statements is true regarding management of pheochromocytoma in this individual?

A. Beta blockade is absolutely contraindicated for tachycardia even after adequate alpha blockade has been attained.
B. Immediate surgical removal of the mass is indicated, because the patient presented with hypertensive crisis with encephalopathy.
C. Salt and fluid intake should be restricted to prevent further exacerbation of the patient's hypertension.
D. Treatment with phenoxybenzamine should be started at a high dose (20–30 mg three times daily) to rapidly control blood pressure, and surgery can be undertaken within 24–48 h.
E. Treatment with IV phentolamine is indicated for treatment of the hypertensive crisis. Phenoxybenzamine should be started at a low dose and titrated to the maximum tolerated dose over 2–3 weeks. Surgery should not be planned until the blood pressure is consistently below 160/100 mmHg.

28. Inhibition of renin activity is a contemporary target mechanism for treatment of hypertension. All of the following physiologic alterations will cause an increase in renin secretion *except*

A. decreased effective circulating blood volume
B. high-potassium diet
C. increased sympathetic activity
D. low solute delivery to the distal convoluted tubules
E. upright posture

29. Which of the following represents the likelihood of finding a pituitary microadenoma at autopsy in the general population?

A. 0.1%
B. 2%
C. 5%
D. 11%
E. 25%

30. A 33-year-old woman presents to the emergency room complaining of headache, palpitations, sweating, and anxiety. These feelings began abruptly about 30 min ago, and she reports intermittent symptoms similar to these that occur perhaps once per month. She has previously been diagnosed with panic attacks and has been prescribed paroxetine 20 mg daily. Her symptoms have not improved since initiation of this drug, and she believes that her episodes

30. *(Continued)*
of palpitations and anxiety have worsened since this time. Her past medical history includes a diagnosis of hypertension, but treatment with amlodipine has recently been discontinued because her blood pressure was 88/50 mmHg with symptomatic orthostasis at her last visit with her primary care provider. Her only other medical history is headaches for the past year for which she has been prescribed ibuprofen, 600 mg, as needed. She believes the headaches accompany her episodes and last for several hours after the sweating has subsided. On physical examination, the patient appears flushed and diaphoretic. Her blood pressure while lying down is 170/100 mmHg with a heart rate of 90 beats/min. Upon standing her blood pressure falls to 132/74 mmHg with a heart rate of 112 beats/min. Her respiratory rate is 22 beats/min, and her temperature is 37.4°C (99.3°F). Her examination is otherwise normal. There is no papilledema. Which of the following is most likely to correctly diagnose this patient?

A. 24-h urine collection for 5-hydroxyindoleacetic acid (5-HIAA)
B. 24-h urine collection for fractionated metanephrines
C. CT scan of the abdomen with IV contrast
D. ^{131}I-metaiodobenzylguanidine scan (MIBG)
E. No testing is necessary; the patient is suffering from a panic attack

31. The mineralocorticoid receptor in the renal tubule is responsible for the sodium retention and potassium wasting that is seen in mineralocorticoid excess states such as aldosterone-secreting tumors. However, states of glucocorticoid excess (e.g., Cushing's syndrome) can also present with sodium retention and hypokalemia. What characteristic of the mineralocorticoid-glucocorticoid pathways explain this finding?

A. Higher affinity of the mineralocorticoid receptor for glucocorticoids
B. Oversaturation of the glucocorticoid degradation pathway in states of glucocorticoid excess
C. Similar, but distinct, DNA-binding sites producing the same metabolic effect
D. Upregulation of the mineralocorticoid-binding protein in states of glucocorticoid excess

32. A 40-year-old female with Graves' disease was recently started on methimazole. One month later she comes to the clinic for a routine follow-up. She notes some low-grade fevers, arthralgias, and general malaise. Laboratories are notable for a mild transaminitis and a glucose of 150 mg/dL. All of the following are known side effects of methimazole *except*

A. agranulocytosis
B. rash
C. arthralgia
D. hepatitis
E. insulin resistance

33. A 60-year-old woman is referred to your office for evaluation of hypercalcemia of 12.9 mg/dL. This was found incidentally on a chemistry panel that was drawn during a hospitalization for cervical spondylosis. Despite fluid administration in the hospital, her serum calcium at discharge was 11.8 mg/dL. The patient is asymptomatic. She is otherwise in good health and has had her recommended age-appropriate cancer screening. She denies constipation or bone pain and is now 8 weeks out from her spinal surgery. Today, her serum calcium level is 12.4 mg/dL, and phosphate is 2.3 mg/dL. Her hematocrit and all other chemistries including creatinine were normal. What is the most likely diagnosis?

A. Breast cancer
B. Hyperparathyroidism
C. Hyperthyroidism
D. Multiple myeloma
E. Vitamin D intoxication

34. A 62-year-old man presents to a local emergency room complaining of chest pressure and feeling "like my heart is fluttering inside my chest." He experienced similar symptoms 1 month ago that resolved spontaneously. He did not seek medical attention at that time. He has no significant past medical history. On review of systems he notes some recent weight loss and excessive sweating. He feels as though his appetite has increased lately. His wife adds that he has recently taken some time off work due to fatigue; despite his time off he has not been able to relax and has not been sleeping well. On physical examination his heart rate is irregular at 140–150 beats/min. Blood pressure is 134/55 mmHg. He is admitted to the hospital and screening tests reveal an undetectable thyroid-stimulating hormone level. Which of the following statements is true?

A. 50% of hyperthyroid patients will convert from atrial fibrillation to normal sinus rhythm with thyroid management alone.
B. A firm, small thyroid on physical examination would be compatible with a diagnosis of Graves' disease.
C. Atrial fibrillation is the most common cardiac manifestation of hyperthyroidism.

34. *(Continued)*

D. His excessive sweating is likely not related to hyperthyroidism.

E. Hyperthyroidism leads to a high-output state for the heart, and narrowing pulse pressure.

35. The patient described above is started on atenolol and his heart rate slows to 80 beats/min. Which of the following additional therapies is indicated?

A. Diltiazem
B. Itraconazole
C. Liothyronine
D. Methimazole
E. Phenoxybenzamine

36. A patient presents to his primary care physician complaining of fatigue and hair loss. He has gained 6.4 kg since his last clinic visit 6 months ago but notes markedly decreased appetite. On review of systems, he reports that he is not sleeping well and feels cold all the time. He is still able to enjoy his hobbies and spending time with his family, and does not believe that he is depressed. His examination reveals diffuse alopecia and slowed deep tendon reflex relaxation. Hypothyroidism is high on the differential for this patient. Which of the statements regarding that diagnosis is correct?

A. A normal thyroid-stimulating hormone (TSH) excludes secondary, but not primary hypothyroidism.
B. T_3 measurement is not indicated to make the diagnosis.
C. The T_3/T_4 ratio is important for determining response to therapy.
D. Thyroid peroxidase antibodies distinguish between primary and secondary hypothyroidism.
E. Unbound T_4 is a better screening test than TSH for subclinical hypothyroidism.

37. Which of the following statements regarding autoimmune hypothyroidism is true?

A. 10% of 40- to 60-year-old adults have subclinical hypothyroidism.
B. Absence of a goiter makes autoimmune hypothyroidism unlikely.
C. Family history of autoimmune disorders does not significantly increase risk.
D. It is more common in the Pacific Rim where diets are lower in iodine.
E. Viral thyroiditis does not induce subsequent autoimmune thyroiditis.

38. You are researching a cell line with an altered membrane structure that makes the cell membrane impermeable to extracellular molecules of all sizes and charges. You then expose the cell line to varying concentrations of various hormones. Of the following hormones, which one should no longer exert an effect on this cell line?

A. Dopamine
B. Gonadotropin-releasing hormone
C. Insulin
D. Vitamin D

39. In regard to Graves' disease, which of the following is true?

A. It accounts for >90% of all causes of thyrotoxicosis.
B. It occurs in 2% of women.
C. It typically occurs in patients between 50 and 60 years of age.
D. Populations with a low iodine intake have an increased prevalence.
E. There is an equal male-to-female prevalence.

40. The parents of a 14-year-old boy want your opinion about treatment of their child's lipid disorder. The family emigrated from South Africa to the United States recently. The child has had cutaneous xanthomas on the hands, elbows, heels, and buttocks since childhood. In South Africa, he underwent thoracotomy for a problem with his aortic valve 3 years ago. He currently experiences exertional dyspnea, and his diet consists mostly of unhealthy, fatty foods. On examination, you appreciate bruits in the femoral arteries and abdominal aorta. His most recent lipid profile shows a total cholesterol of 734 mg/dL and a low-density lipoprotein (LDL) of 376 mg/dL. What is the most appropriate step in this patient's evaluation?

A. Genetic test for familial defective apoB100
B. Rule out congenital syphilis
C. Rule out hypothyroidism
D. Screen the parents for Munchausen-by-proxy syndrome

41. A 16-year-old male is brought to your clinic by his parents due to concern about his weight. He has not seen a physician for many years. He states that he has gained weight due to inactivity and that he is less active because of exertional chest pain. He takes no medications. He was adopted and his parents do not know the medical history of his biologic parents. Physical examination is notable for Stage 1 hypertension and body mass index of 30 kg/m^2. He has xanthomas on his hands, heels, and buttocks. Laboratory testing shows a low-density lipoprotein (LDL) of

41 *(Continued)*
210 mg/dL, creatinine of 0.7 mg/dL, total bilirubin of 3.1 mg/dL, haptoglobin of <6 mg/dL, and a glycosylated hemoglobin of 6.7%. You suspect a hereditary lipoproteinemia due to the clinical and laboratory findings. Which test would be diagnostic of the primary lipoprotein disorder in this patient?

A. Congo red staining of xanthoma biopsy
B. CT scan of the liver
C. Family pedigree analysis
D. Gas chromatography
E. LDL receptor function in skin biopsy

42. A 35-year-old woman presents with amenorrhea over the past 4 months. She has been trying to get pregnant without success. She complains of a thin milky discharge from her nipples and over the past several days has noted some blurry vision. On laboratory testing, her prolactin level is 110 μg/L (normal: 5–20 μg/L). A head MRI is performed and reveals an 11-mm pituitary macroadenoma. What is the next step in management?

A. Follow visual fields; if worse in 1 month, refer for surgery.
B. Reassure the patient and follow up closely.
C. Refer for urgent neurosurgery.
D. Repeat MRI in 4 months.
E. Do visual field testing and initiate a dopamine agonist.

43. A patient is asked to undergo a testing protocol to assess adrenocortical function. After 5 days of severe sodium restriction (10 mmol/d), blood is drawn for analysis. Which hormone abnormality may be detected using this protocol?

A. Hypercortisolism
B. Glucocorticoid deficiency
C. Mineralocorticoid deficiency
D. Mineralocorticoid excess
E. Vasopressin excess

44. A 38-year-old woman presents to her primary care doctor complaining of fatigue and irritability. She thinks these symptoms have been worsening over a period of several months. She has a history of mild intermittent asthma and hypertriglyceridemia. Physical examination reveals a resting heart rate of 105 beats/min, blood pressure of 136/72 mmHg, bilateral proptosis, and warm, moist skin. Screening tests are sent and reveal a thyroid-stimulating hormone (TSH) level that is undetectable and a normal unbound T_4. What should be the next step in diagnosis?

44. *(Continued)*

A. Radionuclide scan of the thyroid
B. Thyroid-stimulating antibody screen
C. Thyroid peroxidase (TPO) antibody screen
D. Total T_4
E. Unbound T_3

45. A 24-year-old female patient returns to your office to review her recent laboratory data. On her last clinic visit, you began an evaluation for secondary amenorrhea. Her vital signs are normal and her body mass index (BMI) is 20 kg/m^2. Her β-human chorionic gonadotropin is negative. Serum follicle-stimulating hormone (FSH) is below the lower limit of normal. Serum testosterone is within normal limits. Morning cortisol is 24 mg/dL. Urinalysis is unremarkable and there is no glucose in the urine. Thyroid-stimulating hormone is 3.7 mU/L. Serum prolactin is elevated. What is the most likely cause of this patient's secondary amenorrhea?

A. Ectopic pregnancy
B. Pituitary tumor
C. Primary ovarian failure
D. Uterine outflow obstruction
E. Malnutrition

46. A couple seeks advice regarding infertility. The female partner is 35 years old. She has never been pregnant and was taking oral contraceptive pills from age 20 until age 34. It is now 16 months since she discontinued her oral contraceptives. She is having menstrual cycles approximately once every 35 days, but occasionally will go as long as 60 days between cycles. Most months, she develops breast tenderness about 2–3 weeks after the start of her menstrual cycle. When she was in college, she was treated for *Neisseria gonorrhoeae* that was diagnosed when she presented to the student health center with a fever and pelvic pain. She otherwise has no medical history. She works about 60 h weekly as a corporate attorney and exercises daily. She drinks coffee daily and alcohol at social occasions only. Her body mass index (BMI) is 19.8 kg/m^2. Her husband, who is 39 years old, accompanies her to the evaluation. He also has never had children. He was married previously from the age of 24–28. He and his prior wife attempted to conceive for about 15 months, but were unsuccessful. At that time, he was smoking marijuana on a daily basis and attributed their lack of success to his drug use. He has now been completely free of drugs for 9 years. He suffers from hypertension and is treated with lisinopril, 10 mg daily. He is not obese (BMI, 23.7 kg/m^2). They request evaluation

46. *(Continued)*
for their infertility and request help with conception. Which of the following statements is true in regard to their infertility and likelihood of success in conception?

A. Determination of ovulation is not necessary in the female partner as most of her cycles occur regularly, and she develops breast tenderness midcycle indicative of ovulation.
B. Lisinopril should be discontinued immediately because of the risk of birth defects associated with its use.
C. The female partner should be assessed for tubal patency by a hysterosalpingogram. If significant scarring is found, in vitro fertilization should be strongly considered to decrease the risk of ectopic pregnancy.
D. The prolonged use of oral contraceptives for >10 years has increased the risk of anovulation and infertility.
E. The use of marijuana by the male partner is directly toxic to sperm motility, and this is the likely cause of their infertility.

47. A 22-year-old male seeks evaluation from his primary care doctor for gynecomastia that has developed over the past 2 years. He states he did not enter puberty until much later than his friends and has only had sparse growth of facial and axillary hair. He continues to have poor libido and rarely desires sexual intercourse, even though he has been in a monogamous relationship for the past 8 months. His girlfriend is increasingly frustrated by his lack of sexual desire and also urged him to seek medical evaluation. He has no other medical history and was born prematurely at 34 weeks' gestation. His birth weight was 2400 g (50th percentile). His early development was normal. During elementary school, he was held back in third grade because of learning difficulties and thereafter was in special educational classes to assist him with reading and mathematics. He is taking no medications. On physical examination, he is 188 cm tall and has eunuchoid features. His facial, axillary, and genital hair is sparse. Gynecomastia is present. The testes are small, measuring 2.8 cm in length. What is the most likely diagnosis in this patient?

A. Androgen insensitivity syndrome (testicular feminization)
B. Klinefelter syndrome
C. Mixed gonadal dysgenesis (45,X/46,XY mosaicism)
D. Testicular dysgenesis
E. True hermaphroditism

48. All of the following drugs may interfere with testicular function *except*

48. *(Continued)*
A. cyclophosphamide
B. ketoconazole
C. metoprolol
D. prednisone
E. spironolactone

49. A 65-year-old man with a central left upper lobe lung mass presents with renal stones and generalized bone pain. He is found to have a calcium level of 16.4 mg/dL with a phosphate level of 1.2 mg/dL. A bone scan is normal. Which of the following laboratory tests is most likely to establish a diagnosis?

A. Adrenocorticotropic hormone (ACTH)
B. Cortisol
C. Magnesium level
D. Parathyroid hormone (intact PTH or PTHi)
E. Parathyroid hormone–related peptide (PTHrp)

50. A biopsy of the lung mass in the patient in Question 49 will most likely show:

A. Bronchoalveolar lung carcinoma
B. Bronchial carcinoid
C. Poorly differentiated adenocarcinoma
D. Small cell carcinoma
E. Squamous cell carcinoma

51. All of the following are direct actions of parathyroid hormone (PTH) *except*

A. increased calcium resorption from bone
B. increased calcium resorption from the kidney
C. increased calcium resorption from the gastrointestinal tract
D. increased synthesis of 1,25-dihydroxyvitamin D
E. decreased phosphate resorption from the kidney

52. A 45-year-old Caucasian woman seeks advice from her primary care physician regarding her risk for osteoporosis and the need for bone density screening. She is a lifelong nonsmoker and drinks alcohol only socially. She has a history of moderate persistent asthma since age 12. She is currently on fluticasone, 44 mg/puff twice daily, with good control currently. She last required oral prednisone therapy about 6 months ago when she had influenza that was complicated by an asthma flare. She took prednisone for a total of 14 days. She has had three pregnancies and two live births at ages 39 and 41. She currently has irregular periods occurring approximately every 42 days. Her follicle-stimulating hormone level is 25 mIU/L and 17β-estradiol level is 115 pg/mL on day 12 of her menstrual cycle. Her mother and

52. *(Continued)*
maternal aunt both have been diagnosed with osteoporosis. Her mother also has rheumatoid arthritis and requires prednisone therapy, 5 mg daily. Her mother developed a compression fracture of the lumbar spine at age 68. On physical examination, the patient appears well and healthy. Her height is 168 cm. Her weight is 66.4 kg. The chest, cardiac, abdominal, muscular, and neurologic examinations are normal. What do you tell the patient about the need for bone density screening?

A. As she is currently perimenopausal, she should have a bone density screen every other year until she completes menopause and then have bone densitometry measured yearly thereafter.
B. Because of her family history, she should initiate bone density screening yearly beginning now.
C. Bone densitometry screening is not recommended until after completion of menopause.
D. Delayed childbearing until the fourth and fifth decade decreases her risk of developing osteoporosis.
E. Her use of low-dose inhaled glucocorticoids increases her risk of osteoporosis threefold, and she should undergo yearly bone density screening.

53. A 62-year-old woman presents to your clinic complaining of fatigue and lethargy over a period of 6 months. She cannot recall exactly when these symptoms started, but feels that they are worsening with time. She describes dry skin and has noted that she is losing hair. On examination she is mildly bradycardic at 52 beats/min with normal blood pressure and has dry, coarse skin. There are areas of alopecia and mild lower extremity edema is noted. Which of the following is the most likely clinical diagnosis and which test would be indicated for screening for the diagnosis?

A. Hyperthyroidism: thyroid-stimulating hormone (TSH)
B. Hyperthyroidism: unbound T_4
C. Hypothyroidism: TSH
D. Hypothyroidism: unbound T_4

54. A 55-year-old male is admitted to the intensive care unit with 1 week of fever and cough. He was well until 1 week before admission, when he noted progressive shortness of breath, cough, and productive sputum. On the day of admission the patient was noted by his wife to be lethargic and unresponsive. 911 was called, and the patient was intubated in the field and then brought to the emergency department. His medications include insulin. The past medical history is notable for alcohol abuse, diabetes mellitus, and chronic renal insufficiency. Temperature is 38.9°C (102°F). He is hypotensive with a blood pressure of 76/40 mmHg. Oxygen saturation is 86% on room air. On examination, the patient is sedated and intubated. Jugular venous pressure is normal. There are decreased breath sounds at the right lung base with egophony. Heart sounds are normal. The abdomen is soft. There is no peripheral edema. Chest radiography shows a right lower lobe infiltrate with a moderate pleural effusion. An electrocardiogram is normal. Sputum Gram stain shows gram-positive diplococci. White blood cell count is $23 \times 10^3/\mu L$, with 70% polymorphonuclear cells and 6% bands. Blood urea nitrogen is 80 mg/dL, and creatinine is 6.1 mg/dL. Plasma glucose is 425 mg/dL. He is started on broad-spectrum antibiotics, IV fluids, omeprazole, and an insulin drip. A nasogastric tube is inserted, and tube feedings are started. On hospital day 2 plasma phosphate is 1.0 mg/dL. All of following are causes of hypophosphatemia *except*

A. sepsis
B. renal failure
C. insulin
D. alcoholism
E. malnutrition

55. A 50-year-old male presents to the clinic for a routine health examination. A comprehensive metabolic panel shows a serum calcium level of 11.2 mg/dL. Serum phosphate is 3.0 mg/dL. Serum creatinine is normal. He denies bone pain, lethargy, weakness, or weight loss. What is the most common cause of hypercalcemia in outpatients?

A. Malignancy
B. Medications
C. Milk-alkali syndrome
D. Primary hyperparathyroidism
E. Granulomatous disease

56. All of the following would be indicated in the workup of infertility *except*

A. endometrial biopsy
B. hysterosalpingogram
C. measurement of testosterone and dehydroepiandrosterone in the female partner
D. measurement of testosterone, follicle-stimulating hormone (FSH), and luteinizing hormone (LH) in the male partner
E. semen analysis

57. You are asked to see a 15-year-old African-American girl because of anovulation. She has never experienced menarche, and her mother is concerned since most women in her family experience menarche around 13 years of age. The patient has prominent nipples and the areolae are part of the breast. Pubic hair is dark, curly, and coarse and is abundant in the pubic area and inner thigh. There is no facial hair, and muscular development is age and sex appropriate. She does have cyclical pelvic pain. What is the next step in her evaluation?

A. Examination with a speculum
B. MRI of the abdomen and pelvis
C. Serum follicle-stimulating hormone (FSH)
D. Serum prolactin

58. The World Health Organization (WHO) recently defined osteoporosis operationally as

A. a patient with a bone density less than the mean of age-, race-, and gender-matched controls
B. a patient with a bone density <1.0 standard deviation (SD) below the mean of race- and gender-matched controls
C. a patient with a bone density <1.0 SD below the mean of age-, race-, and gender-matched controls
D. a patient with a bone density <2.5 SD below the mean of race- and gender-matched controls
E. a patient with a bone density <2.5 SD below the mean of age-, race-, and gender-matched controls

59. All of the following are side effects of HMG-CoA reductase inhibitors (statins) *except*

A. hepatitis
B. myopathy
C. dyspepsia
D. headache
E. pulmonary fibrosis

60. Which of the following is consistent with a diagnosis of subacute thyroiditis?

A. A 38-year-old female with a 2-week history of a painful thyroid, elevated T_4, elevated T_3, low thyroid-stimulating hormone (TSH), and an elevated radioactive iodine uptake scan
B. A 42-year-old male with a history of a painful thyroid 4 months ago, fatigue, malaise, low free T_4, low T_3, and elevated TSH
C. A 31-year-old female with a painless enlarged thyroid, low TSH, elevated T_4, elevated free T_4, and an elevated radioiodine uptake scan

60. *(Continued)*
D. A 50-year-old male with a painful thyroid, slightly elevated T_4, normal TSH, and an ultrasound showing a mass
E. A 46-year-old female with 3 weeks of fatigue, low T_4, low T_3, and low TSH

61. All of the following statements regarding hypoglycemia in diabetes mellitus are true *except*

A. individuals with type 2 diabetes mellitus experience less hypoglycemia than those with type 1 diabetes mellitus.
B. recurrent episodes of hypoglycemia predispose to the development of autonomic failure with defective glucose counterregulation and hypoglycemia unawareness.
C. the average person with type 1 diabetes mellitus has two episodes of symptomatic hypoglycemia weekly.
D. thiazolidinediones and metformin cause hypoglycemia more frequently than sulfonylureas.
E. from 2–4% of deaths in type 1 diabetes mellitus are directly attributable to hypoglycemia.

62. Which of the following forms of contraception have theoretical efficacy of >90%?

A. Condoms
B. Intrauterine devices
C. Oral contraceptives
D. Spermicides
E. All of the above

63. A patient is seen in the clinic for follow-up of type 2 diabetes mellitus. Her hemoglobin A_{1C} has been poorly controlled at 9.4% recently. The patient can be counseled to expect all of the following improvements with improved glycemic control *except*

A. decreased microalbuminuria
B. decreased risk of nephropathy
C. decreased risk of neuropathy
D. decreased risk of peripheral vascular disease
E. decreased risk of retinopathy

64. A healthy 53-year-old man comes to your office for an annual physical examination. He has no complaints and has no significant medical history. He is taking an over-the-counter multivitamin and no other medicines. On physical examination he is noted to have a nontender thyroid nodule. His thyroid-stimulating hormone (TSH) level is checked and is found to be low. What is the next step in his evaluation?

64. *(Continued)*

A. Close follow-up and measure TSH in 6 months
B. Fine-needle aspiration
C. Low-dose thyroid replacement
D. Positron emission tomography followed by surgery
E. Radionuclide thyroid scan

65. During a routine checkup, a 67-year-old male is found to have a level of serum alkaline phosphatase three times the upper limit of normal. Serum calcium and phosphorus concentrations and liver function test results are normal. He is asymptomatic. The most likely diagnosis is

A. metastatic bone disease
B. primary hyperparathyroidism
C. occult plasmacytoma
D. Paget's disease of bone
E. osteomalacia

66. A 78-year-old man presents to your clinic and describes headaches and back pain. These have been chronic complaints, and he thinks they are getting worse despite conservative management. His wife believes he is experiencing some hearing loss. She describes how over the past several months he needs to turn up the volume on the television and has a difficult time talking to his children on the telephone. Physical examination is largely unremarkable; straight leg raise is normal. Based on Rinne and Weber tests, the patient appears to have some mild sensorineural hearing loss on the right side. A comprehensive chemistry panel shows an elevated alkaline phosphatase of 170 U/L. Paget's disease is now high on the differential. Which of the following is true regarding this diagnosis?

A. Family history is not predictive.
B. Hearing loss is the most common symptom.
C. Nuclear medicine bone scan is required for diagnosis.
D. Serum calcium and phosphate are usually abnormal.
E. The pelvis, skull, and vertebrae are most commonly affected.

67. Which of the following is the most common sign of Cushing's syndrome?

A. Amenorrhea
B. Hirsutism
C. Obesity
D. Purple skin striae
E. Skin hyperpigmentation

68. A patient receives CT of the head as part of a "virtual wellness physical exam" he received as a gift certificate from his family. A 7-mm sellar mass "most consistent with a pituitary adenoma" is reported, and he comes to your office very concerned that he has a life-threatening brain tumor. A full panel of endocrine laboratory measurements reveals no abnormalities, and besides his anxiety he reports feeling quite healthy. What is the next step in management?

A. Perform positron emission tomography/CT (PET-CT) to evaluate for metabolic activity.
B. Reassure the patient that this finding is common and benign; take no action.
C. Reassure and repeat laboratory measurements in 6 months.
D. Reassure and repeat head imaging in 1 year.
E. Refer to neurosurgery.

69. Which of the following statements regarding hormone release from the anterior pituitary is true?

A. All hormones are released in a pulsatile manner.
B. Follicle-stimulating hormone (FSH) and luteinizing hormone (LH) release are suppressed prior to puberty and after menopause.
C. Somatostatin acts in a feedback loop to inhibit adrenocorticotropin hormone (ACTH) release.
D. Thyroid-stimulating hormone (TSH) is released primarily at night.
E. With the exception of prolactin, none of the anterior pituitary hormones are present in a fetus until week 28 of gestation.

70. All of the following are features of lipoprotein lipase deficiency *except*

A. low levels of plasma chylomicrons
B. acute pancreatitis
C. hepatosplenomegaly
D. xanthomas
E. autosomal recessive inheritance

71. A 21-year-old female with a history of type 1 diabetes mellitus is brought to the emergency room with nausea, vomiting, lethargy, and dehydration. Her mother notes that she stopped taking insulin 1 day before presentation. She is lethargic, has dry mucous membranes, and is obtunded. Blood pressure is 80/40 mmHg, and heart rate is 112 beats/min. Heart sounds are normal. Lungs are clear. The abdomen is soft, and there is no organomegaly. She is responsive and oriented × 3 but diffusely weak. Serum sodium is 126 meq/L, potassium is 4.3 meq/L, magnesium is 1.2 meq/L, blood urea nitrogen is 76 mg/ dL, creatinine is 2.2 mg/dL, bicarbonate is 10 meq/L, and

71. *(Continued)*
chloride is 88 meq/L. Serum glucose is 720 mg/dL. All of the following are appropriate management steps *except*

A. arterial blood gas
B. IV insulin
C. IV potassium
D. 3% sodium solution
E. IV fluids

72. All of the following are effects of hypercalcemia *except*

A. diarrhea
B. confusion
C. polyuria
D. a shortened QT interval
E. nephrolithiasis

73. All of the following are actions of parathyroid hormone *except*

A. direct stimulation of osteoblasts to increase bone formation
B. direct stimulation of osteoclasts to increase bone resorption
C. increased reabsorption of calcium from the distal tubule of the kidney
D. inhibition of phosphate reabsorption in the proximal tubule of the kidney
E. stimulation of renal 1α-hydroxylase to produce 1,25-hydroxycholecalciferol

74. Which of the following statements regarding hypothyroidism is true?

A. Hashimoto's thyroiditis is the most common cause of hypothyroidism worldwide.
B. The annual risk of developing overt clinical hypothyroidism from subclinical hypothyroidism in patients with positive thyroid peroxidase (TPO) antibodies is 20%.
C. Histologically, Hashimoto's thyroiditis is characterized by marked infiltration of the thyroid with activated T cells and B cells.
D. A low TSH level excludes the diagnosis of hypothyroidism.
E. Thyroid peroxidase antibodies are present in <50% of patients with autoimmune hypothyroidism.

75. You are evaluating a patient for secondary causes of hypertension. The patient is a 39-year-old woman who has hypertension despite using four different classes of antihypertensive medications, including a diuretic at therapeutic doses. She mainly has diastolic hypertension and has been found to have hypokalemia on several routine blood chemistry analyses. You hold her diuretics and provide her with potassium supplementation for 14 days, after which you find the serum potassium is in the normal range. She denies licorice ingestion. Plasma renin activity is low. After days of saline loading, aldosterone levels are elevated. A CT scan of the adrenal glands reveals no masses. An overnight dexamethasone suppression test shows no aldosterone suppression. What is the most likely diagnosis?

A. Conn's syndrome
B. Cortical nodular hyperplasia
C. Glucocorticoid remediable aldosteronism
D. Liddle's syndrome
E. Renin-secreting tumor

76. A 17-year-old woman is evaluated in your office for primary amenorrhea. She does not feel as if she has entered puberty in that she has never had a menstrual period and has sparse axillary and pubic hair growth. On examination, she is noted to be 150 cm tall. She has a low hairline and slight webbing of her neck. Her follicle-stimulating hormone level is 75 mIU/mL, luteinizing hormone is 20 mIU/mL, and estradiol level is 2 pg/mL. You suspect Turner syndrome. All of the following tests are indicated in this individual *except*

A. buccal smear for nuclear heterochromatin (Barr body)
B. echocardiogram
C. karyotype analysis
D. renal ultrasound
E. thyroid-stimulating hormone (TSH)

77. A 30-year-old male, the father of three children, has had progressive breast enlargement during the last 6 months. He does not use any drugs. Laboratory evaluation reveals that both luteinizing hormone (LH) and testosterone are low. Further evaluation of this patient should include which of the following?

A. Blood sampling for serum glutamic-oxaloacetic transaminase (SGOT) and serum alkaline phosphatase and bilirubin levels
B. Measurement of estradiol and human chorionic gonadotropin (hCG) levels
C. A 24-h urine collection for the measurement of 17-ketosteroids
D. Karyotype analysis to exclude Klinefelter syndrome
E. Breast biopsy

78. Obesity is associated with an increased incidence of all of the following *except*

A. diabetes mellitus
B. cancer
C. hypertension
D. biliary disease
E. chronic obstructive lung disease

79. Which of the following statements regarding Paget's disease is true?

A. 1% of patients over the age of 50 have evidence of Paget's disease.
B. A majority of patients with disease will experience symptoms at the time of diagnosis.
C. The disease frequency has decreased over the past 20 years.
D. There is a significant female predominance.
E. While prevalent worldwide, Paget's disease is most common in Asia.

80. Which of the following statements is true about familial hypocalciuric hypercalcemia (FHH)?

A. It is inherited in an autosomal recessive pattern.
B. The cause is a defect in the parathyroid hormone receptor.
C. Clinical symptoms first manifest in the third and fourth decades of life.
D. Treatment is rarely necessary.
E. Renal calcium reabsorption is >99%.

81. A 48-year-old female is undergoing evaluation for flushing and diarrhea. Physical examination is normal except for nodular hepatomegaly. A CT scan of the abdomen demonstrates multiple nodules in both lobes of the liver consistent with metastases in the liver and a 2-cm mass in the ileum. The 24-h urinary 5-hydroxyindoleacetic acid (5-HIAA) excretion is markedly elevated. All of the following treatments are appropriate *except*

A. diphenhydramine
B. interferon-α
C. octreotide
D. ondansetron
E. phenoxybenzamine

82. While undergoing a physical examination during medical student clinical skills, this patient develops severe flushing, wheezing, nausea, and light-headedness. Vital signs are notable for a blood pressure of 70/30 mmHg and a heart rate of 135 beats/min. Which of the following is the most appropriate therapy?

82. *(Continued)*

A. Albuterol
B. Atropine
C. Epinephrine
D. Hydrocortisone
E. Octreotide

83. A 66-year-old Asian woman seeks treatment for osteoporosis. She fell and fractured her right hip, requiring a surgical intervention 3 months ago. She was told while hospitalized that she had osteoporosis but had not previously been evaluated for this. During the hospitalization, she developed a deep-vein thrombosis (DVT) with pulmonary embolus, for which she is currently taking warfarin. She completed menopause at age 52. She is a former smoker, quitting about 6 years ago. She has always been thin, and her current body mass index (BMI) is 19.2 kg/m^2. Her laboratory studies show a calcium of 8.7 mg/dL, phosphate of 3 mg/dL, creatinine of 0.8 mg/dL, and 25-hydroxyvitamin D levels of 18 ng/mL (normal >30 ng/mL). A dual-energy x-ray absorptiometry scan of bone mineral density has a T-score of –3.0. What is the best initial therapy for this patient?

A. Calcitonin, 200 IU intranasally daily
B. Calcium carbonate, 1200 mg, and vitamin D, 400 IU daily
C. Ethinyl estradiol, 5 μg, and medroxyprogesterone acetate, 625 mg daily
D. Raloxifene, 60 mg daily
E. Risedronate, 35 mg once weekly

84. All of the following would be expected to increase prolactin levels *except*

A. chest wall trauma
B. hyperthyroidism
C. pregnancy
D. renal failure
E. sexual orgasm

85. A 35-year-old male is referred to your clinic for evaluation of hypercalcemia noted during a health insurance medical screening. He has noted some fatigue, malaise, and a 4-lb weight loss over the last 2 months. He also has noted constipation and "heartburn." He is occasionally nauseated after large meals and has water brash and a sour taste in his mouth. The patient denies vomiting, dysphagia, or odynophagia. He also notes decreased libido and a depressed mood. Vital signs are unremarkable. Physical examination is notable for a clear oropharynx, no evidence of a thyroid mass, and no lymphadenopathy. Jugular venous pressure is normal. Heart sounds are regular with no

85. *(Continued)*
murmurs or gallops. The chest is clear. The abdomen is soft with some mild epigastric tenderness. There is no rebound or organomegaly. Stool is guaiac-positive. Neurologic examination is nonfocal. Laboratory values are notable for a normal complete blood count. Calcium is 11.2 mg/dL, phosphate is 2.1 mg/dL, and magnesium is 1.8 meq/dL. Albumin is 3.7 g/dL, and total protein is 7.0 g/dL. TSH is 3 μIU/mL, prolactin is 250 μg/L, testosterone is 620 ng/dL, and serum insulin-like growth factor 1 (IGF-1) is normal. Serum intact parathyroid hormone level is 135 pg/dL. In light of the patient's abdominal discomfort and heme-positive stool, you perform an abdominal computed tomography (CT) scan that shows a lesion measuring 2 cm by 2 cm in the head of the pancreas. What is the diagnosis?

A. Multiple endocrine neoplasia (MEN) type 1
B. MEN type 2A
C. MEN type 2B
D. Polyglandular autoimmune syndrome
E. Von–Hippel Lindau (VHL) syndrome

86. Your 60-year-old patient with a monoclonal gammopathy of unclear significance presents for a follow-up visit and to review recent laboratory data. His creatinine is newly elevated to 2.0 mg/dL, potassium is 3.7 mg/dL, calcium is 12.2 mg/dL, low-density lipoprotein (LDL) is 202 mg/dL, and triglycerides are 209 mg/dL. On further questioning he reports 3 months of swelling around the eyes and "foamy" urine. On examination, he has anasarca. Concerned for multiple myeloma and nephrotic syndrome, you order a urine protein/creatinine ratio, which returns at 14:1. Which treatment option would be most appropriate to treat his lipid abnormalities?

A. Cholesterol ester transfer protein inhibitor
B. Dietary management
C. HMG-CoA reductase inhibitors
D. Lipid apheresis
E. Niacin and fibrates

87. All of the following statements regarding asymptomatic adrenal masses (incidentalomas) are true *except*

A. all patients with incidentalomas should be screened for pheochromocytoma.
B. fine-needle aspiration may distinguish between benign and malignant primary adrenal tumors.
C. in patients with a history of malignancy, the likelihood the mass is a metastasis is ~50%.
D. the majority of adrenal incidentalomas are nonsecretory.
E. the vast majority of adrenal incidentalomas are benign.

88. Which of the following studies is most sensitive for detecting diabetic nephropathy?

A. Serum creatinine level
B. Creatinine clearance
C. Urine albumin
D. Glucose tolerance test
E. Ultrasonography

ANSWERS

1. The answer is D.
(Chap. 4) The thyroid produces two related hormones, T_3 and T_4. These hormones act on nuclear receptors inside cells to regulate differentiation during development and maintain metabolic homeostasis in virtually all human cells. T_4 is secreted in excess of T_3 from the thyroid and both are protein-bound in the plasma. Protein binding delays hormone clearance. Unbound protein appears to be more biologically active. T_4 is converted to more active T_3 in peripheral tissues. Two thyroid hormone receptors are bound to specific DNA sequences; when activated by thyroid hormone, these receptors can act to upregulate or downregulate gene transcription. Iodide uptake by the thyroid is the critical first step of thyroid hormone synthesis. Dietary iodine deficiency leads to decreased production of thyroid hormone and represents the most common cause of hypothyroidism worldwide. In areas of iodine sufficiency, autoimmune disease such as Hashimoto's thyroiditis and iatrogenic causes are the most common etiologies for hypothyroidism. Paradoxically, chronic iodine excess can also cause goiter and hypothyroidism via unclear mechanisms. This is the mechanism for the hypothyroidism that occurs in up to 13% of patients taking amiodarone. Graves' disease leads to hyperthyroidism.

2. The answer is A.
(Chap. 2) The diagnosis of Cushing's syndrome relies on documentation of endogenous hypercortisolism. Of the list given, the most cost-effective and precise test is the 24-h urine free cortisol. Failure to suppress plasma A.M. cortisol after overnight suppression with 1 mg

dexamethasone is an alternative. Most ACTH-secreting pituitary adenomas are <5 mm in diameter and approximately half are not detected even with sensitive MRI. Further, because incidental microadenomas are common in the pituitary, the presence of a small pituitary abnormality on MRI may not establish the source of ACTH production. Basal plasma ACTH levels are used to distinguish between ACTH-independent (adrenal or exogenous glucocorticoid) and ACTH-dependent (pituitary, ectopic ACTH) sources of hypercortisolism. Mean basal ACTH levels are higher in patients with ectopic ACTH production than in patients with pituitary ACTH adenomas. There is significant overlap in ACTH levels, however, and this test should not be used as an initial diagnostic test. Rarely, patients have Cushing's syndrome and elevated ACTH due to a CRH-releasing tumor. In this case, CRH levels are elevated. Inferior petrosal venous sampling can be used to identify a pituitary source of ACTH secretion when imaging modalities do not reveal a source.

3. The answer is C.
(Chap. 1) Intermittent pulses of GnRH are necessary to maintain pituitary sensitivity to the hormone. Continuous exposure to GnRH causes pituitary gonadotrope desensitization, which ultimately leads to decreased levels of testosterone. The relationship between GnRH and LH/FSH is a positive feedback loop where GnRH causes secretion of LH and FSH. Receptor translocation from the cytoplasm into the nucleus occurs with certain hormones (e.g., glucocorticoid); however, this receptor phenomenon is not specific to any regulatory mechanism. GnRH does not promote production of sex hormone–binding globulin. Moreover, although binding globulins can decrease the amount of bound hormone measured in the serum, abnormal levels of binding globulins usually do not have any clinical significance because the free hormone levels usually increase.

4. The answer is C.
(Chap. 12) Perimenopause refers to the time period prior to menopause during which menstrual cycles become increasingly irregular and fertility wanes. This period usually lasts for 2–8 years before final menses and menopause. In perimenopause, the interval between menses typically declines by about 3 days because of acceleration of the follicular phase of the menstrual cycle. Measurement of hormone levels in the perimenopausal period can be difficult to interpret because hormone levels are "irregularly irregular." Measurement of follicle-stimulating hormone during the early follicular phase (days 2–5) of the menstrual cycle can rule out perimenopause if the levels are very low, while high levels are suggestive of the perimenopausal state. Perimenopause is generally a hyperestrogenic state, and there is an increased risk of endometrial carcinoma, uterine polyps, and leiomyoma during this period. Because of these risks, low-dose oral contraceptive pills are commonly used during perimenopause. Use of oral contraceptives is also important because the risk of unintended pregnancy in this period rivals that of adolescence. However, the risks of oral contraceptives need to be weighed against the increased risk of thrombosis and breast cancer. Contraindications to the use of oral contraceptives are breast cancer, cigarette smoking, liver disease, history of thromboembolic or cardiovascular disease, or unexplained vaginal bleeding.

5. and 6. The answers are A and E.
(Chap. 28) Osteoporosis is a significant public health problem in the United States affecting 8 million women and 2 million men. An additional 18 million individuals are at risk for development of osteoporosis as measured by low bone density (osteopenia). Most of these individuals are unaware of the presence of osteopenia or osteoporosis. In the United States and Europe, fractures related to osteoporosis are much more common in women than men, although this is not seen in all races. Nonmodifiable risk factors for the development of osteoporosis include a personal history of fracture or a history of fracture in a first-degree relative, female sex, advanced age, and white race. African Americans have approximately one-half the risk of osteoporotic fractures as whites. Diseases that increase the risk of falls or frailty, such as dementia and Parkinson's disease, also increase fracture risk. Cigarette smoking, low body weight, low calcium intake, alcoholism, and lack of physical activity are all associated with increased bone loss and fractures. Multiple drugs are associated with an increased risk of osteoporosis. In addition to those listed, other anticonvulsants, cytotoxic drugs, excessive thyroxine, aluminum, gonadotropin-releasing hormone agonists, and lithium are associated with decreased bone mass and osteoporosis. Histamine antagonists are not associated with osteoporosis.

7. The answer is C.
(Chap. 2) Diagnosis of pituitary insufficiency is made by biochemical demonstration of low levels of trophic hormones in the setting of low target hormone levels. Thus, in a postmenopausal woman, a low FSH and LH would suggest hypopituitarism. Provocative tests may also be used to test reduced pituitary reserve. Growth hormone should elevate during hypoglycemic stress, not during hyperglycemia. Elevation of aldosterone (or cortisol) after cosyntropin, cortisol after insulin-induced hypoglycemia, or TSH after TRH are consistent with intact pituitary function. A summary of tests of pituitary insufficiency is shown in Table 2-3.

8. The answer is A.
(Chap. 20) When an individual presents with profound hypoglycemia and no history of diabetes mellitus, one

must determine the cause expediently and treat accordingly. Immediate treatment of this patient should include ongoing glucose administration while attempting to determine the cause. The initial step for diagnosing this patient is to determine the plasma glucose, insulin, and C-peptide levels. When the plasma glucose level is <55 mg/dL, the plasma insulin levels should be low. If the insulin levels are inappropriately high (≥18 pmol/L or ≥3 μU/mL), the C-peptide level should be assessed simultaneously. C peptide is the protein fragment that remains after proinsulin is cleaved to insulin. C peptide would be high (≥0.6 ng/mL) in individuals with an endogenous source of hyperinsulinemia such as insulinoma. However, C-peptide levels are low or undetectable when the source of insulin is exogenous, such as in surreptitious insulin intake or insulin overdose. One exception to consider in this individual is surreptitious intake or overdose of a sulfonylurea, an insulin secretagogue. In this case, insulin and C-peptide levels would both be elevated, and a sulfonylurea screen is also appropriate in this patient.

9. The answer is D.
(Chap. 4) Sick-euthyroid syndrome can occur in the setting of any acute, severe illness. Abnormalities in the levels of circulating TSH and thyroid hormone are thought to result from the release of cytokines in response to severe stress. Multiple abnormalities may occur. The most common hormone pattern is a decrease in total and unbound T_3 levels as peripheral conversion of T_4 to T_3 is impaired. Teleologically, the fall in T_3, the most active thyroid hormone, is thought to limit catabolism in starved or ill patients. TSH levels may vary dramatically, from 0.1 to >20 mU/L, depending on when they are measured during the course of illness. Very sick patients may have a decrease in T_4 levels. This patient undoubtedly has abnormal thyroid function tests as a result of his injuries from the motor vehicle accident. There is no indication for obtaining further imaging in this case. Steroids have no role. The most appropriate management consists of simple observation. Over the course of weeks to months, as the patient recovers, thyroid function will return to normal.

10. The answer is A.
(Chap. 28) A number of biochemical tests are used to assess the rate of bone remodeling. Bone remodeling is related to the rate of formation and resorption. Remodeling markers do not predict bone loss well enough to be applied clinically. However, measures of bone resorption may help in the prediction of risk of fracture in older patients. In women over 65 years old, even in the presence of normal bone density, a high index of bone resorption should prompt consideration for treatment. Measures of bone resorption fall quickly after the initiation of antiresorptive therapy (bisphosphonates, estrogen, raloxifene, calcitonin) and provide an earlier measure of response than does bone densitometry. Serum alkaline phosphatase is a measure of bone formation, not resorption, as are serum osteocalcin and serum propeptide of type I procollagen.

Biochemical Markers of Bone Metabolism in Clinical Use

Bone formation
- Serum bone-specific alkaline phosphatase
- Serum osteocalcin
- Serum propeptide of type I procollagen

Bone resorption
- Urine and serum cross-linked N-telopeptide
- Urine and serum cross-linked C-telopeptide
- Urine total free deoxypyridinoline
- Urine hydroxyproline
- Serum tartrate-resistant acid phosphatase
- Urine hydroxylysine glycosides

11. The answer is B.
(Chap. 28) Osteoporosis is a common disease affecting 8 million women and 2 million men in the United States. It is most common in postmenopausal women, but the incidence is also increasing in men. Estrogen loss probably causes bone loss by activation of bone remodeling sites and exaggeration of the imbalance between bone formation and resorption. Osteoporosis is diagnosed by bone mineral density scan. Dual-energy x-ray absorptiometry (DXA) is the most accurate test for measuring bone mineral density. Clinical determinations of bone density are most commonly measured at the lumbar spine and hip. In the DXA technique, two x-ray energies are used to measure the area of the mineralized tissues and compared to gender- and race-matched normative values. The T-score compares an individual's results to a young population, whereas the Z-score compares the individual's results to an age-matched population. Osteoporosis is diagnosed when the T-score is –2.5 SD in the lumbar spine, femoral neck, or total hip. An evaluation for secondary causes of osteoporosis should be considered in individuals presenting with osteoporotic fractures at a young age and those who have very low Z-scores. Initial evaluation should include serum and 24-h urine calcium levels, renal function panel, hepatic function panel, serum phosphorous level, and vitamin D levels. Other endocrine abnormalities including hyperthyroidism and hyperparathyroidism should be evaluated, and urinary cortisol levels should be checked if there is a clinical suspicion for Cushing's syndrome. Follicle-stimulating hormone and luteinizing hormone levels would be elevated but are not useful in this individual as she presents with a known perimenopausal state.

12. The answer is D.
(Chap. 29) Despite her lack of symptoms, this patient has enough evidence to diagnose her with Paget's disease. Her radiographs show characteristic changes of active

disease in the pelvis, one of the most common areas for Paget's disease to present. Her elevated alkaline phosphatase provides further evidence of active bone turnover. The normal serum calcium and phosphate levels are characteristic for Paget's disease. Management of asymptomatic Paget's disease has changed since effective treatments have become available. Treatment should be initiated in all symptomatic patients and in asymptomatic patients who have evidence of active disease (high alkaline phosphatase or urine hydroxyproline) or disease adjacent to weight-bearing structures, vertebrae, or the skull. Second-generation oral bisphosphonates such as tiludronate, alendronate, and risedronate are excellent choices due to their ability to decrease bone turnover. The major side effect from these agents is esophageal ulceration and reflux. They should be taken in the morning, on an empty stomach, sitting upright to minimize the risk of reflux. Duration of use depends on the clinical response; typically 3–6 months are needed to see the alkaline phosphatase begin to normalize. IV zoledronate and pamidronate are adequate alternatives to oral bisphosphonates. While their IV administration avoids the risk of reflux, there is a potential of developing a flulike syndrome within 24 h of use. The presence of this side effect does not require drug discontinuation. The same time to response can be expected from these agents.

13. and 14. The answers are E and B.
(Chap. 4) Subacute thyroiditis, also known as de Quervain's thyroiditis, granulomatous thyroiditis, or viral thyroiditis, is a multiphase illness three times more frequent in women than men. Multiple viruses have been implicated, but none have been definitively identified as the trigger for subacute thyroiditis. The diagnosis can be overlooked in patients as the symptoms mimic pharyngitis, and it frequently has a similarly benign course. In this patient, Graves' disease is unlikely given her elevated TSH and negative antibody panel. Autoimmune hypothyroidism should be considered; however, the tempo of her illness, the tenderness of the thyroid on examination, and her preceding viral illness make this diagnosis less likely. Ludwig's angina is a potentially life-threatening bacterial infection of the retropharyngeal and submandibular spaces, often caused by preceding dental infection. Cat-scratch fever is a usually benign illness that presents with lymphadenopathy, fever, and malaise. It is caused by *Bartonella henselae* and is frequently transmitted from cat scratches that penetrate the epidermis. It will not cause an elevated TSH. Subacute thyroiditis can present with hypothyroidism, thyrotoxicosis, or neither. In the first phase of the disease, thyroid inflammation leads to follicle destruction and release of thyroid hormone. Thyrotoxicosis ensues. In the second phase, the thyroid is depleted of hormone and hypothyroidism results. A recovery phase typically follows in which decreased inflammation allows the follicles to heal and regenerate hormone.

Large doses of aspirin (such as 600 mg PO every 4–6 h) or nonsteroidal anti-inflammatory drugs are often sufficient for what is usually a self-limited illness. A glucocorticoid taper can be used if symptoms are severe. Thyroid function should be monitored closely; some patients may require low-dose thyroid hormone replacement. (See Fig. 4-9.)

15. The answer is A.
(Chap. 19) The DCCT found definitive proof that reduction in chronic hyperglycemia can prevent many of the complications of type 1 DM. This multicenter randomized trial enrolled over 1400 patients with type 1 DM to either intensive or conventional diabetes management and prospectively evaluated the development of retinopathy, nephropathy, and neuropathy. The intensive group received multiple administrations of insulin daily along with education and psychological counseling. The intensive group achieved a mean hemoglobin A_{1C} of 7.3% versus 9.1% in the conventional group. Improvement in glycemic control resulted in a 47% reduction in retinopathy, a 54% reduction in nephropathy, and a 60% reduction in neuropathy. There was a nonsignificant trend toward improvement in macrovascular complications. The results of the DCCT showed that individuals in the intensive group would attain up to 7 more years of intact vision and up to 5 more years free from lower limb amputation. Later, the United Kingdom Prospective Diabetes Study (UKPDS) studied over 5000 individuals with type 2 DM. Individuals receiving intensive glycemic control had a reduction in microvascular events but no significant change in macrovascular complications. These two trials were pivotal in showing a benefit of glycemic control in reducing microvascular complications in patients with type 1 and type 2 DM, respectively. Another result from the UKPDS was that strict blood pressure control resulted in an improvement in macrovascular complications.

16. The answer is B.
(Chap. 27) Hypocalcemia can be a life-threatening consequence of thyroidectomy if the parathyroid glands are inadvertently removed during the surgery, as the four parathyroid glands are located immediately posterior to the thyroid gland. This is an infrequent occurrence currently as the parathyroid glands are better able to be identified both before and during surgery. However, hypoparathyroidism may occur even if the parathyroid glands are not removed by thyroidectomy due to devascularization or trauma to the parathyroid glands. Hypocalcemia following removal of the parathyroid glands may begin any time during the first 24–72 h, and monitoring of serial calcium levels is recommended for the first 72 h. The earliest symptoms of hypocalcemia are typically circumoral paresthesias and paresthesias with a "pins-and needles" sensation in the fingers and toes. The development of carpal spasms upon inflation of the

blood pressure cuff is a classic sign of hypocalcemia and is known as Trousseau sign. Chvostek sign is the other classic sign of hypocalcemia and is elicited by tapping the facial nerve in the preauricular area causing spasm of the facial muscles. A prolongation of the QT interval on the ECG suggests life-threatening hypocalcemia that may progress to fatal arrhythmia, and treatment should not be delayed for serum testing to occur in a patient with a known cause of hypocalcemia. Immediate treatment with IV calcium should be initiated. Maintenance therapy with calcitriol and vitamin D is necessary for ongoing treatment of acquired hypoparathyroidism. Alternatively, surgeons may implant parathyroid tissue into the soft tissue of the forearm, if it is thought that the parathyroid glands will be removed. Hypomagnesemia can cause hypocalcemia by suppressing parathyroid hormone release despite the presence of hypocalcemia. However, in this patient, hypomagnesemia is not suspected after thyroidectomy, and magnesium administration is not indicated. Benztropine is a centrally acting anticholinergic medication that is used in the treatment of dystonic reactions that can occur after taking centrally acting antiemetic medications with dopaminergic activity, such as metoclopramide or Compazine. Dystonic reactions involve focal spasms of the face, neck, and extremities. While this patient has taken a medication that can cause a dystonic reaction, the spasms that she is experiencing are more consistent with tetanic contractions of hypocalcemia than dystonic reaction. Finally, measurement of forced vital capacity is most commonly used as a measurement of disease severity in myasthenia gravis or Guillain-Barré syndrome. Muscle weakness is a typical presenting feature but not paresthesias.

17. The answer is C.
(Chap. 22) This patient presents with the classic findings of a VIPoma, including large-volume watery diarrhea, hypokalemia, dehydration, and hypochlorhydria (WDHA, or Verner-Morrison, syndrome). Abdominal pain is unusual. The presence of a secretory diarrhea is confirmed by a stool osmolal gap [2(stool Na + stool K) – (stool osmolality)] <35 and persistence during fasting. In osmotic or laxative-induced diarrhea, the stool osmolal gap is over 100. In adults, over 80% of VIPomas are solitary pancreatic masses that usually are larger than 3 cm at diagnosis. Metastases to the liver are common and preclude curative surgical resection. The differential diagnosis includes gastrinoma, laxative abuse, carcinoid syndrome, and systemic mastocytosis. Diagnosis requires the demonstration of large-volume secretory diarrhea (over 700 mL/d) and elevated serum VIP. CT scan of the abdomen will often demonstrate the pancreatic mass and liver metastases.

18. The answer is E.
(Chap. 27) Malignancy can cause hypercalcemia by several different mechanisms, including metastasis to bone, cytokine stimulation of bone turnover, and production of a protein structurally similar to parathyroid hormone by the tumor. This protein is called parathyroid hormone–related peptide (PTHrp) and acts at the same receptors as parathyroid hormone (PTH). Squamous cell carcinoma of the lung is the most common tumor associated with the production of PTHrp. Serum calcium levels can become quite high in malignancy because of unregulated production of PTHrp that is outside of the negative feedback control that normally results in the setting of hypercalcemia. PTH hormone levels should be quite low or undetectable in this setting. When hypercalcemia is severe (>15 mg/dL), symptoms frequently include dehydration and altered mental status. The electrocardiogram may show a shortened QTc interval. Initial therapy includes large-volume fluid administration to reverse the dehydration that results from hypercalciuria. In addition, furosemide is also added to promote further calciuria. If the calcium remains elevated, as in this patient, additional measures should be undertaken to decrease the serum calcium. Calcitonin has a rapid onset of action with a decrease in serum calcium seen within hours. However, tachyphylaxis develops, and the duration of benefit is limited. Pamidronate is a bisphosphonate that is useful for the hypercalcemia of malignancy. It decreases serum calcium by preventing bone resorption and release of calcium from the bone. After IV administration, the onset of action of pamidronate is 1–2 days with a duration of action of at least 2 weeks. Thus, in this patient with ongoing severe symptomatic hypercalcemia, addition of both calcitonin and pamidronate is the best treatment. The patient should continue to receive IV fluids and furosemide. The addition of a thiazide diuretic is contraindicated because thiazides cause increased calcium resorption in the kidney and would worsen hypercalcemia.

19. The answer is C.
(Chap. 11) Dysmenorrhea refers to the crampy lower abdominal discomfort that begins with the onset of menstrual bleeding and gradually decreases over 12–72 h. Primary dysmenorrhea results from increased stores and subsequent release of prostaglandin precursors. Nonsteroidal anti-inflammatory medications are effective in >80% of cases. Secondary dysmenorrhea is caused by underlying pelvic pathology, the causes of which are many. The differential diagnosis includes endometriosis (ectopic endometrium), mittelschmerz (ruptured Graafian follicle), adenomyosis (ectopic endometrial glands within the myometrium), and cervical stenosis. A history of sexual abuse correlates with dyspareunia more often than dysmenorrhea.

20. The answer is E.
(Chap. 13) Hirsutism is defined as excessive male-pattern hair growth. It may represent a variation on the norm or

be a prelude to a more serious underlying condition. Virilization refers to the state in which androgen levels are elevated enough to cause signs and symptoms of changes in voice, enlargement of genitalia, and increased libido. Virilization is a concerning sign for an ovarian or adrenal cause of excess androgen production. This patient's change in voice and body habitus heightens one's concern about a virilizing process. A thorough medication history is indicated because drugs such as phenytoin, minoxidil, and cyclosporine have been associated with androgen-dependent hair growth. Family history is critical as some families have a higher incidence of hirsutism than others do. Congenital conditions such as congenital adrenal hyperplasia can show distinct patterns of inheritance. Androgens are secreted by both the ovaries and the adrenal glands. An elevation in plasma total testosterone above 12 nmol/L usually indicates a virilizing tumor. A basal DHEAS level above 18.5 μmol/L suggests an adrenal source. Therefore, checking both levels is a useful initial hormonal screen in evaluating virilization. Although polycystic ovarian syndrome is by far the most common cause of ovarian androgen excess, initial screening with ultrasound is not recommended. Polycystic ovaries may be found in females without any evidence of excess androgen secretion. Likewise, females may have an ovarian source of androgen secretion with only slightly enlarged ovaries on ultrasound. Therefore, ultrasound is an insensitive and nonspecific test.

21. The answer is B.
(Chap. 2) The identification of an empty sella is often the result of an incidental MRI finding. Typically these patients will have normal pituitary function and should be reassured. It is likely that the surrounding rim of pituitary tissue is functioning normally. An empty sella may signal the insidious onset of hypopituitarism, and laboratory results should be followed closely. Unless her clinical situation changes, repeat MRI is not indicated. Endocrine malignancy is unlikely, and surgery is not part of the management of an empty sella.

22. The answer is C.
(Chap. 2) Craniopharyngiomas are benign suprasellar cystic masses that typically present with headaches, visual field deficits, and hypopituitarism. They arise near the pituitary stalk and extend into the suprasellar cistern. They are most common in children and often present with signs of increased intracranial pressure. More than half present before the age of 20. Weight gain, cognitive changes, sleep disorders, and visual field defects are common. Hypopituitarism is present in 90% of cases, and diabetes insipidus in 10% of cases. MRI is the test of choice for evaluation. Definitive management includes transcranial or transsphenoidal surgical resection followed by radiation. Meningioma should appear on the differential of this patient; epidemiologically, these tumors are more common in women than men, and tend to occur between the ages of 40 and 70. Congenital panhypopituitarism would not explain his acute worsening nor his increased intracranial pressure. McCune-Albright syndrome consists of polyostotic fibrous dysplasia, pigmented skin patches, and a variety of endocrine disorders including adenomas and pituitary tumors. Carney syndrome consists of myxomas; endocrine tumors including adrenal, testicular, and pituitary adenomas; and skin pigmentation.

23. The answer is D.
(Chap. 1) Positive feedback control is the least understood of the endocrine regulatory systems. The estrogen-LH relationship is a classic example of rising levels of a hormone having a positive effect on the release of another. Paracrine regulation refers to factors released by one cell that act on adjacent cells in the same tissue (e.g., somatostatin released from pancreatic δ cells inhibits secretion of insulin from adjacent β cells). Insulin-like growth factor I released from chondrocytes acts on the cells that produce it, which is an example of autocrine regulation. Negative feedback control is the classic model of an endocrine regulatory system (e.g., high levels of thyroxine inhibit further release of thyroid-stimulating hormone).

24. The answer is D.
(Chap. 28) The epidemiology of fractures follows trends similar to those for loss of bone density. Fractures of the radius increase until age 50 and then plateau by age 60. There are approximately 250,000 wrist fractures each year in the United States. However, there are approximately 300,000 hip fractures annually, with incidence rates doubling every 5 years after age 70. The shift from arm and wrist fractures to hip fractures may be related to the way elderly people fall, with less frequent landing on the hands and more frequent direct hip trauma with increasing age. There are approximately 700,000 vertebral fractures each year in the United States. Most are clinically silent and rarely require hospitalization. They may lead to height loss, kyphosis, and pain secondary to altered biomechanics.

25. The answer is B.
(Chap. 28) The Women's Health Initiative (WHI) demonstrated that estrogen-progestin therapy can reduce the risk of hip fractures by 34%. Other clinical trials have shown a decrease in all osteoporotic fractures, including vertebral compression fractures. The beneficial effect of estrogen appears to be maximal in those who start therapy early and continue taking the medication. The benefit declines after discontinuation, and there is no net benefit by 10 years after discontinuation. These effects are present for oral and transdermal formulations. However, the WHI

also demonstrated that estrogens are associated with a 30% increase in myocardial infarction, a 40% increase in stroke, a 100% increase in venous thromboembolism, and a 25% increase in breast cancer. In the WHI study there was no overall effect of estrogen-progestin therapy on mortality, probably because of the balance between the detrimental cardiovascular effects and the beneficial effects (in addition to fractures, there was a beneficial effect on the development of colon cancer).

26. The answer is D.
(Chap. 28) The selective estrogen receptor modulators (SERMs) tamoxifen and raloxifene act in a fashion similar to that of estrogen in decreasing bone turnover and bone loss in postmenopausal women. These agents have been shown to decrease the risk of invasive breast cancer. Raloxifene, which is approved for the prevention of osteoporosis, reduces the risk of vertebral fractures by 30–50%. There are no data confirming a similar effect on nonvertebral fractures. Optimal calcium intake reduces bone loss and suppresses bone turnover. Vitamin D plus calcium supplements have been shown to reduce the risk of hip fractures by 20–30%. The bisphosphonates alendronate and risedronate are structurally related to pyrophosphate and are incorporated into bone matrix. They reduce the number of osteoclasts and impair the function of those already present. Both have been shown to reduce the risk of vertebral and hip fractures by 40–50%. One trial found that risedronate reduced hip fractures in osteoporotic women in their seventies but not in older women without osteoporosis. Risedronate may be administered weekly. The newer bisphosphonates zoledronate and ibandronate may be dosed yearly or monthly. A daily injection of exogenous parathyroid hormone analogue superimposed on estrogen therapy produced increases in bone mass and decreased vertebral and nonvertebral fractures by 45–65%. There are no published studies of combinations of parathyroid hormone and SERMs or bisphosphonates.

27. The answer is E.
(Chap. 6) Complete removal of the pheochromocytoma is the only therapy that leads to a long-term cure, although 90% of tumors are benign. However, preoperative control of hypertension is necessary to prevent surgical complications and lower mortality. This patient is presenting with encephalopathy in a hypertensive crisis. The hypertension should be managed initially with IV medications to lower the mean arterial pressure by ~20% over the initial 24-h period. Medications that can be used for hypertensive crisis in pheochromocytoma include nitroprusside, nicardipine, and phentolamine. Once the acute hypertensive crisis has resolved, transition to oral α-adrenergic blockers is indicated. Phenoxybenzamine is the most commonly used drug and is started at low doses (5–10 mg three times daily) and titrated to the maximum tolerated dose (usually 20–30 mg daily). Once alpha blockers have been initiated, beta blockade can safely be utilized and is particularly indicated for ongoing tachycardia. Liberal salt and fluid intake helps expand plasma volume and treat orthostatic hypotension. Once blood pressure is maintained below 160/100 mmHg with moderate orthostasis, it is safe to proceed to surgery. If blood pressure remains elevated despite treatment with alpha blockade, addition of calcium channel blockers, angiotensin receptor blockers, or angiotensin-converting enzyme inhibitors should be considered. Diuretics should be avoided as they will exacerbate orthostasis.

28. The answer is B.
(Chap. 5) Control of renin release involves the independent actions of four factors: the juxtaglomerular cells, macula densa cells, the sympathetic nervous system, and circulating factors such as potassium concentration and atrial natriuretic peptide concentration. When effective circulating volume is low, cells in the juxtaglomerular apparatus (JGA) perceive this as a decreased stretch exerted on the afferent arteriole wall, and renin secretion is augmented. Macula densa cells may function as chemoreceptors monitoring the sodium and chloride load delivered to the distal tubule. Under conditions of low solute load delivered to the distal tubule, a signal is conveyed to increase juxtaglomerular release of renin. Increased sympathetic activity stimulates the JGA to release renin when upright posture is assumed. Increased potassium intake and release of atrial natriuretic peptide both decrease renin release.

29. The answer is E.
(Chap. 2) Pituitary adenomas are very common and are the most likely cause of pituitary hormone excess or deficiency states in adults. They make up 10% of all intracranial neoplasms. Pituitary microadenomas are present in ~25% of all autopsies, independent of antemortem clinical disease, and are usually unsuspected. Ten percent of the general population will have a microadenoma on head imaging. The clinical and biochemical phenotype of pituitary adenomas depend on the cell type from which they arise. They may cause hypersecretion or hyposecretion syndromes.

30. The answer is B.
(Chap. 6) This patient has the classic triad of symptoms for pheochromocytoma: headaches, palpitations, and profuse sweating. When this triad of symptoms is found in association with hypertension, pheochromocytoma is the most likely diagnosis. Differential diagnosis for pheochromocytoma includes panic disorder, essential hypertension, cocaine or methamphetamine abuse, carcinoid syndrome, intracranial mass, clonidine withdrawal, and factitious disorder. While episode hypertension is

classically described in association with pheochromocytoma, many patients have sustained hypertension that may be difficult to treat. In addition, 5–15% of individuals may present with normal blood pressure (*WM Manger: J Clin Hypertens 4: 62, 2002*). The patient also exhibits significant orthostatic changes in blood pressure, which is a common finding in pheochromocytoma. Interestingly, there is a case report of treatment with paroxetine unmasking symptoms of pheochromocytoma (*MA Seeler et al: Ann Intern Med 126: 333, 1997*). The cornerstone of diagnosis of pheochromocytoma is the documentation of elevated levels of urine and plasma catecholamines. The usual diagnostic algorithm includes the measurement of vanillylmandelic acid, catecholamines, and fractionated metanephrines in a 24-h urine collection or plasma sample. These tests should be greater than two to three times the upper limit of normal. If metanephrines are elevated, a CT scan or MRI of the chest, abdomen, and pelvis is performed with contrast to localize the site of the pheochromocytoma. Nuclear imaging with ^{123}I or ^{131}Imetaiodobenzylguanidine (MIBG) can also be utilized for localization of the pheochromocytoma after biochemical testing has confirmed elevated levels of catecholamines. Given the classic symptoms of this patient, panic attack is a diagnosis of exclusion because the missed diagnosis of pheochromocytoma increases the risk of adverse outcomes, including death and stroke. Carcinoid syndrome is diagnosed with 24-h urine testing for 5-HIAA, but is unlikely in this patient because carcinoid syndrome is not associated with hypertension.

31. The answer is B.
(Chap. 1) With few exceptions, hormone binding is highly specific for a single type of nuclear receptor. The mineralocorticoid-glucocorticoid hormones are a notable exception because the mineralocorticoid receptor also has a high, but not greater, affinity for glucocorticoid. An enzyme (11β-hydroxysteroid dehydrogenase) located in renal tubules inactivates glucocorticoid, allowing selective responses to mineralocorticoid. When there is glucocorticoid excess, the enzyme becomes oversaturated and glucocorticoid can exhibit mineralocorticoid effects. This effect is in contrast to the estrogen receptor, where different compounds confer unique transcription machinery. Mineralocorticoid hormones do not have serum-binding proteins. Examples of hormones that circulate with serum-binding proteins are T_4, T_3, cortisol, estrogen, and growth hormone. Most binding protein abnormalities have little clinical consequence because the free concentrations of the hormone often remain normal.

32. The answer is E.
(Chap. 4) The thionamides propylthiouracil (PTU), carbimazole, and methimazole are the main antithyroid medications used for the treatment of hyperthyroidism. They all inhibit the function of thyroid peroxidase, reducing oxidation and organification of iodide. PTU also inhibits the deiodination of T_4 to T_3. PTU has a half-life much shorter than that of methimazole. Rash, urticaria, fever, and arthralgias are common side effects, occurring in up to 5% of these patients. They may resolve spontaneously. Major side effects are rare but include hepatitis, agranulocytosis, and a systemic lupus erythematosus (SLE)-like syndrome. If major side effects are noted, it is essential that antithyroid medications be stopped.

33. The answer is B.
(Chap. 27) Hyperparathyroidism is the most common cause of hypercalcemia and is the most likely cause in an adult who is asymptomatic. Cancer is the second most common cause of hypercalcemia but usually is associated with symptomatic hypercalcemia. In addition, there are frequently symptoms from the malignancy itself that dominate the clinical picture. Primary hyperparathyroidism results from autonomous secretion of parathyroid hormone (PTH) that is no longer regulated by serum calcium levels, usually related to development of parathyroid adenomas. Most patients are asymptomatic or have minimal symptoms at the time of diagnosis. When present, symptoms include recurrent nephrolithiasis, peptic ulcers, dehydration, constipation, and altered mental status. Laboratory studies show elevated serum calcium with decreased serum phosphate. Diagnosis can be confirmed with measurement of parathyroid hormone levels. Surgical removal of autonomous adenomas is generally curative, but not all patients need to be treated surgically. It is recommended that individuals <50 undergo primary surgical resection. However, in those >50 years, a cautious approach with frequent laboratory monitoring is often used. Surgery can then be undertaken if a patient develops symptomatic or worsening hypercalcemia or complications such as osteopenia. Breast cancer is a frequent cause of hypercalcemia because of metastatic disease to the bone. In this patient, who has received routine mammography as part of age-appropriate cancer screening and is asymptomatic, this would be unlikely. Multiple myeloma is another malignancy frequently associated with hypercalcemia that is thought to be due to production of cytokines and humoral mediators by the tumor. Multiple myeloma should not present with isolated hypercalcemia and is associated with anemia and elevations in creatinine.

Approximately 20% of individuals with hyperthyroidism develop hypercalcemia related to increased bone turnover. This patient exhibits no signs or symptoms of hyperthyroidism, making the diagnosis unlikely. Vitamin D intoxication is a rare cause of hypercalcemia. An individual must ingest 40–100 times the recommended daily amount in order to develop hypercalcemia. Because vitamin D acts to increase both calcium and phosphate absorption from the intestine, serum levels of both minerals would be elevated, which is not seen in this case.

34. The answer is A.

(Chap. 4) Thyrotoxicosis presents with a characteristic set of signs and symptoms. Common signs include tachycardia and atrial fibrillation, tremor, goiter, and warm, moist skin. Common symptoms include hyperactivity, dysphoria, irritability, heat intolerance, excessive sweating, and fatigue. Weight loss occurs frequently; however, some patients will gain weight as they typically have a marked increase in appetite. The most common cardiac abnormality of thyrotoxicosis is sinus tachycardia. In older patients atrial fibrillation is frequently seen. These arrhythmias are a manifestation of a high-output state, which frequently leads to a widened pulse pressure and a systolic murmur. This can exacerbate underlying heart failure or coronary disease. Up to 50% of patients with atrial fibrillation related to untreated thyrotoxicosis will convert to normal sinus rhythm with management of their thyroid condition.

35. The answer is D.

(Chap. 4) Hyperthyroidism is treated by reducing thyroid hormone synthesis, using antithyroid drugs, reducing the amount of thyroid tissue with radioactive iodine, or thyroidectomy. Antithyroid drugs are used more frequently in Japan and Europe, whereas radioactive thyroid is used more frequently in North America. Propthiouracil and methimazole are the most commonly used antithyroid drugs and act by inhibiting the function of thyroid peroxidase. In Graves' disease, they also reduce thyroid antibody levels. Thyroid function tests and clinical manifestations are reviewed every 3–4 weeks with dose titrated based on unbound T_4 levels. Euthyroidism usually takes 6–8 weeks with this regimen. Agranulocytosis occurs in <1% of patients. Since radioactive iodine is contraindicated in pregnancy, propthiouracil may be used carefully since blocking doses may cause fetal hypothyroidism. Diltiazem may be used to slow heart rate in atrial fibrillation; however, beta blockers are effective in hyperthyroidism to control adrenergic symptoms. Itraconazole is an antifungal agent. Phenoxybenzamine is an α-adrenergic blocker often used to control blood pressure in patients with pheochromocytoma. Liothyronine is the oral form of T_3 and would not be used in hyperthyroidism. Levothyroxine has been used in combination with antithyroid drugs (block-replace regimen) to avoid drug-induced hypothyroidism.

36. The answer is B.

(Chap. 4) While hypothyroidism may be strongly suspected from history and physical examination findings, it is definitively diagnosed with serum laboratory measurements. TSH should be the first test sent. A normal TSH level excludes primary, but not secondary, hypothyroidism. Primary hypothyroidism refers to disease caused by hypofunction of the thyroid gland itself. Secondary hypothyroidism typically arises from disease of the anterior pituitary. If the TSH is low or normal and pituitary disease is suspected, a free T_4 should be sent. If this test is low, the differential includes anterior pituitary dysfunction, sick euthyroid syndrome, and drug effects. TSH, not unbound T_4, is the test of choice for diagnosing subclinical hypothyroidism. In these cases, TSH is elevated and T_4 is normal. Thyroid peroxidase antibodies are present in >90% of patients with autoimmune hypothyroidism; this test helps distinguish autoimmune causes of hypothyroidism from other possibilities. Circulating T_3 levels are normal in ~25% of patients with clinical hypothyroidism and are not indicated for diagnosis. A T_3/T_4 ratio is not helpful for diagnosis or prognosis. (See Fig. 4-6.)

37. The answer is E.

(Chap. 4) Autoimmune hypothyroidism is a common diagnosis, present in 4 per 1000 women and 1 per 1000 men. The mean age of diagnosis is 60 years. It is more prevalent in locations with chronic exposure to a high-iodine diet, such as Japan. Subclinical hypothyroidism (elevated thyroid-stimulating hormone, normal unbound T_4) is present in 6–8% of women and 3% of men. It is present in up to 10% of adults >60 years of age. There is an association between autoimmune hypothyroidism and other autoimmune conditions, and there appears to be a heritable familial risk of developing disease. There are likely environmental triggers other than heavy iodine exposure that predispose to the disease phenotype in susceptible individuals, but these have not been identified. Autoimmune thyroiditis may present with or without a goiter. When a goiter is present, it is termed *Hashimoto's thyroiditis*. The goiter is due to lymphocytic infiltration of the thyroid. Eventually atrophy of thyroid follicles leads to shrinkage of the gland. Atrophic thyroiditis likely represents the end stage of Hashimoto's thyroiditis. There is no evidence that viral thyroiditis induces subsequent autoimmune thyroiditis.

38. The answer is D.

(Chap. 1) Hormones can be broadly divided into five classes: amino acid derivatives, small neuropeptides, large proteins, steroid hormones, and vitamin derivatives. As a rule, amino acid derivatives and peptide hormones interact with cell-surface proteins while steroids, thyroid hormone, vitamin D, and retinoids interact with intracellular nuclear receptors. In a cell line impermeable to passage by extracellular molecules, steroids, thyroid hormone, vitamin D, and retinoids would not be able to exert their effect on the nuclear receptors. Hormones that interact with cell-surface membrane receptors would still be able to initiate their signaling. Dopamine is an amino acid

derivative. Gonadotropin-releasing hormone is a small neuropeptide. Insulin is a large protein.

39. The answer is B.
(Chap. 4) Thyrotoxicosis is a state of hormone excess. It is not synonymous with hyperthyroidism, which is the result of excessive thyroid function. Graves' disease accounts for 60–80% of thyrotoxicosis. Graves' disease is caused by the presence of thyroid-stimulating antibodies, which autonomously activate the thyroid-stimulating hormone receptor and cause overproduction of thyroid hormone. Other common causes of thyrotoxicosis include toxic multinodular goiter and toxic thyroid adenoma. Thyrotoxicosis without hyperthyroidism may occur in subacute thyroiditis, thyroid destruction from amiodarone or radiation, or ingestion of excess thyroid hormone. Graves' disease is common among populations with high iodine intake and occurs in up to 2% of women. It is one-tenth as frequent in men. It rarely presents in adolescence, and is most prevalent in patients between the ages of 20 and 50 years.

40. The answer is C.
(Chap. 21) The child exhibits clinical and laboratory manifestations of homozygous familial hypercholesterolemia (FH). The presence of childhood xanthomas including hands, wrists, elbows, knees, and buttocks with evidence of premature atherosclerosis is characteristic. The atherosclerosis often develops initially in the aortic root, causing valvular or supravalvular stenosis. Drug therapy is often ineffective, and LDL apheresis is usually the necessary therapy. Before initiating therapy to reduce his LDL, it is necessary to rule out hypothyroidism, nephrotic syndrome, and obstructive liver disease. Although parental control of the patient's diet is also partly to blame, deliberate or unintentional ingestion of a poor diet is less likely to be responsible than a genetic disorder. Familial defective apoB100 is a dominantly inherited disorder that may be confused with heterozygous FH, but not homozygous. These patients usually present with cardiovascular disease in adulthood. Syphilis can cause aortitis; however, it does not cause premature coronary artery disease.

41. The answer is D.
(Chap. 21) This patient has signs and symptoms of familial hypercholesterolemia (FH) with elevated plasma LDL, normal triglycerides, tendon xanthomas, and premature coronary artery disease. FH is an autosomal codominant lipoprotein disorder that is the most common of these syndromes caused by a single gene disorder. It has a higher prevalence in Afrikaners, Christian Lebanese, and French Canadians. There is no definitive diagnostic test for FH. FH may be diagnosed with a skin biopsy that shows reduced LDL receptor activity in cultured fibroblasts (although there is considerable overlap with normals). FH is predominantly a clinical diagnosis, although molecular diagnostics are being developed. Hemolysis is not a feature of FH. Sitosterolemia is distinguished from FH by episodes of hemolysis. It is a rare autosomal recessive disorder that causes a marked increase in the dietary absorption of plant sterols. Hemolysis is due to incorporation of plant sterols into the red blood cell membrane. Sitosterolemia is confirmed by demonstrating an increase in the plasma levels of sitosterol using gas chromatography. CT scanning of the liver does not sufficiently differentiate between the hyperlipoproteinemias. Many of the primary lipoproteinemias, including sitosterolemia, are inherited in an autosomal recessive pattern, and thus, a pedigree analysis would not be likely to isolate the disorder.

42. The answer is E.
(Chap. 2) Oral dopamine agonists, cabergoline or bromocriptine, are the mainstay of treatment for prolactinomas, regardless of their size. Patients with macroadenomas (>1 cm in diameter) should undergo visual field testing before starting therapy. MRI and visual field testing should be assessed at 6- to 12-month intervals to evaluate for shrinkage of the mass. Indications for surgery include dopamine agonist resistance or intolerance, invasive tumor, or lack of improvement on visual field testing.

43. The answer is C.
(Chap. 5) Plasma and urine assessment of steroid levels may be misleading due to improper collection or altered metabolism. Moreover, the plasma level depends on the secretion rate and the rate at which the hormone is metabolized. As such, stimulation tests are used to diagnose hormone deficiency states, while suppression tests document hypersecretion of adrenal hormones. One protocol for assessing mineralocorticoid deficiency involves severe sodium restriction, which is a potent stimulator of mineralocorticoid release. Rates of aldosterone secretion should increase two- to threefold. When dietary sodium intake is normal, stimulation testing of mineralocorticoid deficiency may be achieved by injection of a potent diuretic (e.g., 40–80 mg of furosemide) followed by 2–3 h of upright posture. The normal response is a two- to fourfold increase in plasma aldosterone levels.

44. The answer is E.
(Chap. 4) This patient has signs and symptoms of Graves' disease. In patients with thyrotoxicosis due to Graves' disease, the TSH level is low and total and unbound thyroid hormone levels are increased. In 2–5% of patients, only the T_3 levels will be increased. In this patient, with a high pretest probability of Graves' disease, a suppressed TSH and normal T_4 supports Graves'; however, testing of T_3 should be performed to definitively make the diagnosis. A total T_4 level would not provide definitive evidence of Graves' disease. Radionuclide scan of the thyroid is used to evaluate for toxic multinodular goiter and toxic adenoma. Measurement of thyroid-stimulating

antibodies and thyroid peroxidase antibodies will help confirm the diagnosis of Graves' but are not routinely used since the diagnosis may be made with a consistent clinical picture combined with supportive TSH and thyroid hormone results. (See Fig. 4-8.)

45. The answer is B.
(Chap. 11) Pregnancy, whether intrauterine or ectopic, is the most common cause of secondary amenorrhea and should be ruled out early in the evaluation of such patients. In a patient with secondary amenorrhea, uterine outflow tract obstruction is uncommon unless there has been curettage for pregnancy complications or, in an endemic region, genital tuberculosis. Primary ovarian failure is ruled out by the low levels of FSH in that FSH levels should be very elevated if anovulation is caused by ovarian pathology. Malnutrition or extreme weight loss (BMI <18) may cause secondary amenorrhea, but these are not likely in this case. An MRI is indicated in this patient with secondary amenorrhea because she is not pregnant, does not have evidence of primary ovarian failure, and has an elevated prolactin level and a normal thyroid-stimulating hormone level. These results suggest the possibility of central nervous system pathology.

46. The answer is C.
(Chap. 10) Evaluation of infertility should include evaluation of common male and female factors that could be contributing. Abnormalities of menstrual function are the most common cause of female infertility, and initial evaluation of infertility should include evaluation of ovulation and assessment of tubal and uterine patency. The female partner reports an episode of gonococcal infection with symptoms of pelvic inflammatory disease, which would increase her risk of infertility due to tubal scarring and occlusion. A hysterosalpingogram is indicated. If there is evidence of tubal abnormalities, many experts recommend in vitro fertilization for conception as these women are at increased risk of ectopic pregnancy if conception occurs. The female partner reports some irregularity of her menses, suggesting anovulatory cycles, and thus, evidence of ovulation should be determined by assessing hormonal levels. There is no evidence that prolonged use of oral contraceptives affects fertility adversely (*A Farrow et al: Hum Reprod 17: 2754, 2002*). Angiotensin-converting enzyme inhibitors, including lisinopril, are known teratogens when taken by women, but have no effects on chromosomal abnormalities in men. Recent marijuana use may be associated with increased risk of infertility, and in vitro studies of human sperm exposed to a cannabinoid derivative showed decreased motility (*LB Whan et al: Fertil Steril 85: 653, 2006*). However, no studies have shown long-term decreased fertility in men who previously used marijuana.

47. The answer is B.
(Chap. 7) Disorders of sexual differentiation involve both chromosomal disorders as well as gonadal and phenotypic disorders. Klinefelter syndrome classically is associated with a 47,XXY karyotype resulting from meiotic nondisjunction. Clinically, individuals with Klinefelter syndrome present in young adulthood with poor virilization and eunuchoid proportions noted by tall height with long leg length. Secondary sexual development is poor, with decreased facial and axillary hair and low sexual drive. Gynecomastia is frequently present, and the testes have a median length of 2.5 cm with almost all <3.5 cm. It is noted that the testes seem particularly small given the degree of androgenization present. A testicular biopsy would show hyalinization of the seminiferous tubules and azoospermia. Learning difficulties are frequently associated. Individuals with Klinefelter syndrome are also at increased risk of thromboembolic disease, diabetes mellitus, breast tumors, and obesity. Laboratory tests would reveal elevated follicle-stimulating hormone and luteinizing hormone with low plasma testosterone consistent with primary testicular failure. Increased concentrations of estradiol are also commonly encountered and are responsible for the development of gynecomastia. Treatment of the disorder primarily is androgen supplementation. Severe gynecomastia may require surgical reduction of breast tissue.

Androgen insensitivity syndrome (AIS) was previously known as testicular feminization and is a disorder caused by a mutation in the androgen receptor. Complete AIS is characterized by a female phenotype in XY individuals with normal breast development. However, there is no uterus, the vagina is short, and there is minimal axillary and pubic hair development.

Mixed gonadal dysgenesis results from a 45,X/46,XY mosaicism. Phenotype can be either male or female, and most individuals have ambiguous genitalia at birth. If the primary phenotype is male, hypospadias is common, and dysgenetic gonads lead to an increased risk of gonadoblastomas and other malignancies.

Testicular dysgenesis is also known as Swyer syndrome. These individuals have a complete absence of androgenization, and external genitalia is usually female or ambiguous.

True hermaphroditism is now known as ovotesticular DSD (disorder of sexual development). Both ova and testes are found in a single individual, and sometimes this is manifest as an ovotestis. The karyotype is most frequently 46, XX.

48. The answer is C.
(Chap. 8) Many drugs may interfere with testicular function through a variety of mechanisms. Cyclophosphamide damages the seminiferous tubules in a dose- and time-dependent fashion and causes azoospermia within a few weeks of initiation. This effect is reversible

in approximately half these patients. Ketoconazole inhibits testosterone synthesis. Spironolactone causes a blockade of androgen action. Glucocorticoids lead to hypogonadism predominantly through inhibition of hypothalamic-pituitary function. Sexual dysfunction has been described as a side effect of therapy with beta blockers. However, there is no evidence of an effect on testicular function. Most reports of sexual dysfunction were in patients receiving older beta blockers such as propranolol and timolol.

49. and 50. The answers are E and E.
(Chap. 27) Malignancy may cause hypercalcemia by metastasizing to bone or producing ectopic PTHrp. Bone scan is a sensitive test for bone metastasis, making ectopic hormone production more likely in this case. PTHrp is a tumor-associated protein that is most often seen in squamous cell tumors of the lung. There are high concentrations in human breast milk, although the physiologic significance is unknown. At the cellular level it behaves like PTHi binding to receptors on bone and kidney to increase calcium resorption and stimulate synthesis of 1,25-vitamin D. Elevations of PTHrp and PTHi cause an elevated calcium and low phosphate. While primary hyperparathyroidism is the most common cause of hypercalcemia, in the presence of a lung mass, PTHrp is more likely. Serum magnesium is usually normal in primary hyperparathyroidism or in PTHrp-related hypercalcemia. Small cell carcinoma of the lung may secrete ACTH, causing Cushing's syndrome, but this would not present with isolated hypercalcemia. It also may secrete antidiuretic hormone, causing syndrome of inappropriate antidiuretic hormone. Bronchial carcinoids may produce peptide hormones including serotonin, bradykinin, ACTH, or somatostatin. Adenocarcinomas cause hypercalcemia by metastasizing to bone, which would cause an abnormal bone scan. Bronchoalveolar carcinomas do not usually cause ectopic hormone production or metastasize to bone.

51. The answer is C.
(Chap. 27) The four parathyroid glands are located posterior to the thyroid gland. Parathyroid hormone is the primary regulator of calcium. PTH acts directly on bone and the kidney and indirectly, through the action of vitamin D, on the GI tract. Calcium induces calcium absorption from the kidney and bone. It stimulates hydroxylation of 25-hydroxyvitamin D, resulting in the more active form. Vitamin D stimulates calcium resorption from the GI tract. Calcium and vitamin D are part of a feedback loop that inhibits PTH release and synthesis. PTH prevents resorption of phosphate from the kidney.

52. The answer is C.
(Chap. 28) Determination of when to initiate screening for osteoporosis with bone densitometry testing can be complicated by multiple factors. In general, most women do not require screening for osteoporosis until after completion of menopause unless there have been unexplained fractures or other risk factors that would suggest osteoporosis. There is no benefit to initiating screening for osteoporosis in the perimenopausal period. Indeed most expert recommendations do not recommend routine screening for osteoporosis until age 65 or older unless risk factors are present. Risk factors for osteoporosis include advanced age, cigarette smoking, low body weight (<57.7 kg), family history of hip fracture, and long-term glucocorticoid use. Inhaled glucocorticoids may cause increased loss of bone density, but as this patient is on a low dose of inhaled fluticasone and is not estrogen-deficient, bone mineral densitometry cannot be recommended at this time. The risk of osteoporosis related to inhaled glucocorticoids is not well defined, but most studies suggest that the risk is relatively low, and inhaled glucocorticoids do not confer a threefold greater risk of osteoporosis. Delaying childbearing until the fourth and fifth decade does increase the risk of osteoporosis but does not cause early onset of osteoporosis prior to completion of menopause. The patient's family history of menopause likewise does not require early screening for osteoporosis.

53. The answer is C.
(Chap. 4) The main clinical symptoms of hypothyroidism include tiredness, weakness, dry skin, feeling cold, hair loss, difficulty concentrating, constipation with poor appetite, dyspnea, and hoarse voice. Menorrhagia, amenorrhea, paresthesias, and impaired hearing may also occur. Signs of hypothyroidism include dry coarse skin, puffy hands/face/feet (myxedema), diffuse alopecia, bradycardia, peripheral edema, delayed tendon reflex relaxation, carpal tunnel syndrome, and serous cavity effusions. The symptoms of hyperthyroidism include hyperactivity, irritability, dysphoria, heat intolerance, sweating, palpitations, fatigue and weakness, weight loss with increased appetite, diarrhea, loss of libido, polyuria, and oligomenorrhea. Signs include tachycardia, atrial fibrillation (particularly in the elderly), tremor, goiter, warm moist skin, proximal myopathy, lid lag, and gynecomastia. Exophthalmos is specific for Graves' disease. TSH is the most effective screening test for hypothyroidism. If elevated, an unbound T_4 is necessary to confirm clinical hypothyroidism. Testing of unbound T_4 will not detect subclinical hypothyroidism. Subclinical hypothyroidism is present when the TSH is elevated and unbound T_4 is normal. Patients may have minor or early symptoms of hypothyroidism in this stage.

54. The answer is B.
(Chap. 25) Hypophosphatemia results from one of three mechanisms: inadequate intestinal phosphate absorption, excessive renal phosphate excretion, and rapid

redistribution of phosphate from the extracellular space into bone or soft tissue. Inadequate intestinal absorption is rare. Malnutrition from fasting or starvation may result in depletion of phosphate, causing hypophosphatemia during refeeding. In hospitalized patients, redistribution is the main cause. Insulin drives phosphate into cells. Sepsis may cause destruction of cells and metabolic acidosis, resulting in a net shift of phosphate from the extracellular space into cells. Renal failure is associated with hyperphosphatemia, not hypophosphatemia.

55. The answer is D.
(Chap. 27) Primary hyperparathyroidism and malignancy account for over 90% of cases of hypercalcemia. In asymptomatic patients, primary hyperparathyroidism is the most common cause. In patients admitted to the hospital with symptomatic hypercalcemia, malignancy is the most common cause. Calcium is regulated in bone, the gastrointestinal tract, and the kidney. Other causes of increased bone turnover include Paget's disease, immobilization, hyperthyroidism, hypervitaminosis A, and adrenal insufficiency. Causes of increased GI absorption include vitamin D intoxication and milk-alkali syndrome. Hypercalcemia from thiazide diuretics and familial hypocalciuric hypercalcemia result from disordered regulation of calcium in the kidney.

56. The answer is A.
(Chap. 10) Infertility is defined as the inability to conceive after 12 months of unprotected sexual intercourse and affects 14% of couples in the United States. Infertility is attributable to female causes in 58% of cases and male causes in 25% of cases, and 17% remain unexplained after evaluation. Initial evaluation of the infertile couple includes counseling regarding the appropriate timing of intercourse and discussion of modifiable risk factors for infertility, including drug and alcohol use, cigarette smoking, caffeine, and obesity. A semen analysis is performed to determine sperm count, and if the sperm count is low on repeated analysis, measurement of serum testosterone, FSH, and LH is indicated to determine if hypogonadism is contributing to infertility. In the female partner, it is important to confirm ovulation and assess tubal patency. This evaluation includes testing of FSH, LH, prolactin, and estradiol levels in many individuals. A midcycle progesterone level may also be useful to document that the midcycle LH surge has occurred. Polycystic ovarian syndrome can be found in 30% of women who have anovulatory cycle and is associated with androgen excess. If polycystic ovarian syndrome is suspected, the female partner should have levels of testosterone and dehydroepiandrosterone assessed. Determination of patency of the uterine outflow tract and fallopian tubes is also recommended through performance of a hysterosalpingogram. Endometrial biopsy was once a frequent component of the evaluation of infertility to exclude luteal-phase insufficiency, which would affect fetal implantation. However, prior research has a high degree of intraobserver variability in the dating criteria used to assess endometrial biopsies (*TC Li et al: Fertil Steril 51: 759, 1989*). Moreover, out-of-phase biopsies are seen on a single endometrial sample in >30–50% of fertile women and in sequential samples in 7–27% (*OK Davis et al: Fertil Steril 51: 582, 1989*).

57. The answer is A.
(Chap. 11) This patient describes primary amenorrhea. It is important to rule out disorders of the uterus or outflow tract before initiating an exhaustive workup for hormonal causes. On examination, one may find obstruction of the transverse vaginal septum or an imperforate hymen, which should be treated surgically. An MRI may further delineate an abnormal genital tract but should not be performed prior to a physical examination. In a nonpregnant woman with primary amenorrhea, an elevated FSH would suggest primary ovarian failure. An elevated prolactin in such a patient should direct your evaluation toward a neuroanatomic abnormality or hypogonadotropic hypogonadism.

58. The answer is D.
(Chap. 28) Osteoporosis is defined as a reduction of bone mass or density or the presence of a fragility fracture. Operationally, the WHO defines osteoporosis as a bone density >2.5 SD less than the mean for young healthy adults of the same race and sex. Dual-energy x-ray absorptiometry (DXA) is the most widely used study to determine bone density. Bone density is expressed as a T-score, that is, the SD below the mean of young adults of the same race and gender. A T-score >2.5 characterizes osteoporosis, and a T-score <1 identifies patients at risk of osteoporosis. The Z-score compares individuals with those in an age-, race-, and gender-matched population. The figure shows the relationship between Z-scores and T-scores. (See Fig. 28-6.)

59. The answer is E.
(Chap. 21) Statins have emerged over the last decade as one of the most clinically important classes of medications. Numerous studies have indicated important benefits in both primary and secondary prevention of cardiovascular disease. Statins act by inhibiting HMG-CoA reductase, the rate-limiting step in cholesterol biosynthesis. Statins are generally well tolerated, with an excellent safety profile over the years. However, attention must be paid to the side effects, which may be severe. Dyspepsia, headache, fatigue, and myalgias may occur and are generally well tolerated. Myopathy and rhabdomyolysis are rare but serious side effects. The risk of myopathy is increased in the presence of renal insufficiency and with concomitant use of certain medications, including some antibiotics, antifungal agents, some immunosuppressive

drugs, and fibric acid derivatives. Hepatitis is another side effect. Liver transaminases should be checked before therapy is started and 4–8 weeks afterward. Elevations more than three times the normal range may mandate stopping therapy.

60. The answer is B.

(Chap. 4) Subacute thyroiditis, also known as de Quervain's thyroiditis, granulomatous thyroiditis, and viral thyroiditis, is characterized clinically by fever, constitutional symptoms, and a painful enlarged thyroid. The etiology is thought to be a viral infection. The peak incidence is between 30 and 50 years of age, and women are affected more frequently than are men. The symptoms depend on the phase of the illness. During the initial phase of follicular destruction, there is a release of thyroglobulin and thyroid hormones. As a result, there is increased circulating T_4 and T_3, with concomitant suppression of TSH. Symptoms of thyrotoxicosis predominate at this point. Radioiodine uptake is low or undetectable. After several weeks, thyroid hormone is depleted and a phase of hypothyroidism ensues, with low unbound T_4 levels and moderate elevations of TSH. Radioiodine uptake returns to normal. Finally, after 4–6 months, thyroid hormone and TSH levels return to normal as the disease subsides. Patient A is consistent with the thyrotoxic phase of subacute thyroiditis except for the increased radioiodine uptake scan. Patient C is more consistent with Graves' disease with suppression of TSH, an elevated uptake scan, and elevated thyroid hormones as a result of stimulating immunoglobulin. Patient D is consistent with a neoplasm. Patient E is consistent with central hypothyroidism.

61. The answer is D.

(Chap. 20) The most common cause of hypoglycemia is related to the treatment of diabetes mellitus. Individuals with type 1 diabetes mellitus (T1DM) have more symptomatic hypoglycemia than individuals with type 2 diabetes mellitus (T2DM). On average, those with T1DM experience two episodes of symptomatic hypoglycemia weekly; and at least once yearly, individuals with T1DM will have a severe episode of hypoglycemia that is at least temporarily disabling. It is estimated that 2–4% of individuals with T1DM will die from hypoglycemia. In addition, recurrent episodes of hypoglycemia in T1DM contribute to the development of hypoglycemia-associated autonomic failure. Clinically, this is manifested as hypoglycemia unawareness and defective glucose counterregulation, with lack of glucagon and epinephrine secretion as glucose levels fall. Individuals with T2DM are less likely to develop hypoglycemia. Medications that are associated with hypoglycemia in T2DM are insulin and insulin secretagogues, such as sulfonylureas. Metformin, thiazolidinediones, α-glucosidase inhibitors, glucagon-like peptide-1 receptor agonists, and dipeptidyl peptidase-IV inhibitors do not cause hypoglycemia.

62. The answer is E.

(Chap. 10) All of the choices have a theoretical efficacy in preventing pregnancy of >90%. However, the actual effectiveness can vary widely. Spermicides have the greatest failure rate of 21%. Barrier methods (condoms, cervical cap, diaphragm) have an actual efficacy between 82 and 88%. Oral contraceptives and intrauterine devices perform similarly, with 97% efficacy in preventing pregnancy in clinical practice.

63. The answer is D.

(Chap. 19) Tight glycemic control with a hemoglobin A_{1C} of 7% or less has been shown in the Diabetes Control and Complications Trial (DCCT) in type 1 diabetic patients and the United Kingdom Prospective Diabetes Study (UKPDS) in type 2 diabetic patients to lead to improvements in microvascular disease. Notably, a decreased incidence of neuropathy, retinopathy, microalbuminuria, and nephropathy was shown in individuals with tight glycemic control. Interestingly, glycemic control had no effect on macrovascular outcomes. Instead, it was blood pressure control to at least moderate goals (142/88 mmHg) in the UKPDS that resulted in a decreased incidence of macrovascular outcomes, namely, DM-related death, stroke, and heart failure. Improved blood pressure control also resulted in improved microvascular outcomes.

64. The answer is E.

(Chap. 4) Thyroid nodules are found in 5% of patients. Nodules are more common with age, in women, and in iodine-deficient areas. Given their prevalence, the cost of screening, and the generally benign course of most nodules, the choice and order of screening tests have been very contentious. A small percentage of incidentally discovered nodules will represent thyroid cancer, however. A TSH should be the first test to check after detection of a thyroid nodule. A majority of patients will have normal thyroid function tests. In the case of a normal TSH, fine-needle aspiration or ultrasound-guided biopsy can be pursued. If the TSH is low, a radionuclide scan should be performed to determine if the nodule is the source of thyroid hyperfunction (a "hot" nodule). In the case described here, this is the best course of action. "Hot" nodules can be treated medically, resected, or ablated with radioactive iodine. "Cold" nodules should be further evaluated with a fine-needle aspiration. Four percent of nodules undergoing biopsy will be malignant, 10% are suspicious for malignancy, and 86% are indeterminate or benign. (See Fig. 4-14.)

65. The answer is D.

(Chap. 29) Paget's disease of bone is relatively common, and the incidence increases with age. An estimated prevalence of 3% in persons over age 40 years is a generally accepted figure. Most frequently, the disease is

asymptomatic and is diagnosed only when the typical sclerotic bones are incidentally detected on x-ray examinations done for other reasons or when increased alkaline phosphatase activity is recognized during routine laboratory measurements. The etiology is unknown, but increased bone resorption followed by intensive bone repair is thought to be the mechanism that causes increased bone density and increased serum alkaline phosphatase activity as a marker of osteoblast activity. Because increased mineralization of bone takes place (although in an abnormal pattern), hypercalcemia is not present unless a severely affected patient becomes immobilized. Hypercalcemia, in fact, would be an expected finding in a patient with primary hyperparathyroidism, bone metastases, or plasmacytoma, with plasmacytoma typically producing no increase in alkaline phosphatase activity. Osteomalacia resulting from vitamin D deficiency is associated with bone pain and hypophosphatemia; normal or decreased serum calcium concentration produces secondary hyperparathyroidism, further aggravating the defective bone mineralization.

66. The answer is E.
(Chap. 29) Paget's disease, a disorder characterized by increased osteoclastic activity and subsequent bony remodeling with structurally unsound woven bone, is often diagnosed incidentally when screening tests reveal an increased alkaline phosphatase or when a radiograph displays characteristic abnormalities. Serum calcium and phosphate levels are normal in Paget's disease. Rarely, immobilization in a patient with Paget's disease may cause hypercalcemia. The most common symptom of Paget's disease is pain. Hearing loss is very frequent, usually due to bony compression of the eighth cranial nerve. The most commonly affected areas include the pelvis, the skull, and the vertebral bodies. Diagnosis does not require nuclear bone scan. Physical findings of bony deformity such as frontal bossing of the skull or bowing of an extremity, an elevated alkaline phosphatase level, or characteristic findings on plain radiographs, such as cortical thickening and lytic and sclerotic changes, suffice. Increased osteoclastic activity, possibly initiated by viral infection and likely modulated by genetic factors, drives the pathogenesis of Paget's disease. The disease tends to run in families, with a positive family history in 15–25% of patients.

67. The answer is C.
(Chap. 2) Cushing's syndrome is caused by hypercortisolism, typically from an adrenocorticotropic hormone (ACTH)–secreting adenoma, ectopic tumor ACTH production, or iatrogenic ingestion of cortisol. Iatrogenic hypercortisolism is the most common cause of cushingoid features. ACTH-secreting adenomas account for 10–15% of all pituitary tumors. Ectopic ACTH-secreting tumors include bronchial and abdominal carcinoids, small cell lung cancer, and thymoma. In patients with Cushing's syndrome, the frequency of obesity is 80%. Thin skin is also very common and present in up to 80% of patients. Purple skin striae and hirsutism occur 65% of the time in these patients, and amenorrhea about 60% of the time. Skin hyperpigmentation occurs in about 20% of patients. Patients with Cushing's syndrome may also develop hyperglycemia, osteoporosis, proximal muscle weakness, acne, hirsutism, leukocytosis, lymphopenia, and eosinopenia. Patients die of cardiovascular disease, infections, and suicide.

68. The answer is D.
(Chap. 2) Pituitary adenomas, often called "incidentalomas," are commonly discovered on head MRI or CT. At autopsy, unsuspected microadenomas are present in up to 25% of cases. In the absence of symptoms or endocrine laboratory abnormalities, adenomas <1 cm in diameter can be safely monitored with annual MRI. PET-CT is not indicated; laboratory testing is used to evaluate for functional activity. Surgery is not indicated for microadenomas (<1 cm). About one-third of macroadenomas (>1 cm) will become invasive or exert mass effect; surgery should be considered for incidental macroadenomas.

69. The answer is A.
(Chap. 2) The anterior pituitary produces six major hormones: prolactin, growth hormone (GH), ACTH, luteinizing hormone, follicle-stimulating hormone, and TSH. These hormones are all released in a pulsatile manner from the pituitary. GH and ACTH are present in the fetus at 6 and 8 weeks, respectively; the remainder of the anterior pituitary hormones appear by week 12 of gestation. All of the hormones have inhibitors that act in a negative feedback loop to regulate their production and release. Somatostatin, along with insulin-like growth factor I, inhibits GH. ACTH is suppressed by glucocorticoids.

70. The answer is A.
(Chap. 21) Lipoprotein lipase (LPL) and its cofactor apoC-II are required for the hydrolysis of triglycerides in chylomicrons and very low density lipoproteins (VLDLs). A genetic deficiency of either protein impairs lipolysis and results in an elevation in plasma chylomicrons. VLDL is also elevated. The triglyceride-rich proteins persist for days in the circulation, causing fasting levels higher than 1000 mg/dL. The inheritance pattern is autosomal recessive. Heterozygotes have normal or mildly elevated plasma triglyceride levels. Clinically, these patients may have repeated episodes of pancreatitis secondary to hypertriglyceridemia. Eruptive xanthomas may appear on the back, the buttocks, and the extensor surfaces of the arms and legs. Hepatosplenomegaly may result from the uptake of circulating chylomicrons

by the reticuloendothelial cells. The diagnosis is made by assaying triglyceride lipolytic activity in plasma. Dietary fat restriction is the treatment of choice.

71. The answer is D.

(Chap. 19) Diabetic ketoacidosis is an acute complication of diabetes mellitus. It results from a relative or absolute deficiency of insulin combined with a counterregulatory hormone excess. In particular, a decrease in the ratio of insulin to glucagons promotes gluconeogenesis, glycogenolysis, and the formation of ketone bodies in the liver. Ketosis results from an increase in the release of free fatty acids from adipocytes, with a resultant shift toward ketone body synthesis in the liver. This is mediated by the relationship between insulin and the enzyme carnitine palmitoyltransferase I. At physiologic pH, ketone bodies exist as ketoacids, which are neutralized by bicarbonate. As bicarbonate stores are depleted, acidosis develops. Clinically, these patients have nausea, vomiting, and abdominal pain. They are dehydrated and may be hypotensive. Lethargy and severe central nervous system depression may occur. The treatment centers on replacement of the body's insulin, which will result in cessation of the formation of ketoacids and improvement of the acidotic state. Assessment of the level of acidosis may be done with an arterial blood gas. These patients have an anion gap acidosis and often a concomitant metabolic alkalosis resulting from volume depletion. Volume resuscitation with IV fluids is critical. Many electrolyte abnormalities may occur. Patients are total body sodium-, potassium-, and magnesium-depleted. As a result of the acidosis, intracellular potassium may shift out of cells and cause a normal or even elevated potassium level. However, with improvement in the acidosis, the serum potassium rapidly falls. Therefore, potassium repletion is critical despite the presence of a "normal" level. Because of the osmolar effects of glucose, fluid is drawn into the intravascular space. This results in a drop in the measured serum sodium. There is a drop of 1.6 meq/L in serum sodium for each rise of 100 mg/dL in serum glucose. In this case, the serum sodium will improve with hydration alone. The use of 3% saline is not indicated because the patient has no neurologic deficits, and the expectation is for rapid resolution with IV fluids alone.

72. The answer is A.

(Chap. 27) Hypercalcemia manifests in a variety of ways. "Stones, bones, groans, and psychiatric overtones" often is used on rounds as a way to remember the clinical symptoms and signs. Neurologic changes may range from depression to confusion and frank coma. These patients often are constipated and may have nausea, vomiting, and abdominal pain. Increased calcium may affect the genitourinary tract with nephrolithiasis, renal tubular acidosis, and polyuria. A shortened QT interval may result in cardiac arrhythmias.

73. The answer is B.

(Chap. 27) Parathyroid hormone (PTH) is produced by the four small parathyroid glands that lie posterior to the thyroid gland and is the primary hormone responsible for regulating serum calcium and phosphate balance. PTH secretion is tightly regulated with negative feedback to the parathyroid glands by serum calcium and vitamin D levels. PTH primarily affects serum calcium and phosphate levels through its action in the bone and the kidney. In the bone, PTH increases bone remodeling through its actions on the osteoblasts and osteoclasts. It directly stimulates osteoblasts to increase bone formation, and this action of PTH has been utilized in the treatment of osteoporosis. Its action on osteoclasts, however, is indirect and likely is mediated through its actions on the osteoblasts. The osteoclast has no receptors for PTH. It has been hypothesized that cytokines produced by osteoblasts are responsible for increased osteoclastic activity that is seen after PTH administration, as PTH fails to have an effect on osteoclasts in the absence of osteoblasts. The net effect of PTH on the bone is to increase bone remodeling. Ultimately, this leads to an increase in serum calcium, an effect that can be seen within hours of drug administration. In the kidney, PTH acts to increase calcium reabsorption while increasing phosphate excretion. At the proximal tubule, PTH acts to decrease phosphate transport, thus facilitating its excretion. Calcium reabsorption is increased by the action of PTH on the distal tubule. A final action of PTH in the kidney is to increase the production of 1,25-hydroxycholecalciferol, the activated form of vitamin D, through stimulation of 1α-hydroxylase. Activated vitamin D then helps to increase calcium levels by increasing intestinal absorption of both calcium and phosphate.

74. The answer is C.

(Chap. 4) Iodine deficiency is the most common worldwide cause of hypothyroidism. Autoimmune, or Hashimoto's, thyroiditis is a common cause in developed countries with dietary iodine supplementation. Histologically, it is characterized by lymphocytic infiltration of the thyroid with activated T cells and B cells. Thyroid cell destruction is thought to be mediated by cytotoxic CD8+ T lymphocytes. Primary hypothyroidism is characterized by an elevation in TSH as the feedback inhibition of the anterior pituitary is diminished. However, patients with hypothyroidism may have low TSH in the setting of secondary hypothyroidism. In this case, a clinical and radiologic evaluation of the pituitary is required. Subclinical hypothyroidism is characterized by abnormalities in the serum levels of TSH but minimal symptoms and often minimal change in the free T_4 level. The rate of development of overt, symptomatic hypothyroidism is about 4% per year, especially in the case of positive TPO antibodies, which are present in 90–95% of patients with autoimmune hypothyroidism.

75. The answer is B.
(Chap. 5) Primary hyperaldosteronism is suggested by diastolic hypertension without edema, hyposecretion of renin that fails to increase appropriately during volume depletion, and hypersecretion of aldosterone that fails to suppress in response to volume expansion. When signs of hyperaldosteronism are present without a solitary adenoma, these patients have bilateral cortical nodular hyperplasia or nodular hyperplasia. One distinguishing feature between these two conditions is the lack of severe hypokalemia in patients with cortical nodular hyperplasia. After potassium supplementation, patients with cortical nodular hyperplasia, but not patients with primary hyperaldosteronism, may have normal potassium levels. A low-renin state is characteristic of hyperaldosteronism. Conn's syndrome is defined by an aldosterone-secreting adrenal adenoma. Liddle's syndrome resembles hyperaldosteronism clinically and biochemically except that aldosterone levels are low or normal in patients with Liddle's syndrome. The defect in Liddle's syndrome is due to dysregulation of an epithelial Na^+ channel. A rare form of hyperaldosteronism, glucocorticoid-remediable aldosteronism, resembles cortical nodular hyperplasia. Whereas dexamethasone suppression does not affect aldosterone levels in patients with cortical nodular hyperplasia, profound suppression is seen in patients with glucocorticoid-remediable aldosteronism.

76. The answer is A.
(Chap. 7) Turner syndrome most frequently results from a 45,X karyotype, but mosaicism (45,X/46,XX) also can result in this disorder. Clinically, Turner syndrome manifests as short stature and primary amenorrhea if presenting in young adulthood. In addition, chronic lymphedema of the hands and feet, nuchal folds, a low hairline, and high arched palate are also common features. To diagnose Turner syndrome, karyotype analysis should be performed. A Barr body results from inactivation of one of the X chromosomes in women and is not seen in males. In Turner syndrome, the Barr body should be absent, but only 50% of individuals with Turner syndrome have the 45,X karyotype. Thus, the diagnosis could be missed in those with mosaicism or other structural abnormalities of the X chromosome.

Multiple comorbid conditions are found in individuals with Turner syndrome, and appropriate screening is recommended. Congenital heart defects affect 30% of women with Turner syndrome, including bicuspid aortic valve, coarctation of the aorta, and aortic root dilatation. An echocardiogram should be performed, and the individual should be assessed with blood pressures in the arms and legs. Hypertension can also be associated with structural abnormalities of the kidney and urinary tract, most commonly horseshoe kidney. A renal ultrasound is also recommended. Autoimmune thyroid disease affects 15–30% of women with Turner syndrome and should be assessed by screening TSH. Other comorbidities that may occur include sensorineural hearing loss, elevated liver function enzymes, osteoporosis, and celiac disease.

77. The answer is B.
(Chap. 8) Pathologic gynecomastia develops when the effective ratio of testosterone to estrogen is decreased owing to diminished testosterone production (as in primary testicular failure) or increased estrogen production. The latter may arise from direct estradiol secretion by a testis stimulated by LH or hCG or from an increase in peripheral aromatization of precursor steroids, most notably androstenedione. Elevated androstenedione levels may result from increased secretion by an adrenal tumor (leading to an elevated level of urinary 17-ketosteroids) or decreased hepatic clearance in patients with chronic liver disease. A variety of drugs, including diethylstilbestrol, heroin, digitalis, spironolactone, cimetidine, isoniazid, and tricyclic antidepressants, also can cause gynecomastia. In this patient, the history of paternity and the otherwise normal physical examination indicate that a karyotype is unnecessary, and the bilateral breast enlargement essentially excludes the presence of carcinoma and thus the need for biopsy. The presence of a low LH and testosterone suggests either estrogen or hCG production. Because of the normal testicular examination, a primary testicular tumor is not suspected. Carcinoma of the lung and germ cell tumors both can produce hCG, causing gynecomastia.

78. The answer is E.
(Chap. 16) Obesity leads to a major increase in morbidity and mortality. Individuals who are >150% of their ideal body weight have as much as a twelvefold increase in mortality. Insulin resistance leading to diabetes mellitus is one of the most prominent features of obesity. The vast majority of patients with type 2 diabetes are obese. Weight loss to a moderate degree may be associated with improvements in insulin sensitivity. Obesity is an independent risk factor for cardiovascular disease. Obesity is associated with hypertension. The impact of obesity on cardiovascular mortality may be seen in persons with BMIs >25. Obesity is associated with an increased incidence of cholesterol stones. Periodic fasting may increase the supersaturation of bile by decreasing the phospholipid component. Multiple studies have indicated increased mortality from cancer in obese individuals. Some of this increase may result from the increased conversion of androstenedione to estrone in adipose tissue. Obesity decreases chest wall compliance. Restrictive lung defects may occur in these individuals. Sleep apnea and obesity hypoventilation syndrome may occur. Although obesity may be associated with obstructive sleep apnea, it is not typically associated with other forms of chronic obstructive lung disease (COPD).

79. The answer is C.

(Chap. 29) Paget's disease is a disorder of bone remodeling that affects multiple areas of the skeleton. The prevalence increases with age, and it is more common in men than women. There is wide variation in global prevalence; Western Europe and North America are disproportionately and heavily affected. In autopsy series, 3% of those over the age of 40 have evidence of disease. For reasons that are not clear, the frequency of disease appears to be declining over the past 20 years. A majority of patients with Paget's disease are asymptomatic. The etiology of the disease is unknown, though both genetic and environmental factors have been implicated. The central pathophysiology is driven by overactive and overabundant osteoclasts, which erode bone. Accelerated bone formation from recruited osteoblasts leads to woven, poorly structured bone that is prone to fracture and bowing. A viral etiology has been postulated, based on findings of viral inclusion bodies and viral mRNA in osteoclasts of patients with Paget's disease. To date, no full-length viral genes have been recovered, and virus has never been cultured from pagetic bone.

80. The answer is D.

(Chap. 27) FHH is inherited as an autosomal dominant trait. It results from a defect in serum calcium sensing by the parathyroid gland and renal tubule, causing inappropriate secretion of PTH and excessive renal reabsorption of calcium. The calcium-sensing receptor is sensitive to extracellular calcium concentration, suppressing PTH secretion and therefore resulting in negative feedback regulation. Many different mutations in the calcium-sensing receptor have been described in patients with FHH. These mutations lower the ability of the sensor to bind calcium, resulting in excessive secretion of PTH and subsequent hypercalcemia. Urinary excretion of calcium is very low, with reabsorption >99%. The hypercalcemia is often detected in the first decade of life. This contrasts with primary hyperparathyroidism, which rarely occurs before age 10. Few clinical signs or symptoms are present in patients with FHH. These patients have excellent outcomes, and surgery or medical therapy is rarely necessary. Jansen's disease refers to mutations in the PTH receptor.

81. and 82. The answers are E and E.

(Chap. 22) In patients with a nonmetastatic carcinoid, surgery is the only potentially curative therapy. The extent of surgical resection depends on the size of the primary tumor because the risk of metastasis is related to the size of the tumor. Symptomatic treatment is aimed at decreasing the amount and effect of circulating substances. Drugs that inhibit the serotonin 5-HT_1 and 5-HT_2 receptors (methysergide, cyproheptadine, ketanserin) may control diarrhea but not flushing. 5-HT_3 receptor antagonists (ondansetron, tropisetron, alosetron) control nausea and diarrhea in up to 100% of these patients and may alleviate flushing. A combination of H_1 and H_2 receptor antagonists may control flushing, particularly in patients with foregut carcinoid tumors. Somatostatin analogues (octreotide, lanreotide) are the most effective and widely used agents to control the symptoms of carcinoid syndrome, decreasing urinary 5-HIAA excretion and symptoms in 70–80% of patients. Interferon α, alone or combined with hepatic artery embolization, controls flushing and diarrhea in 40–85% of these patients. Phenoxybenzamine is an α_1-adrenergic receptor blocker that is used in the treatment of pheochromocytoma.

Carcinoid crisis is a life-threatening complication of carcinoid syndrome. It is most common in patients with intense symptoms from foregut tumors or markedly high levels of urinary 5-HIAA. The crisis may be provoked by surgery, stress, anesthesia, chemotherapy, or physical trauma to the tumor (biopsy or, in this case, physical compression of liver lesions). These patients develop severe typical symptoms plus systemic symptoms such as hypotension and hypertension with tachycardia. Synthetic analogues of somatostatin (octreotide, lanreotide) are the treatment of choice for carcinoid crisis. They are also effective in preventing crises when administered before a known inciting event. Octreotide 150–250 μg SC every 6–8 h should be started 24–48 h before a procedure that is likely to precipitate a carcinoid crisis.

83. The answer is E.

(Chap. 28) Multiple treatment choices are available to prevent fractures and reverse bone loss in osteoporosis, and the side-effect profiles should be carefully considered when making the appropriate choice for this patient. Risedronate belongs to a family of drugs called bisphosphonates. Bisphosphonates act to inhibit osteoclast activity to decrease bone resorption and increase bone mass. Alendronate, risedronate, and ibandronate are approved for treatment of postmenopausal osteoporosis, and alendronate and risedronate are also approved for the treatment of steroid-induced osteoporosis and osteoporosis in men. In clinical trials, risedronate decreases risk of hip and vertebral fracture by 40–50% over 3 years. However, risedronate is not effective in decreasing hip fracture in women over the age of 80. The major side effect of bisphosphonate compounds taken orally is esophagitis. These drugs should be taken with a full glass of water, and the patient should remain upright for 30 min after taking the drug. Estrogens are also effective in preventing and treating osteoporosis. Epidemiologic data indicate that women taking estrogen have a 50% decreased risk of hip fracture. Raloxifene is a selective estrogen receptor modulator (SERM). The effect of raloxifene on bone density is somewhat less than that of estrogen, but it does decrease the risk of vertebral fracture by 30–50%. However, both drugs are contraindicated in this patient because of the recent occurrence of venous thromboembolic disease. Both estrogen and SERMs increase

the risk of DVT and pulmonary embolus severalfold. If estrogen is to be used, it should be used in combination with a progestin compound in women with an intact uterus to decrease the risk of uterine cancer associated with unopposed estrogen stimulation. Calcium and vitamin D supplementation are recommended, but given the degree of osteoporosis are inadequate alone. Calcitonin is available as an intranasal spray and produces small increases in bone density, but it has no proven effectiveness on prevention of fractures.

84. The answer is B.
(Chap. 2) Hyperprolactinemia is the most common pituitary hormone secretion syndrome in men and women. Prolactin-secreting pituitary adenomas (prolactinomas) are the most common cause of high prolactin levels. Hyperprolactinemia has a wide array of etiologies. Pregnancy and lactation are physiologic causes of increased prolactin levels. Chronic renal failure increases prolactin levels by decreasing clearance. Nipple stimulation and sexual orgasm both can increase prolactin release into the blood. Chest wall trauma, including surgery and herpes zoster infection, can induce prolactin secretion likely by activating a reflex suckling arc. Primary hypothyroidism can cause mild hyperprolactinemia due to compensatory thyrotropin-releasing hormone secretion. Many drugs including dopamine receptor blockers (phenothiazines, haloperidol, metoclopramide), opiates, H_2 blockers, serotonin reuptake inhibitors (fluoxetine), verapamil, estrogens, and antiestrogens are associated with prolactin hypersecretion. Hyperthyroidism is not associated with increased prolactin levels.

85. The answer is A.
(Chap. 23) This patient's clinical scenario is most consistent with MEN 1, or the "3 Ps": parathyroid, pituitary, and pancreas. MEN 1 is an autosomal dominant genetic syndrome characterized by neoplasia of the parathyroid, pituitary, and pancreatic islet cells. Hyperparathyroidism is the most common manifestation of MEN 1. The neoplastic changes affect multiple parathyroid glands, making surgical care difficult. Pancreatic islet cell neoplasia is the second most common manifestation of MEN 1. Increased pancreatic islet cell hormones include pancreatic polypeptide, gastrin, insulin, vasoactive intestinal peptide, glucagons, and somatostatin. Pancreatic tumors may be multicentric, and up to 30% are malignant, with the liver being the first site of metastases. The symptoms depend on the type of hormone secreted. Elevations of gastrin result in the Zollinger-Ellison syndrome (ZES). Gastrin levels are elevated, resulting in an ulcer diathesis. Conservative therapy is often unsuccessful. Insulinoma results in documented hypoglycemia with elevated insulin and C-peptide levels. Glucagonoma results in hyperglycemia, skin rash, anorexia, glossitis, and diarrhea. Elevations in vasoactive intestinal peptide result in profuse watery diarrhea. Pituitary tumors occur in up to half of patients with MEN 1. Prolactinomas are the most common. The multicentricity of the tumors makes resection difficult. Growth hormone–secreting tumors are the next most common, with ACTH- and corticotropin-releasing hormone (CRH)–secreting tumors being more rare. Carcinoid tumors may also occur in the thymus, lung, stomach, and duodenum.

86. The answer is C.
(Chap. 21) This patient has nephrotic syndrome, which is likely a result of multiple myeloma. The hyperlipidemia of nephrotic syndrome appears to be due to a combination of increased hepatic production and decreased clearance of very low density lipoproteins, with increased LDL production. It is usually mixed but can manifest as hypercholesterolemia or hypertriglyceridemia. Effective treatment of the underlying renal disease normalizes the lipid profile. Of the choices presented, HMG-CoA reductase inhibitors would be the most effective to reduce this patient's LDL. Dietary management is an important component of lifestyle modification but seldom results in a >10% fall in LDL. Niacin and fibrates would be indicated if the triglycerides were higher, but the LDL is the more important lipid abnormality to address at this time. Lipid apheresis is reserved for patients who cannot tolerate the lipid-lowering drugs or who have a genetic lipid disorder refractory to medication. Cholesterol ester transfer protein inhibitors have been shown to raise high-density lipoprotein levels and their role in the treatment of lipoproteinemias is still under investigation.

87. The answer is B.
(Chap. 5) Incidental adrenal masses are often discovered during radiographic testing for another condition and are found in ~6% of adult subjects at autopsy. Fifty percent of patients with a history of malignancy and a newly discovered adrenal mass will actually have an adrenal metastasis. Fine-needle aspiration of a suspected metastatic malignancy will often be diagnostic. In the absence of a suspected nonadrenal malignancy, most adrenal incidentalomas are benign. Primary adrenal malignancies are uncommon (<0.01%), and fine-needle aspiration is not useful to distinguish between benign and malignant primary adrenal tumors. Although 90% of these masses are nonsecretory, patients with an incidentaloma should be screened for pheochromocytoma and hypercortisolism with plasma free metanephrines and an overnight dexamethasone suppression test, respectively. When radiographic features suggest a benign neoplasm (<3 cm), scanning should be repeated in 3–6 months. When masses are >6 cm, surgical removal (if more likely primary adrenal malignancy) or fine-needle aspiration (if more likely metastatic malignancy) is preferred.

88. The answer is C.

(Chap. 19; Nathan DM: N Engl J Med 328: 1676–1685, 1993) Nephropathy is a leading cause of death in diabetic patients. Diabetic nephropathy may be functionally silent for 10–15 years. Clinically detectable diabetic nephropathy begins with the development of microalbuminuria (30–300 mg of albumin per 24 h). The glomerular filtration rate actually may be elevated at this stage. Only after the passage of additional time will the proteinuria be overt enough (0.5 g/L) to be detectable on standard urine dipsticks. Microalbuminuria precedes nephropathy in patients with both non-insulin-dependent and insulin-dependent diabetes. An increase in kidney size also may accompany the initial hyperfiltration stage. Once the proteinuria becomes significant enough to be detected by dipstick, a steady decline in renal function occurs, with the glomerular filtration rate falling an average of 1 mL/min per month. Therefore, azotemia begins about 12 years after the diagnosis of diabetes. Hypertension clearly is an exacerbating factor for diabetic nephropathy.

INDEX

Bold number indicates the start of the main discussion of the topic; numbers with "f" and "t" refer to figure and table pages.